Lecture Notes in Computer Science 3565

Commenced Publication in 1973
Founding and Former Series Editors:
Gerhard Goos, Juris Hartmanis, and Jan van Leeuwen

Editorial Board

David Hutchison
  Lancaster University, UK
Takeo Kanade
  Carnegie Mellon University, Pittsburgh, PA, USA
Josef Kittler
  University of Surrey, Guildford, UK
Jon M. Kleinberg
  Cornell University, Ithaca, NY, USA
Friedemann Mattern
  ETH Zurich, Switzerland
John C. Mitchell
  Stanford University, CA, USA
Moni Naor
  Weizmann Institute of Science, Rehovot, Israel
Oscar Nierstrasz
  University of Bern, Switzerland
C. Pandu Rangan
  Indian Institute of Technology, Madras, India
Bernhard Steffen
  University of Dortmund, Germany
Madhu Sudan
  Massachusetts Institute of Technology, MA, USA
Demetri Terzopoulos
  New York University, NY, USA
Doug Tygar
  University of California, Berkeley, CA, USA
Moshe Y. Vardi
  Rice University, Houston, TX, USA
Gerhard Weikum
  Max-Planck Institute of Computer Science, Saarbruecken, Germany

Gary E. Christensen Milan Sonka (Eds.)

Information Processing in Medical Imaging

19th International Conference, IPMI 2005
Glenwood Springs, CO, USA, July 10-15, 2005
Proceedings

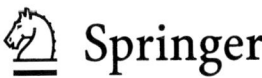
Springer

Volume Editors

Gary E. Christensen
Milan Sonka
The University of Iowa
Department of Electrical and Computer Engineering
Iowa City, IA 52242, USA
E-mail: {gary-christensen,milan-sonka}@uiowa.edu

Library of Congress Control Number: 2005928332

CR Subject Classification (1998): I.4, I.5, I.2.5-6, J.1, I.3

ISSN   0302-9743
ISBN-10   3-540-26545-7 Springer Berlin Heidelberg New York
ISBN-13   978-3-540-26545-0 Springer Berlin Heidelberg New York

This work is subject to copyright. All rights are reserved, whether the whole or part of the material is concerned, specifically the rights of translation, reprinting, re-use of illustrations, recitation, broadcasting, reproduction on microfilms or in any other way, and storage in data banks. Duplication of this publication or parts thereof is permitted only under the provisions of the German Copyright Law of September 9, 1965, in its current version, and permission for use must always be obtained from Springer. Violations are liable to prosecution under the German Copyright Law.

Springer is a part of Springer Science+Business Media

springeronline.com

© Springer-Verlag Berlin Heidelberg 2005
Printed in Germany

Typesetting: Camera-ready by author, data conversion by Scientific Publishing Services, Chennai, India
Printed on acid-free paper   SPIN: 11505730   06/3142   5 4 3 2 1 0

Preface

The nineteenth biennial International Conference on Information Processing in Medical Imaging (IPMI) was held July 11–15, 2005 in Glenwood Springs, CO, USA on the Spring Valley campus of the Colorado Mountain College. Following the successful meeting in beautiful Ambleside in England, this year's conference addressed important recent developments in a broad range of topics related to the acquisition, analysis and application of biomedical images.

Interest in IPMI has been steadily growing over the last decade. This is partially due to the increased number of researchers entering the field of medical imaging as a result of the Whitaker Foundation and the recently formed National Institute of Biomedical Imaging and Bioengineering. This year, there were 245 full manuscripts submitted to the conference which was twice the number submitted in 2003 and almost four times the number of submissions in 2001. Of these papers, 27 were accepted as oral presentations, and 36 excellent submissions that could not be accommodated as oral presentations were presented as posters. Selection of the papers for presentation was a difficult task as we were unable to accommodate many of the excellent papers submitted this year. All accepted manuscripts were allocated 12 pages in these proceedings.

Every effort was made to maintain those traditional features of IPMI that have made this conference a unique and exciting experience since the inaugural meeting in 1969. Papers were presented in single-track sessions, followed by discussions that did not have time limits. Although unlimited discussion ruins carefully planned meal schedules, many participants welcome the rich, detailed descriptions of essential techniques that often emerge from the discussions. For that reason, IPMI is often viewed as a true workshop in contrast to the constrained schedules of most conferences.

The main focus at IPMI has always been to encourage the participation of new investigators, loosely described as students, postdocs, and junior faculty under 35 years of age who are presenting at IPMI for the first time. To broaden participation in the discussion, we continued the "discussion group" idea introduced by Chris Taylor and Alison Noble in 2003. Small groups of new investigators led by Scientific Committee members met before each session to discuss the papers to be presented and formulate questions and comments to be raised during the session. We were lucky to have Carl Jaffe from the National Cancer Institute, to give a plenary talk on recent advances and open problems in cancer imaging research.

The setting and dress have always been casual, which promotes collegiality and an exchange of information unfettered by the usual formalities. This year the conference was held on the Spring Valley campus of the Colorado Mountain College, where attendees stayed together in the university housing. The causal approach helps organizers keep costs low, thus encouraging young investigator participation. The tradition of carrying on discussion into the evening was continued. We provided bus service to downtown Glenwood Springs where attendees enjoyed the local bars, relaxed in the hot springs, and took strolls through the beautiful downtown area. On Wednesday afternoon, attendees bonded during a 13-mile bike ride along the scenic Colorado River, relaxed in the hot springs, or visited the ski resort town of Aspen. Later that evening, everyone enjoyed a pleasant dinner at the elegant Rivers restaurant, and those who wanted stayed late into the night on the porch overlooking the Roaring Fork River.

IPMI is a unique meeting for which we, the members of the IPMI board, and many other participants hold a true affection. While it was a great deal of work, we were delighted to be given the opportunity to organize this meeting and continue the IPMI tradition. We are looking forward to a more relaxed participation at IPMI 2007 in the Rolduc Abbey in The Netherlands!

July 2005

Gary E. Christensen
Milan Sonka

Acknowledgements

The nineteenth IPMI conference was made possible by the efforts of many hard-working individuals and generous organizations. First, the organizers wish to thank the Scientific Committee for their critical reviews that determined the content of the program. We appreciate their detailed and thoughtful comments considering they were asked to review an average of 12 full manuscripts in a little more than 3 weeks' time. We also extend our gratitude to all authors who submitted papers to the conference and our regrets to those we turned down. We are grateful to the members of the Paper Selection Committee who shared with us the difficult task of assimilating the referees' comments and choosing the papers to include in the conference. We greatly appreciate the help, guidance and insights provided by Chris Taylor from his experience with planning the previous IPMI conference.

We thank David Risely for his support of the CAWS Web-based conference administration system that greatly simplified many of the organizational tasks associated with this conference. We gratefully acknowledge the assistance of the Conference and Event Services staff at the Colorado Mountain College, particularly Mary Lehrman and Stephanie Owston who helped coordinate the on-site conference logistics. We would like to thank Kim Sherwood for general administrative support including communication with authors and attendees. We thank Xiujuan Geng, Mona Haeker and Dinesh Kumar for taking time from their research to compile the proceedings.

Finally, we are grateful to the following organizations for their generous financial support:

The Whitaker Foundation
The National Institute of Biomedical Imaging and Bioengineering
The Obermann Center for Advanced Studies, The University of Iowa
Department of Electrical Engineering, The University of Iowa
College of Engineering, The University of Iowa

Francois Erbsmann Prize Winners

1987 (Utrecht, The Netherlands): **John M. Gauch**, University of North Carolina, Chapel Hill, NC, USA
J.M. Gauch, W.R. Oliver, S.M. Pizer: *Multiresolution shape descriptions and their applications in medical imaging*

1989 (Berkeley, CA, USA): **Arthur F. Gmitro**, University of Arizona, Tucson, AZ, USA
A.F. Gmitro, V. Tresp, V. Chen, Y. Snell, G.R. Gindi: *Video-rate reconstruction of CT and MR images*

1991 (Wye, Kent, UK): **H. Isil Bozma**, Yale University, New Haven, CT, USA
H.I. Bozma, J.S. Duncan: *Model-based recognition of multiple deformable objects using a game-theoretic framework*

1993 (Flagstaff, AZ, USA): **Jeffrey A. Fessler**, University of Michigan, Ann Arbor, MI, USA
J.A. Fessler: *Tomographic reconstruction using information-weighted spline smoothing*

1995 (Brest, France): **Maurits K. Konings**, University Hospital, Utrecht, The Netherlands
M.K. Konings, W.P.T.M. Mali, M.A. Viergever: *Design of a robust strategy to measure intravascular electrical impedance*

1997 (Poultney, VT, USA): **David Atkinson**, Guy's Hospital, London, UK
D. Atkinson, D.L.G. Hill, P.N.R. Stoyle, P.E. Summers, S.F. Keevil: *An autofocus algorithm for the automatic correction of motion artifacts in MR images*

1999 (Visegrad, Hungary): **Liana M. Lorigo**, Massachusetts Institute of Technology, Cambridge, MA, USA
L.M. Lorigo, O. Faugeras, W.E.L. Grimson, R. Keriven, R. Kikinis, C.-F. Westin: *Co-dimension 2 geodesic active contours for MRA segmentation*

2001 (Davis, CA, USA): **Viktor K. Jirsa**, Florida Atlantic University, FL, USA
V.K. Jirsa, K.J. Jantzen, A. Fuchs, J.A. Scott Kelso: *Neural field dynamics on the folded three-dimensional cortical sheet and its forward EEG and MEG*

2003 (Ambleside, UK): **Guillaume Marrelec**, INSERM, France.
G. Marrelec, P. Ciuciu, M. Pélégrini-Issac, H. Benali: *Estimation of the hemodyamic response function in event-related functional MRI: directed acyclic graphs for a general Bayesian inference framework*

Conference Committees

Chairs

Gary E. Christensen University of Iowa, USA
Milan Sonka University of Iowa, USA

Paper Selection Committee

James S. Duncan Yale University, USA
Kyle J. Myers United States Food and Drug Administration, USA

Scientific Committee

Craig K. Abbey University of California, Davis, USA
Scott T. Acton University of Virginia, USA
Faiza Admiraal-Behloul Leiden University Medical Center, The Netherlands
Amir A. Amini Washington University in St. Louis, USA
Stephen R. Aylward University of North Carolina, USA
Christian Barillot IRISA/INRIA, France
Horst Bischof Graz University of Technology, Austria
Yves J.C. Bizais Medical School, UBO, France
Johan G. Bosch Erasmus Medical Center Rotterdam, The Netherlands
Djamal Boukerroui Université de Technologie de Compiègne, France
Aaron B. Brill Vanderbilt University, USA
Elizabeth Bullitt University of North Carolina, USA
Ela Claridge University of Birmingham, UK
Timothy F. Cootes University of Manchester, UK
Christos Davatzikos University of Pennsylvania, USA
Marleen de Bruijne IT University of Copenhagen, Denmark
James S. Duncan Yale University, USA
Jeffrey A. Fessler University of Michigan, USA
James C. Gee University of Pennsylvania, USA
Guido Gerig University of North Carolina at Chapel Hill, USA
Ali Gholipour University of Texas at Dallas, USA
Polina Golland Massachusetts Institute of Technology, USA
Michael L. Goris Stanford University School of Medicine, USA

Ghassan Hamarneh	Simon Fraser University, Canada
David J. Hawkes	King's College London, UK
Derek L.G. Hill	University College London, UK
Kenneth R. Hoffmann	State University of New York at Buffalo, USA
Michael F. Insana	University of California, Davis, USA
Sarang C. Joshi	University of North Carolina at Chapel Hill, USA
Nico Karssemeijer	Radboud University Nijmegen, The Netherlands
Frithjof Kruggel	University of Leipzig, Germany
Attila Kuba	University of Szeged, Hungary
Jan Kybic	Czech Technical University, Czech Republic
Rasmus Larsen	Technical University of Denmark, DTU, Denmark
Boudewijn P.F. Lelieveldt	Leiden University Medical Center, The Netherlands
Bostjan Likar	University of Ljubljana, Slovenia
Gabriele Lohmann	Max-Planck Institute of Cognitive Neuroscience, Germany
Sven Loncaric	University of Zagreb, Croatia
Gregoire Malandain	INRIA Sophia-Antipolis, France
Calvin Maurer	Stanford University School of Medicine, USA
François G. Meyer	University of Colorado at Boulder, USA
Michael I. Miga	Vanderbilt University, USA
Wiro Niessen	Erasmus Medical Center Rotterdam, The Netherlands
Alison Noble	University of Oxford, UK
Kalman Palagyi	University of Szeged, Hungary
Jussi P.S. Parkkinen	University of Joensuu, Finland
Stephen M. Pizer	University of North Carolina, USA
Josien Pluim	University Medical Center Utrecht, The Netherlands
Jerry L. Prince	Johns Hopkins University, USA
Anand Rangarajan	University of Florida, USA
Joseph M. Reinhardt	University of Iowa, USA
Torsten Rohlfing	SRI International, USA
Karl Rohr	University of Heidelberg, DKFZ Heidelberg, Germany
Daniel Rueckert	Imperial College London, UK
Andrea Schenk	MeVis — Center for Medical Diagnostic Systems and Visualization, Germany
Julia A. Schnabel	University College London, UK
Oskar Skrinjar	Georgia Institute of Technology, USA
Mikkel B. Stegmann	Technical University of Denmark, DTU, Denmark
Gabor Szekely	Swiss Federal Institute of Technology, Switzerland
Chris Taylor	University of Manchester, UK
Carole J. Twining	University of Manchester, UK
Edwin J.R. van Beek	University of Iowa, USA

Baba C. Vemuri   University of Florida, USA
Bram van Ginneken   Image Sciences Institute, The Netherlands
Ge Wang   University of Iowa, USA
William M. Wells   Harvard Medical School, and Brigham and Women's
                      Hospital, USA
Xiaodong Wu   University of Iowa, USA

IPMI Board

Stephen L. Bacharach
Harrison H. Barrett
Yves J.C. Bizais
Aaron B. Brill
Gary E. Christensen
Alan C.F. Colchester
Frank Deconinck
Robert DiPaola
James S. Duncan
Michael L. Goris
Attila Kuba
Richard M. Leahy
Douglas A. Ortendahl
Stephen M. Pizer
Chris Taylor
Andrew Todd-Pokropek
Max A. Viergever

Table of Contents

Shape and Population Modeling

A Unified Information-Theoretic Approach to Groupwise Non-rigid Registration and Model Building
  Carole J. Twining, Tim Cootes, Stephen Marsland, Vladimir Petrovic, Roy Schestowitz, Chris J. Taylor 1

Hypothesis Testing with Nonlinear Shape Models
  Timothy B. Terriberry, Sarang C. Joshi, Guido Gerig 15

Extrapolation of Sparse Tensor Fields: Application to the Modeling of Brain Variability
  Pierre Fillard, Vincent Arsigny, Xavier Pennec, Paul M. Thompson, Nicholas Ayache 27

Bayesian Population Modeling of Effective Connectivity
  Eric R. Cosman, William M. Wells III 39

Diffusion Tensor Imaging and Functional Magnetic Resonance

Fiber Tracking in q-Ball Fields Using Regularized Particle Trajectories
  Muriel Perrin, Cyril Poupon, Yann Cointepas, Bernard Rieul, Narly Golestani, Christophe Pallier, Denis Rivière, Andre Constantinesco, Denis Le Bihan, Jean-Francois Mangin 52

Approximating Anatomical Brain Connectivity with Diffusion Tensor MRI Using Kernel-Based Diffusion Simulations
  Jun Zhang, Ning Kang, Stephen E. Rose 64

Maximum Entropy Spherical Deconvolution for Diffusion MRI
  Daniel C. Alexander 76

From Spatial Regularization to Anatomical Priors in fMRI Analysis
  Wanmei Ou, Polina Golland 88

Segmentation and Filtering

CLASSIC: Consistent Longitudinal Alignment and Segmentation for Serial Image Computing
  Zhong Xue, Dinggang Shen, Christos Davatzikos 101

Robust Active Appearance Model Matching
  Reinhard Beichel, Horst Bischof, Franz Leberl, Milan Sonka 114

Simultaneous Segmentation and Registration of Contrast-Enhanced Breast MRI
  *Xiaohua Chen, Michael Brady, Jonathan Lok-Chuen Lo,
  Niall Moore* 126

Multiscale Vessel Enhancing Diffusion in CT Angiography Noise Filtering
  Rashindra Manniesing, Wiro Niessen 138

Poster Session 1

Information Fusion in Biomedical Image Analysis: Combination of Data vs. Combination of Interpretations
  *Torsten Rohlfing, Adolf Pfefferbaum, Edith V. Sullivan,
  Calvin R. Maurer* 150

Parametric Medial Shape Representation in 3-D via the Poisson Partial Differential Equation with Non-linear Boundary Conditions
  Paul A. Yushkevich, Hui Zhang, James C. Gee 162

Diffeomorphic Nonlinear Transformations: A Local Parametric Approach for Image Registration
  *Ramkrishnan Narayanan, Jeffrey A. Fessler, Hyunjin Park,
  Charles R. Meyer* 174

A Framework for Registration, Statistical Characterization and Classification of Cortically Constrained Functional Imaging Data
  *Anand A. Joshi, David W. Shattuck, Paul M. Thompson,
  Richard M. Leahy* 186

PET Image Reconstruction: A Robust State Space Approach
  Huafeng Liu, Yi Tian, Pengcheng Shi 197

Multi-dimensional Mutual Information Based Robust Image Registration Using Maximum Distance-Gradient-Magnitude
  Rui Gan, Albert C.S. Chung 210

Tissue Perfusion Diagnostic Classification Using a Spatio-temporal Analysis of Contrast Ultrasound Image Sequences
  *Quentin Williams, J. Alison Noble, Alexander Ehlgen MD,
  Harald Becher MD* 222

Topology Preserving Tissue Classification with Fast Marching and
Topology Templates
  Pierre-Louis Bazin, Dzung L. Pham 234

Apparent Diffusion Coefficient Approximation and Diffusion Anisotropy
Characterization in DWI
  Yunmei Chen, Weihong Guo, Qingguo Zeng, Xiaolu Yan,
  Murali Rao, Yijun Liu 246

Linearization of Mammograms Using Parameters Derived from Noise
Characteristics
  Nico Karssemeijer, Peter R. Snoeren, Wei Zhang 258

Knowledge-Driven Automated Detection of Pleural Plaques and
Thickening in High Resolution CT of the Lung
  Mamatha Rudrapatna, Van Mai, Arcot Sowmya, Peter Wilson 270

Fundamental Limits in 3D Landmark Localization
  Karl Rohr 286

Computational Elastography from Standard Ultrasound Image
Sequences by Global Trust Region Optimization
  Jan Kybic, Daniel Smutek 299

Representing Diffusion MRI in 5D for Segmentation of White Matter
Tracts with a Level Set Method
  Lisa Jonasson, Patric Hagmann, Xavier Bresson,
  Jean-Philippe Thiran, Van J. Wedeen 311

Automatic Prediction of Myocardial Contractility Improvement in
Stress MRI Using Shape Morphometrics with Independent Component
Analysis
  Avan Suinesiaputra, Alejandro F. Frangi, Hildo J. Lamb,
  Johan H.C. Reiber, Boudewijn P.F. Lelieveldt 321

Brain Segmentation with Competitive Level Sets and Fuzzy Control
  Cybèle Ciofolo, Christian Barillot 333

Coupled Shape Distribution-Based Segmentation of Multiple Objects
  Andrew Litvin, William C. Karl 345

Partition-Based Extraction of Cerebral Arteries from CT Angiography
with Emphasis on Adaptive Tracking
  Hackjoon Shim, Il Dong Yun, Kyoung Mu Lee, Sang Uk Lee 357

Small Animal Imaging

Regional Whole Body Fat Quantification in Mice
  *Xenophon Papademetris, Pavel Shkarin, Lawrence H. Staib,
  Kevin L. Behar* 369

Surfaces and Segmentation

Surface Matching via Currents
  Marc Vaillant, Joan Glaunès 381

A Genetic Algorithm for the Topology Correction of Cortical Surfaces
  Florent Ségonne, Eric Grimson, Bruce Fischl 393

Simultaneous Segmentation of Multiple Closed Surfaces Using Optimal
Graph Searching
  *Kang Li, Steven Millington, Xiaodong Wu, Danny Z. Chen,
  Milan Sonka* 406

A Generalized Level Set Formulation of the Mumford-Shah Functional
for Brain MR Image Segmentation
  Lishui Cheng, Jie Yang, Xian Fan, Yuemin Zhu 418

Applications

Integrable Pressure Gradients via Harmonics-Based Orthogonal
Projection
  Yuehuan Wang, Amir A. Amini 431

Design of Robust Vascular Tree Matching: Validation on Liver
  *Arnaud Charnoz, Vincent Agnus, Grégoire Malandain,
  Stéphane Nicolau, Mohamed Tajine, Luc Soler* 443

Image Registration

A Novel Parametric Method for Non-rigid Image Registration
  Anne Cuzol, Pierre Hellier, Etienne Mémin 456

Transitive Inverse-Consistent Manifold Registration
  Xiujuan Geng, Dinesh Kumar, Gary E. Christensen 468

Cortical Surface Alignment Using Geometry Driven Multispectral
Optical Flow
   Duygu Tosun, Jerry L. Prince 480

Inverse Consistent Mapping in 3D Deformable Image Registration:
Its Construction and Statistical Properties
   *Alex Leow, Sung-Cheng Huang, Alex Geng, James Becker,
Simon Davis, Arthur Toga, Paul Thompson* 493

Poster Session 2

Robust Nonrigid Multimodal Image Registration Using Local Frequency
Maps
   Bing Jian, Baba C. Vemuri, José L. Marroquin 504

Imaging Tumor Microenvironment with Ultrasound
   Mallika Sridhar, Michael F. Insana 516

PDE-Based Three Dimensional Path Planning for Virtual Endoscopy
   M. Sabry Hassouna, Aly A. Farag 529

Elastic Shape Models for Interpolations of Curves in Image Sequences
   Shantanu H. Joshi, Anuj Srivastava, Washington Mio 541

Segmenting and Tracking the Left Ventricle by Learning the Dynamics
in Cardiac Images
   *Walter Sun, Müjdat Çetin, Raymond Chan, Vivek Reddy,
Godtfred Holmvang, Venkat Chandar, Alan Willsky* 553

3D Active Shape Models Using Gradient Descent Optimization of
Description Length
   Tobias Heimann, Ivo Wolf, Tomos Williams, Hans-Peter Meinzer ... 566

Capturing Anatomical Shape Variability Using B-Spline Registration
   Thomas H. Wenckebach, Hans Lamecker, Hans-Christian Hege 578

A Riemannian Approach to Diffusion Tensor Images Segmentation
   *Christophe Lenglet, Mikaël Rousson, Rachid Deriche,
Olivier Faugeras, Stéphane Lehericy, Kamil Ugurbil* 591

Coil Sensitivity Estimation for Optimal SNR Reconstruction and
Intensity Inhomogeneity Correction in Phased Array MR Imaging
   *Prashanthi Vemuri, Eugene G. Kholmovski, Dennis L. Parker,
Brian E. Chapman* 603

Many Heads Are Better Than One: Jointly Removing Bias from
Multiple MRIs Using Nonparametric Maximum Likelihood
 Erik G. Learned-Miller, Vidit Jain 615

Unified Statistical Approach to Cortical Thickness Analysis
 Moo K. Chung, Steve Robbins, Alan C. Evans 627

ZHARP: Three-Dimensional Motion Tracking from a Single Image Plane
 *Khaled Z. Abd-Elmoniem, Matthias Stuber, Nael F. Osman,
 Jerry L. Prince* 639

Analysis of Event-Related fMRI Data Using Diffusion Maps
 Xilin Shen, François G. Meyer 652

Automated Detection of Small-Size Pulmonary Nodules Based on
Helical CT Images
 *Xiangwei Zhang, Geoffrey McLennan, Eric A. Hoffman,
 Milan Sonka* 664

Nonparametric Neighborhood Statistics for MRI Denoising
 Suyash P. Awate, Ross T. Whitaker 677

Construction and Validation of Mean Shape Atlas Templates for
Atlas-Based Brain Image Segmentation
 *Qian Wang, Dieter Seghers, Emiliano D'Agostino, Frederik Maes,
 Dirk Vandermeulen, Paul Suetens, Alexander Hammers* 689

Multi-figure Anatomical Objects for Shape Statistics
 *Qiong Han, Stephen M. Pizer, Derek Merck, Sarang Joshi,
 Ja-Yeon Jeong* 701

The Role of Non-overlap in Image Registration
 Jonas August, Takeo Kanade 713

Registration and Segmentation

Multimodality Image Registration Using an Extensible Information
Metric and High Dimensional Histogramming
 Jie Zhang, Anand Rangarajan 725

Spherical Navigator Registration Using Harmonic Analysis for
Prospective Motion Correction
 Christopher L. Wyatt, Narter Ari, Robert A. Kraft 738

Tunneling Descent Level Set Segmentation of Ultrasound Images
  Zhong Tao, Hemant D. Tagare 750

Multi-object Segmentation Using Shape Particles
  Marleen de Bruijne, Mads Nielsen 762

Author Index 775

A Unified Information-Theoretic Approach to Groupwise Non-rigid Registration and Model Building

Carole J. Twining[1], Tim Cootes[1], Stephen Marsland[2], Vladimir Petrovic[1], Roy Schestowitz[1], and Chris J. Taylor[1]

[1] Imaging Science and Biomedical Engineering (ISBE),
Stopford Building, University of Manchester, Manchester, UK
[2] Institute of Information Sciences, Massey University,
Private Bag 11222, Palmerston North, New Zealand

Abstract. The non-rigid registration of a group of images shares a common feature with building a model of a group of images: a dense, consistent correspondence across the group. Image registration aims to find the correspondence, while modelling requires it. This paper presents the theoretical framework required to unify these two areas, providing a groupwise registration algorithm, where the inherently groupwise model of the image data becomes an integral part of the registration process.

The performance of this algorithm is evaluated by extending the concepts of generalisability and specificity from shape models to image models. This provides an independent metric for comparing registration algorithms of groups of images. Experimental results on MR data of brains for various pairwise and groupwise registration algorithms is presented, and demonstrates the feasibility of the combined registration/modelling framework, as well as providing quantitative evidence for the superiority of groupwise approaches to registration.

1 Introduction

Over the past few years, non-rigid registration has been used increasingly as a basis for medical image analysis. Applications include structural analysis, atlas matching and change analysis. There are well-established methods for pairwise image registration(for a review, see e.g., [12]), but often it is necessary to register a group of images. This can be achieved by repeatedly applying pairwise registration, but there is no guarantee that the solution is unique – depending on the choice of reference image, representation of warp, and optimisation strategy, many different results can be obtained for the same set of images. Clearly, this does not form a satisfactory basis for analysis.

In this paper we consider non-rigid image registration as a complementary problem to that of modelling a group of images [2]. A statistical model of a group of images requires that a dense correspondence is defined across the group, which is precisely what non-rigid image registration provides. The key idea explored in this paper is that the best correspondence is that which generates the best model of the data. Building on the optimal shape model approach of Davies et al [3], we define a minimum description length (MDL) criterion for image model quality. We show that a unique correspondence can be defined across a group of images by minimising, explicitly, an MDL objective function.

The combination of non-rigid image registration with modelling was shown previously by Frangi et al. [5], who used non-rigid registration to automatically construct 3D statistical shape models of the left and right ventricles of the heart. However, their method did require an initial manual labelling of every image in the training set. As regards groupwise non-rigid registration, several authors have considered the problem of choosing the best reference image. For instance, Bhatia et al [1] use a fixed intensity reference picked from the training set, but select the spatial frame of the reference so that the sum of deformations from this spatial reference frame is zero. Davis et al [4] concentrate specifically on deriving the most representative template image for a group of images, using sum-of-squared difference on the space of image discrepancies, and a metric on the diffeomorphism group of spatial deformations. Each of these approaches involve defining a series of independant criteria for what constitutes image matching, how image deformation is weighted against spatial deformation and so on. The advantage of our approach is that we use a single criterion – minimum description length – which can in principle determine not just the groupwise correspondence across the set of images, but also the optimal spatial reference frame, the optimal reference image and, potentially, the optimal model parameters (e.g., number of modes of the model retained). It hence combines registration and modelling within a *single* framework.

In this paper, we present a full description of our framework for groupwise registration, defining the MDL objective function and showing how the optimisation can be performed in a principled way by moving between different frames of reference. We validate the MDL objective function experimentally, using a set of annotated 2D MR brain slices. We also address the problem of evaluating different groupwise correspondences, by defining the generalisabilty and specificity of the resulting models. Again, we validate these measures using annotated data. We use these measures to evaluate the performance of a range of pairwise and groupwise approaches to registering a set of brain images, and show that the groupwise approach gives quantitatively better performance than pairwise.

2 Spatial and Pixel/Voxel-Value Transformations

The aim of non-rigid registration is to define a consistent spatial correspondence across a set of training images. One way to ensure a consistent correspondence is to define all correspondences w.r.t. a spatial reference frame – the origin of the space of spatial deformations. We define the following basic notational conventions , taking as our example the simplest case of a spatial warp directly between a training image frame and a reference frame (see Fig. 1):

- X_0 is the regular grid of pixel/voxel positions on which each of our images is defined.
- $\mathcal{R}$ is the spatial frame of the reference. A reference image $I_\mathcal{R}(X_0)$ consists of the set of values of a function $I_\mathcal{R}$, taken at the set of positions X_0.
- The set of N training images is denoted by $\{I_{\mathcal{T}_i}(X_0) : i = 1, \ldots N\}$, where $\mathcal{T}_i$ is the spatial frame of image i, with associated image function $I_{\mathcal{T}_i}$.

The dense correspondence between a training image frame $\mathcal{T}_i$ and the reference frame $\mathcal{R}$ is defined by a spatial warp $\omega_i : x \in \mathcal{T}_i \mapsto \omega_i(x) \in \mathcal{R}$. The warp ω_i also induces a mapping between the function spaces (that is, it warps images between frames). Mathematically, there are two such mappings:

The push-forward: $\omega_i : I_{\mathcal{T}_i} \mapsto I_{\mathcal{T}_i}^{\omega_i} \doteq \omega_i(I_{\mathcal{T}_i}), \quad I_{\mathcal{T}_i}^{\omega_i}(\omega_i(x)) \doteq I_{\mathcal{T}_i}(x)$
The pullback: $\omega_i^* : I_\mathcal{R} \mapsto I_\mathcal{R}^* \doteq \omega_i^*(I_\mathcal{R}), \quad I_\mathcal{R}^*(x) \doteq I_\mathcal{R}(\omega_i(x))$

The pullback ω_i^* is easier to compute, since we resample $I_\mathcal{R}$ in $\mathcal{R}$ from the regular grid X_0 to the irregular, warped grid $\omega_i(X_0)$ to obtain $I_\mathcal{R}^*(X_0)$ in $\mathcal{T}_i$, whereas the push-forward mapping entails resampling $I_{\mathcal{T}_i}^{\omega_i}$ in $\mathcal{R}$ from the irregular grid $\omega_i(X_0)$ to the regular grid X_0, which is computationally more expensive. So, in what follows, we will use the **pullback** mapping wherever possible, where the direction of flow of image information is in the **opposite** direction to that of the spatial mapping.

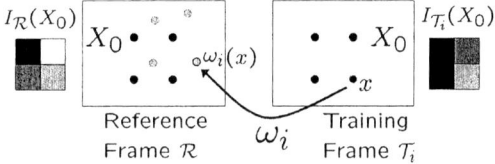

Fig. 1. A spatial warp ω_i from training frame $\mathcal{T}_i$ to reference frame $\mathcal{R}$. X_0 (black filled circles) is the set of regular voxel positions, with the grey filled circles being the warped voxel positions $\omega_i(X_0)$

Once we can map images between frames, we can compare images. We will denote a general image-difference/discrepancy-image by ΔI. So, in the example above, if we define a discrepancy image in the frame $\mathcal{T}_i$:

$$\Delta I_{\mathcal{T}_i}(X_0) = I_{\mathcal{T}_i}(X_0) - I_\mathcal{R}^*(X_0) \implies (\Delta I_{\mathcal{T}_i} \circ \omega_i^*) I_\mathcal{R}(X_0) \equiv I_{\mathcal{T}_i}(X_0), \quad (1)$$

where $(\Delta I_{\mathcal{T}_i} \circ \omega_i^*)$ is taken to denote the composition of a pullback mapping ω_i^* and a voxel-value deformation $\Delta I_{\mathcal{T}_i}(X_0)$. The pixel/voxel-value deformation in this case is defined such that when applied to the warped reference image $I_\mathcal{R}^*(X_0)$ it exactly recreates the training set image $I_{\mathcal{T}_i}(X_0)$. It is important to note that in general these two classes of transformations **do not** commute. We now have a general class of image deformations, composed of a spatial part and a discrepancy image part – we will denote such a general combined deformation by capital greek letters (e.g., Ω_i).

A more complicated situation is shown in Fig. 2. This shows the reference image being transformed into a training image $I_{\mathcal{T}_i}$, by a sequence of two combined transformations Υ_i then Ω_i. We take this approach since, if we are to model combined transformations across the group of images, we need them to be applied

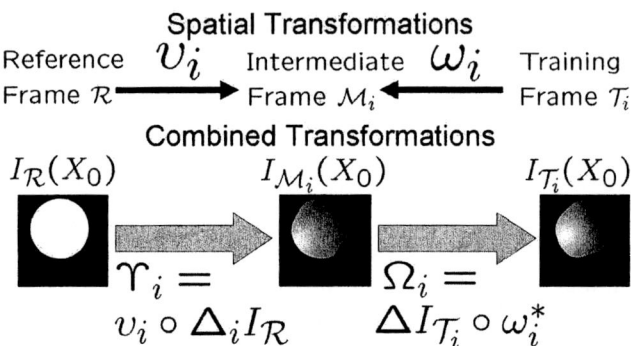

Fig. 2. Top: The spatial transformations (black arrows) between reference, intermediate and training image frames for one image i in the training set. **Bottom:** The corresponding combined (spatial and voxel-intensity) transformations (broad grey arrows) between images

in a **common** frame. So, the spatial transformations $\{v_i\}$ and the discrepancy images $\{\Delta_i I_\mathcal{R}\}$ are all applied in the reference frame $\mathcal{R}$, hence can be modelled across the group. However, the direction of the spatial warp v_i is now in the **same** direction as the combined warp Υ_i (the direction of flow of image information), which means that Υ_i no longer has the simple form given above, but is given by:

$$\Upsilon_i = v_i \circ \Delta_i I_\mathcal{R}, \qquad (2)$$

which uses the push-forward mapping v_i as applied to images, rather than the easier-to-compute pullback. The spatial warp ω_i is now just from the training frame $\mathcal{T}_i$ to the intermediate frame $\mathcal{M}_i$, the corresponding combined warp Ω_i being constructed using the pullback ω_i^* and the discrepancy image $\Delta I_{\mathcal{T}_i}$, which is calculated in a manner analogous to (1), but with the intermediate image $I_{\mathcal{M}_i}$ taking the place of the reference image $I_\mathcal{R}$. This second combined transformation is included because in general the groupwise-modelled transformation will not completely represent the total required transformation.

3 The Objective Function

As we explained in the Introduction, we have chosen to define the optimal groupwise non-rigid registration as that which minimises an objective function based on the minimum description length (MDL) principle [7].

The basic idea behind MDL is that we consider transmitting our dataset to a receiver, encoding the dataset using some model[1]. Using the structure and notation defined in the previous section, the data we have to transmit is the

---

[1] Note that in this paper, we use 'model' in two senses – in terms of an encoding model, which can be something very simple, such as a flat distribution over a known range, and in terms of a groupwise model, explicitly constructed to fit the data.

reference image $I_\mathcal{R}$ and the set of combined deformations $\{\Upsilon_i, \Omega_i\}$ that enable us to exactly reconstruct each training image. Optimising the description length means in principle finding:

- The optimal reference image $I_\mathcal{R}(X_0)$ and optimal reference frame $\mathcal{R}$.
- The optimal set of combined transformations $\{\Upsilon_i, \Omega_i\}$ via:
  - The optimal groupwise encoding of the deformations that act in a common frame, that is, the optimal groupwise model of the set $\{\Upsilon_i\}$,
  - Encoding of the residual deformations $\{\Omega_i\}$, which do not act in a common frame.

The total description length can hence be decomposed thus:

$$\mathcal{L}_{\text{total}} = \underset{\text{Reference frame \& reference image}}{\mathcal{L}_\mathcal{R}(\mathcal{R}, I_\mathcal{R})} + \underset{\text{Parameters of groupwise model}}{\mathcal{L}_{\text{params}}} + \underset{\text{Encoded using groupwise model}}{\mathcal{L}_{\text{group}}(\{\Upsilon_i\})} + \underset{\text{Encoded residuals}}{\mathcal{L}_{\text{residuals}}(\{\Omega_i\})} \quad (3)$$

Actual description lengths are computed using the fundamental result of Shannon [9] – if there are a set of possible, discrete events $\{A\}$ with associated encoding-model probabilities $\{p_A\}$, then the optimum code length required to transmit the occurrence of event A is given by:

$$\mathcal{L}_A = -\ln p_A \text{ nats}^* \quad (4)$$

The encoding lengths for unsigned and signed integers are calculated thus:

$$\mathcal{L}_{\mathbb{Z}^+}(n) = \frac{1}{e} + \ln(n) \text{ nats, } n \in \mathbb{Z}^+, \quad \mathcal{L}_\mathbb{Z}(n) = \frac{2}{e} + \ln(n) \text{ nats, } n \in \mathbb{Z}. \quad (5)$$

As an example, consider the description length for transmitting a discrepancy image $\Delta I(X_0)$ according to the image histogram. The $N_I = \text{size}(X_0)$ voxels of the image are taken to be integers in the range $[-N_{\text{range}}, \ldots N_{\text{range}}]$, N_m voxels having the value m. The associated model probability is then $p(m) = \frac{N_m}{N_I}$. The description length is:

$$\mathcal{L}_{\text{Hist}}(\Delta I) = -\underset{\text{Positions of occupied bins}}{\sum_{m, N_m > 0} \ln\left(\frac{1}{2N_{\text{range}}+1}\right)} + \underset{\text{Bin Occupancies}}{\sum_{m, N_m > 0} \mathcal{L}_{\mathbb{Z}^+}(N_m)} - \underset{\text{Encoded Data}}{\sum_{x \in X_0} \ln p(\Delta I(x))}. \quad (6)$$

See [11, 10] for further details.

4 The Algorithmic Framework

4.1 Initialisation

In [10], an algorithm was presented to find an initial correspondence using MDL. The structure of the algorithm followed that shown in Fig. 1. The free variables

---

* The **nat** is the analogous unit to the **bit**, but using a base of e rather than base 2.

Algorithm 1. MDL NRR Initialisation

1: $\{\omega_i = \mathbb{I}, i = 1, \ldots N\}$ %:Initialize warps to the identity.
2: **Repeat**
3:   Randomize the order of the set of training images $I_{T_i}(X_0)$, indexed by i.
4:   **For** $i = 1$ to N **do**
5:     Optimise $\mathcal{L}_{\text{init}}(\{\omega_k\})$ w.r.t. spatial warp ω_i.
6:     Update Intermediate Images $\{I_{\mathcal{M}_j}(X_0) : j \neq i\}$. %:Using equation (8).
7:   **End**
8: **Until** convergence

were the set of spatial warps $\{\omega_i\}$, initialised to the identity $\mathbb{I}$, and the reference image was taken to be the mean of the training images, pulled-back using the inverses $\{\omega_i^{-1}\}$:

$$I_\mathcal{R}(X_0) = \frac{1}{N} \sum_{i=1}^{N} \left[\omega_i^{-1*}(I_{T_i})\right](X_0). \qquad (7)$$

This algorithm was fully groupwise, in that changes to any of the $\{\omega_i\}$ change the reference, hence change the description length for all of the images in the set. However, the calculation of the inverse warps (or alternatively the push-forward mappings generated by $\{\omega_i\}$) is computationally expensive.

We propose here a computationally cheaper initialisation algorithm, within the structure shown in Fig. 2. We keep the idea from the algorithm presented in [10], of initial image estimates based on averages of pushed-forward training images, but instead choose to populate the intermediate images, using the leave-one-out means:

$$I_{\mathcal{M}_i}(X_0) = \frac{1}{N-1} \sum_{j \neq i} [\omega_j^{-1*}(I_{T_j})](X_0), \qquad (8)$$

with $\{v_i = \mathbb{I}\}$. We do not explicitly assign a value to the reference image. But we would expect the intermediate images to mutually converge as the algorithm progresses and the images are brought into alignment, so that $\{\Delta_i I_\mathcal{R} \mapsto \varnothing\}$. So, we estimate the true description length thus:

$$\mathcal{L}_{\text{init}}(\{\omega_i\}) = \underbrace{\tfrac{1}{N}\sum_i \mathcal{L}_{\text{Hist}}(I_{\mathcal{M}_i}(X_0))}_{\text{Estimate of } \mathcal{L}_{\text{Hist}}(I_\mathcal{R}(X_0))} + \underbrace{\sum_i \mathcal{L}(\omega_i)}_{\text{Spatial Warps}} + \underbrace{\sum_i \mathcal{L}(\Delta I_{T_i}(X_0))}_{\text{Discrepancy Images}}. \qquad (9)$$

The pseudocode for the initialisation algorithm is given in Alg. 1. Note that the update of the Intermediate images $\{I_{\mathcal{M}_i}(X_0)\}$ (line 6) can be carried out less-frequently than at every training image, if required.

4.2 Groupwise Models

We have shown how to initialise the registration algorithm, within the structure shown in Fig. 1. However, when it comes to building groupwise models, we

Algorithm 2. MDL NRR & Groupwise Model Building

1: **Run** Algorithm 1   %:Output is $\{I_{\mathcal{M}_i}(X_0), \omega_i, \Delta I_{\mathcal{T}_i}(X_0)\}$
2: $v_i \Leftarrow \mathbb{I}$ %:Initial Shared frame for all Intermediate Images
3: $I_{\mathcal{R}}(X_0) \Leftarrow \frac{1}{N} \sum_i I_{\mathcal{M}_i}(X_0)$ %:Estimate Reference as Mean
4: $\Delta_i I_{\mathcal{R}} \Leftarrow I_{\mathcal{M}_i}(X_0) - I_{\mathcal{R}}(X_0)$ %:Maintain Intermediate Images
    Build & Test groupwise model of $\{\Upsilon_i \equiv v_i \circ \Delta_i I_{\mathcal{R}}\}$
5: $(I_{\mathcal{R}}, \{\Delta_i I_{\mathcal{R}}, v_i, \omega_i, I_{\mathcal{M}_i}, \Delta I_{\mathcal{T}_i}\}) \Leftarrow$ **TEST-MODEL**$(I_{\mathcal{R}}, \{\Delta_i I_{\mathcal{R}}, v_i, \omega_i\})$
    Main Loop
6: **Repeat**
7:   **Repeat**
8:     Randomize the order of the set of training images $I_{\mathcal{T}_i}(X_0)$, indexed by i
      Optimise warps ω_i
9:     **For** $i = 1$ to N **do**
10:      Optimise $\mathcal{L}_{\text{total}}$ w.r.t. spatial warps ω_i.   %:$\mathcal{L}_{\text{total}}$ calculated from eq. (3)
11:     **End**
12:   **Until** convergence
    Re-Build Model
13: $(I_{\mathcal{R}}, \{\Delta_i I_{\mathcal{R}}, v_i, \omega_i, I_{\mathcal{M}_i}, \Delta I_{\mathcal{T}_i}\}) \Leftarrow$ **TEST-MODEL**$(I_{\mathcal{R}}, \{\Delta_i I_{\mathcal{R}}, v_i, \omega_i\})$
14: **Until** convergence

Function TEST-MODEL: Build & Test Groupwise Model

1: $\mathcal{L}_{\text{old}} \Leftarrow \mathcal{L}_{\text{total}}(I_{\mathcal{R}}, \{\Delta_i I_{\mathcal{R}}, v_i, \omega_i\})$ %:Description Length $\mathcal{L}$ before modelling, eq.(3)
2: $v_i^{\text{new}} \Leftarrow \omega_i^{-1} \circ v_i$ %:Put all spatial warp into v_i
    Build Model
3: $(I_{\mathcal{R}}^{\text{new}}, \{\Delta_i^{\text{new}} I_{\mathcal{R}}, v_i^{\text{new}}\}) \Leftarrow$ **MODEL**$(I_{\mathcal{R}}, \{\Delta_i I_{\mathcal{R}}, v_i^{\text{new}}\})$
4: $\omega_i^{\text{new}} \Leftarrow v_i^{\text{new}} \circ (v_i^{-1} \circ \omega_i)$ %:Reset ω_i^{new} to maintain spatial correspondence
5: $\mathcal{L}_{\text{new}} \Leftarrow \mathcal{L}_{\text{total}}(I_{\mathcal{R}}^{\text{new}}, \{\Delta_i^{\text{new}} I_{\mathcal{R}}, v_i^{\text{new}}, \omega_i^{\text{new}}\})$ %:Description Length after modelling
6: **If** $\mathcal{L}_{\text{new}} \leq \mathcal{L}_{\text{old}}$ **then**
7:   $\omega_i \Leftarrow \omega_i^{\text{new}}, v_i \Leftarrow v_i^{\text{new}}, I_{\mathcal{R}} \Leftarrow I_{\mathcal{R}}^{\text{new}}, \Delta_i I_{\mathcal{R}} \Leftarrow \Delta_i^{\text{new}} I_{\mathcal{R}}$ %:Accept new values
8:   $I_{\mathcal{M}_i}(X_0) \Leftarrow (v_i \circ \Delta_i I_{\mathcal{R}}) I_{\mathcal{R}}(X_0)$ %:Reset Intermediate Images
9:   $\Delta I_{\mathcal{T}_i}(X_0) \Leftarrow I_{\mathcal{T}_i}(X_0) - [\omega_i^*(I_{\mathcal{M}_i})](X_0)$ %:Reset discrepancies in Training frame
10: **End**

have the structure shown in Fig. 2. One method would be to build some default generative model of the set of deformations $\{\Upsilon_i\}$, and then search within the space of this model. However, this approach suffers from two drawbacks; firstly, the use of a default model (such as a gaussian) would bias the results, since it would tend to force the deformations to have a gaussian distribution, rather than finding the best deformations. The second drawback is computational – if we alter Υ_i, we have to then re-calculate Ω_i so that the combined deformation does indeed re-create our target training image $I_{\mathcal{T}_i}(X_0)$. This means that we have to re-calculate the intermediate image $I_{\mathcal{M}_i}(X_0)$, which means either calculating a pushforward mapping via v_i, or a pushback via v_i^{-1}, both of which are computationally expensive.

We take an alternative approach, which is to optimise the $\{\omega_i\}$. As in Alg. 1, this only involves computing the pullback ω_i^*. So, after we have optimised the set $\{\Omega_i\}$, we then transfer of much of this combined deformation as possible from the intermediate frame $\mathcal{M}_i$ to the equivalent deformation applied in the reference frame $\mathcal{R}$. We can then construct a model in the reference frame. The proposed algorithm is given in Alg. 2. Lines 1-5 are just the initialisation stages, which run the previous initialisation algorithm. The transfer between $\{\Omega_i\}$ and $\{\Upsilon_i\}$ is given in lines 2-3 of the function TEST-MODEL. An important point to note is in line 4 of that function – we maintain the spatial correspondence that we have previously found, despite moving spatial warps between frames. We then build a model of the set of combined deformations $\{\Upsilon_i = (v_i \circ \Delta_i I_\mathcal{R})\}$ and the reference image $I_\mathcal{R}(X_0)$. The modelled deformations are not necessarily the same as the input deformations to the modelling process, which is the reason for the resetting in line 5. We then accept this model provided that it decreases the total description length.

5 Implementation Issues

Consider the relation of spatial frames for the groupwise algorithm (e.g., see Fig. 2 and Alg. 2) – it is clear that we require a description of spatial warps $\{\omega_i, v_i\}$ that allows us to efficiently invert and concatenate warps, as well as a description which allows us to represent a set of warps (i.e.,$\{v_i\}$) within a common representation for the purposes of modelling. Such a description is provided by spline-based formulations which interpolate the movement of general points from the movement of a set of nodes/knotpoints, where the knotpoints can take **arbitrary** positions. In the experiments which follow, we use both the clamped-plate spline, and an efficient spline based on the piecewise-linear interpolation of movements across a tesselated set of knotpoints in either 2D or 3D.

The advantages of such a knotpoint based scheme is that it can be applied in both a multi-resolution and a data-driven fashion. Successive optimisations of the set $\{\omega_i\}$ in Alg. 2 are calculated by adding knotpoints to the previously-optimised set (hence increasing the resolution of the spatial warp). These knotpoints are also chosen in a data-driven manner (e.g., image features such as edges, or places of high discrepancy – see [6,8] for further examples of such data-driven techniques). This not only increases the computational efficiency of our implementation but, as will be shown later, also leads to quantitatively better models. We use a coarse-to-fine strategy during the optimisation – at a coarse spatial resolution, node movements can be large, and it is sufficient to use a low-resolution version of the image. As the spatial resolution of the warps increases, so does the spatial resolution of the image used. The optimisation scheme for the nodes is a simple gradient descent – points are moved singly to estimate the gradient direction for the objective function, but moved all at once using a line search.

6 Model Evaluation Criteria

In order to compare different algorithms for non-rigid registration and model building, we need to have some quantitative measures of the properties of a given model. Following Davies et al. [3], we use two measures of model performance:

- **Generalisability:** the ability to represent unseen images which belong to the same class as images in the training set.
- **Specificity:** the ability to only represent images similar to those seen in the training set.

Let $\{I_\mathfrak{a}(X_0) : \mathfrak{a} = 1, \ldots \mathfrak{N}\}$ be some large set of images, generated by the group-wise model, and having a distribution which is the model distribution. Then we define the following:

$$G = \frac{1}{N} \sum_{i=1}^{N} \min_{\text{w.r.t } \mathfrak{a}} \left(|I_{T_i}(X_0) - I_\mathfrak{a}(X_0)| \right), \text{ Generalisability}, \quad (10)$$

$$S = \frac{1}{\mathfrak{N}} \sum_{\mathfrak{a}=1}^{\mathfrak{N}} \min_{\text{w.r.t. } i} \left(|I_{T_i}(X_0) - I_\mathfrak{a}(X_0)| \right), \text{ Specificity}, \quad (11)$$

where the distance $|\cdot|$ is a measure of the distance between two images. This could be taken as the Euclidean distance between images, but this is likely to be very sensitive to quite small shape changes or misalignments, and thus not provide a useful measure of image difference. To deal with this problem, we have used shuffle distance, calculating, for each pixel in one image, the minimum intensity difference to any pixel/voxel within a radius r of the corresponding pixel/voxel in the other image. The shuffle distance is then defined as the sum across all voxels/pixels of the absolute intensity differences, since this is more robust to outliers than sum-of squares. Note that our definition of G is not that used in [3], but a form which is symmetric as regards the form of S; G measures how close each training image is to images in the modelled distribution, whereas S measures how close each model-generated image is to the training data. Standard errors for S and G can be defined similarly to Davies et al.

7 Experiments

We have performed experiments to validate our MDL objective function and model evaluation criteria and investigate the performance of several different non-rigid registration methods, including that presented in this paper. Although all the methods we have described can be used in 3D, it was impractical to run the very large set of experiments required in the time available, thus we present results for 2D images of the brain.

7.1 Behaviour of the MDL Objective Function

The first question to be answered is whether the total description length has a suitable minimum as regards correspondence across a set of images. To investi-

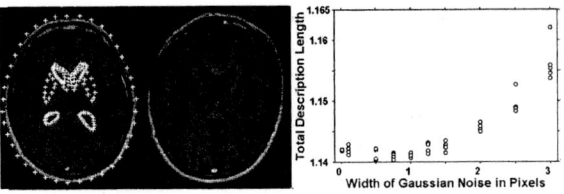

Fig. 3. Left: Two examples of marked-up brains, showing annotation. **Right:** Total description length for this dataset as a function of the size of the perturbation of the points

gate this, we took a dataset which consisted of 2D MR image slices; this dataset had been expertly annotated with 163 points around the skull, ventricles, the caudate nucleus and the lentiform nucleus (see Fig. 3). The clamped-plate spline warp between these points then defined dense image correspondence. We applied a perturbation to the point positions on all the images (independent Gaussian noise of width σ, 5 trials for each value of σ, with 10 images in the dataset). For each value of σ, we constructed the corresponding shape and texture models, the discrepancy between the actual images and the model representations, and hence calculated the total description length. As can be seen from the Figure, there is a general trend that as the perturbation increases, so does the total description length, indicating that the description length does indeed have a minimum in the vicinity of the annotated correspondence.

7.2 Behaviour of the Model Evaluation Criteria

To validate our Generalisability G (10) and Specificity S (11) criteria, we took the same dataset and markup as above, but now with 36 examples. As before, we perturbed the point positions and built the corresponding shape and texture models. We then generated 1000 examples sampled from each model p.d.f., and calculated G and S. The results for various values of the perturbation width σ,

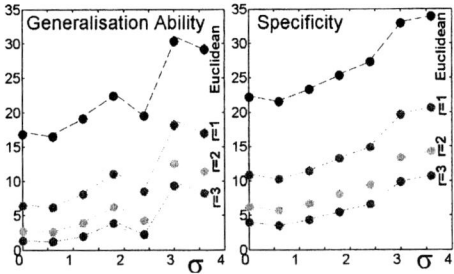

Fig. 4. Left: Generalisation Ability and **Right:** Specificity as a function of the size of the perturbation on the points, for various radii of shuffle distance plus Euclidean distance. Standard errorbars smaller than markers in all cases

and different shuffle distances (r), are shown in Fig. 4. It can be seen that both Generalisability and Specificity increase (get worse) as σ is increased, indicating that they provide useful independent measures of model quality.

The useful range of response is greater for larger shuffle distances (e.g., the slope of the 5×5 ($r = 2$) shuffle distance curve is lower than that of the Euclidian distance curve). In the automatic model building experiments described below we used the 5×5 shuffle distance to calculate G and S.

7.3 Evaluation of Pairwise and Groupwise Registration and Models

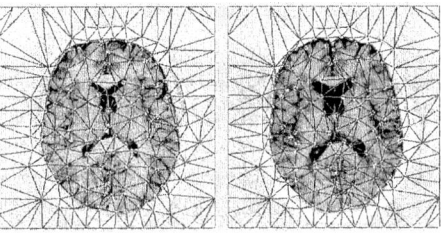

To evaluate different methods of non-rigid registration we used a dataset consisting of 104 2D MR slices of brains taken from normals; the initial 3D data set was affinely-aligned, and then the corresponding slice extracted from each example. Fig. 5 shows examples of the slices. In order to compare different registration strategies, for each technique we registered the entire set of 104 images and built the statistical

Fig. 5. Example images from the brain slice training set, showing the tessellation

models of shape and appearance given by the found correspondence, using the nodes/knotpoints used during the registration. We then computed the Generalisability G (10) and Specificity S (11) for each model (generating 1000 model examples in each case, and using a 5-pixels square sample region for the shuffle distance), enabling a quantitative comparison of the registration strategies from which each model was derived. The strategies tested were:

1 Pairwise Registration:
A Image from training set chosen as reference & 16×16 regular grid of nodes:
  i Residuals calculated in reference frame.
  ii Residuals calculated in training frame.
B As above, but removing points from the grid in regions of low texture variance.
C Ditto, but moving points to nearby strong edges.

2 Groupwise Registration:
A Registering to Intermediate Images estimated as the leave-one-out means (Alg. 1).
B Registering to Intermediate Images estimated using the leave-one-out models.

Note that for **1**, we tried a selection of images from the training set as the reference, and choose that which gave the best results in terms of the evaluation criteria. Strategy **2B** can be viewed as an approximation to the full algorithm given in Alg. 2; in the same way that in the initialisation algorithm (Alg. 1) we estimate the Intermediate Images $\{I_{\mathcal{M}_i}\}$ using the leave-one-out mean, in this case we estimate them by finding the closest fit to the training image $I_{\mathcal{T}_i}$ using the shape model built from all the other examples and the current best estimate of their correspondence. We then optimise the description length of the shape

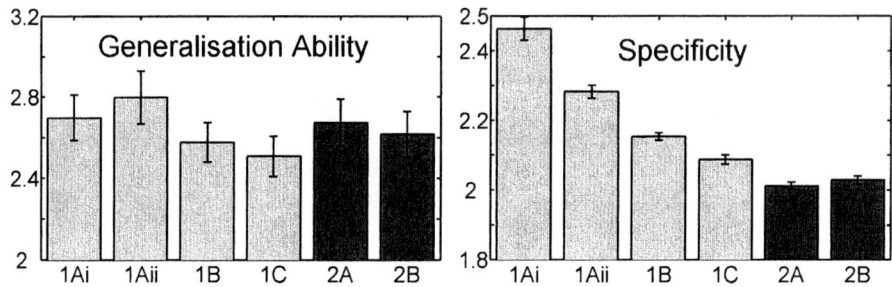

Fig. 6. Generalisation ability and Specificity for the strategies listed in §7.3 – dark bars groupwise, light bars pairwise

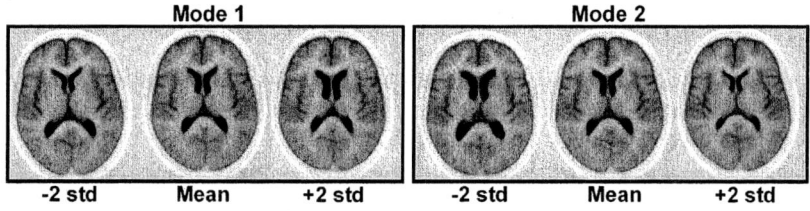

Fig. 7. The first two modes of the shape model built using the results of groupwise registration, acting upon the mean of the texture model

and texture discrepancies between this model estimate and the training image. Note that we do not model the texture at this intermediate stage – this is because in the inner loops of Algs. 1&2, the warps $\{\omega_i\}$ at each spatial resolution are fully optimised, hence can then be modelled, whereas the texture discrepancy is merely continually reduced. The results of this comparison are given in Fig. 6.

8 Discussion and Conclusions

We have presented a principled framework for groupwise non-rigid registration, based on the concept of minimum description length. A groupwise model of shape and appearance is an integral part of the regsitration algorithm, hence the registration also produces an optimal appearance model. We have given a full description of a practical implementation of the basic ideas. Another important contribution is the introduction of objective criteria for evaluating the results of non-rigid registration, based on the properties of the resulting appearance model. The results summarised in Fig. 4 show that the method of evaluation we propose provides a practical method of comparing the quality of different non-rigid registrations. The results summarised in Fig. 3 show that our MDL objective function behaves as expected, with a minimum for a groupwise correspondence close to that given by expert manual annotation. the key results are those summarised in Fig. 6. These show that our groupwise approach achieves better Specificity than several different pairwise approaches. They also show the importance of measuring errors in the correct frame of reference. Further work is required to implement more sophisticated versions of our groupwise approach, and to provide a more comprehensive set of comparisions to alternative approaches. Our initial results are, however, extremely encouraging.

Acknowledgements

This research was supported by the MIAS IRC project, EPSRC grant No. GR/N14248/01, UK Medical Research Council Grant No. D2025/31 (*"From Medical Images and Signals to Clinical Information"*). S. Marsland was supported by the Marsden Fund grant MAU0408, Royal Society of New Zealand, *"A principled approach to the non-rigid registration and structural analysis of groups of medical images"*.

References

1. K. K. Bhatia, J. V. Hajnal, B. K. Puri, A. D. Edwards, and D. Rueckert. Consistent groupwise non-rigid registration for atlas construction. *Proceedings of the IEEE Symposium on Biomedical Imaging (ISBI)*, pages 908–911, 2004.
2. T. F. Cootes, G. J. Edwards, and C. J. Taylor. Active appearance models. *IEEE Transactions on Pattern Analysis and Machine Intelligence*, 23:681–685, 2001.
3. R. H. Davies, C. J. Twining, P. D. Allen, T. F. Cootes, and C. J. Taylor. Shape discrimination in the hippocampus using an MDL model. In *Proceedings of IPMI 2003*, pages 38–50, 2003.
4. B. Davis, P Lorenzen, and S. Joshi. Large deformation minimum mean squared error template estimation for computational anatomy. *Proceedings of the IEEE Symposium on Biomedical Imaging (ISBI)*, pages 173–176, 2004.
5. A. F. Frangi, D. Rueckert, J. A. Schnabel, and W. J. Niessen. Automatic construction of multiple-object three-dimensional statistical shape models: Application to cardiac modelling. *IEEE Transactions on Medical Imaging*, 21(9):1151–1166, 2002.
6. S. Marsland and C. J. Twining. Constructing data-driven optimal representations for iterative pairwise non-rigid registration. *Lecture Notes in Computer Science*, 2717:50–60, 2003.
7. J. Rissanen. *Stochastic Complexity in Statistical Inquiry*. World Scientific Press, 1989.
8. J. A. Schnabel, D. Rueckert, M. Quist, J. M. Blackall, A. D. Castellano-Smith, T. Hartkens, G. P. Penney, W. A. Hall, H. Liu, C. L. Truwit, F. A. Gerritsen, D.L.G. Hill, and D. J. Hawkes. A generic framework for non-rigid registration based on non-uniform multi-level free-form deformations. In *Proceedings of MICCAI 2001*, number 2208 in Lecture Notes in Computer Science, pages 573 – 581, 2001.
9. C.E. Shannon. A mathematical theory of communication. *Bell System Technical Journal*, 27:379–423,623–656, 1948.

10. C. J. Twining, S. Marsland, and C. J. Taylor. Groupwise non-rigid registration: The minimum description length approach. In *Proceedings of the British Machine Vision Conference (BMVC)*, volume 1, pages 417–426, 2004.
11. C.J. Twining, S. Marsland, and C.J. Taylor. A unified information-theoretic approach to the correspondence problem in image registration. In *Proceedings of the International Conference on Pattern Recognition (ICPR)*, 2004.
12. Barbara Zitová and Jan Flusser. Image registration methods: A survey. *Image and Vision Computing*, 21:977 – 1000, 2003.

Hypothesis Testing with Nonlinear Shape Models

Timothy B. Terriberry[1], Sarang C. Joshi[1,2], and Guido Gerig[1,3]

[1] Dept. of Computer Science
[2] Dept. of Radiation Oncology
[3] Dept. of Psychiatry, Univ. of North Carolina, Chapel Hill, NC 27599, USA
{tterribe, joshi, gerig}@cs.unc.edu

Abstract. We present a method for two-sample hypothesis testing for statistical shape analysis using nonlinear shape models. Our approach uses a true multivariate permutation test that is invariant to the scale of different model parameters and that explicitly accounts for the dependencies between variables. We apply our method to m-rep models of the lateral ventricles to examine the amount of shape variability in twins with different degrees of genetic similarity.

1 Introduction

We have been developing methods for statistical shape analysis utilizing medial representations. However, these and many other useful shape models contain a large number of parameters that lie in nonlinear spaces, and so traditional statistical analysis tools designed for Euclidean spaces have to be reformulated. In this paper we formalize the notion of hypothesis testing against data that lies in the direct product of a large number of nonlinear spaces as a tool for understanding growth and disease.

Recently, Fletcher et al. have developed methods for one-sample statistical shape analysis based on medial representations, or *m-reps* [1, 2, 3]. We turn to the problem of two-sample statistics, where we wish to answer the following question: given two samples from two different populations, do they have the same statistical distribution? This is the classic problem of testing the null hypothesis, H_0, that the populations are identical, against its complement, H_1. The main difficulty arises from the fact that m-reps lie on high-dimensional nonlinear manifolds where assumptions of Gaussianity are unreasonable, making traditional parametric or linear methods inapplicable.

We present a true multivariate permutation test approach that is equivalent to traditional nonparametric permutation tests in the univariate case, and converges to the same result as Hotelling's well-known T^2 test in the linear, normally-distributed case. The only tool we require on the underlying space our data lives in is the existence of a metric.

The mechanics of the method are similar to those used in correction for multiple tests [4]. Unlike methods of direct combination, which sum up various

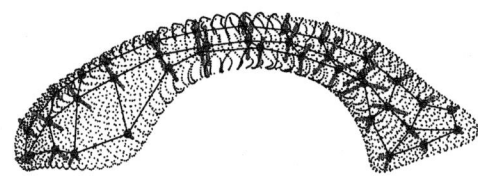 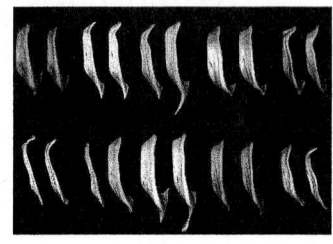

Fig. 1. Left: An example m-rep of a left lateral ventricle. The mesh vertices and off-shooting spokes make up the medial atoms. The shape the m-rep was fit to is shown as a point cloud surrounding it. Right: Ventricle pairs from five monozygotic twin pairs (top) and five dizygotic twin pairs (bottom)

test statistics [5,6], our method is invariant to the scale of each term. This is critical when different shape parameters have different physical units and the choice of weighting between them can be arbitrary. Our test also accounts for the dependencies between model parameters.

1.1 A Metric Space for M-Reps

M-reps are a medial shape model whose parameters provide intuitive descriptions of local object thickness, bending, narrowing, and widening. They have been well-described by previous authors [7], but for completeness we provide a brief summary. An m-rep is a coarse grid of samples that lie on the medial axis of an object. Each sample, called a *medial atom*, consists of a 4-tuple $\underline{m} = (\mathbf{x}, r, \mathbf{n}_0, \mathbf{n}_1)$ of parameters. The 3-D position of the atom is $\mathbf{x} \in \mathbb{R}^3$, the distance to the two closest boundary points is $r \in \mathbb{R}^+$, and $\mathbf{n}_0, \mathbf{n}_1 \in S^2$ are unit vectors that point from the atom position towards the two boundary points. The direct product of these spaces, $\mathbb{R}^3 \times \mathbb{R}^+ \times S^2 \times S^2$, is denoted $\mathcal{M}(1)$, and an entire m-rep with p medial atoms lives in the direct product space $\mathcal{M}(p) = \mathcal{M}(1)^p$. See Fig. 1 for an example of a complete model and a sample of our shape population.

Fletcher et al. treat medial atoms as elements of a Riemannian symmetric space [2]. Such a space is a differentiable manifold and has a Riemannian metric that is invariant to certain transformations of the space. $\mathbb{R}^3$ uses the normal Euclidean metric, while the positive reals, $\mathbb{R}^+$, use the metric $d(r_1, r_2) = |\log(r_1) - \log(r_2)|$, and the unit sphere, S^2, uses distance measured along the surface of the sphere. Every point on the manifold has a tangent plane, which is a vector space, and exponential and log maps that project from the plane to the manifold and back while preserving distances from the tangent point in a local neighborhood. For a more complete treatment, see Fletcher's Ph.D. thesis [3].

1.2 One-Sample Statistics in Nonlinear Spaces

In linear spaces, the most important property of a probability distribution is often its first moment, the mean. Fréchet generalized the notion of an arithmetic mean of a sample of n points x_i drawn from a distribution in a general metric space M as the point which minimizes the sum-of-squared distances [8]:

$$\hat{\mu} = \text{argmin}_{x \in M} \frac{1}{2n} \sum_{i=1}^{n} d(x, x_i)^2 \, . \tag{1}$$

This is sometimes referred to as the Fréchet mean or the *intrinsic mean*, but hereafter will just be called the mean.

In general, this mean may not exist, or may not be unique, and without additional structure on the metric space, the minimization may be difficult to perform. However, for Riemannian manifolds, it is possible to compute the gradient of this functional [9], making a gradient descent algorithm possible [10]. Kendall showed that existence and uniqueness is guaranteed if the data is well-localized [11]. Fletcher et al. extend this, using principal component analysis (PCA) in the tangent plane at the mean to characterize the distribution of one sample [2].

1.3 Two-Sample Statistics

If we assume both of our distributions are identical around the mean, and that they can be characterized entirely by the distance from the mean, then a single global distance value is sufficient to construct a univariate permutation test for equality of the two means. Permutation tests are appealing because they make no other distributional assumptions, requiring only that the data in each group be exchangeable under the null hypothesis that they do in fact come from the same distribution. The interested reader is referred to Bradley [12] or Nichols and Holmes [13] for details.

However, our geometric models contain parameters in nonlinear spaces, like the sphere. Some parameters may have a large variance, masking the effects of other variables with a smaller variance that might provide greater discrimination. Some may be highly correlated, unduly increasing their contribution to the distance over that of parameters with less correlation. Some will have completely different scales, and appropriate scale factors need to be determined to combine them in a single metric. These factors make the assumption that the distance from the mean entirely characterizes the distribution hard to justify.

For example, scaling the model will change the distance between medial atom centers, **x**, without affecting the distance between radii or spoke directions. To combat this, Fletcher et al. propose scaling the latter by the average radius across corresponding medial atoms [2], but this choice is somewhat arbitrary. It does restore invariance to scale, but does nothing to handle differing degrees of variability or correlation. Different choices of scale factors will produce tests with different powers.

In $\mathbb{R}^n$, if we relax our assumption that the distribution is characterized by the distance from the mean, and instead assume only a common covariance, the classic Hotelling's T^2 test provides a test invariant to coordinate transformations. For normally distributed data, it is uniformly the most powerful (see a standard text, such as Anderson's [14], for a derivation). The test is based on the statistic:

$T^2 \propto D^2 = (\hat{\mu}_1 - \hat{\mu}_2)^T \hat{\Sigma}^{-1}(\hat{\mu}_1 - \hat{\mu}_2)$, where $\hat{\mu}_1$ and $\hat{\mu}^2$ are the sample means and $\hat{\Sigma}$ the pooled sample covariance. Any linear change of coordinates yields a corresponding change in metric, but this is absorbed by the $\hat{\Sigma}^{-1}$ term.

2 Multivariate Permutation Tests

The hypothesis test we propose is an attempt to generalize the desirable properties of Hotelling's T^2 test to a nonparametric, nonlinear setting. We cannot take advantage of the vector space structure of the tangent plane, as Fletcher et al. do, to apply Hotelling's test directly, because there is a different tangent space around each sample's mean, and there may be no unique map between them. For example, on the sphere, such a map has one degree of freedom, allowing an arbitrary rotation of the coordinate axes in the vector space. Instead, we take a more general approach, only requiring that our objects lie in a metric space.

Our approach is based upon a general framework for nonparametric combination introduced by Pesarin [15]. The general idea is to perform a set of partial tests, each on a different aspect of the data, and then combine them into a single summary statistic, taking into account the dependence between the variables and the true multivariate nature of the data. We assume that we have two distributions with the same structure around the mean, and develop a test to determine if the means are equal. We now begin describing the details.

2.1 The Univariate Case

We begin by introducing notation and describing the procedure for a single, univariate permutation test. Suppose we have two data sets of size n_1 and n_2, $x_1 = \{x_{1,i}, i \in 1 \ldots n_1\}$ and $x_2 = \{x_{2,i}, i \in 1 \ldots n_2\}$, and a test statistic, $T(x_1, x_2)$. To test for a difference in the means, a natural test statistic is

$$T(x_1, x_2) = d(\hat{\mu}_1, \hat{\mu}_2) , \qquad (2)$$

where $\hat{\mu}_1$ and $\hat{\mu}_2$ are the sample means of the two data sets computed via the optimization in (1). For other tests, other statistics are possible.

Under the null hypothesis, both samples are drawn from the same distribution, and so we may randomly permute the data between the two groups without affecting the distribution of $T(x_1, x_2)$. We pool the data together, and then generate $N = \binom{n_1+n_2}{n_1}$ random partitions into two new groups, still of size n_1 and n_2. We label these $x_{1,i}^k$ and $x_{2,i}^k$, with $k \in 1 \ldots N$, and compute the value of the test statistic, T^k, for all of them. We always include the actual observed groupings among this list, and denote its test statistic T^o. This forms an empirical distribution of the statistic, from which we can calculate the probability of observing T^o under the null hypothesis:

$$p(T^o) = \frac{1}{N} \sum_{k=1}^{N} H(T^k, T^o) , \qquad H(T^k, T^o) = \begin{cases} 1, & T^k \geq T^o \\ 0, & T^k < T^o \end{cases} . \qquad (3)$$

2.2 Partial Tests

If our data can be adequately summarized by a single test statistic, then this is the end of the story. We now turn to the case where we have M test statistics: one for each of the parameters in our shape model. Let $\mu_{1,j}$ and $\mu_{2,j}$ be the means of the jth model parameter for each population. Then we wish to test whether any hypothesis $H_{1,j} : \{\mu_{1,j} \neq \mu_{2,j}\}$ is true against the alternative, that each null hypothesis $H_{0,j} : \{\mu_{1,j} = \mu_{2,j}\}$ is true. The partial test statistics $T_j(x_1, x_2), j \in 1 \ldots M$ are defined analogously to (2), and the values for permutations of this data are denoted T_j^k, , with $j \in 1 \ldots M$, $k \in 1 \ldots N$.

Given that each $T_j(x_1, x_2)$ is significant for large values, consistent, and marginally unbiased, Pesarin shows that a suitable combining function (described in the next section) will produce an unbiased test for the global hypothesis H_0 against H_1 [15]. The meaning of each of these criteria is as follows:

1. **Significant for large values:** Given a significance level α and the critical value of $T_j(x_1, x_2)$ at α—T_j^α—the probability that $T_j^o \geq T_j^\alpha$ is at least α. For a two-sided test $T_j(x_1, x_2)$ must be significant for both large and small values.

2. **Consistent:** As the sample size $n = n_1 + n_2$ goes to infinity, the probability that $T_j^o \geq T_j^\alpha$ must converge to 1.

3. **Marginally unbiased:** For any threshold z, the probability that $T_j^o \leq z$ given $H_{0,j}$ must be greater than the probability that $T_j^o \leq z$ given $H_{1,j}$, irrespective of the results of any other partial test. This implies that T_j^o is positively dependent in $H_{1,j}$ regardless of any dependencies between variables.

Since each of our tests are restricted to the data from a single component of the direct product and we have assumed that the distributions around the means are identical, they are marginally unbiased. We cannot add a test for equality of the distributions about the mean, as then the test for equality of means would be biased on its outcome.

To illustrate these ideas, we present a simple example, which we will follow through the next few sections. We take two samples of $n_1 = n_2 = 10$ data points from the two-dimensional space $\mathbb{R} \times \mathbb{R}^+$, corresponding to a position and a scale parameter. The samples are taken from a multivariate normal distribution by exponentiating the second coordinate, and then scaling both coordinates by a factor of ten. They are plotted together in Fig. 2a. They have the common covariance (before the exponentiation) of $\frac{1}{2} \left(\begin{smallmatrix} 3 & 1 \\ 1 & 3 \end{smallmatrix} \right)$, and the two means are slightly offset in the second coordinate. That is, $\mu_{1,1} = \mu_{2,1}$, but $\mu_{1,2} < \mu_{2,2}$.

We construct $M = 2$ partial test statistics using (2) for each coordinate, and evaluate them using Monte Carlo simulation. To avoid an exponential complexity, we use a fixed $N = 10,000$ permutations, which still provides an unbiased test. The results are shown in Fig. 2b. The first partial test value lies in the middle of the distribution, while the second lies near the edge. However, the scale of the first test is much larger, because no logarithm is involved in its metric.

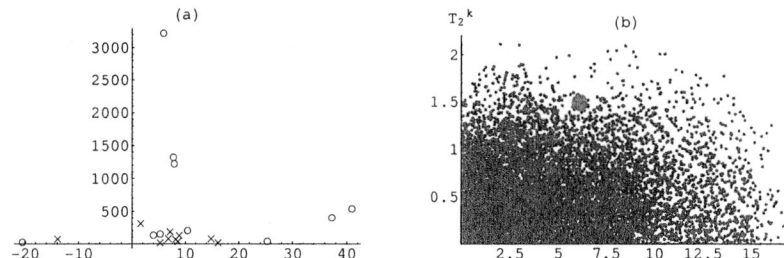

Fig. 2. The observed data and test statistics for our simple example. (a) shows the distribution of our two samples, with ×'s for the first and o's for the second. (b) shows the distribution of the partial test statistics under permutation. The large dot indicates the location of the observed data point

2.3 Multivariate Combination

Given the partial tests from the previous section, we wish to combine them into a single test, while preserving the underlying dependence relations between the tests. This is done in the following manner. We apply the same N permutations to the data when computing each of partial tests, and then compute a p-value using the empirical distribution for that test over all of the other permutations:

$$p(T_j^k) = \frac{1}{N} \sum_{l=1}^{N} H(T_j^l, T_j^k) \ . \tag{4}$$

Thus, for every permutation k we have a column vector of p-values, $p(T^k) = (p(T_1^k), \ldots, p(T_j^k), \ldots, p(T_M^k))^T$. It is critical to use the same permutations for each partial test, as this is what captures the nature of the joint distribution.

We now wish to design a combining function to produce a single summary statistic, $T'(p(T^k))$, from each p-value vector. For one-sided tests, this statistic must be monotonically non-increasing in each argument, must obtain its (possibly infinite) supremum when any p-value is zero, and the critical value T'^α must be finite and strictly smaller than the supremum. If these conditions are satisfied, along with those on the partial tests from the previous section, then $T'(p(T^k))$ will be an unbiased test for the global hypothesis H_0 against H_1 [15].

Our combining function is motivated by the two-sided case, where we can use the Mahalanobis distance. First, we compute a U^k vector for each permutation, where $U_j^k = \Phi^{-1}(p(T_j^k) - \frac{1}{2N})$ and $j \in 1 \ldots M$. Here Φ is the cumulative distribution function for the standard normal distribution. The extra $\frac{1}{2N}$ term keeps the values finite when the p-value is 1, and is negligible as N goes to infinity.

Because the distribution of p-values for each partial test is uniform by construction, the marginal distribution of the U_j^k values over k for a single j is standard normal. Arranging these vectors into a single $N \times M$ matrix U, we can estimate the covariance matrix $\hat{\Sigma}_U = \frac{1}{N} U^T U$, and use the Mahalanobis statistic: $T'^k = (U^k)^T \hat{\Sigma}_U^{-1} U^k$. In the event that the data really is linear and normally distributed, $\hat{\Sigma}_U$ matrix converges to the true covariance as the sample size goes to infinity [16], making it asymptotically equivalent to Hotelling's T^2 test. Even if the sample size is small, the matrix Σ_U is well-conditioned regardless of the number of variables, since it is the covariance over the N permutations.

Typically, our distances are not signed, and so we are interested in a one-sided test. In this case, we use the positive half of the standard normal c.d.f., $U_j^k = \Phi^{-1}(1 - \frac{1}{2}(p(T_j^k) - \frac{1}{2N}))$, and assume the U^k distribution is symmetric about the origin. This assumption, however, implies that the covariance between $U_{j_1}^k$ and $U_{j_2}^k$ when $j_1 \neq j_2$ is exactly zero. The diagonal entries of $\hat{\Sigma}_U$ are 1 by construction, and so $\hat{\Sigma}_U = I$, the identity matrix. The fact that the p-values of the partial tests are invariant to scale obviates the need for arbitrary scaling factors. Thus, our one-sided combining function is:

$$T'^k = (U^k)^T \cdot U^k \ . \tag{5}$$

Note that normality of the partial test statistics is not required, and that the even though the marginal distributions of the U^k vectors are normal, the joint distribution may not be. Therefore, we must use a nonparametric approach to estimating the distribution of the T'^o statistic under the null hypothesis. Just as in the univariate case, this produces a single p-value:

$$p(T'^o) = \frac{1}{N} \sum_{k=1}^{N} H(T'^k, T'^o) \ . \tag{6}$$

It is this nonparametric approach that corrects for correlation among the tests, even without explicit diagonal entries in the covariance matrix.

We return to our example from the previous section. The U^k vectors are plotted in Fig. 3a, along with the $\alpha = 0.95$ decision boundary, and our sample is shown to lie outside of it. As can be seen, equal power is assigned to alternatives lying at the same distance from the origin in this space. Figure 3b shows this boundary mapped back into the space of the original p-values. The p-values of the individual partial tests are 0.36 and 0.022, and the combined result is 0.049.

2.4 Relation to Other Testing Procedures

The entire procedure is very similar to procedures used in correction for multiple tests, such as that proposed by Pantazis et al. [4]. In fact, another alternative for a combining function is Tippet's $T'^k = \max_{j=1}^{M}(1 - p(T_j^k))$, which results in a Bonferroni-style correction [15]. Some authors have suggested methods of direct combination applied to the T_j^k statistics themselves [5,6]. They are more appealing computationally, being $O(nMN)$ instead of our method's $O(nMN \log(N))$, but they do not avoid problems of differing scale or strong correlation.

Consider what happens when $T'^k = \sqrt{(T_1^k)^2 + (T_2^k)^2}$. Now, the first test dominates the results, and the overall p-value becomes 0.34. With $n_1 = n_2 = 100$ samples, our test becomes much more significant ($p = 0.0008$), while the direct combination test becomes even worse ($p = 0.44$).

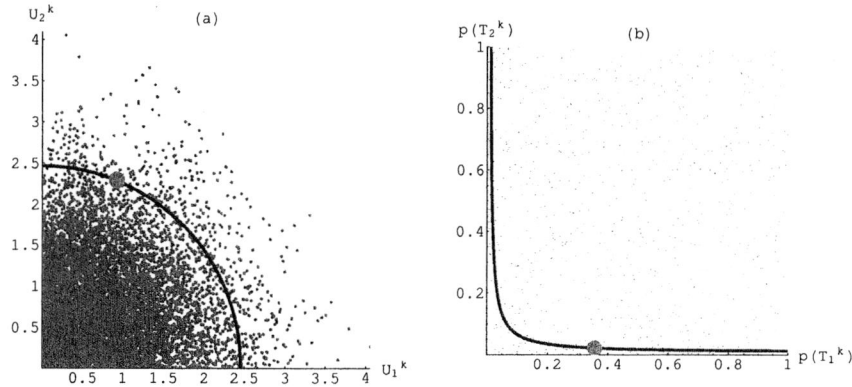

Fig. 3. The empirical distribution of our example plotted against the decision boundary at $\alpha = 0.95$. (a) The distribution of the U^k vectors, where the cutoff is a circle centered around the origin. (b) The distribution of the original p-values with the decision boundary pulled back into this space

3 Experimental Data and Results

The data for our experiments comes from a twin pair schizophrenia study conducted by Weinberger et al. [17]. High resolution ($0.9375 \times 0.9375 \times 1.5$ mm^3) Magnetic Resonance Imaging (MRI) scans were acquired from three different subject groups: 9 healthy monozygotic twin pairs (MZ), 10 healthy dizygotic twin pairs (DZ), and 9 monozygotic twin pairs with one twin discordant for schizophrenia and one twin unaffected. See Fig. 1 for some examples. A fourth group of 10 healthy non-related subject pairs (NR) was constructed by matching unrelated members of the two healthy groups. All four groups were matched for age, gender, and handedness. A tenth healthy, monozygotic twin pair was discarded due to segmentation problems attributed to head trauma suffered by one of the twins in a car accident at age seven. A tenth twin pair discordant for schizophrenia was discarded due to hydrocephaly in the unaffected twin.

The left and right lateral ventricles were segmented using supervised classification and 3-D connectivity [18]. An automatic morphological closing operation was applied to ensure a spherical topology. An area-preserving map was used to map them to a sphere, after which they were converted to a spherical harmonics representation (SPHARM) [19]. Correspondence on the boundary was established using the first order harmonics [20]. Point Distribution Models (PDMs) were constructed by uniformly sampling the boundary at corresponding points. The m-rep models were constructed using a robust method that ensures a common medial topology [21]. For our data, this consists of a single medial sheet with a 3×13 grid of medial atoms, which provides 98% volume overlap with the original segmentations.

From this data set, we wish to determine if the twin pairs that were more closely related had smaller variations in shape. We also wish to see if the shape variations between the discordant and the unaffected twins in the schizophrenic pairs is similar to the normal variation between healthy monozygotic twins. For this purpose, we use the partial test statistics:

$$T_j(x_1, y_1, x_2, y_2) = \frac{1}{n_2} \sum_{i=1}^{n_2} d(x_{2,i,j}, y_{2,i,j}) - \frac{1}{n_1} \sum_{i=1}^{n_1} d(x_{1,i,j}, y_{1,i,j}) \ . \quad (7)$$

Here (x_1, y_1) form the twin pairs for one group, while (x_2, y_2) form the twin pairs for the other. The partial tests are applied separately to all three components of the medial atom location, **x**, as well as the radius and two spoke directions. This gives six partial tests per medial atom, for a total of $M = 3 \times 13 \times 6 = 234$, much larger than the sample size. Each is a one-sided test that the variability in group 2 is larger than that in group 1.

For consistency with previous studies [22], all shapes were volume normalized. After normalization, we also applied m-rep alignment, as described by Fletcher et al. [2], to minimize the sum of squared geodesic distances between models in a medial analog of Procrustes alignment. First, the members of each twin pair were aligned with each other, and then the pairs were aligned together as a group, applying the same transformation to each member of a single pair.

In order to ensure invariance to rotations, we had to choose data-dependent coordinate axes for the **x** component of each medial atom. Our choice was the axes which diagonalized the sample covariance of the displacement vectors from one twin's atom position to the other at each site. While this had some influence on the results, the general trend was the same irrespective of the axes used.

For each pair of twin groups, we generated $N = 50,000$ permutations, and computed their p-value vectors using (4). Following Sect. 2.3, these were mapped into U^k vectors, from which the empirical distribution of the combined test statistic T'^k from (5) was estimated, producing a single global p-value via (6).

The results are summarized in Table 1. For comparison, we list the results of a previous study which used a univariate test on the average distance between corresponding points on the PDMs [22]. While we note that the significance of a p-value on an experimental data set is not a useful metric for comparing different methods, it is interesting to see the differences between the two. Our tests give a consistent ranking: MZ $\approx$ DS $<$ DZ $\approx$ NR, which is fully transitive. The boundary study, however, finds a significant difference between DZ and NR, but fails to identify the difference between DS and DZ.

We also performed local tests, to identify specific medial atoms with with strong differences. A multivariate test was conducted using our procedure on the 6 components of $\mathcal{M}(1)$ for each atom, and the results were corrected for multiple tests using the minimum p-value distribution across the shape, as described by Pantazis et al. [4]. The results are shown in Fig 4.

Table 1. p-values for paired tests for the difference in the amount of shape variability in groups with different degrees of genetic similarity. Results from our method are in the first two columns, while results from a previous study [22] are in the last two for comparison. Groups are: monozygotic (MZ), monozygotic twins with one twin discordant for schizophrenia (DS), dizygotic (DZ), and non-related (NR). Results significant at the $\alpha = 0.95$ level are shown in **bold**

	Our Study		Boundary Study [22]	
	Left	Right	Left	Right
MZ vs. DS	0.12	0.38	0.28	0.68
MZ vs. DZ	**0.00006**	**0.0033**	**0.0082**	**0.0399**
MZ vs. NR	**0.00002**	**0.00020**	**0.0018**	**0.0006**
DS vs. DZ	**0.020**	**0.0076**	0.25	0.24
DS vs. NR	**0.0031**	**0.00026**	**0.018**	**0.0026**
DZ vs. NR	0.16	0.055	**0.05**	**0.016**

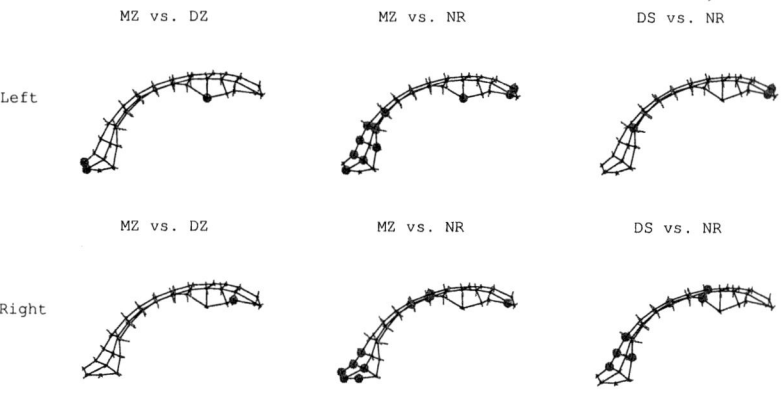

Fig. 4. Results for local tests for the difference in shape variability in groups with different degrees of genetic similarity. Atoms with differences significant at the $\alpha = 0.95$ level are shown in a larger size. Tests not shown had no significant local differences

4 Conclusion

We have presented a true multivariate permutation test approach for hypothesis testing in direct products of metric spaces. The resulting test does not require a priori scaling factors to be chosen, and captures the true multivariate nature of the data. It is well-defined even in the high-dimensional, low-sample size case. The method has been applied to shape discrimination using m-reps, though it is suitable for any type of metric data, including potentially categorical data.

An important area for future research is the design of suitable partial tests to use in each space. Because they cannot be broken into smaller pieces than a single component of the direct product, the distance to the mean and similar tests are limited in the types of distributions they can describe. For example, the distance from the mean can only characterize an isotropic distribution on the sphere. An interesting candidate is the test designed by Hall and Tajvidi, which can test for equality of entire distributions in a single metric space [23]. This would allow us to relax our assumption of identical distribution about the mean. For manifolds, another possibility is the use of tests based on Distance Weighted Discrimination [24]. It is also possible to extend this to different shape models, such as PDMs with surface normals or deformable templates [25].

Acknowledgments

The authors would like to thank Douglas Jones and Daniel Weinberger at NIMH, Clinical Brain Disorder Branch (Bethesda, MD) for providing the MRI for the twin ventricle data set, and Martin Styner for producing the m-rep models.

References

1. Fletcher, P.T., Lu, C., Joshi, S.C.: Statistics of shape via principal component analysis on Lie groups. In: Proceedings of the Conference on Computer Vision and Pattern Recognition (CVPR'03), Los Alamitos, CA (2003) 95–101
2. Fletcher, P.T., Lu, C., Pizer, S.M., Joshi, S.C.: Principal geodesic analysis for the study of nonlinear statistics of shape. IEEE Transactions on Medical Imaging 23 (2004) 995–1005
3. Fletcher, P.T.: Statistical Variability in Nonlinear Spaces: Application to Shape Analysis and DT-MRI. PhD thesis, UNC at Chapel Hill (2004)
4. Pantazis, D., Leahy, R.M., Nichols, T.E., Styner, M.: Statistical surface-based morphometry using a non-parametric approach. In: Proceedings of the IEEE International Symposium on Biomedical Imaging (ISBI'04). (2004) 1283–1286
5. Chung, J.H., Fraser, D.A.S.: Randomization tests for a multivariate two-sample problem. Journal of the American Statistical Association 53 (1958) 729–735
6. Blair, R.C., Higgins, J.J., Karniski, W., Kromrey, J.D.: A study of multivariate permutation tests which may replace Hotelling's T^2 test in prescribed circumstances. Multivariate Behavioral Research 29 (1994) 141–164
7. Joshi, S.C., Fletcher, P.T., Yushkevich, P.A., Thall, A., Marron, J.S.: Multi-scale deformable model segmentation and statistical shape analysis using medial descriptions. IEEE Transactions on Medical Imaging 21 (2002) 538–550
8. Fréchet, M.: Les éléments aléatoires de nature quelconque dans un espace distancié. Annales de L'Institut Henri Poincaré 10 (1948) 215–310
9. Karcher, H.: Riemannian center of mass and mollifier smoothing. Communications on Pure and Applied Math 30 (1977) 509–541
10. Pennec, X.: Probabilities and statistics on Riemannian manifolds: Basic tools for geometric measurements. In Cetin, A., Akarun, L., Ertuzun, A., Gurcan, M.N., Yardimci, Y., eds.: Proceedings of the IEEE-EURASIP Workshop on Nonlinear Signal and Image Processing (NSIP'99). (1999) 194–198

11. Kendall, W.S.: Probability, convexity, and harmonic maps with small image I: Uniqueness and fine existence. In: Proceedings of the London Mathematical Society. Volume 61. (1990) 371–406
12. Bradley, J.V.: Distribution-Free Statistical Tests. Prentice Hall, Englewood Cliffs, New Jersey (1968)
13. Nichols, T.E., Holmes, A.P.: Nonparametric permutation tests for functional neuroimaging: A primer with examples. Human Brain Mapping **15** (2002) 1–25
14. Anderson, T.W.: An Introduction to Multivariate Statistical Analysis. John Wiley & Sons, Inc., New York (1958)
15. Pesarin, F.: Multivariate Permutation Tests with Applications in Biostatistics. John Wiley & Sons, Ltd., Chirchester (2001)
16. Pallini, A., Pesarin, F.: A class of combinations of dependent tests by a resampling procedure. In Jöckel, K.H., Rothe, G., Sendler, W., eds.: Bootstrapping and Related Techniques. Volume 376 of Lecture Notes in Economics and Mathematical Systems., Berlin, Springer-Verlag (1992) 93–97
17. Weinberger, D.R., Egan, M.F., Bertolino, A., Callicott, J.H., Mattay, V.S., Lipska, B.K., Berman, K.F., Goldberg, T.E.: Prefrontal neurons and the genetics of schizophrenia. Biological Psychiatry **50** (2001) 825–844
18. van Leemput, K., Maes, F., Vandermeulen, D., Seutens, P.: Automated model-based tissue classification of MR images of the brain. IEEE Transactions on Medical Imaging **18** (1999) 897–908
19. Brechbühler, C., Gerig, G., Kübler, O.: Parameterization of closed surfaces for 3-D shape description. Computer Vision, Graphics, and Image Processing: Image Understanding **61** (1995) 195–170
20. Gerig, G., Styner, M., Jones, D., Weinberger, D.R., Lieberman, J.A.: Shape analysis of brain ventricles using SPHARM. In: Proceedings of the IEEE Workshop on Mathematical Methods in Biomedical Image Analysis. (2001) 171–178
21. Styner, M., Gerig, G., Joshi, S.C., Pizer, S.M.: Automatic and robust computation of 3-D medial models incorporating object variability. International Journal of Computer Vision **55** (2003) 107–122
22. Styner, M., Lieberman, J.A., McClure, R.K., Weinberger, D.R., Jones, D.W., Gerig, G.: Morphometric analysis of lateral ventricles in schizophrenia and healthy controls regarding genetic and disease-specific factors. Proceedings of the National Academy of Science **102** (2005) 4872–4877
23. Hall, P., Tajvidi, N.: Permutation tests for equality of distributions in high-dimensional settings. Biometrika **89** (2002) 359–374
24. Marron, J.S., Todd, M.J.: Distance weighted discrimination. Technical Report 1339, Operations Research and Industrial Engineering, Cornell University (2002)
25. Grenander, U., Keenan, D.M.: Towards automated image understanding. Advances in Applied Statistics: Statistics and Images **1** (1993) 89–103

Extrapolation of Sparse Tensor Fields: Application to the Modeling of Brain Variability

Pierre Fillard[1], Vincent Arsigny[1], Xavier Pennec[1], Paul M. Thompson[2], and Nicholas Ayache[1]

[1] INRIA Sophia Antipolis - Epidaure Project - France
{Pierre.Fillard, Arsigny, Pennec, Ayache}@sophia.inria.fr
[2] Lab of Neuro Imaging, UCLA School of Medicine, Los Angeles, CA, USA
thompson@loni.ucla.edu

Abstract. Modeling the variability of brain structures is a fundamental problem in the neurosciences. In this paper, we start from a dataset of precisely delineated anatomical structures in the cerebral cortex: a set of 72 sulcal lines in each of 98 healthy human subjects. We propose an original method to compute the average sulcal curves, which constitute the mean anatomy in this context. The second order moment of the sulcal distribution is modeled as a sparse field of covariance tensors (symmetric, positive definite matrices). To extrapolate this information to the full brain, one has to overcome the limitations of the standard Euclidean matrix calculus. We propose an affine-invariant Riemannian framework to perform computations with tensors. In particular, we generalize radial basis function (RBF) interpolation and harmonic diffusion PDEs to tensor fields. As a result, we obtain a dense 3D variability map which proves to be in accordance with previously published results on smaller samples subjects. Moreover, leave one (sulcus) out tests show that our model is globally able to recover the missing information when there is a consistent neighboring variability. Last but not least, we propose innovative methods to analyze the asymmetry of brain variability. As expected, the greatest asymmetries are found in regions that includes the primary language areas. Interestingly, such an asymmetry in anatomical variance could explain why there may be greater power to detect group activation in one hemisphere than the other in fMRI studies.

1 Introduction

Brain structures differ greatly in shape and size even among normal subjects, and these variations make it difficult to identify abnormal differences due to disease. Understanding the degree and quality of brain variation is vital for distinguishing signs of disease from normal variations. Geometric variability of anatomy also makes the automated segmentation and labeling of brain structures difficult. Statistical information on brain variability would make this task easier, and could be used in Bayesian approaches for nonlinear registration as well (which adjust for anatomical variations across subjects). Finally, neuroscientists are interested in identifying the causes of brain variability at a genetic or environmental level. Measuring brain asymmetry (i.e. differences between hemispheres) is of special interest as it sheds light on how the functions of the two hemispheres become specialized. Improved modeling of the range of variations in brain structure could make it easier to isolate specific effects of genetic polymorphisms on these normal variations and asymmetries.

A major class of anatomical variations can be thought of as arising from the smooth deformation of a reference anatomy, where the deformation is represented as a 3D displacement field, after affine (linear) differences are factored out. Ideally, one could model the joint variability of all pairs of points to see how the displacement of one any point in a specific subject w.r.t the reference anatomy covaries with the displacement of neighboring or distant points in the brain (e.g. symmetric ones in the opposite hemisphere). In this article, we simply model the variability of each point independently. Assuming that the mean deformation of the reference anatomy is null, the first moment of the 3D displacement distribution is its covariance matrix, which will be called a *variability tensor*. Thus, our goal is to compute the field of variability tensors within the brain from information that may be sparsely distributed.

However, working with tensors is not so easy as the underlying space is a manifold that is not a vector space. As tensors constitute a convex half-cone in the vector space of matrices, many operations (like computing the mean) are stable. Nonetheless, this Euclidean framework is not satisfactory as one can easily reach the boundary of the space (singular symmetric matrices) with a classical gradient descent. Moreover, the arithmetic mean of a tensor and its inverse is not the identity matrix. This lack of symmetry is unsatisfactory: in many cases, one would like the mean to be geometric.

In Sec. 2.1 we present a consistent Riemannian framework to compute with tensors. Then, we show in Sec. 2.2 how to extend these tools to implement harmonic diffusion PDEs and extrapolate tensors that are sparsely distributed in space. Solving these PDEs is computer intensive, so in Sec. 2.3 we provide a practical but efficient initialization by extending the radial basis functions (RBF) concept to tensors. In Sec. 3, we consider low dimensional but anatomically very readily defined and delineated features (sulcal lines) as a way to obtain meaningful brain variability tensors. We show in Sec. 3.1 how to compute the mean sulcal curve and its correspondence with the sulcal instances of each subject. To extract only the relevant information and minimize the number of parameters, we fit in Sec. 3.2 a parametric tensor model to these data. Then, we come back to our original goal in 3.3 by extrapolating this sparse tensor model to the whole brain. The validity of our extrapolated model is analyzed in Sec. 3.4. In Sec. 3.5 we generalize our statistical model to examine the correlation of the variations observed at symmetric points in the brain.

2 A Mathematical Framework to Extrapolate Tensors

Much of the literature addresses tensor computing problems in the context of diffusion tensor image (DTI) regularization. In these articles, the spectral decomposition of the tensors is exploited. For instance, [1] anisotropically restores the principal direction of the tensors, while [2] independently restores the eigenvalues and eigenvectors. This last approach requires an additional reorientation step of the eigenvectors due to the non-uniqueness of the decomposition.

More recently, differential geometric approaches have been developed to generalize the PCA to tensor data [3], for statistical segmentation of tensor images [4], for computing a geometric mean and an intrinsic anisotropy index [5], or as the basis for a full framework for Riemannian tensor calculus [6]. In this last work, we endowed the space of tensors with an affine invariant Riemannian metric to obtain results that are independent of the choice of the spatial coordinate system. In fact, this metric had already been proposed in statistics [7], and turns out to be the basis of all the previous differential geometric approaches.

2.1 A Riemannian Framework for Tensor Calculus

The invariant metric provides a new framework in which the limitations of Euclidean calculus are fully overcome: it endows the tensor space with a very regular structure where matrices with null or negative eigenvalues are at an infinite distance from any positive definite matrix. Moreover, the geodesic between two tensors is uniquely defined, leading to interesting properties such as the existence and uniqueness of the (geometric) mean [6].

On Riemannian manifolds, geodesics realize a local diffeomorphism, called the exponential map, from the tangent space at a given point to the manifold itself. This allows us to (locally) identify points of the manifold with tangent vectors. With the invariant metric on tensors, the geodesic starting at Σ and with tangent vector W can be expressed simply with the classical matrix exponential and the (Riemannian) exponential map realizes a global diffeomorphism [6]:

$$\exp_\Sigma(W) = \Sigma^{\frac{1}{2}} \exp\left(\Sigma^{-\frac{1}{2}} W \Sigma^{-\frac{1}{2}}\right) \Sigma^{\frac{1}{2}} \quad \text{and} \quad \log_\Sigma(\Lambda) = \Sigma^{\frac{1}{2}} \log\left(\Sigma^{-\frac{1}{2}} \Lambda \Sigma^{-\frac{1}{2}}\right) \Sigma^{\frac{1}{2}}.$$

These two diffeomorphisms are the key to the numerical implementation and generalization to manifolds of numerous algorithms that work on a vector space. For instance, the "difference vector" between two tensors Σ_1 and Σ_2 may be expressed as $Z = \Sigma_1^{-1/2} \log_{\Sigma_1}(\Sigma_2) \Sigma_1^{-1/2} = \log(\Sigma_1^{-1/2} \Sigma_2 \Sigma_1^{-1/2})$ in the tangent space at the identity (i.e. Z is a symmetric but not necessarily positive matrix). The distance between the two tensors is simply given by:

$$\mathrm{dist}^2(\Sigma_1, \Sigma_2) = \|Z\|_2^2 = \mathrm{trace}\left(\log\left(\Sigma_1^{-1/2} \Sigma_2 \Sigma_1^{-1/2}\right)^2\right).$$

Likewise, the Euclidean gradient descent scheme $\Sigma_{t+1} = \Sigma_t - \varepsilon \nabla C(\Sigma_t)$, which could easily lead to a non-positive matrix, is advantageously replaced by the *geodesic marching scheme* $\Sigma_{t+1} = \exp_{\Sigma_t}(-\varepsilon \nabla C(\Sigma_t))$.

2.2 Dense Extrapolation of Sparse Tensors

Let us consider a set of N measures Σ_i of a tensor field $\Sigma(x)$ at spatial positions $x_i \in \mathbb{R}^d$. To access the value of the tensor field at any point, one could think of interpolating or approximating these measures. We proposed in [6] a least square attachment term to the sparsely distributed tensors, combined with a regularization term to perform an estimation of the extrapolated tensor: $C(\Sigma) = \text{Sim}(\Sigma) + \text{Reg}(\Sigma)$. In a continuous setting, the data attachment term is:

$$\text{Sim}(\Sigma) = \tfrac{1}{2} \sum_{i=1}^{N} \text{dist}^2 (\Sigma(x_i), \Sigma_i) = \tfrac{1}{2} \int_{\Omega} \sum_{i=1}^{N} \text{dist}^2 (\Sigma(x), \Sigma_i) \, \delta(x - x_i) \, dx.$$

The Dirac distributions $\delta(x - x_i)$ are problematic when numerically differentiating the criterion. To regularize the problem, we consider them as the limit of a Gaussian function G_σ when σ goes to zero. Practically, σ has to be of the order of the spatial resolution of the grid on which $\Sigma(x)$ is estimated, so that each measure influences its immediate neighborhood. After differentiating the criterion, one obtains: $\nabla \text{Sim}_\sigma (x) = -\sum_i G_\sigma (x - x_i) \log_{\Sigma(x)}(\Sigma_i)$.

Basically, the attachment term prevents the tensor field from deviating too much from the measures at the points x_i. In between these points, we need to add a regularization term that ensures a homogeneous result. The simplest criterion is the harmonic regularization: $\text{Reg}(\Sigma) = \tfrac{1}{2} \int_\Omega \|\nabla \Sigma(x)\|_\Sigma^2$. We showed in [6] that the gradient of this criterion is $\nabla \text{Reg}(\Sigma)(x) = -\Delta \Sigma(x)$, and we provided a practical implementation of this Laplace-Beltrami operator on a tensor field. Using the geodesic marching scheme, we compute at each point x of our estimation grid the following intrinsic gradient descent:

$$\Sigma_{t+1}(x) = \exp_{\Sigma_t(x)} \left(-\varepsilon \nabla \text{Sim}(x) - \varepsilon \nabla \text{Reg}(x) \right). \qquad (1)$$

Finally, we can evaluate the extrapolated field Σ at any point x by tri-linear interpolation of the values at the grid nodes.

However, due to the large number of tensors and the large domain of diffusion used here (see next section), this algorithm converges slowly, even with a multi resolution implementation. To improve the initialization and enable faster convergence, in this paper we develop a RBF interpolation.

2.3 Extending RBFs to Extrapolate Tensors

RBFs provide a family of methods to extrapolate sparsely defined observations [8]. The extrapolated field is expressed as a linear combination of translated versions of a single radial function (the *basis*). Thus, if (y_i) is a set of scalar measures of the field $y(x)$ at points x_i, we find a set of scalar coefficients (λ_i) such that $y(x) = \sum_i \lambda_i h(x - x_i)$. To interpolate the data, the coefficients need to yield $y(x_i) = y_i$, i.e. be solutions of the linear system $\forall j : y_j = \sum_i \lambda_i h(x_j - x_i)$. There is a unique solution for any set of measurements at any set of spatial positions if the symmetric matrix $[H]_{i,j} = h(x_i - x_j)$ is always *positive definite*.

Scalar RBF extrapolation can be extended to vectors by simply running the extrapolation on each component independently. To apply this method to tensors, we map all tensors into the tangent space $T_\Sigma M$ of a reference tensor Σ. We then run the RBF extrapolation on the vectors $\log_\Sigma(\Sigma_i)$ and map the resulting values back into tensor space by the inverse mapping $\exp_\Sigma$. Among the many possible choices for a common reference tensor, we chose the mean $\bar{\Sigma}$ of all tensor measurements. Also, rather than letting the extrapolated values explode at infinity as with Thin Plate Splines, we use an interpolating function that decreases toward zero at infinity, namely from the family $h(x) = 1/\left(1 + (\|x\|^2/\alpha^2)^\gamma\right)$. The asymptotic value for the interpolation will be the reference tensor $\overline{\Sigma}$.

3 Modeling Brain Variability from Sulcal Lines

To model the spatial pattern of variability in brain structure, we chose to focus on anatomically well defined 3D curves that could be manually delineated by neuroanatomists and considered as ground truth data. This choice naturally led us to the primary anatomical landmarks on the cortex: the sulcal lines. Over 70 sulcal curves consistently appear in all normal individuals and allow a consistent subdivision of the cortex into major lobes and gyri [9]. In the absence of individual functional imaging data, sulci also provide an approximate guide to the functional subdivisions of the cortex, for all of the lobes.

We use a dataset of sulcal lines, or *sulci*, manually delineated in 98 subjects by expert neuroanatomists according to a precise protocol[1]. We included the maximal subset of all sulcal curves that consistently appear in all normal subjects (72 in total), with formal rules governing the handling of branching patterns, breaks in sulci, and doubling of specific sulci (e.g. the cingulate). By repeated training on test sets of brain images, the maximum allowed inter- and intra-rater error (reliability) was ensured to be 2mm everywhere, and in most regions less than 1mm, far less than the intersubject anatomical variance. Delineations were made in 3D on cortical surfaces extracted from MR images linearly aligned to the ICBM stereotactic space, thus providing a common coordinate system for all traced curves. Next, we determined the mean curve for each sulcal line by modeling samples as deformations of a single average curve. Based on the mean sulcal line, for each sulcus, and the mapping from this curve to its instance in each subject image, we can easily compute the local covariance matrix to create our second order statistical model of the sulcal line.

3.1 Learning Local Variability from a Sulcal Lines Dataset

Statistical models have frequently been constructed for objects such as open or closed curves and surfaces [10, 11, 12]. In each of these examples, the *aperture problem occurs*: as we do not have landmarks, the point-to-point correspondences between instances of a surface or a curve cannot be recovered exactly. For instance, the correspondences of two instances of a sulcus are intrinsically subject to error, with greater tangential than normal uncertainty. Here, we propose a one-to-one correspondence mapping that minimizes the influence of this error.

First, we denoise the sample lines by approximating them with B-splines. In this setting, the number of degrees of freedom can be adjusted to increase

---

[1] http://www.loni.ucla.edu/~khayashi/Public/medial_surface/

Fig. 1. Sulcal variability. Left: The Sylvian Fissure mean curve (in red) with traces from 98 healthy normal individuals (in green and yellow). Right: 50 covariance matrices (1 σ ellipsoids) are overlaid on the mean sulcus. Note that the very first and last tensors are larger than the interior ones

robustness to noise while avoiding resampling problems [13]. Typically, we reduce the number of control points to one third of the original sampling points.

Many criteria have been proposed in the literature to evaluate the appropriateness of one-to-one correspondences between geometric objects. They usually invoke local differential characteristics such as the tangent space, curvature [14], the local Frenet frame for a curve on a surface, regional shape information [15]. In our case, the variability is so large (see Fig. 1), that using such refined measures is meaningless. Therefore, we simply use the total variance of curve models as a criterion. Minimizing this variance greatly reduces the variability due to inadequate correspondences. Practically, we alternately improve the correspondences between the mean curves and each sample by dynamic programming and optimize the average curve position by a first-order gradient descent with an adaptive step. This optimization strategy converges after a few iterations.

For each of the 72 sulci, we now have the mean curve position $\bar{c}(t)$, parameterized by B-splines, and a one-to-one mapping that gives the corresponding point $c_i(t)$ in each instance. The variability tensor $\Sigma(t)$ along the mean sulcus is: $\Sigma(t) = \sum_{i=1}^{n} [c_i(t) - \bar{c}(t)] [c_i(t) - \bar{c}(t)]^\top / (n-1)$. An example set of covariance tensors estimated along the Sylvian Fissure is shown in Fig. 1. Variability is greater at the extremities of the sulci. These points should be landmarks as they are precisely identifiable by neuro-anatomists. We believe that the main part of their variability is due to a bias when we estimate the position of the end points of the mean curve. To remain consistent, we chose in this paper to remove this information from our model, and focussed only on the interior part of the sulci.

3.2 Model Simplification Using Tensor Interpolation

In the interior part of the sulci, the tensors are highly regular in size and shape. Some of this information is therefore redundant and could be simplified by selecting only a few tensors at specific points along the mean sulcus, and interpolating in between them. We use interpolation along the geodesic joining 2 tensors, because it preserves the monotonic evolution of the determinant. This is crucial when interpolating two probability densities and is in general not possible with direct interpolation. For efficiency reasons, we also selected the tensor values among the observed data rather than optimizing them as free parameters. This operation has been automated in an algorithm called *tensor picking*.

Let $\Sigma(t_i)$ be a set of N covariance tensors defined at parameter t_i along a mean sulcus. Riemannian interpolation between them gives the tensor: $\tilde{\Sigma}(t) = \exp_{\Sigma(t_i)}[(t - t_i)/(t_{i+1} - t_i)\log_{\Sigma(t_i)}(\Sigma(t_{i+1}))]$ for $t_i \leq t < t_{i+1}$. As we are working only on the interior of the sulcus, t takes its values between t_2 and $t_N - 1$, so that the *interpolated variability* $\tilde{\Sigma}(t)$ is always defined. The tensor picking operation consists of finding the optimal t_i such that the least-square error between the observed and interpolated variability tensors is minimized: $C(\Sigma) = \int_{t_1}^{t_N} \text{dist}^2(\Sigma(t), \tilde{\Sigma}(t)) dt$. To minimize this criterion, N points (i.e. tensors) are uniformly chosen along the mean curve. Then, an exhaustive search for the optimal point positions is done. If the criterion value at the optimal set is below a given threshold (0.7 in our experiments), the tensors are picked, otherwise the number of chosen tensors N is increased and the search is repeated.

Results of this operation are presented in Fig. 2 (middle panel): by choosing tensors at adequate positions, one can accurately reconstruct the full variability of each sulcus using 4 to 10 matrices, depending on its length and shape. The variability of all the major sulci can be represented by about 310 variability tensors out of 2000 initially.

3.3 Extrapolating the Variability to the Full Brain

The next step consists of extrapolating these selected tensors to the full brain, using the framework developed in Sec. 2.2. Fig. 2 presents the result of the extrapolation of our 310 tensors on discrete grid of size $91 \times 109 \times 91$ and with a spacing of $2 \times 2 \times 2\,mm^3$ (ICBM 305 space). We used the parameter values $\alpha = 20$ and $\gamma = 0.95$ for the RBF interpolation and $\sigma = 2$ for the discretization of the data attachment term in the extrapolation (Eq. (1)).

The spatial pattern of variability agrees with established neuroanatomical data. For instance, [16] computed the variability of the cortex surface in an independent normal sample (15 controls) using a non-linear surface registration algorithm. Fig. 3 compares his variability map with ours. Our model of variability presents the same high values in the temporo-parietal cortex (red area, marked "b" in Fig. 3) and low values in the superior frontal gyrus (marked "a" in Fig. 3), Broca's language area, and the lower limits of the primary sensorimotor cortices

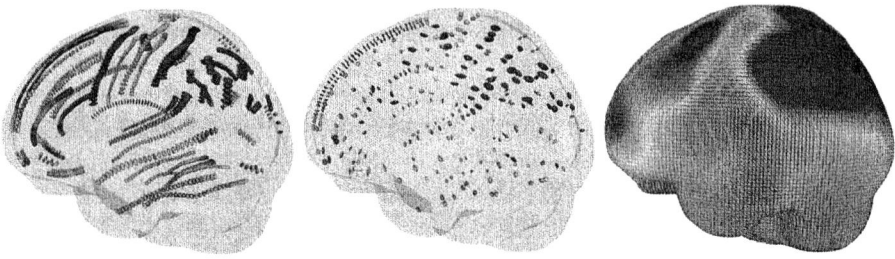

Fig. 2. Accessing the full brain variability step by step. The color bar is the same as in Fig. 3. **Left:** Covariance matrices calculated along the mean sulci. **Middle:** Matrices selected by the tensor picking operation. **Right:** Result of the extrapolation

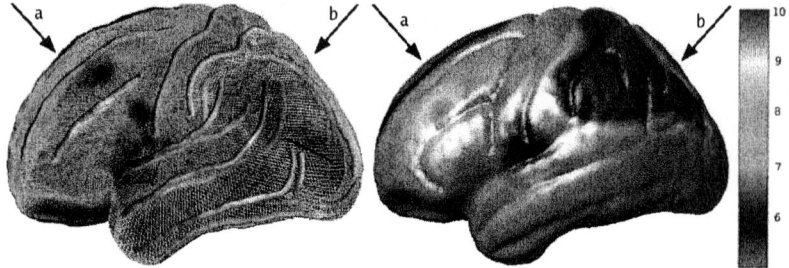

Fig. 3. Comparison of two independent models of brain variability. The scalar value mapped on the mean cortex is the trace of the tensors (the variance). **Left:** Cortical variability map from [16]. **Right:** Extrapolation of our simplified sulci variability model to the full brain (the display is restricted to the cortex). Note the similarity in the superior frontal gyrus (a) and the temporo-parietal cortex [shown in red colors (b)]

in the central and precentral gyri. Phylogenetical older areas (e.g. orbitofrontal cortex), and primary cortices that myelinate earliest (e.g. primary somatosensory and auditory cortex) exhibit least variability. The planum parietale (marked "b" in Fig. 3) consistently shows the highest variance of any cortical area, consistent with the complex pattern of secondary fissures surrounding the supramarginal and angular gyri (the perisylvian language cortex). It is also reasonable that the temporo-parietal areas around the Sylvian fissures are the most variable: they specialize and develop in different ways in each hemisphere, and are also the most asymmetric in terms of gyral patterning and volumes.

3.4 Validation of the Variability Model

Validating our extrapolated variability model is a tough issue. Obviously, using the information given by the sulci is not enough to infer the variability of the full brain, particularly within the brain (e.g. in the white matter, ventricles and deep gray matter nuclei). Moreover, we have no ground truth in these areas to validate the predicted variability. Thus, we restrict the evaluation of the predictive power of our model to the places where we have enough data: on the cortex. The first idea is to see how well our interpolation and extrapolation models fits the observed variability along each sulcus. This yields a root mean square error (RMSe) assessing the fidelity of the approximation. Then, we can perform a "leave one sulcus out" test to see if a group of sulci can correctly predict the variability of another sulcus in their neighborhood. This would mean that the model can effectively find missing data (the measures are independent) and somehow predict the variability of missing structures in our datasets.

Intra-Sulcus Variability Recovery. We computed the "difference" or error vector between the observed variability tensor and the reconstructed one with our interpolation and extrapolation methods. We found that the mean errors were not significantly different from zero (p-value of 0.25 at the Hotelling's test). Second, we found a standard deviation of $\sigma_{ref} = 0.15$ for the interpolation error.

This value gives us a lower bound on the range of the reconstruction errors. The slightly higher value of 0.21 for the extrapolation error could be attributed to the aperture problem: in regions with orthogonal sulci, the normal component of one tensor influences the tangential part of its perpendicular neighbors and vice versa, which misleads the reconstruction. After removing these "outliers", the error distributions after interpolation and extrapolation are comparable.

Leave One Sulcus Out. This test removes one sulcus and its variability tensors from the model and extrapolates the rest of the data to the full brain. Then, the prediction error made on this specific sulcus is compared to the interpolation and extrapolation errors. As the measures are independent, an error below $3\sigma_{ref}$ is not significant and shows that our extrapolation model recovers the missing variability information up to the intrinsic reconstruction uncertainty. However, a RMSe larger than $3\sigma_{ref}$ means that we do not recover a comparable variability *in at least one direction*. We know that an uncertainty in the tangent of the mean sulcus could be induced by the aperture problem. To remove this effect, we "project" the error vector onto the plane perpendicular to the tangent of the mean sulcus. Thus, the error component in this direction is zeroed out. We will call this error the "partial error".

This test is performed on 3 sulci: the Sylvian Fissure, the Superior Temporal Sulcus Main Body and the Inferior Temporal Sulcus. Fig. 4 displays the reconstructed sulci after extrapolation with and without their variability tensors while Table 1 summarizes the global RMSe statistics. The prediction error with missing sulci is globally 2 to 3 times larger than that incurred by interpolating or extrapolating the full model, but the difference is not high enough to be significant. However, errors are locally significant. In some places, like for the Sylvian Fissure, the prediction errors occur primarily in the tangential direction to the mean sulcus. Such behavior was expected due to the aperture problem and is confirmed by the "partial" error that is much lower than the standard error. By contrast, the variability of some sulci like the Central Sulcus cannot be correctly recovered from neighboring sulci: the error is not only due to the

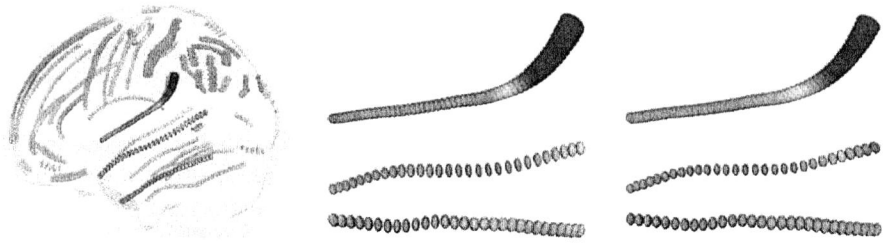

Fig. 4. Result of the "leave one sulcus out" test. Left: Positions of the 3 tested sulci in the ICBM305 space. **Middle:** variability of each sulcus after extrapolation of the complete model. The color bar is the same as in Fig. 3. **Right:** extrapolated variability from the neighboring sulci only. **Top:** the Sylvian Fissure, **middle:** the Superior Temporal Sulcus main body, **bottom:** the Inferior Temporal Sulcus

Table 1. RMSe of reconstruction of 3 sulci with the interpolation, extrapolation and leave one-sulcus out extrapolation methods. * indicates the "partial error" (Sec. 3.4)

Sulcus	Sylvian Fiss.	Sup. Temporal	Inf. Temporal.
Interpolation	0.12 - 0.10*	0.17 - 0.15*	0.17 - 0.14*
Extrapolation	0.18 - 0.13*	0.21 - 0.17*	0.17 - 0.15*
Extrapolation w/o sulcus	0.43 - 0.27*	0.37 - 0.32*	0.27 - 0.22*

aperture problem but spatial correlations between adjacent sulci may be lower in some brain regions, making variations more difficult to predict.

3.5 Analysis of the Asymmetry of Brain Variability

The study of asymmetry in brain variability is of great interest for neuroscientists [17], and measures of structural and functional lateralization are of interest in mapping brain development, and disorders such as dyslexia and schizophrenia. The two brain hemispheres develop according to slightly different genetic programs, and the right hemisphere is torqued forward relative to the left, with greatest volume asymmetries in the planum temporale and language cortex surrounding the Sylvian fissures (typically larger in the left hemisphere). If the types of variation in the two hemispheres could be differentiated, their genetic basis would be easier to investigate. It could also help understand whether there is an asymmetry in the power to detect group activation in functional brain imaging studies, due to structural variance asymmetries.

We therefore measured the symmetry/asymmetry of brain variability using our extrapolation model. The principle is to compute the distance between the variability tensor at one point and the (symmetrized) tensor at the symmetric point in the brain. To define the symmetric point, we simply use the 3D position that is symmetric w.r.t. the mid-sagittal plane in the stereotaxic space (ICBM 305). In that case, we compute a dense asymmetry map from the extrapolated tensor values at each 3D point of a hemisphere (Fig. 5, left). We may also retrieve

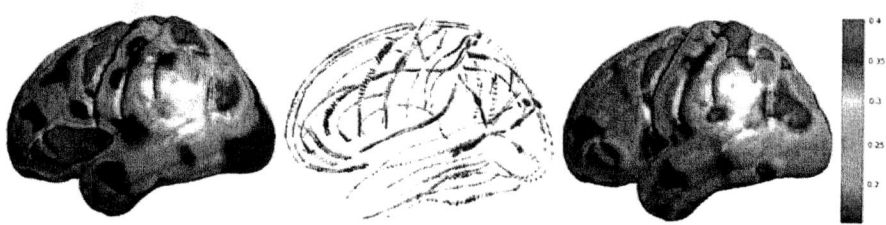

Fig. 5. Maps of the asymmetry of the brain variability. Red to purple colors indicate a significant asymmetry. **Left:** Asymmetry of the 3D extrapolation w.r.t. the mid-sagittal plane. **Middle:** Difference vectors between left-right variability tensors. **Right:** Extrapolation to the volume of the "asymmetry vectors" of the previous figure

the corresponding points between each left and right mean sulcus by mapping the left sulci into the right hemisphere and computing the correspondences using the algorithm of Sec. 3.1. In that case, we end up with an error tensor measuring the asymmetry along each sulcus (Fig. 5 middle). This error is finally extrapolated to the full brain using once again the framework previously developed (Fig. 5, right). A very interesting feature is that the regions with greatest asymmetries in variability include the 2 main language areas, Broca's speech area (see pink colors in the inferior frontal cortex) and Wernicke's language comprehension area (yellow and red colors surrounding the posterior Sylvian fissure). As expected, these areas vary more on the left hemisphere which is dominant for language. The greater left hemisphere variation may be attributable to the greater volumes of structures such as the planum temporale in the left hemisphere. Also as expected, the primary sensorimotor areas (central and pre-central gyri) are relatively symmetric in their variance, as the absolute variability is lower, as is their degree of hemispheric specialization (i.e. they perform analogous functions in each hemisphere, but innervate opposite sides of the body).

4 Discussion

This paper applies a powerful Riemannian framework for tensor computing to extrapolate sparsely distributed tensors. We extend a RBF extrapolation method combined with diffusion PDEs. While the RBF provides a good initialization, the diffusion with attachment to the measures results in a smooth tensor field that stays close to the observed measures and converges in a few iterations. We applied this methodology to model the profile of brain variability, where tensors are measured along sulcal lines that are consistently anatomical landmarks.

When modeling variability, the main weakness is the unknown variability along the direction tangent to the mean sulci (aperture problem). We intend to tackle this point by first improving our sulcal matching algorithm to safely use the landmark information at the ends of sulci, and second by removing the data attachment term in the direction of the sulcal tangent. Doing this, the neighboring information could diffuse freely in that direction and hopefully reconstruct a globally coherent variability. For the model validation, we need to compare to other sources of information, like the variability obtained from the matching of surfaces (e.g. ventricles or basal ganglia), fiber pathways mapped from DTI, or of full 3D images. As these sources of information are also subject to an aperture problem (we mainly retrieve the deformation in the direction of the gradient of the image), we expect to obtain a good fit in some areas, but we require complementary measures in other areas.

These results are also interesting neuroscientifically. Variance and the asymmetry of variability are greatest in language areas, which have fundamentally different developmental programs in each brain hemisphere, leading to volumetric and functional asymmetries (e.g. left hemisphere language dominance). This variance asymmetry was also seen in Broca's area, which is specialized in the left hemisphere for producing speech, but is less commonly associated with structural asymmetries. Lower variance was seen in cortical regions subserving primary brain functions (e.g., touch, motor function, hearing) and these areas are the earliest to mature in utero. The modeling of variance is practically valuable for understanding the genetic and disease related factors that affect brain structure, which are currently hard to identify given the extremely complex patterns of variation in normal anatomy.

References

1. O. Coulon, D. Alexander, and S. Arridge. Diffusion tensor magnetic resonance image regularization. *Medical Image Analysis*, 8(1):47–67, 2004.
2. D. Tschumperlé and R. Deriche. Orthonormal vector sets regularization with pde's and applications. *Int. J. of Computer Vision (IJCV)*, 50(3):237–252, 2002.
3. P.T. Fletcher and S.C. Joshi. Principal geodesic analysis on symmetric spaces: Statistics of diffusion tensors. In *Proc. of CVAMIA and MMBIA Workshops, Prague, Czech Republic, May 15, 2004*, LNCS 3117, pages 87–98. Springer, 2004.
4. C. Lenglet, M. Rousson, R. Deriche, and O. Faugeras. Statistics on multivariate normal distributions: A geometric approach and its application to diffusion tensor MRI. Research Report 5242, INRIA, 2004.
5. P. Batchelor, M. Moakher, D. Atkinson, F. Calamante, and A. Connelly. A rigorous framework for diffusion tensor calculus. *Mag. Res. in Med.*, 53:221–225, 2005.
6. X. Pennec, P. Fillard, and N. Ayache. A Riemannian framework for tensor computing. *IJCV*, 2005. To appear.
7. L.T. Skovgaard. A Riemannian geometry of the multivariate normal model. *Scand. J. Statistics*, 11:211–223, 1984.
8. X. Sun. Conditional positive definiteness and complete monotonicity. In *Approximation Theory VIII*, volume 2, pages 211–234. World Scientific, 1995.
9. J.-F. Mangin, D. Riviere, A. Cachia, E. Duchesnay, Y. Cointepas, D. Papadopoulos-Orfanos, P. Scifo, T. Ochiai, F. Brunelle, and J. Regis. A framework to study the cortical folding patterns. *NeuroImage*, 23(Supplement 1):S129–S138, 2004.
10. T. F. Cootes, C. J. Taylor, D. H. Cooper, and J. Graham. Active shape models-their training and application. *Comput. Vis. Image Underst.*, 61(1):38–59, 1995.
11. A. Trouve and L. Younes. Diffeomorphic matching problems in one dimension: Designing and minimizing matching functionals. In *Proc of ECCV'00, part I.*, LNCS 1842, pages 573–587, 2000.
12. R. R. Paulsen and K. B. Hilger. Shape modelling using markov random field restoration of point correspondences. In *IPMI'03*, LNCS 2732, pages 1–12, 2003.
13. A. Baumberg and D. Hogg. Learning flexible models from image sequences. In *Proc of ECCV'94 (vol. 1), Stocklholm, Sweden*, LNCS 800, pages 299–308, 1994.
14. M. Bakircioglu, U. Grenander, N. Khaneja, and M.I. Miller. Curve matching on brain surfaces using induced Frenet distance metrics. *HBM*, 6(5):329–331, 1998.
15. A. Pitiot, H. Delingette, A. Toga, and P. Thompson. Learning object correspondences with the observed transport shape measure. In *Proc. of IPMI'03*, LNCS 2732, pages 25–37. Springer Verlag, 2003.
16. P.M. Thompson, M.S. Mega, K.L. Narr, E.R. Sowell, R.E. Blanton, and A.W. Toga. Brain image analysis and atlas construction. In M. Fitzpatrick and M. Sonka, editors, *Handbook of Medical Image Proc. and Analysis*, chapter 17. SPIE, 2000.
17. A.W. Toga and P.M. Thompson. Mapping brain asymmetry. *Nature Reviews Neuroscience*, 4(1):37–48, January 2003.

Bayesian Population Modeling of Effective Connectivity*

Eric R. Cosman[1,3] and William M. Wells III[1,2,3]

[1] Computer Science and Artificial Intelligence Laboratory,
Massachusetts Institute of Technology, Cambridge, MA, USA
ercosman@mit.edu, sw@csail.mit.edu
[2] Harvard Medical School, Brigham and Woman's Hospital,
Department of Radiology, Boston, MA, USA
[3] The Harvard Center for Neurodegeneration and Repair, Boston, MA, USA

Abstract. A hierarchical model based on the Multivariate Autoregessive (MAR) process is proposed to jointly model neurological time-series collected from multiple subjects, and to characterize the distribution of MAR coefficients across the population from which those subjects were drawn. Thus, inference about effective connectivity between brain regions may be generalized beyond those subjects studied. The posterior on population- and subject-level connectivity parameters are estimated in a Variational Bayesian (VB) framework, and structural model parameters are chosen by the corresponding evidence criteria. The significance of resulting connectivity statistics are evaluated by permutation-based approximations to the null distribution. The method is demonstrated on simulated data and on actual multi-subject neurological time-series.

1 Introduction

Neuroimaging studies are regularly conducted in which measurements of brain activity are collected simultaneously from multiple, analogous brain regions in multiple subjects. These measurement may be taken by EEG, MEG, fMRI or intracranial electrical monitoring. Such studies are often motivated by hypotheses about the interaction among gross brain regions under particular experimental conditions or due to some neurological disorder. Numerous techniques have been proposed which use such functional data to characterize *Effective Connectivity*, defined as the influence that one brain region exerts on another under a given interaction model. These include Structural Equation Modeling (SEM) [14], Multivariate Autoregressive Modeling (MAR) [9, 16, 7] and Dynamic Causal Modeling (DCM) [4]. The MAR and DCM approaches characterize effective connectivity by modeling particular brain regions as variables in a causal, dynamical system. Model parameters may thereby inform about the influence that each region exerts on the others, either directly or indirectly through other regions.

---

* This research was supported by grants NIH 5 P41 RR13218 and FIRST BIRN.

It is of interest to determine which interactions between modeled brain regions are characteristic under experimental conditions within the population from which studied subjects are drawn. However, to our knowledge, models for effective connectivity have been applied only in subject-independent manner. As such, statistical inference about connectivity is limited to the specific subjects included in a study, except by *post hoc* analysis of the variation in subject-specific connectivity parameters. We propose a hierarchical, or Random Effects (RFX), approach to the analysis of multi-subject functional time-series such that the effective connectivity parameters of all subjects are estimated jointly along with a density describing the variation in those parameters across the population from which studied subjects were drawn. Such joint estimation of connectivity under SEM, MAR, DCM or other models, would be valuable for neuroimaging studies. We have chosen the MAR process as a starting point for investigation of the applicability of such hierarchical modeling to generalize inference about effective connectivity to the population level.

In particular, we present the RFX-MAR model which parameterizes the interactions of specified brain regions for each subject using the MAR process, and describes the variability in those subject-level models by the mean and variance of their MAR coefficients. We estimate population- and subject-specific parameters in a Variational Bayesian (VB) framework, and characterize effective connectivity at the population level by inference on the posterior of the MAR coefficients' means, which we refer to as the population-level MAR coefficients. Specifically, we compute statistics related to evidence of non-zero directional influence between each pair of monitored brain regions under the MAR model, across the sampled population. Structural parameters of the RFX-MAR model are selected by an approximate maximum evidence criteria.

Though Gaussian population models have been used extensively in neuroimaging analysis for the purpose of localizing protocol-related neural activity [5], this work is the first to investigate their utility in modeling of neural connectivity. We describe the results of our analysis on synthetic and EEG time-series collected from multiple subjects.

2 The Multivariate Autoregressive Process

The Multivariate Autoregressive (MAR) process models the temporal dynamics of multivariate systems causally and without hidden state variables, such that multivariate measurements at the present time are a linear function of measurements in the past. This kind of parametric process has been used to identify the linear, time-invariant (LTI) system dynamics and spectra of multichannel time-series data in a number of contexts, including geophysics, economics and neuroimaging [9, 16, 7]. In neuroimaging, the MAR process has been used to model and test effective connectivity based on neurological data collected by fMRI, EEG and direct electrical recording. In general, the MAR process may be used when specialization of a dynamical model, possibly through hidden state variables, is difficult or unnecessary. Since the MAR process is strictly causal, it can model directional influence between channels, and elucidate causal chains and loops.

A MAR(p) process is defined as follows, where $\mathbf{Y}_{n\cdot} \in \Re^d$ is a sample from d channels at time n arranged in a row vector, $\mathbf{A}(l) \in \Re^{d \times d}$, $l = 1, \ldots, p$, is a series of matrices comprising the coefficients of the MAR model, and $\mathbf{E}_{n\cdot} \in \Re^d$ is a temporally-white innovation with stationary distribution $\mathcal{N}(\mathbf{0}, \mathbf{\Lambda}^{-1})$. Note that we replace a matrix or sequence index with a large dot · to refer collectively to elements corresponding to all values of that index.

$$\mathbf{Y}_{n\cdot} = \sum_{l=1}^{p} \mathbf{Y}_{(n-l)\cdot} \mathbf{A}(l) + \mathbf{E}_{n\cdot} = \underbrace{[\mathbf{Y}_{(n-1)\cdot} | \ldots | \mathbf{Y}_{(n-p)\cdot}]}_{\equiv \mathbf{X}_{n\cdot}} \underbrace{\begin{bmatrix} \mathbf{A}(1) \\ \vdots \\ \mathbf{A}(p) \end{bmatrix}}_{\equiv \mathbf{W}} + \mathbf{E}_{n\cdot}. \quad (1)$$

We denote the p coefficients by which channel i directly influences channel j as $A_{ij}(\cdot) \in \Re^p$, and refer to this as the *Direct Influence Function* (DIF) from channel i to j. Stacking these equations for each time sample n, we get the matrix equation $\mathbf{Y} = \mathbf{X}\mathbf{W} + \mathbf{E}$. To highlight that this is a specialized linear regression model, we will henceforth use its vectorized form, where $\mathbf{y} \equiv \text{vec}(\mathbf{Y}) \in \Re^{Nd}$, $\mathbf{w} \equiv \text{vec}(\mathbf{W}) \in \Re^{d^2 p}$, and $\otimes$ denotes the Kronecker product (as defined in [13]):

$$p(\mathbf{y} \mid \mathbf{w}, \mathbf{\Lambda}) = \mathcal{N}(\mathbf{y} \,;\, (\mathbf{I}_d \otimes \mathbf{X})\mathbf{w} \,,\, \mathbf{\Lambda}^{-1} \otimes \mathbf{I}_N) \quad (2)$$

The utility of maximum likelihood (ML) estimates of MAR parameters, $\tilde{\mathbf{w}} = \text{vec}(\mathbf{X}^+\mathbf{Y})$ and $\tilde{\mathbf{\Lambda}} = (\mathbf{Y} - \mathbf{X}\tilde{\mathbf{W}})'(\mathbf{Y} - \mathbf{X}\tilde{\mathbf{W}})/(N - d^2 p)$, is limited by the large amount of data required to fit these $\Theta(d^2)$ parameters reliably. A Variational Bayesian framework for MAR estimation has been proposed which relieves this data requirement to some degree, by means of a prior that regularizes coefficient magnitudes [16].

Neuroimaging experiments are commonly associated with time-varying stimuli or tasks. Encodings of such information can be added as linear terms in Equation 1 without affecting analysis. As such, they account for bias in the innovations, and do not influence system dynamics *per se*, which are assumed to be stationary in the time-series $\mathbf{y}$. Nonlinear coupling between variables can be approximated in the MAR framework by adding new variables which are nonlinear functions of data from other variables (e.g. product terms) [7].

3   The RFX-MAR Model

To generalize inference about effective connectivity to the greater population from which studied subjects were drawn, we propose to model the variation of subject-specific MAR coefficients across that greater population. As is standard in population inference, we approximate the population density as Gaussian, so that its mean characterizes dynamical structure common to the population, and its covariance characterizes the degree of variability in that structure found within that population. Hence, we construct a hierarchical, or *Random Effects* (RFX), model which describes both the subject-specific MAR parameters and the inter-subject variation of those parameters.

$$p(\mathbf{y}_k \mid \mathbf{w}_k, \mathbf{\Lambda}_k) = \mathcal{N}\left(\mathbf{y}_k\,;\, (\mathbf{I}_d \otimes \mathbf{X}_k)\mathbf{w}_k\,,\, \mathbf{\Lambda}_k^{-1} \otimes \mathbf{I}_n\right), \quad k = 1, \ldots, S \quad (3)$$

$$p(\mathbf{w}_k \mid \mathbf{w}_0, \boldsymbol{\gamma}) = \mathcal{N}\left(\mathbf{w}_k;\, \mathbf{w}_0\,,\, \sum_{h=1}^{H} \gamma_h^{-1} \mathbf{Q}_{\gamma_h}\right) \quad (4)$$

$$p(\mathbf{w}_0 \mid \boldsymbol{\alpha}) = \mathcal{N}\left(\mathbf{w}_0;\, \mathbf{0}\,,\, \sum_{g=1}^{G} \alpha_g^{-1} \mathbf{Q}_{\alpha_g}\right) \quad (5)$$

In particular, we model the multivariate time-series $\mathbf{y}_k \in \Re^{N_k d}$ from each subject k as MAR(p) process with coefficients $\mathbf{w}_k$ and innovations precision (inverse covariance) $\mathbf{\Lambda}_k$ (Equation (3)). The data from subject k comprise N_k time samples of dimension d. Each subject-specific MAR coefficient $[\mathbf{w}_k]_i$ is drawn independently about its population mean $[\mathbf{w}_0]_i$ with some precision γ_h (Equation (4)). We group coefficients to reflect similarity in their inter-subject variation, rather than assuming a single variance for all coefficients a priori. Each of these random-effects variance groups are associated with a precision γ_h, $h = 1, \ldots, H$. This "structuring" of inter-subject variation is defined as follows:

$$\text{group}_\gamma(i) \equiv \text{the RFX group of } [\mathbf{w_k}]_i \qquad [\mathbf{Q}_{\gamma_h}]_{ij} \equiv \delta_{ij}\delta(\text{group}_\gamma(i) = h) \quad (6)$$

Additionally, we assume that each population-level coefficient $[\mathbf{w}_0]_i$ is drawn independently from a zero-mean Gaussian, and partitioned into one of G groups with other coefficients with similar magnitudes (Equation (5)). This kind of "structured" prior was used to reduce the effective degrees of freedom in single-subject MAR modeling [16,7], and has been referred to as an *Automatic Relevance Determination* (ARD) prior [11]. This ARD structuring is defined as follows, where $g = 1, \ldots, G$ indexes the groups:

$$\text{group}_\alpha(i) \equiv \text{the ARD group of } [\mathbf{w}_0]_i \qquad [\mathbf{Q}_{\alpha_g}]_{ij} \equiv \delta_{ij}\delta(\text{group}_\alpha(i) = g) \quad (7)$$

In summary, we have a three-level linear Gaussian model. Its first level describes subject-specific variation with the MAR process. Its second level describes variation in subject-specific coefficients across the sampled population by means of a Gaussian density with diagonal precision matrix. The third level regularizes the magnitude of the population-level coefficients. Naturally, care should be taken to look for inconsistency between this model and the qualities of data to which it is applied. Since the data has zero mean under the MAR model, the sample mean is removed from each data channel as a pre-processing step. Furthermore, each channel's signal is individually normalized by its sample variance (we expect to model stable systems). By doing so, the cross-coefficients of $\mathbf{w}_k$, i.e. $[\mathbf{A}_k]_{ij}(\cdot)$ for $i \neq j$, are comparable across subjects, normalized by the ratio between the amplitudes of the "to" and "from" signals $\|[\mathbf{Y}_k]_{\bullet j}\|/\|[\mathbf{Y}_k]_{\bullet i}\|$.

For notational simplicity, we will henceforth refer to the $N \equiv \sum_{k=1}^{S} N_k$ samples of multi-subject data collectively as $\mathbf{y} \equiv [\mathbf{y}_1' \ldots \mathbf{y}_S']'$; the subject-level precisions as $\mathbf{\Lambda} \equiv \{\mathbf{\Lambda}_1, \ldots, \mathbf{\Lambda}_S\}$; and the population and subject-specific coefficients as $\mathbf{w} \equiv [\mathbf{w}_0' \ \mathbf{w}_1' \ldots \mathbf{w}_S']'$.

3.1 Precision Priors

Since we intend to estimate the RFX-MAR model in a Bayesian framework, we set the following "noninformative" priors for the precision parameters in (3)–(5) to represent an absence of prior information.

$$p(\mathbf{\Lambda}) \propto \prod_{k=1}^{s} |\mathbf{\Lambda}_k|^{-\frac{d+1}{2}} \qquad p(\boldsymbol{\alpha}) = \prod_{g=1}^{G} \mathrm{Ga}(\alpha_g\,;\,a_p,\,b_p), \quad a_p,\,b_p \equiv 10^{-3}$$

$$p(\boldsymbol{\gamma}) = \prod_{h=1}^{H} \left(2u\gamma_h^{\frac{3}{2}}\right)^{-1}, \quad \gamma_h \geq u^{-2}, \quad u \equiv 10^3 \tag{8}$$

We subscribe to the view in [6] that "any noninformative prior distribution [is] inherently provisional— after the model has been fit, one should look at the posterior distribution to see if it makes sense." We follow [16] in the form of the priors on precisions $\mathbf{\Lambda}$ and $\boldsymbol{\alpha}$ due to their success in the single-subject MAR modeling and in our experiments on synthetic multi-subject data. The prior on $\boldsymbol{\alpha}$ follows a Gamma density [1], and the prior on $\mathbf{\Lambda}$ is improper. Both were motivated by Jeffreys' Rule [2]; however, they do not follow from its strict application, but rather from its application to the first and third levels of the model in isolation. The prior on $\boldsymbol{\gamma}$ is equivalent to a locally uniform prior on the standard deviation of inter-subject variation $\sigma_h \equiv \gamma_h^{-0.5}$ for each RFX variance group h. This prior is suggested for RFX models as preferable to those of the family $\mathrm{Ga}(\gamma_h;\epsilon,\epsilon)$, under which inference is sensitive to ϵ when σ_h is near zero [6]. We observed this sensitivity in our experiments.

4 Variational Posterior Estimation

In this section, we describe a Variational Bayesian (VB) algorithm [8,10] for estimating the posterior of the RFX-MAR model's real-valued parameters, including the MAR coefficients $\mathbf{w}$ and precision parameters $\mathbf{\Lambda}$, $\boldsymbol{\gamma}$ and $\boldsymbol{\alpha}$. Our choice of this framework for posterior estimation was motivated by its suitability to estimation of a single MAR process [16,7]. In Sect. 5, we address selection of the model's discrete-valued, structural parameters, which include the MAR model order and the RFX and ARD structuring functions.

The VB algorithm proceeds as follows: For a generic statistical model with parameters $\boldsymbol{\theta}$ and observed data $\mathbf{D}$, an approximation to the true posterior $q(\boldsymbol{\theta}) \equiv \hat{p}(\boldsymbol{\theta} \mid \mathbf{D})$ is produced by maximizing a lower bound on the model's log evidence

$$F \equiv \log p(\mathbf{D}) - D(q(\boldsymbol{\theta}) \parallel p(\boldsymbol{\theta} \mid \mathbf{D})) \leq \log p(\mathbf{D}) \tag{9}$$

with the simplifying assumption that the posterior approximation factorizes $q(\boldsymbol{\theta}) \equiv \prod_i q(\boldsymbol{\theta}_i)$ in some way. The quantity F is referred to as the *negative variational free energy*. Maximization proceeds by fixed-point iteration whereby the posterior for each subset of parameters $\boldsymbol{\theta}_i$ is updated sequentially, while holding the posterior of remaining parameters constant. If priors are set to be conditionally-conjugate under such posterior independence assumptions, each VB update step may reduce to a closed-form update of the induced sufficient statistics of $q(\boldsymbol{\theta}_i)$. This is referred to as *Free-Form Variational Bayes*. Alternatively, *Fixed-Form Variational Bayes* refers to a VB update step which follows from assuming additionally that the posterior factor has a particular parametric form. For instance, the *Expectation Maximization* (EM) algorithm [3] is a special case in which the second of two parameter groups is assumed to have a singular posterior $q(\boldsymbol{\theta}_1, \boldsymbol{\theta}_2) \equiv q(\boldsymbol{\theta}_1)\delta(\boldsymbol{\theta}_2 - \widehat{\boldsymbol{\theta}}_2)$ with parameter $\widehat{\boldsymbol{\theta}}_2$.

For the RFX-MAR model, we assume the posterior independence of the precisions parameters and MAR coefficients. With this assumption, it can be shown that precisions' posterior further factorizes, due to the graphical structure of the model and their prior independence:

$$q(\mathbf{w}, \boldsymbol{\Lambda}, \boldsymbol{\gamma}, \boldsymbol{\alpha}) \equiv q(\mathbf{w})q(\boldsymbol{\Lambda}, \boldsymbol{\gamma}, \boldsymbol{\alpha}) = q(\mathbf{w}) \prod_{k=1}^{S} q(\boldsymbol{\Lambda}_k) \prod_{h=1}^{H} q(\gamma_h) \prod_{g=1}^{G} q(\alpha_g) \quad (10)$$

Furthermore, with priors on the precision parameters of the form given in (8), it can be shown that the posterior factors follow Normal, Wishart, Gamma and incomplete Gamma[1] densities (denoted $\mathcal{N}$, $\mathcal{W}$, Ga, and IGa, respectively) [1]. Thus the free-form VB algorithm proceeds by sequential update of the sufficient statistics of each posterior factor until convergence to a fixed point. These updates are given below in (11)–(14). For clarity in these equations, we let $\sum_{i_g}$ denote summation over the κ_g coefficient indices i which are part of ARD prior group g, i.e. $\sum_{i:\text{group}_\alpha(i)=g}$. Similarly, $\sum_{i_h}$ denotes $\sum_{i:\text{group}_\gamma(i)=h}$, where the RFX group h contains ν_h coefficients. We also define $\widetilde{\boldsymbol{\Lambda}}_k \equiv \widehat{\boldsymbol{\Lambda}}_k \otimes \mathbf{X}_k'\mathbf{X}_k$ and $\widetilde{\mathbf{w}}_k \equiv \text{vec}(\mathbf{X}_k^+ \mathbf{Y}_k)$, and let $\widehat{\boldsymbol{\Gamma}} \equiv \sum_{h=1}^{H} \widehat{\gamma}_h \mathbf{Q}_{\gamma_h}$ and $\widehat{\boldsymbol{\Xi}} \equiv \sum_{g=1}^{G} \widehat{\alpha}_g \mathbf{Q}_{\alpha_g}$ denote the estimated precision matrices for the second and third levels of the RFX-MAR model.

Update for $q(\mathbf{w}) \leftarrow \mathcal{N}(\mathbf{w}; \widehat{\mathbf{w}}, \widehat{\boldsymbol{\Sigma}})$: The $(k,l)^{th}$ block of $\widehat{\boldsymbol{\Sigma}}$ of size $d^2p \times d^2p$ is denoted $\widehat{\boldsymbol{\Sigma}}^{(kl)}$, $k, l = 0, \ldots, S$

$$\begin{aligned}
\widehat{\boldsymbol{\Sigma}}^{(00)} &= \left(\widehat{\boldsymbol{\Xi}} + S\widehat{\boldsymbol{\Gamma}} - \widehat{\boldsymbol{\Gamma}}\left[\sum_{k=1}^{S}(\widehat{\boldsymbol{\Gamma}} + \widetilde{\boldsymbol{\Lambda}}_k)^{-1}\right]\widehat{\boldsymbol{\Gamma}}\right)^{-1} \\
\widehat{\boldsymbol{\Sigma}}^{(0k)} &= \widehat{\boldsymbol{\Sigma}}^{(k0)\prime} = \widehat{\boldsymbol{\Sigma}}^{(00)}\widehat{\boldsymbol{\Gamma}}(\widehat{\boldsymbol{\Gamma}} + \widetilde{\boldsymbol{\Lambda}}_k)^{-1}, \quad k = 1, \ldots, S \quad (11) \\
\widehat{\boldsymbol{\Sigma}}^{(kl)} &= \delta_{kl}(\widehat{\boldsymbol{\Gamma}} + \widetilde{\boldsymbol{\Lambda}}_k)^{-1} + (\widehat{\boldsymbol{\Gamma}} + \widetilde{\boldsymbol{\Lambda}}_k)^{-1}\widehat{\boldsymbol{\Gamma}}\widehat{\boldsymbol{\Sigma}}^{(00)}\widehat{\boldsymbol{\Gamma}}(\widehat{\boldsymbol{\Gamma}} + \widetilde{\boldsymbol{\Lambda}}_l)^{-1}, \quad k, l \geq 1
\end{aligned}$$

---

[1] We define the incomplete Gamma density $\text{IGa}(x; a, b, x_{min})$ to be proportional to the Gamma density $\text{Ga}(x; a, b)$ for positive values $x \geq x_{min}$, and zero otherwise.

$$\widehat{\mathbf{w}}' = \begin{bmatrix} \mathbf{0}' & (\tilde{\mathbf{\Lambda}}_1 \tilde{\mathbf{w}}_1)' & \dots & (\tilde{\mathbf{\Lambda}}_S \tilde{\mathbf{w}}_S)' \end{bmatrix} \widehat{\mathbf{\Sigma}}$$

Update for $q(\mathbf{\Lambda}) \leftarrow \prod_{k=1}^{S} \mathcal{W}_d(\mathbf{\Lambda}_k \,;\, a_k,\, \mathbf{B}_k)$:

$$a_k = N_k \qquad \mathbf{\Omega}_k \equiv \sum_{n=1}^{N_k} (\mathbf{I}_d \otimes [\mathbf{X}_k]_{n\bullet}) \widehat{\mathbf{\Sigma}}^{(kk)} (\mathbf{I}_d \otimes [\mathbf{X}_k]_{n\bullet})' \qquad (12)$$

$$\mathbf{B}_k = (\mathbf{Y}_k - \mathbf{X}_k \widehat{\mathbf{W}}_k)'(\mathbf{Y}_k - \mathbf{X}_k \widehat{\mathbf{W}}_k) + \mathbf{\Omega}_k \qquad \widehat{\mathbf{\Lambda}}_k \equiv \mathcal{E}_{q(\mathbf{\Lambda}_k)}\{\mathbf{\Lambda}_k\} = a_k \mathbf{B}_k^{-1}$$

Update for $q(\boldsymbol{\gamma}) \leftarrow \prod_{h=1}^{H} \text{IGa}(\gamma_h \,;\, a_{\gamma_h}, b_{\gamma_h}, u^{-2})$:

$$a_{\gamma_h} = \frac{\nu_h S - 1}{2} \qquad b_{\gamma_h} = \frac{1}{2} \sum_{k=1}^{S} \sum_{i_h} \left[[\widehat{\mathbf{\Sigma}}^{(00)} - 2\widehat{\mathbf{\Sigma}}^{(k0)} + \widehat{\mathbf{\Sigma}}^{(kk)}]_{i_h i_h} + [\widehat{\mathbf{w}}_k - \widehat{\mathbf{w}}_0]_{i_h}^2 \right] \qquad (13)$$

$$\widehat{\gamma}_h \equiv \mathcal{E}_{q(\gamma_h)}\{\gamma_h\} = \frac{1}{b_{\gamma_h}} \left[a_{\gamma_h} + \frac{(b_{\gamma_h} u^{-2})^{a_{\gamma_h}} \exp\{-b_{\gamma_h} u^{-2}\}}{\Gamma(a_{\gamma_h}, b_{\gamma_h} u^{-2})} \right]$$

Update for $q(\boldsymbol{\alpha}) \leftarrow \prod_{g=1}^{G} \text{Ga}(\alpha_g \,;\, a_{\alpha_g}, b_{\alpha_g})$:

$$a_{\alpha_g} = a_p + \frac{\kappa_g}{2} \qquad b_{\alpha_g} = b_p + \frac{1}{2} \sum_{i_g} \left[[\widehat{\mathbf{\Sigma}}^{(00)}]_{i_g i_g} + [\widehat{\mathbf{w}}_0]_{i_g}^2 \right] \qquad (14)$$

$$\widehat{\alpha}_g \equiv \mathcal{E}_{q(\alpha_g)}\{\alpha_g\} = a_{\alpha_g} b_{\alpha_g}^{-1}$$

In our experiments with this algorithm, we found that the sufficient statistics for $q(\mathbf{\Lambda})$ and $q(\boldsymbol{\alpha})$ converge quite rapidly, but that convergence of those for $q(\boldsymbol{\gamma})$ is extremely slow for data in which any RFX group has a large precision γ_h. This observation is consistent with the literature on EM estimation of generic RFX models [15]. However, we found that posterior optimization could be made quite rapid by using Powell's direction set method [17] to estimate the otherwise slow-converging sufficient statistics of $q(\boldsymbol{\gamma})$. In this approach, the optimal negative variational free energy F at each setting of $q(\boldsymbol{\gamma})$ is computed using the relatively rapid VB fixed-point iteration for the remaining parameters (Equations (11), (12) and (14)).

$$\underbrace{\max_{\widehat{\boldsymbol{\gamma}}} \overbrace{\max_{\widehat{\mathbf{w}}, \widehat{\mathbf{\Sigma}}, \widehat{\mathbf{\Lambda}}, \widehat{\boldsymbol{\alpha}}} F(\widehat{\mathbf{w}}, \widehat{\mathbf{\Sigma}}, \widehat{\mathbf{\Lambda}}, \widehat{\boldsymbol{\gamma}}, \widehat{\boldsymbol{\alpha}})}^{\text{VB iteration}}}_{\text{Powell's Method}} \qquad (15)$$

Above, we are able write F above as a function solely of the precision means since only one of the two sufficient statistics of their respective posteriors varies during VB optimization.

We initialize this hybrid algorithm by computing the sample mean and precision of source-independent ML estimates of the source-level coefficients and noise precisions, and then by running the full VB iteration until the change in $\widehat{\mathbf{\Lambda}}$ and $\widehat{\boldsymbol{\alpha}}$ becomes less than 10^{-4}. This quickly produces a posterior estimate $q(\mathbf{\Lambda}, \boldsymbol{\gamma}, \boldsymbol{\alpha})$ which is nearly optimal. We cache the optimal $\widehat{\mathbf{\Lambda}}$ and $\widehat{\boldsymbol{\alpha}}$ for recent evaluations of

$F(\widehat{\gamma})$ to initialize the VB iteration of subsequent evaluations, so that as Powell's method converges, the VB iteration is started very close to its fixed-point. We terminate the hybrid optimization when F is maximized to precision $\pm 10^{-10}$.

The following is an expression for the negative variational free energy F under the RFX-MAR model. Note that we have dropped an infinite constant due to the improper prior on Λ, and have canceled a number of terms by assuming that F is evaluated after the update steps for $q(\Lambda)$ and $q(\alpha)$, but before the next update for $q(\mathbf{w})$. If $q(\gamma)$ is being updated, then the last line also cancels. The block structure of $\widehat{\Sigma}$ can be used to make evaluation of its determinant $|\widehat{\Sigma}| = |\widehat{\Sigma}^{(00)}| \prod_{k=1}^{S} |\widehat{\Gamma} + \widetilde{\Lambda}_k|^{-1}$ computationally manageable.

$$F = \frac{d}{2}\left(\frac{S(d-1)}{2} - N\right)\log \pi + \frac{(S+1)d^2 p}{2} + \frac{1}{2}\log|\widehat{\Sigma}| + \sum_{g=1}^{G} \log \frac{b_{\alpha_g}^{a_{\alpha_g}} \Gamma(\widehat{a}_{\alpha_g})}{\widehat{b}_{\alpha_g}^{\widehat{a}_{\alpha_g}} \Gamma(a_{\alpha_g})}$$

$$+ \sum_{h=1}^{H} \log \frac{\Gamma(\widehat{a}_{\gamma_h}, \widehat{b}_{\gamma_h} u^{-2})}{2u\widehat{b}_{\gamma_h}^{\widehat{a}_{\gamma_h}}} + \sum_{k=1}^{S}\left[\frac{N_k}{2}\log\left(|\widehat{\Lambda}_k| N_k^{-d}\right) + \sum_{i=0}^{d-1} \log \Gamma\left(\frac{N_k - i}{2}\right)\right]$$

$$+ \sum_{h=1}^{H} \widehat{\gamma}_h\left(\widehat{b}_{\gamma_h} - \frac{\widehat{\gamma}_h}{2}\sum_{k=1}^{S}\sum_{i_h}\left[[\widehat{\Sigma}^{(00)} - 2\widehat{\Sigma}^{(k0)} + \widehat{\Sigma}^{(kk)}]_{i_h i_h} + [\widehat{\mathbf{w}}_k - \widehat{\mathbf{w}}]_{i_h}^2\right]\right)$$

5 Model Structure Selection

Since the VB algorithm maximizes a lower bound on the log evidence $p(\mathbf{D}|H)$ of a generic model H, the optimized negative variational free energy $F(H)$ can be used to approximate the posterior on model structure $p(H|\mathbf{D})$ by search over competing models [16, 12]. For the RFX-MAR model, H is parameterized by its discrete-valued structural parameters: the MAR model order p, the RFX structuring function $\text{group}_\gamma()$, and the ARD structuring function $\text{group}_\alpha()$. Thus, inference can proceed either by model averaging (for which $\exp(F(H))$ weights the posterior $q(\boldsymbol{\theta}|H)$ under each H), or by model selection (for which inference proceeds based only on the posterior $q(\boldsymbol{\theta}|\widehat{H})$ under the model $\widehat{H} = \arg\max F(H)$ with maximum approximate evidence). The latter VB model selection criteria is equivalent to the Bayesian Information Criteria (BIC) in the large sample limit, and has been shown superior to BIC for model order selection in single-subject MAR modeling [16]. We choose a model selection framework since in our experience with the RFX-MAR on real and synthetic data, $F(H)$ is typically strongly peaked and the coefficient posterior is very similar under all explored model structures with non-vanishing evidence.

We search the MAR order parameter p exhaustively over positive integer values, up to some maximum. Since exhaustive search is not possible for the RFX and ARD group functions, we follow [16] which suggests a semi-automatic, heuristic search method for finding a structuring function likely to group coefficients appropriately. These may include hand-tailored structurings, or generic ones such as a "global" function which puts all coefficients into the same group.

Another example is an "interaction" function which groups all coefficients corresponding to interactions between channels, $A_{ij}(\cdot)$ for all $i \neq j$, and places the remaining coefficients into a second group. Such functions may also be selected semi-automatically. For instance, an "auto" function for the ARD structuring can be produced by k-means clustering of the MAP coefficient estimates under the "global" structuring. An "auto" function for the RFX variance structuring can be produced by k-means clustering of the sample variances of MAP coefficient estimates from subject-independent MAR modeling.

6 Connectivity Inference

We are principally interested in inferring which direct interactions between modeled brain regions are non-zero within a population under experimental conditions. Inference of this kind will be based on (marginalization of) the posterior of the population-level coefficients $q(\mathbf{w}_0)$. Having selected a model structure by the VB maximum evidence criteria, we can report on the population-level effective connectivity between variables i and j by computing a statistic that relates to the posterior "plausibility" of $A_{ij}^0(\cdot) = \mathbf{0}$ under $q(\mathbf{w}_0)$, where $A_{ij}^0(\cdot)$ are the coefficients in $\mathbf{w}_0$ related to the direct influence of variable i on j. Generally speaking, one can report on the posterior plausibility of a specific parameter value $\boldsymbol{\theta} = \boldsymbol{\theta}_0$ by computing the complementary probability content of the smallest *Highest Probability Density* (H.P.D.) region of the posterior $q(\boldsymbol{\theta})$ that contains the value in question [2]. For a Gaussian posterior $q(\boldsymbol{\theta}) = \mathcal{N}(\boldsymbol{\theta}; \boldsymbol{\mu}, \boldsymbol{\Omega})$ with full-rank covariance $\boldsymbol{\Omega}$, it is readily shown that this connectivity statistic s_0 is a monotonic function of the Mahalanobis distance from the posterior mean $\boldsymbol{\mu} \in \Re^r$ to the specified value $\boldsymbol{\theta}_0$. Note that s_0 decreases as $\boldsymbol{\theta} = \boldsymbol{\theta}_0$ becomes less plausible a posteriori.

$$s_0 = 1 - \chi_r^2\left((\boldsymbol{\theta}_0 - \boldsymbol{\mu})'\boldsymbol{\Omega}^{-1}(\boldsymbol{\theta}_0 - \boldsymbol{\mu})\right) \tag{16}$$

To assess the specificity of a test which rejects the null hypothesis (that $A_{ij}^0(\cdot) = \mathbf{0}$) by thresholding such connectivity statistics, we simulate a null distribution by permutations of the time-series data and re-estimation of the these statistics [9]. In particular, we randomly sample circular translations of each of the d time-series for each subject such that every pair of univariate time-series are shifted by more than $2p_{max}$ lags. Here, p_{max} is the maximum MAR model order entertained in our search. This produces multivariate time-series whose univariate statistics are roughly unaffected, while removing causal interactions between variables.

7 Experiments

The ability of the MAR process to capture inter-regional neural dynamics has been shown on synthetic data from biologically plausible models [9]. We validated our estimation algorithm in terms of its ability to estimate all real-valued and structural RFX-MAR parameters using multivariate time-series sampled from known RFX-MAR models. The scope of our investigation was quite broad and involved varying the number of subjects S, number of samples per subject N_k, and degree of inter-subject variance of MAR coefficients. We considered the cases where the subject-specific coefficients were drawn about a single mean, about two means, and drawn independently. We also compared performance of the RFX-MAR model to the subject-independent MAR estimation of [16], and to a "fixed-effects" model in which all subject-level coefficients were assumed to be identical. In summary, we found parameter estimation and model selection to be robust when the number of subjects $S \geq 10$, and the number of samples per subject N_k was greater than approximately three times the number of parameters per subject at the optimal model order $d^2(p+1)$. Classification error for non-zero direct influences between pairs of variable was less than 5% in general. When the amount of data was more limited, the RFX-MAR model tended to overestimate the model order p, but with little impact on connectivity inference. Subject-independent estimation of p was generally more robust.

RFX-MAR analysis of a small number of fMRI and EEG multi-subject datasets have produced promising results. Here, we detail our analysis of multi-subject EEG time-series from the UCI Knowledge Discovery Database[2]. This dataset contains measurements from 64 electrodes placed on the scalps of healthy subjects and sampled at 256 Hz for 1 second during a picture presentation task. The protocol and data are described in [18]. We performed RFX-MAR modeling of 1 second of data from each of S=20 healthy subjects, having selected d=6 channels from the frontal (F5, F6), temporal (T7, T8), and parietal (P3, P4) regions in each hemisphere. We searched all combinations of the following structural parameter settings: $p = \{1, \ldots, 5\}$, group$_\gamma$ = {global, interaction, auto (H=2, 3, 4)} and group$_\alpha$ = {global, interaction, auto (G=2, 3, 4)}. The MAP model structure was $p = 5$, group$_\gamma$ = group$_\alpha$ = interaction. This model order was consistent with the most common model order estimated by subject-independent analysis of the data. The MAP inter-subject standard deviation of coefficients involved with within-channel predictions was 0.027, whereas that for coefficients involved in cross-channel prediction was 0.007. The posterior of the population-level coefficients is shown in Fig. 1. We computed connectivity statistics using (16) to assess evidence of a non-zero causal interaction between each pair of channels, and estimated the null distribution of these statistics by repeating analysis on 100 randomly, circularly shifted versions of each channel, in each subject. This yielded $100\,d(d-1) = 3000$ samples of connectivity statistics between channels for which there is unlikely to be a causal connection. Figure 2 shows the inferred population-level effective connectivity pattern, the associated connectivity statistics, and their estimated p-values. We note that few variables were found to be interacting when the same data was modeled in a subject-independent manner, except when a larger sample of the data was included for each subject. This points to the cross-subject regularizing effect that joint modeling of multiple

---

[2] *http://kdd.ics.uci.edu* These data were provided by Henri Begleiter at the Neurodynamics Laboratory at the State University of New York Health Center at Brooklyn.

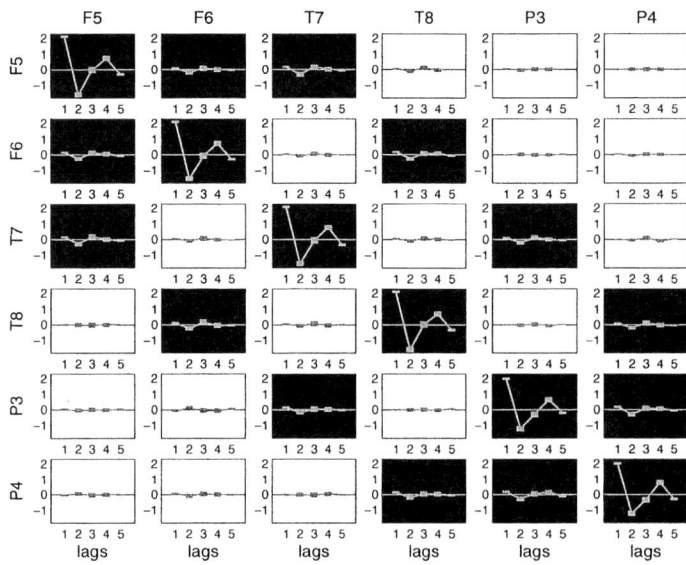

Fig. 1. The posterior mean of the population-level directed influence functions $A_{ij}^0(\cdot)$ (plotted with 99% H.P.D.-content error bars) given the RFX-MAR structural parameters with maximum F for the EEG dataset. The background of plot (i,j) is colored black when the connectivity statistic s_0 for $A_{ij}^0(\cdot) = \mathbf{0}$ is less than 10^{-6}

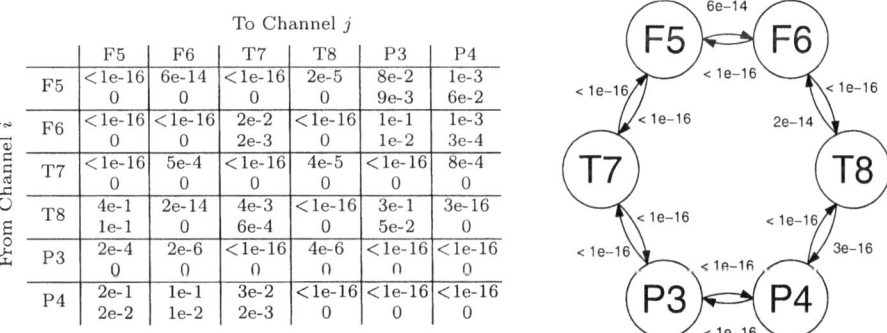

Fig. 2. A graphical representation of the population-level effective connectivity inferred from the EEG data. We only show edges between channels whose connectivity statistic is $\leq 10^{-6}$, and omit self interactions for clarity. EEG channels with odd (even) index are in the left (right) hemisphere. This pattern suggests that regions which are spatially closer interact to a greater degree under the MAR model. The table gives the connectivity statistic (top) and the estimated p-value (bottom) for each interaction

subjects can have to elucidate more subtle connectivity patterns in the data. We repeated this analysis for S=20 different healthy subjects from the same study, and found the population-level posterior and effective connectivity pattern to be very similar.

8 Discussion

We have presented the initial development of a method for population modeling of effective connectivity among brain regions based on neurological time-series. Numerous avenues exist for further elaboration, validation and utilization of this kind of model. We are particularly interested in different ways two populations (distinguished, for example, by the presence of disease) might be compared on the basis of effective connectivity. Certainly, one can perform inference on the population-level coefficients produced by independent RFX-MAR modeling of the two populations. However, the success of classifiers produced from such population models would lend credence to what is necessarily a model-dependent characterization of the interaction among brain regions. It would also be valuable to construct similar population models for more elaborate systems models, such as those not limited to time-invariant connectivity patterns. Finally, we note that the RFX-MAR model can also be used to characterize other types of variation in connectivity parameters, such as that arising from repeated trials under similar experimental conditions.

References

1. J. M. Bernardo and A. F. M. Smith. *Bayesian Theory*. John Wiley & Sons, 1994.
2. G. E. P. Box and G. C. Tao. *Bayesian Inference in Statistical Analysis*. John Wiley & Sons, 1992.
3. A. P. Dempster, N. M. Laird, and D. B. Rubin. Maximum-likelihood from incomplete data via the em algorithm. *J. Royal Statist. Soc. Ser. B*, 39:1–38, 1977.
4. K. J. Friston, L. Harrison, and W. Penny. Dynamic causal modeling. *NeuroImage*, 19, 2003.
5. K. J. Friston, W. Penny, C. Phillips, S. Kiebel, G. Hinton, and J. Ashburner. Classical and bayesian inference in neuroimaging: Theory. *Neuroimage*, 16:465–483, 2002.
6. A. Gelman. Prior distributions for variance parameters in hierarchical models. *Bayesian Analysis*, June 2004.
7. L. Harrison, W. D. Penny, and K. J. Friston. Multivariate autoregressive modeling of fmri time series. *NeuroImage*, 19:1477–1491, 2003.
8. G. E. Hinton and D. V. Camp. Keeping neural networks simple by minimizing the description length of the weights. *Proceedings of the COLT'93*, pages 5–13, 1993.
9. M. Kaminski, M. Ding, W. A. Truccolo, and S. L. Bressler. Evaluating causal relations in neural systems: Granger causality, directed transfer functions and statistical assessment of significance. *Biological Cybernetics*, 85:145–157, 2001.
10. H. Lappalainen and J. W. Miskin. Ensemble learning. *Advances in Independent Components Analysis*, 2000.
11. D. J. C. MacKay. Bayesian non-linear modeling for the energy prediction competition. *ASHRAE Transactions*, 100:1053–10062, 1994.
12. D. J. C. MacKay. *Information Theory, Inference, and Learning Algorithms*. Cambridge University Press, 2003.
13. J. R. Mangus and H. Neudecker. *Matrix Differential Calculus with Applications in Statistics and Econometrics (Revised Edition)*. John Wiley & Sons, 1999.

14. A. R. McIntosh and F. Gonzalez-Lima. The application of structural equation modeling to metabolic mapping of functional neural systems. *HBM*, 2:2–22, 1994.
15. X.-L. Meng and D. van Dyk. Fast em-type implementations for mixed effects models. *J. Royal Statist. Soc. Ser. B*, 60(3):559–578, 1998.
16. W. D. Penny and S. J. Roberts. Bayesian multivariate autoregressive models with structured priors. *IEE Proc.-Vis. Image Signal Process.*, 149(1), February 2002.
17. W. H. Press, S. A. Teukolsky, W. T. Vetterling, and B. P. Flannery. *Numerical Recipes in C*. Cambridge University Press, 1992.
18. X. L. Zhang, H. Begleiter, B. Porjesz, W. Wang, and A. Litke. Event related potentials during object recognition taks. *Brain Research Bulletin*, 38(6), 1995.

Fiber Tracking in q-Ball Fields
Using Regularized Particle Trajectories

M. Perrin[1,3], C. Poupon[1,3], Y. Cointepas[1,3], B. Rieul[1,3], N. Golestani[1,2], C. Pallier[1,2],
D. Rivière[1,3], A. Constantinesco[4], D. Le Bihan[1,3], and J.-F. Mangin[1,3]

[1] Service Hospitalier Frédéric Joliot, CEA, 91401 Orsay, France
perrin@shfj.cea.fr
http://brainvisa.info
[2] INSERM U562 Cognitive Neuro Imaging, Orsay, France
[3] Institut Fédératif de Recherche 49 (Imagerie Neurofonctionnelle), Paris
[4] CHU Hautepierre, Strasbourg

Abstract. Most of the approaches dedicated to fiber tracking from diffusion-weighted MR data rely on a tensor model. However, the tensor model can only resolve a single fiber orientation within each imaging voxel. New emerging approaches have been proposed to obtain a better representation of the diffusion process occurring in fiber crossing. In this paper, we adapt a tracking algorithm to the q-ball representation, which results from a spherical Radon transform of high angular resolution data. This algorithm is based on a Monte-Carlo strategy, using regularized particle trajectories to sample the white matter geometry. The method is validated using a phantom of bundle crossing made up of haemodialysis fibers. The method is also applied to the detection of the auditory tract in three human subjects.

1 Introduction

Brownian motion of water molecules in brain white matter is disturbed by the fiber bundle microscopic structure. Therefore, the anisotropy of the molecule displacements embeds information about the fiber bundle orientations. Hence, diffusion MRI, which probes these water molecule displacements, provides a way to detect the main bundles and to map the large scale connectivity of the brain.

A lot of methods have been proposed for this purpose. Most of them rely on a tensor model of the water diffusion process (Diffusion Tensor Imaging, DTI) [1, 15]. This model, however, is too simple to represent the complex diffusion process occurring in voxels filled by fiber crossing. More sophisticated models have been recently introduced to overcome these difficulties [22, 8, 16]. They usually aim at explaining the MR signal as a mixture of tensor models. They provide convincing results in some crossing areas, but lack the versatility required to untangle any complex diffusion pattern (fan-shaped bundle, bending fibers, kissing fibers, etc.). Therefore, another strategy consists in using iconic representations of the diffusion process, namely an image for each voxel. This point of view alleviates the risk of misinterpreting the MR data because of the narrowness of the model.

Diffusion Spectrum Imaging (DSI), which provides for each voxel a 3D image of the water displacement probability distribution, is the most attractive solution [25, 12]. Unfortunately DSI is based on sampling the 3D Fourier space of the water displacement distribution, which requires large pulsed field gradients and time-intensive acquisition. Therefore DSI can not be used in clinical situations. However, it has been shown recently that the orientation distribution function (ODF) of this probability distribution can be reconstructed from high angular resolution diffusion imaging (HARDI) using a spherical tomographic inversion called the Funk-Radon transform, also known as the spherical Radon transform [21]. This technique called q-ball imaging could resolve intravoxel white matter fiber crossing as well as white matter insertions into cortex [23].

In this paper, we propose a new algorithm to infer fiber bundles from q-ball imaging data. This algorithm combines the idea of performing a probabilistic tractography [4, 3, 16] with regularization of the curvature of the particle trajectories used to sample the white matter organization [17, 24, 13, 5]. The method is first validated with a phantom of fiber crossing made up of haemodialysis fibers. Then, the method is successfully applied to the detection of the auditory tract in 3 human subjects. This tract can not be detected with the standard DTI-based streamline method [14, 6, 2] because of its crossing with a large orthogonal bundle.

2 Method

2.1 QBall Imaging

The QBall model has been introduced by David Tuch in 2002 because performing routine DSI acquisition was too difficult [20]. The MR diffusion signal E is related to the diffusion function P by the Fourier relation $P = F[||E(q)||]$ where q is the diffusion wave-vector. The radial projection of the diffusion function is called the diffusion ODF and is defined as $\psi(u) = \int_0^\infty P(ru)dr$, where u is the unit direction vector. Given a sampling of E on a sphere (HARDI), David Tuch demonstrated that the spherical Radon transform or Funk-Radon Transform (FRT) provides a good approximation of this ODF. Let us consider a function p(w) on a sphere where w is the unit direction vector: for a given direction of interest u, the FRT is defined as the integral over the corresponding equator,

$$S[u] = \int_{w \perp u} p(w)dw. \qquad (1)$$

David Tuch demonstrated that the FRT of E evaluated at a particular radius q' can be written in cylindrical coordinates as :

$$S_{q'}[E] = 2\pi q' \int P(r,\theta,z) J_0(2*\pi*q'r) r dr d\theta dz \qquad (2)$$

where J_0 is the 0th order Bessel Function. If we replace this Bessel function by a delta function, $\delta(r)$, then we obtain the radial projection ODF exactly. Therefore, due to the Fourier relationship between the diffusion MR signal and the diffusion function, we can exploit this finding to measure the displacement probability in a particular direction by simply summing the diffusion MR signal along an equator around that direction [23, 21]. Q-ball field is the result of this summation computed voxel by voxel.

In the following, q-ball data are visualised according to the following rules. Each q-ball is represented by a spherical mesh. Each node of the mesh is moved outward according to the water molecule displacement probability. In order to maximize the information provided by this deformation process, this motion is computed as $(p - min_S(p))/(max_S(p) - min_S(p))$, where p is the node probability and S the sampled sphere of the current voxel. To improve visualisation further, each node is given a color related to its orientation relative to the image axis: red for x axis, green for y axis and blue for z axis, interpolated in between.

2.2 Fiber Direction and ODF

Due to the mathematical approximation mentioned above, the q-ball-based ODF does not match exactly the actual ODF. Moreover, the relationship between the diffusion ODF and the fiber ODF is an open issue governed for instance by the link between the physics of diffusion and some biophysical properties of the tissue such as cell membrane permeability or free diffusion coefficients for the different cellular compartments. This issue corresponds to a crucial research program for the community of diffusion imaging. This program, however, needs time to deliver some answers, which should not stop the development of tracking algorithms. These algorithms, indeed, have the possibility to use contextual knowledge, namely the neighborhood of a voxel, in order to tackle locally the inverse problem: which geometry of fiber can explain such q-ball data. Therefore, in the following, we assimilate the diffusion ODF with the fiber ODF, but the relationship could be refined in the future. One key issue, for instance, when dealing with q-ball imaging will be the optimal choice of the radius q' of the HARDI acquisition. Increasing q', indeed, sharpens the Bessel kernel and increases the ability to resolve distinct diffusion peaks but at the cost of a lower signal to noise ratio.

2.3 Probabilistic Tracking and Curvature Regularization

The simplest approaches for fiber tracking, which are based on DTI, are variants of the "streamline" method. The eigenvector of the tensor associated with the highest eigenvalue is supposed to provide the local fiber direction. Then this local direction is followed step by step in order to build 3D trajectories supposed to correspond to the bundles [14,6,2]. Unfortunately, in case of partial volume (fiber crossing), the diffusion ellipsoid associated to the tensor may be a disk or a sphere. In such cases, the first eigenvector indicates a spurious fiber direction leading to false fork of the tracking process.

Various approaches have been proposed to reduce the bad influence of ambiguous tensors. They all involve the use of the entire tensor information. For instance the tensor is used in [26,9] to deflect the estimated fiber trajectory leading to the reconstruction of "tensorlines". Another approach considers the tensor field as a Riemannian manifold and the fibers as some geodesics of this manifold [10]. Using a regularization point of view leads to define the fibers as a trade-off between high diffusion along fibers and low curvature constraints [17]. The tensor field can also feed a model of uncertainty on the fiber orientation used to perform Monte-Carlo estimations of the connectivity [4,3] or probabilistic tracking [5].

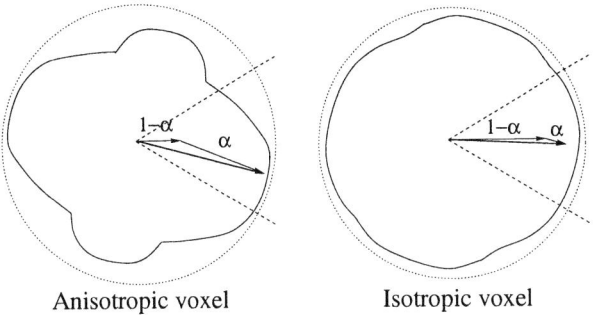

Fig. 1. The normalized standard deviation of the q-ball provides a measure of anisotropy α, that is used to weight the influence of the q-ball on the particle trajectories

All these approaches perform better than the simple streamline idea. However, when getting close to the cortex, they get in touch with large areas of crossing fibers where the reliability of the results drop down. In such areas, the tracking problem becomes ill-posed because of the poor representation of the diffusion process provided by the tensor. There is now a consensus that higher angular resolution data like HARDI is required to untangle such crossing. New approaches are then needed to infer information on the fiber orientation from such data. The multi-tensor point of view converts HARDI into a short list of fiber directions for each voxel that can be used to develop tracking approaches [16]. A weakness of this strategy stems from the potential failures of the process leading to this list, either a standard fitting procedure [22] or more sophisticated approaches from information theory [8]. The q-ball approach, which converts directly the diffusion data into a fiber ODF, overcomes this difficulty. Therefore, this data representation seems the perfect candidate for developing Monte-Carlo estimation of white matter geometry. In the following, we describe such an approach where this geometry is sampled using regularized particle trajectories.

Like most approaches, our method requires a Region of Interest (ROI) as input. Each voxel of this ROI is spatially sampled in order to define the starting points of n particles. These particles move inside a continuous q-ball field defined by linear interpolation. Each particle is endowed with an initial speed in the direction of the q-ball maximum. Then, each particle moves with constant speed according to a simplistic sampling scheme: let us note $p(i)$ the location of the particle at time i, and $\overrightarrow{v(i)}$ the direction of the particle speed at time i:

$$p(i + \delta t) = p(i) + \overrightarrow{v(i)} * \delta t \qquad (3)$$

The behaviour of the particle speed direction can be understood from a simple mechanical analogy: at each step of the trajectory sampling, the new speed $\overrightarrow{v(i+\delta t)}$ results from a trade-off between inertia ($\overrightarrow{v(i)}$) and a force stemming from the local q-ball ($\vec{v_q}$):

$$\overrightarrow{v(i+\delta t)} = \alpha \vec{v_q} + (1-\alpha)\overrightarrow{v(i)} \qquad (4)$$

where α is a parameter ranging between 0 and 1 that will be described latter. The orientation $\vec{v_q}$ of the force acting on the particle is chosen randomly inside a half cone defined from the incident direction $\vec{v(i)}$. The probability distribution driving this sampling corresponds to the restriction of the q-ball to this half cone. Therefore, the maximum of the q-ball inside the half cone has the highest probability.

The parameter α is the standard deviation of the q-ball normalized by its maximum in the field. Hence, this weight depends on the location in the q-ball field. In fact α is a measure of anisotropy [7]. For isotropic voxels, α parameter is small and the algorithm favours incident orientation; while for anisotropic voxels, α parameter is large and the algorithm favours q-ball distribution (see Fig. 1).

The particle trajectory regularization depends on three parameters:

1. the half-cone angle is used to discard the diffusion peaks leading to high curvature of the trajectory. In the following, the cone angle defined from the cone axis is 30 degrees.
2. the q-ball standard deviation (α parameter) tunes the weight of inertia.
3. the constant sampling δt provides another level of tuning: increasing the trajectory sampling decreases curvature regularization. In all the following, δt is set such as the particles do a 0.5 mm move at each iteration.

In this paper, the influence of these ad hoc parameters is not explored. The algorithm proposed in this paper, indeed, aims mainly at studying the inner organization of the q-ball field and its links with the bundle organization. It is too early to address the optimal tuning of such parameters.

The particles propagate throughout a mask computed from the T2 image. Trajectories stop only when they leave the mask. After the propagation, a postprocessing can be applied to keep only the reliable part of a bundle. After selection of a set of particle trajectories, for instance using a second ROI, a meter is used for each voxel accounting for the number of particles which go through that voxel. Then, the trajectories crossing some voxels whose meter is under a given threshold are discarded as non significant.

3 Fiber Crossing Phantom

The lack of knowledge about the white matter organization of the human brain is a huge handicap for the community developing fiber tracking algorithms. Considering the complexity of the MR diffusion signal, it is rather difficult to validate such algorithms using only simulated data. Therefore, the development of phantoms with known geometry is in our opinion crucial for a better understanding of the algorithm behaviours [12].

For this purpose, we have designed a phantom corresponding to two intersecting fiber bundles. It consists of sheets of parallel haemodialysis Fibers (Gambro, Polyflux 210 H) with an inner diameter of 200 micrometers and an outer diameter of 250 micrometers. Sheets of two different orientations intersecting at 90 degrees were stacked on each other in an interleaved fashion [12]. Crossing thickness is above 2cm. Fibers are suspended and hold by two arms as seen in Fig. 2. Fibers are permeable to water. They are dived in pure water mixed with gadolinium.

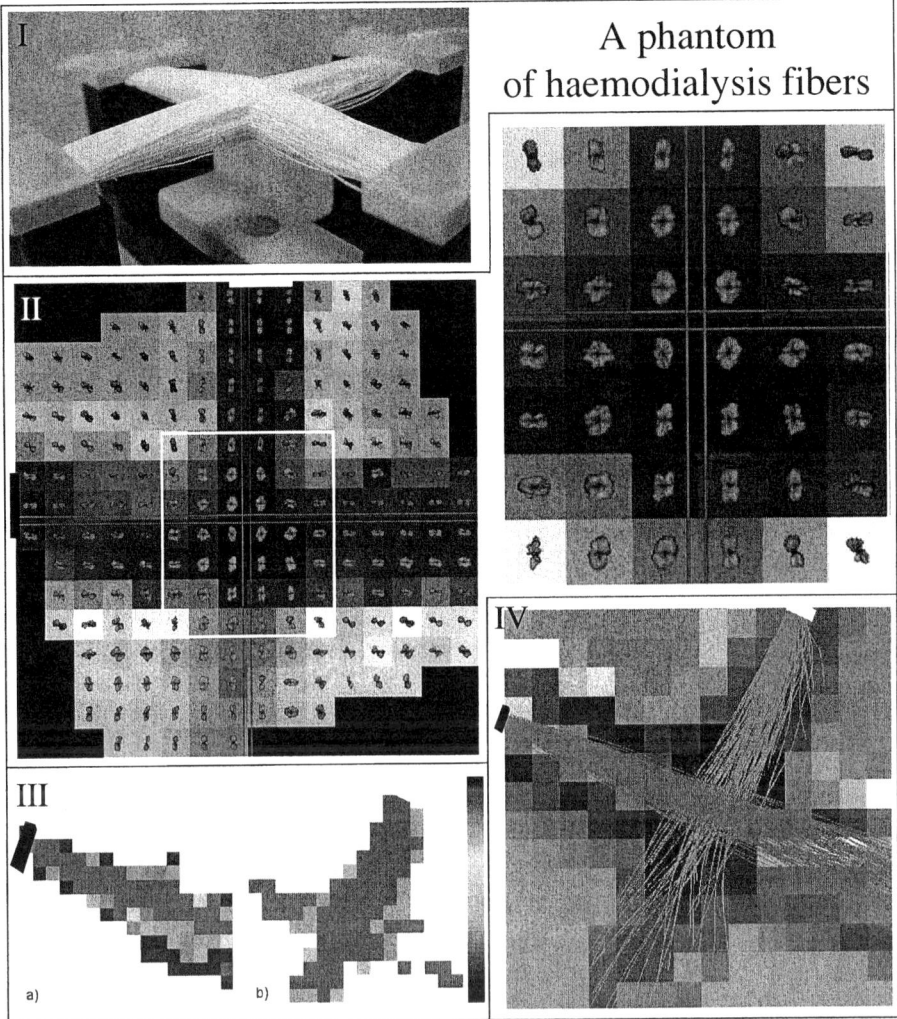

Fig. 2. I: A phantom of fiber crossing. II: A slice of the 512 directions q-ball acquisition with a zoom on the crossing area. q-balls are superimposed on a T2-weighted MR image whose intensity is related to water amount. q-balls and MR data have been slightly rotated in order to simplify the reading of the q-ball 3D color code. Green and blue rectangles denote the regions of interest at the origin of fiber tracking. III: Slices of the number of particles crossing each voxels at the end of the fiber sampling (left: blue bundle, right: green bundle). IV: Trajectories selected by a threshold on the particle density map for each bundle. A T2-weighted slice of the phantom crossing the bundles is used as background and hides some trajectories

We performed MRI acquisitions with a 1.5 Tesla magnet (Signa, General Electrics) with maximal gradient intensity of 40 mT m^{-1}. Acquisitions were performed with Spin echo EPI sequence and Stejskal and Tanner diffusion gradient [19]: b value is

700 s mm^{-2}, equivalent to 2000 s mm^{-2} for diffusion in brain white matter, 512 orientations of the diffusion gradient (HARDI), Matrix 64 x 64, In-plane voxel resolution 3.75 x 3.75 mm, Slice thickness 2.0 mm, TE 66.6 ms, TR 3000 ms, 1 shot, field of view 24 cm. Spatial distortions of the diffusion-weighted images induced by Eddy currents were corrected before estimation of the q-ball field. This correction relies on a slice by slice affine geometric model and maximization of mutual information with the diffusion free T2-weighted image.

A slice of the q-ball field is shown in Fig. 2. Unfortunately, because of a difficult positioning of the phantom due to the shape of its container, the two crossing bundles are not parallel to the slice axes. To clarify the visualisation of the q-ball data based on color encoding, a rotation around the z-axis has been applied to the data before visualization. Then the orientation of each bundle corresponds to a pure color in the q-ball meshes (green and red). A zoom on the crossing area highlights the additional information provided by the q-ball compared to a tensor model. The diffusion peaks, however, would provide a better angular discrimination with higher b value (q').

For each bundle, the tracking algorithm is fed with a ROI made up of 3 voxels, using 3 x 130 particles. The particles propagate throughout a mask defined from the T2-weighted image. This mask corresponds to the part of the field of view including the artificial fibers. It was defined from a high threshold on intensity (the voxels including fibers contain less water, which leads to less signal), followed by a morphological closing in order to fill up spurious holes. A slice of the two resulting particle density maps is shown in Fig. 2. A threshold of 5 particles is applied to these maps in order to create a mask used to select reliable trajectories. The remaining trajectories do not include any spurious fork in the crossing area.

A second experiment was performed to check that the successful result was not only due to the fact that the phantom bundles have a straight geometry. With such a geometry, indeed, curvature regularization is sufficient for the particles to pass through the crossing area without trouble. For this second experiment, a 20 degree rotation around the z axis was applied to the q-balls of the crossing area corresponding to the zoom of Fig. 2. Then the tracking algorithm was triggered with the same set of particles as for the first experiment using first the initial q-ball field and second the modified field. However, the particles could propagate throughout the whole field (no mask) and no filtering of the trajectories was applied using the particle density map. The results shown in Fig. 3 prove that the curvature regularization does not prevent the particle to follow the rotated fiber direction indicated by the q-balls of the crossing area. This observation means that the q-balls of the crossing area are anisotropic enough to oppose the particle inertia.

A last experiment was performed to observe the behaviour of the streamline approach with the same data and the same ROIs. The algorithm was provided by brainVISA software (http://brainvisa.info). Each voxel of the ROI was spatially sampled in order to provide several starting points. The streamlines were sampled with 0.5mm steps. For each step, the tensor is estimated after linear interpolation of the 512 diffusion-weighted images and the streamline follows the direction of the main eigenvector. Streamlines are stopped by a threshold on the angle between two consecutive directions, namely a threshold on the streamline curvature. We performed the experiment

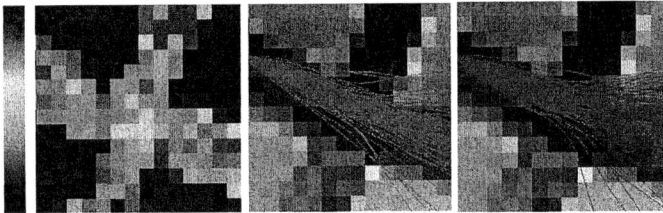

Fig. 3. Left: a slice of the normalized standard deviation of the q-ball (α). **Middle**: particle trajectories in the initial q-ball field (T2-weighted image behind). **Right**: particle trajectories in the field where the q-balls of the crossing area have been rotated around the z axis (20 degrees)

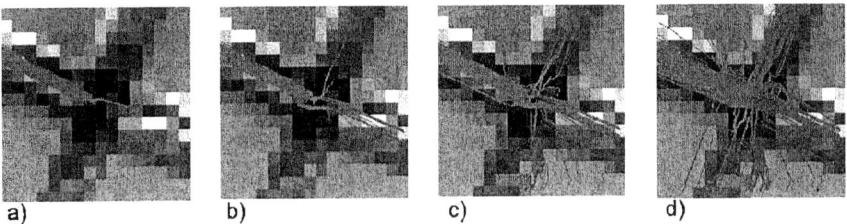

Fig. 4. Streamline algorithm with different thresholds on the angle between two consecutive steps. a) 30 degrees, b) 60 degrees, c) 80 degrees d) 90 degrees

with four different thresholds (30deg, 60deg, 80deg, 90deg). The results are shown in Fig. 4. With a 30deg threshold, the streamlines can not pass through the crossing area. Increasing the threshold allows the streamlines to go further, but the result is uncertain. When the streamlines remains inside the correct bundle, they include questionable high curvature parts. All these difficulties stem from the fact that the directions of the tensor main eigenvectors in the crossing area are not predictable.

4 Human Brain

One of the bundles often used to illustrate the behaviour of tracking methods is the optic tract, which conveys information from the thalamus to the visual cortex in occipital lobe [6]. The optic tract is interesting for validation because it is one of the few well known bundles of brain architecture. A few other primary bundles like the pyramidal tract are used for the same purpose. Surprisingly, the auditory tract, which conveys information from the thalamus to the auditory cortex in temporal lobe, is usually absent from tracking reports. This bundle seems to be lost in a large crossing with orthogonal fibers. To study the potential of the approach described in this paper, the last experiment aims at detecting this primary tract.

The acquisitions used for this last experiment were not initially dedicated to q-ball methodology. Therefore, the angular resolution is low and the b-value is too small to get accurate information on the crossing geometry. Nevertheless, the q-ball approach can

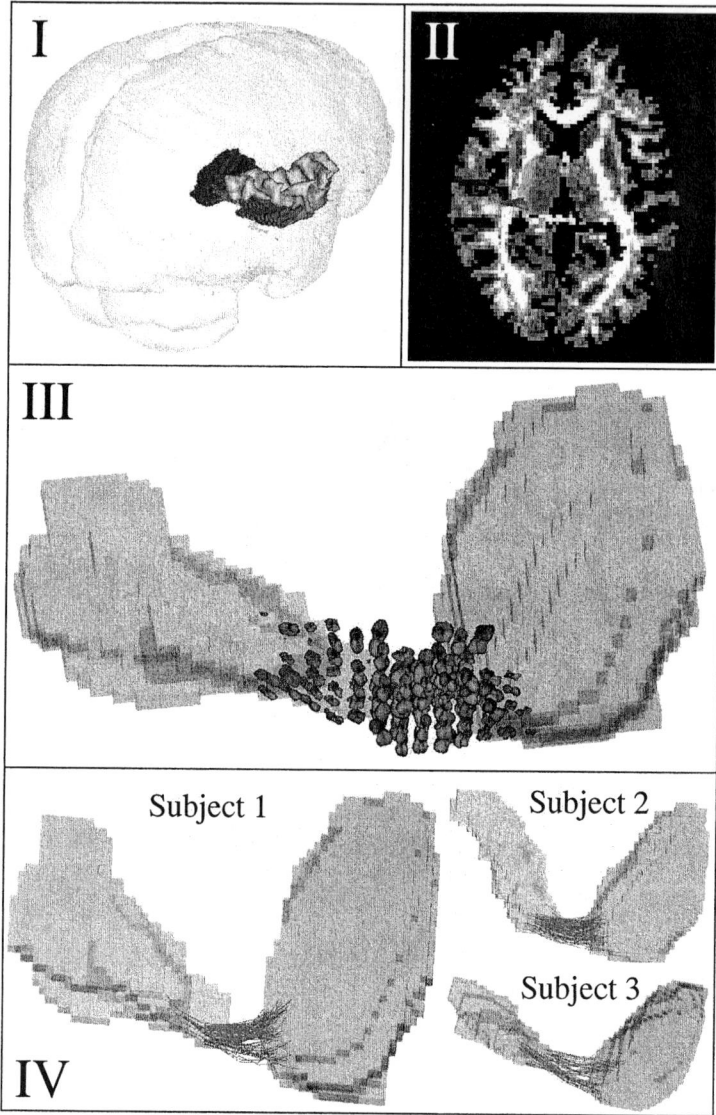

Fig. 5. I: The two regions of interest (ROIs) used to define auditory tract are the thalamus (red) and Heschl gyrus (green), a good landmark of primary auditory area. The yellow object is the grey matter of the lateral fissure surrounding Heschl gyrus. The blue bundle, supposed to correspond to auditory tract, has been inferred from q-ball data. II: Intersection of the ROIs and of the tracked bundle with a slice of the anisotropy map (the parameter α mentioned in the text) computed inside the mask used for tracking. III: The q-balls of the voxels crossed by at least one particle trajectory linking the two ROIs. IV: the representation of the auditory tract obtained after thresholding the particle density map for the subject used above and for two other subjects

be used to analyze such data, which has been done for 3 different subjects. The acquisition parameters are the following: 41 diffusion gradient directions (HARDI), b value is 700 s mm^{-2}, Matrix 128 x 128, In-plane voxel resolution 1.875 x 1.875 mm, Slice thickness 2.0 mm, TE 66.6 ms, TR 2000 ms, single shot, FOV 24 cm. After correction of the spatial distortions induced by Eddy currents, the q-ball field was estimated using a tessellation of the sphere made up of 240 nodes. To improve further 3D visualization, a homothetic factor was applied to the q-ball meshes. This factor corresponds to the normalized standard deviation of the q-ball (α). Hence, anisotropic q-balls are larger than isotropic ones.

A white matter mask was used to prevent the particles to go through cortical folds. The process leading to this mask is the following. A low threshold was applied to the normalized standard deviation of the q-ball in order to get a first mask of anisotropic areas. This mask was used to compute the histogram of intensities of anisotropic areas in the T2-weighted image. A simple histogram analysis provides two thresholds allowing the definition of the white matter mask.

A good landmark of the primary auditory cortex is called Heschl gyrus, a small gyrus hidden in the temporal part of the lateral fissure [18, 11]. This gyrus and the thalamus have been drawn manually in the T2-weighted images (see Fig. 5). Each voxel of Heschl gyrus has been spatially sampled with 20 particles leading to a total of 20000 starting points (1000 voxels in the ROI). After the tracking, the trajectories reaching the thalamus ROI are selected first. Then, these trajectories are split in order to keep only the part linking the two ROIs. A 3D view of the q-balls crossed by the remaining trajectories is proposed in Fig. 5. While the auditory bundle orientation is clear close to Heshl gyrus from the q-ball shapes, the q-balls of the crossing area depict mainly the orthogonal bundle that disturb the streamline approach. A threshold of 3 particles in the density map was used to select further reliable trajectories, which defined a reasonable putative auditory bundle for the three subjects (see Fig. 5).

We performed an additional experiment to compare globally the particle trajectories with streamlines computed for the same data and with the same starting points, using a 80 degrees threshold on angles. The results are shown in Fig. 6. The streamlines are all attracted by the orthogonal bundle.

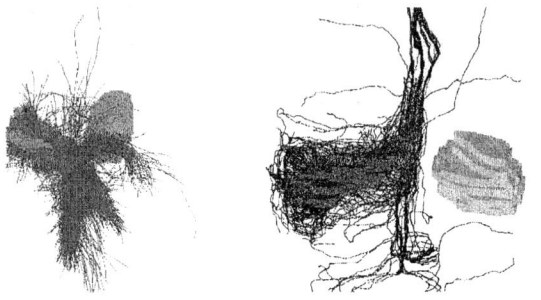

Fig. 6. Left: the entire set of particle trajectories **right:** the equivalent set of streamlines

5 Conclusion

In this paper, we have explored the new possibilities provided by q-ball representations for untangling fiber crossing during tracking. We have shown with the phantom study that the additional information on the fiber ODF provided by the q-ball increases largely the potential of tracking algorithms. In this paper, we advocate the use of probabilistic tracking approaches, which can embed uncertainty about the fiber ODF. The potential of this kind of approaches had already been shown in previous work using tensor [4, 3, 5] and multi-tensor models [16]. Here, we have shown that the probabilistic framework fits perfectly the information provided by the q-ball, even if some more work has to be done in order to convert q-ball data into a more reliable fiber ODF. For instance, the proportions of the different fiber orientations included in a voxel influence the q-ball in a way that should be corrected in the fiber ODF. This could largely bias the algorithm described in this paper. This algorithm was kept deliberately simple to prevent the need for sophisticated theoretical development that would be meaningless because of our lack of understanding of the link between the two ODFs. The development of new phantoms could be of great help to improve this understanding. Some of the key parameters whose influence on q-ball should be studied are the proportions of the bundles, the angle between the bundles and the bending of the bundles.

While the experiments with the human brain data may be discussed, because the acquired data are far to optimize the q-ball representation, they show that gathering some of the most advanced ideas of the diffusion community (q-ball, probabilistic tracking, curvature regularization) allows the tracking to get closer to the few a priori anatomical knowledge about the brain connectivity. The next stage will imply to use higher angular resolution data and higher b-value, in order to address the tracking of longer bundles.

References

1. P. J. Basser, J. Mattiello, and D. LeBihan. MR Diffusion Tensor Spectroscopy and Imaging. *Biophysical Journal*, 66:259–267, January 1994.
2. P. J. Basser, S. Pajevic, C. Pierpaoli, J. Duda, and A. Aldroubi. In vivo fiber tractography using DT-MRI data. *MRM*, 44(4):625–32, 2000.
3. T.E.J Behrens, H. Johansen-Berg, M.W Woolrich, S.M.Smith, C.A.M Wheeler-Kingshott, P.A. Boulby, G.J. Barker, E.L. Sillery, K. Sheehan, O. Ciccarelli, A.J. Thompson, J.M. Brady, and P.M. Matthews. Non-invasive mapping of connections between human thalamus and cortex using diffusion imaging. *nature neuroscience*, 6(7):750–7, 2003.
4. T.E.J Behrens, M.W. Woolrich, M. Jenkinson, H. Johansen-Berg, R.G. Nunes, S. Clare, P.M. Matthews, J.M. Brady, and S.M. Smith. Characterization and propagation of uncertainty in diffusion-weighted mr imaging. *Magnetic Resonance in Medicine*, 50:1077–1088, 2003.
5. M. Björnemo, A. Brun, R. Kikinis, and C.-F. Westin. Regularized stochastic white matter tractography using diffusion tensor mri. In *MICCAI'02, LNCS 2488, Springer Verlag*, pages 435–442, 2002.
6. T. E. Conturo, N. F. Lori, T. S. Cull, E. Akbudak, A. Z. Snyder, J. S. Shimony, R. C. McKinstry, H. Burton, and M. E. Raichle. Tracking neuronal fiber pathways in the living human brain. *Proc. Natl. Acad. Sci. USA*, 96:10422–10427, August 1999.
7. L.R Frank. Anisotropy in high angular resolution diffusion-weighted mri. *Magnetic Resonance in Medicine*, 45:935–939, 2001.

8. K.M. Jansons and D.C. Alexander. Persistent angular structure: new insights from diffusion magnetic resonance imaging data. *Inverse Problems*, 19(5):1031–1046, 2003.
9. M. Lazar, J. S. Tsuruda D. Weinstein, K. Arfanakis K. M. Hasan, M. E. Meyerand, B. Badie, H. A. Rowley, V. Haugton, A. Field, and A. Alexander. White matter tractography using diffusion tensor deflection. In *Hum Brain Mapp*, volume 18, pages 306–321, 2003.
10. C. Lenglet, R. Deriche, and O. Faugeras. Inferring white matter geometry from diffusion tensor mri: Application to connectivity mapping. In *8th European Conference on Computer Vision*, 2004.
11. C.M. Leonard, C. Puranik, J. Kuldau, and L.J. Lombardino. Normal variation in the frequency and location of human auditory cortex landmarks. heschl's gyrus: where is it? *Cereb Cortex.*, 8(5):397–406, 1998.
12. C.P Lin, V.J. Wedeen, J.H. Chen, C. Yao, and W.Y.I Tseng. Validation of diffusion spectrum magnetic resonance imaging with manganese-enhanced rat optic tracts and ex vivo phantoms. *NeuroImage*, 2003.
13. J.-F. Mangin, C. Poupon, Y. Cointepas, D. Rivière, D. Papadopoulos-Orfanos, C. A. Clark, J. Régis, and D. Le Bihan. A framework based on spin glass models for the inference of anatomical connectivity from diffusion-weighted MR data. *NMR in Biomedicine*, 15:481–492, 2002.
14. S. Mori, B.J. Crain, V. P. Chacko, and P. C. M. van Zijl. Three dimensional tracking of axonal projections in the brain by magnetic resonance imaging. *Ann. Neurol.*, 45:265–269, 1999.
15. S. Mori and P.C. van Zijl. Fiber tracking: principles and strategies - a technical review. *NMR Biomed*, 15(7-8):468–80, 2002.
16. G. J. M Parker and D. C. Alexander. Probabilistic Monte Carlo based mapping of cerebral connections utilising whole-brain crossing fibre information. In *IPMI, Ambleside*, volume 18, pages 684–95, 2003.
17. C. Poupon, C.A. Clark, V. Frouin, J. Régis, I. Bloch, D. Le Bihan, and J-F. Mangin. Regularization of diffusion-based direction maps for the tracking of brain white matter fascicles. *NeuroImage*, 12(2):184–195, 2000.
18. J. Rademacher, P. Morosan, T. Schormann, A. Schleicher, C. Werner, H-J Freund, and K. Zilles. Probabilistic mapping and volume measurement of human primary auditory cortex. *NeuroImage*, 13:669–683, 2001.
19. E.O Stejskal and T.E Tanner. Spin diffusion measurements: spin echoes in the presence of a time dependent field gradient. *The journal of Chemical Physics*, 42:288–92, 1965.
20. D. S. Tuch. *Diffusion MRI of complex tissue structure*. PhD thesis, MIT, 2002.
21. D. S. Tuch. Q-ball imaging. *Magn Reson Med*, 52(6):1358–72, 2004.
22. D. S. Tuch, T. G. Reese, M. R. Wiegell, N. Makris, J.W. Belliveau, and V. J. Wedeen. High angular resolution diffusion imaging reveals intravoxel white matter fiber heterogeneity. *Magn Reson Med*, 48(4):577–82, 2002.
23. D. S. Tuch, T. G. Reese, M. R. Wiegell, and V. J. Wedeen. Diffusion MRI of complex neural architecture. *Neuron*, 40(5):885–895, 2003.
24. D. S. Tuch, M. R Wiegell, T. G. Reese, J. W. Belliveau, and J Van Wedeen. Measuring corticocortical connectivity matrices with diffusion spectrum imaging. In *ISMRM*, page 502, 2001.
25. J. Van Wedeen, T. G. Reese, D. S. Tuch, M. R. Weigel, J.-G. Dou, R.M. Weiskoff, and D. Chessler. Mapping fiber orientation spectra in cerebral white matter with fourier-transform diffusion. In *ISMRM*, page 82, 2000.
26. David M. Weinstein, Gordon L. Kindlmann, and Eric C. Lundberg. Tensorlines: Advection-diffusion based propagation through diffusion tensor fields. In David Ebert, Markus Gross, and Bernd Hamann, editors, *IEEE Visualization '99*, pages 249–254, San Francisco, 1999.

Approximating Anatomical Brain Connectivity with Diffusion Tensor MRI Using Kernel-Based Diffusion Simulations

Jun Zhang[1], Ning Kang[1], and Stephen E. Rose[2]

[1] Laboratory for High Performance Scientific Computing and Computer Simulation,
Department of Computer Science, University of Kentucky,
Lexington, KY 40506-0046, USA
{jzhang, nkang2}@cs.uky.edu
http://www.cs.uky.edu/~jzhang
[2] Centre for Magnetic Resonance, University of Queensland,
Brisbane, QLD, 4072 Australia
stephen.rose@cmr.uq.edu.au

Abstract. We present a new technique for noninvasively tracing brain white matter fiber tracts using diffusion tensor magnetic resonance imaging (DT-MRI). This technique is based on performing diffusion simulations over a series of overlapping three dimensional diffusion kernels that cover only a small portion of the human brain volume and are geometrically centered upon selected starting voxels where a seed is placed. Synthetic and real DT-MRI data are employed to demonstrate the tracking scheme. It is shown that the synthetic tracts can be accurately replicated, while several major white matter fiber pathways in the human brain can be reproduced noninvasively as well. The primary advantages of the algorithm lie in the handling of fiber branching and crossing and its seamless adaptation to the platform established by new imaging techniques, such as high angular, q-space, or generalized diffusion tensor imaging.

1 Introduction

A number of fiber tracking algorithms have been developed since the appearance of diffusion tensor magnetic resonance imaging (DT-MRI). Typical fiber tracking schemes, including the streamline-based technique [1,2,10], reconstruct the white matter tracts by tracing down in a voxel-by-voxel manner, using an estimate of the local fiber orientation determined by the principal eigenvector in each voxel that is assumed to align with the mean fiber direction in that voxel. These techniques appear to give excellent results in many instances if the principal eigenvector field is smooth. However, it suffers from several significant limitations. The vector field is error prone in the sense that the noise of DT-MRI data will influence the direction of the principal eigenvector, yielding an accumulation of orientational errors and thus an erroneous fork of the trajectory. Another major restriction is that these techniques may also be affected by partial volume effects [19], leading to unstable tracking through the primary eigenvector field in regions of fiber crossing, branching, or merging.

Under the diffusion tensor imaging platform, a variety of methods have been proposed aiming to palliate the difficulties with more information incorporated from the diffusion tensor data. The algorithm presented in [8] uses a deflection term obtained from the diffusion tensor to improve the image noise immunity. Other schemes [7, 15] use predefined knowledge to group together neighboring voxels based on a similarity measure. Taking into account the uncertainty of fiber direction, probabilistic and statistical approaches [3, 5, 12] have been developed to mitigate the effects of fiber crossing and diverging as well as the sensitivity to noise. The level set theory is also utilized to find fiber paths connecting different brain regions [13]. Another front evolution algorithm proposed in [17] utilizes the fiber orientation function to reconstruct fiber tracts.

As the measured quantity in DT-MRI is for water diffusion, an intuitive way to gain insights from the diffusion tensor data is to treat the brain volume as a physical system and simulate a virtual water diffusion process over it, which is anisotropic and governed by the diffusion equation. The shape of the anisotropic diffusion, represented by diffusion fronts, can be used to estimate the directional arrangement of the underlying white matter fiber bundles. This reflection is based upon the principle that the faster the diffusion, the longer the distance will be traveled on average by water molecules within the same amount of diffusion time. The fiber tracts are thus expected to proceed along the direction where the diffusion is the greatest. The fiber tractography presented in this paper performs simulations of the diffusion process stemming from a series of diffusion starting voxels, within corresponding overlapped 3D diffusion kernels. The diffusion simulation initiated from a diffusion root node is utilized to construct a diffusion front in its associated kernel. The next set of diffusion root nodes, where a seed will be placed, are located on the diffusion front which is generated by the diffusion process initiated from a previous seeded root voxel. They are picked up according to the created distance map and the local orientation information involving these voxels and the diffusion root node. For the next round, each of the newly selected diffusion root voxels will be used to generate a front by starting a diffusion process in its own kernel. Given below is the detailed description of the diffusion-based fiber tractography theory and algorithm.

2 Methods

2.1 The Anisotropic Diffusion Equation

The anisotropic diffusion process simulated in this work is governed by the equation

$$\frac{\partial C}{\partial t} = \nabla \cdot (D \nabla C), \quad (1)$$

where D is the so-called diffusion coefficient, which is a second-order tensor in the presence of anisotropy, C the concentration, and t the independent time variable. The coefficient used in the anisotropic diffusion simulation is the diffusion tensor calculated from the diffusion-weighted imaging data, which is represented by a three-by-three symmetric positive definite matrix,

$$D = \begin{pmatrix} D_{xx} & D_{xy} & D_{xz} \\ D_{yx} & D_{yy} & D_{yz} \\ D_{zx} & D_{zy} & D_{zz} \end{pmatrix},$$

where the subscripts xx, xy, xz, etc., denote the values of the individual coefficients in the matrix.

2.2 Extracting Front in Diffusion Kernel

The first step to reconstruct fiber pathways starting from a pre-chosen root node s involves simulating the diffusion process in its associated diffusion kernel, initiated from a seed (an initial concentration value) in this voxel. A diffusion kernel defined here is a cube with six rectangular sides, which covers only a small bulk of the whole 3D data volume and is geometrically centered upon the diffusion starting voxel. The virtual concentration seed of water spreads from the root node through the neighboring nodes, within a limited amount of time, forming a diffusion front which is the surface of a diffusion volume containing nodes with nonzero concentration values. The expansion of the diffusion volume originated from the root node is achieved by integrating Eq. (1) over a certain amount of time, subject to the following initial condition,

$$C\Big|_{t=0} = \begin{cases} 1 \text{ at the root node,} \\ 0 \text{ elsewhere in the diffusion kernel.} \end{cases} \quad (2)$$

The boundary of the diffusion kernel is assumed to be insulated, i.e.,

$$(D\nabla C) \cdot \boldsymbol{n} = 0, \quad (3)$$

where $\boldsymbol{n}$ is the direction normal to the boundary. This condition implies that the normal part of the gradient of the concentration on the boundary is zero, in other words, nothing escapes out of the domain.

We have developed an unsteady state anisotropic diffusion solver framework, which is adapted to the cerebral circumstance and runs in both sequential and parallel computing environments. In the current paper, (1) was solved sequentially under the initial condition (2) and boundary condition (3) by resorting to the established computational framework. We used a diffusion kernel with dimensions $11 \times 11 \times 7$ and a voxel size same as in the original data volume, which proved to be very efficient in time cost and showed no impairment on tracking performance. Fig. 1 shows a concentration distribution map of the anisotropic diffusion simulated in a diffusion kernel using the human brain tensor data.

Once the time integration for solving (1) is done, a discrete approximation to the diffusion front can be calculated in terms of whether the concentration value is zero in a voxel. Thus all nodes in the diffusion kernel can be partitioned into two groups, one with zero concentration and the other with nonzero values. Since only one seed is diffused over the root node, the diffusion-swept volume, denoted

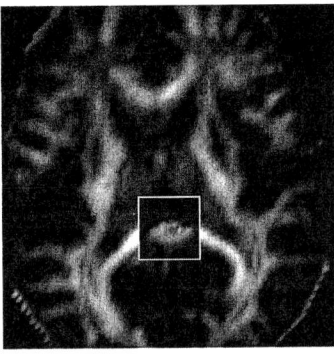

Fig. 1. The concentration distribution map of the anisotropic diffusion simulated in a diffusion kernel (bounded by the white rectangle). The profile is superimposed on a grey-scale axial map of the fractional anisotropy

as $V(r)$, is comprised of voxels with nonzero concentration values, where r is the position of the root node. For each member of $V(r)$, we consider its surrounding 26 closest neighboring nodes in a $3 \times 3 \times 3$ cube. Let i, j, k index the relative coordinates of the 26 nearest neighbors of r with $i, j, k \in \{-1, 0, 1\}$. If $F(r)$ is the set of voxels that form the diffusion front of r, then for any node $p \equiv (p_x, p_y, p_z) \in V(r)$, we define $p \in F(r)$ if $\exists\, (i, j, k)$, such that $(p_x - i, p_y - j, p_z - k) \notin V(r)$, which implies that if any of the 26 nodes is not in $V(r)$, then $p \in F(r)$.

2.3 The Criteria Set

In order to store and handle the front nodes dynamically produced in each diffusion kernel, we set up a queue Q, a first-in first-out data structure. Q is initialized to contain just the starting node s, i.e., $Q = \{s\}$, thereafter, Q always contains the set of diffusion front nodes which will be the subsequent diffusion root voxels. Once $F(r)$ is computed for the root node r, we further apply the criteria in the set C (see below) to the nodes of $F(r)$ and pick up those that meet the corresponding thresholds. We define $I(r)$ to be the set of nodes selected from $F(r)$ that satisfy the criteria in C, i.e., $I(r) = \{\, p \in F(r) \mid p$ meets all the criteria in $C\, \}$. The qualified nodes in $F(r)$ are inserted into $I(r)$ in a non-ascending order of α (see the first criteria c_1 below). $I(r)$ is then appended to the tail of the queue Q.

The set C bears a number of criteria, which determine the connection of fiber pathways. There are five criteria in C used to evaluate the information about distance and orientation between the root r and its front nodes in $F(r)$. Let $C = \bigcup_{i \in \{1, \cdots, 5\}} \{c_i\}$. The first criterion, c_1, is the threshold for distance ratio measure α, which is defined as $\alpha = d/d_{max}$, where $d = \|v(r)\|$ is the Euclidean distance in $\mathbb{R}^3$ of two points, connected by the vector $v(r)$ pointing from r to a node in $F(r)$, while d_{max} is the maximum value among the d's. We set c_2 to be a threshold of an invariant anisotropy index, the fractional anisotropy (fa) [14]. The next criterion, c_3, is a curvature constraint introduced to secure the tracks yielded moving forward consistently and smoothly without erratically turning back on themselves. A threshold is used to restrain the angle between $v(\pi(r))$ and the current direction of tracking, $v(r)$. Here, $\pi(r)$ is the predecessor voxel of r, i.e., $r \in I(\pi(r))$. $v(\pi(r))$ is an established vector pointing from $\pi(r)$ toward r, which implies the presence of a trajectory passing in this direction. c_4 is used to judge the coherence of fiber directions along the reconstructed trajectories passing through r. One threshold is set on three inner products, ϕ_1, ϕ_2, and ϕ_3, where $\phi_1 = |\hat{v}(r) \cdot e_1(r)|$, $\phi_2 = |\hat{v}(r) \cdot e_1(f)|$, and $\phi_3 = |e_1(r) \cdot e_1(f)|$. Here, $\hat{v}(r) = v(r)/\|v(r)\|$; $e_1(r)$ and $e_1(f)$ are principal eigenvectors (corresponding to the largest eigenvalue of D) at the voxel r and $f \in F(r)$, respectively. The last criterion, c_5, specifies the maximum number of voxels $I(r)$ allowed to have if there are more voxels than expected satisfying all previous four criteria, which controls the overall computational time for simulating the diffusion process in diffusion kernels.

2.4 Recovering Fiber Pathways

When Q is not empty, the current head node of Q is removed off the queue and is considered to be a new root r' where a seed is diffused. r' is positioned at the geometrical center of the diffusion kernel, which is then initialized using the global-to-local mapping to retrieve necessary information from the original data volume for carrying out the new diffusion simulation. The diffusion front $F(r')$ is calculated in the same way as that of $F(r)$. As in the derivation of $I(r)$, the set $I(r')$ is determined as well by checking each member of $F(r')$ based upon the criteria in C, then it is added to the tail of Q. We continue in this way by repeatedly taking off the head node of Q and processing it as a new root to diffuse a seed over it, until the queue becomes empty.

Aimed at recovering the fiber pathways after constructing the diffusion front in each kernel, each voxel p in the global data grid owns a memory of its predecessor voxel, $\pi(p)$, where $p \in I(\pi(p))$. Since every voxel in the grid can be taken as a diffusion root no more than once, $\pi(p)$ is the sole predecessor of p if there is one. Thus, back propagation from the voxels on diffusion fronts by following continuously the corresponding predecessor voxels leads to paths that merge to the starting voxel s. This merging corresponds to the procedure that can be viewed in the reverse direction as fiber tracts branch outwards from s. Finally, the pathways are smoothed out using B-spline least-square approximations. The diffusion equation-based fiber tractography procedure is outlined in Alg. 1.

2.5 Connectivity Index

Since the size of the set $I(r)$ can be larger than one for any root r, there may exist a bunch of reconstructed fiber pathways that branch outwards from the voxel where tracking starts. We utilize a heuristic connectivity index, ξ, as a confidence measure to estimate the odds that any generated path well approximates a true anatomical connection. For a given putative pathway, the index is defined as $\xi = \prod_{i=1}^{n}(\frac{\alpha_i + \beta_i}{2})$, where α is the distance ratio, $\beta = (\phi_1 + \phi_2 + \phi_3)/3$, and n the number of diffusion kernels used to produce the pathway. The definition of ξ may

Algorithm 1. Fiber tracking using kernel-based diffusion simulations
---
1: specify a starting node s and initialize Q such that $Q = \{s\}$
2: **while** Q is not empty **do**
3:     remove the head node r off Q and take it as a root
4:     initialize the 3D diffusion kernel that is geometrically centered on r
5:     get $V(r)$ by solving the diffusion equation (1) over the diffusion kernel with the initial and boundary conditions (2) and (3) imposed
6:     compute $F(r)$, then determine $I(r)$ and append it to the tail of Q
7: **end while**
8: record π values for voxels during front construction
9: retrieve fiber pathways using back propagation
---

be construed as evaluating how faithful the computed pathways are to follow the fastest diffusion direction, yet adjusted by coherence with local fiber orientations.

3 Data Acquisition

3.1 Synthetic Tensor Fields

In order to assess fidelity and robustness of the tracking algorithm, we generated synthetic DT-MRI data with a uniform voxel size of 1 mm^3, where the true path of a fiber tract is known. The tensor field was constituted upon an anisotropic and an isotropic tensors taken out of real DT-MRI data. The shape of the diffusion tensor in synthetic fibers was described by the anisotropic one such that $\lambda_1 : \lambda_2 : \lambda_3$ was approximately 2.5 : 1 : 1, while the isotropic one was used to forge the background of the simulated tensor field. The vector field for fiber orientations was derived by sampling discretely the trajectories which were analytically defined. To make the simulated field more realistic, an approximation to Rician noise [4] was added in the diffusion-weighted images which were calculated from the Stejskal-Tanner equation using the gradient sequence in [18] and a b-value of 1000. The noisy realization led to a signal-to-noise ratio of 10. A compact analytic solution to the Stejskal-Tanner equation [18] was employed to yield the desired noisy synthetic diffusion tensor data.

3.2 Real Diffusion Tensor Data

Real diffusion tensor imaging data were acquired from a single healthy male subject. A 1.5T Siemens Sonata scanner was used to do the measurement using an optimized diffusion tensor imaging sequence described in [6]. The imaging parameters were 43 axial slices, FOV = 230 mm, TR = 6000 ms, TE = 106 ms, 2.5 mm slice thickness with 0.25 mm gap, acquisition matrix 128 × 128, and 60 images acquired at each location consisting of 16 with low diffusion weighting ($b = 0$) and 44 diffusion images in which the encoding gradient vectors were uniformly distributed in space ($b = 1100$ s/mm^2) using the electrostatic approach described elsewhere. The reconstruction matrix was 256 × 256, resulting in an in-plane resolution of 0.898×0.898 mm^2. The diffusion tensor was calculated according to the Stejskal-Tanner equation [16]. The resolution of the original calculated tensor data volume was $256 \times 256 \times 43$ with a voxel size of $0.898 \times 0.898 \times 2.75$ mm^3 defined on a Cartesian mesh. It has been recomputed using trilinear interpolation, leading to a uniform voxel size of $(0.898$ mm$)^3$.

4 Results

Five single-turn helical fiber bundles were synthetically generated with radius being 25 mm, 20 mm, 15 mm, 10 mm, and 5 mm, respectively. For each helix, trajectories were traced from a single voxel at the lower end of the tract. In Fig. 2, the tracking result is presented, showing the simulated helical curves are closely reproduced. Fig. 3 delineates the tracing results on crossing fiber tracts synthetically constructed with two straight-line fiber bundles. It can be seen that the algorithm is capable of getting through the crossing area with planar tensors.

Fig. 4 demonstrates the capability of the tracking algorithm on real human brain DT-MRI data, showing computed tracks launched from two starting voxels that are placed in the corticospinal tract approximately at the level of the left and right pons area, respectively. It is apparent that the calculated tracks emerging from the starting points branch into different cortical motor regions. In Fig. 5, the pathways reconstructed stem from three starting voxels located approximately in the midline of the corpus callosum, which interconnect the two hemispheres. Depicted in Figure 6 is another tracking example, which shows computed fiber pathways of the cingulum. We also generated pontocerebellar tracts with two different settings of the criteria set C, as shown in Figs. 7 and 8, respectively. One can observe that with appropriate selection of the thresholds, the medial lemniscus erroneously yielded in Fig. 7 can be eliminated when segmenting the pontocerebellar tracts in the pons which bear an entangled fiber crossing structure.

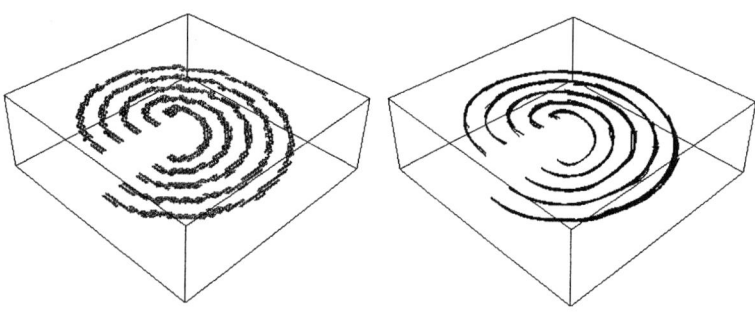

Fig. 2. Synthetic helical fiber tracts with varying radii (left, shown as diffusion tensor ellipsoid map) and the tracing results (right) yielded by the fiber tracking algorithm

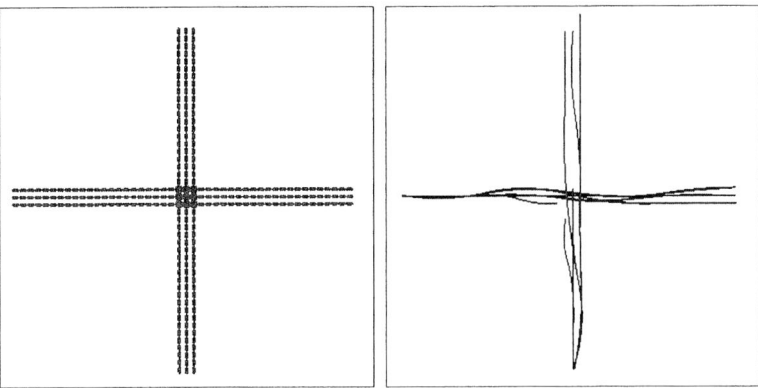

Fig. 3. Synthetic crossing fiber tracts (left, shown as diffusion tensor ellipsoid map) and the tracing results (right) yielded by the fiber tracking algorithm

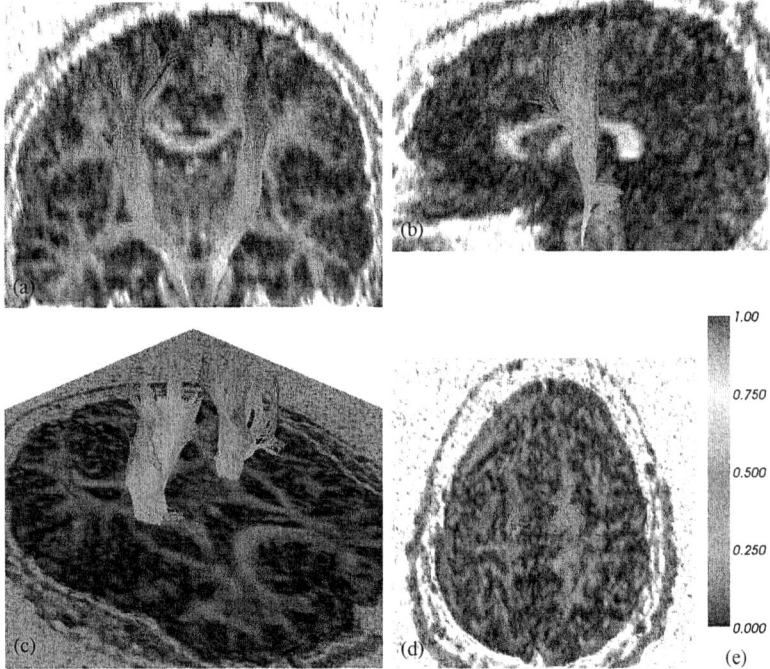

Fig. 4. Fiber pathways of corticospinal tract computed from a starting voxel positioned approximately at the level of the left pons. The colors on tracks correspond to the connectivity index as shown in (e), the color bar legend. Fibers are incorporated into grey-scale fractional anisotropy (fa) maps for anatomical reference, where bright grey-scale regions reflect high diffusion anisotropy. (a) Viewed from front, superimposed on a coronal fa map. (b) Viewed from left, overlaid on a midline sagittal fa map. (c) A 3D view, shown together with an axial fa map at the level of the internal capsule. (d) Viewed from top, overlaid on an axial fa map at the level of the motor cortex

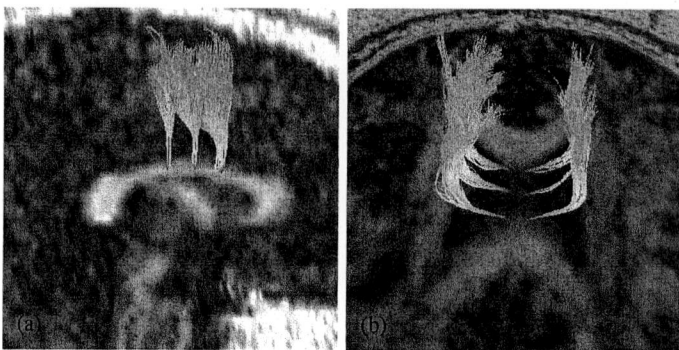

Fig. 5. Fiber pathways generated from three starting voxels located in the midline of the body of the corpus callosum. The tracks are color-scaled as in Fig. 4. (a) Viewed from right, overlaid on a sagittal fa map at the midline. (b) Viewed from top-front, overlaid on an axial fa map

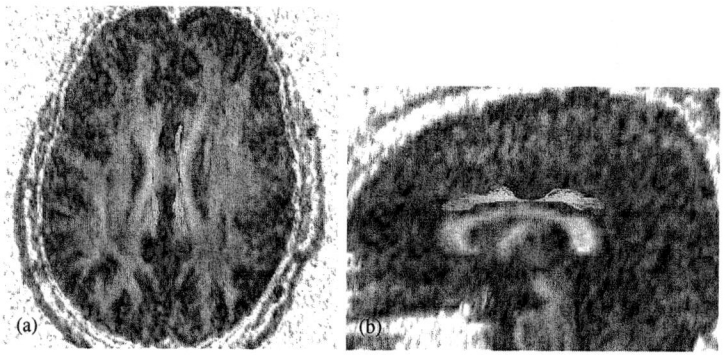

Fig. 6. Fiber pathways of cingulum calculated from two starting voxels which are slightly above the body of the corpus callosum. The tracks are color-coded as in Fig. 4. (a): Viewed from top, shown together with an axial fa map. (b): A lateral view from left, overlaid on a midline sagittal fa map

5 Discussion and Conclusion

We have conducted tracking experiments on synthetic as well as on real human brain diffusion tensor data, utilizing the tractography algorithm based on simulating the diffusion process in diffusion kernels. An accurate replication of the ideal track geometries has been presented in the tracing results on simulated tensor fields, while the estimated pathways on several major white matter tracts are faithful to the corresponding neuroanatomy performed with postmortem dissections and compatible to those obtained by using other reported tracking techniques. The demonstration shows that with the diffusion tensor imaging data, it is possible to employ the diffusion equation-based tracking technique to

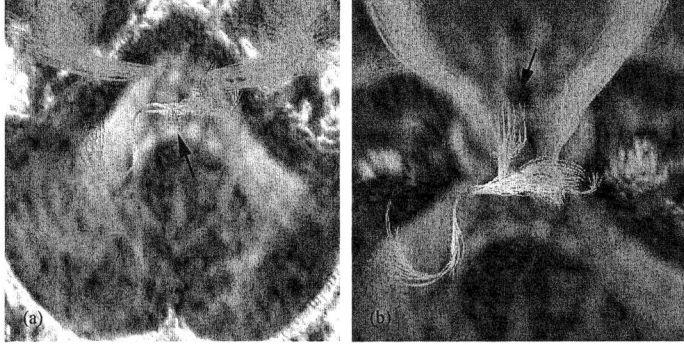

Fig. 7. Fiber pathways of pontocerebellar tract. The tracks are color-coded as in Fig. 4. Here $C = \{0.8, 0.25, 0.7, 0.65, 4\}$. The pink pathways are corticospinal tracts as in Fig. 4. The tracks pointed to by the black arrow belong to medial lemniscus. (a): Viewed from top, shown together with an axial fa map. (b): A 3D projection with an axial and a coronal fa map superimposed

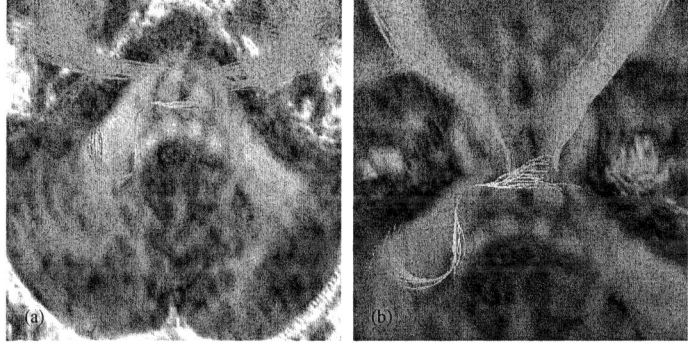

Fig. 8. Fiber pathways of pontocerebellar tract. The tracks are color-coded as in Fig. 4. Here $C = \{0.8, 0.2, 0.7, 0.7, 4\}$. The pink pathways are corticospinal tracts as in Fig. 4. (a): Viewed from top, shown together with an axial fa map. (b): A 3D projection with an axial and a coronal fa map superimposed

noninvasively follow the major white matter fiber tracts and construct maps of connectivity in the living human brain.

The demonstrations have shown that the tracking algorithm has the capability of elucidating branched fiber pathways naturally from a single starting voxel, without using multiple interpolated starting points within the starting voxel or specifying regions of interest defined from anatomical landmarks. It relies on simulating the diffusion process to construct diffusion front in kernels, which is truly a physical phenomenon and the magnitude of the tensor contributes to fiber tracking, instead of fully relying on the orientation of the tensor in each voxel. So the primary advantage of the algorithm is its ability to accommodate branching fibers with the connectivity index assigned representing uncertainty.

Another desirable feature is its capability to behave correctly in crossing regions with reduced tensor information. It also reveals that the properties of the generated tracts are dependent on the threshold values in the criterion set C, which bears flexibility to improve the tracking reliability and robustness to noise.

In fact, diffusion tensor imaging (DTI), as used by our diffusion equation-based tracking method, is unable to truly resolve the crossing of multiple axon directions within a single voxel. However, it has been suggested to get around the inadequacy by using newly developed imaging approaches, like high angular resolution diffusion imaging (HARDI), q-space imaging (QSI), or generalized diffusion tensor imaging (GDTI). An outstanding feature of fiber reconstruction using diffusion simulations is that it can be seamlessly adapted to the platform established by the new imaging techniques. Studies have shown that the generalized diffusion tensor model is able to not only accommodate HARDI and GDTI methods but QSI as well, due to the relationships among DTI, HARDI, GDTI, and QSI [9, 11]. This makes it possible for the diffusion simulation based tractography to become independent of the imaging techniques used, while the fiber tracking will require a more sophisticated diffusion simulation, which is governed by a generalized diffusion equation associated with generalized diffusion tensors, according to a generalization of Fick's second law.

References

1. Basser, P.J., Pajevic, S., Pierpaoli, C., Duda, J., Aldroubi, A.: In vivo fiber tractography using DT-MRI data. Magn. Reson. Med. **44** (2000) 625-632
2. Conturo, T.E., Lori, N.F., Cull, T.S., Akbudak, E., Snyder, A.Z., Shimony, J.S., McKinstry, Burton, H., Raichle, M.E.: Tracking neuronal fiber pathways in the living human brain. Proc. Natl. Acad. Sci. USA **96** (1999) 10422-10427
3. Gössl, C., Fahrmeir, L., Pütz, B., Auer, L.M., Auer, D.P.: Fiber tracking from DTI using linear state space models: detectability of the pyramidal tract. NeuroImage **16** (2002) 378-388
4. Gudbjartsson, H., Patz, S.: The Rician distribution of noisy MRI data. Magn. Reson. Med. **34** (1995) 910-914
5. Hagmann, P., Thiran, J.P., Jonasson, L., Vandergheynst, P., Clarke, S., Maeder, P., Meuli, R.: DTI mapping of human brain connectivity: statistical fibre tracking and virtual dissection. NeuroImage **19** (2003) 545-554
6. Jones, D.K., Horsefield, M.A., Simmons, A.: Optimal strategies for measuring diffusion in anisotropic systems by magnetic resonance imaging. Magn. Reson. Med. **42** (1999) 515-525
7. Jones, D.K., Simmons, A., Williams, S.C.R., Horsfield, M.A.: Non-invasive assessment of axonal fiber connectivity in the human brain via diffusion tensor MRI. Magn. Reson. Med. **42** (1999) 37-41
8. Lazar, M., Weinstein, D.M., Tsuruda, J.S., Hasan, K.M., Arfanakis, K., Meyerand, M.E., Badie, B., Rowley, H.A., Haughton, V., Field, A., Alexander, A.L.: White matter tractography using diffusion tensor deflection. Human Brain Mapping **18** (2003) 306-321
9. Liu, C., Bammer, R., Acar, B., Moseley, M.E.: Characterizing non-Gaussian diffusion by using generalized diffusion tensors. Magn. Reson. Med. **51** (2004) 924-937

10. Mori, S., Crain, B., Chacko, V.P., van Zijl, P.C.M.: Three dimensional tracking of axonal projections in the brain by magnetic resonance imaging. Ann. of Neurol. **45** (1999) 265-269
11. Özarslan, E., Mareci, T.H.: Generalized diffusion tensor imaging and analytical relationships between diffusion tensor imaging and high angular resolution diffusion imaging. Magn. Reson. Med. **50** (2003) 955-965
12. Parker, G.J.M., Alexander, D.C.: Probabilistic Monte Carlo based mapping of cerebral connections utilising whole-brain crossing fibre information. LNCS 2737 (2003) 684-695
13. Parker, G.J.M., Wheeler-Kingshott, C.A.M., Barker, G.J.: Estimating distributed anatomical connectivity using fast marching methods and diffusion tensor imaging. IEEE Trans. Med. Imag. **21** (2002) 505-512
14. Pierpaoli, C., Basser, P.J.: Toward a quantitative assessment of diffusion anisotropy. Magn. Reson. Med. **36** (1996) 893-906
15. Poupon, C., Clark, C.A., Frouin, V., Regis, J., Bloch, I., Le Bihan, D., Mangin, J.: Regularization of diffusion-based direction maps for the tracking of brain white matter fascicles. NeuroImage **12** (2000) 184-95
16. Stejskal, E.O., Tanner, J.E.: Spin diffusion measurements: spin echoes in the presence of a time-dependent field gradient. J. Chem. Phys. **42** (1965) 288-292
17. Tournier, J.-D., Calamante, F., Gadian, D.G., Connelly, A.: Diffusion-weighted magnetic resonance imaging fibre tracking using a front evolution algorithm. NeuroImage **20** (2003) 276-288
18. Westin, C.-F., Maier, S.E., Mamata, H., Nabavi, A., Jolesz, F.A., Kikinis, R.: Processing and visualization for diffusion tensor MRI. Med. Imag. Anal. **6** (2002) 93-108
19. Wiegell, M.R., Larsson, H.B., Wedeen, V.J.: Fiber crossing in human brain depicted with diffusion tensor MR imaging. Radiology **217** (2000) 897-903

Maximum Entropy Spherical Deconvolution for Diffusion MRI

Daniel C. Alexander

Department of Computer Science,
University College London, Gower Street, London, WC1E 6BT, UK
D.Alexander@cs.ucl.ac.uk

Abstract. This paper proposes a maximum entropy method for spherical deconvolution. Spherical deconvolution arises in various inverse problems. This paper uses the method to reconstruct the distribution of microstructural fibre orientations from diffusion MRI measurements. Analysis shows that the PASMRI algorithm, one of the most accurate diffusion MRI reconstruction algorithms in the literature, is a special case of the maximum entropy spherical deconvolution. Experiments compare the new method to linear spherical deconvolution, used previously in diffusion MRI, and to the PASMRI algorithm. The new method compares favourably both in simulation and on standard brain-scan data.

1 Introduction

Diffusion MRI has exploded over the last decade, since the introduction of diffusion-tensor MRI (DT-MRI) by Basser et al [1]. Diffusion MRI measures the displacement of particles, usually water molecules, within a material over a fixed time interval. The material microstructure controls the scatter pattern of particles within and, conversely, measurements of the particle displacement reveal information about the microstructure. The current standard diffusion MRI technique is DT-MRI, which provides two unique insights into material microstructure. First, DT-MRI provides quantitative measurements of the anisotropy of particle displacements and, second, it provides an estimate of the dominant orientation of particle displacements. In fibrous material, such as white matter in the brain, the dominant orientations of particle displacements are similar to the dominant fibre directions. Diffusion MRI is particularly useful for brain imaging, because it reveals the orientations of white-matter fibres in each voxel of an image volume. Tractography algorithms use these fibre-orientation estimates to determine the connectivity of the whole brain.

A well-documented problem with DT-MRI is that it fails at fibre crossings. Recent trends in the field are towards a new generation of reconstruction algorithm that can resolve the orientations of multiple fibre populations within each voxel, see [2] for a review. One such technique [3, 4] views the diffusion MRI signal as the convolution of the response from a single fibre with specific orientation with the distribution of fibre orientations. A deconvolution of the signal by the single-fibre response yields the fibre-orientation distribution (FOD). The implementations of this deconvolution technique in [3,4] use a linear basis for spherical functions to represent the FOD. Although the literature shows nice results from the technique in certain regions of high-quality data, the methods are reknowned for instability and, in performance comparisons such as [5], they perform worse than rival methods such as PASMRI [6] and q-ball imaging [7].

Maximum entropy methods [8] have proved useful in a variety of reconstruction and inverse problems. In particular, the methods have proved effective for deconvolution. This paper constructs a maximum-entropy formulation of the spherical deconvolution problem and demonstrates its application to reconstruction of the FOD from diffusion MRI measurements. Experiments show that the maximum-entropy spherical-deconvolution (MESD) improves on a linear implementation and produces results comparable to the PASMRI algorithm on data from a standard diffusion MRI acquisition sequence. Further analysis shows that the PASMRI algorithm is a special case of the MESD method. Performance of the method depends on the choice of response function (deconvolution kernel). Here we use only a simple kernel to show efficacy of the approach. We can expect further improvements in the method through better choices of deconvolution kernel. Although particularly useful for diffusion MRI, the method extends naturally to any spherical deconvolution problem.

Section 2 gives some background on the diffusion MRI reconstruction problem and existing techniques. Section 3 outlines the MESD method and compares it analytically to other reconstruction techniques used in diffusion MRI. Section 4 shows results from using the new methods on diffusion MRI data acquired from a standard brain imaging sequence and compares them with results from linear spherical deconvolution (SD) and PASMRI on the same data. Simulation experiments compare the methods further. Finally, section 5 concludes and outlines areas for further work.

2 Background

Diffusion-tensor MRI models the particle displacements in each image voxel with a zero-mean Gaussian distribution with covariance $2tD$, where t is the diffusion time and D is the diffusion tensor. The diffusion MRI measurement is approximately proportional to the Fourier transform of the particle-displacement density function p:

$$A(\mathbf{q}) = (A^\star(\mathbf{0}))^{-1} A^\star(\mathbf{q}) = \int_{\mathbb{R}^3} p(\mathbf{x}) \cos(\mathbf{q} \cdot \mathbf{x}) d\mathbf{x}, \qquad (1)$$

where $A^\star(\mathbf{q})$ is the MR signal with wavenumber $\mathbf{q}$, which depends on the strength and direction of the magnetic gradient pulses in the diffusion MR imaging sequence [9]. The MRI measurements also vary spatially, although we omit the spatial dependence from the notation for simplicity. Substituting the Gaussian model for p in (1) and taking logs shows that each measurement provides a linear constraint on the six elements of the diffusion tensor, D. We can estimate

D from seven or more measurements with independent **q**. Since the contours of the Gaussian model are ellipsoidal, DT-MRI can only reveal a single dominant fibre orientation in each voxel. At fibre crossings, however, p has multiple peaks at fixed radii and the Gaussian model is poor. We can also fit other models for p using (1), such as mixtures of Gaussians, e.g. [10, 11], which can reveal the directions of multiple fibre orientations.

Although DT-MRI extends to handle multiple fibre populations through the use of mixture models, fitting becomes non-linear with mixtures of two or more Gaussians and is often unstable. Furthermore, model fitting procedures require a choice of the number of fibres in each voxel prior to fitting. A new generation of *multiple-fibre reconstruction* techniques [2, 12], including PASMRI [6], **q**-ball imaging [7] and spherical-deconvolution methods [3, 4] all compute objects that provide the number of fibres, together with an orientation estimate for each, without requiring prior specification of the number of fibres present.

Spherical-deconvolution methods assume that the diffusion MRI signal in each voxel is the convolution of the FOD (fibre-orientation distribution) f, which is a real-valued function of the unit sphere, with the signal $R(\cdot; \hat{\mathbf{x}})$ from a single fibre with orientation $\hat{\mathbf{x}}$:

$$A(\mathbf{q}) = \int R(\mathbf{q}; \hat{\mathbf{x}}) f(\hat{\mathbf{x}}) d\hat{\mathbf{x}}, \qquad (2)$$

where the integration is over the unit sphere in three-dimensional space. Note that (2) assumes that $R(\cdot; \hat{\mathbf{x}})$ has rotational symmetry about $\hat{\mathbf{x}}$ and does not vary spatially. The methods aim to deconvolve the signal, using a model for $R(\cdot; \hat{\mathbf{x}})$, to obtain f. The function f can have multiple pairs of equal and opposite peaks and each pair provides a separate fibre-orientation estimate.

To implement the method, the standard approach represents f using a linear basis:

$$f(\hat{\mathbf{x}}) = \sum_{k=1}^{K} \beta_k \theta_k(\hat{\mathbf{x}}). \qquad (3)$$

We substitute for f in (2) and reverse the order of the integral and sum to obtain

$$A(\mathbf{q}) = \sum_{k=1}^{K} \left(\beta_k \int R(\mathbf{q}; \hat{\mathbf{x}}) \theta_k(\hat{\mathbf{x}}) d\hat{\mathbf{x}} \right). \qquad (4)$$

Diffusion MRI sequences usually acquire a set of measurements with wavenumbers $\mathbf{q}_i$, $i = 1, \cdots, N$, together with some number of measurements with $\mathbf{q} = \mathbf{0}$ for normalization. The set of $\mathbf{q}_i$ is the same in each voxel. For a set of measurements with wavenumbers $\mathbf{q}_i$, $i = 1, \cdots, N$, we can summarize the set of equations from (4) as $\mathbf{A} = \mathbf{XB}$, where $\mathbf{A} = (A(\mathbf{q}_1), \cdots, A(\mathbf{q}_N))^T$ is the vector of normalized measurements, $\mathbf{B} = (\beta_1, \cdots, \beta_K)^T$ is the vector of basis-function weights and $\mathbf{X}$ is the matrix with ik-th entry

$$X_{ik} = \int R(\mathbf{q}_i; \hat{\mathbf{x}}) \theta_k(\hat{\mathbf{x}}) d\hat{\mathbf{x}}.$$

We solve the matrix equation to obtain the set of basis-function weights that define f via a linear transformation of the measurements: $\mathbf{B} = \mathbf{X}'\mathbf{A}$, where $\mathbf{X}' = (\mathbf{X}^T\mathbf{X})^{-1}\mathbf{X}^T$ is the pseudoinverse of $\mathbf{X}$. Since the set of $\mathbf{q}_i$ is identical in each voxel, we need to compute $\mathbf{X}'$ only once. The computational burden of the method is therefore light (a single matrix multiplication in each voxel) and comparable to that of diffusion-tensor MRI.

Following the general method outlined in [13], references [3, 4] use the spherical harmonics as the basis for f. References [3, 11] use Gaussian models of the particle displacement within single fibres to obtain R. Tournier et al [4] derive R directly from the data by taking an average signal from the most anisotropic voxels.

The PASMRI algorithm [6] aims to compute a feature of p called the persistent angular structure (PAS) by assuming independence of the angular and radial structure of p, so that $p(\mathbf{x}) = g(|\mathbf{x}|)\hat{p}(\hat{\mathbf{x}})$, where g is a model for the radial structure of p and $\hat{p}$ is the PAS. Jansons and Alexander [6] take $g(|\mathbf{x}|) = \delta(|\mathbf{x}|-r)$ for some scalar r, so that (1) becomes

$$A(\mathbf{q}_i) = r^{-2} \int \hat{p}(\hat{\mathbf{x}}) \cos(r\mathbf{q}_i \cdot \hat{\mathbf{x}}) d\hat{\mathbf{x}}. \tag{5}$$

Jansons and Alexander derive a maximum-entropy parametrization of $\hat{p}$:

$$\hat{p}(\hat{\mathbf{x}}) = \exp\left(\lambda_0 + \sum_{j=1}^{N} \lambda_j \cos(r\mathbf{q}_j \cdot \hat{\mathbf{x}})\right), \tag{6}$$

which they fit to the measurements in each voxel using a Levenberg–Marquardt algorithm. The recovered PAS reflects the angular structure of p that persists over a wide range of radii. Like the FOD, the PAS is a real-valued function of the sphere with peaks that provide fibre-orientation estimates.

Another class of method, including q-ball imaging [7], diffusion spectrum imaging [14], and the methods in [15, 16], all compute or estimate the *orientation distribution function* (ODF) ϕ, which is the projection of p onto the unit sphere:

$$\phi(\hat{\mathbf{x}}) = \int_0^\infty p(\alpha\hat{\mathbf{x}}) d\alpha. \tag{7}$$

The ODF is also a real-valued function of the sphere with peaks that provide fibre-orientation estimates. If we represent ϕ using a linear basis, recovery of the ODF in each voxel comes from multiplication of the measurements by the same matrix in each voxel so computation time is similar to linear SD, see [7, 12].

3 Maximum Entropy Spherical Deconvolution

This section outlines the new MESD method. Since the literature already contains a variety of multiple-fibre reconstruction algroithms, we begin with some motivation for the development of the new technique.

The literature contains little evaluation and comparison of multiple-fibre reconstructions, but early indications [5, 12] suggest that the PASMRI algorithm recovers fibre directions more accurately and consistently than spherical deconvolution and the q-ball algorithm. The PASMRI algorithm has two fundamental differences to the other methods that may account for differences in performance: it computes a different object, the PAS, and it uses a non-linear basis to represent that object. Comparison of Eq. (2) with Eq. (5) reveals that the PASMRI inversion is a deconvolution with $R(\mathbf{q}; \hat{\mathbf{x}}) = r^{-2} \cos(r\mathbf{q} \cdot \hat{\mathbf{x}})$. If we replace the maximum-entropy representation of the PAS in Eq. (6) with a linear combination of basis functions, as used for f in Eq. (3), the method reduces to a single matrix multiplication in each voxel like the linear SD method. However, experiments with this linearized version of PASMRI (not shown) reveal that performance is signficantly worse than the non-linear implementation in [6]. This suggests that the power of the method lies in the non-linear maximum-entropy representation of the PAS. In fibrous tissue, the PAS function often has very sharp peaks, which linear bases cannot capture accurately but the product of exponential waves in Eq. (6) is better equipt to represent.

Spherical-deconvolution methods have some advantages over the PASMRI method and methods that estimate the ODF. First, the output of the spherical deconvolution, the FOD, is a readily understandable object with well-defined meaning. The PAS is more arcane and it is less obvious why its peaks should correspond to fibre orientations. Second, spherical deconvolution does not rely on the Fourier relationship between the MRI measurements and p, which is only approximate. Third, the peaks of the FOD, at least in theory using an ideal deconvolution kernel, correspond genuinely to fibre orientations rather than the directions of ridges in p. The peaks of p at a fixed radius may not correspond exactly to fibre directions particularly if the fibre orientations are not orthogonal. If p is a mixture of Gaussians, for example, the peaks at fixed radii (or ridge directions) are more closely aligned than the peaks of the individual Gaussian components when the peaks are not orthogonal. The effect is similar in mixtures of Gaussians in one dimension where the peaks of the mixture are closer than those of the mixed components.

The observation that the linear representation of the PAS produces worse performance than the non-linear representation suggests that the poor performance of spherical-deconvolution methods in diffusion MRI may arise from the linear basis representation of the FOD. Like the PAS, we may expect the FOD to have sharp peaks in fibrous tissue regions where the distribution of fibre directions is highly concentrated. This section derives an alternative non-linear representation for the FOD using a maximum-entropy argument similar to that used by Jansons and Alexander [6] to derive the PAS representation in Eq. (6). We aim to determine a representation for f that imposes the minimum information on the reconstructed f. The information content of the FOD, f, is

$$I[f] = \int f(\hat{\mathbf{x}}) \log f(\hat{\mathbf{x}}) \, d\hat{\mathbf{x}}. \tag{8}$$

We shall minimize the information content of f subject to the constraints from the measurements and that f is a probability density function and so integrates to one:

$$\int f(\hat{\mathbf{x}})\mathrm{d}\hat{\mathbf{x}} = 1. \tag{9}$$

Each measurement provides a constraint on f given by Eq. (2). We incorporate each constraint into the expression for the information content of f using the method of Lagrange multipliers to yield

$$I[f] = \int \left(f(\hat{\mathbf{x}}) \log f(\hat{\mathbf{x}}) - f(\hat{\mathbf{x}}) \sum_{i=1}^{N} (\lambda_i R(\mathbf{q}_i; \hat{\mathbf{x}})) - f(\hat{\mathbf{x}})\mu \right) \mathrm{d}\hat{\mathbf{x}}, \tag{10}$$

where $\mathbf{q}_i$, $i = 1, \cdots, N$, are the wavenumbers of the MRI measurements, the λ_i are Lagrange multipliers for the constraints from the data and the Lagrange multiplier μ controls the normalization of f. Taking a variational derivative $\delta I[f]$ and solving $\delta I[f] = 0$, we find that the information content, $I[f]$, is minimum when

$$f(\hat{\mathbf{x}}) = \exp\left(\lambda_0 + \sum_{i=1}^{N} \lambda_i R(\mathbf{q}_i; \hat{\mathbf{x}})\right), \tag{11}$$

where $\lambda_0 = \mu - 1$.

We need to solve

$$\int f(\hat{\mathbf{x}}) R(\mathbf{q}_i; \hat{\mathbf{x}}) \mathrm{d}\hat{\mathbf{x}} = A(\mathbf{q}_i) \tag{12}$$

for the λ_i. We implement the method following Jansons and Alexander's implementation of the PASMRI algorithm in [6]. We use a Levenburg–Marquardt algorithm to search for a set of λ_i that minimize

$$\sum_{i=1}^{N} \left(A(\mathbf{q}_i) - \int f(\hat{\mathbf{x}}) R(\mathbf{q}_i; \hat{\mathbf{x}}) \mathrm{d}\hat{\mathbf{x}} \right)^2. \tag{13}$$

In all the experiments in the next section we use the simple deconvolution kernel

$$R(\mathbf{q}; \hat{\mathbf{x}}) = \exp\left(-t|\mathbf{q}|^2 d^{-1}(\hat{\mathbf{x}} \cdot \hat{\mathbf{q}})^2\right), \tag{14}$$

following [11], where d is the diffusivity in the fibre direction; we take $t|\mathbf{q}|^2 d^{-1} = 1$, since the $|\mathbf{q}_i|$ are all equal in the test data we use. The kernel in Eq. (14) is the signal we expect from a material in which particles displace only in direction $\hat{\mathbf{x}}$.

4 Experiments and Results

We begin by comparing the output of the MESD algorithm with linear SD and the PASMRI algorithm. Figure 1(a) shows the maximum entropy FOD in each voxel of the image region spanning the two highlighted regions of interest on the

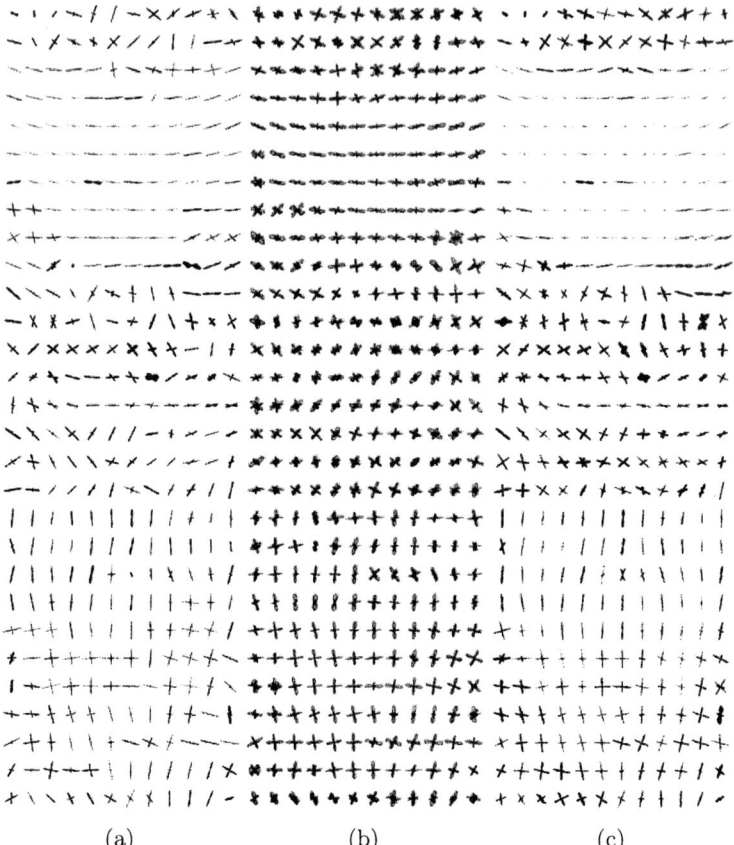

Fig. 1. Reconstructions over the region spanning the two highlighted regions in figure 2 for (a) MESD and (b) linear SD and (c) PASMRI

coronal slice in figure 2. Figure 1(b) shows the linear FOD over the same region and figure 1(c) shows the PAS. The diffusion MRI data comes from a standard acquisition sequence with $N = 54$, $t = 0.04$ s, $|\mathbf{q}_i| = 2.00 \times 10^5$ m^{-1}, $i = 1, \cdots, N$, and the $\hat{\mathbf{q}}_i$ minimize the electrostatic energy with equal charges at each $\hat{\mathbf{q}}_i$ and $-\hat{\mathbf{q}}_i$. The signal to noise ratio with $|\mathbf{q}| = \mathbf{0}$ in white matter is approximately 16, which is lower than for the test data used to introduce many multiple-fibre reconstructions in the literature but is typical for whole-brain diffusion MRI acquisitions.

In the linear SD, we use a radial-basis-function representation with

$$\theta_k(\hat{\mathbf{x}}) = \exp(-(\cos^{-1}(|\hat{\mathbf{x}} \cdot \hat{\mathbf{y}}_k|))^2/\sigma^2), \tag{15}$$

where σ is a constant scaling parameter and the $\hat{\mathbf{y}}_k$, $k = 1, \cdots, K$, are unit vectors evenly distributed on the unit sphere. The method is simpler to control using radial basis functions than spherical harmonics. We take $K = 120$ and $\sigma = 20.0$.

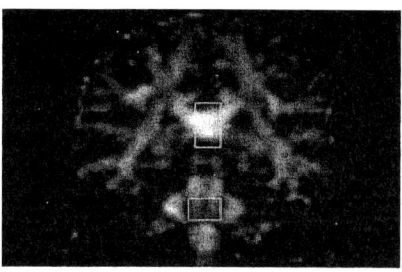

Fig. 2. Fractional anisotropy over a coronal slice of the brain data set with two highlighted regions of interest: the corpus callosum (top) and the fibre crossing at the pons (bottom)

The value of σ controls the smoothness of the output of the linear SD method. With $\sigma > 50$, the basis functions are too broad for the linear combination to support two orthogonal peaks reliably. With $\sigma < 10$ spurious peaks dominate the real peaks both in simulation and on the brain data and the method gives no sensible output. In the PASMRI algorithm, we set $r = 1.4$ following the suggestion in [6].

The image region in figure 1 contains part of the corpus callosum (top), where we expect a single fibre with left-right orientation, and part of the pons, where we expect two approximately orthogonal fibres with left-right and superior-inferior orientations. All three methods produce peaks in the expected fibre directions in both regions. In the corpus callosum, the linear SD method consistently produces false-positive fibre directions approximately orthogonal to the correct fibre direction; PASMRI and MESD rarely generate false positives in the corpus callosum. In the pons, PASMRI and linear SD show two peaks more consistently than MESD. However, linear SD produces extra peaks pointing in the posterior-anterior direction (out of the page) in a significant proportion of voxels in the pons region; PASMRI produces similar false positives to a lesser extent; MESD rarely shows these false positives.

Further experiments compare the methods in simulation. We synthesize measurements from the imaging sequence for the brain data using a simple test function for p, which models the particle displacement in tissue containing two distinct fibre orientations. We set

$$p(\mathbf{x}) = aG(\mathbf{x}; \mathcal{D}_1, t) + (1-a)G(\mathbf{x}; \mathcal{D}_2, t) \qquad (16)$$

where $a \in [0,1]$ is the mixing parameter, $G(\cdot; \mathcal{D}, t)$ is a zero-mean trivariate Gaussian function with covariance matrix $2t\mathcal{D}$ and the diffusion tensors are

$$\mathcal{D}_1 = \mathrm{diag}(\lambda_1, \lambda_2, \lambda_2) \text{ and} \qquad (17)$$
$$\mathcal{D}_2 = \mathbf{R}^T(\phi)\mathrm{diag}(\lambda_2, \lambda_1, \lambda_2)\mathbf{R}(\phi), \qquad (18)$$

where $\mathbf{R}(\phi)$ is a rotation about the z-axis through angle ϕ and $\mathrm{Tr}(\mathcal{D}_i) = \lambda_1 + 2\lambda_2 = 2.1 \times 10^{-9}\,\mathrm{m^2 s^{-1}}$ (typical for brain tissue).

Table 1. Summary of simulation results for the MESD, PASMRI and linear SD. The angle $\alpha = \cos^{-1}(\mu_1 \cdot \mathbf{n})$ is the bias in recovered directions. Each set of trials produces two direction concentrations, $\gamma(\kappa_1)$, and two bias angles, one from each component. The table shows the lowest diresction concentration and the highest bias angle of each pair

$\lambda_1/10^{-12}$ $m^2 s^{-1}$	a	ϕ deg	MESD C	MESD $\gamma(\kappa_1)$	MESD α/deg	PAS C	PAS $\gamma(\kappa_1)$	PAS α/deg	Lin. SD C	Lin. SD $\gamma(\kappa_1)$	Lin. SD α/deg
100	0.5	0	1.000	5.9	0.2	1.000	5.6	0.2	0.012	3.9	1.7
100	0.5	22.5	0.980	5.5	9.2	0.758	2.5	10.4	0.008	4.0	7.9
100	0.6	0	1.000	5.6	0.2	1.000	5.3	0.2	0.024	3.7	1.9
100	0.6	22.5	0.964	5.2	12.6	0.832	3.4	9.0	0.020	3.6	11.5
300	0.5	0	0.996	4.7	0.4	0.996	4.3	0.4	0.063	3.0	3.2
300	0.5	22.5	0.773	4.0	10.0	0.949	3.7	1.9	0.020	2.5	10.0
300	0.6	0	0.996	4.4	0.4	1.000	4.2	0.5	0.043	2.7	4.1
300	0.6	22.5	0.727	3.8	13.2	0.906	3.7	3.6	0.020	2.3	13.4
500	0.5	0	0.504	2.3	3.1	0.270	2.1	2.2	0.012	1.7	8.6
500	0.5	22.5	0.176	2.0	15.1	0.211	1.8	9.8	0.008	1.5	17.4
500	0.6	0	0.492	2.3	2.5	0.273	2.0	2.1	0.012	1.6	9.0
500	0.6	22.5	0.156	1.9	15.2	0.180	1.6	12.8	0.012	1.5	21.0

For various settings of a, ϕ and λ_1, we synthesize 256 voxels of data with independent noise and estimate the fibre orientations using MESD, linear spherical deconvolution and PASMRI. We use the peak-finding algorithm in [6] to determine the fibre directions from each method in each trial. In each set of trials, we compute the following performance statistics:

- The consistency fraction C, which is the fraction of trials in which the reconstruction algorithm finds the right number of fibres (two) to within a small angular tolerance of the principal directions of $\mathcal{D}_1$ and $\mathcal{D}_2$. We set the tolerance to $\cos^{-1} 0.95$.
- The direction concentration of each population of recovered fibre directions. The concentration of a collection of directions $\hat{\mathbf{x}}_i$, $i = 1, ..., n$, is $\gamma(\kappa_1) = -\log(1-\kappa_1)$, where κ_1 is the largest eigenvalue of the mean dyadic tensor $\mathbf{Y} = n^{-1} \sum_{j=1}^{n} \hat{\mathbf{x}}_i \hat{\mathbf{x}}_i^T$. To group corresponding peak directions from separate trials, we cluster the directions to maximize the concentration of each population.
- The direction bias of each recovered population. The bias is $\mu_1 \cdot \mathbf{n}$, where μ_1 is the principal eigenvector of $\mathbf{Y}$ and $\mathbf{n}$ is the closest of the principal directions of $\mathcal{D}_1$ and $\mathcal{D}_2$.

Table 1 shows the performance statistics for each algorithm with each combination of settings in the test function. Some observations from table 1 are:

- The consistency fraction is much greater for PASMRI and MESD than for linear SD. The linear method produces false positives in most trials, although it rarely produces false negatives. Reducing σ can reduce the false positive rate slightly, but the effect is not significant until a sudden change when

the basis functions become too smooth to support two peaks and the false negative count increases sharply.
- The peak directions are more consistent using MESD than linear SD, since the direction concentrations are higher for MESD than linear SD.
- The bias in the mean reconstructed directions is lower for MESD than linear SD apart from when the test function is very anisotropic (low λ_1). At very high anisotropy, some of the measurements hit the noise floor, which corrupts the reconstruction.
- The PASMRI method shows better results than both spherical deconvolutions. Both deconvolution methods show greater bias in the mean reconstructed directions than PASMRI, particular when the test-function principal directions are non-orthogonal. The consistency fraction is generally slightly greater for PASMRI than for MESD. Further examination of the output reveals that PASMRI tends to have a greater false-positive rate than MESD, which has greater false-negative rate. However, we note that the false-positive false-negative trade off is easy to control in PASMRI by varying the parameter r.

In fact, we might expect that the PASMRI algorithm performs better in this simulation. To generate the synthetic data we use the Fourier model in Eq. (1), which is also the basis of the PASMRI algorithm. Since both deconvolution algorithms show similar trends in the bias of the reconstructed directions, it seems likely that the bias is a product of the choice of deconvolution kernel. The deconvolution kernel we use in the deconvolution methods does not match the components of the test function. We might expect that the spherical-deconvolution methods are more robust to the departures from the Fourier model in the measurement process from which the brain data comes; see [9, 17] for some discussion of the nature of the departures from the Fourier model in diffusion MRI data.

5 Conclusions

This paper introduces a maximum-entropy spherical-deconvolution method and demonstrates efficacy within the diffusion MRI application. The method improves on a linear implementation of the spherical deconvolution method. With the chosen deconvolution kernel, the method does not quite match the performance of PASMRI in simulation, but the spherical deconvolution method, which generalizes the PASMRI method, potentially has theoretic advantages, which warrant its use and further investigation. Many avenues of future work may extend and improve the basic MESD implementation here. Better choices of deconvolution kernel surely exist. In [4], Tournier et al estimate R directly from the input data. In more recent work [18], they improve the robustness to noise of linear SD by choosing a deconvolution kernel that minimizes the entropy of the output FOD. The MESD method is simple to adapt to use the kernels in [4, 18] or any other kernel.

A disadvantage of MESD is that computation time is much greater than for linear SD and is similar to that of the PASMRI algorithm. The numerical integration in (12) dominates the computation time. The numerical integration scheme is naive, however, and approximates the integral with a summation over points evenly distributed over the sphere. A better approach would sample the integrand more densely around its sharp peaks and avoid unnecessary evaluations where the integrand is near zero.

Other possible areas for improvement are the optimization algorithms that fit the non-linear FOD to the measurements. We use a single starting point for the optimization and do not guarantee to find the global minimum of the least-squares objective function. Other choices for the objective function itself may also improve results. For example, we may extend the maximum-entropy analogy by maximizing the entropy of the FOD subject to the data constraints rather than minimizing the least-squares fit to the data. Other regularization techniques may also improve stability.

Acknowledgements

The author thanks Claudia Wheeler-Kingshott at the Institute of Neurology, UCL, for providing the human brain data used in this work.

References

1. Basser P J, Matiello J and Le Bihan D 1994 MR diffusion tensor spectroscopy and imaging *Biophysical Journal* **66** 259–67
2. Alexander D C 2005 An introduction to computational diffusion MRI: the diffusion tensor and beyond *Visualization and Image Processing of Tensor Fields* ed Weichert J and Hagen H (Springer)
3. Anderson A and Ding Z 2002 Sub-voxel measurement of fiber orientation using high angular resolution diffusion tensor imaging *Proc. 10th Annual Meeting of the ISMRM (Honolulu)* (Berkeley, USA: ISMRM) 440
4. Tournier J-D, Calamante F, Gadian D G and Connelly A 2004 Direct estimation of the fiber orientation density function from diffusion-weighted MRI data using spherical deconvolution *NeuroImage* **23** 1176–1185
5. Alexander D C 2005 Monte-Carlo studies of multiple-fibre reconstructions for diffusion MRI *Proc. 13th Annual Meeting of the ISMRM (Miami)* (Berkeley, USA: ISMRM) Accepted
6. Jansons K M and Alexander D C 2003 Persistent Angular Structure: new insights from diffusion MRI data *Inverse Problems* **19** 1031–1046
7. Tuch D S 2004 Q-ball imaging *Magnetic Resonance in Medicine* **52** 1358–1372
8. Skilling J and Gull S F 1985 Algorithms and applications *Maximum Entropy and Bayesian methods in Inverse Problems* ed Smith C R and Grandy W T (Dordrecht: Reidel publishing company) 83–132
9. Callaghan P T 1991 *Principles of Magnetic Resonance Microscopy* (Oxford, UK: Oxford Science Publications)

10. Tuch D S 2002 *Diffusion MRI of Complex Tissue Structure* (Doctor of Philosophy in Biomedical Imaging at the Massachusetts Institute of Technology)
11. Behrens T E J, Woolrich M W, Jenkinson M, Johansen-Berg H, Nunes R G, Clare S, Matthews P M, Brady J M and Smith S M 2003 Characterization and propagation of uncertainty in diffusion-weighted MR imaging *Magnetic Resonance in Medicine* **50** 1077–1088
12. Alexander D C 2005 Multiple-fibre reconstruction algorithms for diffusion MRI *Annals of the NYAS* In Press
13. Healy D M, Hendriks H and Kim P T 1998 Spherical deconvolution *Journal of Multivariate Analysis* **67** 1–22
14. Wedeen V J, Reese T G, Tuch D S, Dou J-G, Weiskoff R M and Chessler D 1999 Mapping fiber orientation spectra in cerebral white matter with Fourier-transform diffusion MRI *Proc. 7th Annual Meeting of the ISMRM (Philadelphia)* (Berkeley, USA: ISMRM) 321
15. Lin C P, Tseng W Y I, Kuo L, Wedeen V J and Chen J H 2003 Mapping orientation distribution function with spherical encoding *Proc. 11th Annual Meeting of the ISMRM (Toronto)* (Berkeley, USA: ISMRM) 2120
16. Ozarslan E, Vemuri B C and Mareci T H 2004 Fiber orientation mapping using generalized diffusion tensor imaging *Proc. IEEE International Symposium on Biomedical Imaging (Arlington)* (IEEE)
17. Mitra P P and Halperin B I 1995 Effects of finite gradient-pulse widths in pulsed-field-gradient diffusion measurements *Journal of Magnetic Resonance* **113** 94–101
18. Tournier J-D, et al 2005 *Proc. 13th Annual Meeting of the ISMRM (Miami)* (Berkeley, USA: ISMRM) Accepted

From Spatial Regularization to Anatomical Priors in fMRI Analysis

Wanmei Ou and Polina Golland

Computer Science and Artificial Intelligence Laboratory, MIT, Cambridge, MA

Abstract. In this paper, we study Markov Random Fields as spatial smoothing priors in fMRI detection. Relatively high noise in fMRI images presents a serious challenge for the detection algorithms, creating a need for spatial regularization of the signal. Gaussian smoothing, traditionally employed to boost the signal-to-noise ratio, often removes small activation regions. Recently, the use of Markov priors has been suggested as an alternative regularization approach. In this work, we investigate fast approximate inference algorithms for using MRFs in fMRI detection, propose a novel way to incorporate anatomical information into the detection framework, validate the methods through ROC analysis on simulated data and demonstrate their application in a real fMRI study.

1 Introduction

Functional magnetic resonance imaging (fMRI) provides a non-invasive dynamic method for studying brain activation by capturing the change in the blood oxygenation level. Most fMRI detection algorithms operate by comparing the time course of each voxel with the experimental protocol, labelling the voxels whose time courses correlate significantly with the protocol as "active". The commonly used general linear model (GLM) [9] further assumes that the fMRI signal possesses linear characteristics with respect to the stimulus and that the temporal noise is white. Application of GLM to an fMRI time series results in the so-called statistical parametric map (SPM), which is often thresholded to produce a binary map of active areas. However, because of a low signal-to-noise ratio (SNR), the binary maps typically contain many small false positive islands.

A common approach to reducing such false detections employs a Gaussian filter to smooth the fMRI signal prior to applying the GLM detector. Unfortunately, Gaussian smoothing, though intended to combat low SNR, leads to overly smoothed SPMs and a loss of detail in the resulting binary activation maps. A number of alternative approaches have explicitly incorporated spatial and temporal correlations into the estimation procedure. Examples include autoregressive spatio-temporal models [4, 24], Markov Random Fields (MRFs) [5, 8, 7], Bayesian models inferring hidden psychological states [15], adaptive thresholding methods that adjust statistical significance of active regions according to their size, based on the Gaussian Random Field theory [10]. In this paper, we focus on MRFs for modeling spatial coherency, study their performance and develop several increasingly rich spatial prior models. Following the formulation in [5], we assume that, given the activation state of each voxel, the time courses of different voxels are conditionally independent and can be reduced to a sufficient statistic. This work therefore concentrates on spatial regularization of the activation maps. Temporal regularization models can be easily incorporated into our framework by changing the activation statistic.

For MRFs with binary states, exact solution can be obtained in polynomial time. An fMRI detection algorithm based on the GLM statistic and the binary activation states was demonstrated in [5]. However, if one wants to go beyond binary states (e.g., treating positively and negatively activated voxels differently), the problem of estimating the optimal activation states becomes intractable and approximation algorithms must be used. Prior work in MRF-based fMRI detection employed simulated annealing [8, 21] and the iterated conditional mode algorithm [22]. We adopt the Mean Field solver, introduced in statistical physics [18], which has been widely used for image segmentation [16, 17, 20, 25]. In our experiments with binary MRFs, the Mean Field algorithm produced results comparable to those of the exact solver while reducing computation time by one to two orders of magnitude[1].

We further refine the activation priors by incorporating anatomical information. Similarly to segmentation, where a probabilistic atlas serves as a spatially varying prior on the tissue types, the anatomical information can provide a prior on the activation map. Intuitively speaking, we want the prior to reflect the fact that activation is much more likely to occur in gray matter than in white matter, and not at all in cerebrospinal fluid (CSF) or bone. In addition, the spatial coherency of activation is strong within each tissue and not across tissue boundaries. In this model, the hidden nodes encode both the tissue type and the activation state. Segmentation provides an additional, potentially noisy, observation at each node. We derive the detection algorithm for this model and evaluate it on simulated and real data, achieving high detection accuracy with significantly shorter time courses compared to the standard GLM detector.

Anatomical scans have certainly been used in fMRI analysis and visualization before. Hartvig [14] used the anatomical information in his marked point process spatial prior. Moreover, in some systems (e.g., BrainVoyager [1]), the subject's anatomical image is transformed into a standard coordinate frame (such as Talairach) and the functional activation map is displayed on the surface that corresponds to the cortical sheet in that coordinate frame. Other systems (e.g., FSL [2]) rely on sophisticated segmentation algorithms to extract a topologically correct representation of the cortical surface from the anatomical scan [6]. Performing Gaussian smoothing on the surface eliminates irrelevant voxels from the weighted average for the cortical locations. In contrast, our approach does not require a surface extraction algorithm, but instead utilizes anatomical information to inject the anatomically based coherency bias into the detection algorithm

---

[1] We also experimented extensively with the Belief Propagation algorithm, which often produces better approximations, but did not find it to be more accurate in this application. We therefore present the results of the Mean Field solution only.

while performing the computation directly on the volumetric data. The inspiration for this work comes from the success enjoyed by MRFs in providing spatial smoothing priors for image segmentation [16, 17, 20, 25].

In the next section, we briefly outline how the GLM detector can be augmented with an MRF prior closely following the derivation presented in [5], review the Mean Field algorithm, and present the empirical evaluation of the detector on simulated data. In Section 3, we extend the Markov priors to incorporate the anatomical information and show the empirical evaluation of this new, refined model. Section 4 illustrates the proposed detectors on a real fMRI data set.

2 Markov Priors for Activation Maps

Background. An fMRI scan contains a time course $y_i \in \mathbb{R}^T$ for each voxel i ($i = 1, ..., N$), where T is the number of time samples and N is the number of voxels in the scan. GLM models the fMRI signal as a linear combination of the protocol-dependent component B, and the protocol-independent component A, such as cardiopulmonary factors. The presence of the protocol-dependent signal indicates that the corresponding voxel is active due to the stimulus. Let H_1 be the hypothesis that a voxel is active and H_0 be the null hypothesis. Under GLM,

$$H_0: y_i = A\alpha_i + \epsilon_i \qquad H_1: y_i = A\alpha_i + B\beta_i + \epsilon_i$$

for $i = 1, ..., N$. For white temporal noise, $\epsilon_i \sim \mathcal{N}(0, \sigma_i^2 I)$. Least squares estimates of the activation response β_i and the protocol-independent factors α_i are found through a linear regression on the design matrix $C = [A\ B]$:

$$[\hat{\alpha}_i\ \hat{\beta}_i] = (C^T C)^{-1} C^T y_i, \qquad (1)$$

and the corresponding F-statistic is given by $F_i = \hat{\beta}_i^T \hat{\Sigma}_{\beta_i}^{-1} \hat{\beta}_i / N_\beta$, where N_β is the number of the regression coefficients in β_i and $\hat{\Sigma}_{\beta_i}$ is their estimated covariance.

Let random variable $X = [X_1, ..., X_N]$ represent an activation configuration of all voxels in the volume, and $x = [x_1, ..., x_N]$ be one possible configuration i.e., the activation map. In the case of binary hypothesis testing, the random variable X_i, which represents the activation state of voxel i, is also binary. Given an fMRI scan $[y_1, ..., y_N]$, the GLM estimate of the activation map x^* is obtained by thresholding the statistic value F_i for all voxels in the volume at a certain user-specified level.

It can be shown that the maximum log-likelihood ratio

$$z_i = \log \frac{\max_{\alpha_i, \beta_i, \sigma_i^2} p(y_i | H_1)}{\max_{\alpha_i, \sigma_i^2} p(y_i | H_0)} = \log \frac{\max_{\alpha_i, \beta_i, \sigma_i^2} \mathcal{N}(y_i; B\beta_i + A\alpha_i, \sigma_i^2 I)}{\max_{\alpha_i, \sigma_i^2} \mathcal{N}(y_i; A\alpha_i, \sigma_i^2 I)} \qquad (2)$$

is a monotonic function of the F statistic (see [5] for a detailed derivation). We can therefore consider z_i as an alternative statistic indicative of the activation state of voxel i. We will use this fact in the derivations of the MRF-based detection. If a different model of fMRI activation is proposed, it can be easily incorporated into our algorithm by formulating the corresponding maximum log-likelihood ratio and using it in place of z_i.

Markov Priors. A Markov prior on the activation configuration X, $P_X(x) = \frac{1}{\lambda} \prod_{<i,j>} \Psi_{ij}(x_i,x_j) \prod_i \Psi_i(x_i)$, is defined in terms of the singleton potentials $\Psi_i(x_i)$ that provide bias over state values x_i for voxel i, and the pairwise potentials $\Psi_{ij}(x_i, x_j)$ (often referred to as the compatibility matrices) that evaluate the compatibility of voxel i being in state x_i and voxel j being in state x_j for each pair $<i,j>$ of neighboring voxels. λ is a normalization constant, also called the partition function. Given the activation statistic values z, we seek the maximum *a posteriori* (MAP) estimate of the activation configuration:

$$x^* = \arg\max_x P_{X|Z}(x|z) = \arg\max_x P_{X,Z}(x,z) = \arg\max_x P_X(x)P_{Z|X}(z|x)$$

$$= \arg\max_x \frac{1}{\lambda} \prod_{<i,j>} \Psi_{ij}(x_i,x_j) \prod_i \Psi_i(x_i) P_{Z_i|X_i}(z_i|x_i) \quad (3)$$

The last equality is based on the assumption that the observations at different voxels are independent given the activation state of each voxel, and the likelihood over the volume can therefore be written as a product of the individual likelihood terms for each voxel. Fig. 1 depicts the corresponding graphical model, using a two-dimensional grid for illustration purposes only. The estimation is performed

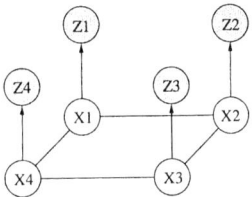

Fig. 1. Graphical model for $P_{X,Z}$

fully in 3D in all experiment reported here. We assume a spatially stationary generative model, i.e., $P_{Z_i|X_i}$, Ψ_i, and Ψ_{ij} are identical for all voxels in the volume. The observations (the fMRI signal, and in Section 3, the anatomical information) move the MAP estimate away from the spatially stationary configurations.

Direct search for the optimal activation configuration is intractable in general. However, a polynomial-time algorithm for exact MAP estimation exists for binary MRFs [13], based on a reduction to the Minimum-Cut-Maximum-Flow problem. We refer to this exact solver as Min-Max throughout this paper. Min-Max is still computationally intensive when applied to the volumetric data: in our experiments, it took 1-3 hours, depending on the pairwise potential settings and the initial threshold applied to the GLM statistic. On the other hand, the Mean Field approximation for MRFs is fast (ten to hundred times faster than Min-Max on the 3D grids we consider in this paper) and reasonably accurate, as our results in the remainder of this section indicate.

Mean Field Solution. The Mean Field algorithm approximates $P_{X|Z}(x|z)$ by a product distribution $Q(x) = \prod_i b_i(x_i)$ through minimization of the KL-Divergence between the two distributions:

$$D(Q\|P_{X|Z}) = \sum_x Q(x) \log(Q(x)) - \sum_x Q(x) \log(P_{X|Z}(x|z)) \quad (4)$$

$b_i(x_i)$ denotes the probability of voxel i being in state x_i (often called the belief), therefore $\sum_{x_i=1}^{M} b_i(x_i) = 1$, where M is the number of possible states of X_i. The KL-Divergence measures how closely Q approximates $P_{X|Z}$; it is non-negative and is equal to zero only for $Q = P_{X|Z}$. It is easy to see that the minimum of $D(\cdot)$ is achieved for the same state configuration x that minimizes the so called *free energy*, $F_{MF} = D(Q||P_{X|Z}) - \log(P_Z(z)) - \log(\lambda)$, since the last two terms of the latter function are independent of x. Substituting the product form for Q, we obtain,

$$F_{MF}(b) = -\sum_i \sum_{j \in \mathcal{N}(i)} \sum_{x_i=1}^{M} \sum_{x_j=1}^{M} b_i(x_i) b_j(x_j) \log(\Psi_{ij}(x_i, x_j))$$
$$+ \sum_i \sum_{x_i=1}^{M} b_i(x_i) \left[\log(b_i(x_i)) - \log(P_{Z_i|X_i}(z_i|x_i) \Psi_i(x_i)) \right] \quad (5)$$

Setting $\partial F_{MF}(b)/\partial b_i = 0$ under the constrains $\sum_{x_i=1}^{M} b_i(x_i) = 1 \ \forall i$ yields the following iterative update rule:

$$\boxed{b_i^{t+1}(x_i) \leftarrow \gamma \, P_{Z_i|X_i}(z_i|x_i) \, \Psi_i(x_i) \, e^{\sum_{j \in \mathcal{N}(i)} \sum_{x_j=1}^{M} b_j^t(x_j) \log \Psi_{ij}(x_i, x_j)}} \quad (6)$$

The normalization constant γ ensures the solution is a valid probability distribution. $\mathcal{N}(i)$ is the set of voxel i's neighbors. In each iteration of the Mean Field algorithm, the voxel's belief is updated according to the linear combination of its neighbors' beliefs in the previous iteration. The probability model (i.e., $P_{Z_i|X_i}$, Ψ_i, and Ψ_{ij}) determines the exact form of the update rule. Each voxel is assigned the state value with the highest belief at the end of the procedure (for binary MRFs, the voxel is set active if $b_i(1) > b_i(0)$).

Estimating Model Parameters. The potential functions Ψ_i, and Ψ_{ij} and the observation likelihood $P_{Z_i|X_i}$ must correspond to our notions of the appropriate bias toward desired solutions. In this work, we follow a common practice of setting the potential functions (same for all voxels) to the corresponding marginal probability distributions estimated from data: $\Psi_i(x_i)$ is set to the expected percentage of voxels in state x_i, $\Psi_{ij}(x_i, x_j)$ is set to the joint frequency of the states x_i and x_j, and $P_{Z_i|X_i}$ is approximated by a smoother version of a class-conditional histogram. Other forms of potential functions have also been explored [7, 11, 12].

Lack of training data or ground truth necessary for estimating the marginal frequencies is a more serious problem. Unlike the segmentation application, where manual segmentations by experts can be used to construct priors on the frequencies and co-occurrences of tissue types, in most fMRI experiments even the experts cannot provide such information. Model parameters in the currently used detectors are either set using researcher's intuition on the underlying activation properties (e.g., the threshold in GLM or the kernel width in Gaussian smoothing) or estimated from the input images (e.g., the noise variance in GLM). We take a similar approach of first running the GLM detector without smoothing and using the resulting SPM at a user-chosen threshold to estimate the probability model. To study the sensitivity of the method to the parameter

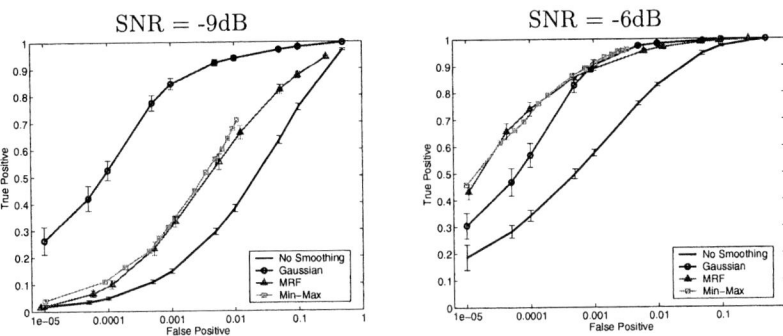

Fig. 2. ROC curves for different smoothing techniques, at two noise levels. False positive rate is shown on the log scale

settings, we ran experiments where the values of the singleton potentials and the compatibility matrices varied substantially (0.1 to 2 times the estimated frequencies). The variability in the detection accuracy (3-7%) was within the variability across different data sets as reported below.

Empirical Evaluation. To quantitatively evaluate the performance of the method, we generated realistic phantom data by applying EM segmentation [19] to an anatomical MRI scan and placing activation areas of variable size (average diameter of 15mm) randomly in the gray matter. We then downsampled the scan to an fMRI resolution. The gray matter voxels represent 10% of the total number of voxels in the volume, and the active voxels represent about 10% of the gray matter voxels in these images. We then created simulated fMRI scans based on a fixed parametric hemodynamic response function, an event-related protocol, and varying levels of noise. We used the estimated SNR, $\widehat{\text{SNR}} = -10\log_{10}(|B\hat{\beta}|^2)/\hat{\sigma}^2$, to determine a realistic level of the simulated noise as the true SNR is unaccessible for real fMRI scans. Since the signal and the noise overlap in some frequency bands, part of the noise energy is assigned to the estimated signal during detection. The estimated SNR is therefore an optimistic approximation of the true SNR, which can still be used as a monotonic upper bound of the true SNR. In our real fMRI studies, the estimated SNR is about -5dB. Here, we illustrate the results for two levels of true SNR, -6dB and -9dB, which correspond to estimated SNR of -4.3dB and -6.2dB respectively.

In all experiments, we used the same GLM detector based on a 10-bin nonparametric hemodynamic response function. To create a baseline for comparison, we ran the GLM detector with and without Gaussian smoothing. To evaluate the Markov priors, we ran GLM coupled with the exact Min-Max solver and with the approximate Mean Field solver on the same raw images. Fig. 2 shows the ROC curves created for the four methods by varying the threshold applied to the GLM statistic. Due to the large number of voxels in the volume and the relatively small number of active voxels, only very low false positive rates are of interest (we focus on the false positive rates below 0.1%, which corresponds to about 10% of the total number of the active voxels, or approximately 250 voxels). The error bars indicate the standard deviation of the true detection rate over 15 different, independently created and processed, data sets. The Min-Max ROC curve does not have the error bars, as the estimation takes too long (1 to 3 hours for a single run). Moreover, the Min-Max ROC curve is incomplete because extreme threshold values cause it to run even longer (we stopped the runs after 3 hours).

The Mean Field detection accuracy is very close to the exact Min-Max solution, providing a reasonable approximation to the exact solution that also takes much less time to compute (most Mean Field runs finished in a few minutes). The Min-Max accuracy is sometimes lower than the Mean Field accuracy, which appears to contradict the optimality of Min-Max. However, we note that both algorithms solve a particular estimation problem that does not necessarily describe the ground truth precisely but rather approximates it using a Markov model. Thus, the lowest energy state under this model might not be the best detector in practice. It is still reassuring to see that the approximate solver performs as well as the exact algorithm. It also suggests that more realistic spatial priors could further improve the detection accuracy.

As expected, the accuracy of all methods improves with increasing SNR. At high noise levels (low SNR), Gaussian smoothing outperforms MRFs. As the simplest smoothing technique, Gaussian smoothing is more robust to noise. We also believe that our current way of constructing the likelihood term in the MRF model over-emphasizes the data evidence over the prior. We are investigating ways to compensate for this in the estimation of the model. As the SNR increases, MRFs provide better regularization of the activation state (for example, at SNR=-6dB, at the false positive rate of 0.01%, the MRF outperforms the Gaussian smoothing by about 15% in true detection accuracy; at 70% true detection, the MRF approximately halves the false detections compared to the Gaussian smoothing). With the improving scanning technology, we believe MRFs will become even more helpful in reducing spurious false detection islands.

3 Anatomical Priors for Spatial Regularization

The general nature of the Mean Field algorithm allows straightforward extension of the probabilistic model in the previous section to include the tissue type for each voxel. We define $V = [V_1, ..., V_N]$ to be the tissue types of all voxels, and $W = [W_1, ..., W_N]$ the tissue type observations, such as a result of an automatic segmentation procedure. W_i's are noisy observations due to imperfect registration between the fMRI image and the anatomical scan, the mismatch in their resolution and the noise in the segmentation itself. Now each voxel has two

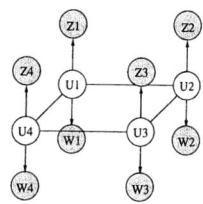

Fig. 3. Graphical model for $P_{U,Z,W}$

hidden attributes: the activation state X_i and the tissue type V_i. We combine these attributes into a single hidden node U_i, as illustrated in Fig. 3. For example, for a binary activation states (active or not active) and three tissue types (gray matter, white matter, or other), U_i has six possible states. Similarly to the derivations in the previous section, the MAP estimate in this case is as follows:

$$\boldsymbol{u}^* = \arg\max_{\boldsymbol{u}} P_{U|Z,W}(\boldsymbol{u}|\boldsymbol{z},\boldsymbol{w}) = \arg\max_{\boldsymbol{u}} P_U(\boldsymbol{u})P_{Z|U}(\boldsymbol{z}|\boldsymbol{u})P_{W|U}(\boldsymbol{w}|\boldsymbol{u})$$

$$= \arg\max_{\boldsymbol{u}} \frac{1}{\lambda}\prod_{<i,j>}\Psi_{ij}(u_i,u_j)\prod_i \Psi_i(u_i)P_{Z_i|U_i}(z_i|u_i)P_{W_i|U_i}(w_i|u_i) \quad (7)$$

We assume that the segmentation W and the fMRI observation Z are conditionally independent given the state of the voxel since they are obtained from two different images. Similarly to the previous section, we derive the iterative update step in the estimation procedure:

$$\boxed{b_i^{t+1}(u_i) \leftarrow \gamma P_{W_i|U_i}(w_i|u_i)P_{Z_i|U_i}(z_i|u_i)\Psi_i(u_i)e^{\sum_{j\in\mathcal{N}(i)}\sum_{u_j=1}^M b_j^t(u_j)\log\Psi_{ij}(u_i,u_j)}}$$

(8)

This update rule is similar to Eq. (6), with the exception of the extra likelihood term $P_{W_i|U_i}(w_i|u_i)$ for the tissue type observation. The compatibility matrix $\Psi_{ij}(x_i,x_j)$ is $M \times M$, where M is the number of states in U_i.

Empirical Evaluation. We used the same phantom data sets described earlier to evaluate the performance of the anatomically-guided detectors. The basic GLM with anatomical prior suppresses activations outside of the gray matter using segmentation as a guidance ("soft" masking could also account for misregistration and errors in segmentation). To incorporate the anatomical information into the Gaussian filter, we adjust the weights of the filter based on the tissue types of the voxel's neighbors: when evaluating the filter at voxel i, we assign higher weights to the neighbors sharing the same segmentation results as voxel i. Fig. 4 illustrates the ROC analysis for the three regularization methods investigated in the previous section (solid lines) and their anatomically-based variants (dashed lines). We omit the Min-Max solver for the MRF model, as it cannot handle multi-valued states.

In addition to the trends observed before, we note that the anatomical information significantly boosts the performance of all detectors at all noise levels. At high noise levels (SNR = -9dB) and false positive rates between 0.01% and 0.1%, all methods gain at least 10% in true detection rate when using the anatomical information. The MRF model benefits more than the Gaussian smoothing, but its detection accuracy is still lower. At the lower noise level (SNR = -6dB), the basic GLM detector augmented with anatomical information approaches the performance of the Gaussian smoothing. At 0.01% false positive rate, the anatomically-guided MRF outperforms the anatomically-guided

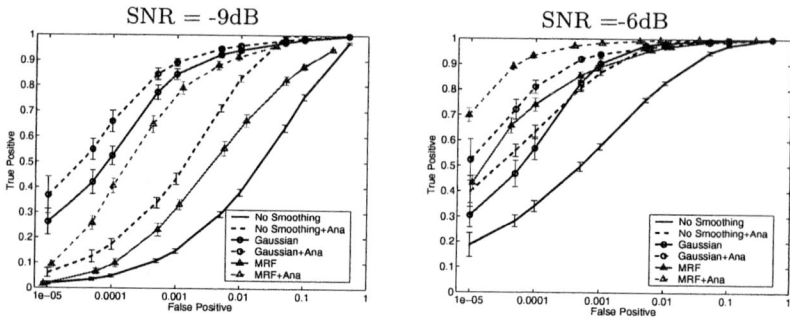

Fig. 4. ROC curves for different smoothing techniques augmented with the anatomical information, at two noise levels. False positive rate is shown on the log scale

Gaussian smoothing by about 15% in true detection rate, achieving over 90% detection accuracy. The large boost experienced by the basic GLM when augmented with anatomical information is easy to understand: since false detections occur relatively uniformly throughout the volume, masking the gray matter improves the performance substantially.

In addition to the quantitative analysis presented above, we find it useful to visually inspect the resulting activation maps. Fig. 5 illustrates the detection results by showing one axial slice of the estimated activation map. The top image shows the phantom activation areas that were placed in the volume and used to generate the simulated fMRI scan. The middle and the bottom rows show the same slice in the reconstructed volume at two different noise levels. All the reconstructions were performed at 0.05% false positive rate. In other words, each image in Fig. 5 shows one slice in the reconstructed volume that corresponds to a point on the ROC curve of the respective detector at 0.05% false positive rate.

The basic GLM produces a fragmented activation map that contains a number of false detection islands at high SNR and shows very little of the original activation at low SNR. Given either of these maps, the users would have troubles inferring the true activation areas and disambiguating them from spurious false detections. The Gaussian smoothing leads to a reasonable estimate of the ground truth. Gaussian smoothing tends to make the detections "spherical", which may change the shape of the detected activations. The smoothing effectively overestimates the extent of the regions. Consequently, many false positive voxels in the Gaussian smoothing occur at the boundaries of the activation regions. Imposing anatomical information reduces this over-smoothing effect for some of the areas. At low SNR (-9dB), the MRF model fills in many of the active pixels that were missed by the GLM, but as we saw before, it does not produce as accurate result as Gaussian smoothing. At higher SNR (-6dB), MRF produces a relatively accurate result. Not all of the scatter activation islands are removed through regularization, but the activation map looks more similar to the ground truth. The activation map is further improved when the anatomical information is incorporated into the model.

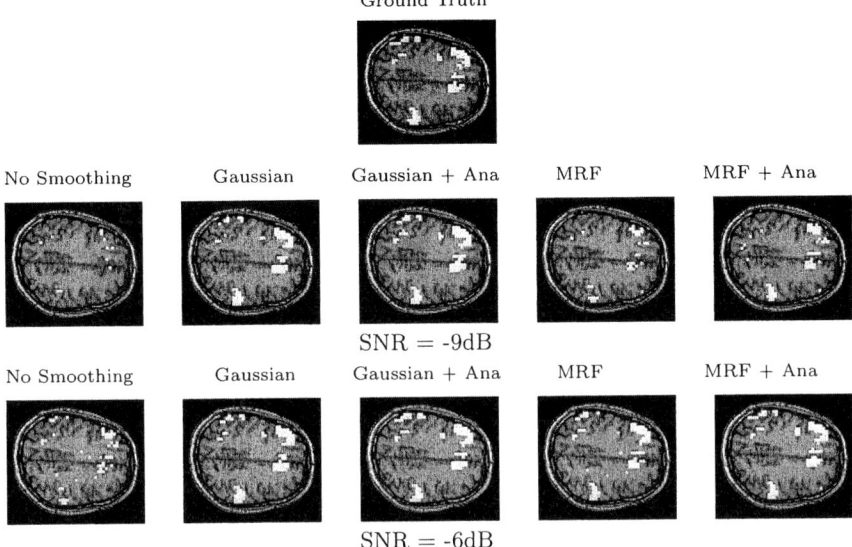

Fig. 5. One slice from estimated activation maps for the same ground truth at 0.05% false positive rate. True and false detections are shown in yellow. The on-line version shows true and false detections in different colors

4 Real fMRI Experiment

In real fMRI experiments, the ground truth is unavailable, and ROC analysis is not possible. Instead, we visually compare the resulting activation maps produced by different detectors to evaluate their performance on reduced-length time courses. This effectively evaluates the ability of each method to reconstruct the true activation areas with less evidence on the strength of the signal.

In this fMRI study [23], the original scans were obtained during an auditory "two-back" word experiment. Each experiment consisted of five rest epochs and four task epochs, each epoch 30 seconds long. In the rest condition, the subjects were instructed to concentrate on the noise of the scanner and lie still. In the task condition, the subjects were presented with a series of pre-recorded single-digit numbers, one number every three seconds. The subjects were asked to tap their index finger to the thumb when hearing a number that was the same as the one spoken two numbers before. The experiment was repeated ten times for each subject. The anatomical images were acquired on a 1.5 Tesla GE signa clinical MR scanner (T1-weighted SPGR, 256×256, 124 slices, 1.5mm slice thickness). The EPI images were acquired on the same scanner (axial, TR/TE=2500/50msec, FA90, 64×64, 24 slices, 6mm slice thickness, no gap). The original study contains nine subjects, but for the purposes of voxel by-voxel comparison of the detectors, we present the results for one subject across all detectors. The estimated SNR when averaging over all voxels in the brain was -4.7dB (-2.3dB when averaging voxels in selected ROIs relevant to the task).

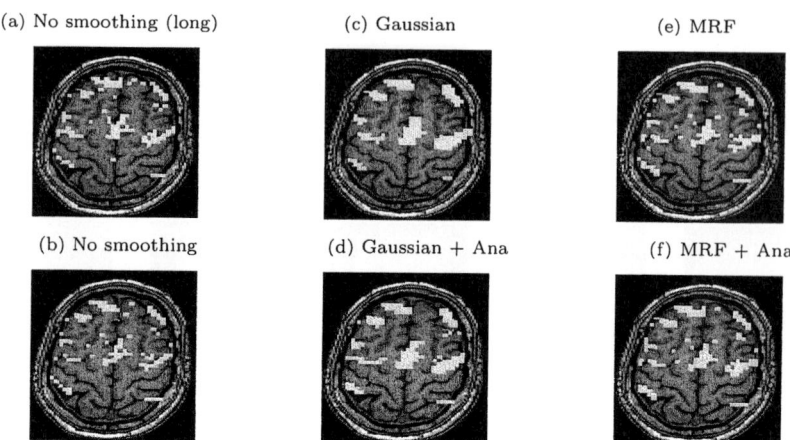

Fig. 6. Real fMRI study. One slice in the estimated activation map. (a) No spatial smoothing, using the entire time course. (b)-(f) Estimation based on the first five epochs of the time course using different spatial smoothing methods

Fig. 6a shows one axial slice in the reconstructed activation map using GLM without any spatial smoothing on the full-length fMRI signal (all 9 epochs). The ground truth for this scan is unknown, but we can use this map as a visual reference when evaluating the performance of the detectors on the time course of reduced length. For example, Fig. 6b shows the result of applying the same GLM detector to the first 5 epochs of the time course. This map is more fragmented due to loss in SNR from reducing the length of the signal. The other four images illustrate the results of applying GLM with the Gaussian smoothing and the MRF priors, as well as their anatomically augmented versions. Although Gaussian smoothing removes most of the single voxel activation islands, its activation map (Fig. 6c) is an overestimate compared with Fig. 6a. Anatomical weighting slightly reduces the overestimate in the Gaussian smoothing. MRF regularization (Fig. 6e,f) yields reconstruction results that are close to the activation map estimated from the full-length signal, but do not look overly smoothed. This highlights the potential benefit of using the Markov priors in fMRI detection. Similarly to the Gaussian smoothing, the MRF model benefits from using anatomical information to remove spurious activations.

5 Discussion and Conclusions

Our experiments confirm the importance of spatial regularization in reducing fragmentation of the activation maps. This paper investigates two improvements in spatial modelling for fMRI detection: Markov priors and anatomical bias. An MRF provides a spatial prior that refines the structure of the resulting activation map over the Gaussian smoothing, as demonstrated by our experiments on phantom and real data. In this work, we explored fast approximate solvers in application to MRF-based fMRI detection and showed that they provide reasonably accurate approximations to the exact solution while taking substantially less time to evaluate. We also note that since the Markov model itself is an approximation of the real geometry of the activation regions, we should not dwell on the small differences in the activation maps introduced by the approximate solvers but rather focus on their performance relative to the ground truth.

A separate insight of this paper is that we can use anatomical information to bias the fMRI detector. Gaussian smoothing can be straightforwardly augmented with the anatomical prior by rescaling the coefficients of the smoothing kernel. Moreover, we derived an algorithm for anatomically-guided MRF estimation. One of the problems that should be investigated in the future is the partial voluming effects. The anatomical information comes at much higher resolution than the fMRI signals. Right now, we downsample the anatomical scan to match the resolution of the functional scan. A better solution would be to use the high-resolution anatomical scans to resolve the activation in the functional voxels that are on the boundary of the gray matter, leading to a "super-resolution" detector.

We evaluated the methods on phantom data by performing ROC analysis and on real data by studying their ability to recover activation from significantly shorter time courses. While in high noise settings the Gaussian smoothing outperformed other methods, as the SNR in the images increased, the Markov priors offered a substantial improvement in the detection accuracy. Using this smoothing prior enabled us to shorten fMRI scan length by half while retaining the detection power comparable with the full-length fMRI scan. We expect a similar effect to occur with respect to the spatial resolution when we extend the method to utilize the anatomical information at the original scan resolution. As the quality of the scanning equipment improves, the sophisticated spatial models, such as MRFs, will become even more important in recovering the details of the activation regions.

Acknowledgement. We thank Sandy Wells for suggesting we look at the MRF regularization for fMRI applications, Eric Cosman and Kilian Pohl for help on this paper, and Dr. L.P. Panych for providing fMRI data. This work was partially supported by the NIH National Center for Biomedical Computing Program, National Alliance for Medical Imaging Computing (NAMIC), Fund No. 1U54 EB005149, the NSF IIS 9610249 grant. fMRI acquisition was supported by the NIH R01 NS37922 grant.

References

1. BrainVoyager software package. http://www.brainvoyager.de.
2. FMRIB software library. http://www.fmrib.ox.ac.uk/fsl.
3. Besag, J. Spatial interaction and statistical analysis of lattice systems. *Acad. R. Statistical Soc. Series B*, 36:721–741, 1974.
4. Burock, M.A., and Dale, A.M. Estimation and detection of event-related fmri signals with temporally correlated noise: A statistically efficient and unbiased approach. *Human Brain Mapping*, 11:249–260, 2000.

5. Cosman, E.R., Fisher, J. and Wells, W.M. Exact MAP activity detection in fMRI using a GLM with an spatial. *In Proc. MICCAI'04*, 2:703–710, 2004.
6. A. M. Dale, *et al.* Cortical Surface-Based Analysis I: Segmentation and Surface Reconstruction. *NeuroImage*, 9:179-194, 1999.
7. Descombes, X., Kruggel, F., and Von Cramon, D.Y. fMRI signal restoration using a spatio-temporal Markov random field preserving transitions. *NeuroImage*, 8:340–349, 1998.
8. Descombes, X., Kruggel, F. and Von Cramon, D.Y. Spatio-temporal fMRI analysis using Markov random fields. *IEEE TMI*, 17(6):1028–1039, 1998.
9. Friston, K.J., *et al.* Statistical parametric maps in functional imaging: a general linear approach. *Human Brain Mapping*, 2:189–210, 1995.
10. Friston, K.J., *et al.* Assessing the significance of local activations using their spatial extent. *Human Brain Mapping*, 1:210–220, 1994.
11. Geman, S. and McClure, D. Statistical methods for tomographic image reconstruction. *Proc. 46th Session of ISI*, 51:22–26, 1987.
12. Geman, S. and Reynolds, G. Constrained restoration and recovery of discontinuities. *IEEE Trans. PAMI*, 14:367–383, 1992.
13. Greig, D.M., Porteous, B.T. and Gramon, D.Y. Exact maximum a posteriori estimation for binary images. *J. R. Statistical Society*, 51:271–279, 1989.
14. Hartvig, N.V. A stochastic Geometry model for functional Magnetic resonance images *Scandinavian Journal of Statistics*, 29:333–253, 2002.
15. Hojen-Sorensen, F., Hansen, L.K. and Rasmussen, C.E. Bayesian modeling of fMRI time series. *Adv. Neuroinform. Processing Syst.*, Vol.12:754–760, 2000.
16. Kapur, T., *et al.* Enhanced spatial priors for segmentation of magnetic resonance imagery. *Proc. MICCAI'98*, 148-157, 1998.
17. Langan, D.A., *et al.* Use of the mean-field approximation in an EM-based approach to unsupervised stochastic model-based image segmentation. *Proc. ICASSP*, 3:57–60, 1992.
18. G. Parisi. *Statistical Field Theory.* Addison-Wesley, 1998.
19. Pohl, K.M., *et al.* Anatomical guided segmentation with non-stationary tissue class distributions in an expectation-maximization framework. *Proc. IEEE ISBI*, 81–84, 2004.
20. Pohl, K.M., *et al.* Incorporating non-rigid registration into expectation maximization algorithm to segment MR images. *Proc. MICCAI'02*, 508-515, 2002.
21. Rajapakse, J.C. and Piyaratna, J. Bayesian modeling of fMRI time series. *IEEE Transactions on Biomedical Engineering*, 48:1186–1194, 2001.
22. Salli, E., *et al.* Contextual clustering for analysis of functional MRI data. *IEEE TMI*, 20:403–413, 2001.
23. Wei, X., *et al.* Functional MRI of auditory verbal working memory: long-term reproducibility analysis. *NeuroImage*, 21:1000-1008, 2004.
24. Woolrich, M.W., *et al.* Fully Bayesian spatio-temporal modeling of fMRI data. *IEEE TMI*, 23(2):213–231, 2004.
25. Zhang, J. The mean-field theory in EM procedures for markov random field. *IEEE Trans. on Signal Processing*, 40:2570–2583, 1992.

CLASSIC: Consistent Longitudinal Alignment and Segmentation for Serial Image Computing

Zhong Xue, Dinggang Shen, and Christos Davatzikos

Section of Biomedical Image Analysis, Department of Radiology,
University of Pennsylvania, Philadelphia, PA 19104
{zhong.xue, dinggang.shen, christos.davatzikos}@uphs.upenn.edu

Abstract. This paper proposes a temporally-consistent and spatially-adaptive longitudinal MR brain image segmentation algorithm, referred to as CLASSIC, which aims at obtaining accurate measurements of rates of change of regional and global brain volumes from serial MR images. The algorithm incorporates image-adaptive clustering, spatiotemporal smoothness constraints, and image warping to jointly segment a series of 3-D MR brain images of the same subject that might be undergoing changes due to development, aging or disease. Morphological changes, such as growth or atrophy, are also estimated as part of the algorithm. Experimental results on simulated and real longitudinal MR brain images show both segmentation accuracy and longitudinal consistency.

1 Introduction

MR brain image segmentation is a key processing step in many brain image analysis applications, *e.g.* morphometry, automatic tissue labeling, tissue volume quantification, image registration, and computer integrated surgery [1, 2, 3, 4, 5, 6, 7, 8]. Analysis of a series of 3-D data of the same subject captured at different time-points, *i.e.* of a 4-D image, is important in many neuroimaging studies that concentrate on normal development, aging, and evolution of pathology [9]. Consistent segmentation is particularly important in the literature of aging and Alzheimer's Disease (AD) since subtle brain changes that might be indicative of early stages of underlying pathology must be estimated from serial MR images. However, existing 3-D segmentation algorithms may not provide adequate longitudinal stability for serial brain images since they process each image at a time. Herein, we propose a 4-D segmentation method that overcomes this limitation and significantly improves longitudinal stability of segmentation.

Fuzzy algorithms [1, 2, 3, 4, 5, 10] have been proven to be more suitable for 3-D MR images than hard segmentation algorithms since the intensity of each voxel of an MR image may represent a combination of different tissues. Fuzzy C-Means (FCM) algorithms have been used in many segmentation applications often accounting for intensity inhomogeneity [6, 7, 11, 12] and incorporating spatial information among voxels [8, 13, 14]. The intensity inhomogeneity can be well modeled by the product of the original image and a gain field [12] or by the summation of them [6]. It is also desirable that the clustering algorithm be spatially-adaptive to relatively local image intensity variations in order to adaptively segment tissues of different structures. Different methods have been proposed to incorporate the spatial image context information, including the methods using smoothness constraints of the spatially varying centroid [8], using intensity dissimilarities of neighboring voxels [13], and using smoothing operations of fuzzy membership functions [14]. By combining [6] and [14], Pham and Prince proposed a Fuzzy And Noise Tolerant Adaptive Segmentation Method (FANTASM), which is robust to the effects of both intensity inhomogeneities and noise, while providing a soft segmentation [http://iacl.ece.jhu.edu/projects/fantasm/]. The advantage of FANTASM is that it uses the intermediate information of the segmentation results while compensating the gain field and performing smoothness on the membership functions. However, in FANTASM, the spatial smoothness constraints of fuzzy membership functions are the same for all the locations in an image, which can result in an "over smoothing" effect across tissue boundaries. More importantly, FANTASM and other existing segmentation methods are designed for segmentation of 3-D images, and they might yield inconsistent results when applied to serial scans of the same subject, thereby rendering estimations of rates of brain atrophy and growth noisy.

In this paper, we propose a novel algorithm for longitudinal MR brain image segmentation based on FANTASM, which we refer to as CLASSIC (Consistent Longitudinal Alignment and Segmentation for Serial Image Computing). CLASSIC not only jointly segments longitudinal 3-D MR brain images of the same subject, but also estimates the longitudinal deformations in the image series, *e.g.* tissue atrophy. It iteratively performs two steps: *(1)* it jointly segments serial 3-D images using a 4-D image-adaptive clustering algorithm based on the current estimate of the longitudinal deformations in the image series, *(2)* it then refines these longitudinal deformations using a 4-D elastic warping algorithm [15, 16]. In this way, we obtain both a longitudinally-consistent segmentation result and an estimate of longitudinal deformation of anatomy in a series of 3-D images. The 4-D image-adaptive clustering algorithm used in CLASSIC extends FANTASM in three aspects. First, a new temporal consistency constraint term on the fuzzy membership functions is used in order to obtain temporally-consistent segmentation results. Second, the spatiotemporal constraints of fuzzy membership functions are made adaptive to the smoothness of the image, *i.e.* they are stronger in the regions that have more uniform image intensities, and vice versa, thus fuzzy membership functions are not necessarily overly smooth across tissue boundaries. Third, the clustering centers at each voxel location are adaptive to local image intensity variations. In this way, the proposed algorithm not only provides temporally-consistent segmentation results, but also adapts to local image intensity variations.

Experiments are performed to segment simulated and real longitudinal MR brain images. The longitudinal 3-D T1-SPGR MR images of healthy, older adults from the Baltimore Longitudinal Study of Aging (BLSA) [9] are used in the experiments, which display both brain atrophy and changes of tissue contrast due to vascular and possibly other pathologies. In all the experiments, we focused on evaluating the performance of the CLASSIC and FANTASM algorithms in terms of obtaining temporally-consistent segmentation, capturing global and local intensity/contrast changes, as well as estimating longitudinal deformations. The results demonstrate that CLASSIC gives consistent segmentation results across different years and adapts to image intensity variations.

2 Serial Image Segmentation

2.1 The Framework of CLASSIC

A 4-D MR brain image in the context of this work is a series of 3-D MR brain images obtained from the same subject at different times. Because the brain changes that we might be interested in can be extremely small, for example in early stages of Alzheimer's Disease (AD), temporally-inconsistent segmentation can significantly reduce the statistical power of longitudinal neuroimaging studies aiming at determining early structural changes as markers of AD. In this paper, we focus on jointly segmenting a 4-D image and follow the underlying temporal changes in anatomical structures, in order to provide more stable and consistent tissue segmentation across different years. Our idea is to classify the tissue of each voxel according to the intensities around that voxel, plus incorporating image-adaptive spatiotemporal constraints at that location. Therefore, a 4-D image segmentation framework, referred to as CLASSIC, is proposed, which iteratively performs the following two steps: *(1)* given a current estimate of the longitudinal deformations necessary to align 3-D images, it jointly segments the image series using a 4-D image-adaptive clustering algorithm, *(2)* it then refines the longitudinal deformations using a 4-D HAMMER registration algorithm [15].

The pre-processing of the input 3-D image series include: correct global intensity inhomogeneity [6] and globally normalize the intensities of each image according to the histogram of the first image [17]; transfer the subsequent images onto the space of the first image using rigid transformations. After pre-processing, CLASSIC is applied to consistently segment the rigidly aligned serial images $I_t, t \subset T = \{t_1, t_2, ..., t_Y\}$, with initial longitudinal deformations from the first image I_{t_1} to other images I_t as $F_{t_1 \to t}$, $t = t_2, t_3, ..., t_Y$, and Y being the total number of the serial images. If no initial longitudinal deformations among the images are available, $F_{t_1 \to t}(i) = 0$, where i refers to a voxel location in the first image I_{t_1}, i.e. initially there is no deformation at all. The standard FCM algorithm is also performed on each image I_t to give initial values of the clustering centroids. Then, CLASSIC iteratively performs the following two steps:

1. Apply the proposed 4-D image-adaptive clustering algorithm to the image series $I_t, t \in T$, based on the current estimate of the longitudinal deformations $F_{t_1 \to t}$, $t = t_2, t_3, ..., t_Y$, and obtain the segmented images $I_t^{(seg)}, t \in T$ (The algorithm will be described in Section 2.2 in detail).
2. Use the 4-D HAMMER [15], to register the segmented images $I_t^{(seg)}$, $t = \{t_2, t_3, ..., t_Y\}$ onto the reference image series formed by repeating the first

segmented image $I_{t_1}^{\text{seg}}$ for $Y-1$ times, i.e. $I_{t_1}^{(\text{seg})}, I_{t_1}^{(\text{seg})}, ..., I_{t_1}^{(\text{seg})}$. After performing 4-D registration, the longitudinal deformations $F_{t_1 \to t}, t = t_2, t_3, ..., t_Y$ are refined according to the 4-D segmentation results of step (1). Go to step (1) if the amount of deformation changes between two iterations is larger than a prescribed threshold; otherwise terminate with $I_t^{(\text{seg})}$ and $F_{t_1 \to t}$ as the final segmentation results and the final estimate of the longitudinal deformations, respectively.

These two steps are performed iteratively so that consistent segmentation results can be obtained. In practice, we find that a few iterations are enough to obtain stable segmentation results. In Section 2.2, we describe the 4-D image-adaptive clustering algorithm used in step (1) of CLASSIC in detail.

2.2 The 4-D Image-Adaptive Clustering Algorithm

Algorithm Formulation. Given image series $I_t, t \in T$ and the longitudinal deformations $F_{t_1 \to t}, t = t_2, ..., t_Y$, the purpose of the 4-D segmentation is to calculate the segmented images $I_t^{(\text{seg})}, t \in T$. Since $F_{t_1 \to t}$ is the deformation from I_{t_1} to I_t, the corresponding point of voxel i of image I_{t_1} will be $F_{t_1 \to t}(i)$ in image I_t. For simplicity, we denote point $F_{t_1 \to t}(i)$ in image I_t as (t, i), and $x_{(t,i)}$ as its intensity. According to the 4-D image-adaptive clustering algorithm, $x_{(t,i)}(t \in T, i \in \Omega)$ is classified into different tissue types by finding $c_{(t,i),k}$, the kth clustering center at location (t,i), and $\mu_{(t,i),k}$, the fuzzy membership function of $x_{(t,i)}$ belonging to class k, and by minimizing the objective function in Eq.(1), which includes three terms: the weighted squared error between the intensities around each voxel and the clustering centroids, the spatially-adaptive smoothness constraints, and temporally-adaptive smoothness constraints.

$$E(\mu, c) = \sum_{t \in T} \sum_{i \in \Omega} \{ \frac{1}{S(N_{(t,i)})} \sum_{k=1}^{K} \sum_{(\tau,j) \in N_{(t,i)}} [\mu_{(\tau,j),k}^q (x_{(\tau,j)} - c_{(t,i),k})^2] \}$$

$$+ \frac{\alpha}{2} \sum_{t \in T} \sum_{i \in \Omega} \{ \rho_{(t,i)}^{(s)} \sum_{k=1}^{K} [\mu_{(t,i),k}^q \bar{\mu}_{(t,i),k}^{(s)}] \}$$

$$+ \frac{\beta}{2} \sum_{t \in T} \sum_{i \in \Omega} \{ \rho_{(t,i)}^{(t)} \sum_{k=1}^{K} [\mu_{(t,i),k}^q \bar{\mu}_{(t,i),k}^{(t)}] \}, \quad (1)$$

where $\bar{\mu}_{(t,i),k}^{(s)} = \frac{1}{N_1} \sum_{(t,j) \in N_{(t,i)}^{(s)'}} \sum_{m \in M_k} \mu_{(t,j),m}^q$, $\bar{\mu}_{(t,i),k}^{(t)} = \frac{1}{N_2} \sum_{(\tau,i) \in N_{(t,i)}^{(t)'}} \sum_{m \in M_k} \mu_{(\tau,i),m}^q$.

The fuzzy membership functions are subject to

$$\sum_{k=1}^{K} \mu_{(t,i),k} = 1, \text{ for all } i \in \Omega, t \in T. \quad (2)$$

In Eq.(1), $N_{(t,i)}$ is the spatiotemporal neighborhood of point (t,i). It is a combination of its spatial neighborhood $N_{(t,i)}^{(s)}$ and temporal neighborhood $N_{(t,i)}^{(t)} =$

$\{(\tau, i) : |\tau - t| \leq T_N\}$, thus $N_{(t,i)} = N_{(t,i)}^{(s)} \cup N_{(t,i)}^{(t)}$. $S(N_{(t,i)})$ represents the number of voxels within $N_{(t,i)}$. In the first term of Eq.(1), the centroids $c_{(t,i),k}$ are adaptively changed at different image locations based on local image intensity variations within the spatiotemporal neighborhood $N_{(t,i)}$ of each location. The second term of Eq.(1) reflects the spatial constraints of the fuzzy membership functions, which is analogous to the FANTASM algorithm. The difference is that an additional factor $\rho_{(t,i)}^{(s)}$ is used as an image-adaptive weighting coefficient, thus stronger smoothness constraints are applied to the fuzzy membership functions in the image regions that have more uniform intensities, and vice versa. The third term of Eq.(1) reflects the temporal consistency constraints. Similar to $\rho_{(t,i)}^{(s)}$, $\rho_{(t,i)}^{(t)}$ is a weighting coefficient that reflects the temporal smoothness of the image. $\bar{\mu}_{(t,i),k}^{(s)}$ and $\bar{\mu}_{(t,i),k}^{(t)}$ are the means of $\mu_{(\tau,l),k}^{q}$ in the spatial and temporal neighborhoods $N_{(t,i)}^{(s)'}$ and $N_{(t,i)}^{(t)'}$ of the current position (t,i), respectively ($N_{(t,i)}^{(s)'}$ and $N_{(t,i)}^{(t)'}$ do not include the point (t,i)). α and β are the weighting coefficients and N_1 and N_2 are the numbers of addends for normalization.

$\rho_{(t,i)}^{(s)}$ is the spatial smoothness factor of image I_t at voxel (t,i). The value of $\rho_{(t,i)}^{(s)}$ is close to 1 when the image around voxel (t,i) is spatially-smooth, and close to 0 when the image around voxel (t,i) is not spatially-smooth. Using a spatial difference operator D_r along each of 3 spatial axis r, $\rho_{(t,i)}^{(s)}$ is defined as

$$\rho_{(t,i)}^{(s)} = \exp\{-\sum_r [(D_r * I_t)_{(t,i)}^2 / 2\sigma_s^2]\}, \qquad (3)$$

where $(D_r * I_t)_{(t,i)}$ refers to first calculating the spatial convolution $(D_r * I_t)$, and then taking its value at location (t,i). $\rho_{(t,i)}^{(t)}$ is the temporal smoothness factor,

$$\rho_{(t,i)}^{(t)} = \exp\{-(D_t * x_{(t,i)})_t^2 / 2\sigma_t^2\}, \qquad (4)$$

where D_t is the temporal difference operator, and $(D_t * x_{(t,i)})_t$ refers to first calculating the temporal convolution $(D_t * x_{(t,i)})$ and then taking its value at t.

Notice the size of the spatiotemporal neighborhood $N_{(t,i)}$ at each location (t,i) can also be adaptively adjusted. A smaller neighborhood size will make the algorithm much adaptive to local image intensity variations, while a larger neighborhood size has to be used to capture adequate intensity information of different tissues around that location in order to label that voxel correctly. No spatiotemporal smoothness constraints on c were used in Eq.(1), because we have found that the image-adaptive constraints of μ along with reasonably large and smooth neighborhood sizes are adequate for yielding smoothly varying centroids.

Finding the Solutions of the 4-D Clustering Algorithm. Using Lagrange multipliers to enforce the constraint in Eq.(2), the new objective function is,

$$J = E(\mu, c) + \sum_{t \in T} \sum_{i \in \Omega} \lambda_{(t,i)} (1 - \sum_{k=1}^{K} \mu_{(t,i),k}). \qquad (5)$$

Setting the partial derivative of Eq.(5) with respect to $\mu_{(t,i),k}$ to zero, and using Eq.(2), we get the equation to update the fuzzy membership functions,

$$\mu_{(t,i),k} = \frac{[\sum_{(\tau,j)\in \bar{N}_{(t,i)}} \frac{(x_{(t,i)}-c_{(\tau,j),k})^2}{S(N_{(\tau,j)})} + \alpha \rho^{(s)}_{(t,i)} \bar{\mu}^{(s)}_{(t,i),k} + \beta \rho^{(t)}_{(t,i)} \bar{\mu}^{(t)}_{(t,i),k}]^{\frac{-1}{q-1}}}{\sum_{k=1}^{K} [\sum_{(\tau,j)\in \bar{N}_{(t,i)}} \frac{(x_{(t,i)}-c_{(\tau,j),k})^2}{S(N_{(\tau,j)})} + \alpha \rho^{(s)}_{(t,i)} \bar{\mu}^{(s)}_{(t,i),k} + \beta \rho^{(t)}_{(t,i)} \bar{\mu}^{(t)}_{(t,i),k}]^{\frac{-1}{q-1}}}. \quad (6)$$

Since different spatiotemporal neighborhood sizes are used for different image locations, in Eq.(6), $\bar{N}_{(t,i)} = \{(\tau,j) : (t,i) \in N_{(\tau,j)}\}$.

Setting the partial derivative of Eq.(5) with respect to $c_{(t,i),k}$ to zero, the equation to update the centroids can be acquired,

$$c_{(t,i),k} = \frac{\sum_{(\tau,j)\in N_{(t,i)}} \mu^q_{(\tau,j),k} x(\tau,j)}{\sum_{(\tau,j)\in N_{(t,i)}} \mu^q_{(\tau,j),k}}. \quad (7)$$

Given a series of 3-D images and the longitudinal deformations among them, the 4-D image-adaptive clustering algorithm then jointly segments them by iteratively calculating the fuzzy membership functions using Eq.(6) and the centroids using Eq.(7) until convergence. In order to determine adaptively the size of each neighborhood $N_{(t,i)}$, we first initialize an identical neighborhood size for all the locations, and then adaptively adjust these sizes in every iteration: we segment the images using the current fuzzy membership functions, and then calculate the Fractional Anisotropy (FA) [18] of point (t,i) within the current neighborhood $N_{(t,i)}$, denoted as $a_{(t,i)}$. Since FA describes difference proportions of three tissue classes, the size of neighborhood $N_{(t,i)}$ is increased if its $a_{(t,i)}$ is greater than a prescribed threshold a_{high}, or is decreased if $a_{(t,i)}$ is smaller than a threshold a_{low}, or remains unchanged if $a_{(t,i)}$ is between the two thresholds. Finally, the neighborhood sizes are spatially smoothed across the images.

The 4-D image-adaptive clustering algorithm can be summarized as follows:

1. Set α, β, σ_s, σ_t, a_{high}, a_{low} and neighborhoods $N_{(t,i)}$, $N^{(s)'}_{(t,i)}$ and $N^{(t)'}_{(t,i)}$.
2. Compute fuzzy membership functions using Eq.(6).
3. Compute centroids using Eq.(7). In order to accelerate the calculation speed, we only calculate the centroids on down-sampled grid points and linearly interpolate the values at other locations.
4. Segment the images using the current fuzzy membership functions. If the algorithm were converged (the difference of the values of the objective function between two iterations is smaller than a prescribed threshold), then output the segmentation results, otherwise update the size of each spatiotemporal neighborhood $N_{(t,i)}$ and back to step (2).

3 Experimental Results

3.1 Segmentation of Simulated MR Brain Images

In this section, the simulated longitudinal MR brain images are used to evaluate the performance of CLASSIC. Three sets of simulated data are generated,

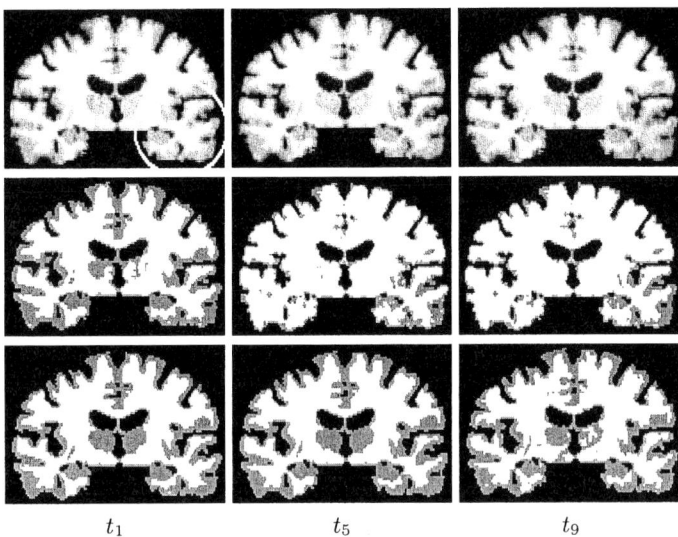

t_1 t_5 t_9

Fig. 1. An example of the segmentation results for simulated 4-D images with local (see the white circle) longitudinal intensity/contrast changes. Top: simulated images, middle: FANTASM results, bottom: CLASSIC results. It can be seen that for FANTASM, because of the intensity and contrast decrease in the spherical region, the overall centroid for WM becomes lower, which results in "over segmentation" of WM

including *(1)* global intensity/contrast decrease; *(2)* local intensity/contrast decrease; and *(3)* local atrophy with intensity/contrast decrease. To generate simulated longitudinal images, starting from a 3-D segmented template image, we set the means of CerebroSpinal Fluid (CSF), Gray Matter (GM) and White Matter (WM) to prescribed intensity values and insert random spatially correlated noise to the image. The initial values of the means of CSF, GM and WM of the first image I_{t_1} were set to 25, 85 and 105, respectively, and the standard deviation of the noise was set to 2. The intensity/contrast decrease is simulated by changing the means of GM and WM (m_g and m_w) with time t. The change rate of GM is defined as $r_g = (m_g(t_Y) - m_g(t_1))/m_g(t_1)/(Y - 1)$ and that of WM is defined as $r_w = (m_w(t_Y) - m_w(t_1))/m_w(t_1)(Y - 1)$. Different combinations of r_g and r_w yield different simulation results. r_g, r_w, $m_g(t_1)$ and $m_w(t_1)$ determine the change rate of contrast $r_c = (m_w(t_Y) - m_g(t_Y) - m_w(t_1) + m_g(t_1))/(m_w(t_1) - m_g(t_1))/(Y - 1)$. Local intensity/contrast changes are achieved by setting r_g and r_w to some values within a prescribed spherical region and setting them to zero outside that region. Gaussian function is used to smooth the change rates across the boundary of this spherical region in order to obtain smooth simulated images. The local atrophy is simulated by matching the Jacobian of the simulated deformation to the desired volumetric changes subject to smoothness and topology preserving constraints [19]. The amount of atrophy can be described by the shrinkage rate, $0 < r_s <= 1$. For example, $r_s = 0.9$ implies a 10% atrophy within the spherical area.

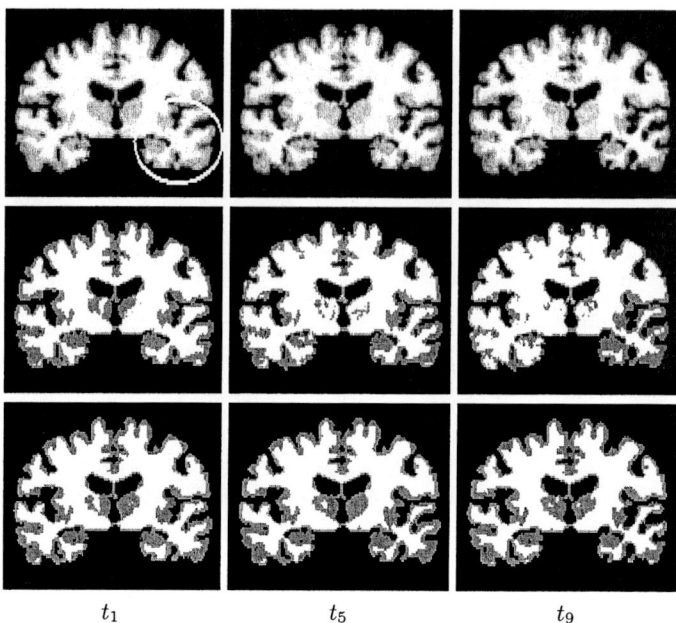

Fig. 2. An example of segmenting the simulated longitudinal data with local atrophy and intensity/contrast decrease. Top: the simulated images, the white circle indicates the spherical area within which atrophy and intensity decrease are simulated, middle: segmentation results of FANTASM, bottom: segmentation results of CLASSIC

CLASSIC and FANTASM were then used to segment these simulated images. In all the experiments, the parameters of CLASSIC were set as follows, $\alpha = 150$, $\beta = 200$, $\sigma_s = 25$, $\sigma_t = 35$, $a_{\text{high}} = 0.3$, $a_{\text{low}} = 0.1$, the initial size of $N_{(t,i)}^{(s)}$ was set to 35 (radius), and $N_{(t,i)}^{(t)}$, $N_{(t,i)}^{(s)'}$ and $N_{(t,i)}^{(t)'}$ were set as the immediate spatial or temporal neighborhoods of (t,i). A quantitative measure of the Correct Classification Rate (CCR) was used to evaluate the similarity between the segmented images and the ground truth. CCR is defined as the percentage of the number of brain voxels that have been correctly labeled according to the ground truth with respect to the total number of brain voxels.

Because of space limitation, we only illustrate some examples of the segmentation results of the simulated images with local intensity/contrast decrease, and with local atrophy. Fig.1 is an example of simulated local intensty/contrast decrease with $r_g = 0$, $r_w = -0.013$ and $r_c = -0.066$. Fig.2 shows an example of simulated local atrophy and intenstiy/contrast decrease, where the shrinkage rate $r_s = 0.8$, and the rates of intensity decrease are $r_g = -0.006$, $r_w = -0.013$, $r_c = -0.035$. The white circles in the images reflect the spherical area within which the atrophy and/or intensity decrease were simulated.

The results of CCR of these two examples are reported in Fig.3 and Fig.4 respectively. Comparing the segmentation results of FANTASM and those of CLASSIC, it can be seen that CLASSIC yields more temporally-consistent seg-

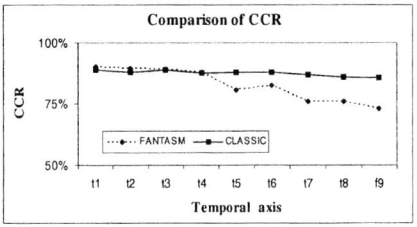 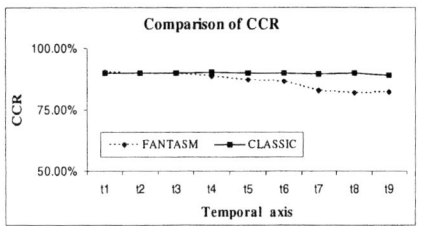

Fig. 3. CCR for the results in Fig.1   **Fig. 4.** CCR for the results in Fig.2

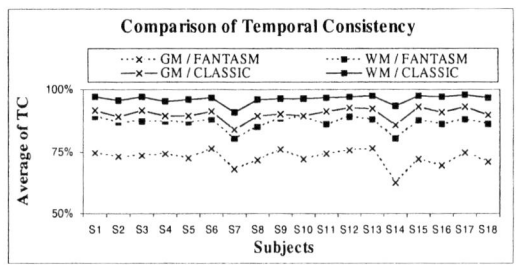

Fig. 5. Temporal consistency of GM and WM of different subjects. Small values indicate relatively less temporally-consistent segmentation

mentation results, while capturing the longitudinal deformations at the same time. Also, comparing either Fig.1 and Fig.2 or Fig.3 and Fig.4, we find that the results of FANTASM in Fig.2 are better than those of Fig.1. This is because their rates of contrast decrease are different. It can also be seen that CLASSIC adapts to local intensity variations quite well. For FANTASM, some larger local intensity variations, e.g. contrast decrease, may affect the segmentation results at other image locations. The reason is that FANTASM models the intensity changes through a very smooth gain-field, whereas the 4-D clustering algorithm of CLASSIC is fully-adaptive to local image intensity variations.

3.2 Segmentation of Real Longitudinal MR Brain Images

In this experiment, we used CLASSIC to segment 18 sets of longitudinal MR brain images from the BLSA data [9]. The nine serial scans of each subject were obtained during a period or nine consecutive years. In order to quantitatively analyze the segmentation results, we used a Temporal Consistency (TC) factor to reflect the temporal consistency of the segmentation results. Suppose $x_{(t,i)}^{\mathrm{seg}}$ is the segmentation result (label) of $x_{(t,i)}$, the segmentation results of voxel i across different times can be denoted as $x_{(t_1,i)}^{\mathrm{seg}}, x_{(t_2,i)}^{\mathrm{seg}}, ..., x_{(t_Y,i)}^{\mathrm{seg}}$. Denote L_i as the number of label changes of corresponding voxels across time, then the segmentation of the corresponding voxels is consistent if L_i is small, and vice versa. Therefore, the TC of segmentation results is measured by $TC = 1/S(\Omega') \sum_{i \in \Omega'} (1 - L_i/(Y-1))$,

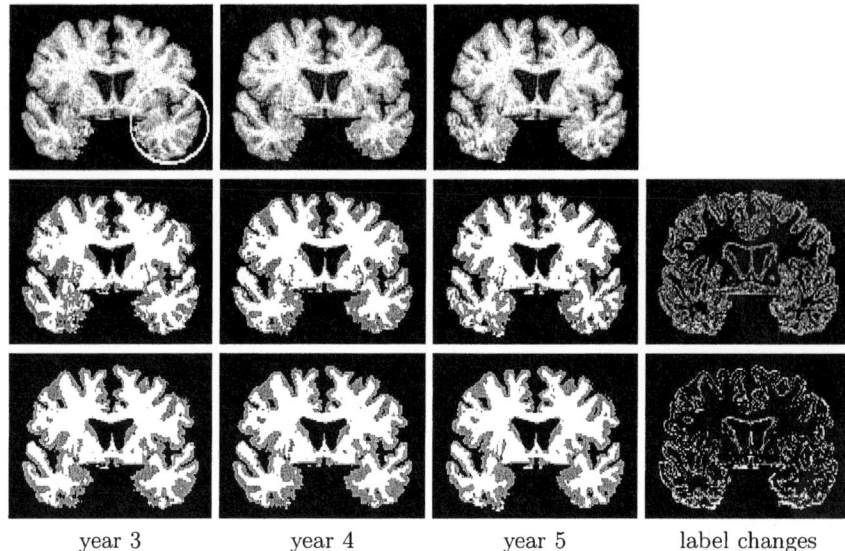

Fig. 6. Comparison of a typical segmentation result of BLSA data using CLASSIC and FANTASM. The top row shows the original serial scans after rigid transformations, the middle row indicates the segmentation results using FANTASM, and the bottom row gives the results of CLASSIC. The two images in the right column show the number of label changes L_i. It can be seen that CLASSIC gives not only spatially-smooth but also temporally-consistent segmentation results. It is worth noting that some atrophy is present between serial scans, thereby contributing to the label changes on the right

where Ω' is the voxel set of the region of interest, and $S(\Omega')$ is the number of voxels in Ω'. Fig.5 gives the TCs of GM and WM of the entire brains calculated from the segmentation results of CLASSIC and FANTASM on the 18 image series respectively. The figure shows that TCs of CLASSIC are much higher than those of FANTASM, which indicates CLASSIC achieves more temporally-consistent results. Fig.6 shows a typical segmentation result using CLASSIC and FANTASM respectively. For comparative purposes, the images shown are the aligned images using rigid transformations. The two images on the right illustrate the number of label changes L_i of corresponding voxels projected on the first image, where white indicates many label changes, and black means no changes across time. In summary CLASSIC got relatively smoother and temporally-consistent segmentation results than FANTASM for real MR image series.

Finally, it is worth noting that although the proposed CLASSIC incorporates temporal smoothness constraints of the segmentation results, it still maintains longitudinal change information. Moreover, CLASSIC captures these changes in a more stable and smooth way by means of the longitudinal deformations among the images and the parameters of the clustering algorithm. For example, Fig.7 shows the GM and WM volumes of the brains of 13 subjects using CLASSIC and FANTASM. Fig.8 gives similar plots calculated within a local spherical region

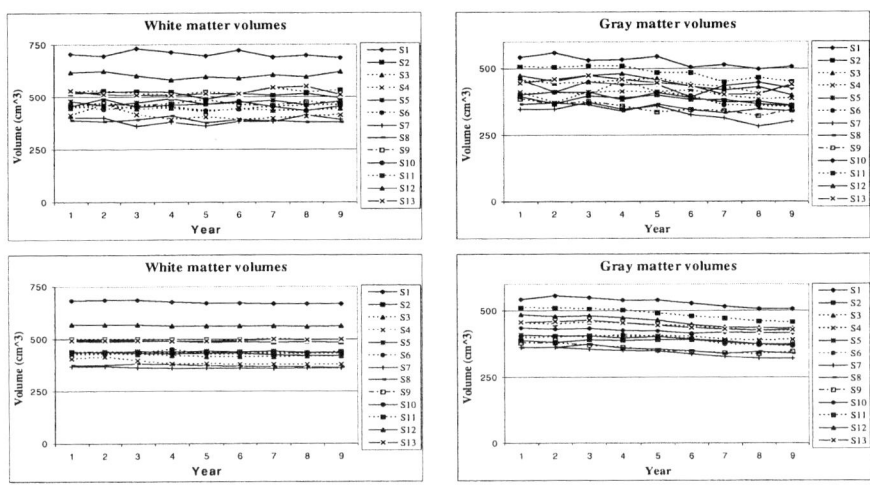

Fig. 7. GM and WM volumes of entire brains. Top: FANTASM, bottom: CLASSIC

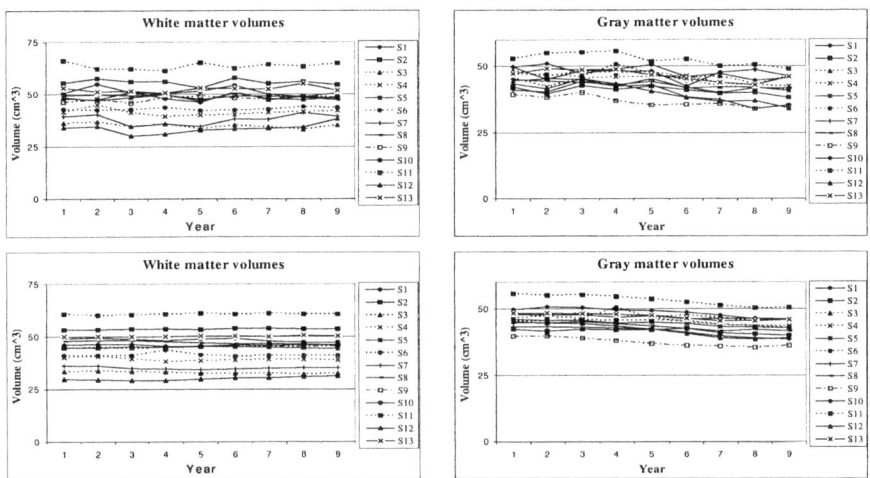

Fig. 8. GM and WM volumes in a local sphere. Top: FANTASM, bottom: CLASSIC

(see Fig.6). It can be seen that the curves of CLASSIC are quite smooth. Moreover, the GM and WM volumes calculated from the results of CLASSIC steadily decrease with time, which suggests tissue loss with aging. Although longitudinal analysis of MR brain images is much more complex, the experiments indicate that CLASSIC is a promising tool for longitudinally-consistent segmentation without compromising measurement of longitudinal atrophy.

4 Conclusion

We proposed an algorithm for segmentation of serial MR brain images, which yields spatially-adaptive and temporally-consistent segmentation results. The longitudinal deformations among the image series that reflect the underlying structural changes across time are also estimated. Experiments with simulated and real longitudinal MR brain images have confirmed the advantages of CLASSIC over more conventional 3-D segmentation analogous formulation.

References

1. Bezdek, J., Hall, L., Clarke, L.: Review of MR image segmentation techniques using pattern recognition. Medical Physics **20** (1993) 1033–1048
2. Pappas, T.: An adaptive clustering algorithm for image segmentation. IEEE Trans. on Signal Processing **40** (1992) 901–914
3. Udupa, J., Samarasekera, S.: Fuzzy connectedness and object definition: theory, algorithms and applications in image segmentation. Graph. Models Images Processing **58** (1996) 246–261
4. Brandt, M., Bohan, T., Kranmer, L., Fletcher, J.: Estimation of CSF, white and gray matter volumes in hydrocephalic children using fuzzy clustering of MR images. Comput. Med. Imag. Graph. **18** (1994) 25–34
5. Lim, K., Prefferbaum, A.: Segmentation of MR brain images into cerebrospinal fluid, white and gray matter. Journal of Comput. Assisted Tomogr. **13** (1989) 588–593
6. Pham, D., Prince, J.: Adaptive fuzzy segmentation of magnetic resonance images. IEEE Trans. on Medical Imaging **18** (1999) 737–752
7. Chen, W., Giger, M.: A fuzzy c-mean (FCM) based algorithm for intensity inhomogeneity correction and segmentation of MR images. In: IEEE International Symposium on Biomedical Imaging (ISBI 2004), Arlington, VA (2004) 1307–1310
8. Rezaee, M., van der Zwet, P., , Lelieveldt, B., van der Geest, R., Reiber, J.: A multiresolution image segmentation technique based on pyramidal segmentation and fuzzy clustering. IEEE Trans. on Image Processing **9** (2000) 1238–1248
9. Resnick, S., Goldszal, A., Davatzikos, C., Golski, S., Kraut, M., Metter, E., Bryan, R., Zonderman, A.: One-year age changes in MRI brain volumes in older adults. Cerebral Cortex **10** (2000) 464–472
10. Bezdek, J., Ehrlich, R., Full, W.: FCM: the fuzzy c-means clustering algorithm. Computers and Geosciences **10** (1984) 191–203
11. Guillemaud, R., Brady, M.: Estimating the bias field of MR images. IEEE Trans. on Medical Imaging **20** (1998) 57–68
12. Ahmed, M., Yamany, S., Mohamed, N., Farag, A., Moriarty, T.: A modified fuzzy c-means algorithm for bias field estimation and segmentation of MRI data. IEEE Trans. on Medical Imaging **21** (2002) 193–199
13. Liew, A., Leung, S., Lau, W.: Fuzzy image clustering incorporating spatial continuity. IEE Proc. Vis. Image Signal Process. **147** (2000) 185–192
14. Pham, D.: Spatial model for fuzzy clustering. Computer Vision and Image Understanding **84** (2001) 285–297
15. Shen, D., Davatzikos, C.: Measuring temporal morphological changes robustly in brain MR images via 4-D template warping. NeuroImage **21** (2004) 1508–1517

16. Shen, D., Davatzikos, C.: HAMMER: Hierarchical attribute matching mechanism for elastic registration. IEEE Trans. on Medical Imaging **21** (2002) 1421–1439
17. Nyul, G., Udupa, J., Zhang, X.: New variants of a method of MRI scale standardization. IEEE Trans. on Medical Imaging **19** (2000) 143–150
18. Zhu, C., Liu, F., Zhu, L., Jiang, T.: Anatomy dependent multi-context fuzzy clustering for separation of brain tissues in mr images. In: 2nd International Workshop on Medial Imaging and Augmented Reality, China (2004) 197–203
19. Karacali, B., Davatzikos, C.: Simulation of tissue atrophy using a topology preserving transformation model. Submit to IEEE Trans. on Medical Imaging (2004)

Robust Active Appearance Model Matching

Reinhard Beichel[1], Horst Bischof[1], Franz Leberl[1], and Milan Sonka[2]

[1] Institute for Computer Graphics and Vision, Graz University of Technology,
Inffeldgasse 16/2, A-8010 Graz, Austria
beichel@icg.tu-graz.ac.at
[2] Department of Electrical and Computer Engineering, The University of Iowa,
Iowa City, IA 52242 USA

Abstract. A novel robust active appearance model (AAM) matching algorithm is presented. The method consists of two main stages. First, initial residuals are clustered by a non parametric mean shift mode detection step. Second, modes without gross outliers are selected using an objective function. Robustness of the matching procedure is demonstrated on a variety of examples with different noise conditions. The proposed algorithm outperformed the conventional AAM matching on images with gross disturbances and can tolerate up to 40% of disturbed data.

1 Introduction

Active Appearance Models (AMMs) introduced by Cootes et al. [1,2] have proven to be a useful method for the segmentation of medical image data. Applications reported in the literature include the segmentation of knee parts in MRI data [1], the heart in MRI data [3,4,5] and stress echocardiograms [6], parts of the human brain in MR images [7], or the diaphragm in CT data [8], to name a few. One reason for the popularity of AAMs is that knowledge learned in the training phase about object shape and texture (appearance) is utilized for segmentation.

Despite the success of AAMs in medical image analysis and other application domains, problems are encountered in cases where the object gray-value appearance is significantly changed due to gross disturbances. Here, the learned model will fail to describe the whole object to be segmented correctly. Such cases occur quite frequent in clinical routine and may have several reasons including artificial changes of organ appearance (e.g. implants), pathological changes of organ appearance (e.g. tumors), missing data, or image acquisition artifacts. The impact of disturbances in gray-value appearance can range from a partially erroneous result to a complete failure to match the target object. Consequently, another (manual) procedure may have to be used for segmentation.

In cases of gross disturbances, the AAM based segmentation method should match undisturbed portions of input data and utilize a priori knowledge gained in the learning phase of the AAM to estimate the plausible object shape and appearance in the disturbed regions. Such a robust behavior can be obtained by treating missing or abnormal information (outliers) differently compared to undisturbed information (inliers) during the model matching process. The goal of the matching step is to minimize the difference between model and image data (residual) in order to achieve a good segmentation. In the standard AAM framework proposed by Cootes et al. [1,2], matching is treated as a least-squares optimization problem. Because of the quadratic error measure (L_2 norm), it is sensitive to outliers and limits the performance of AAMs.

Approaches to make AAMs more robust have been reported by Edwards et al. [9], Stegmann at al. [10], and Gross et al. [11]. All reported methods try to reject outliers solely based on the magnitude of residuals observed during the AAM matching. In general, a large residual is not an information that should be discarded a priori. For example, the error might be due to an initial model displacement. In this case, the error is a valuable information. If discarded, a slower convergence of the AAM or a complete failure to match image data might result. Therefore, treating the error information of an AAM only in terms of its magnitude is not a generally viable solution.

In this paper we propose a novel robust AAM matching algorithm. Residuals are analyzed by means of a Mean Shift based mode detection step and selected according to the impact on the matching process. This allows an individual adaptation to disturbances in input data. Compared to other methods, no assumptions regarding "normal" residuals are made. This translates into a higher flexibility regarding the types of disturbances that can be handled without adjusting the algorithm.

2 Methods

2.1 Robust Active Appearance Models (RAAMs)

The proposed robust AAM matching method builds on the AAM framework described by Cootes et al. in [1,2] and requires that training data is free of disturbances. During standard AAM matching, updates of model parameter vector $\mathbf{p}$ are obtained by evaluating

$$\delta \mathbf{p} = - \left([\mathbf{J}(\mathbf{r})^T \mathbf{J}(\mathbf{r})]^{-1} \mathbf{J}(\mathbf{r})^T \right) \mathbf{r}(\mathbf{p}) = -\mathbf{R}\mathbf{r}(\mathbf{p}) \qquad (1)$$

based on the observed actual residual $\mathbf{r}$, calculated by comparing the gray-values of the model and the image data underneath [1,2]. In Eq. (1), $\mathbf{J}(\mathbf{r}) = \partial \mathbf{r}/\partial \mathbf{p}$ denotes the Jacobian of $\mathbf{r}$ and $\mathbf{R}$ is the prediction matrix. To increase the robustness of AAMs to gross disturbances (outliers) in the input image, "misleading" coefficient updates (incorrect $\delta \mathbf{p}$) must be avoided. Therefore, inliers and outliers must be identified. If the outliers in $\mathbf{r}(\mathbf{p})$ are known, Eq. (1) can be adjusted accordingly. Let $\mathbf{v}_{sel} = (v_1, \ldots, v_M)^T$ be the selection vector with respect to the residual $\mathbf{r} = (r_1, \ldots, r_M)^T$ with the following property:

$$v_i = \begin{cases} 1 & : \quad r_i \in \mathcal{I}(\mathbf{r}) \\ 0 & : \quad r_i \in \mathcal{O}(\mathbf{r}) \end{cases} \qquad (2)$$

where the set of inliers is denoted as $\mathcal{I}(\mathbf{r})$ and the set of outliers as $\mathcal{O}(\mathbf{r})$. Then the rows of the Jacobian $\mathbf{J}(\mathbf{r})$ are rearranged into the vector $\mathbf{J}(\mathbf{r})_{sel}$. $\mathbf{J}(\mathbf{r})_{sel}$ denotes the components of $\mathbf{J}(\mathbf{r})$ for which $\mathbf{v}_{sel}$ is equal to one:

$$\mathbf{J}(\mathbf{r})_{sel} = \mathbf{J}(\mathbf{r})_{[\mathbf{v}_{sel}==1,:]} \ . \tag{3}$$

According to Eq. (1), a new matrix $\mathbf{R}_{sel}$ and a new parameter update vector $\delta \mathbf{p}_{sel}$ can be calculated, assuming that $\mathcal{I}(\mathbf{r})$ consists of at least one element. By using $\delta \mathbf{p}_{sel}$ instead of $\delta \mathbf{p}$, only inliers are used for the update of model parameters $\mathbf{p}$ during matching. A successive degeneration of the model, due to outliers, can be avoided. Note, that $\mathbf{R}_{sel}$ has to be recalculated in each iteration of the matching procedure, since the residual $\mathbf{r}(\mathbf{p})$ changes during matching.

The crucial step in this procedure is the classification of the residual into inliers and outliers. As explained in the introduction, classifying outliers only according to the magnitude of the residual $\mathbf{r}(\mathbf{p})$ is not sufficient. Therefore, we propose a robust AAM matching procedure based on optimization of an objective function:

1. *Initialize the AAM with the parameter vector $\mathbf{p}_0$ based on an initial estimate.*
2. *Calculate the initial residual $\tilde{\mathbf{r}}(\mathbf{p}_0)$ by roughly aligning the texture vector of the model $\mathbf{g}_m(\mathbf{p}_0)$ to the image texture vector $\mathbf{g}_i(\mathbf{p}_0)$ (model frame):*

$$\tilde{\mathbf{r}}(\mathbf{p}_0) = \mathbf{g}_i(\mathbf{p}_0) - a(\mathbf{g}_m(\mathbf{p}_0)) \ , \tag{4}$$

where $a(\mathbf{g})$ denotes the alignment function.
3. *Analyze the modes of the initial residual $\tilde{\mathbf{r}}(\mathbf{p}_0)$ (Section 2.2).*
4. *Choose an optimal (outlier-free) combination of modes based on the optimization of an objective function (Section 2.3).*
5. *Utilize only pixels covered by the finally selected mode combination in the intrinsic iterative AAM matching process.*

Steps 1 and 2 are similar to the standard AAM matching steps. In step 3 the initial residual $\tilde{\mathbf{r}}(\mathbf{p}_0)$ is partitioned into modes by using a Mean Shift based algorithm (Section 2.2). Based on the partitioning, the combination of modes is optimized according to an objective function. The goal is to select only the modes associated with $\mathcal{I}(\mathbf{r})$ and to reject the modes associated with $\mathcal{O}(\mathbf{r})$. Mode combinations are tested by running an *intrinsic AAM matching* followed by the evaluation of the objective function (Section 2.3). Finally, the best mode combination is selected. The results obtained with this selection are taken as the final matching result.

Intrinsic AAM matching deviates from the standard AAM matching in two ways:

1. Prior to each parameter update during *intrinsic AAM matching*, a selection vector $\mathbf{v}_{sel}$ is generated and utilized for calculating $\mathbf{r}_{sel}$, $\mathbf{R}_{sel}$ and $\delta \mathbf{p}_{sel}$, respectively. The generation of $\mathbf{v}_{sel}$ is based on an estimate $\tilde{\mathbf{r}}$ for the residual $\mathbf{r}$. $\tilde{\mathbf{r}}$ is calculated in an analogous way to Eq. (4) using the rough alignment function $a(\mathbf{g})$. The components of $\mathbf{v}_{sel}$ are set to one, if the corresponding value in $\tilde{\mathbf{r}}$ is covered by the actual mode combination under evaluation.

2. A z-score function $z(\mathbf{x}) = [\mathbf{x} - \mu(\mathbf{x})\mathbf{i}]/\sigma(\mathbf{x})$ is applied during residual calculation for the alignment of the image and the model texture vectors

$$\mathbf{r}(\mathbf{p}) = z\left(\mathbf{g}_i(\mathbf{p})\right) - z\left(\mathbf{g}_m(\mathbf{p})\right), \qquad (5)$$

where the mean of the components of vector $\mathbf{x}$ is denoted as $\mu(\mathbf{x})$, the standard deviation as $\sigma(\mathbf{x})$ and the unit vector as $\mathbf{i}$. Based on $\mathbf{r}(\mathbf{p})$ and $\mathbf{v}_{sel}$, $\mathbf{r}_{sel}(\mathbf{p})$ is generated by taking only components of $\mathbf{r}(\mathbf{p})$ for which $\mathbf{v}_{sel}$ is equal to one and used in combination with $\mathbf{R}_{sel}$ for a parameter update: $\delta \mathbf{p}_{sel} = -\mathbf{R}_{sel}\mathbf{r}_{sel}(\mathbf{p})$.

2.2 Mode Analysis of Residuals

To find the modes of the initial residual $\tilde{\mathbf{r}}(\mathbf{p}_0)$, the mean shift algorithm is utilized [12, 13]. Given a set of points $X = \{\mathbf{x}_i \in \mathbf{R}^d | i = 1, \ldots, n\}$, the mean shift vector at point $\mathbf{x}$ is defined as

$$\mathbf{m}_{h,G}(\mathbf{x}) = \frac{\sum_{i=1}^{n} g\left(\left\|\frac{\mathbf{x}-\mathbf{x}_i}{h}\right\|^2\right) \mathbf{x}_i}{\sum_{i=1}^{n} g\left(\left\|\frac{\mathbf{x}-\mathbf{x}_i}{h}\right\|^2\right)} - \mathbf{x} \qquad (6)$$

where h is the bandwidth parameter of the radial symmetric kernel $G(\mathbf{u}) = c_{k,d}g(\|\mathbf{u}\|^2)$ with the profile function g; $c_{k,p}$ is a normalization constant. The mean shift vector has the following property: $\mathbf{m}_{h,G}(\mathbf{x})$ always points in the direction of the maximum probability density function (PDF) ascent.

For our application, the boundaries between modes are of interest to partition the residual $\tilde{\mathbf{r}}(\mathbf{p}_0) = (r_1, \ldots, r_M)^T$ into modes. Therefore, the valleys between the modes need to be found. Following the mean shift vector $\mathbf{m}_{h,G}(\mathbf{x})$ would lead to a mode (local maximum of PDF). However, by reversing the direction of $\mathbf{m}_{h,G}(\mathbf{x})$ local minima, representing the boundaries between modes, can be found by the following procedure:

1. Repeat for each $\mathbf{x}_l \in X$ with $X = \{r_i\}_{i=1,\ldots,M}$, the set of all components of residual $\tilde{\mathbf{r}}(\mathbf{p}_0)$, and $l = 1, \ldots, n$:
   (a) Set $\mathbf{y}_0 = \mathbf{x}_l$.
   (b) Shift each point proportionally to the negative gradient of the PDF (mean shift) until it converges to a valley point by iteratively computing:

$$\mathbf{y}_{j+1} = \mathbf{y}_j - \mathbf{m}_{h,G}(\mathbf{y}_j) \quad j = 0, 1, 2, \ldots \qquad (7)$$

   (c) Store the obtained valley point: $\mathbf{p}_{\mathbf{x}_l} = \mathbf{y}_{end}$.
2. Quantize all valley points into bins: $\tilde{\mathbf{p}}_{\mathbf{x}_i} = q(\mathbf{p}_{\mathbf{x}_i})$.
3. Find all the different valley points in $P = \{\tilde{\mathbf{p}}_{\mathbf{x}_i}\}_{i=1,\ldots,n}$ and store them as a list of scalars ($d = 1$) in $B_X = [b_1, \ldots, b_{o+1}]$ where $b_i \leq b_j$ for $i < j$. Modes are stored in $M_X = \{\mathcal{M}_1, \ldots, \mathcal{M}_o\}$, whereas mode $\mathcal{M}_i$ is limited by the valley points b_i and b_{i+1}.

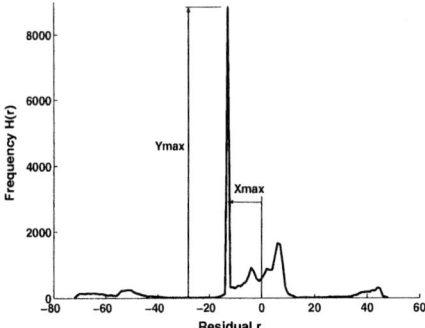

Fig. 1. Histogram $H(\mathbf{r})$ of a residual $\mathbf{r}$. $Y_{max}(\mathbf{r})$ denotes the maximum value of $H(\mathbf{r})$ and $X_{max}(\mathbf{r})$ the magnitude of the corresponding residual

Modes consisting only of a few data points are of secondary importance, since they have hardly any influence on the result. Therefore, modes with less than $T = \gamma \max_{i=1,\ldots,o}\{|\mathcal{M}_i|\}$ ($0 \leq \gamma < 1$) data points can be merged with neighboring modes, and B_X and M_X are updated accordingly. The number of remaining modes is denoted by $\tilde{o}$. The choice of γ depends on the selected kernel bandwidth h, which defines the sensitivity regarding small modes.

2.3 Mode Selection

The main idea behind the objective function for mode selection is as follows: gross outliers in images usually lead to a degeneration of AAMs during matching. For the evaluation of the AAM matching performance, an objective function is utilized for the selection of a mode combination. A suitable objective function should consider two criteria. First, the quality of the match should be high. Ideally, a matched AAM would result in a residual vector $\mathbf{r}$ equal to $\mathbf{0}$. Therefore, the histogram $H(\mathbf{r})$ would show a single peak at the residual value of 0 with the peak height equaling to M. Peak heights lower than M or a peak occurring at other residual values than zero indicate a less desirable match (Fig. 1). Second, the match should be based on as many (inlier) points as possible. It is also crucial that no assumptions regarding a "normal" magnitude of residuals are made, since large residual values might provide important information for AAM matching. The objective function described below takes this into account. It weights the peak height with a combination of the peak offset and the number of data points used for matching. Let $S = \wp(M_X) \setminus \{\emptyset\} = \{\mathcal{S}_1, \ldots, \mathcal{S}_l\}$ be the set of all possible mode combinations with at least one mode selected where $\wp$ denotes the power set and $l = |S| = 2^{\tilde{o}} - 1$. Given S, our goal is to find an optimal mode combination $\mathcal{S}_j$ with $\mathcal{Q}(\mathcal{S}_j) = \max_{i=1,\ldots,l}\{\mathcal{Q}(\mathcal{S}_i)\}$.

Let $\mathbf{r}_{\mathcal{S}_i}$ be the final residual (Eq. 5) after the *intrinsic AAM matching* based on the actual selected modes $\mathcal{S}_i$. The distribution of residual $\mathbf{r}_{\mathcal{S}_i}$ is analyzed by calculating the histogram $H(\mathbf{r}_{\mathcal{S}_i})$. The maximum value $Y_{max}(\mathbf{r}_{\mathcal{S}_i})$ of $H(\mathbf{r}_{\mathcal{S}_i})$

is calculated and the magnitude of the corresponding residual is denoted as $X_{max}(\mathbf{r}_{S_i})$ (Fig. 1). We define the following objective function

$$Q(S_i) = Y_{max}(\mathbf{r}_{S_i}) f_{and}(w_o, w_s) , \tag{8}$$

where $f_{and}(w_o, w_s) = 2w_o w_s / (w_o + w_s)$ represents an AND-conjunction of two weighting functions w_o and w_s. The peak offset (quality of match) is taken into account by the weighting function $w_o = \alpha^{-|X_{max}(\mathbf{r}_{S_i})|}$ and the number of residual components used is reflected in $w_s = 1/M \sum_{\mathcal{M}_j \in S_i} |\mathcal{M}_j|$. The values of both weighting functions range between zero and one. The relative influence of w_o and w_s is adjusted by the factor α. Both weights are combined by the function f_{and} and attenuate the peak value $Y_{max}(\mathbf{r}_{S_i})$.

Since the number of modes is usually rather small, an exhaustive search is used to find the best mode combination. In the case where a lot of modes are found, the use of a greedy search strategy is possible, but may yield suboptimal results. If a priori knowledge about the disturbance is available (e.g. disturbance is dark), it can be incorporated into the search strategy.

3 Case Studies

To evaluate the performance of the RAAM, segmentation results obtained with a standard AAM (with z-score alignment; see Eq. 5) were compared to RAAM results on proximal phalanx (Fig. 2(a)) and metacarpal bone (Fig. 2(b)) X-ray images of the small finger. Forty images showing both bones were available. Reference tracings were made manually by a physician, and landmarks used for model building were placed automatically by using the method proposed by Thodberg [14]. The gray-values of the images were scaled to $[0, 255]$. Image data is disturbed by natural or artificially generated outliers. The following RAAM parameters were used in all experiments: $g(x) = \exp(-x/2)$, $h = 4$, $\gamma = 0.05$, and $\alpha = 1.03$. For model building, the number of principal component analysis (PCA) modes used to represent shape, texture, and the final model were selected to explaining 99% of the variation present in training data.

Matching performance was measured by the relative overlap error $E_{rol\%} = 100\% (|A_{ref} \oplus A_{model}|)/|A_{ref}|$ where A_{ref} and A_{model} are object masks for the

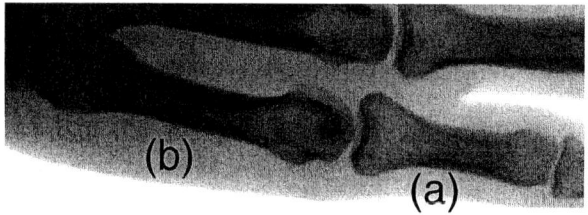

Fig. 2. Example of a X-ray image of the small finger. (a) Proximal phalanx. (b) Metacarpal bone

reference segmentation and the matched model, respectively. The operator ⊕ denotes the XOR operation between masks and the number of object pixels is denoted by $|A|$. Reference masks were generated by converting reference tracings of the object contours. The relative overlap error is suitable to measure not only the success of the matching process, but also the degree of failure.

For interpreting the distribution of the relative overlap errors of test series, box-and-whisker plots were used [15]. The box has lines at the lower quartile, median, and upper quartile values. The whiskers show the extent of the rest of the data. Outliers are displayed by a '+' symbol.

Both, AAM and RAAM matching started with identical initial model parameters. Images, showing original information and disturbances, have been grayvalue transformed for better visibility.

3.1 Proximal Phalanx X-Ray Images with Synthetic Disturbances

Performance of AAMs and RAAMs was compared using the undisturbed original data and the artificially corrupted images (Fig. 3) using a leave-one-out approach. Models were generated and trained on 39 complete proximal phalanx images, and matching performance was subsequently evaluated on the left-out image. The training process was repeated 40 times, always leaving out a different data set for evaluation.

Results. Full object masks were used for error calculation with the exception of the test case occlusion pattern n (Fig. 3(a)), where the occluded part was ignored for error calculation. Full masks allow to measure the degree of model degeneration caused by local disturbances, but are not meaningful if only dis-

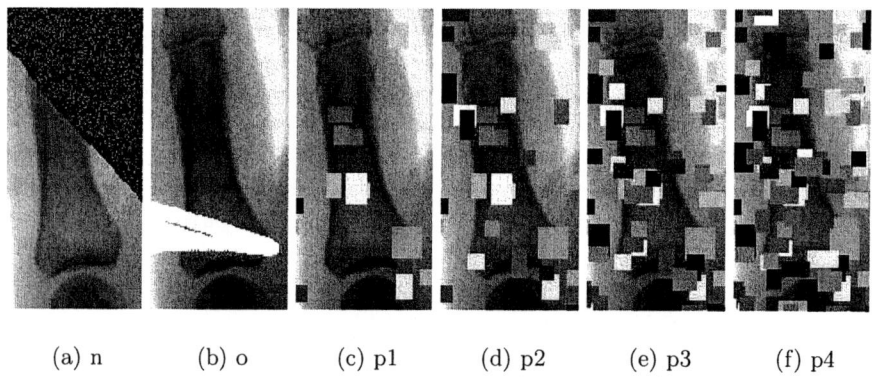

(a) n (b) o (c) p1 (d) p2 (e) p3 (f) p4

Fig. 3. Occlusion patters used in combination with proximal phalanx X-ray images (Section 3.1). Disturbance patterns were fixed in all 40 proximal phalanx images. (a) Occlusion noise (normally distributed within range of $[-50, 50]$). (b) Constant disturbance (gray-value: 255). (c)–(f) Occlusion with varying density. Gray-values of occluding boxes are chosen randomly between [0,255]. (a)–(f) Effective mean occlusion of the 40 target objects: $n : 29.2\%$, $o : 15.5\%$, $p1 : 8.2\%$, $p2 : 19.8\%$, $p3 : 39.5\%$, and $p4 : 64.4\%$

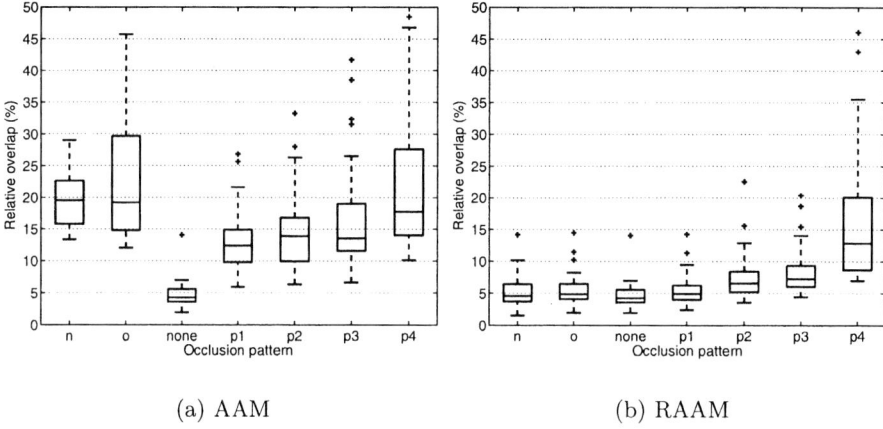

Fig. 4. Box-and-whisker plots of the relative overlap error for AAM and RAAM on proximal phalanx X-ray images (Section 3.1). Each plot is based on leave-on-out experiments using 40 cases. (a) Standard AAM. (b) Robust AAM

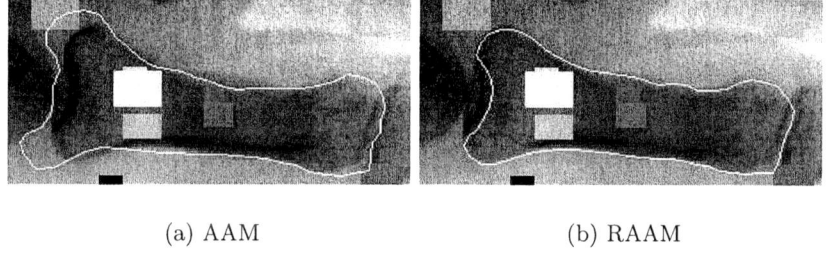

Fig. 5. Example of matching results on images with synthetic disturbances (Section 3.1). The pattern p1 was used to occlude the image

turbed image data is available in a larger area (pattern n). A comparison of the relative overlap error for AAM and RAAM algorithms is given in Fig. 4. For the case with no occlusion pattern applied, the results are essentially the same. In all other cases with disturbed image data (patterns n, o, p1–p4), the RAAM algorithm had a considerably lower median of the overlap error than the standard AAM (see also example in Fig. 5). The RAAM algorithm tolerates occlusion rates of up to 40% well, and fails in the cases of the occlusion pattern p4 with an average object occlusion rate of 64.4%.

3.2 Proximal Phalanx X-Ray Image with Implants

A proximal phalanx X-ray image with a disturbance, caused by a medical intervention, was used for comparison of the AAM and RAAM methods. Fig. 6(a) shows the test image with a reference tracing of the bone contour. When compared to a normal proximal phalanx (Fig. 2), several differences can be observed.

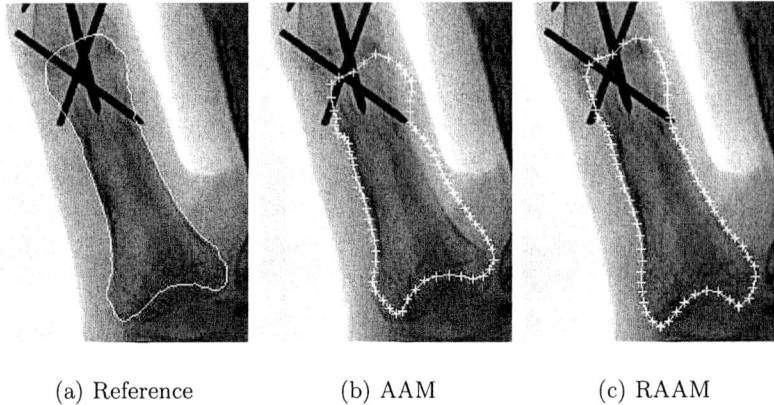

(a) Reference   (b) AAM   (c) RAAM

Fig. 6. Proximal phalanx X-ray image with implants. (a) Manual reference tracing. (b) AAM and (c) RAAM matching result. Landmarks are represented by '+' symbols and are connected by white lines

First, the patient is suffering from rheumatoid arthritis, causing lower bone density and pathological changes of the joints, compared to normals. Second, an arthrodesis of the proximal interphalangeal joint (top of bone in Fig. 6(a)) of the finger with wires for fixation, leading to union of the of the bones, has been carried out. This and the data set presented in Section 3.3 (metacarpal bone data) are of particular interest, since model-based segmentation techniques are promising for the automated assessment of rheumatoid arthritis [16]. Training of AAM and RAAM was performed on the 40 segmented (normal) data sets available. After training, models were applied to the test case.

Results. The AAM and RAAM matching result is shown in Fig. 6(b) and Fig. 6(c), respectively. The relative overlap error was calculated as 33.66% for the AAM and 15.53% for the RAAM. The AAM is severely influenced by the changed object appearance and fails to deliver an acceptable result. The RAAM does not show such a behavior. In case of the RAAM, segmentation errors mainly occur in the region of the joint which is affected by rheumatoid arthritis.

3.3 Metacarpal Bone X-Ray Image with Implant and Severely Changed Shape

The metacarpal bone X-ray image of the small finger that was used for comparison is depicted in Fig. 7. In the area of the metacarpophalangeal joint, a silicone-spacer-implant for metacarpophalangeal arthroplasty in rheumatoid arthritis is present. The implant causes a gross disturbance in gray-value appearance combined with a severe shape change of the metacarpal joint (parts of the bone are missing). In addition, the carpometacarpal joint shows pathological changes caused by rheumatoid arthritis (compare with Fig. 2(b)). Learning and training of the AAM and the RAAM was performed on the 40 healthy metacarpal bone contours as described above. Testing was done on the image shown in Fig. 7.

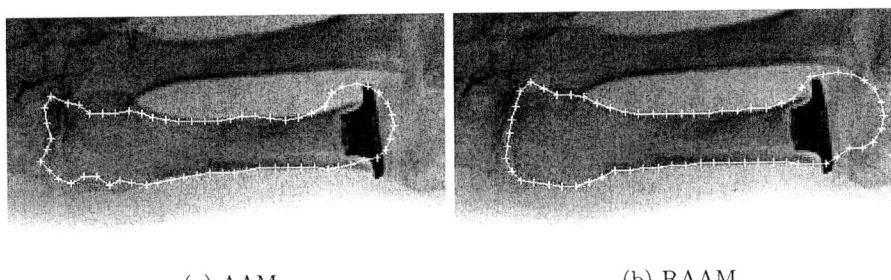

(a) AAM (b) RAAM

Fig. 7. Metacarpal bone data. (a) AAM and (b) RAAM matching result. Landmark points are represented by '+' symbols and are connected by white lines

Results. The standard AAM matching result is shown in Fig. 7(a). The contour is atypical for a metacarpal bone (Fig. 2(b)). Areas without shape changes (adjacent joints) are not well segmented. The gray-value disturbance has a clear impact on the segmentation result. In contrast, the RAAM correctly segments the bone structures without severe shape changes (Fig. 7(b)). This example also demonstrates the inherent limits of RAAM matching—and more generally all model based segmentation approaches (including standard AAMs)—the model can not compensate for severe pathological/artificial changes in object shape not learned previously. However, in case of the RAAM result (Fig. 7(b)) a priori knowledge is utilized plausibly. Hence, the contour in the carpometacarpal joint area can for example be used as a starting point for the quantification of the stage of the rheumatoid arthritis based on a snake approach (see [16]).

4 Discussion and Conclusion

While the presented RAAM method has many advantages, a decrease of image analysis speed is experienced due to the increase of the computation complexity. The search for an optimal mode combination requires that all $2^{\tilde{o}} - 1$ individual combinations be tested, where $\tilde{o}$ denotes the final number of modes after mode merging (Section 2.2). The average for $\tilde{o}$ was 2.2 in case of the 40 undisturbed proximal phalanx images. This number increased with the increased image disturbance level. The more modes are found in the process, the more mode combinations need to be analyzed (*intrinsic AAM matching* and objective function evaluation). Hence, a trade-off between selectivity (kernel size) and processing time has to be made. If processing speed is of the utmost importance, the RAAMs may be employed selectively to improve performance in cases known to include metal implants, tumors, or image artifacts as described above while conventional AAMs can be used in the standard situations. The method selection can easily be done interactively when reviewing the images prior to the analysis.

A fully automated robust active appearance model matching approach was presented and compared to the standard matching method. No a priori assumptions regarding the kind of disturbance were made. The RAAM algorithm was universally applicable to different types of segmentation tasks. The performed experiments demonstrated that the RAAM segmentation method outperformed the standard AAM technique in all tested cases exhibiting gross outliers of grayvalue appearance. This is an expected outcome, since gross outliers severely influence the least squares optimization of the standard matching algorithm causing segmentation failures. In comparison, RAAMs tolerated disturbances up to approximately 40% of the object-of-interest area, as demonstrated by the reported experiments.

Acknowledgment

The authors thank Philipp Peloschek (Medical University of Vienna) and Georg Langs (Graz University of Technology) for contributing segmented X-ray images of the small finger. This work was supported in part by the Austrian Science Fund (FWF) under Grants P14897-N04, P17066-N04, and P17083-N04; and by NIH-NHLBI R01-HL071809.

References

1. Cootes, T.F., Edwards, G.J., Taylor, C.J.: Active appearance models. In Burkhardt, H., Neumann, B., eds.: Proc. European Conference on Computer Vision. Volume 2., Springer (1998) 484–498
2. Cootes, T.F., Taylor, C.J.: Statistical models of appearance for computer vision. Technical report, Division of Imaging Science and Biomedical Engineering, University of Manchester (2004) available at http://www.isbe.man.ac.uk/~bim/refs.html.
3. Mitchell, S.C., Lelieveldt, B.P.F., van der Geest, R., Schaap, J., Reiber, J.H.C., Sonka, M.: Segmentation of cardiac MR images: An active appearance model approach. In: Proceedings SPIE, Medical Imaging - Image Processing, Vol. 3979, Bellingham WA, SPIE (2000) 224–234
4. Stegmann, M.B.: Analysis of 4D cardiac magnetic resonance images. Journal of The Danish Optical Society, DOPS-NYT (2001) 38–39
5. Mitchell, S.C., Bosch, J.G., Lelieveldt, B.P.F., van der Geest, R.J., Reiber, J.H.C., Sonka, M.: 3-D Active Appearance Models: Segmentation of cardiac MR and ultrasound images. **21** (2002) 1167–1178
6. Bosch, H.G., Mitchell, S.C., Lelieveldt, B.P.F., Sonka, M., Nijland, F., Reiber, J.H.C.: Feasibility of fully automated border detection on stress echocardiograms by active appearance models (abstract). Circulation **102, No. 18 (Suppl II)** (2000) II-633
7. Cootes, T.F., Beeston, C., Edwards, G.J., Taylor, C.J.: A unified framework for atlas matching using active appearance models. In: Proc. Int. Conf. on Image Processing in Medical Imaging, Springer (1999) 322–333
8. Beichel, R., Gotschuli, G., Sorantin, E., Leberl, F., Sonka, M.: Diaphragm dome surface segmentation in CT data sets: A 3D active appearance model approach. In Sonka, M., Fitzpatrick, J.M., eds.: SPIE: Medical Imaging: Image Processing. Volume 4684. (2002) 475–484

9. Edwards, G.J., Cootes, T.F., Taylor, C.J.: Advances in active appearance models. In: Proc. International Conference on Computer Vision. (1999) 137–142
10. Stegmann, M.B., Fisker, R., Ersbøll, B.K.: Extending and applying active appearance models for automated, high precision segmentation in different image modalities. In Austvoll, I., ed.: Proc. 12th Scandinavian Conference on Image Analysis - SCIA 2001, Bergen, Norway, Stavanger, Norway, NOBIM (2001) 90–97
11. Gross, R., Matthews, I., Baker, S.: Constructing and fitting active appearance models with occlusion. In: Proceedings of the IEEE Workshop on Face Processing in Video. (2004)
12. Fukunaga, K., Hostetler, L.: The estimation of the gradient of a density function, with applications in pattern recognition. **21** (1975) 32–40
13. Comaniciu, D., Meer, P.: Mean shift: a robust approach toward feature space analysis. **24** (2002) 603–619
14. Thodberg, H.H.: Shape modelling and analysis minimum description length shape and appearance models. In: Information Processing in Medical Imaging - IPMI2003, Springer (2003) 51 – 62
15. Tukey, J.W. In: Exploratory Data Analysis. Addison-Wesley (1977)
16. Langs, G., Peloschek, P., Bischof, H.: ASM driven snakes in rheumatoid arthritis assessment. In: Proceedings of 13th Scandinavian Conference on Image Analysis, SCIA 2003, Goeteborg, Sweden, Lecture Notes in Computer Science, LNCS2749. (2003) 454–461

Simultaneous Segmentation and Registration of Contrast-Enhanced Breast MRI

Chen Xiaohua[1], Michael Brady[1], Jonathan Lok-Chuen Lo[1], and Niall Moore[2]

[1] Wolfson Medical Vision Laboratory,
Robotics Research Group,
University of Oxford, Oxford, UK
{xchen, jmb, jlo}@robots.ox.ac.uk
[2] MRI unit, John Radcliffe Hospital,
Oxford, UK

Abstract. Breast Contrast-Enhanced MRI (ce-MRI) requires a series of images to be acquired before, and repeatedly after, intravenous injection of a contrast agent. Breast MRI segmentation based on the differential enhancement of image intensities can assist the clinician detect suspicious regions. Image registration between the temporal data sets is necessary to compensate for patient motion, which is quite often substantial. Although segmentation and registration are usually treated as separate problems in medical image analysis, they can naturally benefit a great deal from each other. In this paper, we propose a scheme for simultaneous segmentation and registration of breast ce-MRI. It is developed within a Bayesian framework, based on a *maximum a posteriori* estimation method. A pharmacokinetic model and Markov Random Field model have been incorporated into the framework in order to improve the performance of our algorithm. Our method has been applied to the segmentation and registration of clinical ce-MR images. The results show the potential of our methodology to extract useful information for breast cancer detection.

1 Introduction

The use of contrast-enhanced magnetic resonance imaging (ce-MRI) has gained considerable attention in recent years, not least for the early detection of breast cancer [1]. Conventional MRI often yields little or no contrast difference between abnormalities and normal tissue. Contrast agents, commonly gadolinium diethylene triamine pentaacetic acid (Gd-DTPA), are used to improve the sensitivity to cancerous tissue, because they highlight areas with increased vascular density, which correlate with tumors. Regular scans of the breast (approximately every one minute) are made before, during and after the administration of the contrast agent. In this paper, a total of 7 scans were made for all the experiments. The resulting signal enhancement-time curve is in the basis for differentiating various tissue types within the breast [2][3][4][5].

The goal of our work is to segment the breast into different regions, each corresponding to a different tissue, and to identify tissue regions judged abnormal, based on the signal enhancement-time information. There are a number of problems that render this task complex. Not least, the images are often noisy, and patient movement occurring during the scan can be rapid and substantial.

In this paper, we propose a simultaneous segmentation and registration method to solve both the segmentation and patient motion correction problems for breast ce-MRI. We show that interleaving segmentation and registration in the way that we propose, is mutually beneficial for both problems; we get better results both for segmentation and for registration. Our simultaneous segmentation and registration (SSR) algorithm is developed within a Bayesian framework, based on a *maximum a posteriori* (MAP) estimation method. We use a pharmacokinetic model of the dynamic MR signal change to gain a more anatomically meaningful measurement of tissue at each voxel in the breast for quantitative analysis. A Markov Random Field (MRF) model is incorporated into our framework to reduce the effects of random noise.

2 Method

2.1 The Hayton-Brady Pharmacokinetic Model

Currently, most radiologists analyze breast MR scans from subtraction images from time slices relative to a baseline and then plot graphs of signal enhancement vs time. The relative enhancement is calculated according to the enhancement formula: $E(t)\% = (SI(t) - SI(t=0))/SI(t=0) * 100\%$, where $SI(t>0)$ is the post-contrast signal intensity at time t and $SI(t=0)$ is the pre-contrast signal intensity.

Hayton[4] proposed a pharmacokinetic model based on the empirical observation that relative signal increase is proportional to the concentration of contrast agent. This is used to relate the observed MR signal to Gd-DTPA concentration in the extracellular space of breast tissue at a particular pixel. The model can be represented by:

$$C(t) = \frac{A}{a-b}(\exp^{-bt} - \exp^{-at}). \qquad (1)$$

By measuring the relative signal increase at each breast pixel, we can fit the model to the temporal data sequences. The pharmacokinetic model provides a mathematical model of the ce-MRI signal time course, which gives quantitative measurement of tissue characteristics at each pixel.

2.2 Segmentation of Breast ce-MRI

We aim to develop algorithms for segmenting the breast into different tissue regions and thus to identify abnormal tissue. Here, we assume that the breast is comprised of four major tissue types: fat, normal tissue, benign lesions and malignant lesions. Due to the strong signal intensity contrast between fat and the non-fat tissue types and the largely undetectable contrast between non-fat tissue types in the pre-contrast scan, we initially use K-means clustering to segment the breast image into two classes: fat vs non-fat. In the following section, the non-fat tissues (normal, benign and malignant) are the areas of interest (ROI) to be segmented.

The Pixel Attribute Vector. Because normal tissue, benign lesion and malignant lesion tend to have similar intensities, a single pre-contrast breast MRI is generally not capable of distinguishing between them. As mentioned above, the shape of the signal enhancement-time curve is an important criterion in differentiating these tissue types in ce-MRI.

Although the parameters A, a and b found for each pixel contain the curve shape information, experiments show that there are substantial overlaps in the parameter values for these physiologically different tissue types. This leads directly to the failure of using these three parameters for segmentation. Instead, we need to identify different parameters to represent each pixel within non-fat breast tissue.

In [5] two criteria were suggested to describe the curve shapes. First, the behavior of signal intensity in the early phase, immediately after the administration of contrast material, is evaluated from the steepness of the post-contrast signal intensity curve; one descriptor is early-phase enhancement rate: which can be calculated by the enhancement for the first post-contrast image using

$$f^1 = C(t=1) = \frac{A}{a-b}(exp^{-bt} - exp^{-at}). \qquad (2)$$

Second, the behavior of signal intensity in the intermediate and late post-contrast periods may be traced to derive diagnostic information. The shape of this part of curve can be evaluated: whether the signal intensity continues to increase after the initial upstroke, whether it is cut off and reaches a plateau, or whether it washes out. The slope of the pharmacokinetic curve at an intermediate and late stage can be used to describe this shape. Due to the lack of curvature at this period, the slope can be represented by

$$f^2 = (C(t=TL) - C(t=TM))/(TL - TM), \qquad (3)$$

where TL is the time when the last scan was taken and TM is the time when the middle scan was taken. The formulation of an attribute vector for each pixel is defined as: $f = [f^1, f^2]$.

MRF Model-Based Segmentation. In this section, an MRF model segmentation method based on [8] is proposed to segment the breast non-fat tissue into three classes: normal, benign and malignant. An attribute vector provides the information for each pixel. From the previous section, we see that the attribute vector calculations can be derived from curve fitting the dynamic time-dependent signal intensity data on a pixel-by-pixel basis, segmentation based only on the attribute vector has an intrinsic limitation – no spatial information is taken into account. In order to minimize the effect of random noise, an MRF model is used in which the spatial information is taken into account through the mutual influences of neighboring sites.

Let us denote the pixels' attribute vectors in the breast region of interest by $\boldsymbol{F} = \{\boldsymbol{f}_1, \boldsymbol{f}_2, \cdots, \boldsymbol{f}_n\}$, where n is the number of pixels. Let $\boldsymbol{S} = \{s_1, s_2, \cdots, s_n\}$ denote the underlying segmentation, where $s_i \in \mathcal{L} = \{1, 2, \cdots, K\}$ and K (3 in our case) is the number of tissue classes. $s_i = k$ indicates that pixel i belongs to tissue type k. We define the probability that pixel i belongs to tissue type k by a non-negative quantity w_i^k, so $P(s_i = k) = w_i^k$. With this notation, the probability vectors describing the image can be written as follows:

$$\boldsymbol{W} = \{\boldsymbol{w}_1, \boldsymbol{w}_2, \cdots, \boldsymbol{w}_n\},$$

where $\boldsymbol{w}_i = [w_i^1, w_i^2, \cdots, w_i^K]^T$ with $\sum_{k=1}^{K} w_i^k = 1$.

The optimal segmentation, given the image attribute data $\boldsymbol{F}$, can be represented by the MAP estimation:

$$s_i = \arg\max_k \tilde{w}_i^k, \tag{4}$$

where

$$\tilde{\boldsymbol{W}} = \arg\max_{\boldsymbol{W}} P(\boldsymbol{W}|\boldsymbol{F}). \tag{5}$$

Using Bayes' rule, we can form the posterior distribution $P(\boldsymbol{W}|\boldsymbol{F})$ by the combination of a data model $P(\boldsymbol{F}|\boldsymbol{W})$ and a prior distribution $P(\boldsymbol{W})$: the former provides a description of the observed data $\boldsymbol{F}$ given the underlying unobserved data $\boldsymbol{W}$; the latter is a probabilistic model for our *a priori* beliefs about the data $\boldsymbol{W}$. Thus, we have:

$$\tilde{\boldsymbol{W}} = \arg\max_{\boldsymbol{W}} P(\boldsymbol{F}|\boldsymbol{W}) P(\boldsymbol{W}). \tag{6}$$

In order to maintain spatial coherence and smoothness, $\boldsymbol{W}$ is considered as a realization of an MRF, and its prior probability can be derived from

$$P(\boldsymbol{W}) = Z^{-1} \exp(-\beta U(\boldsymbol{W})), \tag{7}$$

where Z is a normalizing constant, β is the neighborhood parameter, which controls the granularity of the segmentation result and $U(\boldsymbol{W}) = \sum_{c \in C} V_c(\boldsymbol{W})$, which is a sum of clique potentials $V_c(\boldsymbol{W})$ over all possible cliques C. A clique c is defined as a subset of sites in image domain in which every pair of distinct sites are neighbors, except for single-site cliques. In this paper, we use a second order neighborhood system, in which there are eight neighbors for each site. We also consider only two-site cliques which include horizontal, vertical and diagonal pair-site cliques. The clique potential function V_c is determined by the distance measure:

$$V_c(\boldsymbol{w}_i, \boldsymbol{w}_j) = |\boldsymbol{w}_i - \boldsymbol{w}_j|^2, \tag{8}$$

where i and j are neighboring sites in image domain.

If we assume conditional independence and suppose that the ce-MRI signal enhancement follows a Gaussian distribution, then since the attribute vector is linear with signal enhancement, f_i^j also follows a Gaussian distribution, we have:

$$P(\boldsymbol{F}|\boldsymbol{W}) = \prod_i \prod_{j=1}^{2} P(f_i^j|\boldsymbol{w}_i) =$$

$$\prod_i \prod_{j=1}^{2} (\sum_{k=1}^{K} P(f_i^j|s_i = k, \boldsymbol{w}_i) P(s_i = k|\boldsymbol{w}_i)) =$$

$$\prod_i \prod_{j=1}^{2} \{ \sum_{k=1}^{K} \frac{w_i^k}{\sqrt{2\pi\sigma_{j,k}^2}} \exp[-\frac{(f_i^j - \mu_{j,k})^2}{2\sigma_{j,k}^2}] \}, \quad (9)$$

where $\mu_{j,k}$ and $\sigma_{j,k}$ are the mean and variance of each attribute vector element for tissue class k. These values are unknown and can be estimated either with an EM [6] algorithm or we can use a simple typical sample data method to estimate: based on our prior knowledge of the data, we choose all the pixels with $f^1 > 0.5$ and $f^2 < 0$ as typical malignant data, $f^1 > 0.3$ and $f^2 > 0$ as typical benign data, and $f^1 < 0.3$ and $|f^2| < 0.05$ as typical normal tissue data. We calculate the mean and variance for each group of typical sample data, and get the values μ and σ. From a computational point of view, EM method will be more expensive and may depends on the initialization, and this may favor also the sample method.

Equation 9 may be written as

$$P(\boldsymbol{F}|\boldsymbol{W}) = Z^{-1}\exp(-U(\boldsymbol{F}|\boldsymbol{W})) \quad (10)$$

with the likelihood energy:

$$U(\boldsymbol{F}|\boldsymbol{W}) = \sum_i \sum_{j=1}^{2} \log\{ \sum_{k=1}^{K} \frac{w_i^k}{\sqrt{2\pi\sigma_{j,k}^2}} \exp[-\frac{(f_i^j - \mu_{j,k})^2}{2\sigma_{j,k}^2}] \}.$$

It is easy to show that

$$P(\boldsymbol{W}|\boldsymbol{F}) \propto \exp(-U(\boldsymbol{W}|\boldsymbol{F})), \quad (11)$$

where $U(\boldsymbol{W}|\boldsymbol{F}) = U(\boldsymbol{F}|\boldsymbol{W}) + \beta U(\boldsymbol{W})$ is the posterior energy. MAP estimation is equivalent to minimizing the posterior energy function:

$$\tilde{\boldsymbol{W}} = \arg\min_{\boldsymbol{W}} \{ U(\boldsymbol{F}|\boldsymbol{W}) + \beta U(\boldsymbol{W}) \}. \quad (12)$$

Since the energy function is differentiable, we can use an iterative gradient descent optimization technique to find a local minimum for $\boldsymbol{W}$.

2.3 Simultaneous Segmentation and Registration (SSR)

The signal enhancement-time curve used to describe each pixel is based on the assumption that the patient either makes no motion or that any motions are small enough to be negligible. In reality, due to the breathing of the patient, or other movements made during the examination, the signal enhancement-time curve will be degraded. Image registration should be used to correct for any patient movement that occurs during the scan. This ensures that the images through time always contain the same anatomical volume of tissue at each position within the scan.

Although segmentation and registration are usually considered separately in medical image analysis, they can benefit a great deal from each other. In this section, we propose a novel scheme for simultaneously solving for segmentation and registration.

General Framework. We have a serial observed images from ce-MRI time sequences: $I = \{I_0, I_1, \cdots, I_6\}$. We assume $I_1, \cdots, I_6$ corresponds to some unknown geometric transformation of reference image I_0. "Segmentation", or labelling of each pixel to one tissue types can be regarded as a model of the underlying anatomy. The problem can be formulated as follows: given observed images I, we wish to simultaneously estimate the label field S of the images and recover the geometric transformation $T = \{T_1, T_2, \cdots, T_6\}$ that register the images $I_1, \cdots, I_6$ with I_0. The MAP estimate is to find S and T to maximize $P(S, T|I)$.

The problem can be separated into a 2-step procedure, in which the best T is found given the correct estimate for S, and then the best estimate for S is found, given the correct estimate for the transformation T:

1. Set an initial estimate $\tilde{T} = 0$;
2. Repeat until convergence or often enough:
   (a): Set $\tilde{S} = \arg \max_{S} P(S|\tilde{T}, I)$
   (b): Set $\tilde{T} = \arg \max_{T} P(T|\tilde{S}, I)$

Segmentation Based on Registration. We now analyze step (a). Given the observed data I and a known transformation T between images, we can compute the attribute vector F for each pixel r after applying the transformations on the post-contrast images and calculate the parameters from fitting the curve $C(r,t)$ of data $E(r,t)\% = (SI(T(r),t) - SI(r, t=0))/SI(r, t=0) * 100\%$. Since our segmentation is only based on the attribute vector information of each pixel, we have $P(S|\tilde{T}, I) = P(S|F)$, where the same method described in section 2.2 can be used.

Registration Based on Segmentation. For step (b), we consider image I_0 to be the reference image, transformation T_i to be a spatial mapping from I_i to I_0. The transformation type is a displacement vector per point. Using Bayes' rule, we have:

$$P(T|\tilde{S}, I) \propto P(I|\tilde{S}, T)P(T) = \prod_{i=1}^{6} P(I_i|\tilde{S}, T_i)P(T_i). \tag{13}$$

In order to maintain spatial coherence and smoothness, the transformation T may be required to be similar to its value at its spatial neighbors. We assume a Gibbs distribution on the expected deformations: $P(T) = \exp(-E(T))$, where $E(T)$ is T in the form of an energy. We choose a second order neighborhood system, and consider only two-site cliques which include horizontal, vertical and diagonal pair-site cliques. The energy is the sum of clique potentials over all possible cliques C: $E(T) = \sum_{c \in C} V_c(T)$ where

$$V_c(T(r), T(q)) = |T(r) - T(q)|^2. \tag{14}$$

with r and q are neighboring sites in image domain.

The likelihood of the observations can then be rewritten:

$$P(I_i|\tilde{S}, T_i) = \prod_{r \in \Omega_{I_0}} P(I_i(T_i(r))|\tilde{s}_r). \tag{15}$$

For a Gaussian noise distribution, we have:

$$P(I_i(T_i(r))|\tilde{s}_r) = \frac{1}{\sqrt{2\pi\sigma^2_{i,\tilde{s}_r}}} \exp[-\frac{|E(T_i(r), i) - \mu_{i,\tilde{s}_r}|^2}{2\sigma^2_{i,\tilde{s}_r}}], \tag{16}$$

where $\mu_{i,k}$ and $\sigma_{i,k}$ are the fitted contrast enhancement curve mean and variance for tissue class k at time i. These values are unknown but can be estimated either using an EM algorithm or by the simple typical sample method.

Finally we get:

$$P(T|\tilde{S}, I) \propto \exp[-U(T)], \tag{17}$$

where

$$U(T) = \sum_i \sum_{r \in \Omega_{I_0}} \frac{|E(T_i(r), i) - \mu_{i,\tilde{s}_r}|^2}{2\sigma^2_{i,\tilde{s}_r}} + E(T). \tag{18}$$

The first term of $U(T)$ is the similarity measure, and is proportional to $|I_i - I_0 * M(r)|^2$, with $M(r)$ as adaptive intensity correction factor depends on the segmentation result of pixel r.

Our registration method addresses the fundamental problem associated with ce-MRI registration: contrast enhancement is an intensity inconsistency between two images, which is what intensity-based registration algorithms are designed to minimize. Given that the image intensity might change after injection of the contrast agent, one cannot use a direct comparison of image intensities. With adaptive intensity correction, our algorithm can achieve registration without causing shrinking problem [7].

Step (b) is equivalent to minimizing of $U(T)$. Since the energy function is differentiable, we can use an iterative gradient descent optimization technique to find a local minimum for T.

3 Experiments

Our initial experiments have been on clinical breast MR images. To date, data from fifteen patients have been analyzed using our method. The 3-D MR scans were performed on General Electric Medical Systems (Genesis Signa). The slice is coronal orientation, with thickness of $3mm$ and $1.5mm$ space between slices. The flip angle is 10 degrees. The Repetition Time: $TR = 8.9ms$; Echo Time: $TE = 4.2ms$.

Figure 1 shows scans from one patient dataset. A total of 7 scans were taken. Figure 1(a) is the pre-contrast scan, and Figure 1(b)-(g) are post-contrast scans from 1 minute to 6 minute after injection of Gd-DTPA.

Figure 2 shows the registration results using our SSR method. Figure 2(a)(c)(e) shows the subtraction between the Figure 1(e)(f)(g) and the pre-contrast image: the effect of the breast motion is clearly visible, especially on the edge of the different tissue types. Figure 2(b)(d)(f) show the subtraction between the transformed images of Figure 1(e)(f)(g) after SSR and the pre-contrast image, the amount of mis-registration is significantly reduced. We use a new measure to assess the quality of the registration. We calculate the residual norm value of curve fitting before and after registration. We show in Figure 2(g) and (h) those pixels with large residual norm value (larger than 0.1) before and after SSR. From the significant reduction in large residual norm after SSR, we can see that the pixels' signal-time profiles are much smoother and the changes that occur in the image over time can be better explained mathematically by our pharmacokinetic model.

We segment the images into 4 tissue classes in the breast: fat, normal tissue, benign lesions and malignant lesions. The fat tissue and non-fat tissues are segmented using the K-Means method, while the 3 non-fat tissues are segmented using an MRF-based method according to their attribute vectors which reflect the pixel's signal profile over time. We use grey to indicate fat tissue, blue for normal tissue, red for benign lesions and green for malignant lesions. Figure 3(a) and (c) show the left and right breast segmentation results without considering patient's movement. Figure 3(b) and (d) show the left and right breast segmentation results with our SSR method. Figure 3(e) shows the typical pixel's signal-time profile for each non-fat tissue after SSR, we can see the quick take-up and a wash-out procedure for malignant lesion pixel, a steady growing in intensity of benign lesion and a relatively flat pattern for normal tissue. Figure 3(f) shows the pixels whose segmentation results are changed, which is achieved by our SSR method. This SSR segmentation result shows the reduction of misclassification pixels, whose signal-time profile pattern were distorted by patient movement.

4 Summary

In this paper, we have developed a framework to achieve simultaneous segmentation and registration for breast ce-MRI. With registration, the patient's motion during the 6 minutes examination is corrected, providing a better reflection of

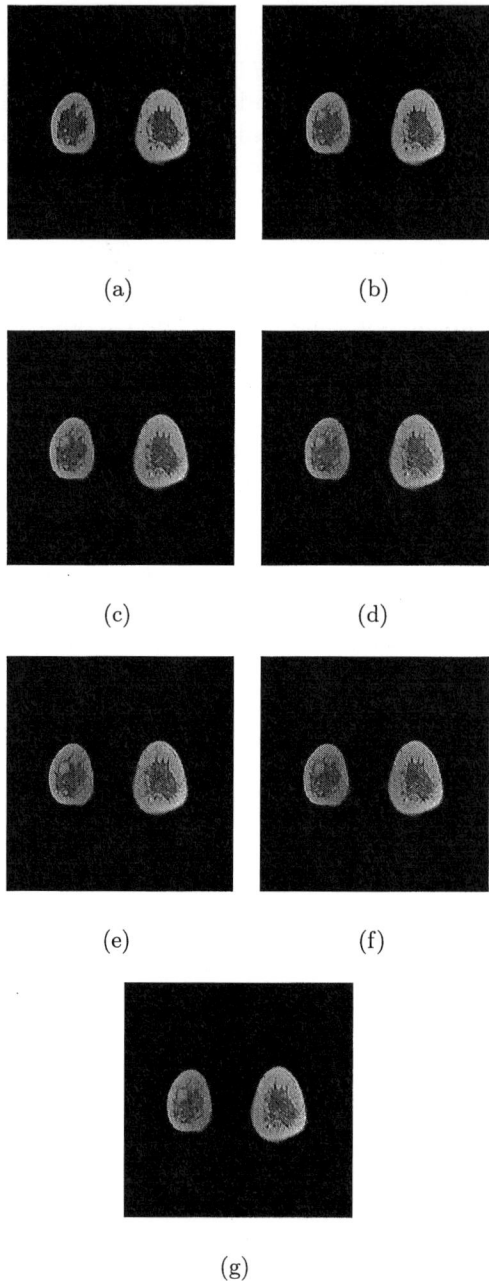

Fig. 1. Example of breast ce-MRI data. (a)Pre-contrast image. (b)Post-contrast image at one minute after contrast agent injection. (c)Post-contrast image at two minutes after injection. (d)Post-contrast image at three minutes after injection. (e)Post-contrast image at four minutes after injection. (d)Post-contrast image at five minutes after injection. (d)Post-contrast image at six minutes after injection

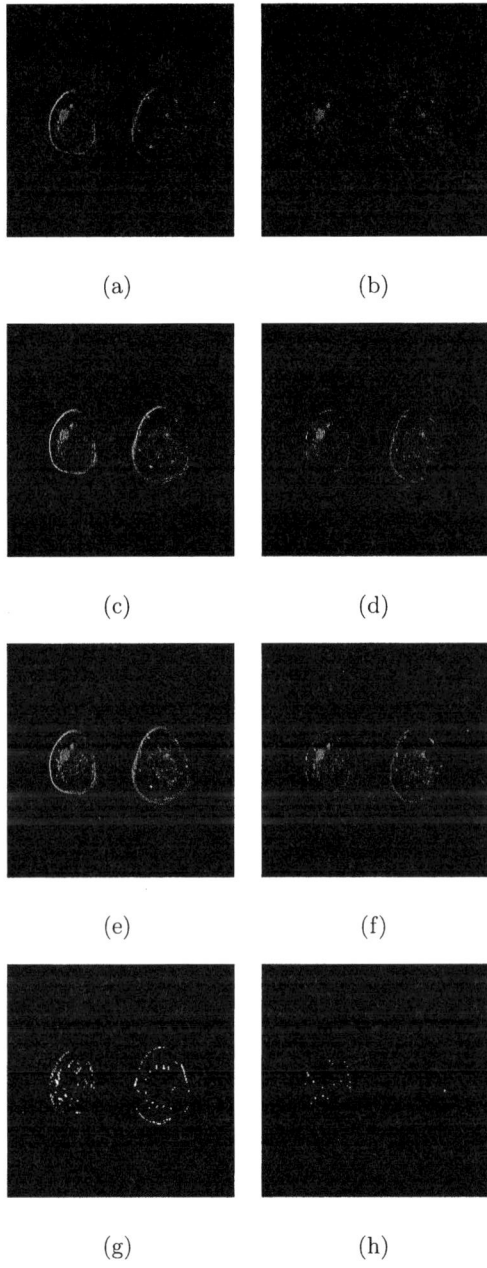

Fig. 2. SSR registration results. (a)Subtraction image of Fig.1(e) and (a). (b)Subtraction image of motion corrected Fig.1(e) and (a). (c)Subtraction image of Fig.1(f) and (a). (d)Subtraction image of motion corrected Fig.1(f) and (a). (e)Subtraction image of Fig.1(g) and (a). (f)Subtraction image of motion corrected Fig.1(g) and (a). (g)Pixels with large residue of curve fitting before registration. (h)Pixels with large residue of curve fitting after SSR

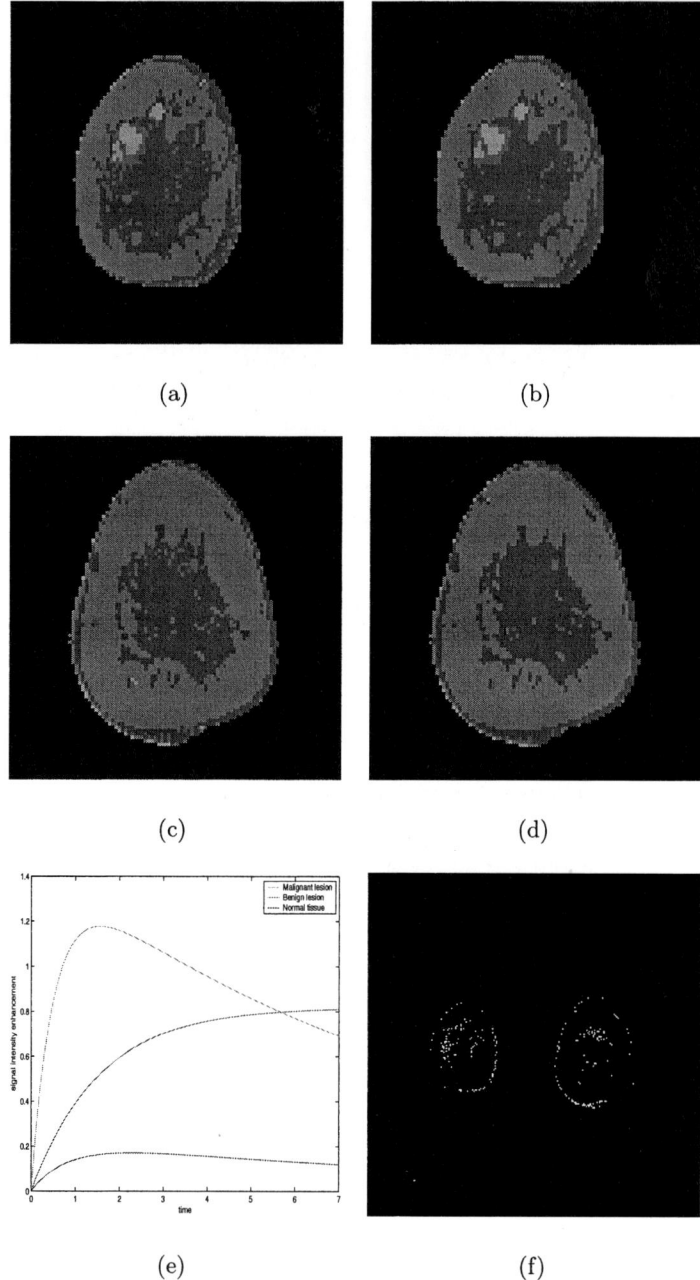

(a) (b)

(c) (d)

(e) (f)

Fig. 3. SSR segmentation results. (a)The left breast segmentation result without registration. (b)The left breast segmentation result after SSR. (c)The right breast segmentation result without registration. (d)The right breast segmentation result after SSR. (e)The signal-time curve of a typical sample chosen from Malignant, Benign, Normal tissue separately. (f)The pixels with different segmentation results before and after SSR

the signal change over time for each pixel, thus we achieve a better segmentation, since the segmentation is based on the signal enhancement pattern. Segmentation enables the predication of intensity enhancement of each pixel at different time, and it is particular useful for dynamic MR images due to the non-uniform signal enhancement in different tissue types. With segmentation information, the intensity of each pixel in the pre-contrast image was adapted, and compared with the post-contrast images, to achieve better registration result. By interleaving segmentation and registration in one framework, the two problems' solution can be benefit to each other, thus achieve better results for both problems.

The pharmacokinetic model used for curve fitting can provide a mathematical measure to calculate the attribute vector for each pixel. The MRF model used for SSR incorporate the neighborhood information into the pixel-based method, the segmentation and registration are smooth and random noise effect is also reduced greatly.

The regions detected by this algorithm are intended to be presented to the clinician as suspicious regions. The computational analysis yields information that is of diagnostic and prognostic value, but further study is needed to better understand the true biological meaning of ce-MRI enhancement curves and the accuracy and specificity of this method should be assessed in a retrospective clinical trial, which will be our future work.

References

1. http://www.icr.ac.uk/cmagres/maribs/maribs.html
2. Orel, S.G.: Differentiating Benign from Malignant Enhancing Lesioins Identified at MR Imaging of the Breast: Are Time-Signal Intensity Curves an Accurate Predictor? Radiology, 1999, 211(1): 5–7
3. Kuhl, C.K, Mielcareck, P., Klaschik, S., Leutner, C., Wardelmann, E., Gieseke, J., Schild, H.: Dynamic Breast MR Imaging: Are Signal Intensity Time Course Data Useful for Differential Diagnosis of Enhancing Lesions? Radiology, 1999, 211: 101–110
4. Hayton, P., Brady, J.M, Tarassenko, L., Moore, N.: Analysis of Dynamic MR Breast Images Using a Model of Contrast Enhancement. Medical Image Analysis, Vol. 1. Num. 3. (1996/7) 207–224
5. Choyke, P.L, Dwyer, A.J., Knopp, M.V.: Functional Tumor Imaging with Dynamic Contrast Enhanced Magnetic Resonance Imaging, Journal of Magnetic Resonance Imaging, 17:509-520 (2003)
6. Zhang, Y., Brady, M., Smith, S.: Segmentation of Brain MR Images Through a Hidden Markov Random Field Model and the Expectation Maximization Algorithm. IEEE Trans. Medical Imaging, Vol. 20. Num. 1. (2001) 45–57
7. Rohlfing, T, Maurer, C.R: Volume-Preserving Nonrigid Registration of MR Breast Images Using Free-Form Deformation With an Incompressibility Constraint. IEEE Trans. Medical Imaging, Vol. 22. Num.6. (2003) 730–741
8. Marroquin, J.L., Santana, E.A., Botello, S.: Hidden Markov Measure Field Models for Image Segmentation . IEEE Trans. Pattern Analysis and Machine Intelligence, Vol. 25. Num. 11. (2003) 1380–1387

Multiscale Vessel Enhancing Diffusion in CT Angiography Noise Filtering

Rashindra Manniesing and Wiro Niessen

Image Sciences Institute, University Medical Center Utrecht,
P.O. Box 85500, 3508 GA, Utrecht The Netherlands
{rashindra, wiro}@isi.uu.nl

Abstract. Filtering of vessel structures in medical images by analyzing the second order information or the Hessian of the image, is a well known technique. In this work we incorporate Frangi's multiscale vessel filter [4], which is based on a geometrical analysis of the Hessian' eigenvectors, into a nonlinear, anisotropic diffusion scheme, such that diffusion mainly takes place along the vessel axis while diffusion perpendicular to this axis is inhibited. The multiscale character of the vesselness filter ensures an equally good response for varying vessel radii. The first, theoretical contribution of this paper is the modification of the original formulation of this vessel filter, such that it becomes a smooth function on its domain which is a necessary condition imposed by the diffusion process to ensure well-posedness. The second contribution concerns the application of noise filtering of 3D synthetic, phantom computed tomography (CT) and patient CT data. It is shown that the method is very effective in noise filtering, illustrating its potential as a preprocessing step in the analysis of low dose CT angiography.

1 Introduction

Vessel analysis in medical images is important both for diagnostic and intervention planning purposes. Vessel centerline extraction can be used to generate specific visualizations, such as endovascular views or multiplaner reformats. Vessel segmentation can be used for quantification, e.g. stenosis grading, or to determine the dimension of stents to be used in interventions. In many approaches for vessel analysis, images are first preprocessed to enhance vascular structures. Vessel enhancement improves vessel visualization, e.g. in volume rendering techniques or maximum intensity projections, and has the potential to facilitate the task of centerline extraction and segmentation.

In this paper a method is proposed to enhance vascular structures within the framework of scale space theory. In scale space theory, a family of images is generated by evolving the image according to the diffusion equation, with the original image as the initial condition. Consider the general diffusion equation in divergence form $L_t = \nabla \cdot (D\nabla L)$, which states that the change in luminance L is the divergence of some flow $D\nabla L$. The *diffusion tensor* D enables us to control the flow such that features of interested are blurred or preserved. The simplest form is by taking the identity matrix for D which results in the linear isotropic heat equation, used in linear scale space theory. The first nonlinear variant was proposed by Perona and Malik [8], in which the diffusion tensor is replaced by a scalar function of the gradient magnitude. Note that the Perona and Malik equation is isotropic, despite its original characterization as being anisotropic. Weickert [14, 16] goes one step further by using not only the gradient magnitude but also the orientation or average gradient direction to enhance small edges and coherent structures by analyzing the structure tensor of the image, obtaining truly anisotropic behaviour. For an overview of these and other diffusion equations, we refer to [11] and [15].

The objective of this work is to extend these types of diffusion equations by replacing the diffusion tensor by a function of the second order information or the Hessian of the image. In the context of vessel analysis, the Hessian has direct geometrical interpretation when analyzing its eigenvectors, and in particular, Frangi's [4] vesselness measure is taken to steer the diffusion process. This combination, coined *vessel enhancing diffusion* - VED, has been explored before by Cañero and Radeva in [1], which is, to the best of our knowledge, the only other work combining vesselness filtering with diffusion. While their incorporation of the vesselness measure into the diffusion process has much resemblance, an important difference is found in our tensor function which satisfies a smoothness constraint; a necessary condition imposed by the diffusion process to ensure well-posedness. Furthermore, compared to [1], the method is extended to 3D.

The second half of this paper is devoted to the application of noise filtering of 3D synthetic, phantom computed tomography (CT) and patient CT data.

2 Method

2.1 Diffusion Filter Class

It can be shown that under fairly mild conditions on the diffusion tensor, the resulting diffusion equations exhibit well-posedness, regularity and a minimum-maximum principle. Well-posedness means that the problem has a solution which is unique and that continuously depends on the initial image. Regularity implies that the solution belongs to the class of smooth functions. The extremum principles states that the range of the intensity values becomes smaller - in fact, the intensity range converges to the average gray value of the image if the number of iterations goes to infinity. The derivation can be found in [16, 14] where the results from [2] and [13] are generalized. Here, only the three conditions imposed on the diffusion tensor $D = (d_{ij})$ are given, which are repeated from [16]:

Smoothness $D \in C^\infty(\mathbb{R}^{m \times m}, \mathbb{R}^{m \times m})$ with m denoting the dimension.
Symmetry $d_{ij}(H) = d_{ji}(H)$ for all (symmetric) Hessian matrices $H \in \mathbb{R}^{m \times m}$.
Uniformly positive definite Let $\Omega \in \mathbb{R}^m$ be the open, bounded subset of $\mathbb{R}^m$ denoting the image domain. If $w : \Omega \to \mathbb{R}^2$, satisfies $|w(x)| \leq K$ on $\overline{\Omega}$ ($\overline{\Omega}$ is the closure of Ω), then there exists a positive lowerbound $v(K)$ for the eigenvalues of $D(H)$.

We aim at constructing a D which fulfills these requirements and allows for vessel preserving diffusion.

2.2 Vesselness Filter

In the context of vessel analysis, we use the second order information or the Hessian matrix $\mathcal{H}$ of the image. Since the Hessian is symmetric and real, by the *Principal Axis Theorem* from linear algebra, it can be decomposed into $\mathcal{H} = Q \Lambda Q^T$, in which Q forms an orthonormal base of eigenvectors, and Λ denotes its corresponding eigenvectors. These eigenvectors and values have a direct geometrical interpretation: the eigenvectors point in the direction in which the curvature takes extremal values, the eigenvalues give these extremal values. These eigenvalues are also called the *principal curvatures*.

In the case of bright vessels on a dark background, and with the following ordering of eigenvalues $|\lambda_1| \leq |\lambda_2| \leq |\lambda_3|$, the direction along the vessel is given by v_1 when $|\lambda_1| \approx 0$ and $|\lambda_1| \ll |\lambda_2| \approx |\lambda_3|$. Several vesselness filters have been proposed based on the eigenvalues of the Hessian [6, 10, 4]. Selected is Frangi's filter [4], because it consists of exponential functions, which turns out to be advantageous when modifying the function (in Section 2.3). The formulation of the vesselness measure by Frangi et al. [4], calculated at scale σ, is as follows:

$$\mathcal{V}_F(\sigma) \triangleq \begin{cases} 0 & \text{if } \lambda_2 > 0 \text{ or } \lambda_3 > 0 \\ \left(1 - e^{-\frac{A^2}{2\alpha^2}}\right) e^{-\frac{B^2}{2\beta^2}} \left(1 - e^{-\frac{S^2}{2\gamma^2}}\right) \end{cases} \quad (1)$$

with

$$A = \frac{|\lambda_2|}{|\lambda_3|} \quad (2)$$

$$B = \frac{|\lambda_1|}{\sqrt{|\lambda_2 \lambda_3|}} \quad (3)$$

$$S = \sqrt{\lambda_1^2 + \lambda_2^2 + \lambda_3^2} \quad (4)$$

in which A differentiates between plate and line like structures, B accounts for deviation from a blob like structure, and S differentiates between foreground (vessel) and background (noise). This function is used as starting point to construct the diffusion tensor D.

2.3 Smoothed Vesselness Filter

Unfortunately, this vesselness function $\mathcal{V}_F$ is not smooth at the origin, and thus can not directly by used in the diffusion equation. Smoothness implies that the nth-order derivative exists and is continuous (since continuity is necessary prerequisite for the next derivative). The following modifications are proposed to remedy this issue. The first modification applies to the domain definition: by testing for $\lambda_{\{2,3\}}$ larger equal zero instead of larger zero, the function becomes continuous at the limit $\lambda_2 \uparrow 0$ and $\lambda_3 \uparrow 0$. Also, for $\boldsymbol{\lambda} \to \boldsymbol{0}$, the function goes to zero since the third term (the contrast term) goes to zero while the other two terms are bounded. Still, the resulting function is not smooth. This is basically due to the appearance of the ratio of polynomial functions in λ_i, which has the same order in the nominator as well as in the denominator, which occur in the first two terms of the vesselness function. It goes wrong first for the second order partial derivatives in λ_1, $\mathcal{V}_{F\lambda_1\lambda_1} = \partial^2 \mathcal{V}_F / \partial \lambda_1^2$. Suppose $\lambda_2 = \lambda_3 \triangleq \alpha\lambda_1$ with $\alpha \in \mathbb{R}$ and $\alpha \geq 1$ and letting $\lambda_1 \to 0$, results in $\mathcal{V}_{F\lambda_1\lambda_1} = (2+4\alpha^2)(1-1/e)e^{(-1/\alpha^2)}$. A similar argument can be applied in the 2D case for the first order derivative in λ_1; thus the diffusion tensor proposed in [1] is not smooth either. To resolve, observe that $\mathcal{V}_F$ and $\mathcal{V}_F^{(n)}$, consist of terms of the form

$$T(\boldsymbol{\lambda}) = \left(\frac{P}{Q}\right) e^{-\left(\frac{R}{S}\right)} \qquad (5)$$

with $\{P, Q\}$ some polynomial function in $\boldsymbol{\lambda}$, and $\{R, S\}$ some polynomial functions in $\boldsymbol{\lambda}$ without any constant terms. Obviously, $\{R, S\}$ remain the same for any order derivative, only $\{P, Q\}$ change. Therefore, if $\boldsymbol{\lambda} \to \mathbf{0}$ then $\{R, S\} \to \{0, 0\}$, making T undefined. Multiplying T with $e^{(-1/S)}$ gives

$$\left(\frac{P}{Q}\right) e^{-\left(\frac{R+1}{S}\right)} \qquad (6)$$

which always goes to zero if $\boldsymbol{\lambda} \to \mathbf{0}$, making this new term properly defined around the origin. By collecting the exponential terms of $\mathcal{V}_F$, it immediately follows that the 'largest' denominator is $|\lambda_2|\lambda_3^2$. Therefore, multiplying $\mathcal{V}_F$ with

$$e^{-\left(\frac{2c^2}{|\lambda_2|\lambda_3^2}\right)} \qquad (7)$$

with c some constant, will result in a smoothed version of the vesselness function. It resembles a Gaussian function with its argument inverted, and is controlled by the standard deviation c. This constant c should be chosen very small to only have influence around the origin, when $\boldsymbol{\lambda} \to \mathbf{0}$. Intuitively, the vesselness function is multiplied by a term which is one everywhere except at the origin and rapidly goes to zero in a small neighborhood around the origin. The new vesselness function $\mathcal{V}_s$ then reads:

$$\mathcal{V}_s(\sigma) \triangleq \begin{cases} 0 & \text{if } \lambda_2 \geq 0 \text{ or } \lambda_3 \geq 0 \\ e^{-\frac{2c^2}{|\lambda_2|\lambda_3^2}} \left(1 - e^{-\frac{A^2}{2\alpha^2}}\right) e^{-\frac{B^2}{2\beta^2}} \left(1 - e^{-\frac{S^2}{2\gamma^2}}\right) \end{cases} \qquad (8)$$

Similar as in the original vesselness function, a multiscale approach is adopted, i.e. the vesselness function is calculated at multiple scales - normalized by σ^2 [5], and the maximum response is selected.

$$\mathcal{V} = \max_{\sigma_{min} \leq \sigma \leq \sigma_{max}} \mathcal{V}_s(\sigma) \qquad (9)$$

2.4 Vessel Enhancing Diffusion

With the new smoothed vesselness function $\mathcal{V}$ in Equation 9, the diffusion tensor D can now be defined such that diffusion mainly takes place in the direction along the vessel, while diffusion perpendicular to this direction is inhibited. A straightforward definition of D is as follows

$$D \triangleq Q\Lambda'Q^T \qquad (10)$$

with Q the eigenvectors of $\mathcal{H}$ and Λ' having the following entries on its diagonal

$$\lambda'_1 \triangleq \epsilon + (1-\epsilon) \cdot \mathcal{V} \qquad (11)$$
$$\lambda'_2 \triangleq \epsilon \qquad (12)$$
$$\lambda'_3 \triangleq \epsilon \qquad (13)$$

That is, for all structures blurring is small and (roughly) isotropic, except within a vessel where the vesselness is high and blurring is maximal in the minimal curvature direction. It easily follows that this definition of the diffusion tensor satisfies the filter conditions from Section 2.1.

3 Experiments and Results

In this section, VED filtering is applied to 3D synthetic, phantom CT and patient CT data and evaluated with respect to improvement in visualization and signal-to-noise ratio.

3.1 Acquisition and Parameters

Patient data, used in Sections 3.2 and 3.5, are acquired on a 16-slice CT scanner, resulting in voxel sizes of $0.3125 \times 0.3125 \times 0.5$ mm. The voxel size of the synthetic data used in Section 3.3 is set to $0.3125 \times 0.3125 \times 0.5$ mm, the same as the voxel sizes of the patient data. The parameters of the method are fixed for all experiments except for the number of iterations n, unless specified otherwise. Following [4], the smoothed vessel filter has the following parameters: $\alpha = \beta = 0.5$ and $\gamma = 50$ (in the patient data, the vessel intensity vary in the range [200...600] HU - Hounsfield Units). Also, $c = 0.000001$, $\sigma_{min} = 0.1$ mm and $\sigma_{max} = 2.0$ mm, with 10 different scales, exponentially distributed between σ_{min} and σ_{max}. Diffusion was performed with $\epsilon = 0.01$ and time step $t = 0.02$. The smoothed vesselness response is calculated every time step t. Furthermore, a quantitative measure is needed for evaluation. To this end, the signal-to-noise ratio is used, defined as

$$\text{SNR} = \left(\frac{\langle I \rangle_\mathcal{V} - \langle I \rangle_\mathcal{B}}{\sigma_\mathcal{B}}\right)^2 \qquad (14)$$

with $\langle I \rangle$ the mean intensity of vessel $\mathcal{V}$ or background $\mathcal{B}$, and with $\sigma_\mathcal{B}$ the standard deviation of background. Background and vessel regions are selected manually.

3.2 Illustration of Performance

For illustration purposes, the method is first applied to a 3D synthetic data set representing a bifurcation (Figure 1), and a real 3D patient data set representing a small part of the cerebral vasculature (Figure 2). The bifurcation model consists of three tubes with equal intensity of 200 (background is set to 0) and radii of 1.7, 2.0 and 2.6 voxels. Gaussian noise is added with a standard deviation of $\eta = 200$, letting the original structure almost completely disappear in noise. Shown are the results after $n = 800$ and $n = 3000$ iterations. Clearly, VED filtering is capable of retrieving tube like structures in the image, and also, increasing the number of iteration results in further blurring over the tube edges of the image, as was expected. It means, that for the signal-to-noise ratio an optimum in the number of iterations exists, as function of the noise η. The method applied to patient data (Figure 2, $n = 800$ iterations) resulted in smoothed vessel like structures while the background (noise) is suppressed.

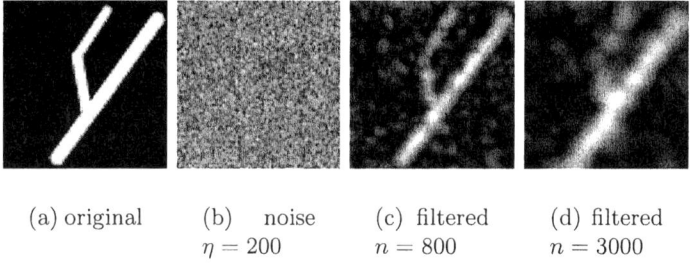

(a) original   (b) noise $\eta = 200$ (c) filtered $n = 800$ (d) filtered $n = 3000$

Fig. 1. A synthetic 3D example of size $64 \times 64 \times 64$ voxels, of a bifurcation consisting of tubes of varying radii. Shown are the maximum intensity projections (mips) of the original data (a), the data with Gaussian noise ($\eta = 200$) added (b) and the results of VED filtering after $n = 800$ (c) and $n = 3000$ (d) iterations

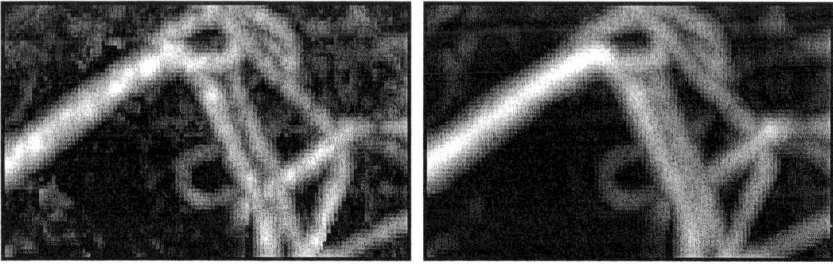

Fig. 2. A small part of the cerebral vasculature from 3D CTA data of size $106 \times 65 \times 261$ voxels. Left a mip of the original, showing some overlapping arteries, and right a mip of the result of VED filtering ($n = 800$)

3.3 Synthetic Data and Noise

The purpose of this experiment is to investigate the relation between the diameter of the vessel, the noise η and the SNR as function of the number of iterations n. Additionally, mips of the filtering results are visually evaluated to determine the influence of filtering on small vessels. A synthetic test bed of tubes is generated with diameters of 1, 2, 3, 4 and 5 voxels and intensity of 200, the background is set to intensity 0. The results are shown in Figures 3 and 4.

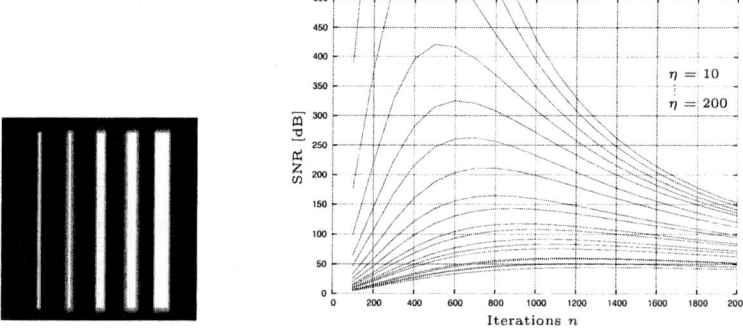

Fig. 3. Left the original test bed of tubes with varying diameters. Right the SNR after filtering for different η of the Gaussian noise

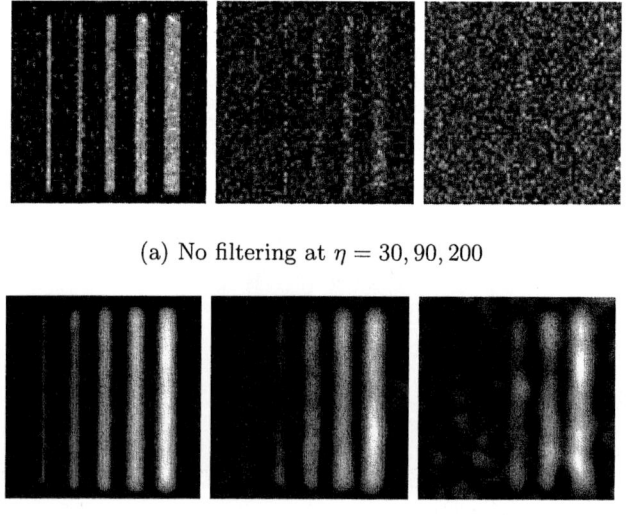

(a) No filtering at $\eta = 30, 90, 200$

(b) Optimal filtered with respect to SNR

Fig. 4. The results of filtering of the test bed for varying η of the Gaussian noise. The optimal results according to the SNR (Figure 3), are obtained after 400, 900 and 1300 iterations, respectively

Figure 3 clearly shows an optimum for different noise values η. This optimum is rapidly achieved for increasing number of iterations n, and the SNR slowly decreases after this optimum. The optimal SNR lies between 200 and 1000 iterations. Figure 4 shows the optimal results for $\eta = 30, 90$ and 200. The visibility of the smallest diameter deteriorate only for relatively small η; shown is the noise level for which the diameters of one and two voxels still was visible (first two columns). From the right column in Figure 4 can be concluded that the smallest diameter that remains visible after filtering even for extremely noisy images, is three voxels.

3.4 Phantom Data and Noise

In CT imaging, X-ray exposure forms a risk to the patient. Attempts to lower this risk usually comes at the expense of a degraded quality of the reconstructed image. The following simple and important relation holds. Both the patient dose and the detector dose (i.e. the image quality), are linear related to the *tube current*, or the mAs setting of the scanner [9]. There are other parameters that are of influence, e.g. the tube voltage, but these are ignored for now by keeping them constant. The purpose of this experiment, is to investigate the capability of VED filtering to improve visualization in low dose CT, by applying the technique to images scanned at decreasing mAs. The image quality is measured by the SNR (Equation 14) and is evaluated visually.

A phantom of the cerebral vasculature [3] is used, which models the most important arteries in the brain, including the Circle of Willis. The phantom was filled with 50 mgI/ml contrast agent, and data was acquired on a Philips 40-slice scanner. A standard head protocol was selected with 120 kV and six different mAs settings [245, 200, 150, 100, 50, 21] - 245 mAs is the standard setting, resulting in data sets of 512×512 by approximately 350 voxels, with almost isotropic voxel sizes of approximately $0.404 \times 0.404 \times 0.33$ mm. A region of interest is selected that includes the Circle of Willis, of $89 \times 84 \times 46$ voxels to run the experiments on. The results are shown in Figures 5 and 6.

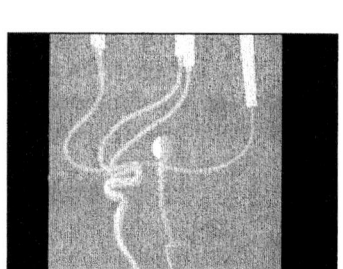
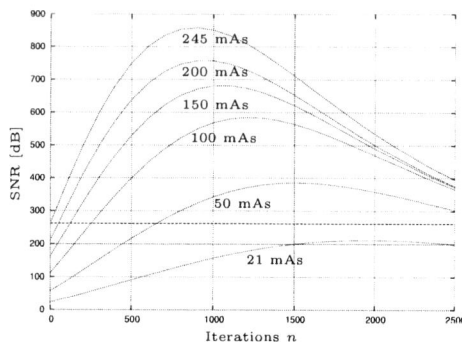

Fig. 5. Left the phantom scanned at the protocol standard and highest current setting of 245 mAs. Right, the results of VED filtering

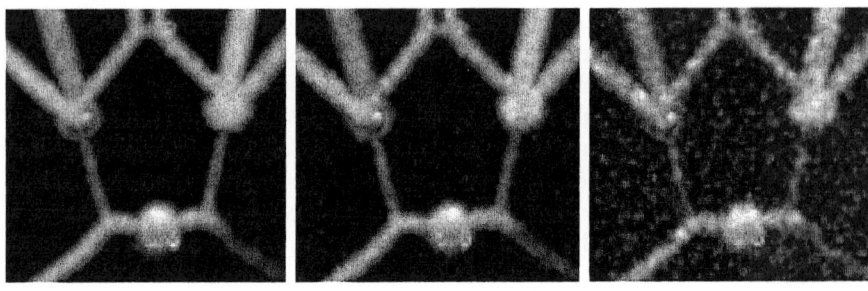

(a) No filtering at 245, 100 and 21 mAs

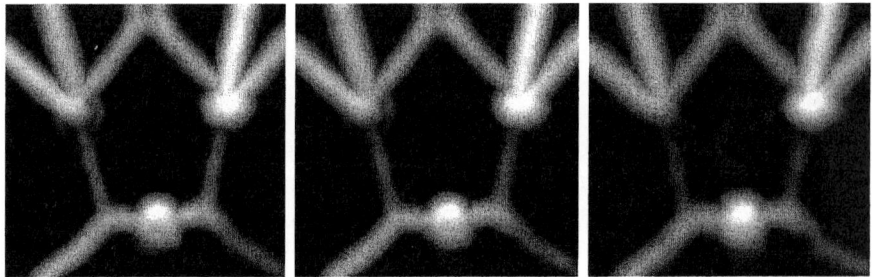

(b) Optimal filtered with respect to SNR

Fig. 6. Zooming in on the Circle of Willis. The optimal results according to the SNR (Figure 5), are obtained after 900, 1200 and 2000 iterations, respectively. Observe that vessels of varying radii are smoothed, while background noise is suppressed

First, a strong similarity with the results obtained in the synthetic data set can be observed; the SNR increases rapidly for increasing n, and decreases slowly after the optimum has been reached. Secondly, all data sets can be improved considerably by VED filtering, even the data scanned at the highest mAs settings. And finally, the mAs setting can be lowered to 100 mAs - more than a factor 2.4, while the SNR is significantly better than at 245 mAs without filtering, achieved already for $n < 500$ iterations (confirm by the horizontal line in Figure 5). Some results for qualitative evaluation are shown in Figure 6, for 245, 100 and 21 mAs settings, for both the unfiltered data sets (first row), and the results after reaching the optimal SNR value (second row). The data show mips of the axial view of the Circle of Willis. Clearly, VED filtering is capable of smoothing the tubular structures of varying sizes. Even in the case of the lowest mAs setting, the results after filtering seem 'acceptable'.

3.5 Patient Data and Visualization

Finally, the method is applied to 3D CT patient data. Before filtering, the bone structures are masked [12] for improved projection visualizations. Bone masking requires an additional, low dose scan of the patient without contrast fluid which is rigidly registered to the high dose scan with contrast. After registration and bone segmentation in the low dose scan by thresholding, bone structures in the

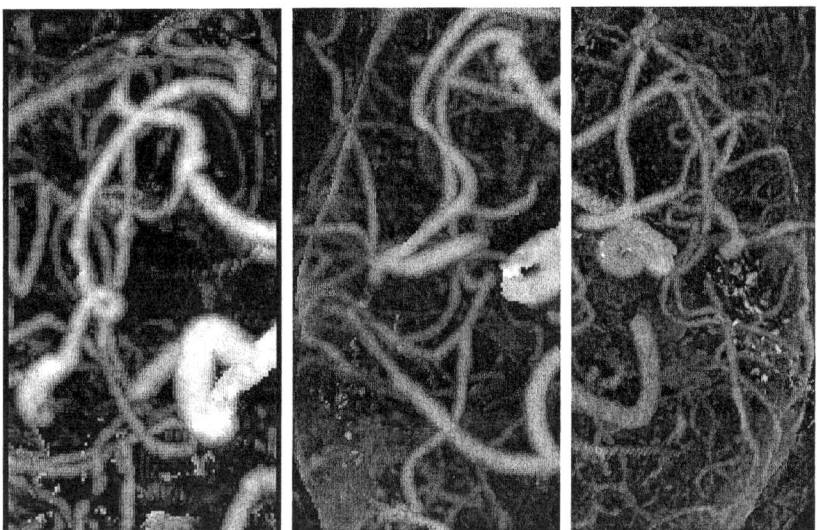

(a) Original patient data, after bone masking

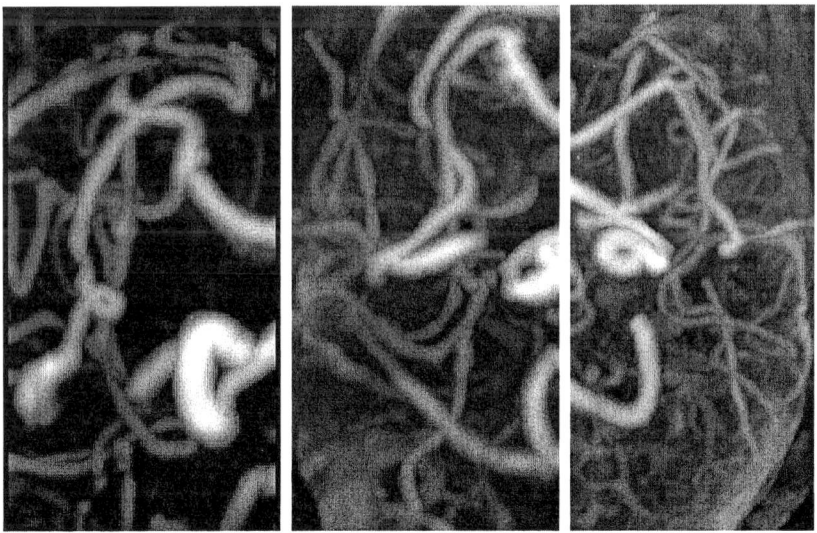

(b) Results after $n = 800$ iterations

Fig. 7. Results of filtering on 3D CT patient data sets

high dose scan are masked. For further details on this technique, we refer to [12] and [7]. Subsequently, the data is chunked to get a smaller roi to reduce computation time and memory requirements.

The results of filtering of three different patient data, after $n = 800$ iterations, are shown in Figure 7. We observe that background noise is suppressed, while the vessels of varying radii are smoothed.

4 Discussion and Conclusion

A nonlinear, anisotropic diffusion scheme has been proposed in which the diffusion tensor is defined from the Hessian of the image, such that diffusion along the vessel axis is encouraged, while diffusion perpendicular to this direction is inhibited. To this end Frangi vesselness filter is adopted and modified such that this function becomes smooth on its domain. A naturally extension is, besides including the Hessian, to include intensity and gradient information into the diffusion tensor. Based on experiments with synthetic data, it is shown that, in the case of extremely noisy data (Gaussian noise of $\eta = 200$ with vessel structures having the same intensity levels), the smallest diameter which still can be made visible has size of three voxels. The phantom experiments showed the potential of the method in decreasing CT dosage while retaining or even improving the signal-to-noise ratio and having visually acceptable results. This is a preliminary conclusion and extensive clinical validation is appropriate. The results of real patient CT data showed the method's capability in smoothing vessel structures of varying radii, while suppressing the background noise level. Comparison with other, well established filtering techniques (such as Gaussian, Perona-Malik, Coherence-Enhanced and Edge-Enhanced filtering), allows for a better characterization and placing of the vessel enhanced diffusion method, which is subject of future work.

References

1. C. Canero and P. Radeva. Vesselness enhancement diffusion. *Pattern Recognition Letters*, 24:3141–3151, 2003.
2. F. Catté, P-L. Lions, J-M. Morel, and T. Coll. Image selective smoothing and edge detection by nonlinear diffusion. *SIAM J. Numer. Anal.*, 29(1):182–193, 1992.
3. R. Fahrig, H. Nikolov, A.J. Fox, and D.W. Holdsworth. A three dimensional cerebrovascular flow phantom. *Medical Physics*, 8(26):1589–1599, 1999.
4. A.F. Frangi, W.J. Niessen, K.L. Vincken, and M.A. Viergever. Multiscale vessel enhancement filtering. In *Medical Image Computing and Computer-Assisted Intervention*, pages 130–137, 1998.
5. T. Lindeberg. Edge detection and ridge detection with automatic scale selection. *Int. J. of Computer Vision*, 30(2):117–154, 1998.
6. C. Lorenz, I.-C. Carlsen, T.M. Buzug, C. Fassnacht, and J. Weese. Multi-scale line segmentation with automatic estimation of width, contrast and tangential direction in 2d and 3d medical images. In *CVRMed*, pages 233–242, 1997.

7. R. Manniesing, B.K. Velthuis, M.S. van Leeuwen, and W.J. Niessen. Skeletonization for re-initialization in level set-based vascular tree segmentation. In J.M. Fitzpatrick and M. Sonka, editors, *SPIE Medical Imaging*, volume 5370, pages 506–514, 2004.
8. P. Perona and J. Malik. Scale-space and edge detection using anisotropic diffusion. *IEEE Transactions on Pattern Analysis and Machine Intelligence*, 12(7):629–639, 1990.
9. M. Prokop and M. Galanski. *Spiral and Multislice Computed Tomography of the Body*. Thieme Verlag Stuttgart, 2003.
10. Y. Sato, S. Nakajima, N. Shiraga, H. Atsumi, S. Yoshida, T. Koller, G. Gerig, and R. Kikinis. Three-dimensional multi-scale line filter for segmentation and visualization of curvilinear structures in medical images. *Medical Image Analysis*, 2(2):143–168, June 1998.
11. B.M. ter Haar Romeny, editor. *Geometry-Driven Diffusion in Computer Vision*, volume 1. Kluwer Academic Publishers, 1994.
12. H.W. Venema, F.J.H. Hulsmans, and G.J. den Heeten. CT angiography of the Circle of Willis and intracranial internal carotid arteries: Maximum intensity projection with matched mask bone elimination - feasibility study. *Radiology*, 218(3):893–898, 2001.
13. J. Weickert. Theoretical foundations of anisotropic diffusion in image processing. In *Theoretical Foundations of Computer Vision*, pages 221–236, 1994.
14. J. Weickert. *Anisotropic Diffusion in Image Processing*. PhD thesis, University of Kaiserslautern, 1996.
15. J. Weickert. A review of nonlinear diffusion filtering. In B. ter Haar Romeny, L. Florack, J. Koenderink, and M. Viergever, editors, *Scale-Space Theory in Computer Vision*, volume 1252 of *Lecture Notes in Comp. Science*, pages 3–28. Springer, 1997.
16. J. Weickert. Coherence-enhancing diffusion filtering. *International Journal of Computer Vision*, 31:111–127, 1999.

Information Fusion in Biomedical Image Analysis: Combination of Data vs. Combination of Interpretations

T. Rohlfing[1], A. Pfefferbaum[1,2], E.V. Sullivan[2], and C.R. Maurer[3]

[1] Neuroscience Program, SRI International, Menlo Park, CA 94025, USA
{torsten, dolf}@synapse.sri.com
[2] Department of Psychiatry and Behavioral Science, Stanford University,
Stanford, CA 94305, USA
edie@stanford.edu
[3] Department of Neurosurgery, Stanford University, Stanford, CA 94305, USA
crmaurer@stanford.edu

Abstract. Information fusion has, in the form of multiple classifier systems, long been a successful tool in pattern recognition applications. It is also becoming increasingly popular in biomedical image analysis, for example in computer-aided diagnosis and in image segmentation. In this paper, we extend the principles of multiple classifier systems by considering information fusion of classifier inputs rather than on their outputs, as is usually done. We introduce the distinction between combination of data (i.e., classifier inputs) vs. combination of interpretations (i.e., classifier outputs). We illustrate the two levels of information fusion using four different biomedical image analysis applications that can be implemented using fusion of either data or interpretations: atlas-based image segmentation, "average image" tissue classification, multi-spectral classification, and deformation-based group morphometry.

1 Introduction

Combinations of multiple independent classifiers can be substantially more accurate than the individual classifiers alone. Numerous applications of this principle have been reported in the pattern recognition literature over the past dozen years. Xu *et al.* [1] evaluated different combination schemes of classifiers for the recognition of unconstrained handwritten numerals. Similarly, Kittler *et al.* [2] combined four classifiers for optical character recognition of uppercase letters and digits. In biomedical image analysis and computer-aided diagnosis, multiple classifier systems have been applied to classification of microcalcifications in breast magnetic resonance (MR) images [3, 4], diagnosis of skin melanomas [5], and classification of breast lesions in ultrasound images [6].

Xu *et al.* [1] point out that classifiers and classifier fusion can operate on three different levels of output information: the abstract level (which assigns a unique output label to each input), the rank level (which assigns a ranking of all available labels to each input), and the measurement level (which assigns a confidence value for each label and to each input). However, their and all other papers referenced above, as well as the vast majority of publications in general, only consider information fusion in the domain of *classifier outputs*, which we refer to in this paper as the *interpretation domain*.

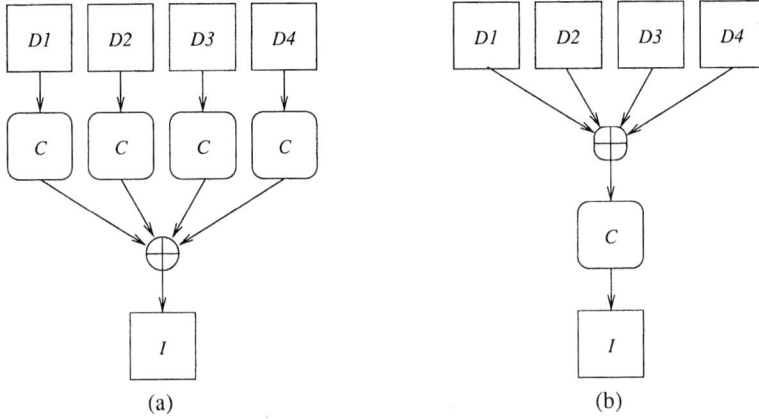

Fig. 1. Illustration of principles of (a) COI approach vs. (b) COD approach. (a) The data from each source are classified separately by the classifier C, and the outputs are combined into a final interpretation I. (b) The data from all sources are first combined and classified by a single classifier C. Note that the combination operators in (a) and (b) typically work on different data types and are, therefore, usually different operators (which are symbolized by different shapes in the illustration)

If the multiple classifiers are generated using different instantiations of their inputs, then we observe that information fusion is possible on the *classifier inputs*, which we refer to as the *data domain*. In fact, there are many applications where we can choose between a combination of interpretations (COI) and a combination of data (COD). The general principle is illustrated in Fig. 1. In this paper, we describe four examples of biomedical image analysis tasks that can each be performed using techniques from either group of information fusion approaches. In each case, we describe examples of such techniques and evaluate and discuss their respective advantages and disadvantages. While typically the data domain is a continuous space and the interpretation domain is a discrete space (set of labels), the interpretation domain can also be a continuous space, as the application in Section 5 shows.

2 Atlas-Based Segmentation

Atlas-based image segmentation generates a segmentation of an image by registering it to an already segmented image, the atlas [7]. We have shown in previous work [8] that the segmentation accuracy can be improved substantially by using multiple atlases. For each atlas a nonrigid transformation from the unsegmented image to the atlas is computed. This transformation maps each pixel of the image to the atlas, where the pixel's label can be looked up, thus producing a segmentation of the entire image.

When combining multiple such segmentations in a COI approach, the labels j assigned by K individual segmentations to a given voxel x are counted, and the one with the most "votes" is assigned to the voxel in the final, combined segmentation:

$$x \mapsto \arg\max_j \#\{k \,|\, 0 \leq k < K, A_k(\mathbf{T}_k(x)) = j\} \tag{1}$$

Note that partial volume interpolation [9] can be used to interpolate smoothly between labels, and it also reduces the frequency of "undecided votes" without a unique winner label.

We have also shown previously that a similar improvement, albeit of smaller magnitude, can be achieved using a single atlas with different nonrigid registration algorithms, or different parameterizations of the same algorithm [10]. This corresponds to replacing $A_k(\mathbf{T}_k(x))$ in Eq. (1) with $A(\mathbf{T}_k(x))$, where there are K different transformations into a single atlas A.

The single-atlas, multi-transformation case is particularly interesting, because all coordinate transformations map from the same source coordinate system (the unsegmented image) to the same target coordinate system (the atlas). They can therefore be averaged numerically in the target image domain, and the average transformation can be used to obtain a segmentation.

$$x \mapsto A(\mathbf{T}^*(x)) \text{ with } \mathbf{T}^* \equiv \frac{1}{K} \sum_k \mathbf{T}_k \tag{2}$$

While Eq. (1) describes a COI approach (i.e., the labels assigned to each voxel), Eq. (2) is a COD approach (i.e., the nonrigid deformation fields). The practical differences between both approaches are illustrated in Fig. 2. In this application, COD, because it is a simple arithmetic averaging operation, can be performed using as few as two deformation fields. In the interpretation domain, however, we need at least three classifiers (and therefore deformation fields) in order to assign an unambiguous label when the individual classifiers disagree. Also, the COI approach tends to work better with odd numbers of classifiers, since this reduces the frequency of voting ties. There is, however, no substantial difference in terms of computational performance, since the rate-limiting step in atlas-based segmentation remains the nonrigid registration.

Table 1 shows the recognition rates (i.e., fraction of correctly classified voxels) for atlas-based segmentations of seven three-dimensional confocal microscopy images of

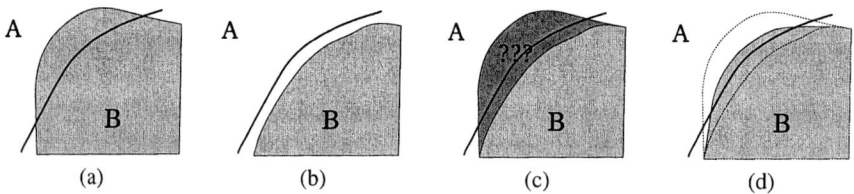

Fig. 2. Atlas-based segmentation using COI vs. COD. We consider two segmentations (a) and (b) of the boundary between structures A and B, where the bold line in all figures represents the true boundary between the two structures. Panel (c) shows the result of COI with an area (dark gray) where the two segmentations disagree so that no unambiguous label assignment is possible. The ambiguity will generally disappear with additional segmentations, especially when using partial volume interpolation. Panel (d) shows the result of COD, with the combined boundary estimate approximately halfway between the two boundary estimates. The gray lines represent the two individual segmentations in (a) and (b)

Table 1. Recognition rates for three atlas-based segmentations and their combinations using label voting (COI) and deformation averaging (COD) in seven subjects. The different individual segmentations were produced using different smoothness constraint weights of the nonrigid registration between subject image and atlas

Subject	Recognition Rates				
	Three Individual Segmentations			Combined Segmentation	
	Min	Max	Mean	Label Voting	Avg. Deformation
1	0.9562	0.9598	0.9585	0.9602	0.9591
2	0.9547	0.9582	0.9566	0.9590	0.9567
3	0.9681	0.9708	0.9695	0.9711	0.9673
4	0.9637	0.9652	0.9643	0.9658	0.9645
5	0.9490	0.9549	0.9519	0.9555	0.9519
6	0.9621	0.9665	0.9647	0.9671	0.9650
7	0.9797	0.9802	0.9800	0.9806	0.9801

bee brains [8]. For each subject, three different nonrigid transformations to a single atlas were computed, each using a different smoothness constraint weight for the registration algorithm [11, 12]. For details of the segmentation and evaluation methods, we refer the interested reader to [10]. The results in Table 1 show that both information fusion approaches achieved improvements over the individual segmentations. However, while label voting (COI) achieved recognition rates better than the *best* individual segmentation, averaging of the deformation fields (COD) produced recognition rates slightly better than the *mean* recognition rate of the individual segmentations.

3 Average Image Segmentation

Population average images [13] have become popular for obtaining images of normal anatomy with high signal-to-noise ratio [14], morphometric comparisons between subjects in different groups [15], as a reference anatomy for integration of sparse data from different subjects [16], and for atlas-based segmentation [8].

When segmented subject images are combined into an average shape image, there are two possible approaches to segment the average image: the individual segmentations (deformed into the average coordinate system) can be combined using label voting as described in the previous section (COI approach). Alternatively, because the average image resembles an actual image of a hypothetical "average" subject, it can be segmented directly (COD approach).

For this paper, we evaluated both strategies using MR brain images from 9 male control subjects that took part in an ongoing longitudinal study on the effects of alcoholism [17, 18]. All images were acquired at 1.5 T using SPoiled Gradient Recalled (SPGR) echo volumetric acquisitions of 94 slices, each 2 mm thick with no inter-slice spacing, collected in the coronal plane ($T_R = 25$ ms; $T_E = 5$ ms, flip angle = 30 degrees, matrix = 256×192, pixel size = 0.94×0.94 mm). Non-brain tissue in all images was removed using the Brain Extraction Tool [19] from the FMRIB Software Library (http://www.fmrib.ox.ac.uk/fsl/).

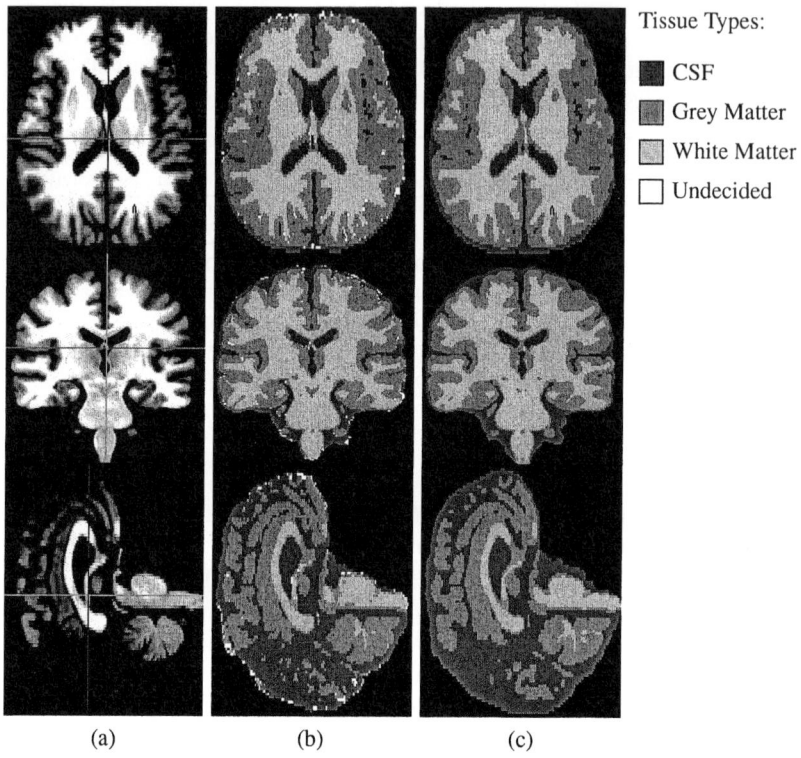

Fig. 3. Comparison of combined individual segmentations (COI) vs. segmentation of average image (COD). (a) Anatomical slice from the shape and intensity average image. The horizontal and vertical lines show the locations of the other orthogonal slices. (b) Combination of individual subject segmentations by label voting (COI). White dots represent voxels with undecided votes. (c) Direct segmentation of the shape and intensity average image (COD)

All subject images were registered, first rigidly and then nonrigidly [11, 12], to a reference subject [20]. They were then combined into a shape and intensity average image by determining the mean deformation of the population [21], deforming all images into this space, and averaging their corresponding image intensities (after an inter-subject intensity normalization).

For segmentation of the anatomical images, individual and average, into tissue types we used FMRIB's Automated Segmentation Tool [22] (FAST), also available from the aforementioned website. We performed segmentation on the intensity-normalized images in the shape average coordinate space, because MR images are more easily deformed and interpolated than label images resulting from segmentation. A combined segmentation of the average brain was generated by label voting, analogous to the method described for atlas-based segmentation in Section 2.

The results of combined individual segmentations (COI) vs. direct segmentation of the average image (COD) are shown in Fig. 3. Since we have no ground truth segmentation for either the subject images or the average, we limit ourselves to some general observations. First of all, the two segmentations appear very similar and both seem quite reasonable. It seems, however, that the direct segmentation of the average image did a slightly better job of capturing the anatomical details of complex and small structures (see for example the cerebellum and the cortical structure in the sagittal slices).

On a more technical level, in the combination of the individual segmentations there are voxels that could not be assigned a unique label due to equal numbers of votes for more than one winning label (voxels without uniquely assigned labels are shown as white dots in Fig. 3(b)). This problem is easily corrected by morphological operators, or greatly reduced by using fractional class weights rather than hard class assignments. It is, however, an issue that needs to be dealt with in the combination of segmentations, whereas it is avoided altogether by segmenting the average image. Finally, for a combination of individual segmentations each subject image has to be segmented separately (which for our data took about 4 minutes on a 3 GHz Pentium 4 CPU per case), whereas segmenting the average image requires only one segmentation step.

4 Multi-spectral Classification

A multi-channel image is one that contains a vector of values for each voxel, rather than a single scalar value. One way of generating such data is the acquisition of multiple aligned MR images with different imaging parameters. The advantage of such data for the purpose of segmentation is that, while tissue intensity distributions typically overlap substantially in scalar images, they are better separated in the higher-dimensional space of multi-channel data.

Tissue type classification of multi-channel MR images typically uses algorithms like k means clustering, which finds the centers of k clusters in the space of multi-dimensional intensity vectors. This is a COD method, where the data combination operator maps intensities of corresponding voxels from the three separate sets I_{T_1}, I_{PD}, and I_{T_2} to the product space of 3-tuples:

$$(I_{T_1}, I_{PD}, I_{T_2}) \mapsto I_{T_1} \times I_{PD} \times I_{T_2}. \quad (3)$$

A straight forward COI method for multi-spectral classification is to segment each channel separately, followed by vote fusion of the classifications for each voxel.

We apply both classification strategies to a three-channel MR image (T_1-weighted, T_2-weighted, proton density (PD)-weighted) from a single male subject. The T_1-weighted channel was acquired at 3 T using a 3D axial inversion recovery-prepared spoiled gradient recalled echo (IRPrep SPGR) pulse sequence with the following parameters: $T_I = 300$ ms, $T_R = 6.5$ ms, $T_E = 1.54$ ms, slice thickness = 1.25 mm, no inter-slice spacing, 124 slices, 0.94 mm pixel size. The PD and T_2-weighted channels were simultaneously acquired in a single 2D axial dual-echo Fast Spin-Echo (FSE) acquisition with the following parameters: $T_R = 10$ s, $T_E = 14/98$ ms (PD/T_2), slice thickness = 2.5 mm, no inter-slice spacing, 62 slices, 0.94 mm pixel size. To account for a small shift between the data sets, the T_1-weighted image was registered and reformatted to the PD-weighted channel using a nine-parameter affine registration algorithm [23, 24].

As in the previous section, tissue types are classified in the single MR images using FMRIB's Automated Segmentation Tool [22] (FAST), whereas the multi-spectral

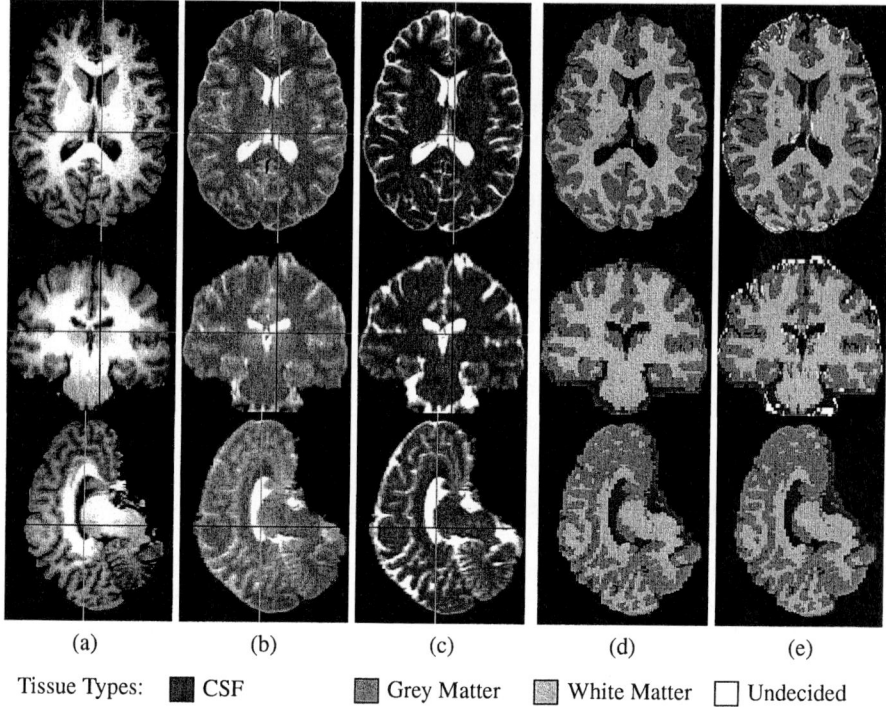

Fig. 4. Multi-spectral MR image and comparison of COD vs. COI tissue classification. (a) T_1-weighted image. (b) PD-weighted image. (c) T_2-weighted image. (d) Tissue classes from multi-spectral classification (COD). (e) Tissue classes from vote fusion of separate classifications of multi-spectral MR images (COI)

segmentation tool (MFAST) from the same software library is used for multi-spectral segmentation.

Orthogonal slices from the three MR images and segmentation results are shown in Fig. 4. Overall, the COD and the COI approaches produce comparable results. As before, there are some voxels for which the COI approach by itself cannot determine an output label, which could be fixed by a morphological correction step. On the other hand, the COI method seems to be better able to identify thin structures, e.g., the *septum pellucidum* that separates the two lateral ventricles, and most CSF-filled cortical folds.

5 Deformation-Based Group Morphometry

Deformation-based morphometry quantifies anatomical differences between groups of subjects, or within subjects over time [25]. A particular technique pioneered by Studholme *et al.* [20, 26] analyzes Jacobian determinant maps derived from nonrigid registrations of subject images to a reference image. The Jacobian maps quantify the local volume differences between the two registered images. By averaging such maps within groups of subjects, distinguishing characteristics between the groups can be identified.

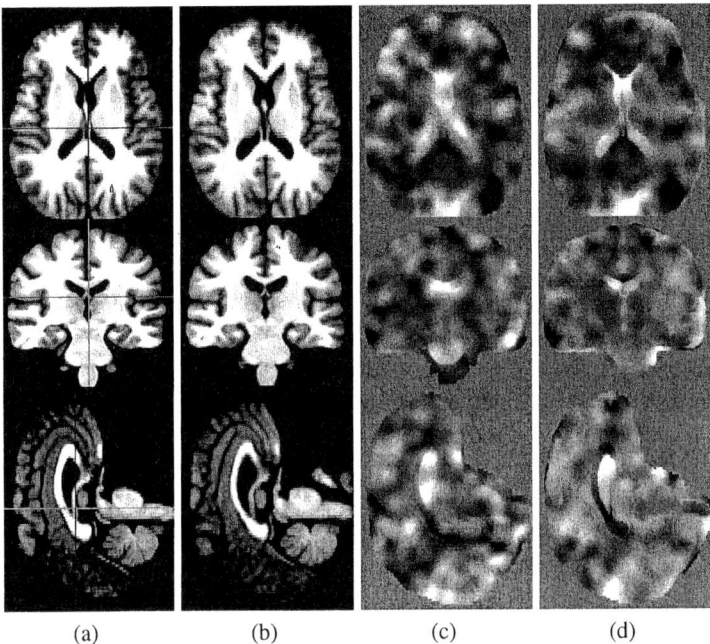

(a)　　　　　(b)　　　　　(c)　　　　　(d)

Fig. 5. Comparison of deformation morphometry based on individual Jacobian maps vs. non-rigid registration of two shape average images. (a) Anatomical slices from control group average image. The horizontal and vertical lines show the locations of the other orthogonal slices. (b) Anatomical slices from alcoholic group average image. (c) COI strategy: Group average of Jacobian maps between individual alcoholics and anatomical control group average. (d) COD strategy: Jacobian map between control group average and alcoholics group average. All Jacobian maps were filtered using Studholme's intensity-consistent filter [26] based on a Gaussian kernel with $\sigma = 4$ mm and cut-off radius $r = 2\sigma$. The Jacobian maps are shown with a logarithmic color scale, where bright colors correspond to increased, and dark colors correspond to decreased, relative volume in subjects in the alcoholic group

In the present context, we can look at the Jacobian map generation as a classification operation, where the classifier output is a local estimate of the volume difference between corresponding regions in two subjects. This example application is particularly interesting because the interpretation domain here is the continuous space of Jacobian determinant values rather than a discrete label set.

Consider the comparison of a group of diseased subjects to a group of normals using an inter-group Jacobian map. There are two alternatives. Given an average shape image [13, 27] of the normals group, we can compute a separate Jacobian map for each subject in the disease group. Each such map is based on the nonrigid transformation between the image from the respective diseased subject to the control group average shape image. All these maps are computed in the same coordinate space, the space of the control average, so they can be numerically averaged [20]. This, in our framework, is a COI strategy.

On the other hand, we can also generate an average shape image from the diseased subjects group and register it to the average image of the control group. The inter-group Jacobian map can then be computed from the resulting transformation, which is a COD strategy.

The group average images of, and the Jacobian maps between, a group of alcoholic men and a group of age-matched control subjects are shown in Fig. 5. These were computed from the image data acquired in the MR brain imaging study mentioned in Section 3 above. Before averaging the individual maps, we applied an intensity-consistent filter introduced by Studholme *et al.* [26], which is based on a Gaussian kernel ($\sigma = 4$ mm, cut off radius $r = 2\sigma$). The same type of filter was also applied to the Jacobian map between the two group average images.

Again, in the absence of ground truth data, we visually assess the Jacobian maps in Fig. 5. It is apparent that the Jacobian values are more specific to certain anatomical structures (e.g., corpus callosum, fourth ventricle, inter-hemispheric fissure) in the map computed using the COD strategy (Fig. 5(d)). In the COI map (Fig. 5(c)), despite applying the intensity-consistent filter, the averaging of Jacobian maps seems to blur the boundaries of structures. It is worth pointing out, however, the fairly specific regions of agreement between the two maps, for example the relative volume increase in the posterior inter-hemispheric fissure and the volume decrease in the left occipital lobe. Note that we are not addressing the question whether the maps are factually correct; we are merely comparing the results obtained through different processing paths.

A fundamental advantage of the COI method is that it allows voxel-wise statistical tests and modeling (c.f., [20]). In addition, a potential problem with the COD approach is that the single nonrigid registration between the group average images creates a single point of failure. That is, in regions where the registration computes an inaccurate[1] transformation, the resulting Jacobian map will almost certainly be incorrect as well. When combining individual Jacobian maps from all subjects in a group, such errors are more likely to be averaged out in the process. Note, however, that registration between two average images is typically less likely to fail than registration between two subjects, so the registration failure issue may not be a serious problem.

6 Discussion

In this paper, we have developed a new view of information fusion, distinguishing between combination of information in the data domain and in the interpretation domain. In four common biomedical image analysis tasks, we have illustrated that problems can often be approached by algorithms operating in either of these domains, with specific advantages and disadvantages. Table 2 gives a brief summary of our examples and the respective COI and COD methods applied to them.

---

[1] The accuracy of a volumetric inter-individual nonrigid transformation between two different subjects is not a particularly well-defined concept. Because of this, and because of the difficulty of inter-subject registration, such a transformation is typically somewhat inaccurate pretty much everywhere.

Table 2. Overview of the biomedical applications of information fusion discussed in this paper

Application	Combination of Interpretations	Combination of Data
Atlas-Based Segmentation	Label voting among individual segmentations generated using different nonrigid coordinate transformations	Averaging of nonrigid transformation in the atlas coordinate system
Average Image Segmentation	Classification of the original individual images with subsequent label voting	Classification of the average image
Multi-Spectral Classification	Classification of each channel with subsequent voting	Classification of multi-spectral data
Deformation Morphometry	Separate Jacobian maps for each individual image based on its registration to the reference image, followed by averaging of the maps for each group	Generation of shape average images, followed by nonrigid registration of averages and Jacobian map computation

In atlas-based segmentation, we found that the COI method (i.e., label voting) appears to be more accurate than the COD method (i.e., deformation averaging), but the differences are relatively small. Recall, however, that COD here preserves the continuity and smoothness of the underlying B-spline transformation, which can be an advantage.

Segmenting a group average image, the COD method (i.e., direct segmentation of the average image) lead to segmentations that were slightly more consistent with the image data than the COI method (i.e., label voting). It was also more computationally efficient, as it required only a single application of the tissue segmentation algorithm.

In the multi-spectral MR segmentation example, the observed differences between the commonly applied COD method and the COI method are fairly subtle. Of course the theoretical advantage of the COD method is that in multi-spectral data clusters of different tissue classes typically overlap much less than in any of the marginal distributions, so that the classes can be more reliably separated. Another advantage of the COD method is its insensitivity to replication of channels. When applied to data that contains the same channel more than once, k-means clustering likely produces very similar results as it would with each channel occurring only once. This, however, is a situation that can heavily bias the COI technique and thereby reduce its usefulness.

In the group morphometry application, we again found that the COD method (i.e., computation of the Jacobian map between group average images) seemed to produce output that was more consistent with the image data than the COI method (i.e., averaging of the individual Jacobian maps). However, depending on a single nonrigid registration step between the group average images creates potential reliability problems due to the single point of failure. Also, the COI approach is more versatile in that it allows voxel-wise statistical tests between the individual Jacobian maps in each group.

We note that information fusion can exist on multiple levels within a single application. For example, the atlas-based segmentation in Section 2 is a single atlas case with multiple transformations generated with different registration parameters (constraint weights). An alternative approach, which we have previously published, is the multiple-atlas case. The multiple-atlas case with many individuals vs. the single-atlas case where the single atlas is an average image of those many individuals is also a COI vs. COD situation. Information fusion exists on two levels within this application, in the sense that the average atlas itself can be constructed with either a COI or a COD approach (as discussed in Section 3). (We used a COI approach to construct the average atlas because we had manually segmented individuals.)

In summary, we conclude that information fusion is a valuable concept in many image analysis tasks. By considering different domains in which information can be combined and analyzed, its benefits may be increased and better adjusted to the specific requirements of a given problem. The primary point of this paper is to provide a framework for thinking about information fusion. The examples we explored illustrate some of the many potential applications of information fusion in biomedical image analysis. A detailed comparison and evaluation of COD and COI approaches is beyond the scope of this paper. Nonetheless, whereas most reported work on information fusion uses COI approaches, the very preliminary results in our work suggest that COD approaches are also useful and worth considering.

Acknowledgments

This work was in part supported by the National Institute on Alcohol Abuse and Alcoholism, Grants No. AA05965, AA12388, AA12999, and AA13521. The authors thank R. Brandt (Mercury Computer Systems, Berlin, Germany) and R. Menzel (Freie Universität Berlin, Berlin, Germany) for providing bee brain microscopy images and ground truth segmentations. Nonrigid registrations were performed on an SGI Origin 3800 supercomputer in the Stanford University Bio-X core facility for Biomedical Computation.

References

1. Xu, L., Krzyzak, A., Suen, C.Y.: Methods of combining multiple classifiers and their applications to handwriting recognition. IEEE Trans. Syst. Man Cybern. **22** (1992) 418–435
2. Kittler, J., Hatef, M., Duin, R.P.W., Matas, J.: On combining classifiers. IEEE Trans. Pattern Anal. Machine Intell. **20** (1998) 226–239
3. De Santo, M., Molinara, M., Tortorella, F., Vento, M.: Automatic classification of clustered microcalcifications by a multiple expert system. Pattern Recognit. **36** (2003) 1467–1477
4. Rogova, G.L., Stomper, P.C.: Information fusion approach to microcalcification characterization. Inform. Fusion **3** (2002) 91–102
5. Sboner, A., Eccher, C., Blanzieri, E., Bauer, P., Cristofolini, M., Zumiani, G., Forti, S.: A multiple classifier system for early melanoma diagnosis. Artif. Intell. Med. **27** (2003) 29–44
6. Gefen, S., Tretiak, O.J., Piccoli, C.W., et al.: ROC analysis of ultrasound tissue characterization classifiers for breast cancer diagnosis. IEEE Trans. Med. Imag. **22** (2003) 170–177
7. Miller, M.I., Christensen, G.E., Amit, Y., Grenander, U.: Mathematical textbook of deformable neuroanatomies. Proc. Natl. Acad. Sci. USA **90** (1993) 11944–11948
8. Rohlfing, T., Brandt, R., Menzel, R., Maurer, Jr., C.R.: Evaluation of atlas selection strategies for atlas-based image segmentation with application to confocal microscopy images of bee brains. NeuroImage **21** (2004) 1428–1442

9. Maes, F., Collignon, A., Vandermeulen, D., Marchal, G., Suetens, P.: Multimodality image registration by maximisation of mutual information. IEEE Trans. Med. Imag. **16** (1997) 187–198
10. Rohlfing, T., Maurer, Jr., C.R.: Multi-classifier framework for atlas-based image segmentation. Pattern Recogn. Lett. (2005) In press.
11. Rueckert, D., Sonoda, L.I., Hayes, C., et al.: Nonrigid registration using free-form deformations: Application to breast MR images. IEEE Trans. Med. Imag. **18** (1999) 712–721
12. Rohlfing, T., Maurer, Jr., C.R.: Nonrigid image registration in shared-memory multiprocessor environments with application to brains, breasts, and bees. IEEE Trans. Inform. Technol. Biomed. **7** (2003) 16–25
13. Guimond, A., Meunier, J., Thirion, J.P.: Average brain models: A convergence study. Comput. Vision Image Understanding **77** (2000) 192–210
14. Collins, D.L., Zijdenbos, A.P., Kollokian, V., et al.: Design and construction of a realistic digital brain phantom. IEEE Trans. Med. Imag. **17** (1998) 463–468
15. Park, H.J., Westin, C.F., Kubicki, et al.: White matter hemisphere asymmetries in healthy subjects and in schizophrenia: a diffusion tensor MRI study. NeuroImage **23** (2004) 213–223
16. Brandt, R., Rohlfing, T., Ryback, J., et al.: An average three-dimensional atlas of the honeybee brain based on confocal images of 20 subjects. J. Comp. Neurol. (2005) In press.
17. Pfefferbaum, A., Lim, K.O., Desmond, J.E., Sullivan, E.V.: Thinning of the corpus callosum in older alcoholic men: a magnetic resonance imaging study. Alcohol. Clin. Exp. Res. **20** (1996) 752–757
18. Pfefferbaum, A., Rosenbloom, M., Serventi, K.L., Sullivan, E.V.: Corpus callosum, pons, and cortical white matter in alcoholic women. Alcohol. Clin. Exp. Res. **26** (2002) 400–406
19. Smith, S.M.: Fast robust automated brain extraction. Hum. Brain Map. **17** (2002) 143–155
20. Studholme, C., Cardenas, V., Blumenfeld, R., et al.: Deformation tensor morphometry of semantic dementia with quantitative validation. NeuroImage **21** (2004) 1387–1398
21. Rueckert, D., Frangi, A.F., Schnabel, J.A.: Automatic construction of 3-D statistical deformation models of the brain using nonrigid registration. IEEE Trans. Med. Imag. **22** (2003) 1014–1025
22. Zhang, Y., Brady, M., Smith, S.: Segmentation of brain MR images through a hidden Markov random field model and the expectation-maximization algorithm. IEEE Trans. Med. Imag. **20** (2001) 45–57
23. Studholme, C., Hill, D.L.G., Hawkes, D.J.: Automated three-dimensional registration of magnetic resonance and positron emission tomography brain images by multiresolution optimization of voxel similarity measures. Med. Phys. **24** (1997) 25–35
24. Studholme, C., Hill, D.L.G., Hawkes, D.J.: An overlap invariant entropy measure of 3D medical image alignment. Pattern Recognit. **32** (1999) 71–86
25. Chung, M.K., Worsley, K.J., Paus, T., et al.: A unified statistical approach to deformation-based morphometry. NeuroImage **14** (2001) 595–606
26. Studholme, C., Cardenas, V., Maudsley, A., Weiner, M.: An intensity consistent filtering approach to the analysis of deformation tensor derived maps of brain shape. NeuroImage **19** (2003) 1638–1649
27. Rohlfing, T., Brandt, R., Maurer, Jr., C.R., Menzel, R.: Bee brains, B-splines and computational democracy: Generating an average shape atlas. In Staib, L., ed.: IEEE Workshop on Mathematical Methods in Biomedical Image Analysis, Kauai, HI, IEEE Computer Society, Los Alamitos, CA (2001) 187–194

Parametric Medial Shape Representation in 3-D via the Poisson Partial Differential Equation with Non-linear Boundary Conditions

Paul A. Yushkevich, Hui Zhang, and James C. Gee

Department of Radiology, University of Pennsylvania

Abstract. This paper presents a new shape representation for a special class of 3-D objects. In a generative approach to object modeling inspired by m-reps [15], skeletons of objects are explicitly defined as continuous manifolds and boundaries are derived from the skeleton by a process that involves solving a Poisson PDE with a non-linear boundary condition. This formulation helps satisfy the equality constraints that are imposed on the parameters of the representation by rules of medial geometry. One benefit of the new approach is the ability to represent different instances of an anatomical structure using a common parametrization domain, simplifying the problem of computing correspondences between instances. Another benefit is the ability to continuously parameterize the volumetric region enclosed by the representation's boundary in a one-to-one and onto manner, in a way that preserves two of the three coordinates of the parametrization along vectors normal to the boundary. These two features make the new representation an attractive candidate for statistical analysis of shape and appearance. In this paper, the representation is carefully defined and the results of fitting the hippocampus in a deformable templates framework are presented.

1 Introduction and Overview of Prior Work

The popularity of Active Shape Models (ASM) [3] and Active Appearance Models (AAM) [4] in the medical image processing community underscores the importance of analytic tools that combine shape and appearance. These two types of features are related in a non-linear way and are both essential for characterizing and comparing anatomical structures. Shape features can detect growth and decay processes or physical deformation, while appearance features can describe a diverse set of local properties, such as tissue contrast, diffusion or blood perfusion. In this paper, we present a novel continuous parametric medial object representation that offers a unique approach to establishing correspondences between shape and appearance features and promises to be useful for statistical analysis of anatomy. We begin this section with a review of the state of the art in shape and appearance modeling; we then motivate the use of medial axes and medial representations and explain the need for continuous medial modeling; and, finally, we summarize the contributions of our method.

A natural way to associate shape and appearance features is to parameterize the image intensities inside and outside of an object using the same set of coordinates that parameterize the boundaries themselves. This is roughly the approach taken by ASM, where appearance features are obtained by sampling the image along fixed-length profiles projected orthogonally from the boundary [3]. When the boundary is represented by a parameterized surface, as in the related spherical harmonics model [7], each profile is associated with two parameter values, and the distance along the profile can serve as a third 'depth' coordinate for parameterizing the space around the boundary [10]. However, since the profiles have fixed length, they are not guaranteed to span the whole interior of the object and they may intersect, causing ambiguity in the parametrization. In contrast, AAM offers a one to one and onto parametrization of space enclosed by the object [4], but it no longer associates internal points with the nearest boundary points because it is based on warps that do not preserve the orthogonality of the vectors normal to the boundary.

We can make the ASM-like parametrization of points inside of an object one to one and onto by making every profile extend all the way to the medial axis of the object (in 3-D, the *medial scaffold*), where it would touch a profile extended from a boundary point on the opposite side. Since it is likely that the medial axis would have a different number and configuration of branches for every instance of a given type of object, it would be seemingly difficult to apply such a parametrization in statistical analysis. However, if we are willing to trade off the accuracy of the representation for consistency, the m-rep approach pioneered by Pizer et al. [15, 12] would allow us to model populations of objects using a prescribed medial branching topology. In this approach, objects are represented by first explicitly defining their medial axes or scaffolds and then deriving the corresponding boundary curve or surface. The medial definition in m-reps is discrete, consisting of a set of rich primitives. Attempts to continuously interpolate these primitives have failed to strictly adhere to the rules of medial geometry, disallowing the kind of object parametrization that we seek [21]. The attempt by [22] to model the medial scaffold and the associated radius field as continuous functions, which is described in more detail in Sec. 2.2, did allow proper object parametrization, but suffered from the inability to define these functions on a prescribed domain, making statistical analysis difficult. This method was also inherently limited to single-manifold medial scaffolds.

In this paper, a new approach to continuous parametric medial representation is presented. Unlike the earlier approach [22], it allows different instances of an anatomical structure to be represented using a common domain of parametrization. In doing so, it overcomes the key limitation of [22] that made the extension of the method to branching medial scaffolds infeasible. In the new method, the radial field on the medial scaffold is defined as the solution of a Poisson PDE with a non-linear boundary condition that seamlessly incorporates the equality constraints that hold at special points on the medial scaffold. This approach allows us to 'transfer' second order properties of the radial field from one medial scaffold to another, opening the door for statistical analysis.

The paper is organized as follows. Sec. 2 summarizes the key results from medial geometry, examines the limitations of the implicit domain solution to continuous medial representation, defines the PDE-based approach and describes its use in deformable templates modeling. Sec. 3 presents the results of fitting a hippocampus template to segmentations from a schizophrenia study. The paper's contributions are summarized in Sec. 4.

2 Methods

2.1 Elements of Medial Geometry

Blum and Nagel [1] pioneered the use of medial axes for 2-D shape analysis. In this paper, we are interested in modeling medial geometry in 3-D. The *medial scaffold*, shown in Fig. 1, is the 3-D analogy of Blum's medial axis and it has been studied rigorously in the recent literature [14, 16, 6], and in this subsection we summarize some of the results. We begin with a formal definition of objects and medial scaffolds.

Definition 1. *A geometric object (or just object) is a bounded set in $\mathbb{R}^3$ that is homeomorphic to a unit ball and whose boundary is a generic surface.*

Definition 2. *A ball with center $\mathbf{x}$ and radius r is called a* maximal inscribed ball *with respect to an object $\mathcal{O}$ if $\{\mathbf{y} : \|\mathbf{x} - \mathbf{y}\| \leq R\} \subset \mathcal{O}$ and $\forall R' > R$, $\{\mathbf{y} : \|\mathbf{x} - \mathbf{y}\| \leq R'\} \not\subset \mathcal{O}$. The* medial scaffold *of an object $\mathcal{O}$ is the set of points in $\mathbb{R}^3 \times \mathbb{R}^+$ formed by the centers and radii of maximal inscribed balls of $\mathcal{O}$.*

According to Damon [6] the medial scaffold is a Whitney stratified set, i.e., a collection of manifolds with boundary that are connected. Giblin and Kimia [14] give a complete taxonomy of the types of points that form the medial scaffold. There are five types of points, each with different order and multiplicity of the tangency between the maximal inscribed ball and the object's boundary. The five point types correspond to five different places on the medial scaffold; a point may lie on a medial manifold; it may lie at an edge of a medial manifold; it may lie at a curve shared by two medial manifolds (we shall call this the *seam curve*); it may lie at an intersection of a seam curve and an edge of a manifold; and it may lie at an intersection of two seam curves.

Our intention in this paper is to model the medial scaffold and the radial field of an object as a parametric function from a domain in $\mathbb{R}^2$ to $\mathbb{R}^3$ and $\mathbb{R}^+$; and then to generate the boundary of the object as a function of the medial scaffold. Given some parametric expression for a single medial surface $(\mathbf{x}(u^1, u^2), R(u^1, u^2))$, the expression for the boundary can be found by observing that the boundary is the envelope of a two-parameter family of spheres defined implicitly by the equation

$$S(\mathbf{y}; u^1, u^2) = \|\mathbf{x}(u^1, u^2) - \mathbf{y}\|^2 - R(u^1, u^2)^2 = 0 . \qquad (1)$$

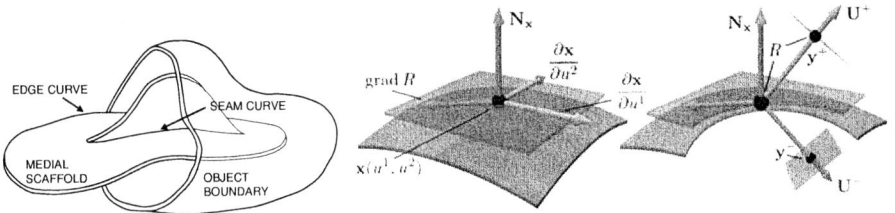

Fig. 1. Left: the medial scaffold with a fin-like branching configuration. Right: the local geometry of a point on the medial scaffold

Thus any point **y** on the boundary of an object must satisfy the following envelope equations:
$$S = 0 \; ; \qquad \frac{\partial S}{\partial u^i} = 0 \, , \quad i = 1, 2 \, . \tag{2}$$

By solving these equations for a vector $\mathbf{U} = \frac{\mathbf{y}-\mathbf{x}}{R}$, we obtain the following system:
$$\mathbf{U} \cdot \mathbf{U} = 1; \qquad \mathbf{U} \cdot \frac{\partial \mathbf{x}}{\partial u^i} = -\frac{\partial R}{\partial u^i} \, , \quad i = 1, 2 \, . \tag{3}$$

By decomposing **U** into a component in the tangent plane of the medial scaffold and a normal component, we find that the tangential component is directly related to the Riemannian gradient of R on the medial surface:
$$\operatorname{proj}_{\mathbf{N_x}} \mathbf{U} = -g^{ij} \frac{\partial \mathbf{x}}{\partial u^i} \frac{\partial R}{\partial u^j} = -\operatorname{grad} R \, , \tag{4}$$

where g^{ij} denotes the contravariant metric tensor on the medial surface and the Einstein summation notation is used. The fact that **U** has unit length allows one to compute the magnitude of its normal component, producing the following expression for **U**:
$$\mathbf{U}^{\pm} = -\operatorname{grad} R \pm \sqrt{1 - \|\operatorname{grad} R\|^2} \, \mathbf{N_x} \, . \tag{5}$$

At points where the argument of the square root is non-zero, **U** takes two distinct values. The pair of boundary points **y** associated with a medial point $(\mathbf{x}, R)$ are then given by
$$\mathbf{y}^{\pm}(u^1, u^2) = \mathbf{x} + R\,\mathbf{U}^{\pm} \, . \tag{6}$$

It is easy to verify that the sphere defined by $S = 0$ is tangent to the object's boundary at the points $\mathbf{y}^{\pm}$ and that the unit normal vectors to the boundary at $\mathbf{y}^{\pm}$ are given by $\mathbf{U}^{\pm}$. This geometry is summarized on Fig. 1.

It is a remarkable fact of medial geometry that the expressions for the boundary **y** and for the boundary normal **U** only involve the first order derivatives of **x** and R. This fact implies that the metric tensor, the second fundamental form and the shape operator on the boundary surface can be computed using derivatives of the medial scaffold of up to the second order. This is great news from the point of view of geometrical modeling: if we were to represent medial surfaces by C^2 functions, then the generated boundaries would also be C^2 continuous.

We will be especially interested in this paper in the situation that occurs at the edges of medial sheets. As shown by [14], at these points the maximal inscribed ball is tangent to the boundary at a single point but with a higher order of contact. Note that in general, (4) is valid only at points on the interior of medial surfaces, where the partial derivatives with respect to u^i can be taken. Points on edges and seams of medial surfaces are typically treated as the limit case of interior medial points [6, 14]. However, in the medial modeling paradigm, we can ignore this issue by simply extending the parametric model definition slightly past the domain on which the medial scaffold is given. Along the medial edge, $\mathbf{y}^-$ and $\mathbf{y}^+$ in (6) must coincide, thus either R or the normal component of $\mathbf{U}$ in (5) must vanish, leading to the following equality constraint:

$$\|\text{grad}\, R\|^2 = g^{ij} \frac{\partial R}{\partial u^i} \frac{\partial R}{\partial u^j} = 1 \quad \text{if } R > 0 \,. \tag{7}$$

A similar equality constraint can be given along the seam curve where three medial surfaces meet; in this case the constraint is a non-linear expression relating vectors $\text{grad}\, R$ on all three surfaces [22].

2.2 Geometric Modeling of Medial Scaffolds

Suppose we were to represent each medial surface in a medial scaffold using twice differentiable functions $\mathbf{x}: \Omega \to \mathbb{R}^3$ and $R: \Omega \to \mathbb{R}$ defined on a regular domain Ω in $\mathbb{R}^2$. These functions must satisfy certain constraints in order for Eqns. 4 - 6 to define a *valid* boundary surface, i.e., a generic surface whose medial scaffold coincides with $(\mathbf{x}, R)$. Damon [6] derives a small number of such constraints and shows that they are necessary and sufficient. In addition to the equality constraints for medial edges and seams described in the previous section, which relate to Damon's *compatibility* constraints, there is a set of inequality constraints that ensure that the boundary surface does not have singularities.

We are interested in modeling medial surfaces using basis functions such as splines or wavelets, which allow us to specify a surface using a finite set of coefficients. From this point of view, equality constraints pose much more of a problem than inequality constraints. The latter can be dealt with by restricting the set of possible coefficient values to a region of Euclidean space. However, when equality constraints are non-linear, there may not be any combination of coefficients that would produce a surface that satisfies the constraints. In other words, the above equality constraints hold at an infinite number of points along medial edges and seams, yet there is only a finite number of coefficients used to define the medial surfaces. Hence, the problem is overconstrained.

Earlier work in continuous medial modeling [22] addressed this problem for single-surface medial scaffolds by computing the domain on which a medial surface is defined implicitly. The coefficients of the representation were chosen in such a way that $\|\text{grad}\, R\|$ would be greater than 1 on the boundary of a regular domain $\Omega \in R^2$, while holding $\|\text{grad}\, R\| < 1$ on some subset of Ω. Then the actual domain on which the medial surface was defined was taken to be the set $\Omega' = \{\mathbf{u} \in \Omega : ||\text{grad}\, R(\mathbf{u})|| \leq 1\}$. By construction, the constraint (7) would hold on $\partial\Omega'$. While this approach made it possible to represent and deform single-surface medial scaffolds, it suffered from a severe limitation: the implicit domain Ω' depends on the values of the coefficients and changes as the model deforms, and it is not possible to generate models of different instances of the same anatomical structure with the same domain. This makes it very difficult to establish point correspondences and perform statistical analysis on such models. Moreover, the implicit domain solution has no obvious extension to handle the equality constraints that hold along seam curves of medial scaffolds with multiple medial surfaces.

2.3 Parametric Medial Surfaces with Fixed Domains

The main contribution of this paper is the derivation of an alternative model that allows the domain Ω to be determined *a priori* and to stay fixed as the model deforms. We achieve this by defining the function R using a partial differential equation. We present here the results for modeling of single-surface medial scaffolds; the extension to seam modeling is the subject of ongoing research.

Suppose that the medial surface $\mathbf{x}$ is a twice differentiable function from a fixed domain $\Omega \in \mathbb{R}^2$ to $\mathbb{R}^3$. For instance, below we let $\mathbf{x}$ be the weighted sum of N basis functions. The key idea of this work is to define the function $R : \Omega \to \mathbb{R}^+$ as the solution of a PDE of the form

$$\mathcal{L}(R;\mathbf{x}) = \rho(u^1, u^2); \qquad ||\text{grad}\, R||^2 = 1 \text{ on } \partial\Omega, \tag{8}$$

where $\mathcal{L}$ is a suitable Riemannian differential operator and $\rho : \Omega \to \mathbb{R}$ is a function defined parametrically, e.g., using basis functions. A suitable choice of $\mathcal{L}$ would be one that would lead to a PDE with provable existence, uniqueness and stability properties. Ideally, the quantity $\mathcal{L}(R;\mathbf{x})$ will have geometric meaning and will be invariant under shape-preserving similarity transformations.

We have examined several possible choices of the operator $\mathcal{L}$ and the only suitable and attractive option that we discovered was the curved-space analog of the Laplacian, the Laplace-Beltrami operator, applied to R^2:

$$\mathcal{L}(R;\mathbf{x}) = \widetilde{\triangle} R^2, \tag{9}$$

$$\widetilde{\triangle} f = \text{div}\, \text{grad}\, f = \frac{1}{\sqrt{g}} \frac{\partial}{\partial u^\eta} \left(\sqrt{g}\, g^{\mu\eta} \frac{\partial f}{\partial u^\mu} \right), \qquad ([13], \text{p. } 231). \tag{10}$$

If we set $\phi = R^2$ and rewrite (8) for ϕ, we obtain a Poisson elliptic partial differential equation with a non-linear boundary condition:

$$\widetilde{\triangle}\phi = \rho; \qquad ||\text{grad}\, \phi||^2 = 4\phi \text{ on } \partial\Omega. \tag{11}$$

There are several ways to justify this particular choice of $\mathcal{L}$. First, we can formally prove that the solution of this PDE is unique if $\rho < 0$ on $\partial\Omega$. The converse of

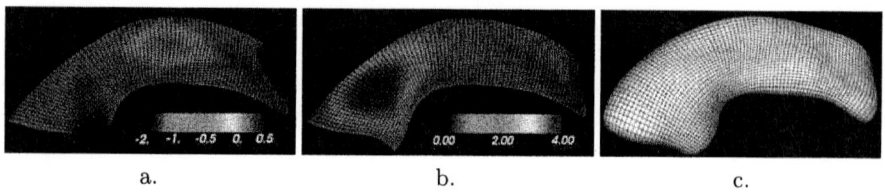

Fig. 2. The three steps of constructing a cm-rep. **a.** A medial manifold **x** with the radial conductance function ρ. **b.** The radial function R computed by solving the Poisson equation (11) on the manifold. **c.** Boundary surface **y** computed using (5)

this condition implies that R increases on the approach to the edge of a medial manifold, which is not possible geometrically. The existence and stability of the solution are demonstrated by empirical evidence, i.e., by our ability to repeatedly solve the PDE for different ρ and **x** in the course of template deformation. The operator $\mathcal{L}$ is intrinsic and it is invariant under similarity transformations.

Finally, $\mathcal{L}(R; \mathbf{x})$ has a definite geometric meaning because it is proportional to the divergence of the vector field $R \operatorname{grad} R$, which is in turn the projection of the vector $\mathbf{y} - \mathbf{x}$ on the tangent plane of the medial surface. The operator $\mathcal{L}$ captures second order properties of the radius field that are independent of the choice of parametrization. It is notable that on the medial scaffold of an ellipsoid $\widetilde{\triangle} R^2$ is constant.

We use the finite difference method to solve (11) numerically on a regular sampling grid in a rectangular or circular domain. The metric tensor and the Christoffel symbols, which are needed to express $\operatorname{grad} \phi$ and $\widetilde{\triangle} \phi$, are computed analytically from the medial surface formulation. The partial derivatives of the unknown function ϕ are expressed as finite differences. The PDE (11) reduces to a system of first and second order equations with values of ϕ on the sampling grid as the unknowns. The roots of this system can be found iteratively using Newton's method [18–pp. 142-147]. Each Newton iteration involves solving a non-symmetric sparse linear system. At each iteration we use the state of the art PARDISO direct sparse solver [17]. On a 100×100 sampling grid, the numerical solution is computed in less than a second on a modern CPU.

The overall process of defining an object from functions **x** and ρ is illustrated on Fig. 2. First, the medial manifold **x** and the scalar field ρ are defined parametrically. Next, the PDE (11) is solved, yielding the scalar field R. Finally, equations (5) and (6) are used to define a closed continuous boundary surface.

2.4 Deformable Modeling Using CM-Reps

Following the example of discrete m-reps [15], we are interested in deforming templates with single-surface medial scaffolds to instances of human anatomy, in particular the hippocampus. This will eventually allow us to build a model of the shape and appearance of the hippocampus, which could serve as a prior for shape-based image segmentation. The model could also be useful for detecting group differences between patients with different medical conditions and controls.

We define the deformable template as a finite set of coefficients that together with a set of orthogonal basis functions give a parametric definition of a smooth medial surface and a smooth function ρ that appears in the right hand side of the PDE (11). In the present implementation, following [19], we use the real-valued Fourier transform as our basis:

$$\mathbf{x}(u^1, u^2; \{\mathbf{C}\}_{j,k}) = \sum_{j,k=0}^{N} \mathbf{C}_{j,k} \cos(2\pi j\, u^1) \cos(2\pi k\, u^2)\,, \qquad (12)$$

and ρ is also defined this way. The advantage of using the Fourier basis is the ability to easily increase the number of high frequency components in the model; the disadvantage is the lack of local control over the surface. In future implementations we will likely switch to the wavelet basis, which allows both frequency and location components to be modulated. Parameters u^1, u^2 are defined on a rectangular domain (we do not use the unit square domain because the metric tensor of $\mathbf{x}$ would vanish at its corners). In the future we anticipate using the unit circle as the domain, in order to generate medial surfaces without corners. Both of these extensions are easy to implement within our framework. Changes in basis functions are virtually transparent to most aspects of parametric medial representation, and a change to the circular domain is a matter of reformulating the finite difference equations.

To construct a hippocampus template, we used a discrete m-rep [15] of the hippocampus (graciously provided by Prof Stephen M. Pizer's group at UNC) and densely interpolated the medial atom positions. We used a least squares fit to the interpolated points to obtain the initial values of the coefficients $\mathbf{C}_{j,k}$. The function ρ was initialized as a negative constant. To deform the medial surface and ρ of the template, we modify the values of the coefficients and solve (11) to generate the radius function R and its derivatives, from which the boundary can be computed using (5) and (6). To be considered *valid*, a set of coefficients values must generate a medial surface and a ρ function that satisfy a set of inequality constraints. While the exhaustive set of constraints is given by Damon [6] could have been implemented, we have found that in practice, only two constraints must be 'kept track of' during template deformation. First, ρ must be negative on $\partial\Omega$ - assuring that R decreases when approaching the edge of a medial surface. Second, the Jacobian of the function $\mathbf{y}(u^1, u^2)$ must be positive at every point in Ω in order to prevent cusps from forming on the boundary.

As in the case of discrete m-reps, we pose the problem of fitting a deformable template to a binary characteristic image of a structure as a Bayesian problem of finding a maximum posterior estimate. This problem is solved by concurrent minimization of a weighted sum of a likelihood, or image match term, and a prior term that incorporates the above constraints in a 'fuzzy' manner using exponential penalty functions. In the future, when a statistical shape model constructed from training data will be available, we will use it as a prior, similar to the way ASM, AAM, and m-reps incorporate existing knowledge [3, 4, 15].

We represent objects such as the hippocampus using real-valued characteristic images in which the object itself is the zeroth level set. These images are computed by smoothing a binary characteristic image with a Gaussian kernel. The variance of the kernel is decreased over the course of the fitting. Two image match terms are used: the less accurate but more globally sensitive relative volume overlap term is used throughout most of the multi-resolution fitting procedure. At the late stages, we switch to a term that integrates the squared image intensity along the template's boundary. Volume overlap is approximated by computing the template's volume and the volume of the template-object intersection by integrating over template's interior. The integration is efficient because vectors **U** span the interior of the template.

Maximum *a posteriori* estimation is implemented as a multi-resolution schedule of conjugate gradient descent optimizations. Each step in the schedule involves using more and more coefficients (we start with 2x4 and finish with 8x10 4-tuples of coefficients), and, from time to time, reducing the aperture of the kernel that is used to smooth the binary characteristic image.

Gradient methods are an appropriate choice because the cost of computing the central difference approximation of the partial derivatives of ϕ with respect to the coefficients is lower than the cost of computing ϕ at arbitrary points. This is the case because the solution of (11) at the central point can be used to initialize Newton's method at points located an ϵ away, reducing the number of iterations needed to solve the equation. The derivatives of ϕ could also be computed directly by solving a Poisson equation with a different non-linear boundary condition; we will explore this option in future work. The partial derivatives of the volume overlap match can be computed very efficiently using Green's theorem; however, the approximation error becomes a detractor at late stages of the optimization. Our results, presented in the following section, indicate that our deterministic approach is not severely hampered by spurious local minima. The fitting is initialized by a global localization that matches the moments of inertia between the template and the image and by an optimization over the space of affine transforms (with ρ scaling), which further improves the initialization.

3 Results and Discussion

To test the representational ability of the parametric medial representation, we fitted the hippocampus template to 174 (87 right, 87 left) segmentations of the hippocampus from a MRI schizophrenia study [2]. The segmentation was computed using the Joshi et al. [11] algorithm for large deformation diffeomorphic registration with manually placed anatomic landmarks. This approach is used extensively in brain morphometry [5] and was shown to be more accurate and reliable than manual segmentation [9]. The data in the form of boundary meshes was graciously provided by Profs. Guido Gerig (UNC Depts. of Comp. Sci. and Psychiatry) and Sarang Joshi (UNC Dept. of Rad. Onc.).

The 174 hippocampus segmentations were fitted on a 14-CPU Linux cluster over approximately 24 hours. The quality of the fit between a template T and an image I was evaluated using the following criteria: robust volume overlap $\text{Vol}(T \cap I)/\text{Vol}(T \cup I)$; 'biased' volume overlap $\text{Vol}(T \cap I)/\text{Vol}(I)$; mean and

Table 1. The results of fitting a template T to 174 hippocampus segmentations I. For each of the six error metrics, the mean and the standard deviation are given. All distances are in millimeters

'Biased' vol. overlap	0.91 (0.016)	Robust vol. overlap	0.88 (0.018)
Mean dist. from T to I	0.20 (0.030)	Mean dist. from I to T	0.33 (0.063)
Max. dist. from T to I	1.58 (0.31)	Max. dist. from T to I	2.56 (0.86)

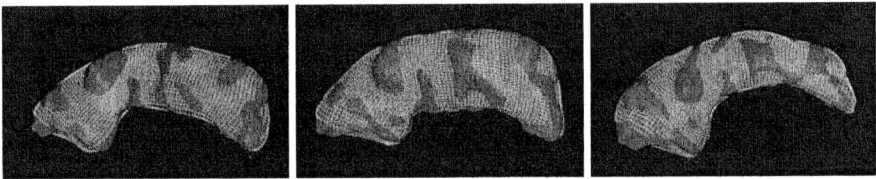

Fig. 3. Examples of a template fitted to instances of the hippocampus. The solid blue surface is the boundary of the subject hippocampus, and the white mesh is the boundary of the fitted cm-rep template

maximum distance from T to I; and mean and maximum distance from I to T. Volume overlaps were computed by digitizing the template and the target segmentation at a 0.1mm voxel resolution; distance metrics were computed using the distance transform at this resolution.

These error measurements are reported in Table 1. Notably, the mean distance from T to I was 0.20mm, on average. This is 0.03mm greater the mean distance reported by Styner et al. [20] in a similar experiment that fitted discrete m-reps to hippocampus segmentations in the same MRI dataset. This is encouraging because discrete m-reps are less constrained by the strict rules of medial geometry and, theoretically, they should produce better fits than continuous parametric m-reps. Fig. 3 presents representative examples of the template fitted to the hippocampus data.[1]

The pilot results leave room for improvement, especially in terms of the maximum distance from I to T. The large variance in this metric shows that there are some poorly fitted outliers that are affecting it. We expect that accuracy can be gained by adopting the wavelet basis, improving the multi-resolution schedule, switching to a domain without corners, and fine-tuning the optimization. These improvements, plus an extension to objects with branching medial scaffolds, as well as development of statistical methods for parametric m-reps will be addressed in our future work.

4 Conclusion

We have presented a new algorithm for generative modeling of 3-D objects that starts with a definition of a single-surface medial scaffold and a second-order

---

[1] Attached demos 1 and 2 show corresponding animations.

property of the radius field, and produces a definition of the object's boundary that is geometrically congruent (in a loose sense of the term) with the medial scaffold. To find a way around a non-linear equality constraint defined along the edge of the medial surface, we posed the problem as a Poisson PDE with a non-linear boundary condition. We applied the method in a deformable templates framework and presented pilot results where the template was fitted to 174 hippocampi from a schizophrenia study.

The PDE-based approach to continuous parametric medial representation is a significant and non-trivial improvement on previous attempts to explicitly model continuous medial geometry because it allows the domain of the medial representation to be specified *a priori*. Previously, the problem of finding continuous medially-based correspondences between objects has been hampered by either the difficulty of interpolating discrete medial atoms in 3-D or by the transient nature of the implicit-domain continuous m-reps approach. The method presented here is relevant because it opens the door to computing such correspondences and through them, to statistical analysis of shape and appearance, to a type of analysis that leverages the descriptive nature of features derived from medial structures (evidenced by [8, 15, 23]) and their unique ability to parameterize object interiors in a way that can be said to combine the attractive features of Active Shape and Active Appearance Models.

Acknowledgements

This work was supported by the NIH grant NS045839. We thank Prof. Charles L. Epstein, Prof. Jean Gallier and Marcelo Siqueira (Penn) for insightful discussions. We are indebted to Profs. Guido Gerig, Stephen M. Pizer, Sarang Joshi, and Martin Styner (UNC) for providing data and inspiration for this work. The term *medial scaffold* was recommended to us by Prof. D. Mumford (Brown).

References

1. H. Blum and R.N. Nagel. Shape description using weighted symmetric axis features. *Pattern Recognition*, 10(3):167–180, 1978.
2. M. H. Chakos, S. A. Schobel, H. Gu, G. Gerig, D. Bradford, C. Charles, and J. A. Lieberman. Duration of illness and treatment effects on hippocampal volume in male patients with schizophrenia. *Br J Psychiatry*, 186(1):26–31, 2005.
3. T. F. Cootes, C. J. Taylor, D. H. Cooper, and J. Graham. Active shape models – their training and application. *Computer Vision and Image Understanding*, 61(1):38–59, 1995.
4. T.F. Cootes, G.J. Edwards, and C.J. Taylor. Active appearance models. In *European Conference on Computer Vision*, volume 2, pages 484–498, Freiburg, Germany, June 1998.
5. J. Csernansky, S. Joshi, L. Wang, J. Haller, M. Gado, J. Miller, U. Grenander, and M. Miller. Hippocampal morphometry in schizophrenia via high dimensional brain mapping. In *Proc. National Academy of Sciences*, volume 95, pages 11406–11411, 1998.

6. James Damon. Determining the geometry of boundaries of objects from medial data. *International Journal of Computer Vision*, 63(1):45–64, 2005. in print.
7. G. Gerig, M. Styner, M.E. Shenton, and J. Lieberman. Shape versus size: Improved understanding of the morphology of brain structures. In W Niessen and M Viergever, editors, *Medical Image Computing and Computer-Assisted Intervention (MICCAI)*, volume 2208, pages 24–32, New York, October 2001. Springer.
8. P. Golland, W.E.L. Grimson, and R. Kikinis. Statistical shape analysis using fixed topology skeletons: Corpus callosum study. In *International Conference on Information Processing in Medical Imaging*, LNCS 1613, pages 382–388. Springer Verlag, 1999.
9. J.W. Haller, A. Banerjee, G.E. Christensen, M. Gado, S. Joshi, M.I. Miller, Y.I. Sheline, M.W. Vannier, and J.G. Csernansky. Three-dimensional hippocampal MR morphometry by high-dimensional transformation of a neuroanatomic atlas. *Radiology*, 202:504–510, 1997.
10. Sean Ho and Guido Gerig. Profile scale-spaces for multiscale image match. In *MICCAI*, pages 176–183, 2004.
11. S. Joshi, U. Grenander, and M. Miller. On the geometry and shape of brain sub-manifolds. *IEEE Transactions on Pattern Analysis and Machine Intelligence*, 11:1317–1343, 1997.
12. S. Joshi, S. Pizer, P.T. Fletcher, P. Yushkevich, A. Thall, and J.S. Marron. Multiscale deformable model segmentation and statistical shape analysis using medial descriptions. *IEEE Transactions on Medical Imaging*, 21(5):538–550, 2002.
13. Erwin Kreyszig. *Differential Geometry*. University of Toronto Press, 1959.
14. B. B. Kimia P. J. Giblin. On the intrinsic reconstruction of shape from its symmetries. *IEEE PAMI*, 25(7):895–911, 2003.
15. S. M. Pizer, P. T. Fletcher, S. Joshi, A. Thall, J. Z. Chen, Y. Fridman, D. S. Fritsch, A. G. Gash, J. M. Glotzer, M. R. Jiroutek, C. Lu, K. E. Muller, G. Tracton, P. Yushkevich, and E. L. Chaney. Deformable m-reps for 3D medical image segmentation. *International Journal of Computer Vision*, 55(2):85–106, Nov 2003.
16. S. M. Pizer, K. Siddiqi, G. Székely, J. N. Damon, and S. W. Zucker. Multiscale medial loci and their properties. *International Journal of Computer Vision*, 55(2-3):155–179, 2003.
17. O. Schenk and K. Gärtner. Solving unsymmetric sparse systems of linear equations with PARDISO. *Journal of Future Generation Computer Systems*, 20(3):475–487, 2004.
18. G.D. Smith. *Numerical Solution of Partial Differential Equations: Finite Difference Methods*. Oxford University Press, 1985.
19. L.H. Staib and J.S. Duncan. Boundary finding with parametrically deformable models. *IEEE PAMI*, 14(11):1061–1075, November 1992.
20. M. Styner, G. Gerig, S. Joshi, and S.M. Pizer. Automatic and robust computation of 3D medial models incorporating object variability. *International Journal of Computer Vision*, 55(2):107–122, November 2003.
21. A. Thall. *Deformable Solid Modeling via Medial Sampling and Displacement Subdivision*. PhD thesis, Dept. of Comp. Sci., UNC Chapel Hill, 2004.
22. P. Yushkevich, P. T. Fletcher, S. Joshi, A. Thall, and S. M. Pizer. Continuous medial representations for geometric object modeling in 2D and 3D. *Image and Vision Computing*, 21(1):17–28, 2003.
23. P. Yushkevich, S.M. Pizer, S. Joshi, and J.S. Marron. Intuitive, localized analysis of shape variability. In *International Conference on Information Processing in Medical Imaging*, pages 402–408, Berlin, Germany, 2001. Springer-Verlag.

Diffeomorphic Nonlinear Transformations: A Local Parametric Approach for Image Registration

R. Narayanan[1], J.A. Fessler[1,2,3], H. Park[3], and C.R. Meyer[1,3]

[1] Department of Biomedical Engineering, University of Michigan,
Ann Arbor, Michigan 48109-2099
[2] Department of Electrical Engineering and Computer Science,
University of Michigan, Ann Arbor, Michigan 48109-2122
[3] Department of Radiology, University of Michigan,
Ann Arbor, Michigan 48109-0553
{rnz, fessler, hyunjinp, cmeyer}@umich.edu

Abstract. Many types of transformations are used to model deformations in medical image registration. While some focus on modeling local changes, some on continuity and invertibility, there is no closed-form nonlinear parametric approach that addresses all these properties. This paper presents a class of nonlinear transformations that are local, continuous and invertible under certain conditions. They are straightforward to implement, fast to compute and can be used particularly in cases where locally affine deformations need to be recovered. We use our new transformation model to demonstrate some results on synthetic images using a multi-scale approach to multi-modality mutual information based image registration. The original images were deformed using B-splines at three levels of scale. The results show that the proposed method can recover these deformations almost completely with very few iterations of a gradient based optimizer.

1 Introduction

Methods for image registration have three main components: the geometric transformation used to model deformations, the objective function, and the optimization algorithm. While using Mutual Information (MI) as the objective function has been successfully explored and validated [1], finding a simple transformation possessing the useful qualities of smoothness, compact support, and the existence of an inverse has been an ongoing effort. Rigid or affine transformations cannot be used to recover local warps. Deformation fields that are solutions to Ordinary Differential Equations (ODEs) [2, 3] have been proposed because of their ability to recover large deformations while still being invertible. These methods have large number of degrees of freedom except Arsigny's Polyrigid transforms [4] and geodesic spline representations of diffeomorphisms [5]. In contrast the parametric transformation proposed here is a more parsimonious approach in that it can be applied only in regions that need correction.

Different types of radial basis functions with global e.g., Thin Plate Splines [6], and local support [7] are used as well. This is because they have fewer degrees of freedom and can be used to recover local warps. But these types of deformations are not invertible in general. In addition, functions with global support change distant regions of the image that may not require correction while attempting to change local regions that do. B-Splines [8] have been used successfully because of their C^2 continuity and local support, but injectivity conditions are non-trivial [9]. In Arsigny's Polyrigid transforms [4] using ODEs, the deformation vector is obtained by integrating the velocity vector that is a distance weighted sum of individual vectors corresponding to 'action' points whose solution is the trajectory equation. This method always ensures that the transform is continuous and invertible. However these weights are normalized, so the transform is global. Furthermore, methods that use ODEs do not have a closed form and the deformation is computed by integrating the velocity vector in a finite number of time steps to obtain the transformation. This paper was motivated by the ideas discussed in [4]. We introduce a nonlinear transformation that possesses the properties discussed by modifying the affine transformation, so that at the center of the region that needs correction we have an affine transform described by all the parameters of the transform, and gradual convergence to identity as we move away from the center. This convergence can be controlled using our transform model. Also our transform has a closed form and is easy and fast to compute because it is characterized by few parameters and always ensures that an inverse exists under certain trivial conditions.

We show some preliminary results using a multi-scale approach to image registration by applying corrections starting from the coarsest level of scale to the finest. We applied synthetic B-Spline based deformations to images and then corrections were applied at three levels of scale using only one seed point at each. A seed point is the center of the region that we are trying to correct. They are picked based on finding high gradients of local MI with respect to local affine transformation parameters. Results show that using these transforms could be a good alternative to current methods used in image registration.

We used normalized mutual information (NMI), first proposed by Studholme [10] as the objective function and a simultaneous perturbation based gradient optimizer [11] to maximize NMI.

2 The Locally Affine Transformation Model

A global affine transformation without shear in $\mathbb{R}^n$ for any vector $\mathbf{x}$ about the center $\mathbf{x}_0$ is

$$T(\mathbf{x}) = e^{sA} e^{sS} (\mathbf{x} - \mathbf{x}_0) + s\mathbf{t} + \mathbf{x}_0, \quad (1)$$

where $\mathbf{x} = \begin{bmatrix} x_1 \ x_2 \ \ldots \ x_n \end{bmatrix}^T$, $\mathbf{x}_0 = \begin{bmatrix} x_{01} \ x_{02} \ \ldots \ x_{0n} \end{bmatrix}^T$, $\mathbf{t} = \begin{bmatrix} t_1 \ t_2 \ \ldots \ t_n \end{bmatrix}^T$ (translation), A is the skew symmetric matrix corresponding to the rotation matrix, S is the symmetric matrix corresponding to the scale matrix and $s \in [0, 1]$.

At $s = 1$ we get the complete affine transformation about the center $\mathbf{x}_0$. Many such centers will be chosen from the image as requiring correction. The parameter s in the above equation can be parameterized in space in the form of a continuous function, say $\lambda(r)$ where $r = \|\mathbf{x} - \mathbf{x}_0\|$ so that at $r = 0$, $s = 1$ and as r increases $s \to 0$. The elegance of writing it this way is that as we move towards the center of the region that we are attempting to correct, we have an affine transformation, but the transformation converges to an identity map as we move away. The region of influence can be controlled by a parameter of the continuous function. So any function with the above properties can be used. Although the Gaussian does not have a compact support it was used because it could be treated as being almost local for small σ. We used the Gaussian because of its C^∞ smoothness and loose bounds for an inverse to exist. The proposed transformation $(T : \mathbb{R}^n \to \mathbb{R}^n)$ is

$$T(\mathbf{x}) = e^{\lambda(r)A} e^{\lambda(r)S}(\mathbf{x} - \mathbf{x}_0) + \lambda(r')\mathbf{t} + \mathbf{x}_0 \qquad (2)$$

where

$$r' = \|e^{\lambda(r)A} e^{\lambda(r)S}(\mathbf{x} - \mathbf{x}_0)\| = \|e^{\lambda(r)S}(\mathbf{x} - \mathbf{x}_0)\|$$

and

$$s \equiv \lambda(r) = e^{-\frac{r^2}{2\sigma^2}}. \qquad (3)$$

One can also write T in Eq. (2) as

$$T(\mathbf{x}) = (T_T \circ T_{RS})(\mathbf{x}) + \mathbf{x}_0 \qquad (4)$$

where

$$T_{RS}(\mathbf{x}) = e^{\lambda(r)A} e^{\lambda(r)S}(\mathbf{x} - \mathbf{x}_0) \qquad (5)$$

and

$$T_T(\mathbf{x}) = \mathbf{x} + \lambda(\|\mathbf{x}\|)\mathbf{t}. \qquad (6)$$

Above, σ^2 is the variance of the Gaussian modulation function. It sets the scale at which we are working in the registration step and is also fine tuned (optimized along with the affine parameters) to match the scale at which the deformations were induced. The transformation is nonlinear and can be applied to each region individually. A region is picked if it has a large gradient of local MI. The center of this region is $\mathbf{x}_0$ about which the transformation is applied.

The transform also satisfies many desirable properties discussed in the following subsections. These properties depend on the choice of λ which can be chosen to be local and smooth. The properties discussed here are for $\lambda(r)$ chosen to be gaussian in Eq. (3). One may select the function λ based on what properties one seeks to satisfy.

2.1 Continuity and Locality

Continuity is determined by the choice of the function λ. The Gaussian ensures C^∞ continuity. Locality also depends on λ. The Gaussian function has "nearly" local support. Functions with strictly local support may also be used to arrive at different conditions for an inverse to exist.

2.2 Existence of Inverse

Current methods using spline-based deformation models have either difficult conditions to incorporate in the optimizer to prevent folding, i.e not invertible or use regularization methods that discourage folding by adding an additional smoothness term in the objective function [8]. In our method we derive loose bounds for the transformation parameters which are straightforward to implement and always ensure invertibility.

The Jacobian matrix for a transformation $T : \mathbb{R}^n \to \mathbb{R}^n$ must be positive definite everywhere to ensure invertibility. We have found the conditions for which the determinant of the Jacobian of the transformation is positive to always guarantee an inverse (see Appendix). We picked λ to be Gaussian because of its loose bounds, infinite continuity and an easily controllable region of influence. Other functions like inverse multiquadratics or differentiable local support functions of the type proposed by Wendland [12] may also be used and lead to similar conditions.

As shown in Eq. (2) the transformation T has an inverse as long as

$$\|\mathbf{t}\| < \sigma e^{\frac{1}{2}}$$

and

$$0 < a < e^{e^{0.5}} \approx 5.2003,$$

where $\mathbf{t}$ is the translation vector and $a = max(a_x, a_y)$, the larger of the two anisotropic scales in the x and y direction. These bounds in practice were found to be very loose and we never experienced any folding in our simulations.

3 Initialization and Registration

3.1 Initialization

We implement a multi-scale approach to image registration starting from the coarsest level of scale and proceeding to the finest.

At each level of scale we pick only regions that are mis-registered and apply the algorithm. Rohde et al. [7] picked regions with large gradient of cost function with respect to radial basis function coefficients while Park et al. [13] used a mismatch measure to quantify mis-registration.

Here we pick regions based on its sensitivity to local affine deformations. Since we apply corrections based on a locally affine transformation model, the gradients computed give us a meaningful estimate on the extent of mis-registration. The way these gradients are computed is as follows. A rectangular window is picked with dimensions in correspondence with the scale and three control points are placed in a triangular fashion spanning the area of the window. The window is placed in the reference and the floating image and the control points in the floating image are perturbed and the gradient of NMI with respect to the affine coefficients is found. This window is moved over the complete reference and floating image in an overlapping fashion. If the gradients of the cost in a region is not small, then it is likely that this region is mis-registered. Regions with large magnitude of gradient norm above a selected threshold are picked and the centers of these regions denoted as seed points are used in the global registration step. If p_i are the parameters that define our affine transformation, the gradient of local NMI is computed as

$$\hat{\mathbf{g}} = \left[\frac{\partial NMI}{\partial p_1} \frac{\partial NMI}{\partial p_2} \cdots \frac{\partial NMI}{\partial p_6} \right]^T$$

We apply transformations about these points and correct for them locally using the transformation model at different levels of scale. Since these points are also fed as parameters to the optimizer they will also be allowed to move to model the deformation better.

3.2 Multi-scale Nonrigid Registration

The final deformation is computed iteratively across different levels of scale. Since the spatial support of the deformation can be constrained to be local, seed points are picked in the initialization step at these different scales, and they serve as the centers for our locally affine transformation model. Global registration is then initiated at the coarsest level of scale (large σ) and optimization is performed over all the seed points with large to smallest σ. The final transform is computed as a composition of individual transformations.

After optimizing over each region, the geometric maps are stored and this is repeated over other regions of the image. Since each of these transforms correct for only one region at a time, they have very few parameters and high local sensitivity yielding their ability to model local changes accurately. Also, only regions that are mis-registered are picked and corrected instead of placing a grid of control points and picking which ones are active (needing optimization) and inactive. This gives us a finer control over the region we are trying to correct. E.g. if we have N seed points, the final transformation is

$$T(\mathbf{x}) = (T_N \circ T_{N-1} \ldots T_2 \circ T_1)(\mathbf{x}), \tag{7}$$

where each seed point 'i' is associated with a transformation T_i.

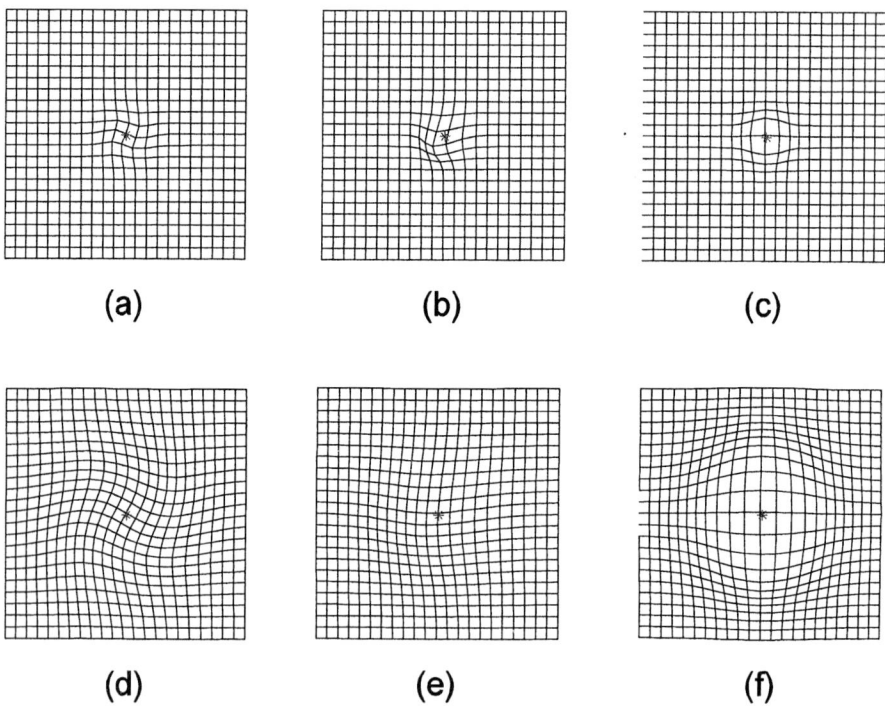

Fig. 1. Deformations applied to a uniform grid at two different levels of scale (σ). The figure shows the same amount of rotation (a and d), translation (b and e) and scale (c and f) applied individually for a small and large σ respectively

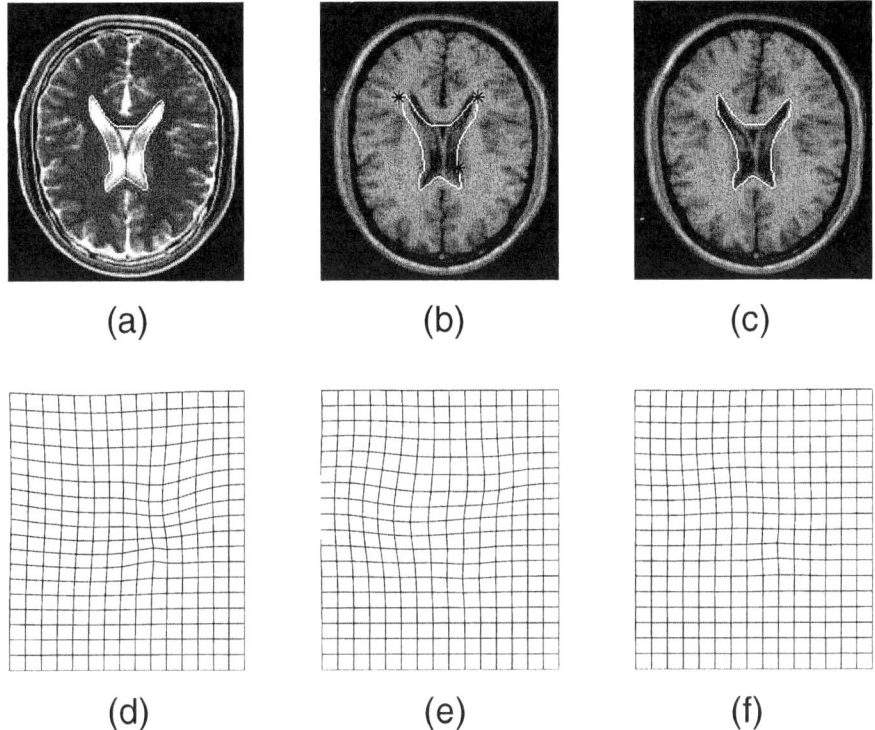

Fig. 2. Registration of T1 and T2 weighted slices using three seed points (a) Original T2 weighted reference image. (b) artificially deformed T1 weighted floating image. (c) T1 weighted floating image after registration. (d) Applied Deformation (e) Estimated inverse after registration (f) Estimated inverse applied to the induced deformation

The reference and the floating image are assumed to be already affine registered with each other before we begin the algorithm. The individual transformation parameters are computed for each seed point. There may be several seed points identified at a level of scale. Global normalized mutual information was used as the objective function and a simultaneous perturbation based gradient optimizer proposed by Spall [11] was used to arrive at the final solution. All eight parameters corresponding to the transformation were optimized: i.e. two translation parameters (t_x and t_y), rotation angle (θ), two anisotropic scale parameters in the scale matrix (a_x and a_y), two center coordinates (C_x and C_y) and a variance parameter (σ from the Gaussian function).

Algorithm

1: Initialize reference (A) and floating images (B) and set T_0 to an identity map
2: **for** $i = 1$ *to Levels of Scale* **do**
3:    $M = $ # of seed points picked based on high local gradients
4:    **for** $k = 1$ *to M* **do**
5:       $\hat{T}_{i,k} = argmax_{T_{i,k}} \ NMI(A(\bullet), B((T_{i,k} \circ \hat{T}_{i,k-1} \ldots \hat{T}_{i,2} \circ \hat{T}_{i,1} \circ \hat{T}_{i-1} \circ \hat{T}_{i-2} \ldots \hat{T}_0)(\bullet)))$

6: **end for**
7: $\hat{T_i} = \hat{T}_{i,k}$
8: **end for**
9: $\hat{T} = \hat{T_i}$

4 Results

4.1 Examples of Locally Affine Deformations

Fig. (1) shows examples of rotate, translate and scale applied individually about one seed point for two different σ. This is to show that we can model all kinds of local and global changes using a combination of these parameters.

4.2 Registration Experiments

Fig. (2) shows a head registration example using an axial slice from T1 and T2 weighted images from Brainweb [14]. They were artificially deformed using B-Splines at three

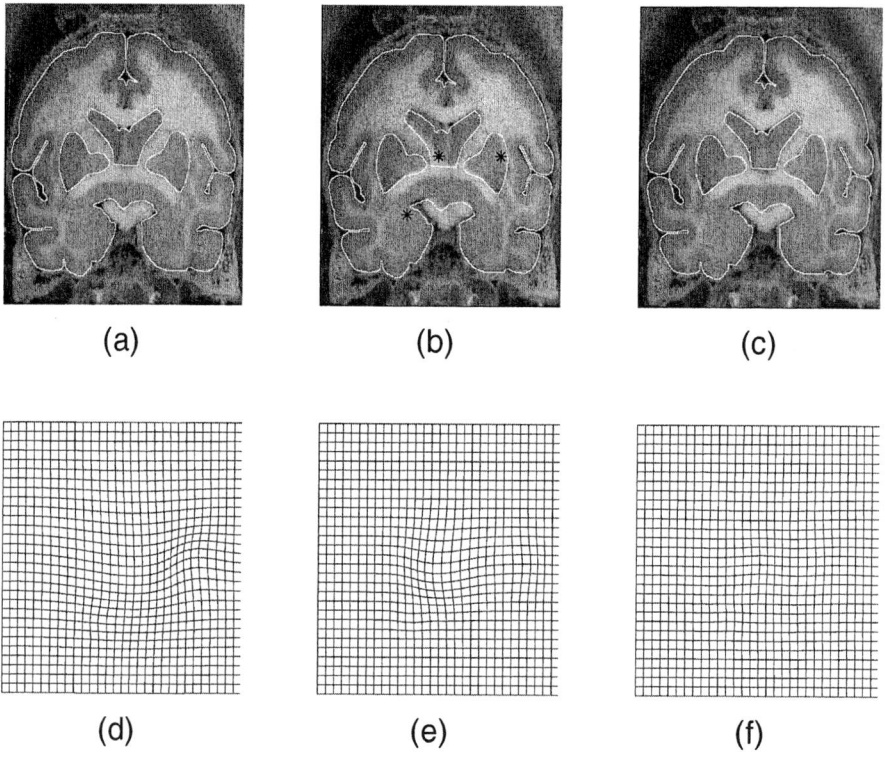

Fig. 3. Registration of a coronal slice of a vervet monkey using three seed points. (a) Original reference image. (b) artificially deformed floating image. (c) Reconstructed floating image after registration. (d) Applied Deformation (e) Estimated inverse after registration (f) Estimated inverse applied to the induced deformation

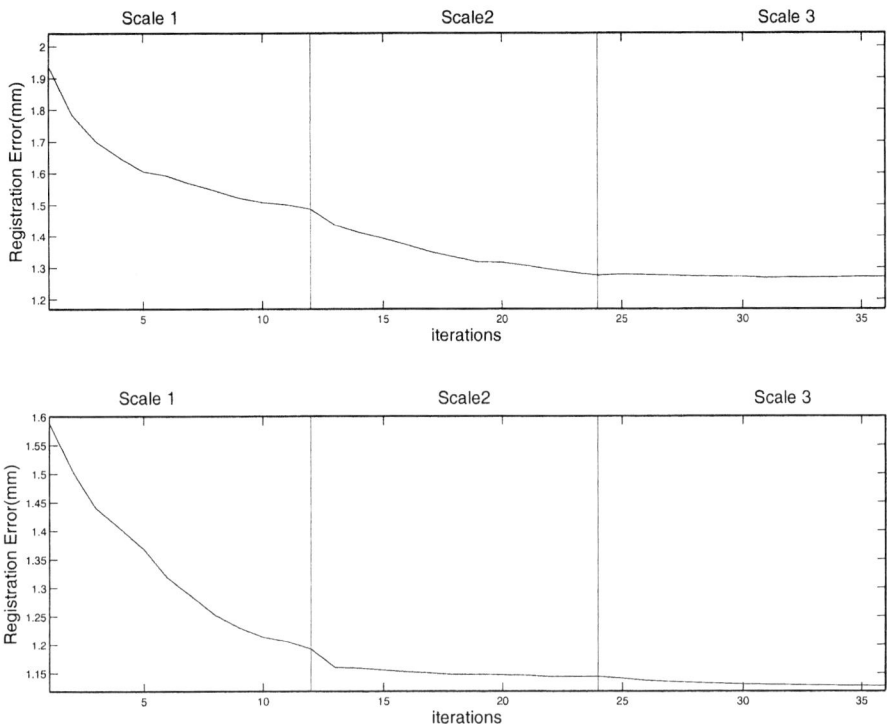

Fig. 4. Average norm of registration error vs. iterations at three different levels of scale (σ). (a) Human brain - T1, T2 weighted registration. (b) Monkey brain registration

different levels of scale. This was done by moving one knot in the B-Spline grid by a known amount at each scale, refining the grid and repeating the procedure at the next level. Registration was performed using three seed points each working at a different scale. i.e different σ. The outline for the ventricle was marked manually so that the registration performance could be visually assessed. In Fig. (2), (a) is the original T2-weighted reference image and (b) is the deformed floating image with three seed points marked. The seed points from left to right are in decreasing levels of scale (σ), i.e. three optimizations were performed, one at each scale. The registered T1 image in (c) shows that the ventricles follow the contours more tightly after registration. (d) shows the applied deformation, (e) is the estimated inverse obtained via registration and (f) shows the deformation computed(e) applied to the induced deformation(d) which should resemble a uniform grid as best as possible.

Fig. (3) shows a coronal slice from a vervet monkey atlas developed at UCLA's Laboratory of Neuroimaging [15]. The slice was deformed using B-Splines similar to the procedure described in the previous paragraph. Seed points were placed at exactly three locations each with a different variance ($\sigma_{center} > \sigma_{right} > \sigma_{left}$) for the Gaussian function that controls the support of the transformation. The contours in (c) shows that the boundaries of the caudate and putamen hug the manually segmented boundaries more tightly, a marked improvement from (b).

Fig. (4) shows the registration error versus iterations at three different levels of scale for the first and second example respectively. Only twelve iterations were performed at each scale and each experiment took less than three minutes to run on a 3.2 Ghz PC with 2 Gb memory running MATLAB 7.

5 Discussion

We have demonstrated and tested a new local nonlinear transformation using a multi-scale approach to multi-modality image registration. This transformation has good local properties and affine behavior near the region of interest. The parameters controlling the support of this transform (σ) can be initialized and changed (by the optimizer) during the course of the registration to match the level of scale of the induced deformation. Furthermore, the transformation has a closed form and there is no need to integrate the velocity vector over time as in the case of methods using ODEs, making it very fast. Since each region is optimized for one at a time, only eight parameters are used in the optimization which makes it very fast. Although we can always guarantee that folding does not occur, finding a direct inverse is not straightforward. A numerical inverse could be found finally using the optimized parameters. Since this is computed only after estimating the transformation (T in Eq. (7)), it could be easily done using any numerical method at the end if required.

5.1 Translation

Consider the case where the vector $\mathbf{x}$ is subjected to pure translation with no rotation or scaling (i.e. $T(\mathbf{x}) = \mathbf{x} + \lambda(\|\mathbf{x} - \mathbf{x}_0\|)\mathbf{t}$). Using the condition that $det(J) > 0$ we get,

$$\bar{\mathbf{x}}^T \mathbf{t} < \frac{1}{d}.$$

Applying the Cauchy-Schwarz inequality to the left hand side and substituting $\|\bar{\mathbf{x}}\| = 1$ we get the sufficient condition

$$\|\mathbf{t}\| < \sigma e^{\frac{1}{2}}, \tag{8}$$

where $\sigma e^{\frac{1}{2}}$ is the smallest value that $\frac{1}{d}$ can assume.

5.2 Rotation

For $\mathbf{x} \in \mathbb{R}^n$, the rotation matrix can be constructed as the composition of elementary rotations in planar subspaces. Each of these matrices is a Jacobi rotation matrix. The rotation matrix is invertible as long as each of these matrices has an inverse. The Jacobian for a Jacobi matrix corresponding to the planar subspace containing axes 'i' and 'j' is given by

$$J = Q_{ij} \begin{bmatrix} p_1 & p_2 & 0 \\ p_3 & p_4 & \\ 0 & & I_{n-2} \end{bmatrix} Q_{ij}$$

where
Q_{ij} is the permutation matrix
$p_1 = \cos(\lambda\theta) + r\theta d\bar{x}_i^2 \sin(\lambda\theta) + r\theta d\bar{x}_i\bar{x}_j \cos(\lambda\theta)$,
$p_2 = -\sin(\lambda\theta) + r\theta \bar{x}_i\bar{x}_j d \sin(\lambda\theta) + r\bar{x}_j^2 \theta d \cos(\lambda\theta)$,
$p_3 = \sin(\lambda\theta) - r\bar{x}_i^2 \theta d \cos(\lambda\theta) + r\bar{x}_i\bar{x}_j \theta d \sin(\lambda\theta)$ and
$p_4 = \cos(\lambda\theta) - r\bar{x}_i\bar{x}_j \theta d \cos(\lambda\theta) + r\bar{x}_j^2 \theta d \sin(\lambda\theta)$.
The determinant of this matrix is always 1. The volume is always preserved under rotation. So the transformation $(T(\mathbf{x}) = e^{\lambda(r)A}(\mathbf{x} - \mathbf{x}_0) + \mathbf{x}_0)$ always has an inverse

5.3 Scale

Finally consider the case when the transformation consists of only scaling. (i.e. $T(\mathbf{x}) = e^{\lambda(r)S}(\mathbf{x} - \mathbf{x}_0) + \mathbf{x}_0$). One can show that the determinant of the Jacobian is $1 - rd\sum_{j=1}^{n} \bar{x}_j^2 \log(a_j)$. Applying the conditions for an inverse to exist(i.e $det(J) > 0$) we get

$$rd \sum_{j=1}^{n} \bar{x}_j^2 \log(a_j) < 1$$

where a_j are the anisotropic scales in each dimension. Let $a = max(a_1, a_2, \ldots, a_n)$. Replacing a_j above with a we get a more stringent inequality

$$rd \log(a) \|\bar{\mathbf{x}}\|^2 < 1.$$

Substituing $\|\bar{\mathbf{x}}\|^2 = 1$ and rearranging above we get

$$a < e^{\frac{1}{rd}}.$$

Since the minimum value that $\frac{1}{rd}$ can assume is easily shown to be $e^{0.5}$, the sufficient condition is

$$0 < a < e^{e^{0.5}} \approx 5.2003. \tag{9}$$

5.4 Conditions for Inverse

We have derived the bounds so that an inverse always exists for rotation, translation and scale each individually applied. Let T_R be the isomorphism for pure rotation (i.e. no scale or translation) so that $T_R(\mathbf{x}) = e^{\lambda(r)A}(\mathbf{x} - \mathbf{x}_0) + \mathbf{x}_0$ and let $T_{R'}(\mathbf{x}) = T_R(\mathbf{x}) - \mathbf{x}_0$. We need to show that T in Eq. (4) has an inverse. Let us first show that T_{RS} in Eq. (5) is invertible. The transformation T_{RS} is

$$T_{RS}(\mathbf{x}) = e^{\lambda(r)A} e^{\lambda(r)S}(\mathbf{x} - \mathbf{x}_0)$$
$$= P\, T_{R'}(\mathbf{x})$$

where

$$P = e^{\lambda(r)A} \begin{bmatrix} a_x^{\lambda(r)} & 0 \\ 0 & a_y^{\lambda(r)} \end{bmatrix} e^{-\lambda(r)A}.$$

Being similar to a diagonal matrix P is invertible. Also $T_{R'}$ is always invertible since T_R is. So T_{RS} always has an inverse as long as $a < e^{e^{0.5}} \approx 5.2003$.

We have already proved that T_T in Eq. (4) has an inverse as long as $\|\mathbf{t}\| < \sigma e^{\frac{1}{2}}$.(See Eq. (8)). So the transformation $T(\mathbf{x}) = (T_T T_{RS})(\mathbf{x}) + \mathbf{x}_0$ has an inverse as long as

$$\|\mathbf{t}\| < \sigma e^{\frac{1}{2}} \tag{10}$$

and

$$0 < a < e^{e^{0.5}} \approx 5.2003. \tag{11}$$

References

1. Viola, P., Wells, W.M.: Alignment by maximization of mutual information. Int. J. Comput. Vision **24** (1997) 137–154
2. Joshi, S.C., Miller, M.I.: Landmark matching via large deformation diffeomorphisms. IEEE Trans. Medical Imaging **9** (2000)
3. Hotel, C.C., Hermosillo, G., Faugeras, O.: Flows of diffeomorphisms for multimodal image registration. In: ISBE. (2002) 753–756
4. Arsigny, V., Pennec, X., Ayache, N.: Polyrigid and polyaffine transformations: A new class of diffeomorphisms for locally rigid or affine registration. In: MICCAI (2). (2003) 829–837
5. Marsland, S., Twining, C.J.: Constructing diffeomorphic representations for the groupwise analysis of nonrigid registrations of medical images. IEEE Trans. Medical Imaging **23** (2004)
6. Meyer, C.R., Boes, J.L., Kim, B., Bland, P.H., Zasadny, K.R., Kison, P.V., Koral, K., Frey, K.A., Wahl, R.L.: Demonstration of accuracy and clinical versatility of mutual information for automatic multimodality image fusion using affine and thin-plate spline warped geometric deformations. Med. Image. Anal. **1** (1997) 195–206
7. Rohde, G.K., Aldroubi, A., Dawant, B.M.: The adaptive bases algorithm for intensity based nonrigid image registration. IEEE Trans. Med. Imaging **22** (2003) 1470–1479
8. Ruckert, D., Sonoda, L.I., Hayes, C., Hill, D.L.G., Leach, M.O., Hawkes, D.J.: Nonrigid registration using free-form deformations: Application to breast MR images. IEEE Trans. Med. Imaging **18** (1999) 712–721
9. Choi, Y., Lee, S.: Injectivity conditions of 2D and 3D uniform cubic B-Spline functions. Graphical Models (**62**)
10. Studholme, C., Hill, D., Hawkes, D.: An overlap invariant entropy measure of 3D medical image alignment. Pattern Recognition **32** (1999) 71–86
11. Spall, H.C.: Multivariate stochastic approximation using a simultaneous perturbation gradient approximation. IEEE Trans. Autom. Control **37** (1992) 332–341
12. Wendland, H.: Piecewise polynomial positive definite and compactly supported radial basis functions of minimal degree. AICM **4** (1995) 389–396
13. Park, H., Bland, P.H., Brock, K.K., Meyer, C.R.: Adaptive registration using local information measures. Medical Image Analysis **8** (2004) 465–473
14. Cocosco, C.A., Kollokian, V., Kwan, R.K.S., Evans, A.C.: Brainweb: Online interface to a 3D MRI simulated brain database. NeuroImage **5** (1997)
15. Rubins, D.J., Ambach, K., Toga, A.W., Melega, W.P., Cherry, S.R.: Development of a digital brain atlas of the vervet monkey. BrainPET **4** (1999)

Appendix

Here we derive conditions under which an inverse exists for a Gaussian weighting function. The conditions have been derived for a vector $\mathbf{x} \in \mathbb{R}^n$ (i.e. $\mathbf{x} = \begin{bmatrix} x_1 & x_2 & \ldots & x_n \end{bmatrix}^T$) for rotation and scale about $\mathbf{x}_0 = \begin{bmatrix} x_{01} & x_{02} & \ldots & x_{0n} \end{bmatrix}^T$. The bounds for 2D and 3D that we are interested in will turn out to be the same as the N dimensional case.

We will derive the conditions for translation, rotation and scale each treated individually and will show that these are sufficient conditions for an inverse to always exist.

For λ gaussian,

$$\frac{\partial \lambda(r)}{\partial x_i} = -\frac{r}{\sigma^2} e^{-\frac{r^2}{2\sigma^2}} \frac{(x_i - x_{0i})}{r} = -d\bar{x}_i,$$

where $d = \frac{r}{\sigma^2} e^{-\frac{r^2}{2\sigma^2}}$ and $\bar{x}_i = \frac{x_i - x_{0i}}{r}$. Let $\bar{\mathbf{x}}$ be the direction cosine vector so that $\bar{\mathbf{x}} = \begin{bmatrix} \bar{x}_1 & \bar{x}_2 & \ldots & \bar{x}_n \end{bmatrix}^T$ and $\|\bar{\mathbf{x}}\| = 1$.

A Framework for Registration, Statistical Characterization and Classification of Cortically Constrained Functional Imaging Data*

Anand A. Joshi[1], David W. Shattuck[2], Paul M. Thompson[2], and Richard M. Leahy[1]

[1] Signal and Image Processing Institute,
University of Southern California,
Los Angeles, CA90089
[2] Laboratory of Neuro Imaging, Brain Mapping Division,
Dept. of Neurology, UCLA School of Medicine,
Los Angeles, CA90095

Abstract. We present a framework for registering and analyzing functional neuroimaging data constrained to the cortical surface of the brain. We assume as input a set of labeled data points that lie on a set of parameterized topologically spherical surfaces that represent the cortical surfaces of multiple subjects. To perform analysis across subjects, we first co-register the coordinates from each surface to a cortical atlas using labeled sulcal maps as constraints. The registration minimizes a thin plate spline energy function on the deforming surface using covariant derivatives to solve the associated PDEs in the intrinsic geometry of the individual surface. The resulting warps are used to bring the functional data for multiple subjects into a common surface atlas coordinate system. We then present a novel method for performing statistical analysis of points on this atlas surface. We use the Green's function of the heat equation on the surface to model probability distributions and thus demonstrate the use of PDEs for statistical analysis in Riemannian manifolds. We describe methods for estimating the mean and variance of a set of points, such that the mean also lies in the manifold. We demonstrate the utility of this framework in the development of a maximum likelihood classifier for parcellation of somatosensory cortex in the atlas based on current dipole fits to MEG data, simulated to represent a somatotopic mapping of S1 sensory areas in multiple subjects.

1 Introduction

Studies of brain activity often result in the detection of focal activated regions constrained to the cerebral cortex. For instance, current dipoles, representing

---

* This work is supported by NIBIB under Grant No: R01 EB002010 and NCRR under Grant No: P41RR013642.

focal neural current sources localized using MEG, can be constrained to lie on the cortical surface [1]. Meaningful analysis of these data requires methods that take into account the non-Euclidean geometry of the surface. For multiple subject analysis, assuming that parameterized representations of the surfaces are available, the problem can be reduced to two stages: (i) coregistration of the coordinate systems of each subject to a cortical atlas; and (ii) statistical analysis of the variability of these registered point sources in the intrinsic geometry of this atlas. For the purposes of this paper we select one representative cortical surface as the target or "atlas". To register other individual cortical surfaces to this atlas, we solve the biharmonic equation using covariant derivatives to obtain a thin-plate spline warp from subject to atlas coordinates. The warp is constrained by a set of sulcal landmarks. Through use of covariant derivatives when solving the PDEs we make the resulting warp dependent only on the intrinsic geometry of the surface and independent of the specific parameterization. This approach is similar to that in [2] except that here we use a thin-plate spline rather than linear elastic energy resulting in a pair of decoupled PDEs, one for each component of the warping field. The resulting warp provides point to point correspondence between subject and atlas cortices by aligning their coordinate systems.

Once the surfaces have been registered, we can apply the same transformation to the functional point-source data so that we have a collection of points, all lying on the atlas surface, which we wish to analyze. The example we will use later in the paper is the location of the primary somatsensory area S1 for digits of the right hand as determined using magnetoncephalography. Mapping these areas for each subject to the atlas will give a collection of points for each digit reflecting the degree of variability of these functional areas in the surface space of the atlas. Our goal is to perform a statistical analysis of this variability.

Since the data are constrained to lie in a manifold, it makes sense to talk about an 'average' that is also constrained to lie in the manifold. Such an average can be called the 'intrinsic mean' [3, 4]. More generally, we would like to define statistical distributions with respect to the manifold [5, 6]. Since there is no simple notion of distance on the surface, averaging and quantifying variance in the intrinsic geometry is not straightforward. Note that geodesic distances are global rather than local attributes. We base our scheme on local attributes by using covariant PDEs, since in local neighborhoods, surfaces look like Euclidean spaces. Consequently it is possible to solve PDEs in the intrinsic geometry of the surfaces [7, 8]. We use this idea to define statistical distributions on a manifold using the Green's function of the heat equation or the *heat kernel*. The heat kernel can be computed on any Riemannian manifold and reduces to a Gaussian function in Euclidean space. In this respect, our approach is a generalization of the use of Gaussian distributions from Euclidean to Riemannian spaces. Using this framework we describe methods for computing the mean and standard deviation of a set of points such that the mean itself lies on the surface. We then describe how to use these ideas to generate a maximum likelihood classifier in the intrinsic geometry of the cortical surface.

2 Surface Registration in the Intrinsic Geometry

2.1 Surface Extraction and Parameterization

We first extract cortical surfaces from MRI for each subject using the Brainsuite software [9], which includes a 6 stage cortical modeling sequence. First the brain is extracted from the surrounding skull and scalp tissues using a combination of edge detection and mathematical morphology. Next the intensities of the MRI are corrected for shading artifacts. Each voxel in the corrected image is labeled according to tissue type using a statistical classifier. Coregistration to a standard atlas is then used to automatically identify the white matter volume, fill ventricular spaces and remove the brain stem and cerebellum, leaving a volume whose surface represents the outer white-matter surface of the cerebral cortex. It is likely that the tessellation of this volume will produce surfaces with topological handles. Prior to tessellation, these handles are identified and removed automatically using a graph based approach. The resulting mask is then tessellated to produce a genus zero surface.

We use our p-harmonic functional minimization scheme to map each cortical hemisphere onto a unit square. Our cortical flat maps are computed as described in [10]. Each brain hemisphere is mapped onto a unit square while constraining the interhemispheric fissure to lie on the boundary of the unit square. Let S denote the cortical surface. We assign a vector in R^2 to every point in the surface such that the two components denote the u and v coordinates assigned to that point, i.e. we define a vector-valued function $\phi : S \to R^2$. We chose the function ϕ to minimize the integral $\int_M \|\nabla \phi\|^p$ where M denotes the integral over the hemisphere. The integral is discretized and minimized numerically using a conjugate gradient method to obtain a bijective p-harmonic map [10,11].

The square maps for each hemisphere are then resampled on a regular 256x256 grid, as illustrated in Fig 1. Because the interhemispheric fissure is fixed on the boundary of the square for each hemisphere, one can visualize the parameter space as two squares placed on each other and connected at the boundaries of the squares. This allows us to calculate partial derivatives across the two hemispheres and explicitly include the connectivity of the two cortical hemispheres in subsequent analysis. This boundary-less space is then used for solving the

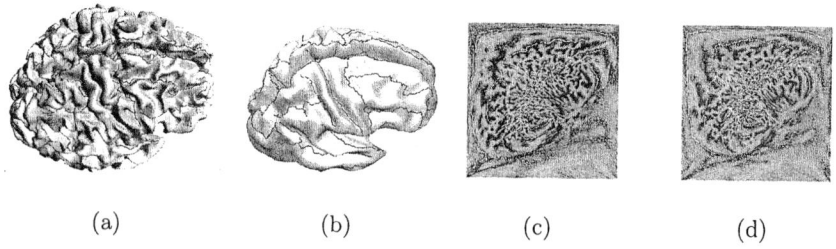

Fig. 1. (a) A cortical surface with hand labeled sulci; (b) a smoothed version of the surface; (c) and (d) square p-harmonic maps of the left and right hemispheres. The interhemispheric fissure is constrained to lie on the boundary of the square

differential equations that will align the (u, v) coordinates of the sulcal features from the subject to the atlas space.

The maps described above serve two purposes. First, they set up an initial alignment of the features across multiple subjects. Second, they are used as our computational space to align the cortices. However, thin plate spline based alignment uses covariant derivatives, and therefore is invariant with respect to the specific parameterization [12].

2.2 Thin Plate Splines in the Intrinsic Geometry of the Cortical Surface

Having parameterized each of the cortical surfaces, we now align coordinate systems between one surface, which we denote the "atlas", and each of the other brain surfaces. The alignment uses a set of interactively labeled sulci, sampled uniformly along their lengths, as a set of point constraints [13]. To compute a smooth warping field ϕ from one coordinate system to the other we use the thin plate spline bending energy on the atlas surface as a regularizing function.

Thin plate (biharmonic) splines [14] have become a very popular method for landmark registration of 2D or 3D images. These splines are a generalization of the 1D cubic spline and correspond to the bending energy E_b of a thin metal plate:

$$E_b = \int \left(\frac{\partial^2 \phi}{\partial x^2}\right)^2 + 2\left(\frac{\partial^2 \phi}{\partial x \partial y}\right)^2 + \left(\frac{\partial^2 \phi}{\partial y^2}\right)^2 dx dy \tag{1}$$

We minimize this bending energy subject to the point landmark constraints, implemented here using a quadratic penalty function approach. Since we wish to minimize the bending energy in the surface, we must account for the intrinsic geometry of the surface when computing the integral. While we use the parameter space for doing the calculations required for evaluation of the bending energy, we account for the effect of the parameterization while calculating the integral. This is achieved using covariant derivatives which results in the property that given a set of homologous landmarks (initial alignment), the deformation is independent of the parameterization used for the computation of the TPS deformation field. The the use of covariant derivatives eliminates the effect of the initial parameterization on the resulting warping field.

We note that the eigenfunctions of the biharmonic operator on the surfaces are dependent on the surface itself. Therefore we cannot expand the deformations in terms of a common eigenfunction basis as in [14]. Instead we take a more direct approach and minimize the integral numerically. The bending energy is minimized in the intrinsic geometry after replacing the first and second partial derivatives in (1) by the corresponding covariant derivatives. This is explained in more detail in the Appendix. Integration over the surface can be carried out by integration in the parameter space while compensating with the surface metric g. The differential form ds^2 for the integration in the surface S is related to its counterpart in the parameter space (u, v) by $ds^2 = gdudv$. Let S be the set of all vertices, and let S_c denote the set of constrained vertices (landmarks). Let d_j^1 and d_j^2 denote the u and v displacements required at the jth landmark,

$1 \leq j \leq N$, to take it to its location in the atlas space. The warping field (ϕ^1, ϕ^2) with respect to the parameter space (u, v) that minimizes bending energy in the surface while matching the constraints is then given by:

$$\phi^1 = \arg\min_{\psi^1} \int_P \left((\psi^1_{,11})^2 + (\sqrt{2}\psi^1_{,12})^2 + (\psi^1_{,22})^2\right) g\, du\, dv, \text{ with } \phi^1(u_j, v_j) = d^1_j, \forall j \in S_c$$

$$\phi^2 = \arg\min_{\psi^2} \int_P \left((\psi^2_{,11})^2 + (\sqrt{2}\psi^2_{,12})^2 + (\psi^2_{,22})^2\right) g\, du\, dv, \text{ with } \phi^2(u_j, v_j) = d^2_j, \forall j \in S_c$$

We discretized the above integral in the parameter space over a 256x256 regular grid for each hemisphere. We denote the covariant differential operator in the above equations by L. As described previously, our parameter space takes into account the neighborhood relationships between the two hemispheres and thus the covariant operator L is discretized in such a way that derivatives at the interhemispheric fissure are calculated correctly. In our current implementation our constraints are enforced by adding a quadratic penalty term rather than the exact matching constraints in (2). Let $\Phi = (\phi^1, \phi^2)$ denote the deformation field. The discretized cost function then takes the form

$$\Phi = \arg\min \sum_{i \in S} \|\sqrt{g} L_i \Phi_i\|^2 + \sigma^2 \sum_{j \in S_c} \|\sqrt{g}(L_j \Phi_j - d_j)\|^2$$

The resulting least squares problem is very high-dimensional (256x256x2x2 parameters), but it can be solved directly since the matrix L is sparse. However, we reduce the dimensionality of the problem by projecting onto a subset of the discrete cosine transform (DCT) basis functions. Provided the constraints can be satisfied with a relatively smooth deformation, this approach will work with fewer basis functions than the original 256x256 samples in (u, v) space. Let B denotes the DCT basis matrix, $T = LB$, $\Psi = B^T \Phi$ and $T_i = L_i B$. The optimization problem reduces to:

$$\Phi = \arg\min \sum_{i \in S} \|\sqrt{g} L_i B B^T \Phi_i\|^2 + \sigma^2 \sum_{i \in S_c} \|\sqrt{g} L_i B B^T \Phi_i - d_i\|^2$$

$$\Psi = \arg\min \sum_{i \in S} \|\sqrt{g} T \Psi\|^2 + \sigma^2 \sum_{i \in S_c} \|\sqrt{g} T_i \Psi - d_i\|^2$$

In this way, we calculate the deformations in DCT transform space. Use of this basis leads to a significant increase in speed. The warps thus obtained are then applied to the (u, v) coordinates of each cortical surface to coregister them to the template. This process is illustrated in Fig. 2 where we show the sulci traced on the original cortical surface and their corresponding locations in flat space. We then show the relative locations of these sulcal features in flat space for the subject and atlas before and after matching. Note that we use a quadratic penalty function to match the landmarks so that they do not exactly align after registration. Note also that cortical regions near the boundary of the unit square exhibit larger metric distortion relative to the cortical surface than do regions near the center. Since the warp bending energy is computed with respect to the intrinsic geometry of the surface rather than flat space, we see that the warp in flat space exhibits larger deformations near the boundaries than at the center, following the pattern of metric distortion.

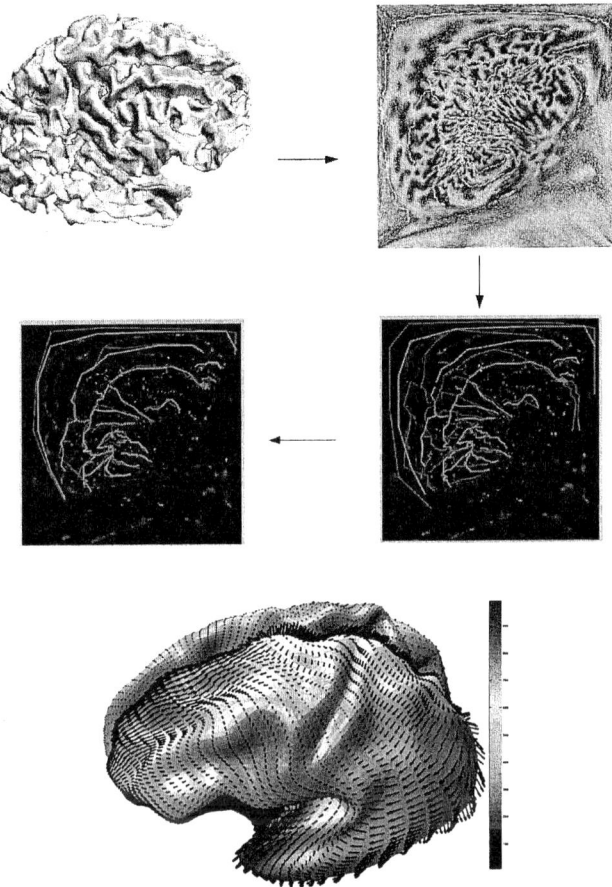

Fig. 2. The intrinsic TPS warping process. The figure show the extracted cortex, its p-harmonic map, and sulci of the subject and atlas mapped to the parameter space before (right) and after (left) warping. The figure at the bottom shows the warping field computed on the surface. The color indicates the magnitude of the deformation

3 Statistical Analysis in Riemannian Spaces

We now turn to the problem of statistical analysis in the space of the cortical surface atlas. We describe a general approach to modeling statistical variability of points on this surface, and illustrate its application to pattern classification. In functional brain imaging, localized regions of activation can be constrained to lie on the cortical surface. Pattern classification of this data requires a classification scheme that considers the intrinsic geometry of the cortical surface. Here we present such a scheme based on a parametric model that extends the Gaussian distribution to Riemannian surfaces [15]. This approach uses the heat kernel to replace the Gaussian distribution so that a probability density function on the surface can be defined by analogy to heat propagation on a surface.

3.1 The Heat Equation in the Intrinsic Geometry

The heat equation in the intrinsic geometry of the surface is given by:

$$(\Delta - \frac{\partial}{\partial t})\zeta = 0 \quad \text{where} \quad \Delta = \frac{1}{\sqrt{g}} \frac{\partial}{\partial u^i} \sqrt{g} g^{ij} \frac{\partial}{\partial u^j}$$

where Δ denotes the Laplace-Beltrami operator and ζ is the scalar field being diffused. We discretized the operator using the metric tensor calculations described in the Appendix. Using this discretized operator, we set up the Crank-Nicolson scheme [16] for solving the heat equation since it is known to be stable. We illustrate the differences between using the usual Laplacian and the Laplace-Beltrami operator in Fig. 3. In the former, diffusion is computed with respect to the 2D Euclidean space and produces a 2D Gaussian distribution in the flat parameter space which maps to a clearly anisotropic distribution on the surface. Conversely, the Laplace-Beltrami form computes the diffusion directly on the surface, on which it produces an isotropic distribution while exhibiting anisotropic behavior with respect to the parameter space. Solutions of linear partial differential equations, such as the heat equation, can be characterized by Green's functions. The Green's function of the heat equation, also known as the *heat kernel*, has been a topic of extensive research in spectral theory [17]. Though the heat kernel can only be implicitly defined in arbitrary surfaces, several of its properties in Euclidean spaces extend to Riemannian spaces and, in particular, to surfaces.

Here we list a few properties we will use later in this paper. Proofs can be found in [17]. Let M be a geodesically complete Riemannian manifold. Then the heat kernel $K_t(x, y)$ exists and satisfies

1. $K_t(x, y) = K_t(y, x)$
2. $\lim_{t \to 0} K_t(x, y) = \delta_x(y)$
3. $(\Delta - \frac{\partial}{\partial t})K = 0$
4. $K_t(x, y) = \int_M K_{t-s}(x, z) K_s(z, y) dz$
5. $K_t(x, y) = \sum_{i=0}^{\infty} e^{-\lambda_i t} \phi_i(x) \phi_i(y)$

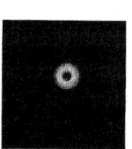 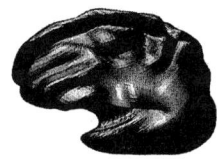 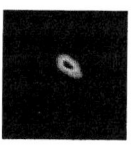 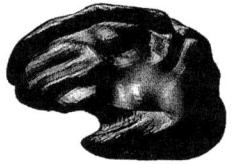

(a) The heat kernel computed using the Laplacian in the (u, v) parameter space

(b) The heat kernel computed using the Laplace-Beltrami operator on the cortical surface

Fig. 3. The heat kernels are displayed in the parameter space and on the surface. It can be seen that when the Laplace-Beltrami operator is used instead of the Laplacian, the heat kernel is not isotropic in the parameter space, however it is isotropic on the surface

3.2 The Heat Kernel as a Pdf

We know that the heat kernel is positive everywhere. It integrates to one on the manifold [18] and therefore it is a suitable candidate for modeling the probability density function of sample points lying in the manifold. Moreover, in Euclidean space, the heat kernel is identical to the Gaussian pdf. Therefore we propose replacing the Gaussian density with the covariant heat kernel in our surface-based analysis [15].

Just as we can characterize an isotropic Gaussian distribution in the Euclidean plane through its mean and standard deviation, so we can characterize distributions on the surface through mean and variance-like parameters that characterize the location of the heat kernel and the 'time' at which it is observed. Estimation of these parameters is in turn analogous to maximum likelihood parameter estimation, i.e. parameter estimation for a set of sample points on the surface can be viewed as the problem of finding the kernel of a covariant differential operator that best fits these points.

For isotropic distributions the corresponding heat kernel $K(m,t)$ on a Riemannian manifold can be completely specified by two parameters: m, the location of the initial impulse, and the time t. Parameters m and t play the role of the mean and variance in the Gaussian case. Thus the probability of finding a sample at x is modeled as $p(x|m,t) = K_t(m,x)$. So the problem of fitting the heat kernel in the given sample points can be reduced to the problem of estimating these two parameters of the heat kernel.

If the sample points are x_i, we define the likelihood function for m and t as:

$$L(m,t) = \prod_{n=1}^{N} K_t(m, x_i)$$

Because of property 2 above, $K_t(m,x)$ can be calculated explicitly by placing a delta function at point m and solving the heat equation up to time t. The problem with this approach is that the parameter m (the location of the mean) is unknown. However, since the heat kernel is symmetric (property 1), we can instead place the delta function at the sample points x_i whose locations are known, rather than at the unknown mean location m, and running the heat equation up to time t. This allows us to explicitly compute the likelihood function (2) for a set of sample points x_i for any time point t. The values of m and t for which the likelihood function $L(m,t)$ attains its maximum are then our estimates of the mean and variance.

To use this scheme for supervised classification of two clusters of points, we first compute ML estimates of the parameters (m_1, t_1) and (m_2, t_2) for the two clusters. We then define a likelihood ratio as the ratio of the two heat kernels: $R = K_1(m_1, t_1)/K_2(m_2, t_2)$ and compute this ratio at each point on the surface. The surface is then partitioned into two regions $R > 1$ and $R \leq 1$.

4 Applications and Results

We illustrate the technique presented above for classification of point localizations of S1 somatosensory regions. For each of 5 subjects we simulated 6 points each representing locations of thumb and index figure on the postcentral gyrus; the 6 points could, for example, represent localizations from 6 separate studies on a single subject. We brought the cortical surfaces for all subjects into register, using one of the subjects as the atlas, as described above. We then used the pooled data from all subjects in the atlas-coordinates to compute the mean and standard deviation for the thumb and index finger respectively as illustrated in Fig. 4. We then applied the likelihood ratio statistic to partition the cortex as illustrated in Fig. 5. Note that this two-class problem classifies the entire brain, including both hemispheres, into two regions. With more somatosensory areas involved we could perform a finer partitioning of somatsensory cortex producing maps of the most probable areas to which each sensory unit would map. While this is a somewhat artificial problem, it is clear that an extension of this analysis would allow us to produce probabilistic maps of functional localization in the atlas space.

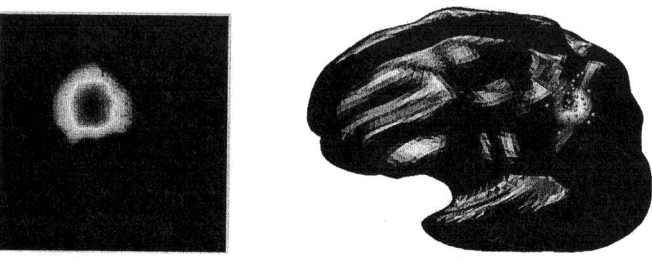

(a) pdf estimated for digit 1

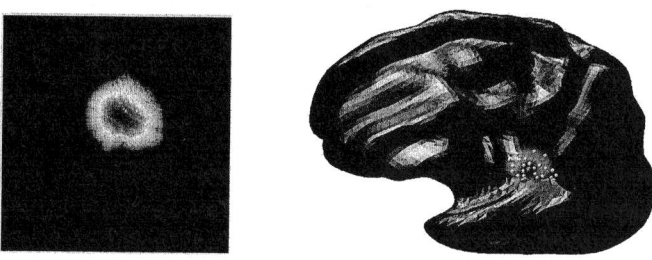

(b) pdf estimated for digit 5

Fig. 4. The figures shows the heat kernels estimated to fit the two datasets for MEG somatosensory data. For each of the datasets the estimated pdf is displayed in the parameter space and on the cortical surface

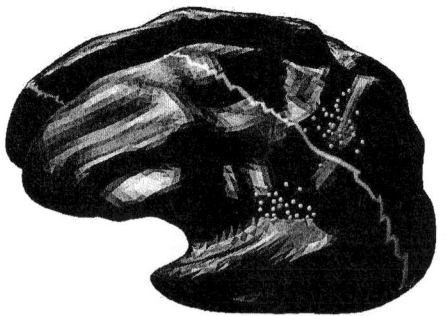

Fig. 5. The classifier: Red and Blue regions shows the two decision regions

5 Conclusion

We have presented a unified framework for analyzing cortically constrained functional data from multiple subjects where the analysis is performed in the intrinsic geometry of the surface. This allows us, for example, to compute the mean with respect to a cluster of points, such that the mean also lies in the surface. We have illustrated this framework by applying the analysis to produce functional parcellation of somatosensory cortex based on (simulated) MEG source localizations across multiple subjects. The method is currently limited to isotropic distributions and to point-wise analysis, but the idea of using the intrinsic heat equation, and kernels of covariant differential operators in place of the Gaussian distribution generalizes to the development of multivariate statistical analysis tools for data constrained to Riemannian manifolds.

References

1. George, J.S., Aine, C.J., Mosher, J.C., Schmidt, D.M., Ranken, D.M., H. A. Schlitt, C.C.W., Lewine, J.D., Sanders, J.A., Belliveau, J.W.: Mapping function in the human brain with magnetoencephalography, anatomical magnetic resonance imaging, and functional magnetic resonance imaging. J Clin Neurophysiol **12** (1995) 406–431
2. Thompson, P.M., Hayashi, K.M., de Zubicaray, G., Janke, A.L., Rose, S.E., Semple, J., Doddrell, D.M., , Cannon, T.D., Toga, A.W.: Detecting dynamic and genetic effects on brain structure using high dimensional cortical pattern matching. In: Proceedings of ISBI. (2002)
3. Fletcher, P.T., Lu, C., Joshi, S.C.: Statistics of shape via principal geodesic analysis on Lie groups. In: Conference on Computer Vision and Pattern Recognition. Volume 1. (2003) 95–101
4. Pennec, X.: Probabilities and statistics on riemannian manifolds: Basic tools for geometric measurements. In Cetin, A., Akarun, L., Ertuzun, A., Gurcan, M., Yardimci, Y., eds.: Proc. of Nonlinear Signal and Image Processing (NSIP'99). Volume 1., June 20-23, Antalya, Turkey, IEEE-EURASIP (1999) 194–198
5. Pennec, X., Ayache, N.: Randomness and geometric features in computer vision. In: IEEE Conf. on Computer Vision and Pattern Recognition (CVPR'96), San Francisco, CA, USA (1996) 484–491 Published in J. of Math. Imag. and Vision 9(1), july 1998, p. 49-67.
6. Srivastava, A., Klassen, E.: Bayesian and geometric subspace tracking. Adv. in Appl. Probab. **36** (2004) 43–56
7. Kreyzig, I.: Differential Geometry. Dover (1999)
8. Do Carmo, M.: Differential Geometry of Curves and Surfaces. Prentice-Hall (1976)
9. Shattuck, D.W., Leahy, R.M.: Brainsuite: An automated cortical surface identification tool. In Delp, S.L., DiGioia, A.M., Jaramaz, B., eds.: MICCAI. Volume 1935 of Lecture Notes in Computer Science., Springer (2000) 50–61
10. Joshi, A.A., Leahy, R.M., Thompson, P.M., Shattuck, D.W.: Cortical surface parameterization by p-harmonic energy minimization. In: ISBI. (2004) 428–431
11. Eells, J., Sampson, J.H.: Harmonic mappings of Riemannian manifolds. Ann. J. Math. (1964) 109–160
12. Thompson, P.M., Mega, M.S., Vidal, C., Rapoport, J., Toga, A.W.: Detecting disease-specific patterns of brain structure using cortical pattern matching and a population-based probabilistic brain atlas. In: Proc. 17th International Conference on Information Processing in Medical Imaging (IPMI2001), Davis, CA, USA. (2001) 488–501

13. Thompson, P.M., Toga, A.W.: A surface based technique for warping 3-dimensional images of the brain. IEEE Transactions in Medical Imaging **15** (1996) 1–16
14. Bookstein, F.L.: Principal warps: Thin-plate splines and the decomposition of deformations. IEEE Transactions in Pattern Analyis and Machine Intelligence **11** (1989) 567–585
15. Hsu, E.P.: Stochastic Analysis on Manifolds. American Mathematical Society, Providence, RI (2002)
16. Smith, G.D.: Numerical solution of partial differential equations: Finite difference methods. 3 edn. Oxford Applied Mathematics and Computing Science Series. Oxford : Clarendon Press (1985)
17. Rosenberg, S.: The Laplacian on a Riemannian manifold. Cambridge University Press (1997)
18. Davies, E.B.: Heat kernels and spectral theory. Cambridge University Press (1989)
19. Thompson, P.M., Mega, M.S., Toga, A.W.: Disease-specific probabilistic brain atlases. In: Procedings of IEEE International Conference on Computer Vision and Pattern Recognition. (2000) 227–234

Appendix

Let $\mathbf{x}$ denote the 3-D position vector of a point on the cortical surface. Let u^1, u^2 denote the coordinates in the parameter space. The metric tensor coefficients required in the computation are given by:

$$g_{11} = \left\| \frac{\partial \mathbf{x}}{\partial u^1} \right\|^2, \ g_{22} = \left\| \frac{\partial \mathbf{x}}{\partial u^2} \right\|^2, \ g_{12} = g_{21} = \left\langle \frac{\partial \mathbf{x}}{\partial u^1}, \frac{\partial \mathbf{x}}{\partial u^2} \right\rangle, \ g = g_{11}g_{22} - (g_{12})^2$$

Cartesian tensors suffice for flows in 2D or 3D Euclidean spaces. However the cortical surface is a two dimensional non-Euclidean space and from the outset demands a full tensorial treatment. We do this by replacing the usual partial derivatives by covariant derivatives. Although we want the deformation field with respect to the cortical surface to be independent of the specific choice of parameterization, the deformation field expressed in the 2D parameter space invariably does depend on the parameterization. Small deformations expressed in the parameter space can be modeled as contravariant vectors [19,7] since, with respect to two different parameterizations u and $\bar{u}$, the respective values of the deformations ϕ and $\bar{\phi}$ are related by $\bar{\phi}^\beta = \phi^j \frac{\partial \bar{u}^\beta}{\partial u^\alpha}$. In order to preserve their tensorial nature, we need to use covariant derivatives instead of the usual partial derivatives. The covariant derivative $\phi^\beta_{,\sigma}$ of a contravariant tensor ϕ^β is given by:

$$\phi^\beta_{,\sigma} = \frac{\partial \phi^\beta}{\partial u^\sigma} + \phi^\kappa \Gamma_{\kappa\sigma}{}^\beta \text{ where } \alpha, \beta, \kappa \in \{1, 2\}$$

where $\Gamma_{\kappa\sigma}$ denote the Christoffel symbols of the second kind [7]. The first covariant derivative of a contravariant tensor ϕ^ζ is a mixed tensor $\phi^\zeta_{,\beta}$. Covariant derivatives $\phi^\zeta_{,\beta\sigma}$ of such a tensor is given by:

$$\phi^\zeta_{,\beta\sigma} = \frac{\partial \phi^\zeta_{,\beta}}{\partial u^\sigma} - \phi^\zeta_{,\mu} \Gamma_{\beta\sigma}{}^\mu + \phi^\nu_\beta \Gamma_{\nu\sigma}{}^\zeta \text{ where } \sigma, \beta, \zeta, \mu, \kappa \in \{1, 2\}$$

PET Image Reconstruction: A Robust State Space Approach

Huafeng Liu[1], Yi Tian[1], and Pengcheng Shi[2]

[1]State Key Laboratory of Modern Optical Instrumentation,
Zhejiang University, Hangzhou, China
[2]Medical Image Computing Group,
Department of Electrical and Electronic Engineering,
Hong Kong University of Science and Technology, Hong Kong
{eeliuhf, eeship}@ust.hk

Abstract. Statistical iterative reconstruction algorithms have shown improved image quality over conventional nonstatistical methods in PET by using accurate system response models and measurement noise models. Strictly speaking, however, PET measurements, pre-corrected for accidental coincidences, are neither Poisson nor Gaussian distributed and thus do not meet basic assumptions of these algorithms. In addition, the difficulty in determining the proper system response model also greatly affects the quality of the reconstructed images. In this paper, we explore the usage of state space principles for the estimation of activity map in tomographic PET imaging. The proposed strategy formulates the organ activity distribution through tracer kinetics models, and the photon-counting measurements through observation equations, thus makes it possible to unify the dynamic reconstruction problem and static reconstruction problem into a general framework. Further, it coherently treats the uncertainties of the statistical model of the imaging system and the noisy nature of measurement data. Since H_∞ filter seeks minimum-maximum-error estimates without any assumptions on the system and data noise statistics, it is particular suited for PET image reconstruction where the statistical properties of measurement data and the system model are very complicated. The performance of the proposed framework is evaluated using Shepp-Logan simulated phantom data and real phantom data with favorable results.

1 Introduction

PET image reconstruction algorithms largely fall into analytic strategies and iterative statistical methods. The first group most frequently uses the deterministic filtered backprojection (FBP) principles, or modifications thereof [1, 9], based on inversion of the Radon transform through the central slice theorem. While they are fast and inexpensive as they operate entirely linearly on the projection data, FBP algorithms do not produce high quality reconstructed images because of their disregarding of the spatially-variant PET system response and treating measurement noise in a post-hoc manner. Iterative statistical methods have thus been the primary focus of many recent efforts, including notable examples of maximum likelihood–expectation maximization (ML–EM) [14], *maximum a posteriori* (MAP) [4], and penalized weighted least-squares (PWLS) [2] algorithms. Unlike conventional FBP methods, iterative methods are based on specific models for the measurement statistics and the physical systems, and thus have the potential to improve bias-variance performance. For any statistical framework, it is then clear that appropriate models for the measurement and the system response play essential roles in achieving good reconstruction [6].

During PET emission scans, one wishes to include only *true coincidences* that are related to gamma rays from the same annihilation and that have not scattered in the body prior to detection. In reality, however, the coincidence events also include the *scattered coincidences* (SC) and the *accidental coincidences* (AC), both being primary sources of background noise in PET. Since the introduction of the ML-EM algorithm, statistical reconstruction methods have heavily relied on the idealized PET system model with Poisson statistics for the measurements. However, due to AC events substraction, the measured data do not actually meet the Poisson distribution requirement in most commercial PET scanners [5]. Several recent works have attempted to derive statistical models that best fit the measurement data under some assumptions, such as the shifted Poisson (SP) model [17] and the saddle point (SD) model [16]. Nevertheless, in practical situations it is almost impossible to have the exact model information *a priori* as these works demand. The accuracy of the system response model, or the *system probability matrix*, also greatly affects the quality of the reconstruction results [11]. Some of the most interesting research efforts in system probability matrix estimation include the use of analytic detector response function [12], the consideration of the voxel position relative to the detectors [10], and the Monte Carlo simulations [15]. While nearly all model-based image reconstruction methods assume that the system response model is known exactly, either *a priori* or once it has been estimated, real imaging systems are subject to a number of physical effects that make the system response space-variant and image-dependent. Proper understanding and handling of system probability matrix uncertainties remains a challenging issue [9].

In this paper, we present a general PET reconstruction paradigm which is based on the state space principles. Given the uncertainties inherently associated with the system response and data measurements, we believe that a state space strategy offers an alternative to achieve robust and optimal image reconstructions. Compared to earlier statistical works, our effort has three significant novel aspects. First, this approach undertakes the uncertainties on both the imaging system model and the measurement data model. Secondly, it unifies the dynamic and the static reconstruction problems into a general framework, allows negative Sinogram values, and can simultaneously estimate the attenuation map and the activity map. Finally, two solutions are proposed for the framework: the Kalman filtering (KF) solution that adopts the minimum-mean-square-error criterion and the H_∞ filter which seeks the minimum-maximum-error estimates. Since the H_∞

principle makes no assumptions on the system and measurement statistics, it is particular suited for PET imaging where the statistical properties of measurement data and the system uncertainty remain difficult to acquire. We realize that several additional efforts in PET/SPECT image reconstruction are of relevance to our work. The noise equivalent counts (NEC) scaled and NEC-shifted ML-EM algorithms aim to transform arbitrary sinogram noise into approximately Poisson distributed one [8] for further processes, although it does not attempt to handle the system response model uncertainties. We believe, however, that we are presenting the first attempt to formulate PET reconstruction as a state estimation problem, to deal with noisy measurement data and uncertain system model in a coordinated effort, and to recursively estimate the activity map with the aid of the robust H_∞ filter.

2 PET Reconstruction: A State-Space Formulation

2.1 Modeling of PET Measurement

In the PET measurement process, a coincidence event indicates that two gamma rays interact with the opposite detector pairs within a small coincidence timing window. The true coincidences are contaminated by the AC and SC events, and the measured PET data Y is usually precorrected for AC events using delayed coincidence timing windows. The emission sinogram data $Y = \{Y_j | j = 1, ..., m\}$ is represented as one-dimensional vectors of dimension m, obtained by scanning all detector bins at each angle. Let vectors Y_p and Y_d be the number of coincidences detected within the prompt and delayed windows, the probability distributions for Y_p and Y_d then follow independent Poisson distributions with mean $y_p = \{y_{pj} | j = 1, ..., m\}$ and $y_d = \{y_{dj} | j = 1, ..., m\}$, respectively. $x = \{x_i | i = 1, ..., n\}$ is a n x 1 vector, with n the total number of image voxels, which represents the unknown radioactivity of emission object in voxel i.

Denoting the additive contributions of AC events with mean r and SC events with mean s, we have $y_d = r$. Further, the relationship between the projection data and emission object is given through affine transform $y_p = Dx + r + s$, where D is the m x n system matrix that gives the probability of a photon emitted from voxel i being detected in projection bin j. The detection probability matrix D depends on various factors: the geometry of the detection system, detector efficiency, attenuation effects, dead time correction factors, and the extent of scattering between source and detector.

Assuming that the expected value of the projection data is y, we have:

$$y = y_p - y_d = Dx + s \tag{1}$$

2.2 Modeling of Tracer Kinetics

To quantitatively obtain measurements of tissue metabolic function, it is necessary to model the relationship between the tracer activity and the metabolic parameter of interest. Since compartmental models are generally used to describe tracer kinetics, there have been many efforts focusing on describing compartmental models and their applications. In general, the dynamic equation for a compartmental system can be expressed as [3] $\dot{x}(t) = \mathcal{A}x(t) + \mathcal{B}\mathcal{U}(t)$, where $\mathcal{A}$ is combinations of the rate constants denoting the transfer of material between compartments, $\mathcal{B}$ is the delivery of the tracer to the tissue, and $\mathcal{U}(t)$ is the blood input function.

In this paper, we focus on static imaging of steady states, assuming that the distribution of the radioisotopes in the body is temporally stationary corresponding to the autoradiographic (ARG) model. The ARG assumption is the equilibrium of the metabolic ratio, which means:

$$\dot{x}(t) = 0 \qquad (2)$$

2.3 State Space Representation for PET Imaging

In more general form, Equation (1) can be rewritten as $y = Dx + e$ where e is the noise vector that represents *unknown* measurement errors including other noise except SC events. Making the time-dependence in the equation gives:

$$y(t) = Dx(t) + e(t) \qquad (3)$$

where t denotes the time steps. The equation can be interpreted as the observation equation of the state-space representation of the PET system, where the measurement noise e models the uncertainty of the measurement data.

Since the state $x(t)$ is temporally stationary for static imaging, we discretize Equation (2) and arrive at $x(t+1) = x(t)$. The state space representation is completed by a more general system equation:

$$x(t+1) = Ax(t) + v(t) \qquad (4)$$

with some initial activity x_0. Here, the state noise v models the statistical uncertainty of the imaging process, and the transition matrix A relates to our knowledge and assumptions about the compartmental model parameters. While Equation (4) represents the system equation of static PET imaging when the transition matrix A is an identity matrix, in general, A can be time invariant, time varying, linear, or nonlinear functions.

Equations (3) and (4) constitute a so-called state-space representation of PET imaging system, and the goal is now to estimate state $x(t)$ based on the observations $y(t)$. If we assume that the noise properties are known (Gaussian or Poisson) for e and v, many classical estimation techniques can be applied to recover the activity state x. However, the results can be sub-optimal or even divergent due to possible mismatch between the actual noise properties and the assumptions. Hence, we will mainly focus on the H_∞ estimation strategy in this paper where no *a priori* knowledge of noise statistics is required.

3 MMSE Estimation with Gaussian Noise

A general solution to the state-space PET system is through the Kalman filter, which has been the standard method for state-space models with Gaussian noise. It adopts a form of feedback control in estimation: the filter estimates the process state at some time and then obtains the feedback in the form of (noisy) measurements. Hence, the reconstruction technique updates state $x(t)$ at time t into an optimal estimate based on: (i) the prediction of the time update equations of the Kalman filter from the previous state and error covariance estimates. The solution to this problem is called the Kalman predictor. (ii) the Kalman filter is completed by adding the update based on the noisy measurements $y(t)$ to the predicted state– i.e. for incorporating measurements into the *a priori* estimate to obtain an improved *a posteriori* estimate. And the final estimation algorithm resembles that of a predictor-corrector algorithm for solving numerical problems. In our implementation, a recursive procedure is used to perform the state estimation of Equations (4) and (3):

1. Initial estimates for state $\hat{x}_0$ and error covariance $P(0)$.
2. Time update equations, *the predictions*, for the state $\hat{x}^-(t) = A\hat{x}(t-1)$ and for the error covariance $P^-(t) = AP(t-1)A^T + Q_v(t)$.
3. Measurement update equations, *the corrections*, for the Kalman gain $L(t) = P^-(t)D^T(DP^-(t)D^T + R_e(t))^{-1}$, for the state $\hat{x}(t) = \hat{x}^-(t) + L(t)(y - D\hat{x}^-(t))$, and for the error covariance $P(t) = P^-(t) - L(t)(DP^-(t)D^T + R_e(t))L^T(t)$.

Here, P is the covariance matrix describing the uncertainty of the state, Q_v is the covariance matrix associated with the process noise $v(t)$, R_e is the covariance of the observation errors $e(t)$, and L incorporates the model and the measurements and is termed the Kalman gain. In this notation the superscript '$-$' refers to the intermediate state and covariance predictions provided by the Kalman predictor, which are then modified by the measured data to produce the next state value.

Discussion. Estimation of radioactivity distribution with the Kalman filter bears strong ties with several existing methods. When A is set to be zero, $x^-(t)$ vanishes and $P^-(t)$ is equal to Q_v. Then the state estimate becomes $\hat{x}(t) = Q_v D^T [DQ_v D^T + R_e]^{-1} y$, the equivalent form of a least square solution.

In developing Kalman-based algorithms, the external excitation has to be assumed with Gaussian distribution, which may be unreasonable for PET measurements. Fortunately, Anscombe transformation can covert Poisson distributed noise into Gaussian distributed one [7], which gives the possibility to describe a clear relationship among these methods. Consider the joint likelihood $p(x,y)$ for the state space equations (3) and (4). Using the Markovian structure of the state space equations, we apply the chain rule and readily see that:

$$p(x,y) = p(x(0))p(x(t+1)|x(t))p(y(t)|x(t)) \qquad (5)$$

where $p(x(0))$ is the *a priori* state (the image) distribution, $p(x(t+1)|x(t))$ is the conditional probability for the next state, and $p(y(t)|x(t))$ the conditional probability for the observations. Taking the logarithm of the joint likelihood:

$$\Phi = lnp(x,y) = lnp(x(0)) + lnp(x(t+1)|x(t)) + lnp(y(t)|x(t)) \qquad (6)$$

the estimation solution is then the state variable that maximizes the objective function. If one chooses the state values that maximize $p(y(t)|x(t))$ by setting the other two terms to be constant, the traditional ML estimate is achieved. Similarly, the MAP estimate is the state value for which $lnp(x(0))$ and $lnp(y(t)|x(t))$ are maximized.

4 Robust Estimation Without Assumptions on Noise

Previous studies have assumed that the noise in PET is Poisson (or shifted Poisson, Gaussian) processes in order to develop the estimation algorithms such as ML-EM and MAP. Similarly, Kalman filter also requires prior knowledge on the statistical properties of the Gaussian state variables and noise. However, in practice, the PET measured data is affected by random coincidence, scatter coincidence, scanner sensitivity and dead time, and thus its distribution is very complicated. The Gaussian, Poisson, or shifted Poisson assumptions may not agree with the actual nature of PET measurement exactly. In the following, we present a robust estimation strategy for the PET state-space estimation, based on the mini-max H_∞ principles that do not impose *any restrictions* on the unknown disturbances $v(t)$ and $e(t)$ but only assume finite disturbance energy. It is thus more robust and less sensitive to noise variations and model assumptions [13].

Along with the state and measurement equations (4) and (3), the required output equation for the H_∞ filter is constructed as:

$$z(t) = Fx(t) \qquad (7)$$

where the output variable $z(t)$ is the linear combination $x(t)$, and the entries of the known output matrix F are problem- and system- specific. In this paper, F is just an identity matrix.

While the Kalman filter calculates the estimation error using the H_2 norm and minimizing the mean-square error, the H_∞ filter aims to provide a small estimation error, $w(t) = z(t) - \hat{z}(t)$, for any types of noises $e(t)$ and $v(t)$. Specifically, the measure of the performance is given by:

$$J = \frac{\|w(t)\|^2_{Q(t)}}{\|x_o - \hat{x}_o\|^2_{p_o^{-1}} + (\|v(t)\|^2_{N(t)^{-1}} + \|e(t)\|^2_{V(t)^{-1}})} \qquad (8)$$

where the notation $\|x\|^2_G$ is defined as the square of the weighted (by G) L_2 norm of x, i.e. $\|x\|^2_G = x^T Gx$. Here, $N(t)$, $V(t)$, $Q(t)$ and p_o are the weighting matrices for the process noise, the measurement noise, the estimation error and the initial conditions respectively, and $\hat{x}_o$ is the *a priori* estimate of the state. These weighting matrices are user-specified and dependent on the performance requirement. The optimal estimate $z(t)$ among all possible $\hat{z}(t)$ should satisfy:

$$\|J\|_\infty = \sup J < \gamma^2 \qquad (9)$$

where $\gamma^2 > 0$ is a prescribed level of disturbance attenuation. It is assumed that the L_2 norms of $e(t)$ and $v(t)$ exist (i.e. finite energies). The robustness of the H_∞ estimator arises from the fact that it yields an energy gain less than γ^2 for all bounded energy disturbances no matter what they are.

As a solution to the H_∞ estimation problem keeps the H_∞ norm less than a prescribed value, an H_∞ filter has been derived for state space PET model (4) and (3). Since the disturbance inputs $e(t)$ and $v(t)$, as well as the uncertainty of the initial state vector x_0, tend to increase the performance index J, while the estimation error $w(t)$ is designed to minimize J, Equation (9) can be further equivalently represented as

$$min_w max_{v,e,x_0} J =$$
$$\|w(t)\|^2_{Q(t)} - \gamma^2 \|x_o - \hat{x}_o\|^2_{p_o^{-1}} - \gamma^2(\|v(t)\|^2_{N(t)^{-1}} + \|e(t)\|^2_{V(t)^{-1}}) \qquad (10)$$

where *min* and *max* stand for minimization and maximization respectively. With this expression, the H_∞ filter represents a typical min-max problem where the worst situation is first induced by the disturbances and the estimator is then introduced for improvement. In other words, the H_∞ filter is in fact a two-person game between the external disturbances and the estimator $w(t)$ [13]. This can be solved by using a game theoretic algorithm which can be implemented through recursive updating of the filter gain $K(t)$, the Riccati difference equation solution $P(t)$, and the state estimates $\hat{x}(t)$:

$$K(t) = AP(t)S(t)D^T V(t)^{-1} \qquad (11)$$
$$P(t+1) = AP(t)S(t)A^T + N(t) \qquad (12)$$
$$\hat{x}(t+1) = A\hat{x}(t) + K(t)(y(t) - D\hat{x}(t)) \qquad (13)$$

where

$$S(t) = (I - \gamma^{-2}\bar{Q}(t)P(t) + D^T V(t)^{-1} DP(t))^{-1}$$
$$\bar{Q}(t) = F^T Q(t) F$$
$$P(0) = (p_0^{-1} + \gamma^{-2} Q)^{-1}$$

This H_∞ filtering formulation has a similar structure to the Kalman filter but with different optimizing criteria. Let the weighting matrices $N(t)$, $V(t)$ and p_0 be the same as the covariances matrices Q_v, R_e and $P(0)$ of Kalman filtering. In the limiting case, when the parameter γ approaches ∞, the H_∞ approaches the Kalman filter. Note that although when $\gamma = \infty$ the H_∞ filter is identical to that of the Kalman filter in form, the meanings of optimality are different. The Kalman filter has quite a large H_∞ norm, which means that the maximum energy gain of the Kalman filter algorithm has no upper bound. This leads to the observation that the Kalman filter will be more sensitive to the variations in the initial state and noise issues.

Detailed computational issues are omitted here because of page limit.

5 Experiments and Discussions

5.1 Digital Phantom Simulation

The synthetic emission phantom with known radioactivity concentrations is used, as shown in Fig. 1. The resolution of the original image is 34 by 32 pixels, and 720 projections over 180 degrees are simulated. To generate realistic data, we simulate the emission coincidence events during prompt windows and delayed windows respectively. The prompt data has to be modified to subtract the effects of the AC events. Taking these effects into account, the measured sinogram y is created based on the equations $y_{prompt} = Poisson\{y_{true}\} + Poisson\{60\%.y_{true}\} + Poisson\{10\%.y_{true}\}$, $y_{delay} = Poisson\{60\%.y_{true}\}$, and $y = y_{prompt} - y_{delay}$. Here, we model the random and scatter events to be uniform field of 60 percents and 10 percents respectively. y_{prompt} is the number of coincident photon pairs collected in the prompt windows. y_{delay} is the number of coincident photon pairs collected in the delay windows. The total number of photon counts in the reconstruction plane is set to be 20,000 (low) and 2,000,000 (high) respectively. Then, a set of 50 separate realizations of pseudorandom emission projection data are generated for each case. These 100 sinograms are then reconstructed using the following four different reconstruction algorithms, in order to quantitatively evaluate the performance of each reconstruction method:

1. ML-EM (OP) algorithm [16]: ideal Poisson measured data, and the resulting logarithm of the likelihood is solved by ordinary EM algorithm.
2. ML-EM (SP) algorithm [16]: the measured data is modeled by shifted Poisson process, and the resulting logarithm of the likelihood is solved by the EM algorithm.
3. State-space KF algorithm: $P(0)$, Q_v, and R_e are all set to diagonal matrices, and the values are fixed during the estimation process.
4. State-space H_∞ algorithm: the H_∞ weighting parameters $N(t)$, $V(t)$, $Q(t)$ and p_o are all set to diagonal matrices.

Convergence is checked using two consecutive errors such that $\|\chi(t+1) - \chi(t)\| < \varsigma$, with ς being a small constant. Let x be the ground truth image and $\hat{x}$ be a single reconstruction, then χ defines the error between the estimated and the exact activity values as $\chi = \left(\frac{1}{n}\sum_{i=1}^{n}|x_i - \hat{x}_i|^2\right)^{0.5}$. Please recall that n are the known sets of image pixels. If the criteria is satisfied, the estimated activity map distribution is considered to be final. No smoothing algorithm is applied.

The system matrix is generated using the MATLAB toolbox developed by Jeff Fessler and his students. In order to investigate how the noise in the system matrix affects the reconstructed image, we have also reconstructed images

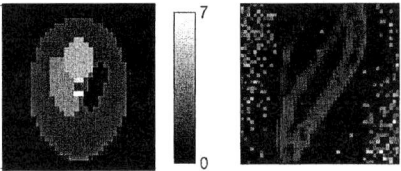

Fig. 1. Digital Shepp-Logan phantom for PET reconstruction experiments (left), and emission sinogram of the phsyical phantom obtained from the SHR-22000 (right)

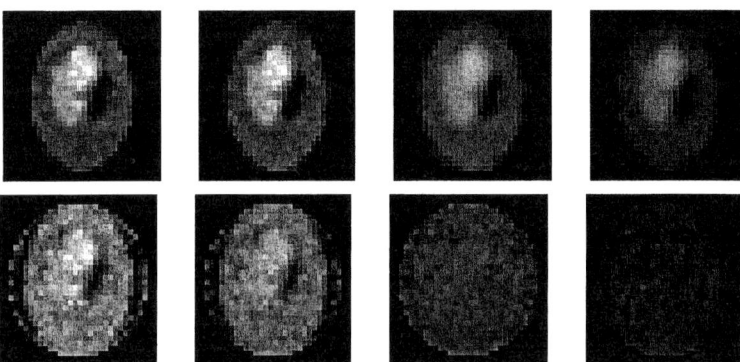

Fig. 2. Mean (top row) and pixel-variance (bottom row) images (Shepp-Logan phantom) reconstructed using low counts measurement with noisy system matrix. From left to right: OP, SP, KF, and H_∞ results

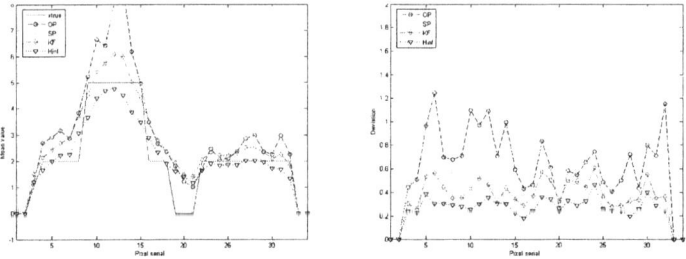

Fig. 3. Vertical profiles through sample mean (left) and standard-deviation (right) of estimators for low counts measurement using noisy system matrix

for different methods based on a noisy system matrix. In our current simulation, we generate a noisy matrix D with the mean relative error in the range of 35%. The reconstructions are evaluated quantitatively in terms of bias and variance estimator performance for each reconstruction technique. We calculate the relative errors bias and variance through $bias = \frac{1}{n}\sum_{i=1}^{n}(x_i - \hat{x}_i)$ and $variance = \frac{1}{n-1}\sum_{i=1}^{n}(x_i - \hat{x}_i)^2$. The errors $bias$ and $variance$ are averaged over

Table 1. Comparative studies of estimated activity distribution on synthetic data. Each data cell represents reconstruction error: bias ± variance

Conditions	Methods	bias ± variance
With exact known system matrix (High Counts)	ML-EM-OP	+0.0044 ± 0.2115
	ML-EM-SP	+0.0046 ± 0.1331
	KF	-0.0417 ± 0.2782
	H_∞	+0.0006 ± 0.1167
With noisy system matrix (High Counts)	ML-EM-OP	+1.1643 ± 1.2913
	ML-EM-SP	+0.5830 ± 0.6454
	KF	+0.4293 ± 0.4027
	H_∞	+0.5743 ± 0.5625
With exact known system matrix (Low Counts)	ML-EM-OP	+0.0189 ± 1.8614
	ML-EM-SP	+0.0239 ± 0.7261
	KF	-0.0060 ± 1.0160
	H_∞	-0.0507 ± 0.5213
With noisy system matrix (Low Counts)	ML-EM-OP	+1.1859 ± 4.2465
	ML-EM-SP	+0.6109 ± 1.7007
	KF	+0.4342 ± 0.7576
	H_∞	+0.0045 ± 0.5103

the 50 reconstructions to give the estimates $E[bias]$ and $E[variance]$ for OP, SP, KF and H_∞ reconstruction methods, and the analysis results are summarized in Table 1. Images of the mean pixel values and the variances obtained by the four algorithms (OP, SP, KF, and H_∞) with noisy system matrix and low counts measurement are shown in Fig. 2, with their sample vertical profiles plotted versus the corresponding pixel positions shown in Fig. 3.

These quantitative results and figures illustrate that both OP and SP results show large positive biases when using a noisy system matrix, while the KF and H_∞ frameworks seem free of such biases. However, the KF result shows significantly large variances for high counts case. Further, because the KF method is sensitive to modeling mismatch problem, it is capable of good performance under Gaussian statistics assumptions, which unfortunately is unrealistic for the PET image reconstruction problem. H_∞ framework is nearly unbiased to known or noisy system matrix cases. Also, it gives the good variance performance.

5.2 Real PET Data

The real data set used in this study was acquired on the Hamamatsu SHR-22000 scanner using a 6-spheres phantom, which has six circular regions of different diameters. These sphere objects have diameters of $37mm$, $28mm$, $22mm$, $17mm$, $13mm$ and $10mm$ respectively, and are each inserted in a circular cylinder with diameter of $200mm$ corresponding to a volume of $9300ml$, as shown in Fig. 4. The phantom filled with pure water was located at the center of both transaxial and axial FOV in the scanner using the patient bed. We injected F-18 concentration

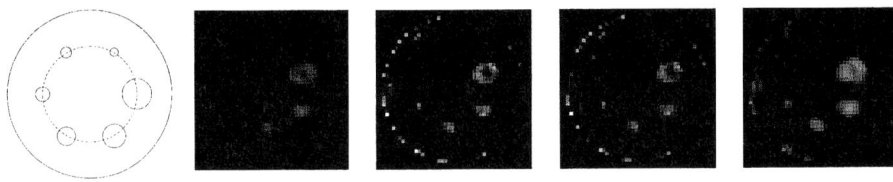

Fig. 4. The geometry of real phantom, and the FBP, OP, SP and H_∞ estimation results (left to right)

with initial activity of 107.92 Bq/ml into the six spheres. A 120-minutes scan was then performed. Fig. 1 (right) shows the sinograms obtained from the emission scan with 48 radial bins uniformly sampled over a $450mm$ transaxial FOV, and 48 angles uniformly sampled over 180 degrees.

Here, system matrix D_{ij} is computed by using a single ray approximation model. For more accurate modeling, physical effects such as attenuation, positron range, and non-collinearity must be accounted for in the D matrix. The random events have been removed by using delayed window coincidence technique. Conventional FBP method, OP, SP and $H\infty$ algorithms as described in the previous sections have been applied to recover images from the noisy data. The reconstruction image size is cropped to 48x48 pixels. For FBP, we choose ramp window type and the cutoff frequency is set to be 1/2. The FBP result in Fig. 4 shows significant noise and streak artifacts. In terms of visibility, four spheres can be visualized in both OP and SP methods, while five spheres are appeared when using the H_∞ framework.

6 Discussion

We want to point out that, in our current implementation, the noise covariance matrices Q_v and R_e (KF framework), as well as the weighting matrices in H_∞ framework are set to some empirically fixed values which are obviously not optimal. Ideally, these parameters should be adaptively updated during the estimation process.

In order to provide more accurate image reconstructions, all physical factors including detector response, attenuation, positron range et al, must be modeled in the reconstruction process. However, establishing an exact system model is a challenging problem, not least because of the system response being space-variant and image-dependent. In the state space representation, the system model parameters can be treated as random variable with known prior statistics. A joint estimation framework can then possibly be applied to *simultaneously estimate* the image and the system matrix D from observations.

In particular, attenuation correction is a well-documented research topic due to the requirement of quantitative analysis. The attenuation and activity distributions from emission data can be simultaneously reconstructed based on the state space framework. The unknown state vector x can be augmented by the unknown attenuation coefficients θ to form the new state vector $z(t) = [x(t)\ \theta(t)]^T$. Thus, we may explicitly construct the state space equations accounting for attenuation effects. This form of formulation may lead to a solution of the filtering problem either based on the extended Kalman filter algorithm (Gaussian models) or iterative sequential H_∞ filter framework (robust solution).

As a straightforward extension, based on the tracer kinematics equation and the measurement equation, we can recover dynamic changes of tracer density in a continuous time domain for dynamic PET. On the other hand, the purpose of dynamic PET imaging is to estimate physiological parameters associated with compartmental model. Thus, joint estimation of the physiological parameters and tracer density can be achieved. Because this integration allows image reconstruction and physiological parameters estimation in a coherent framework, we believe that it will help achieve more robust results from noisy data. Detailed investigations on these issues are underway.

Acknowledgement. Thanks to Dr. T. Yamashita and Dr. E. Yoshikawa of Hamamatsu Photonics K.K. for useful discussions. This work is supported by the National Basic Research Program of China (No. 2003CB716104), by HKUST6151/03E, and by the NSF of China for Innovative Research Groups (No. 60021201).

References

1. H.H. Barrett and W. Swindell. *Radiological Imaging: The Theory of Image Formation, Detection, and Processing.* Academic Press, San Diego, CA, 1981.
2. J. A. Fessler. Penalized weighted least-squares image reconstruction for positron emission tomography. *IEEE Transactions on Medical Imaging*, 13(2):290–300, 1994.
3. R.N. Gunn, S.R. Gunn, F.E. Turkheimer, J.A.D. Aston, and V.J. Cunningham. *Tracer Kinetic Modeling via Basis Pursuit.* Academic Press, In M. Senda, Y. Kimura, and P. Herscovitch, editors, Brain Imaging using PET, 2002.
4. T. Hebert and R. Leahy. A generalized EM algorithm for 3-D Bayesian reconstruction from Poisson data using Gibbs priors. *IEEE Transactions on Medical Imaging*, 8:194–202, 1989.
5. E.J. Hoffman, S.C. Huang, M.E. Phelps, and D.E. Kuhl. Quantitation in positron emission computed tomography: 4. effect of accidental coincidences. *Journal of Computerized Assisted Tomography*, 5:391–400, 1981.
6. R. M. Lewitt and S. Matej. Overview of methods for image reconstruction from projections in emission computed tomography. *Proceedings of the IEEE*, 91:1588–1611, 2003.
7. H. Lu, G. Han, D. Chen, L. Li, and Z. Liang. A theoretically based pre-reconstructing filter for spatio-temporal noise reduction in gated cardiac SPECT. In *IEEE Nuclear Science Symposium*, pages 141–145, Lyon, France, October 2000.
8. J. Nuyts, C. Michel, and P. Dupont. Maximum-likelihood expectation-maximization reconstruction of sinograms with arbitrary noise distribution using NEC-transformations. *IEEE Transactions on Medical Imaging*, 20:365–375, 2001.
9. J.M. Ollinger and J. A. Fessler. Positron emission tomography. *IEEE Signal Processing Magazine*, 14(1):43–55, 1997.

10. J. Qi, R.M. Leahy, S.R. Cherry, A. Chatziioannou, and T.H. Farquhar. High resolution 3D Bayesian image reconstruction using the microPET small-animal scanner. *Physics in Medicine and Biology*, 43:1001–1013, 1998.
11. M. Rafecas, G. Boning, B.J. Pichler, E. Lorenz, M. Schwaiger, and S.I. Ziegler. Effect of noise in the probability matrix used for statistical reconstruction of PET data. *IEEE Transactions on Nuclear Science*, 51:149–156, 2004.
12. V. Selivanov, Y. Picard, J. Cadorette, S. Rodrigue, and R. Lecomte. Detector response models for statistical iterative image reconstruction in high resolution FBI. *IEEE Transactions on Nuclear Science*, 47:1168–1175, 2000.
13. X. Shen and L. Deng. A dynamic system approach to speech enhancement using the $\mathcal{H}_\infty$ filtering algorithm. *IEEE Transactions on Speech and Audio Processing*, 7(4):391–399, 1999.
14. L.A. Shepp and Y. Vardi. Maximum likelihood reconstruction for emission tomography. *IEEE Transactions on Medical Imaging*, 1:113–122, 1982.
15. E. Veklerov, J. Llacer, and E.J. Hoffman. MLE reconstruction of a brain phantom using a Monte Carlo transition matrix and a statistical stopping rule. *IEEE Transactions on Nuclear Science*, 35:603–607, 1988.
16. M. Yavuz and J.A. Fessler. New statistical models for randoms precorrected PET scans. *Lecture Notes in Computer Science:IPMI'97*, 1230:190–203, 1997.
17. M. Yavuz and J.A. Fessler. Statistical image reconstruction methods for randoms-precorrected PET scans. *Medical Image Analysis*, 2(4):369–378, 1998.

Multi-dimensional Mutual Information Based Robust Image Registration Using Maximum Distance-Gradient-Magnitude

Rui Gan and Albert C.S. Chung

Lo Kwee-Seong Medical Image Analysis Laboratory,
Department of Computer Science,
The Hong Kong University of Science and Technology, Hong Kong
{raygan, achung}@cs.ust.hk

Abstract. In this paper, a novel spatial feature, namely *maximum distance-gradient-magnitude (MDGM)*, is defined for registration tasks. For each voxel in an image, the MDGM feature encodes spatial information at a global level, including both edges and distances. We integrate the MDGM feature with intensity into a two-element attribute vector and adopt multi-dimensional mutual information as a similarity measure on the vector space. A multi-resolution registration method is then proposed for aligning multi-modal images. Experimental results show that, as compared with the conventional mutual information (MI)-based method, the proposed method has longer capture ranges at different image resolutions. This leads to more robust registrations. Around 1200 randomized registration experiments on clinical 3D MR-T1, MR-T2 and CT datasets demonstrate that the new method consistently gives higher success rates than the traditional MI-based method. Moreover, it is shown that the registration accuracy of our method obtains sub-voxel level and is acceptably high.

1 Introduction

A key issue in the medical imaging field is multi-modal image registration, which can integrate complementary image information from different modalities. The task of image registration is to reliably identify a geometric transformation to accurately align two images.

A crucial element in the registration process is a similarity measure to determine how well the images match with each other through a hypothesized spatial transformation. General promising results have shown that mutual information (MI) as a voxel intensity-based similarity measure is well-suited for multi-modal image registration [1, 2]. However, it has been suggested that the conventional MI-based registration can result in misalignment for some cases [3, 4] and then room for improvement exists. The standard MI measure only takes intensity values into account. Therefore, a known disadvantage is the lack of concern on any spatial information (neither local nor global) which may be present in individual images to be registered [5, 6]. As a simple illustration, a random perturbation of image points identically on both images results in unchanged MI value as that of the original images.

Several researchers have proposed adaptations of the MI-based registration framework to incorporate spatial information of individual images. Butz et al. [7] applied MI to edge measure (e.g., gradient magnitude) space, which was meant to align object surfaces in images. However, MI based on edge measure is sensitive to the sparseness of joint edge feature histograms. This may increase the difficulty of the optimization procedure. Pluim et al. [4] incorporated spatial information by multiplying the conventional MI measure with an external local gradient term to ensure the alignment of locations of tissue transitions in images. The probing results indicated that the registration function of the combined measure was smoother than that of the standard MI measure. But this approach does not actually extend the MI based similarity measure. Moreover, Rueckert et al. [6] exploited higher-order mutual information for 4D joint histograms. To include local spatial information present by neighboring point pairs, the 4D joint histograms were built on the co-occurrence of intensity pairs of adjacent points. This method was shown to be robust with respect to local intensity variation. However, only one neighbor is considered at a time in this approach and plenty of spatial information which may be present globally or within large neighborhood system has been ignored.

In this paper, a new spatial feature, namely *maximum distance-gradient-magnitude (MDGM)*, is defined for registration tasks. The MDGM feature encodes spatial information for each voxel in an image at a global level, which is about the distance of a voxel to a certain object boundary. In order to improve the conventional MI-based registration framework, we integrate the MDGM feature with intensity to form a two-element attribute vector for each voxel in individual images. Then, multi-dimensional mutual information is exploited as a similarity measure on the attribute vector space. To increase computation efficiency and robustness of the proposed method, the registration procedure is a multi-resolution iterative process.

Based on the results on clinical 3D MR-T1, MR-T2 and CT image volumes, it is experimentally shown that the proposed method has relatively longer capture ranges [1] than the conventional MI-based method at different image resolutions. This can obviously make the multi-resolution image registration more robust. Moreover, the results of around 1200 randomized registration experiments reveal that our method consistently gives higher success registration rates than the traditional MI-based method. Finally, it is demonstrated that our method can obtain acceptably high registration accuracy in sub-voxel level.

The organization of the paper is as follows. Section 2 formulates spatial information as a novel MDGM feature. Our multi-modal image registration method is proposed in Section 3. Some implementation details are given in Section 4.

---

[1] Capture range represents the range of alignments from which a registration algorithm can converge to the correct maximum.

Section 5 presents the experimental results and discussions. The conclusion is drawn in Section 6.

2 Spatial Feature Definition

Given an image pair and a geometric transformation, we aim at evaluating a novel multi-dimensional mutual information based registration criterion. In our proposed approach, each voxel in the image has a two-element attribute vector. The first element is the conventional voxel intensity, while the second one is a newly designed spatial feature term, namely *maximum distance-gradient-magnitude (MDGM)*, for incorporating spatial information at a global level within individual images. Compared with the traditional local gradient magnitude feature, the MDGM feature can encode local edge information, as well as globally defined spatial information about the distance of a voxel to a certain object boundary. Although it can be similar to the distance transform [8], the distance transform is normally applied to binary images, while the proposed MDGM feature directly processes original intensity images and does not rely on segmentation. Moreover, unlike the sparseness of gradient magnitude feature, the MDGM feature varies smoothly and gradually from object boundaries towards homogeneous image regions.

2.1 Maximum Distance-Gradient-Magnitude (MDGM)

Gradient magnitude represents spatial information in an image. However, the traditional gradient magnitude operator is locally defined and normally used to detect the amplitude object boundaries where voxels change their gray-level suddenly. By deriving gradient magnitude map, voxels at object boundaries, which may only occupy a very small proportion of the whole image volume, would give large values. On the other hand, a large amount of voxels (i.e. voxels within background regions and anatomical structures) would give small and almost constant values. Consequently, such gradient magnitude feature of an image can be sparse and insufficient for voxel-based image registration [9].

In this section, we define a new spatial feature, maximum distance-gradient-magnitude (MDGM). It contains not only local edge information, but also spatial information at a global level, which is about the distance of a voxel to a certain object boundary. Moreover, the MDGM feature varies smoothly and gradually from object boundaries towards homogeneous image regions.

We begin by defining a *distance-gradient* operator, ∇_d, on two voxels in an image. Given an image $I(\mathbf{v})$, where $\mathbf{v} = (x, y, z)$ denotes voxel position, the distance-gradient of two different voxels, $\mathbf{v}_1$ and $\mathbf{v}_2$, is defined as

$$\nabla_d I(\mathbf{v}_1, \mathbf{v}_2) = \big(I(\mathbf{v}_1) - I(\mathbf{v}_2)\big) \frac{\mathbf{v}_1 - \mathbf{v}_2}{|\mathbf{v}_1 - \mathbf{v}_2|^2}. \tag{1}$$

Then, a *MDGM map*, $G(\mathbf{v})$, of the image can be derived by using

$$G(\mathbf{v}) = \max_{\mathbf{v}' \in \Omega} |\nabla_d I(\mathbf{v}', \mathbf{v})|, \tag{2}$$

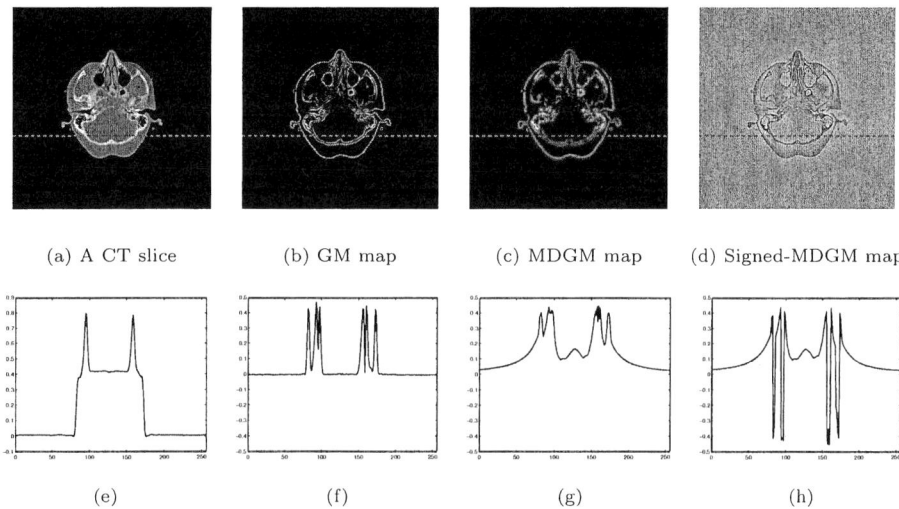

Fig. 1. (a) - (d) are slices respectively selected from a clinical CT image volume and its corresponding GM, MDGM and signed-MDGM maps. (e) - (g) are value profiles of lines in (a) - (d), which are marked as dashed lines

where Ω is the image domain. Following this formulation, when a voxel is at or very close to object boundary, its MDGM value would be large and can approximate the traditional local gradient magnitude. On the other hand, when voxel position varies from boundaries towards interiors of homogenous regions (either background regions or anatomical structures), the MDGM value smoothly and gradually decreases. With this property, the MDGM map of homogenous regions can provide global and detailed spatial information (which is about the distance of a voxel to a certain object boundary), and therefore is superior to the local gradient magnitude map.

As a comparative illustration, we individually computed the traditional local gradient magnitude (GM) and MDGM maps of a clinical CT image volume obtained from the Retrospective Registration Evaluation Project (RREP) [2]. A slice from the volume is shown in Figure 1a, while Figures 1b and 1c respectively present the corresponding slices from the GM and MDGM maps. (Note that values from individual images are re-scaled to [0, 1] for a fair comparison.) It is observed that the GM map can only exhibit sharp edge information. In addition, much more structural information can also be found in the MDGM map. For instance, regions close to boundaries in Figure 1c suggest much more information than those in Figure 1b. However, due to the limitation of image quality, smooth changes within the background regions and anatomical structures may not be clearly displayed in Figure 1c.

---

[2] Images were provided as part of the project, "Evaluation of Retrospective Image Registration", National Institutes of Health, Project Number 1 R01 NS33926-01, Principle Investigator, J. Michael Fitzpatrick, Vanderbilt University, Nashville, TN.

For a detailed description, Figures 1e - 1g respectively present the value profiles of the same line (marked as dashed lines) in Figures 1a - 1c. As suggested by the figures, feature values in Figure 1f are very sparse, where the overwhelming majority are small and constant. Contrarily, for Figure 1g, the value variation from boundaries towards homogenous regions is smooth and gradual. It is worth noting that, although there is little intensity variation at the middle of the line in Figure 1e, an evident and smooth saddle can be found in Figure 1g located at the corresponding position. The raised white boundary slightly below the line cause this saddle. It is because, unlike the local gradient magnitude operator, the MDGM operator is globally defined.

2.2 Signed-MDGM

In order to make the MDGM map be capable of distinguishing voxels of objects with different intensities, we further introduce the *signed-MDGM* map, $\hat{G}(\mathbf{v})$, as follows,

$$\hat{G}(\mathbf{v}) = sign(I(\hat{\mathbf{v}}) - I(\mathbf{v})) \cdot |\nabla_d I(\hat{\mathbf{v}}, \mathbf{v})|, \qquad (3)$$

where $\hat{\mathbf{v}} = arg\max_{\mathbf{v}'} |\nabla_d I(\mathbf{v}', \mathbf{v})|$, and the function $sign(\cdot)$ indicates the sign of the difference. According to this modified definition, a voxel of relatively low intensity would have a positive MDGM value and vice versa. (It should be noticed that, for a fixed $\mathbf{v}$, $|\hat{G}(\mathbf{v})| = G(\mathbf{v})$.)

As a comparison, Figures 1d and 1h respectively show the corresponding slice and value profile from the signed-MDGM map of the aforementioned CT image volume. Obviously, the signed-MDGM map presents all the properties shown in the MDGM map. Furthermore, as shown in Figure 1h, voxels of objects with different intensities are distinguishable. Hereafter, we adopt the signed-MDGM feature to represent spatial information for registration tasks.

3 Multi-modal Image Registration

As we have discussed above, the signed-MDGM feature encodes spatial information at a global level. We associate it with voxel intensity to form a two-element attribute vector for registration. Given two images, in order to measure the degree of dependence of the attribute vector space, multi-dimensional (i.e. 4D) mutual information (MI) is exploited as a similarity measure.

3.1 Multi-dimensional Mutual Information

Suppose that I^r and I^f are the intensity domains for the *reference* and *floating* images respectively, and $\hat{G}^r$ and $\hat{G}^f$ are their signed-MDGM domains. Given a rigid transformation $\mathbf{T}$, the 4D joint histogram $h_{\mathbf{T}}(I^f, \hat{G}^f, I^r, \hat{G}^r)$ over the sampling set $\mathcal{V}$ [3] can be approximated by either Parzen windowing or histogramming [10]. Histogramming is employed in this paper because the approach is

---
[3] The sampling set $\mathcal{V}$ can be all voxels in the floating image or a subset.

computationally efficient. That is, $h_\mathbf{T}(I^f, \hat{G}^f, I^r, \hat{G}^r)$ is constructed by binning the attribute vector pairs $(I^f(\mathbf{v}), \hat{G}^f(\mathbf{v}), I^r(\mathbf{T} \cdot \mathbf{v}), \hat{G}^r(\mathbf{T} \cdot \mathbf{v}))$ for all $\mathbf{v} \in \mathcal{V}$. The trilinear partial volume distribution interpolation [1] is exploited to update the joint histogram for non-grid alignment.

Then the 4D mutual information registration criterion is evaluated by using

$$\mathrm{MI}(\mathbf{T}) = \sum_{I^f, \hat{G}^f, I^r, \hat{G}^r} p_\mathbf{T}(I^f, \hat{G}^f, I^r, \hat{G}^r) \log_2 \frac{p_\mathbf{T}(I^f, \hat{G}^f, I^r, \hat{G}^r)}{p_\mathbf{T}(I^f, \hat{G}^f) \cdot p_\mathbf{T}(I^r, \hat{G}^r)}, \quad (4)$$

where

$$p_\mathbf{T}(I^f, \hat{G}^f, I^r, \hat{G}^r) = \frac{h_\mathbf{T}(I^f, \hat{G}^f, I^r, \hat{G}^r)}{\sum_{I^f, \hat{G}^f, I^r, \hat{G}^r} h_\mathbf{T}(I^f, \hat{G}^f, I^r, \hat{G}^r)},$$

$$p_\mathbf{T}(I^f, \hat{G}^f) = \sum_{I^r, \hat{G}^r} p_\mathbf{T}(I^f, \hat{G}^f, I^r, \hat{G}^r),$$

$$p_\mathbf{T}(I^r, \hat{G}^r) = \sum_{I^f, \hat{G}^f} p_\mathbf{T}(I^f, \hat{G}^f, I^r, \hat{G}^r).$$

3.2 Multi-resolution Optimization

In the proposed registration approach, the optimal transformation $\hat{\mathbf{T}}$ can be estimated by

$$\hat{\mathbf{T}} = arg \max_{\mathbf{T}} \mathrm{MI}(\mathbf{T}). \quad (5)$$

In order to accelerate the registration process and ensure the robustness of the proposed method, we exploit a multi-resolution approach based on the Gaussian Pyramid representation [11, 2, 12]. Rough estimates of $\hat{\mathbf{T}}$ can be found using downsampled images and treated as starting values for optimization at higher resolutions. Then the fine-tuning of the solution can be derived at the original image resolution. In this paper, the value of multi-dimensional mutual information at each resolution is maximized via the Powell's direction set method in multidimensions [13].

4 Implementation Details

Signed-MDGM Map: In our implementation, the signed-MDGM map is computed by separating it into the positive and negative components. Then the two components are calculated by sequentially processing voxels in intensity-decreasing and intensity-increasing orders respectively.

During either procedure, we keep updating a Voronoi diagram and a (positive or negative) MDGM map. When a voxel $\mathbf{v}$ is processed, the Voronoi diagram is locally reconstructed by adding $\mathbf{v}$ into the Voronoi sites. We then update the MDGM map within the Voronoi cell $V(\mathbf{v})$ of $\mathbf{v}$. The reason for ignoring the exterior is illustrated as follows: Let $\mathbf{v}_0$ be a voxel in another Voronoi cell $V(\mathbf{v}')$ (i.e. $|\mathbf{v} - \mathbf{v}_0| > |\mathbf{v}' - \mathbf{v}_0|$). Since $\mathbf{v}'$ has been processed prior to $\mathbf{v}$, we have $I(\mathbf{v}') \geq I(\mathbf{v})$ (for decreasing order) or $I(\mathbf{v}') \leq I(\mathbf{v})$ (for increasing order). Therefore, we have $|\nabla_d I(\mathbf{v}', \mathbf{v}_0)| > |\nabla_d I(\mathbf{v}, \mathbf{v}_0)|$ and the MDGM value of $\mathbf{v}_0$ remains unchanged.

Finally, the positive and negative components of the signed-MDGM map are combined together according to their absolute values.

Multi-dimensional Mutual Information: For calculating multi-dimensional mutual information, the number of 4D joint histogram bins should be limited, due to the relatively high dimensionality. In practice, we have found that 4D histograms with 32 bins both for intensity and signed-MDGM dimensions performs good for registering two images of size $256 \times 256 \times 26$. (Note that the number of histogram bins may be tuned for downsampled images in multi-resolution registration process.)

5 Experimental Results and Discussions

To evaluate the multi-dimensional mutual information similarity measure on the novel two-element attribute vector space (hereafter referred to as *MI-4D*) and the proposed multi-resolution registration method, we have performed three categories of experiments on different image modalities: MR-T1, MR-T2 and CT. Comparisons on capture range of the traditional mutual information similarity measure on intensity (hereafter referred to as *MI-2D*) [1,2] and MI-4D will be presented in Section 5.1. Section 5.2 will show the performance comparisons on registration robustness between the proposed method and the conventional MI-2D based method. The registration accuracy of the two methods will be demonstrated in Section 5.3.

5.1 Comparisons on Capture Range

T1 – T2 (3D – 3D) Registration: Three pairs of clinical MR-T1 and MR-T2 image volumes (datasets #1, #2 and #3) were obtained from RREP. All these images have been rectified for intensity inhomogeneity and scaling, and hereafter they are referred to as T1-rec and T2-rec respectively. The size of these image volumes is $256 \times 256 \times 26$ voxels and the voxel size is around $1.26 \times 1.26 \times 4.1$ mm^3. Note that all image pairs used in our experiments (T1-rec, T2-rec and CT) were first registered by the conventional multi-resolution MI based registration method and were then examined by an experienced consultant radiologist to ensure that the final alignments are correct and acceptable. This procedure was employed for a better presentation of the probing results and also for further facilitating the experiments that will be described in Section 5.2.

Figures 2a and 2d respectively plot the translational probes for registering the low resolution [4] (Level 2) testing image pairs from three datasets for MI-2D

---

[4] The definition of resolution levels in the Gaussian Pyramid representation follows the same line as in [11]. The smoothing filter was $\{1, 4, 6, 4, 1\}$ in our experiments.

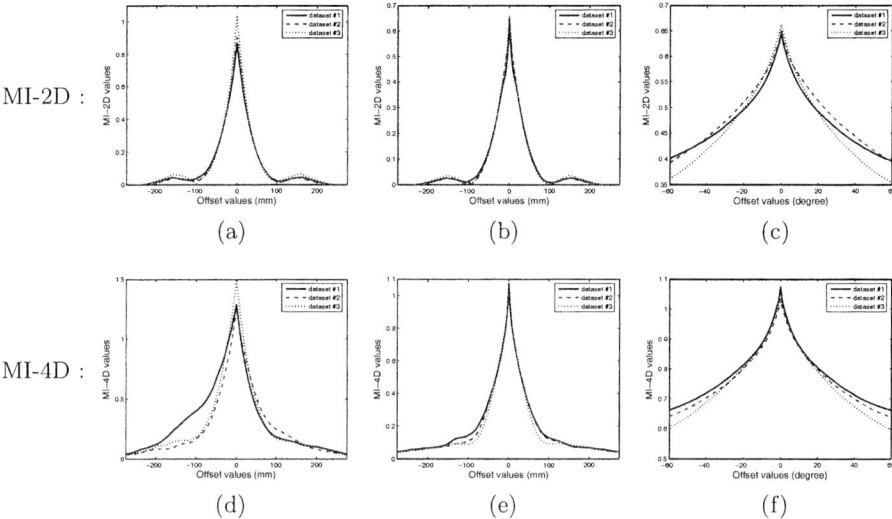

Fig. 2. Probing curves for 3D – 3D registration on three T1-rec and T2-rec datasets (#1, #2 and #3). Translational probes for registering the low resolution (Level 2) image pairs: (a) MI-2D and (d) MI-4D. Translational probes for registering the original resolution (Level 0) image pairs: (b) MI-2D and (e) MI-4D. Rotational probes for registering the original resolution (Level 0) image pairs: (c) MI-2D and (f) MI-4D

and MI-4D. At the original image resolution (Level 0), Figures 2b and 2e plot the translational probes and Figures 2c and 2f plot the rotational probes based on MI-2D and MI-4D respectively. (Note that the number of histogram bins for MI-2D was set to 32×32 at all resolutions while that for MI-4D at Level 2 was set to 32×32×8×8, where 8 was for the signed-MDGM feature.)

As observed in Figures 2a and 2b, for the translational probes of MI-2D at different image resolutions, obvious local maxima occur when the misalignment of two images is relatively large. On the contrary, Figures 2d and 2e suggest that the shape of the probing curves based on MI-4D is improved and the capture ranges of MI-4D can be relative longer than those of MI-2D. This is because, with the proposed two-element attribute vector, regions with homogenous intensities (including the anatomical structures and background regions) can provide varying information related to the distance of a voxel to a certain object boundary. Therefore, when the misalignment increases, the MI-4D values would keep decreasing. With this finding, it is expected that the optimization procedure for registration will be benefited and the registration robustness can be increased. On the other hand, for the rotational probes, the capture ranges of MI-2D and MI-4D are comparable (see Figures 2c and 2f).

CT – T1 (3D – 3D) Registration: Three pairs of clinical CT (around 512×512×30 voxels and 0.65×0.65×4 mm^3) and T1-rec image volumes (datasets #1, #2 and #3) obtained from RREP were used for the experiments. The results

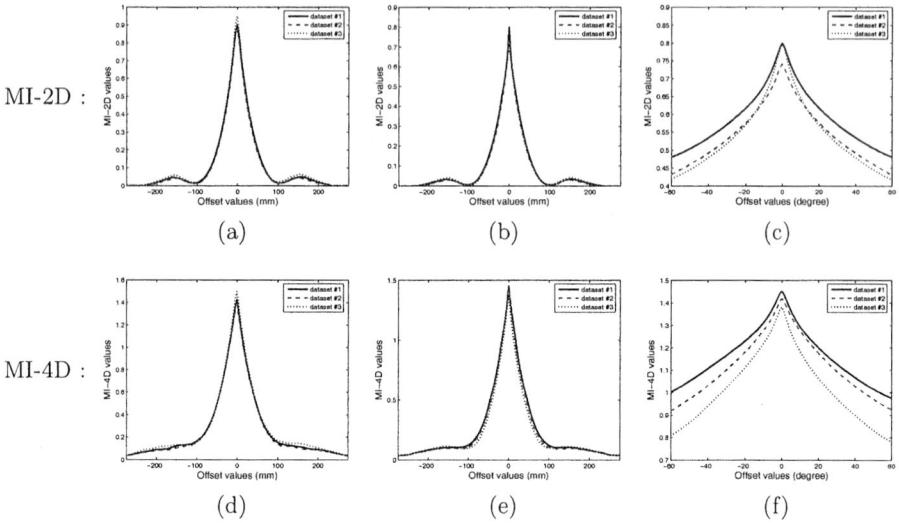

Fig. 3. Probing curves for 3D – 3D registration on three CT and T1-rec datasets (#1, #2 and #3). Translational probes for registering the low resolution (Level 2) image pairs: (a) MI-2D and (d) MI-4D. Translational probes for registering the original resolution (Level 0) image pairs: (b) MI-2D and (e) MI-4D. Rotational probes for registering the original resolution (Level 0) image pairs: (c) MI-2D and (f) MI-4D

of translational probes are shown in Figures 3a (MI-2D) and 3d (MI-4D) for the low resolution (Level 2) registration and in Figures 3b (MI-2D) and 3e (MI-4D) for the original resolution (Level 0) registration. Figures 3c and 3f respectively plot the rotational probes based on MI-2D and MI-4D for the original resolution (Level 0). Similar results of the capture ranges are obtained as compared with T1 – T2 registrations.

5.2 Performance Comparisons on Registration Robustness

In order to study and compare the registration robustness of the proposed MI-4D based method and the conventional MI-2D based method, we have designed a series of randomized experiments for these two methods. The testing image pairs were the aforementioned three T1 – T2 datasets (#1, #2 and #3) and three CT – T1 datasets (#1, #2 and #3). The experiments took 100 tests on each testing image pair for either method. At each trial, the pre-obtained ground truth registration (see Section 5.1) of the testing image pair was perturbed by 6 uniformly distributed random offsets for all translational and rotational axes. The perturbed registration was then treated as the starting alignment. The random offsets for X and Y axes were drawn between [-150, 150] mm, while those for Z axis and each rotational axis were respectively drawn between [-70, 70] mm and [-0.35, 0.35] radians (i.e. [-20, 20] degrees). (Note that for any testing dataset the same set of randomized starting alignments was used for both methods as a fair comparison.)

Table 1. The success rates with the MI-2D based method and the MI-4D based method for all testing image pairs (T1 – T2 and CT – T1)

	Testing dataset	Success rate MI-2D	Success rate MI-4D
T1	#1	68%	89%
|	#2	65%	95%
T2	#3	66%	81%
CT	#1	66%	94%
|	#2	63%	88%
T1	#3	70%	94%

To evaluate each derived registration with respect to the ground truth registration, the translational error (which was the root-sum-square of the differences for three translational axes) and the rotational error (which was the real part of a quaternion) were computed. In our experiments, the threshold vector for assessing registration success was set to ($2mm$, $2°$), because registration errors below $2mm$ and $2°$ are generally acceptable by experienced clinicians [14,15].

The success rates of the MI-2D based method and the MI-4D based method for all testing image pairs are listed in Table 1. It is suggested that the MI-4D based method (Column **MI-4D**) consistently has higher success rates as compared with the MI-2D based method (Column **MI-2D**) for all testing image pairs. (Note that, due to the space limitation, we do not show the registration results of these 1200 randomized experiments in details.)

Based on these experiments, we also observed that the majority of failed cases for the MI-4D based method had about $180°$ misalignment for one rotational axis, while registration errors for other axes were quite small. (It is meant that, after registration, the brain in the floating image was inverted along a rotational axis.) Oppositely, for the MI-2D based method, most of the failed cases had large translational and rotational misalignments simultaneously. This observation somehow implies that, along the translational axes, the capture ranges of MI-4D are longer than those of MI-2D.

5.3 Registration Accuracy

To precisely demonstrate the registration accuracy of the proposed registration method, similar randomized experiments described in Section 5.2 were performed on a pair of T1 and T2 image volumes obtained from the BrainWeb Simulated Brain Database [16] ($181 \times 217 \times 181$ voxels, $1 \times 1 \times 1$ mm^3 and the noise level was 3%). Note that this image pair is perfectly aligned. The experiments took 50 tests for the MI-4D based method, as well as for the MI-2D based method as a comparison. For perturbation, the random offsets for each translational axis were drawn between [-30, 30] mm, and those for each rotational axis were drawn

Table 2. The means and standard deviations of the registration accuracies of the MI-2D based method and the MI-4D based method for a BrainWeb T1 – T2 image pair with 3% noise level

Method	Translation (10^{-3}mm)			Rotation (10^{-3} degrees)		
	Δt_x	Δt_y	Δt_z	$\Delta \theta_x$	$\Delta \theta_y$	$\Delta \theta_z$
MI-2D	-0.40 ± 0.71	-0.62 ± 1.41	4.15 ± 1.88	0.63 ± 1.85	0.47 ± 1.78	0.04 ± 1.55
MI-4D	-1.09 ± 0.60	-1.10 ± 0.79	4.14 ± 2.05	1.02 ± 1.72	0.85 ± 1.61	0.02 ± 1.82

between [-0.17, 0.17] radians (i.e. [-10, 10] degrees). It should be noticed that all registrations obtained by either method are successful.

The means and standard deviations of the registration accuracies for each transformation parameter for these 100 experiments are lists of in Table 2, where Row **MI-2D** is for the MI-2D based method and Row **MI-4D** is for the MI-4D based method. According to the table, the accuracies of the MI-2D based method and the MI-4D based method are comparable and acceptably high. Both methods can achieve sub-voxel level registration accuracy.

6 Conclusion

To conclude, this paper has designed a new spatial feature, namely maximum distance-gradient-magnitude (MDGM), for registration tasks. The MDGM feature encodes spatial information for each voxel in an image at a global level. Then, we have improved the conventional mutual information (MI)-based registration framework by integrating the MDGM feature with intensity and setting a two-element attribute vector to each voxel in individual images. Multi-dimensional mutual information has been adopted as a similarity measure to the attribute vector space. To increase computation efficiency and robustness of the proposed method, the registration procedure has been a multi-resolution iterative process.

The experimental results on clinical 3D MR-T1, MR-T2 and CT datasets have indicated that the proposed method has relatively longer capture ranges than the conventional MI-based method at different image resolutions. Moreover, a large number of (around 1200) randomized experiments on precisely registered clinical image pairs have demonstrated that the success rates of our method are consistently higher than those of the traditional MI-based method. It has been also shown that the registration accuracy of the new method is acceptably high and obtains sub-voxel level.

Acknowledgements

The authors would like to acknowledge the support from the Hong Kong Research Grants Council (HK RGC) under grant (HKUST6155/03E).

References

1. Maes, F., Collignon, A., et al.: Multimodality Image Registration by Maximization of Mutual Information. IEEE Trans. Med. Img. **16** (1997) 187–198
2. Wells, W., Viola, P., et al.: Multi-Modal Volume Registration by Maximization of Mutual Information. Medical Image Analysis **1** (1996) 35–51
3. Penney, G., Weese, J., et al.: A Comparison of Similarity Measures for Use in 2D-3D Medical Image Registration. IEEE Trans. Med. Img. **17** (1998) 586–595
4. Pluim, J., Maintz, J., Viergever, M.: Image Registration by Maximization of Combined Mutual Information and Gradient Information. IEEE Trans. Med. Img. **19** (2000) 809–814
5. Pluim, J., Maintz, J., Viergever, M.: Mutual-Information-Based Registration of Medical Images: A Survey. IEEE Trans. Med. Img. **22** (2003) 986–1004
6. Rueckert, D., Clarkson, M., et al.: Non-rigid registration using higher-order mutual information. In: Proc. SPIE, Medical Imaging: Image Processing. Volume 3979. (2000) 438–447
7. Butz, T., Thiran, J.P.: Affine registration with feature space mutual information. In: MICCAI. (2001) 549–556
8. Borgefors, G.: Distance transformations in arbitrary dimensions. Comput. Vision, Graphics, and Image Processing **27** (1984) 321–345
9. Maes, F., Vandermeulen, D., Suetens, P.: Medical Image Registration Using Mutual Information. Proceedings of the IEEE **91** (2003) 1699–1722
10. Bishop, C.: Neural Networks for Pattern Recognition. Oxford U. Press (1995)
11. Burt, P., Adelson, E.: The Laplacian Pyramid as a Compact Image Code. IEEE Trans. Comms. **31** (1983) 532–540
12. Cole-Rhodes, A., Johnson, K., et al.: Multiresolution Registration of Remote Sensing Imagery by Optimization of Mutual Information Using a Stochastic Gradient. IEEE Trans. Image Processing **12** (2003) 1495–1511
13. Press, W., Teukolsky, S., et al.: Numerical Recipes in C, 2nd Edition. Cambridge University Press (1992)
14. Hajnal, J.V., Hill, D.L.G., Hawkes, D.J.: Medical Image Registration. CRC Press LLC (2001)
15. Zhu, Y., Cochoff, S.: Likelihood Maximization Approach to Image Registration. IEEE Trans. Image Processing **11** (2002) 1417–1426
16. Collins, D., Zijdenbos, A., et al.: Design and Construction of a Realistic Digital Brain Phantom. IEEE Trans. Med. Img. **17** (1998) 463–468

Tissue Perfusion Diagnostic Classification Using a Spatio-temporal Analysis of Contrast Ultrasound Image Sequences

Quentin Williams[1], J. Alison Noble[1], Alexander Ehlgen MD[2], and Harald Becher MD[2]

[1] Wolfson Medical Vision Lab, University of Oxford, UK
{quentin, noble}@robots.ox.ac.uk
http://www.robots.ox.ac.uk/~mvl/
[2] John Radcliffe Hospital, Oxford, UK

Abstract. The analysis of tissue perfusion in myocardial contrast echocardiography (MCE) remains a qualitative process dependent on visual inspection by a clinician. Fully automatic techniques that can quantify tissue perfusion accurately has yet to be developed. In this paper, a novel spatio-temporal technique is described for segmenting the myocardium into differently perfused regions and obtaining quantitative perfusion indices, representing myocardial blood flow and blood flow reserve. Using these indices, Myocardial segments in 22 patients were classed as either healthy or diseased and results compared to coronary angiogram analysis and an experienced clinician. The results show that the automatic method works as well as a human at detecting areas of ischaemia, but in addition localizes the spatial extent of each perfused region as well. To our knowledge this is the first reported spatio-temporal method developed and evaluated for MCE assessment.

1 Introduction

The evaluation of tissue perfusion in various parenchymatous organs is important in the diagnosis, determination of severity, and localisation of ischemic disease. In echocardiography, the assessment of myocardial perfusion by means of ultrasound contrast agents is a valuable adjunct to wall motion analysis although considered today of secondary importance in terms of automatic quantification. The literature in this area is surprisingly sparse although clinically there is great interest in perfusion assessment, as perfusion abnormalities are an earlier indicator of coronary disease than abnormal wall motion.

Both quantitative and qualitative measurements of tissue perfusion can be made by injecting a contrast agent (microbubbles) intravenously and then imaging the changes in signal intensity as the contrast agent makes its pass through an organ. This has permitted the application of myocardial contrast echocardiography (MCE) to the evaluation of myocardial blood flow and, thus, detection of obstructive coronary artery disease([1, 2, 3]). However, interpretation of MCE studies have mostly been qualitative and subjectively based upon a clinician's visual inspection of the image sequences.

Recent advances in contrast ultrasound have made it possible to develop quantitative analysis systems capable of extracting clinical meaningful information from MCE studies. These are mostly based on the *destruction-replenishment* principle introduced by Wei et al. [4]. During a constant intravenous infusion of a contrast agent the microbubbles within the myocardium are depleted using high power ultrasound (mechanical index = 1.0) and their replenishment is assessed using low power ultrasound (mechanical index = 0.1). The replenishment kinetics allow the calculation of myocardial blood flow by estimating blood volume and mean blood velocity within the regions of interest (ROI) placed in the myocardium. Linka et al. ([5]) took the processing a step further by analysing replenishment curves within the entire left ventricular myocardium and displaying the calculated parameters (blood flow, blood volume and mean blood velocity) with different hues in parametric colour maps. Each parameter is displayed in a separate image whose colours display the quantities calculated by the replenishment model. Lower colour hues will indicate lower perfusion rates, and elucidate possible diseased areas. However, these semi-automatic techniques still require user intervention and visual interpretation, while they suffer from ad hoc smoothing in space and time.

Recently, we have developed a new approach for perfusion quantification ([6]) in which a novel spatio-temporal method is used to classify the MCE sequences into different regions of perfusion. Classification is done by analysing the temporal pattern of relationships between pixels in a global manner, using a Bayesian Factor Analysis (BFA) model, and incorporating spatial information through a Markov Random Field (MRF). That paper presented only a preliminary version of the algorithm and no clinical validation.

This paper, however, goes on to further develop the quantification algorithm and shows how the BFA-MRF method can be used to obtain quantitative perfusion indices that can aid the clinician in the diagnosis and assessment of diseased tissues. Two different indices, blood flow and blood flow reserve, are extracted for each region and used to identify the region as normal, abnormal or non-diagnostic. A clinical validation of the methodology based on 22 patient studies, is also presented, and the results are compared to coronary angiogram analysis as well as diagnosis from a clinician experienced in MCE. The results show that the automatic method works as well as a human at detecting areas of ischaemia, but in addition localizes the spatial extent of each perfused region as well.

2 Methods

2.1 Image Data

All patients were referred to the John Radcliffe Hospital for standard dobutamine stress echocardiography for evaluation of inducible ischemia. Only patients, with a scheduled coronary angiogram were included in this study. 12 patients had a normal angiogram or insignificant coronary artery disease and 10 patients showed various degrees of stenosis (>50%) in one or more of the three main coronary arteries.

All datasets were obtained using the replenishment principle of Wei et al. [4] during a constant intravenous infusion of the contrast agent SonoVue® (Bracco International B-V). The contrast agent is routinely used in our hospital to enhance the endocardial border for wall motion analysis and to assess myocardial perfusion visually. Images were acquired using the real-time Power Modulation technique on the SONOS5500 ultrasound machine (Philips, Andover, MA, USA) and afterwards transferred to a computer for off-line analysis. Here, image sequences were cut according to the acquired ECG to keep just end-systolic (end of T-wave) frames and to extract the replenishment sequence. In this study, only standard apical views were used to evaluate the replenishment sequences (apical 4-chamber view, apical 2-chamber view, and apical long-axis view) to allow visualisation of the entire left ventricular myocardium and to minimise artefacts. Images were included into the study if the entire myocardium was visible, free of severe artefacts, and the cavity sufficiently opacified. Most MCE sequences were acquired at peak stress and therefore only 8 rest sequences were available. These resulted in 50 different image sequences consisting of various apical 4-chamber views (4 at rest and 21 at stress), apical 2-chamber views (1 at rest and 9 at stress) and apical long axis views (3 at rest and 11 at stress). For the automatic algorithm analysis, half the image sequences available in each view were randomly selected to form a control group of 25, with the remaining used as a test group. This was done so that the quantification measures could be trained on the control group and then 'blindly' tested on the remaining 25.

2.2 Clinical Reference

The reference (ground truth) for this study was coronary angiography with visually assessed stenosis >50% quoted as abnormal. The left ventricular myocardium for each dataset was divided using the 16-segment anatomical heart model proposed by the American Society of Echocardiography [13] (i.e. each wall was sub-divided in an apical, mid and basal segment). The same model was used to assign each segment to one of the 3 major coronary arteries (LAD, LCX, RCA) as is the clinical practice for assessing heart function. If coronary angiography revealed abnormality in the assigned artery, the segment was designated abnormal and normal otherwise. In total 246 myocardial segments were tagged in this manner. Although there is tremendous variability in the coronary artery blood supply to myocardial segments, it was felt appropriate to assign indivual segments to coronary artery territories to allow for standardisation and comparison to the other methods.

An experienced MCE reader (AE) analysed each dataset qualitatively by visual assessment of myocardial perfusion during the replenishment sequence, and scored each segment as normal, abnormal or non-diagnostic. The MCE reader was completely blinded to any patient information and the outcome of the coronary angiogram. The image quality of each dataset was also graded by the MCE reader as poor, medium or high.

2.3 Review of Automatic BFA-MRF Method

We have previously proposed a novel spatio-temporal technique to assess tissue perfusion by automatically classifying the ultrasound images into different regions of perfusion. This Bayesian Factor Analysis - Markov Random Field (BFA-MRF) method is described in detail in [6], and is summarized below. Briefly, it treats the classification as a statistical problem, which involves assigning to each pixel a class label taking a value from the set $L = \{1, 2, \ldots, l\}$, where each pixel is indexed by a two-dimensional rectangular lattice $S = \{1, 2, \ldots, n\}$ and characterised by a p-variate vector of intensity values $\mathbf{y}_i = \{y_{i1}, \ldots, y_{ip}\}, i \in S$. In this case each observation vector $\mathbf{y}_i$ represents an intensity-time curve for a single pixel location. The problem of classification is then to estimate the true but unknown labeling configuration, $\mathbf{x}^*$, given the observed intensity time vectors, $\mathbf{Y}' = \{\mathbf{y}_1, \ldots, \mathbf{y}_n\}$. In particular, the maximum a posteriori (MAP) estimate of $\mathbf{x}$ is used:

$$\hat{\mathbf{x}} = \arg\max_{\mathbf{x} \in X} \{P(\mathbf{Y}|\mathbf{x})P(\mathbf{x})\}. \tag{1}$$

The right-hand side of the above equation contains two parts: $P(\mathbf{Y}|\mathbf{x})$ and $P(\mathbf{x})$, which are defined as a Bayesian Factor Analysis likelihood distribution and a Markov Random Field prior distribution, respectively. What remains is the estimation of the parameters of these two distribution functions, where the BFA model is constructed as a generative latent variable model,

$$(\mathbf{y}_i | (\mu, \Lambda, \mathbf{f}_i)) = \mu + \Lambda \mathbf{f}_i + \epsilon_i, \tag{2}$$

for each observation vector $\mathbf{y}_i (i = 1, \ldots, n)$, where μ is the overall population mean, Λ is a matrix of constants called the factor loading matrix; $\mathbf{f}_i = (f_{i1}, \ldots, f_{il})$, is the factor score vector for pixel i; and the ϵ_i's are noise variables assumed to be mutually uncorrelated and Normally distributed N(0,Ψ). The factor loading matrix, Λ, expresses how each latent factor loads onto the observed variables, therefore giving an indication of how the hidden factors might look. In the case of a perfusion study, each column in the factor loading matrix will represent an intensity-time curve associated with each different type of perfusion present in the dataset. The factor scores give the estimated value ("weight") of the observations on the hidden factors. Therefore, if each hidden factor represents a class, the factor score vector gives an indication of how much an observation belongs to each class. Since the parameters μ, Λ, the $\mathbf{f}'_i s$, and Ψ are all unobservable, a Normal likelihood distribution for each $\mathbf{y}_i$ is assumed, and written as:

$$p(\mathbf{y}_i | \mu, \Lambda, \mathbf{f}_i, \Psi) = (2\pi)^{-\frac{p}{2}} |\Psi|^{-\frac{1}{2}} e^{-\frac{1}{2}(\mathbf{y}_i - \mu - \Lambda \mathbf{f}_i)' \Psi^{-1} (\mathbf{y}_i - \mu - \Lambda \mathbf{f}_i)}. \tag{3}$$

The probability of an MRF realisation, $\mathbf{x}$, is given by the Gibbs distribution:

$$P(\mathbf{x}) = Z^{-1} e^{(-\omega U(\mathbf{x}))}, \tag{4}$$

where

$$U(\mathbf{x}) = \sum_{c \in C} V_c(\mathbf{x}) \tag{5}$$

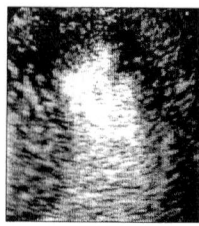 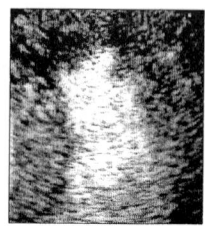 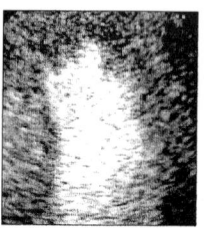 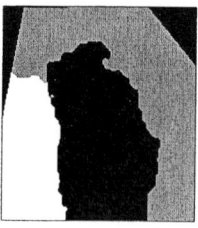

Fig. 1. Frames 1, 3 and 12 of a 4-chamber image sequence and the classification result. White = normal, Gray = abnormal, black = cavity.

is the energy function which is a sum of *clique potentials* $V_c(\mathbf{x})$ over all possible cliques C. Z is a normalisation term and ω is a positive constant which controls the size of clustering. The potential function used is, $V_c(x_i) = -\delta_{x_i = x'_i}$ where $\delta_{x_i = x'_i} = 1$, if $x_i = x'_i$, and 0 otherwise.

The novelty of this particular algorithm stems from the way it interlinks the factor scores in the BFA model to the prior probability of the MRF model. The factor score vector indicates how much an observation belongs to a particular class. It is therefore assumed that the prior probability of the factor scores matrix, $\mathbf{F}' = (\mathbf{f}_1, \ldots, \mathbf{f}_n)$, follows the same prior probability of the classification configuration, $\mathbf{x}$, and in fact that the factor score for each hidden factor (or class) is equivalent to the posterior probability of the class label. For every $l \in L$ and $i \in S$

$$f_{il} = P(\mathbf{y}_i|l) P(x_i = l). \qquad (6)$$

Using the prior probability (4) and the likelihood function (3) with respect to x_i and f_{il} gives

$$f_{il} = Z^{-1} e^{(-\omega U(x_i))} \times (2\pi)^{-\frac{p}{2}} |\Psi|^{-\frac{1}{2}} e^{-\frac{1}{2}(\mathbf{y}_i - \mu - \Lambda_l \mathbf{f}_{il})' \Psi^{-1} (\mathbf{y}_i - \mu - \Lambda_l \mathbf{f}_{il})}. \qquad (7)$$

Therefore the posterior probability values obtained through the MRF-MAP classification can directly be used as the factor scores. Thus, the strategy underlying this algorithm can be summarized as follows: (1) With the Gibbs function estimate the labelling configuration, $\hat{\mathbf{x}}$, using the current estimate of the parameters; (2) use it to specify the factor scores matrix, $\mathbf{F}$; (3) and then estimate the new values of the parameters μ, Λ, and Ψ, using an iterative conditional modes (ICM) approach as described in [6]. These steps are iteratively repeated until suitable convergence is reached. The BFA-MRF algorithm was initiated using a simple K-Means Clustering method that provides the initial estimate for the labelling configuration, $\hat{\mathbf{x}}$. The algorithm was implemented in a multiscale framework to improve convergence, first executed at a 1/4 of the resolution, then at 1/2, and finally at full resolution.

The above method was applied to each dataset to divide the left ventricle into regions with different perfusion characteristics. The number of regions (factors) to search for was set to three, corresponding to cavity, normal and abnormal classes (see Fig. 1). However, it can be expected to find datasets where only 2

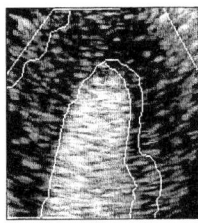 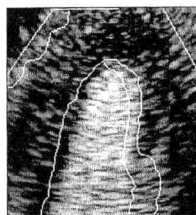 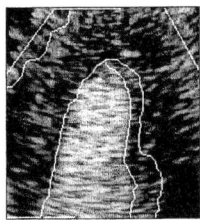 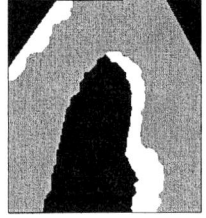

Fig. 2. Frames 3, 7 and 8 of a 4-chamber image sequence affected by motion. White shows the 3rd region found due this artefact. The classification boundaries are overlayed in each frame

classes should be present. This happens when the whole of the myocardium is either completely healthy; or a similar abnormality is found throughout the myocardium (i.e. comparable stenosis in all of the coronary arteries). Nonetheless, it was found that for these datasets, looking for a third class did not alter the results. The reason for this is that when a 3rd class is sought the algorithm does not divide the myocardium any further (because there is no further distinction to be made), but instead will find a third separate region where motion might have caused misalignment (Fig. 2); or the papillary muscles appeared in the cavity. Setting the number of factors to three does mean that for cases where there are indeed three classes present, extra smaller classes like the two mentioned above, will be absorbed by more significant classes that have characteristics close to itself. To determine the exact number of physiological important regions (i.e. perfusion types) present in the data has always been a difficult problem for any Factor Analysis approach (see [7, 8]). A better strategy would be to find this number automatically using prior physiological knowledge. This will be the subject of future work. For this study the number was kept at 3 for all datasets, and it can be seen from the results that this choice works well.

2.4 Quantification

Having divided the myocardium into differently perfused regions, the next step is to find clinically meaningful quantitative parameters that can be used to identify each region as either normal, abnormal or non-diagnostic. Non-diagnostic, in this case, is defined as regions that were caused by ultrasound artefacts (motion, blooming, shadowing, etc.) and therefore have nothing to do with the disease state of the tissue.

The Measures. The mean intensity time curves for each region are calculated. These intensity curves, representing the microbubble replenishment, can then be used to obtain 'perfusion indices' that represent myocardial blood flow and relative blood flow reserve within each region. Before comparisons can be done between datasets based upon the intensity curves, these curves need to be normalised to compensate for variability of intensity amongst the datasets. This variability is usually due to heterogeneity of acoustic power, attenuation and differences in ultrasound acquisition between the datasets. To do this, the cavity curve is first identified as the curve with the highest mean intensity. The rest of the curves are then normalised by additively raising/lowering all intensity levels so that the mean intensity of the cavity curve is always at the same level. In the results shown here, this level was set to 200 which was found to be approximately the mean of the cavity class for all datasets.

The normalised intensity curves are then fit to the exponential model as suggested by Wei et al. [4]:

$$\mathbf{y}_m(t) = A(1 - e^{-\beta t}) + C \qquad (8)$$

In the above equation, A is the plateau of the exponential curve, β the initial slope and C a constant representing the start value of the curve. The constant C was added to the establised Wei et al. model because due to incomplete microbubble destruction, the mean intensity level of myocardial regions in real perfusion data seldom starts with a zero intensity. Curve fitting was only done for myocardial intensity curves, and not for the LV cavity. Wei et al. showed that for the exponential model, the saturation value $(A + C)$ is equivalent to myocardial blood volume, the gradient β to myocardial blood velocity, and that the multiple of the two $(A+C)\beta$ represents myocardial blood flow; which is the first perfusion index used in this paper.

A second parameter available from the intensity curves is the area under the curve. For each myocardial intensity curve ($\mathbf{y}_m$), the ratio of the integral of the curve to the integral of the cavity curve ($\mathbf{y}_c$) was calculated,

$$index_2 = \frac{\int \mathbf{y}_m dt}{\int \mathbf{y}_c dt}. \qquad (9)$$

where the integral is taken over the same time interval. Since the concentration of the microbubbles within the LV cavity stays at roughly the same level, the intensity 'curve' for the cavity will essentially be a straight line and is an indicator of the total blood reserve in circulation. Therefore, the ratio as calculated above represents relative myocardial blood flow reserve and is comparable to the perfusion index proposed by Christian et al. [9] and Klocke et al. [10], for Magnetic Resonance Imaging (MRI) contrast perfusion studies.

Analysis. First, a distinction needs to be made between non-diagnostic regions and other regions. This was done using the goodness-of-fit measure obtained during curve fitting. Based on the assumption that any region severely affected by artefacts will not fit the exponential model, all regions with a low goodness-of-fit value ($\epsilon < x$) were classified as non-diagnostic, and excluded from subsequent analysis.

For the remaining regions, the two measures were used for further classification. Although these perfusion indices do not provide absolute values of coronary blood flow and flow reserve[1], they are still clinically meaningful and can be used

---

[1] To calculate absolute values, both the ultrasound beam width as well as the exact microbubble concentration is needed, see [4].

to identify healthy and diseased tissue. Each index was used separately to classify a region as either normal or abnormal, and the results compared to the clinician's analysis. The combination of the two indices, simple calculated by multiplying the two values, was also evaluated as an index.

To be able to do this classification the indices were learned empirically to find the values at which a distinction can be made between normal and abnormal regions. For all the perfusion indices low values indicate diseased tissue, while high values correspond to healthy tissue. Therefore a certain cut-off value needed to be found for each index, where regions that have a value below the cut-off are classed as abnormal and regions with a value above as normal. Using the datasets in the control group a search was conducted where the cut-off value was changed, in suitable steps, from the minimum value to the maximum value found in the group. At each step, sensitivity and specificity values were calculated, and the value that gave the best combination of the two, was kept. This cut-off value is then also used to classify the myocardial segments in the test group, so that the quantitative method can be properly evaluated.

In practice, an abnormal region does not only fall in one heart segment, but may cross multiple segments or may be constrained to part of a segment only. This type of distinction is not picked up by a clinician, but it is made by the BFA-MRF algorithm which localizes the spatial extent of the regions. Therefore, to make comparisons between the two approaches, the same 16-segment model was used for the BFA-MRF method. After each perfused region (class) is found, the myocardium for each dataset is divided into six equal segments starting from the left basal part of the myocardium and going around until the right basal part (as described in 2.2). The class of each segment is then equal to the class which had the most pixels present in that segment. Comparison was then done by calculating sensitivity and specificity values for the expert, as well as for each one of the indices. Using the angiogram analysis as the ground truth, sensitivity is defined as the percentage of abnormal myocardial segments correctly identified, while specificity is the percentage of normal segments correctly identified. Non-diagnostic segments were not included in the calculation of these values.

A short summary of the complete algorithm is given below:

1. Use the BFA-MRF algorithm to divide the LV into 3 regions with different perfusion characteristics
2. Obtain the mean intensity-time curve for each region
3. Identify the cavity curve as the one with the highest mean intensity and normalise all the curves by additively raising/lowering the intensity levels so that the mean intensity of the cavity curve is equal to 200.
4. Fit the normalised intensity curves to the exponential function $\mathbf{y}_i = A(1 - e^{-\beta t}) + C$
5. Calculate the blood flow index $= (A+C)\beta$.
6. Calculate the blood flow reserve index $= \dfrac{\int \mathbf{y}_m dt}{\int \mathbf{y}_c dt}$
7. Use these values separately to classify myocardial segments as either normal or abnormal.

3 Results

Using the angiogram analysis, the myocardial segments were divided into a normal and abnormal batch. For each of these batches the first order statistics of the blood flow index (BFI), blood flow reserve index (BFRI), and the multiple of the two, are shown in Table 1; first for all the datasets together, then for the control group and lastly for the test group.

All of the 246 myocardial segments were analysed by the clinician and the automatic algorithm. The clinician was only able to make a diagnostic decision for 193 (78.39%) of these segments, while the BFA-MRF algorithm performed much better and quantitative analysis (those not classified as non-diagnostic by the algorithm) was possible in 215 (87.40%) segments. The non-diagnostic segments found by the automatic method had a mean and standard deviation (σ) for

Table 1. First order statistics for Perfusion indices. (BFI = blood flow index, BFRI = blood flow reserve index)

	BFI	BFRI	BFI×BFRI
All datasets			
Normal	48.83±22.25	0.5066±0.1225	25.55±15.68
Abnormal	23.36± 3.98	0.3686±0.0633	8.72± 2.16
Control Group			
Normal	47.03±20.83	0.5109±0.1006	24.20±13.19
Abnormal	23.61± 4.69	0.3697±0.0620	8.96± 2.46
Test Group			
Normal	51.12±23.74	0.5021±0.1418	27.27±18.21
Abnormal	22.99± 2.64	0.3672±0.0649	8.40± 1.60

Table 2. Evaluation percentages for Test Group

	Clinician	BFI	BFRI	BFI×BFRI
Cut-off Value	—	24.75	0.3884	9.61
Sensitivity (%)	48.84	54.76	57.14	52.38
Specificity (%)	79.66	87.67	79.45	87.67
Correctly classed (%)	68.48	75.65	71.30	74.78

Table 3. Evaluation percentages for All Datasets

	Clinician	BFI	BFRI	BFI×BFRI
Sensitivity (%)	49.37	55.91	56.99	54.84
Specificity (%)	79.82	90.78	78.72	92.20
Correctly classed (%)	67.02	76.92	70.09	77.35

the goodness of fit values equal to 0.1555±0.1536. For all of the other segments goodness of fit values had a mean and standard deviation of 0.8935±0.1161. Therefore a distinction can be clearly made and all curves with goodness of fit values smaller than 0.46 (mean + 2σ) were classed as non-diagnostic.

Table 2 (for the test group) and Table 3 (for all the datasets), shows the sensitivity and specificity values, as well as the percentage of segments correctly identified (compared to angiogram analysis), for the clinician and the three perfusion indices. The cut-off value obtained using the optimisation above is also shown.

4 Discussion

In all cases, diagnosis done using the automatic method performed better than the experienced MCE reader. The method was capable of satisfactory sensitivity and specificity values despite a range of image quality (of the 22 patients the MCE reader graded 5 as having poor image quality, 8 as medium, and 9 as high). The study showed that even with simple perfusion indices the method can, with an acceptable degree of accuracy, distinguish between healthy and diseased myocardial segments. It is also capable of excluding regions affected by imaging artefacts such as motion and shadowing, ensuring that these regions do not alter the results. Apart from just scoring a specific segment of the myocardium, the algorithm can also show the full spatial extent of a region (as in Fig. 3(d)) and is not confined to the normal 16-segment heart model. This means that a more accurate localisation of a defect is possible.

However, there are some remaining technical limitations that need to be addressed. Real perfusion curves are very noisy (see Fig. 3(e)) and any quantitative parameter based on the intensity curves will therefore be sensitive to the amount of noise present. Intensity variation within the cavity (due to attenuation, poor acquisition, etc.) will also affect the normalisation step and therefore the intensity curves. Using the mean intensities as well as curve-fitting alleviates some of the noise and intensity variation found, but it is difficult to completely compensate for both. We are working towards an attenuation correction ultrasound contrast imaging protocol in separate work [12]. The algorithm also assumes correspondence between pixel locations from frame to frame in an image sequence. This might not be true in cases affected by motion, and a pre-processing registration step might align the images more effectively than just using ECG-triggering and improve classification results. However preliminary assessment has shown that on the data, alignment did not improve results [11]. Grossly mis-aligned data also invalidates the assumption of pixel correspondence across time as it is likely that tissue has gone out of plane.

This study has identified a number of interesting questions regarding tissue perfusion quantification. In this paper, only the stress image sequences were used, and a simple decision was made between healthy and diseased tissue. A more precise evaluation of the disease state of the myocardium might be possible if the results of the algorithm was compared between the rest and stress datasets

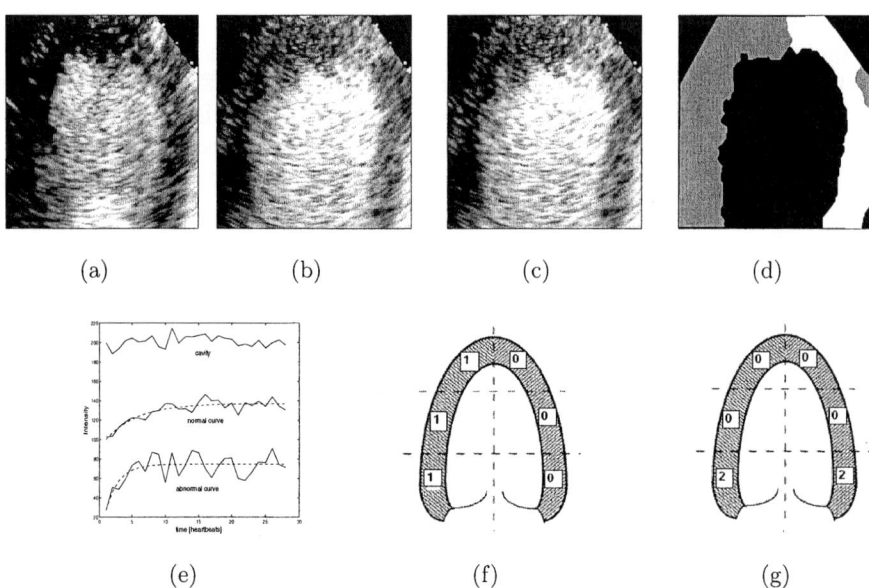

Fig. 3. Frames (a) 1, (b) 10 and (c) 20 along with (d) the classification result (White = normal, Gray = abnormal, black = cavity) for a stress 2-chamber view of an abnormal patient with occlusion in all three main coronary arteries. The associated normalised intensity curves is shown in (e), while (f) shows the diagnosis from the computer algorithm (note the error made in anterior wall) and (g) the clinician's diagnosis (error in whole myocardium) (0 = Normal, 1 = Abnormal). This dataset was graded as 'poor', but is shown here as an example of the strength as well as weakness of the computer algorithm

of a patient. In this way, reversible as well as fixed defects can be studied and the perfusion indices more accurately determined. It would also be interesting to study the correlation of the perfusion indices with true values of tissue perfusion, as well as varying grades of severity of stenosis. This type of analysis might permit a more complicated separation of the degrees of perfusion/stenosis and allow distinction between milder/severe abnormalities.

5 Conclusion

Although several problems regarding quantitative analysis of tissue perfusion using MCE still remain uncertain, this study has documented that the BFA-MRF method can provide a reliable and accurate evaluation of myocardial disease in an ordinary clinical setting. The results have shown that the automatic method performs as well as an experienced clinician, and provides additional information regarding the spatial extent of a tissue defect. This technique can therefore provide a valuable supplementary diagnostic tool, alongside wall motion analysis, for the detection and assessment of coronary artery disease.

References

1. Becher, H., Burns, P.: *Handbook of Contrast Echocardiography*. Berlin: Springer Verlag (2000)
2. Frinking, P.J.A., Bouakaz, A., Kirkhorn, J., et al.: Ultrasound Contrast Imaging: Current and new potential methods. Ultrasound Med. Biol. **26** (2000) 965–975
3. Kaul, S.: Myocardial contrast echocardiography. Curr. Probl. Cardiol. **22** (1997) 549–640
4. Wei, K., Jayaweera A.R., Firoozan S., et al.: Quantification of myocardial blood flow with ultrasound-induced destruction of microbubbles administered as a constant venous infusion. Circulation **98** (1998) 473–483
5. Linka, A., Sklenar, J., Wei, K., Jayaweera A.R., Kaul, S.: Assessment of transmural distribution of myocardial perfusion with contrast echocardiography. Circulation **98** (1998) 1912–1920
6. Williams, Q., Noble, J.A.: A Spatio-Temporal Analysis of Contrast Ultrasound image sequence for assessment of Tissue Perfusion. Proceedings MICCAI **II** (2004) 899–906
7. Martel, A.L., Moody, A.R., Allder, S.J., et al.: Extracting parametric images from dynamic contrast-enhanced MRI studies of the brain using factor. Medical Image Analysis **5** (2001) 29–39
8. Martel, A.L., Moody, A.R.: The use of PCA to smooth functional MR images. Proceedings MIUA, Oxford, July (1997) 13–16
9. Christian, T.F., et al.: Absolute Myocardial Perfusion in canines measured by using dual bolus first-pass MR Imaging. Radiology (2004) 232–677
10. Klocke, F.J., Simonetti, O.P., Judd, R.M., et al.: Limits of detection of regional differences in vasodilated flow in viable myocardium by first-pass MR perfusion imaging. Circulation (2001) 2412
11. Noble, J.A., Dawson, D., Lindner, J., Sklenar, J., Kaul, S.: Automated, non-rigid alignment of clinical myocardial contrast echocardiographic image sequences: comparison with manual alignment. Ultrasound in Medicine and Biology **28(1)** (2002) 115–123
12. Tang, M-X., Eckersley, R.J., Noble, J.A.: Pressure-dependent attenuation with microbubbles at low mechanical index. accepted to Ultrasound in Medicine and Biology (2004)
13. Schiller, N., Shah, P., Crawford, M., et al.: Recommendations for quantitation of the left ventricle by two-dimensional echocardiography. Journal of the American Society of Echocardiography **5** (1989) 358–367

Topology Preserving Tissue Classification with Fast Marching and Topology Templates

Pierre-Louis Bazin and Dzung L. Pham

Laboratory of Medical Image Computing, Neuroradiology Division,
Department of Radiology and Radiological Science,
Johns Hopkins University, Baltimore, MD 21287, USA

Abstract. This paper presents a novel approach for object segmentation in medical images that respects the topological relationships of multiple structures as given by a template. The algorithm combines advantages of tissue classification, digital topology, and level-set evolution into a topology-invariant multiple-object fast marching method. The technique can handle any given topology and enforces object-level relationships with little constraint over the geometry. Applied to brain segmentation, it sucessfully extracts gray matter and white matter structures with the correct spherical topology without topology correction or editing of the sub-cortical structures.

1 Introduction

The topological properties of 2D and 3D objects are often very simple, regardless of the complexity of the geometric object. The cortex of the human brain is a striking example; despite its intricate folds, it is considered to have the topology of a sphere, without any hole or handle-like junction. Most organs and sub-structures found in the human body also share this spherical topology.

Ideally, segmentation algorithms that extract objects from 2D or 3D images should respect the object topology. A major problem is that topology is a *global* property of the object, whereas most extraction techniques operate locally on the voxels or pixel of an image. Two approaches to addressing this issue are to correct the extracted object to obtain the desired topology, or to start from a template object, with the correct topology, and deform it with topology-preserving deformations.

Topology correction techniques alter a segmented object to enforce a spherical topology by removing all holes, sub-parts and handles [16, 7, 18]. However, changes in the resulting object are generally unrelated to the underlying image data and non-spherical topologies cannot be obtained systematically. Topology preserving deformations are more flexible in that they can start from a template with any arbitrary topology. In most surface-based methods, the object of interest is initialized as a sphere, or its topology is corrected using the previous set of methods. Then, a surface evolution algorithm, either explicit [10] or implicit [8, 3] deforms the original surface using forces inherited from a tissue classification technique. This approach still seems limited to spherical topology. Another limitation is that the topology constraints are enforced on one object at a time. When applied simultaneously to multiple objects, the level set method must use a combinatorial composition of level set functions [23] that makes the handling of topology more difficult if not impossible.

In this paper, we address these limitations with a new technique that simultaneously segments multiple objects in an image, while constraining the segmentation to be consistent with the topology of a given template. Our algorithm interweaves tissue classification and topology-invariant object segmentation in an iterative, multi-object fast marching method. The method can enforce spherical or non-spherical topology constraints on a set of objects. Moreover, segmenting these objects simultaneously permits us to encode global object relationships in the topology template: neighboring objects of the template must remain neighbors in the segmented image, separate objects have to stay separated.

The proposed method is somewhat related to some non-linear registration techniques [4, 14] that register a template image to the subject image and preserve the topology using diffeomorphic transformations. However, the approaches are actually very different: our algorithm assumes an object-level class structure and estimates its statistics from the data instead of deforming the image to establish point correspondences. Similarity metrics and deformation models are not required. The result we obtain is truly a tissue segmentation, and two adjacent structures with the same intensity will not be separated.

The paper is organized as follows. In Section 2, we introduce the necessary concepts from tissue classification, level sets and fast marching methods, and digital topology. Section 3 describes how these components are combined into our new segmentation algorithm. Section 4 presents experimental results on the problem of brain segmentation, along with a discussion of the main features of the algorithm.

2 Background

2.1 Definition of the Problem

We are interested in retrieving a collection of objects with a given topology from a digital image I in $\mathbb{Z}^3$. The objects are represented as digital volumes $V_k \in I$, and completely cover the image: $\bigcup V_k = I$ (i.e. there is no background, or the background is itself an object).

Each object V_k, ideally, is characterized by a constant intensity c_k in the image. A topology template, defined as a segmentation of the image in objects that has the correct topology, but not necessarily the correct geometry, is assumed to be given. For instance, if we have one object with spherical topology and its background, this template could be the image of a sphere. For each object, we can compute a membership function $u_{j,k}$ that will attribute a normalized score between zero and one (eg. a probability value) that measures whether pixel j belongs to the object k.

2.2 Pixel Classification and Membership Functions

Tissue classification methods can be used to segment an image by assigning each pixel to an object, defined by some statistical properties. A common assumption is that the object can be modeled as a Markov Random Field with a Gaussian distribution for the intensity. These methods are fast, accurate, and can incorporate prior information, spatial regularization, adaptation to signal inhomogeneities, and other properties [9, 19, 13, 25]. A major drawback for enforcing topological constraints is that the classification of each voxel is made simultaneously and almost independently. There is no concept of a global object one can easily manipulate with these methods.

Most classification techniques estimate a membership function that reflects the probability for each pixel to belong to a given class. We use the Fuzzy C-means (FCM) classification paradigm, although most other classification techniques would also be suitable. The basic FCM algorithm iterates the two steps:

1. compute the membership functions $u_{j,k} = \frac{(\|I_j - c_k\|^2)^{1/1-q}}{\sum_k (\|I_j - c_k\|^2)^{1/1-q}}$ given the centroids c_k,
2. compute the centroids $c_k = \frac{\sum_j u_{j,k}^q I_j}{\sum_j u_{j,k}^q}$ given the membership functions $u_{j,k}$,

until it converges. It minimizes the energy $E = \sum_{j,k} u_{j,k}^q \|I_j - c_k\|^2$. The centroids c_k correspond to the mean intensity for the object k.

2.3 Fast Marching Methods

Fast marching methods, along with their related level set evolution approaches, offer an alternative to independent pixel-based computations. These methods evolve a 3D implicit surface embedded into a 3D volume, using efficient computation techniques [12, 17]. Surface evolution techniques, commonly used in image segmentation [22, 15, 8], iteratively evolve a surface according to image and smoothness forces, until an equilibrium is reached. Fast marching methods propagate an initial surface over all the image in one iteration, but only in one direction (the surface cannot move over points previously visited).

Fast marching methods are implemented through a binary tree sorting technique [17]: all points in front of the initial surface are ranked into a binary tree depending on image and smoothness properties, then the surface is brought in front of the first of those points. Its neighbors (now in front of the surface) are added to the binary tree, and the surface is moved again until the tree is empty. This algorithm performs in $N \log N$, with N the number of visited points. It is commonly used in many tasks involving the propagation of a boundary condition (e.g. distance function computations).

2.4 Digital Topology

The topology of 3D objects can only be characterized globally, by the Euler Number of the surface at their boundary. However, topology changes in evolving scalar fields only occur at critical points [5, 24, 1], which can be detected without computing a global measure. In binary images, these points are locally the singular points of the surface bounding the digital volume (regular and critical points are also referred to as simple and non-simple points in the binary case).

To identify a critical point j in a binary image, we compute the number of regions inside and outside of the object, respectively $N_{in}(j)$ and $N_{out}(j)$. The regions are defined as the sets of 6,18 or 26-connected neighbors to the point of interest. It is enough

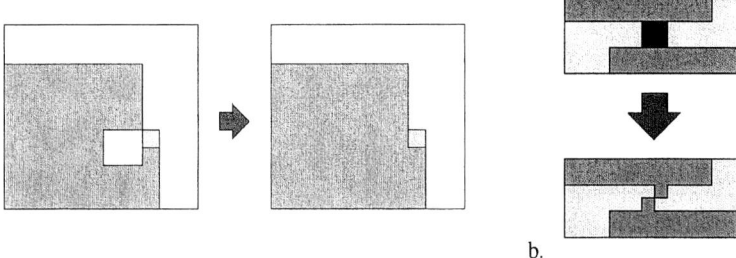

Fig. 1. Critical points and connectivity: a) an example of critical or regular point depending on the connectivity, b) an example of unclassified point with (6,6) connectivity. In (a), the light gray pixel is critical for the gray object with our (6,6) connectivity (left). It would be regular for (6,26) or (6,18) connectivity. With a (18,18) or (26,26) connectivity, the object would have a handle but the background object would stay connected into one piece, so they would intersect. When other points are attributed to the object, the critical point can become regular (right). In (b), the unclassified point (in black) cannot be attributed to either the light or the dark gray object without changing the topology (top). However, a subdivision of the pixel into four half resolution pixels brings a viable solution, without changing the topology (bottom)

to know if a point is regular or critical (although there are different categories of critical points):

$$j \text{ is regular} \equiv N_{in}(j) = N_{out}(j) = 1$$

An important issue when dealing with digital topology is to specify the connectivity of the object and the background. With multiple objects, this becomes a difficult issue because the background for one object must contain the other objects as well. This constraint prohibits two adjacent objects to have 18- or 26-connectivity, because they could go through each other without making a hole (see Figure 1-a). The only viable option is for all objects to have 6-connectivity. This connectivity prevents objects from crossing each other, but can create artificial background points at their interface. These points will remain unclassified in the segmentation, and require a sub-pixel resolution to be properly attributed to the objects (see Fig. 1-b). In practice, very few of these points appear in the computations, so we currently leave them unclassified.

3 Segmentation Algorithm

3.1 Algorithm Outline

To compute the topology preserving tissue classification, the topology template is first aligned to the image to be segmented. This is used as an initialization for one iteration of a modified FCM algorithm. We next remove from each object the pixels with low membership values through a process we call "thinning", leaving only a skeleton of the original object with the same topology and high membership values. We then reverse the process, which we call "joint marching"; starting from the skeleton, new points are added to all objects until there is no outside point left. Pixels with high membership values are recovered first in the joint marching process. This procedure will modify the template to better match the image I, but it will not completely displace the template, as the skeleton remains fixed. We have to iterate these two steps until the objects stabilize. The membership function is re-computed at each iteration, to take into account the extra constraints given by the topology.

3.2 Initialization: Image Alignment

In the two steps of the algorithm, the objects are reduced to their skeleton, then expanded again. To properly segment the objects, we implicitly assume that the template segmentation is close enough to the image segmentation to roughly share the same skeleton.

We enforce this assumption at the beginning of the algorithm by registering the image to segment to the topology template, using a rigid transformation. In the case of brain segmentation, we created our templates in Talairach space, so the images can be registered by AC-PC or Talairach alignment [20, 2], as well as automated rigid alignment. Note that we need to register the image to the template, as resampling the template may affect its topology.

3.3 Membership Functions

We require membership functions for defining the objects within the image, similar to how distance functions are used in level set approaches. The membership function must be bounded and yield comparable membership values for the different objects. The FCM membership function fulfills these requirements. However, the FCM algorithm is sensitive to noise, so we add a regularization term [13] to improve the smoothness of the membership:

$$u_{j,k} = \frac{(\|I_j - c_k\|^2 + \beta \sum_{l \in N_j, m \neq k} u_{l,m}^q)^{1/1-q}}{\sum_k (\|I_j - c_k\|^2 + \beta \sum_{l \in N_j, m \neq k} u_{l,m}^q)^{1/1-q}}.$$

In our algorithm, c_k is computed using only the pixels inside the object V_k, and the topology constraints influence the results. However, we still obtain a result that minimizes the same energy E, given the constraints, as the two marching algorithms follow the lowest energy path on the memberships surface.

3.4 Topology-Preserving Thinning

Topology-preserving fast marching methods are a key component of our algorithm. In the thinning step, the algorithm is the following:

Algorithm 1. Object thinning

1. start from the object V_k in the template,
2. sort all the points j on the inside boundary of V_k into a binary tree, ranked by their membership $u_{j,k}$,
3. extract the point j with lowest membership from the tree,
4. if the point is regular for the object V_k, remove it from the object

5. if the point is *critical* for the object V_k, keep it in the object
6. if j is removed, insert its neighbors that were inside the volume or previously critical into the tree,
7. go back to step 3, until the tree is empty.

The fast marching technique propagates from the boundary to a skeleton, the minimal set of critical points inside V_k, with the ordering given by $u_{j,k}$. Regular points are points that can be removed without changing the topology, while critical points need to be kept to preserve the object's topology. Certain points may or may not remain critical while the object is thinning (see Figure 1), so it is necessary to check them whenever the object changes in their neighborhood. The idea is similar to the level set evolution method of the TGDM algorithm [8], but the fast marching method is non-iterative and handles critical points in a principled way. More importantly, the fast marching technique extends naturally to joint, multiple object segmentation, a key advantage of our method.

3.5 Topology-Preserving Joint Marching of Multiple Objects

After the objects are thinned into skeletons, we perform the opposite operation and grow them again to cover the entire image. The algorithm is again a fast marching method, similar to the previous one:

Algorithm 2: Object growing
1. start from the skeletons of objects $\{V_k\}$,
2. sort all the points j on the outside boundary of all objects into a binary tree, ranked by their membership $u_{j,k}$,
3. extract the point j with highest membership from the tree, and retrieve the associated object V_k,
4. if the point is *regular* for the object V_k, add it to the object V_k,
5. if the point is *critical* for the object V_k, keep it outside,
6. if j is added, insert its neighbors that were outside the object or previously critical into the tree,
7. go back to step 3, until the tree is empty.

Once again, an important property of this approach is that the objects are grown together simultaneously. The segmentation criterion then, is that a point j belongs to object V_k if and only if V_k is the first of all objects to reach j. The objects are all competing, and will try to cover as much as possible of the image, following the ordering of $u_{j,k}$ to grow faster in certain directions. The algorithm ends when the only remaining points are background points generated by the connectivity constraint.

Even if our technique is based on a volumetric representation, the objects grow along their boundaries. We can compute curvature estimates on these boundaries using a simplified level set representation: points inside the object have the level set $+1$, points on the boundary have the level set 0 and points outside the object have the level set -1. Level set techniques have been very successful at regularizing the geometry of surfaces using their curvature κ. We add curvature regularization in our method by replacing the membership $u_{j,k}$ by $u'_{j,k} = u_{j,k} - \gamma \kappa_j$. Note that this modified membership must be computed as the object evolves.

3.6 Segmentation Algorithm

The complete algorithm is as follows:

Algorithm 3: Topology-preserving Fast Marching Segmentation
1. align the image to the topology template and set the initial segmentation $\{V_k\}$ to be the template,
2. compute the classification parameters $c_k = \frac{\sum_{j \in V_k} u_{j,k}^q I_j}{\sum_{j \in V_k} u_{j,k}^q}$ and
$u_{j,k} = \frac{(\|I_j - c_k\|^2 + \beta \sum_{l \in N_j, m \neq k} u_{l,m}^q)^{1/1-q}}{\sum_k (\|I_j - c_k\|^2 + \beta \sum_{l \in N_j, m \neq k} u_{l,m}^q)^{1/1-q}}$ using the current segmentation $\{V_k\}$,
3. reduce each object to its topology skeleton using the Object Thinning algorithm,
4. expand jointly the objects using the Object Growing algorithm,
5. loop to step 2 until convergence.

The convergence criterion is the number of changed labels per iteration. The curvature regularization is computed during the thinning and growing steps.

4 Experimental Results

Topology constraints are particularly relevant to the problem of brain segmentation. It is often desirable to map the cortex of the brain to a sphere, as it provides a coordinate system and unfolds the deep structure of the sulci [21]. We study here the use and performance of our algorithm for brain segmentation.

4.1 Spherical Brain Templates

To apply our algorithm to brain images, we first need to obtain a brain template with the correct topology. This problem is far from trivial. Simple geometric templates, like spheres, are difficult to align well with the images under study and provide poor estimates for the classification parameters. On the other hand, anatomically accurate templates like the Talairach atlas [20] usually have a very complex topology, due to the lack of constraints imposed on the manual segmentation.

Moreover, the anatomy may be in conflict with the topology assumption. The hypothesis of a spherical brain assumes that the cortical gray matter surrounds entirely the white matter of the brain, which in turn surrounds the sub-cortical gray matter and cerebro-spinal fluid. In reality, sub-cortical and cortical gray matter are linked through the base of the brain, near the brainstem, and so are the inner and outer CSF. Previous works assumed a post-processing step after the segmentation to 'fill in' the white matter membership [6].

Here, we use similar rules to separate cortical and sub-cortical gray matter and CSF at the top of the brainstem. We also make the common assumption that the brain has been pre-processed to remove extra-cranial tissues, and that both the brainstem and cerebellum have been removed. Our template possesses outer CSF, gray matter and white matter, all with a spherical topology. To enforce this, an extra layer of gray and white matter has been included in the area on top of the brainstem, to separate sub-cortical and cortical gray matter. We assume the sub-cortical gray matter has spherical

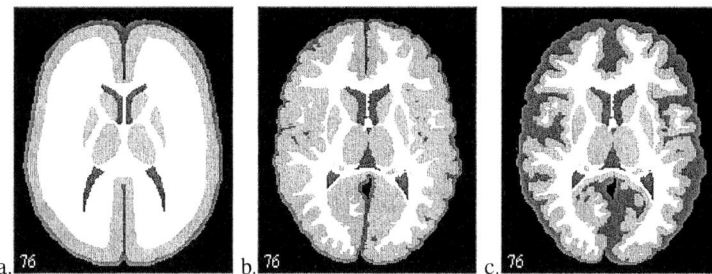

Fig. 2. Topology templates for the spherical brain hypothesis: a) a simplistic template created from the Talaraich atlas, b) a very detailed template created from the MNI/ICBM atlas, c) a simplified version of (b) that preserves more of the CSF. Very simplified templates like (a) are easier to create but they match poorly the structures involved, making the initialization more difficult and increasing the number of needed iterations. On the other hand, very detailed templates may not comply well with the topology constraints: in (b), the folds of cortical gray matter are not respected (the sulci are often isolated) and the template needs much editing. We settled for (c), where the cortical gray matter is obtained by morphological dilatation of the white matter. This last template is more accurate than (a) and better describes the topology constraints than (b)

topology, and the inner CSF has a more complex topology that includes two loops. In practice, the topology constraints are enforced only on the white and gray matter, mostly because the pre-processing affects the CSF outer layer (one could also argue that CSF, being a fluid, has a free topology). We tested several options for the template shape, as shown in Fig. 2. All templates were created from atlas data obtained from a digital version of the Talairach atlas and the MNI/ICBM atlas [2], edited through semi-automatic procedures until reaching the desired topology for each object.

4.2 Experiments

We tested the algorithm on six different examples of brain images from different sources. All images used have been pre-processed to isolate the cerebrum, and then registered to the template of Fig. 2-c using an automated registration technique in MIPAV [11]. The segmentation algorithm has been run with the same parameters for each brain. The results of figures 3 and 4 show that the segmentation closely follows the image data. We have verified that the volumes extracted all have the correct topology. Different brains with large variations in shape have all been processed successfully using the same template, even when variations in shape limited the initial registration accuracy.

The algorithm is rather computationally intensive, but it is efficient. It is composed of two fast marching methods, both using $N \log(N)$ time, with N the number of visited points. For each object, we visit at most the N_k points of the object V_k and its boundary, not the entire image, so the global cost is $2 \sum_k N_k \log(N_k)$ for a complete iteration. The number of iterations depends on the convergence of the algorithm, measured by the number of changed voxels per iteration. In our experiments, the number of iterations needed to reach 0.5% of changed voxels ranges between 8 and 12, with a mean of 10. The mean time for one iteration of the algorithm, which is written in JAVA, is currently

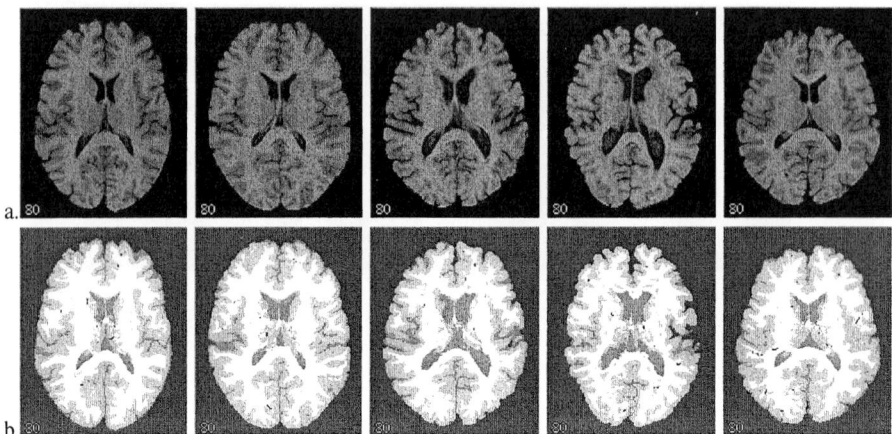

Fig. 3. Segmentation of candidate brains with variations in shape: a) original image, b) hard segmentation. Dark gray corresponds to CSF, medium gray is gray matter, and white is white matter. Black voxels inside the brain correspond to unclassified voxels where the topology constraints of the three classes could not be reconciled at the original resolution

118s on a 3 GHz Pentium 4 PC, with little code optimization, bringing the complete procedure under half an hour.

Noise in the original image translates into noise in the membership functions. As the fast marching evolution follows the order of the memberships, this could create artificial critical points where the object becomes non-convex. The two regularization terms, however, promote a convex ordering limiting this problem. The topology constraints enforce another form of regularization: they prohibit isolated misclassified points in objects, as that would change the topology. They also enforce adjacency at the object level, as objects in contact must stay in contact, and separated areas must stay separated (e.g. the sub-cortical and cortical gray matter is separated by the white matter in the template, it is also separated in the results. The same goes for the inner and outer CSF, because the white and gray matter separate them). Nevertheless, topology constraints alone have little control over the object geometry, and complicated, convoluted shapes can arise. In some cases, the topology constraints can lead to results that do not necessarily correspond to the data. This is a good feature in areas where the template deviates from the anatomy to enforce a certain topology (e.g. the white and gray matter layer added in the area near the top of the brainstem), but it is not desirable everywhere. For instance, had we not enforced topology constraints on the outer CSF, it would be forced to be at least a one voxel thick 6-connected volume, potentially gouging into some of the gray matter. Similarly, the topology constraints can strongly affect other thin structures that are one or two voxels wide. The connectivity constraints generate few unclassified points, and this issue should be settled easily with a subdivision of the unclassified voxels, or when extracting continuous surfaces from the segmentation, as illustrated in Fig. 1-b. Overall, the segmentation closely follows the image data and respects the highly convoluted geometry of cortical surfaces (c.f. Fig.4-f,g).

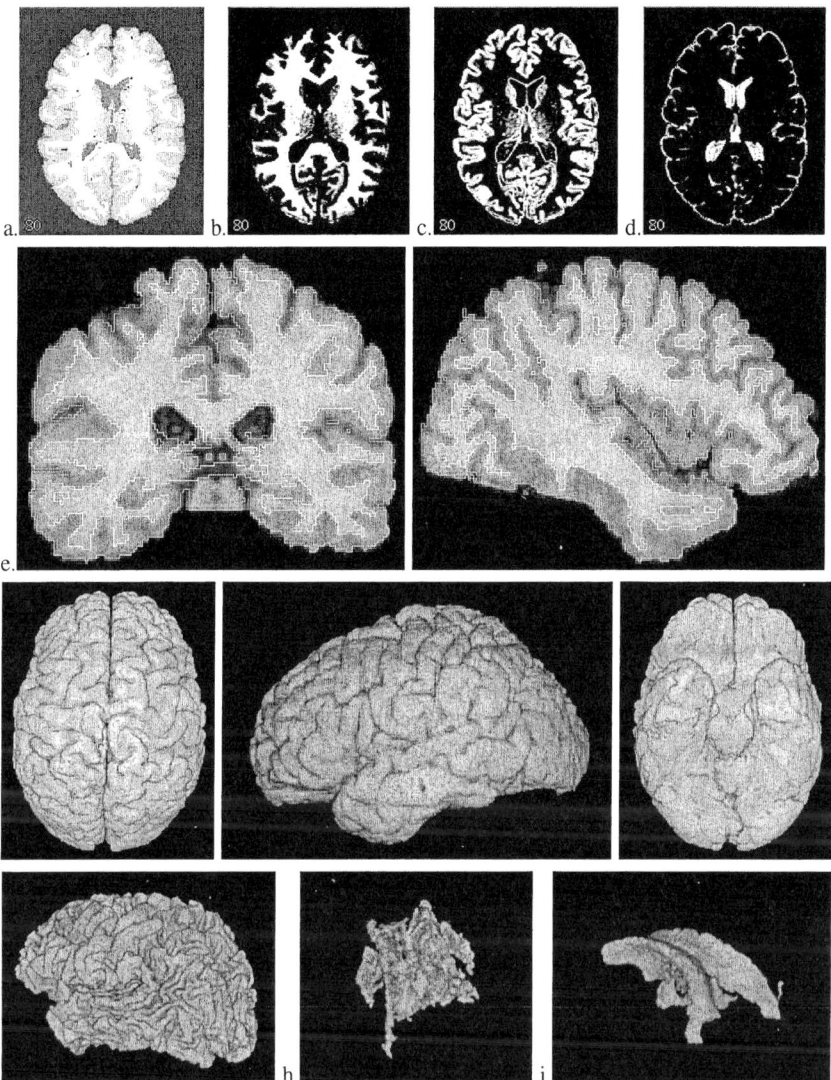

Fig. 4. A detailed example of segmentation: hard segmentation (a), membership functions for each tissue (white matter (b), gray matter (c), CSF (d)), coronal and sagittal views of the original image with superimposed gray and white matter boundaries (e), 3D renderings of the separate structures: cortical gray matter (f), white matter (g), sub-cortical gray matter (h) and ventricles (i)

5 Conclusions

In this paper, we have introduced a technique for joint multiple object segmentation in 3D images with topological constraints. The algorithm is based on a new idea for multiple objects segmentation that combines the advantages of tissue classification techniques and fast marching methods. The topology constraints are maintained simultaneously for all objects in the image, and can be of any nature, not just spherical.

Our preliminary experiments show that the method is well adapted to the brain segmentation problem under the spherical topology hypothesis, which has complex topology requirements. No specific pre-processing is required, and all structures are obtained at once. In our experiments, the computations always converge to a stable result, within a few iterations. Topology constraints and regularization limit the effects of noise. The overall accuracy of the results is visually good for most structures, although it can degrade over very thin structures, where the topology constraints are in balance with the image data. Further tests are under way to alleviate this problem and validate the technique. The creation of topology templates, central to the method, also needs to be studied further. In particular, we need to establish a more precise definition of anatomically approximative assumptions like the spherical brain hypothesis, and to create standardized atlases with both meaningful geometry and topology.

References

1. P.-L. Bazin and D. L. Pham. Topology smoothing for segmentation and surface reconstruction. In *Proceedings of the 7th International Conference on Medical Image Computing and Computer-Assisted Intervention (MICCAI'04)*, St Malo, september 2004.
2. P.-L. Bazin, M. McAuliffe, W. Gandler and D. L. Pham. Free software tools for atlas-based volumetric neuroimage analysis. In *Proceedings of the SPIE Medical Imaging Conference*, San Diego, february 2005.
3. S. Bischoff and L. Kobbelt. Sub-voxel topology control for level-set surfaces. *Computer Graphics Forum*, 22(3):273–280, 2003.
4. G. E. Christensen, S. C. Joshi, and M. I. Miller. Volumetric transformation of brain anatomy. *IEEE Transactions on Medical Imaging*, 16(6):864–877, December 1997.
5. M. Couprie, F. Bezerra, and G. Bertrand. Topological operators for grayscale image processing. *Journal of Electronic Imaging*, 10(4):1003–1015, 2001.
6. X. Han, D. Pham, D. Tosun, M. Rettmann, C. Xu, and J. Prince. Cruise: Cortical reconstructiong using implicit surface evolution. *NeuroImage*, 23(3):997–1012, 2004.
7. X. Han, C. Xu, U. Braga-Neto, and J. L. Prince. Topology correction in brain cortex segmentation using a multiscale, graph-based algorithm. *IEEE Transactions on Medical Imaging*, 21(2):109–121, 2002.
8. X. Han, C. Xu, and J. L. Prince. A topology preserving level set method for geometric deformable models. *IEEE Transactions on Pattern Analysis and Machine Intelligence*, 25(6):755–768, june 2003.
9. K. V. Leemput, F. Maes, D. Vandermeulen, and P. Suetens. Automated model-based tissue classification of mr images of the brain. *IEEE Transactions on Medical Imaging*, 18(10):897–908, 1999.
10. J.-F. Mangin, V. Frouin, I. Bloch, J. Regis, and J. Lopez-Krahe. From 3d magnetic resonance images to structural representations of the cortex topography using topology preserving deformations. *Journal of Mathematical Imaging and Vision*, 5:297–318, 1995.
11. M. McAuliffe, F. Lalonde, D. McGarry, W. Gandler, K. Csaky, and B. Trus. Medical image processing, analysis and visualization in clinical research. In *Proceedings of the 14th IEEE Symposium on Computer-Based Medical Systems (CBMS 2001)*, 2001.
12. S. J. Osher and R. P. Fedkiw. *Level Set Methods and Dynamic Implicit Surfaces*. Springer-Verlag, 2002.

13. D. L. Pham. Spatial models for fuzzy clustering. *Computer Vision and Image Understanding*, 84:285–297, 2001.
14. G. K. Rohde, A. Aldroubi, and B. M. Dawant. Tha adaptative bases algorithm for intensity-based nonrigid image registration. *IEEE Transactions on Medical Imaging*, 22(11):1470–1479, 2003.
15. M. Rousson, N. Paragios, and R. Deriche. Implicit active shape models for 3d segmentation in mri imaging. In *Proceedings of the International Conference on Medical Image Computing and Computer Assisted Intervention (MICCAI)*, 2004.
16. F. Segonne, E. Grimson, and B. Fischl. Topological correction of subcortical segmentation. In *Proceedings of the 6th International Conference on Medical Image Computing and Computer Assisted Intervention (MICCAI'03)*, pages 695–702, Montreal, november 2003.
17. J. Sethian. *Level Set Methods and Fast Marching Methods*. Cambridge University Press, 1999.
18. D. W. Shattuck and R. M. Leahy. Automated graph-based analysis and correction of cortical volume topology. *IEEE Transactions on Medical Imaging*, 20(11), november 2001.
19. D. W. Shattuck, S. R. Sandor-Leahy, K. A. Schaper, D. A. Rottenberg, and R. M. Leahy. Magnetic resonance image tissue classification using a partial volume model. *NeuroImage*, 13(5):856–876, 2001.
20. J. Talairach and P. Tournoux. *Co-Planar Stereotaxic Atlas of the Human Brain*. Thieme, 1988.
21. D. Tosun, M. E. Rettmann, and J. L. Prince. Mapping techniques for aligning sulci across multiple brains. In *Proceedings of The Sixth Annual International Conference on Medical Image Computing and Computer-Assisted Interventions(MICCAI)*, Montral, November 2003.
22. A. Tsai, A. J. Yezzi, W. M. W. III, C. Tempany, D. Tucker, A. Fan, W. E. L. Grimson, and A. S. Willsky. A shape-based approach to the segmentation of medical imagery using level sets. *IEEE Transactions on Medical Imaging*, 22(2):137–154, 2003.
23. L. A. Vese and T. F. Chan. A multi-phase level set framework for image segmentation using the mumford and shah model. *International Journal of Computer Vision*, 50(3):271–293, 2002.
24. G. H. Weber, G. Scheuermann, and B. Hamann. Detecting critical regions in scalar fields. In *Proceedings of the Joint EUROGRAPHICS - IEEE TCVG Symposium on Visualization*, Grenoble, may 2003.
25. Y. Zhang, M. Brady, and S. Smith. Segmentation of brain mr images through a hidden markov random field model and the expectation-maximisation algorithm. *IEEE Transactions on Medical Imaging*, 20(1):45–57, 2001.

Apparent Diffusion Coefficient Approximation and Diffusion Anisotropy Characterization in DWI

Y. Chen[1], W. Guo[1], Q. Zeng[1], X. Yan[1], M. Rao[1], and Y. Liu[2]

[1] Dept. of Mathematics, University of Florida
[2] Dept. of Psychiatry and McKnight Brain Institute, University of Florida

Abstract. We present a new approximation for the apparent diffusion coefficient (ADC) of non-Gaussian water diffusion with at most two fiber orientations within a voxel. The proposed model approximates ADC profiles by product of two spherical harmonic series (SHS) up to order 2 from High Angular Resolution Diffusion-weighted (HARD) MRI data. The coefficients of SHS are estimated and regularized simultaneously by solving a constrained minimization problem. An equivalent but non-constrained version of the approach is also provided to reduce the complexity and increase the efficiency in computation. Moreover we use the Cumulative Residual Entropy (CRE) as a measurement to characterize diffusion anisotropy. By using CRE we can get reasonable results with two thresholds, while the existing methods either can only be used to characterize Gaussian diffusion or need more measurements and thresholds to classify anisotropic diffusion with two fiber orientations. The experiments on HARD MRI human brain data indicate the effectiveness of the method in the recovery of ADC profiles. The characterization of diffusion based on the proposed method shows a consistency between our results and known neuroanatomy.

1 Introduction

Diffusion-weighted magnetic resonance imaging (DWI) adds to conventional MRI the capability of measuring the random motion of water molecules, referred to as water diffusion. The mobility of water molecules within tissue depends on the microstructure of the tissue. For instance, in most gray matter in the brain, the mobility of water molecules is the same in all directions and is termed isotropic diffusion. However, in fibrous tissues, such as cardiac muscle and brain white matter, water diffusion is with preferred direction along the dominant fiber orientation, and hindered to different degrees in different directions, causing diffusion anisotropy. The anisotropy of water diffusion in tissue, and the sensitivity of water diffusion to the underlying tissue microstructure form the basis for the utilization of DWI to infer neural connectivity [1], and to probe tissue structures [2, 1].

Water diffusion in tissue over a time interval t can be described by a probability density function (PDF) p on the displacement $\mathbf{r}$. The PDF $p(\mathbf{r}, t)$ is related to DWI echo signal $s(\mathbf{q})$ via a Fourier transformation (FT) with respect to the diffusion sensitizing gradients $\mathbf{q}$ by

$$s(\mathbf{q}) = s_0 \int p(\mathbf{r}, t) e^{-i\mathbf{q}\cdot\mathbf{r}} d\mathbf{r}, \qquad (1)$$

where s_0 is the MRI signal in the absence of any gradient [3]. From equation (1), the PDF $p(\mathbf{r},t)$ can be estimated by the inverse FT of $s(\mathbf{q})/s_0$. However, it requires a large number of measurements of $s(\mathbf{q})$ over a wide range of $\mathbf{q}$. Recently, Tuch et al. [4] developed q-space imaging method to obtain high angular resolution diffusion (HARD) measurements. In [5] Wedeen et al. succeed in acquiring 512 measurements of $s(\mathbf{q})$ in each scan to perform a stable inverse FT.

However, a more common approach to estimate the PDF of diffusion over time t from much sparser set of measurements $s(\mathbf{q})$ is by assuming $p(\mathbf{r},t)$ to be of Gaussian distribution, whose covariance matrix is the diffusion tensor, that is a 3×3 positive definite matrix. This technique is known as diffusion tensor imaging (DTI). Based on the theory that the principle eigenvector (PE) of D parallels to the mean fiber orientation, it is possible to infer the orientation of the diffusion within a voxel. DTI is in particular useful for creating white matter fiber tracts. Numerous algorithms have been developed to perform a robust estimation, regularization of the tensor field and fiber tracts reconstruction [3, 6, 7, 8, 9, 10, 11, 12].

However, it has been recognized that the single Gaussian model is inappropriate for assessing multiple fiber tract orientations, when complex tissue structure is found within a voxel [13, 14, 15, 16, 4, 5]. A simple extension to non-Gaussian diffusion is to assume that the multiple compartments within a voxel are in slow exchange and the diffusion within each compartment is a Gaussian [14, 15, 17, 18]. Under these assumption the diffusion can be modelled by a mixture of n Gaussians:

$$p(\mathbf{r},t) = \sum_{i=1}^{n} f_i((4\pi t)^3 det(D_i))^{-1/2} e^{\frac{-\mathbf{r}^T D_i^{-1} \mathbf{r}}{4t}}, \qquad (2)$$

where f_i is the volume fraction of the voxel with the diffusion tensor D_i, $f_i \geq 0$, $\sum_i f_i = 1$, and t is the diffusion time. Inserting (2) into equation (1) yields

$$s(\mathbf{q}) = s_0 \sum_{i=1}^{n} f_i e^{-b\mathbf{u}^T D_i \mathbf{u}}, \qquad (3)$$

where $\mathbf{u} = \mathbf{q}/|\mathbf{q}|$, and $b = t|\mathbf{q}|^2$ is the diffusion-weighting factor. To estimate D_i and f_i, at least $7n - 1$ measurements $s(\mathbf{q})$ plus s_0 are required. In [18, 17, 19] the model of a mixture of two Gaussians were used to estimate the PDF. This estimation requires at least 13 diffusion weighted images from 13 different directions.

An alternative method for the characterization of diffusion anisotropy is to use apparent diffusion coefficient(ADC) profiles. The ADC in DWI is defined as a function $d(\theta,\phi)$ in the Stejskal-Tanner equation:

$$s(\mathbf{q}) = s_0 e^{-bd(\theta,\phi)}, \qquad (4)$$

where (θ,ϕ) $(0 \leq \theta < \pi, 0 \leq \phi < 2\pi)$ represents the direction of $\mathbf{q}$ in spherical coordinates, the b-factor is defined as $b = 4\pi^2 |\mathbf{q}|^2 t$. For Gaussian diffusion the PE of D indicates the direction of the diffusion. The fractional anisotropy (FA) defined as

$$FA = \sqrt{\frac{3}{2}} \sqrt{\frac{(\lambda_1 - \lambda_2)^2 + (\lambda_2 - \lambda_3)^2 + (\lambda_3 - \lambda_1)^2)}{(\lambda_1 + \lambda_2 + \lambda_3)^2}}, \qquad (5)$$

has become the most widely used measure of diffusion anisotropy. In (5) λ_i's ($i = 1, 2, 3$) are the eigenvalues of D. If fibers are strongly aligned within a voxel, the FA is high, and the diffusion is anisotropic at that voxel.

For non-Gaussian diffusion the ADC profiles are more complex. Tuch et al. [4] recognized that HARD imaging with high b-values is able to exhibit the variance of the signal as a function of diffusion gradients. This admitted a generation of the concept of DTI to higher order tensors [20] or spherical harmonic series (SHS) approximation of the ADC to characterize complex diffusion properties [21, 22, 16].

To quantify diffusion anisotropy Frank [16] first proposed approximating the ADC profiles by its SHS. Later this idea was applied and more developed in [21, 22]. In these works the ADC profiles were represented by a truncated SHS:

$$d(\mathbf{x}, \theta, \phi) = \sum_{l=0,2,4} \sum_{m=-l}^{l} A_{l,m}(\mathbf{x}) Y_{l,m}(\theta, \phi), \qquad (6)$$

where $Y_{l,m}(\theta, \phi)$ are the spherical harmonics, which are complex valued functions defined on the unit sphere. The SHS in (6) doesn't have odd-order terms. Since the measurements are made by a serie of 3-d rotation, $d(\theta, \phi)$ is antipodal symmetric.

The $A_{l,m}$'s can then be used for the characterization of diffusion anisotropy. In [21, 16] the voxels with significant 4th order ($l = 4$) components were characterized as anisotropic with two fiber orientations (shortened as two-fiber diffusion), while voxels with significant 2nd order ($l = 2$) but not the 4th order components were classified as anisotropic with single fiber orientation (shortened as one-fiber diffusion). Voxels with significant 0th order ($l = 0$) but not the 2nd or the 4th order components are classified as isotropic. The truncated order is getting higher as the structure complexity increases. However, Fig.3 in [21] indicated that there was significant difference in overall ADC profile shape between the order 4 and order 2 models for non-Gaussian diffusion, but no significant change among models with order greater than 4. In [22] Chen et al. realized that the SHS with significant 4th order may not necessarily only describe two-fiber diffusion. Hence, they used the number of local maxima of the ADC, together with the weights of the variances at the local maxima to determine whether the diffusion is isotropic, one-fiber, two-fiber, or even more than two-fiber. This procedure is precise, but the drawback is that there are many measures involved and thus a lot of thresholds to be set subjectively.

In this note we will further study the SHS approximation model for ADC profiles, and develop a new algorithm based on information theory for characterizing the diffusion anisotropy under the assumption that there are at most two fiber orientations within a voxel.

Both the SHS model (6) and the mixture model (3) have been used to reveal intra voxel information with two-fiber diffusion. Model (6) involves 15 unknown complex valued functions $A_{l,m}$. Since $d(\theta, \phi)$ is real and $Y_{l,m}$ satisfies $Y_{l,-m} = (-1)^m \overline{Y_{l,m}}$, each complex valued $A_{l,m}$ is constrained by $A_{l,-m} = (-1)^m \overline{A_{l,m}}$, where $\overline{A_{l,m}}$ denotes the complex conjugate of $A_{l,m}$. This constraint transforms the 15 unknown complex valued functions in (6) to 15 real valued functions: $A_{l,0}(\mathbf{x})$, ($l = 0, 2, 4$), $ReA_{l,m}(\mathbf{x})$, $ImA_{l,m}(\mathbf{x})$, ($l = 2, 4; m = 1, \ldots, l$). Therefore, to use SHS model (6) to approximate d in (4), and hence to detect two-fiber diffusion, at least 15 diffusion weighted measurements $s(\mathbf{q})$ over 15 carefully selected directions are required. However, to use the mixture model (2) with n=2 to detect two-fiber diffusion only 13 unknown functions: f, 6 entries of each of D_1, D_2 need to be solved. This motivated us to study what is the minimum number of the diffusion weighted measurements required for detecting diffusion with no more than two fiber orientations within a voxel, and what is the corresponding model to approximate the ADC profiles in this case. In this note we propose to approximate the ADC profiles from high angular resolution diffusion-weighted (HARD) MRI by the product of two up to the second order spherical SHS instead of a SHS up to order four. We also show that the product of two up to the second order spherical SHS describes only the diffusion with at most two fiber orientations, while the SHS up to order four may also reveals the diffusion with three fiber orientations. The details will be given in the next section.

Moreover, we will introduce an information measurement developed in [23], and termed as CRE (see definition (13)) to characterize the diffusion anisotropy. CRE differs from Shannon entropy in the aspect that Shannon entropy depends only on the probability of the event, while CRE depends also on the magnitude of the change of the random variable. We observed that isotropic diffusion has either no local minimum or many local minima with very small variation in the denoised $s(\mathbf{q})/s_0$, i.e., e^{-bd} profiles in comparing with one fiber or two-fiber diffusions, which implies the corresponding CRE to be small. We also found that one fiber diffusion has only one local minimum with larger variation in the $s(\mathbf{q})/s_0$ profiles, which leads to larger CRE. Therefore, we propose to properly threshold the CRE for the regularized $s(\mathbf{q})/s_0$ profiles to characterize the diffusion anisotropy. Details will be provided in section 3.

2 New Approximation Model for ADC Profiles

In[16, 21, 22] to detect the diffusion with at most two fiber orientation the ADC profiles were represented by a truncated SHS up to order 4 in the form of (6). In [16] the coefficients $A_{l,m}$'s (l is even) were determined by inverse spherical harmonic transform of $-\frac{1}{b}\log\frac{s(\mathbf{q})}{s_0}$ and in [21] they were estimated as the least-squares solutions of

$$-\frac{1}{b}\log\frac{s(\mathbf{q})}{s_0} = \sum_{l=0}^{l_{max}} \sum_{m=-l}^{l} A_{l,m} Y_{l,m}(\theta, \phi). \quad (7)$$

Regularization on the raw data or $A_{l,m}$ wasn't considered in these two work. In [22] $A_{l,m}$'s were considered as a function of $\mathbf{x}$, and estimated and smoothed simultaneously by solving a constrained minimization problem:

$$\min_{A_{l,m}(\mathbf{x}), \tilde{s}_0(\mathbf{x})} \int_\Omega \{\sum_{l=0,2,4} \sum_{m=-l}^{l} |\nabla A_{l,m}(\mathbf{x})|^{p_{l,m}(\mathbf{x})} + |\nabla \tilde{s}_0(\mathbf{x})|^{p(\mathbf{x})}\} d\mathbf{x}$$

$$+ \frac{\lambda}{2} \int_\Omega \{\int_0^{2\pi} \int_0^{\pi} |s(\mathbf{x}, \mathbf{q}) - \tilde{s}_0(\mathbf{x}) e^{-bd(\mathbf{x},\theta,\phi)}|^2 \sin\theta d\theta d\phi + |\tilde{s}_0 - s_0|^2\} d\mathbf{x}, \quad (8)$$

with the constraint $d > 0$. In this model $p_{l,m}(\mathbf{x}) = 1 + \frac{1}{1+k|\nabla G_\sigma * A_{l,m}|^2}$, $q(\mathbf{x}) = 1 + \frac{1}{1+k|\nabla G_\sigma * s_0|^2}$, and d takes the form (6). By the choice of $p_{l,m}$ and q, the regularization is total variation based near edges, isotropic in homogeneous regions, and between isotropic and total variation based that varies depending on the local properties of the image at other locations, In these work since the ADC profile was approximated by (6), at least 15 measurements of $s(q)$ were required to to estimate the 15 coefficients $A_{l,m}$.

However, the mixture model (2) with $n = 2$, which is also able to detect two-fiber diffusion involves only 13 unknown functions. This motivates us to find a model that is able to detect non-Gaussian diffusion with the minimum number of unknowns. In this paper we only discuss the diffusion with no more than two fiber orientations within a voxel. The significance of this study is clear: less number of unknowns lead to less requirement for number of HARD measurements. This will significantly reduce the scan time and thus is important in clinical application.

Our basic idea is to approximate the ADC profiles MRI by the product of two second order SHS's instead of a SHS up to order four. This can be formulated as

$$d(\mathbf{x}, \theta, \phi) = (\sum_{l=0,2} \sum_{m=-l}^{l} b_{l,m}(\mathbf{x}) Y_{l,m}(\theta, \phi)) \cdot (\sum_{l=0,2} \sum_{m=-l}^{l} c_{l,m}(\mathbf{x}) Y_{l,m}(\theta, \phi)). \quad (9)$$

In this model there are only 12 unknowns: $b_{l,m}, c_{l,m}$ ($l = 0, 2$ and $-l \leq m \leq l$).

To estimate the ADC profile from the raw HARD MRI data, which usually contains a certain level of noise, we propose a simultaneous smoothing and estimation model similar to (8) for solving $b_{l,m}, c_{l,m}$, that is the following constrained minimization problem:

$$\min_{b_{l,m}(\mathbf{x}), c_{l,m}(\mathbf{x}), \tilde{s}_0(\mathbf{x})} \int_\Omega \{ \sum_{l=0,2} \sum_{m=-l}^{l} \alpha(|\nabla b_{l,m}(\mathbf{x})| + |\nabla c_{l,m}(\mathbf{x})| + \beta |\nabla \tilde{s}_0(\mathbf{x})| dx$$

$$+ \frac{1}{2} \int_\Omega \{ \int_0^{2\pi} \int_0^\pi |s(\mathbf{x}, \mathbf{q}) - \tilde{s}_0(\mathbf{x}) e^{-bd(\mathbf{x},\theta,\phi)}|^2 \sin\theta d\theta d\phi + |\tilde{s}_0 - s_0|^2 \} dx, \quad (10)$$

with constraint $d \geq 0$, where d is in the form of (9). α, β are constants. The first 3 terms are the regularization terms for $b_{l,m}, c_{l,m}$ and s_0 respectively. The last two terms are the data fidelity terms based on the original Stejskal-Tanner equation(4).

Next, feasibility of this model will be explained. Denote $B := \sum_{l=0,2} \sum_{m=-l}^{l} b_{l,m} \cdot Y_{l,m}(\theta, \phi)$, $C := \sum_{l=0,2} \sum_{m=-l}^{l} c_{l,m} Y_{l,m}(\theta, \phi)$ and $A := \sum_{l=0,2,4} \sum_{m=-l}^{l} A_{l,m} Y_{l,m}$. Define sets $SBC = \{d : d(\theta, \phi) = B \cdot C\}$, $SA = \{d : d(\theta, \phi) = A\}$. Since each $d(\theta, \phi)$ in SBC is a function defined on S^2, it can be approximated by SHS, simple calculation shows that coefficients of the approximated SHS of even order larger than 4 are all zeros, so $SBC \subset SA$. On the other hand, numerous experiments show that when a voxel is not more complicated than 2-fiber diffusion, its ADC is always a function in set SBC. But if a voxel is of 3-fiber diffusion or even more complicated, its ADC can not be described accurately by a function in SBC. This implies that SBC is a real subset of SA. Fig.1 depicts how functions in set SBC and SA differ in representing ADC.

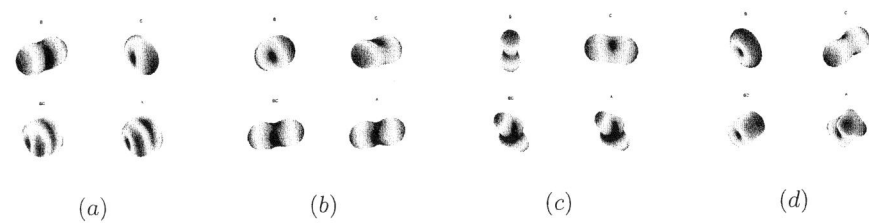

Fig. 1. Comparison of the ADC's approximated by (6) and (9) in four cases: (a) isotropic diffusion, (b) one-fiber diffusion, (c) two-fiber diffusion, (d) three-fiber diffusion. In (a)-(d) from left to right, top to bottom, we show shapes of B, C, $B \cdot C$, and A, respectively

It is observed that the ADC in the form A can not be well approximated by $B \cdot C$ only in 3-fiber diffusion case (see Fig. 1 below). Therefore, if we focus only on characterizing at most two-fiber diffusion, which is the most interesting case, model (9) is reasonable and sufficient to represent ADC.

Model (10) is a minimization problem with constraint $d(\theta, \phi) \geq 0$ for all $0 \leq \theta < \pi, 0 \leq \phi < 2\pi$ which is usually difficult to implement. To improve the efficiency of computation we used the idea that any second order SHS $\sum_{l=0,2}\sum_{m=-l}^{l} b_{l,m} Y_{l,m}(\theta, \phi)$ is equivalent to a tensor model $u^T D u$ for some semi-positive definite 3×3 matrix D, where $u(\theta, \phi) = (sin\theta cos\phi, sin\theta sin\phi, cos\theta)$. This means that the coefficients $b_{l,m}$, $(l = 0, 2, m = -l, ..., l)$ in SHS and the entries $D(i,j)$, $(i, j = 1, ..., 3)$ in D can be computed from each other explicitly. Here are two examples: $b_{00} = \frac{2}{3}\sqrt{\pi}(D_{11} + D_{22} + D_{33})$. $D(1,1) = -\frac{\sqrt{5}b_{20} - 2b_{00} - \sqrt{30}Re(b_{22})}{4\sqrt{\pi}}$, where $Re(b_{22})$ is the real part of b_{22}. Hence, we could let $B = uD_1u^T$, $C = uD_2u^T$, then $d = (uD_1u^T)(uD_2u^T)$. And for $i = 1, 2$ decomposed D_i into $D_i = L_i L_i^T$ with L_i a lower triangular matrix to guarantee semi-positiveness of D_i. The ADC is finally approximated by

$$d(\mathbf{x}, \theta, \phi) = [u(\theta, \phi)L_1(\mathbf{x})L_1(\mathbf{x})^T u(\theta, \phi)^T][(u(\theta, \phi)L_2(\mathbf{x})L_2(\mathbf{x})^T u(\theta, \phi)^T]. \quad (11)$$

Furthermore we substituted model (10) by

$$\min_{L_1^{jk}(\mathbf{x}), L_2^{jk}(\mathbf{x}), \tilde{s}_0(\mathbf{x})} \int_\Omega (\alpha \sum_{i=1}^{2}\sum_{j=1}^{3}\sum_{k=1}^{j} |\nabla L_i^{j,k}| + \beta|\nabla \tilde{s}_0|)d\mathbf{x}$$

$$\frac{1}{2}\int_\Omega \{\int_0^{2\pi}\int_0^{\pi} |s - \tilde{s}_0 e^{-bd}|^2 sin\theta d\theta d\phi + |\tilde{s}_0 - s_0|^2\}d\mathbf{x}, \quad (12)$$

where $d = (uL_1L_1^T u^T)(uL_2L_2^T u^T)$. All the $b_{l,m}, c_{l,m}, l = 0, 2, m = -l...l$ are smooth functions of $L_i^{jk}, i = 1, 2; j = 1, 2, 3; k \leq j$, smoothness of L_i^{jk} guarantees that of $b_{l,m}$'s, $c_{l,m}$'s. The first term in model (12) thus works equivalently as the first two terms in model (10) do, while all the other terms are the same as those left in (10). Hence, (12) is equivalent to (10), but it is a non-constrain minimization problem and is thus easy to implement. After we get L_1 and L_2, $b_{l,m}$ and $c_{l,m}$ in (10) can be obtained by the one to one relation between them.

We apply model(12) to a set of human brain HARD MRI data to reconstruct and characterize ADC profiles. The data set consists of 55 diffusion weighted images $S_k : \Omega \to R, k = 1, ..., 55$, and one image S_0 in the absence of a diffusion-sensitizing field gradient(b=0 in (4)). 24 evenly spaced axial planes with 256×256 voxels in each slice are obtained using a 3T MRI scanner with single shot spin-echo EPI sequence. Slice thickness is $3.8mm$, gap between two consecutive slices is $1.2mm$, repetition time $(TR) = 1000ms$, echo time $(TE) = 85ms$ and $b = 1000s/mm^2$. The field of view (FOV) $=220mm \times 220mm$. We first applied the model(12) to the data to get L_i, and then used L_i to compute $b_{l,m}$ and $c_{l,m}$, $l = 0, 2, m = -l...l$, and the ADC $d = B \cdot C$. On the other hand, we used the model (8) to estimate $A_{l,m}$ and get A. The comparison for the shapes of ADC in the form of $B \cdot C$ and A is demonstrated in Fig.1(a)-(d) at four specific voxels. The diffusion at these 4 voxels are isotropic (a), one-fiber (b), two-fiber (c), and three-fiber (d), respectively. In each sub figure, the up left, up right, down left, down right ones are the shapes of $B, C, B \cdot C$ and A, respectively. It is evident that if the diffusion is isotropic, one-fiber or two-fiber, $B \cdot C$ and A are the same. However, if the diffusion is three-fiber, A can't be well approximated by $B \cdot C$.

To show the effectiveness of the proposed model in recovering ADC, in Fig.2(a)-(d) we compared images of R_2 (defined in section 3) with coefficient $A_{l,m}$ estimated by 4 different methods. The voxels with higher value of R_2 were considered as one-fiber diffusion. The $A_{l,m}$'s in (a), (b) and (c) were estimated using least-squares method in [21], model (8), and model(12) with the diffusion-sensitizing gradient applied to 55 directions, respectively. The $A_{l,m}$'s in (d) are estimated by the same way as that in (c), but from the HARD data with 12 carefully chosen directions. The model (12) applied on 55 measurements worked as good as the model (8) in getting higher value of R_2. Both of them worked better than the least-squares method that does not consider regularization. Although the result from 12 measurements was not as good as that from 55 measurements, they are are still comparable. We will show in Fig.5(a) and (b) that the anisotropy characterization results based on the ADC presented in (c) and (d) are also close. These experimental results indicated that by using the proposed model the voxels with two-fiber diffusion can be detected reasonably well from 12 HARD measurements in carefully selected directions.

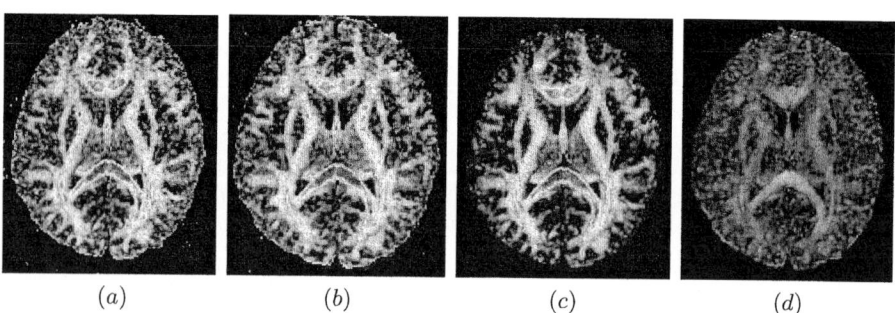

(a)   (b)   (c)   (d)

Fig. 2. (a)-(d) are images of R_2 with $A_{l,m}$'s calculated using least-squares method, model (8), model (12) applied on 55 measurements, and model (12) applied on 12 measurements, respectively

3 Use of CRE to Characterize Anisotropy

As mentioned, FA is only able to detect Gaussian diffusion. For non-Gaussian diffusion, Frank and Alexander et.al. used the order of significant component in SHS to characterize anisotropy. They considered voxels with significant 4th order components as two-fiber diffusion. In [22] Chen et al. realized that such a voxel could have isotropic or one-fiber diffusion. They defined $R_0 := \frac{|A_{0,0}|}{\sum_{l=0,2,4}\sum_{m=-l}^{l}|A_{l,m}|}$, $R_2 := \frac{\sum_{m=-2}^{m=2}|A_{2,m}|}{\sum_{l=0,2,4}\sum_{m=-l}^{l}|A_{l,m}|}$. Higher values of R_0 and R_2 are corresponding to isotropic and one-fiber diffusion, respectively. For the rest of points, the number of local maxima of ADC, together with the weights of the variances at the local maxima were used to classify voxels as isotropic, one-fiber or two-fiber diffusion. This procedure is more precise, but there are many measures involved and thus more thresholds needed to be set subjectively. In this section, we will introduce a simple scheme using only one measurement CRE and two thresholds.

CRE is a measure of uncertainty/information in a random variable. Let X be a random variable in R, CRE of X is defined by

$$CRE(X) = -\int_{R_+} P(X > \lambda) log P(X > \lambda) d\lambda, \qquad (13)$$

where $R_+ = \{X \in R | X \geq 0\}$.

We use CRE of e^{-bd} rather then d to characterize diffusion anisotropy, where d is recovered from HARD measurements through(12). The magnitude of ADC is usually in the order of 10^{-3}, while the magnitude of e^{-bd} is in the order of 10^{-1}, which is larger than that of ADC itself. Moreover, e^{-bd} is a smooth approximation of the data s/s_0.

The weak convergence property of CRE proved in [23] makes empirical CRE computation based on the samples converges in the limit to the true CRE. This is not the case for the Shannon entropy. We define empirical CRE of e^{-bd} as

$$CRE(e^{-bd}) = -\sum_{i=2}^{M} P(e^{-bd} > \lambda_i) log P(e^{-bd} > \lambda_i) \triangle \lambda_i \qquad (14)$$

where $\{\lambda_1 < \lambda_2 < ... < \lambda_M\}$ is range of e^{-bd} at voxel x. $\triangle \lambda_i = \lambda_i - \lambda_{i-1}$ is the absolute difference between two adjacent e^{-bd}, note this term is not shown in Shannon entropy. In most of the cases, the variation of e^{-bd} is the largest for one-fiber diffusion voxels, smaller for two-fiber diffusion and smallest for isotropic voxels. This also explains why CRE is the largest for one-fiber, medium for two-fiber and smallest for isotropic diffusion voxels. In our experiment, we choose M=1000 uniformly distributed directions (θ, ϕ) in (14).

Define the decreasing distribution function $F(\lambda) := P(e^{-bd} > \lambda)$. Fig.3 (a) demonstrate the graphs of $-F(\lambda) log F(\lambda)$ at the same three voxels. It is evident that the area under the right solid curve(one-fiber) is much larger than that under the middle dotted curve(two-fiber), while the area under the left curve is the smallest. Since CRE is exactly the area under curve $-F(\lambda) log F(\lambda)$, we can conclude that measure $CRE(e^{-bd})$

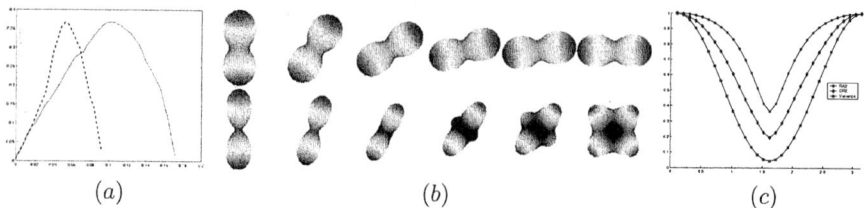

Fig. 3. (a) Graph of $-F(\lambda)\log F(\lambda)$ at three voxels corresponding to isotropic (left), two-fiber (middle dotted), one-fiber (right solid) diffusion.(b) Form left to right, shapes of uD_2u^T (top) and $uD_1u^T \cdot uD_2(\psi)u^T$ (bottom) for $\psi = i\pi/10, i = 0...5$. (c) Graphs of R_2 (top), CRE (middle), variance (bottom) as functions of $\psi \in [0, \pi]$

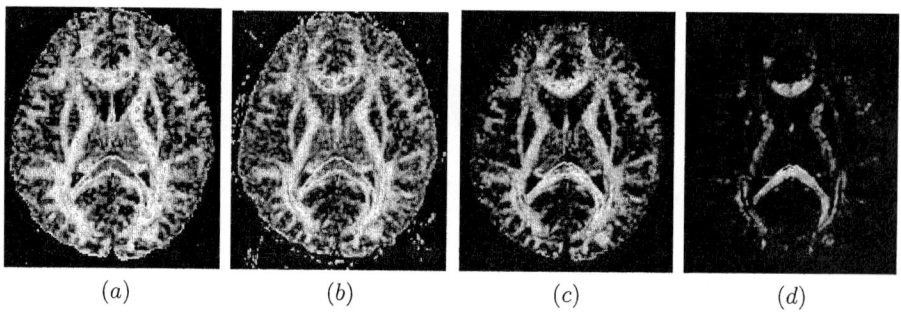

Fig. 4. Images of four measures: (a) R_2, (b) FA, (c) CRE of e^{-bd}, (d) Variance of e^{-bd}

is the largest at the voxels with one-fiber diffusion, medium with two-fiber diffusion, and smallest with isotropic diffusion. Thus measure $CRE(e^{-bd})$ could be used to discern isotopic, one-fiber and two-fiber diffusion with two thresholds T_1 and T_2, with $T_1 < T_2$. Set up 3 intervals:$(0, T_1)$, (T_1, T_2), (T_2, ∞). Voxels with CRE fall into the first, second, and third intervals are classified as isotropic, two-fiber and one-fiber diffusion respectively.

Fig.3(c) on synthetic data and Fig.4 on human brain HARD MRI data further show the strength of CRE over the three popularly used measures R_2, FA and variance in characterizing diffusion anisotropy. The human data is the same as that used in Fig.2. The synthetic data is constructed as follows: Set D_1 and D_2 to be two diagonal matrix with diagonal elements $4 \times 10^{-2}, 10^{-2}, 2 \times 10^{-2}$ and $8 \times 10^{-2}, 10^{-2}, 3 \times 10^{-2}$, respectively. Then fix D_1 but rotate the two eigenvectors corresponding to the first two diagonal entries of D_2 in the plane perpendicular to the third eigenvector by angle ψ to get $D_2(\psi)$. Let $B(\theta, \phi) = u^T D_1 u$, $C_\psi(\theta, \phi) := u^T D_2(\psi) u$ with $u = (\sin\theta\cos\phi, \sin\theta\sin\phi, \cos\theta)$. In Fig.3(b), from left to right, we show figures of $C_\psi(\theta, \phi)$ (top row) and $B(\theta, \phi) \cdot C_\psi(\theta, \phi)$ (bottom row) for $\psi = i\pi/10, i = 0...5$. When ψ varies from 0 to $\pi/2$, $B \cdot C$ changes from a typical one fiber diffusion to a two fiber diffusion. By symmetry, when ψ varies from $\pi/2$ to π $B \cdot C$ changes back to the same shape as $\psi = 0$. Fig.3(c) represents the graphs of R_2 of $B \cdot C$ (top), CRE of $e^{-bB \cdot C}$ (middle), variance of $e^{-bB \cdot C}$ (bottom) as a function of $\psi \in [0, \pi]$. The three measures are normalized by dividing by their corresponding maxima. Values of the three measures decrease when $B \cdot C$ varies from one-fiber diffusion to two-fiber diffusion, and increase when $B \cdot C$ gradually changes from two-fiber diffusion backs to one-fiber diffusion. But the graph CRE is much steeper than others. This implies CRE difference between adjacent voxel is much larger than that of R_2 and variance, thus image of CRE will have better contrast than the other two. This is verified in Fig.4, where figure (c) has better contrast than figure (a)and (d). R_2 cannot detect multi-fiber diffusion as it measures the significance of the second order components in SHS. Nonsignificant difference between R_2 and FA is observed from the images in Fig.4(a) and (b). But CRE differs much from R_2 and FA. Furthermore, the smallness of magnitude of R_2 or FA is unable to distinguish between isotropic and two-fiber diffusion, while that of CRE does better job. Note, CRE is comparable to FA or RA_2 in detecting Gaussian diffusion.

Next we discuss from the theoretical point of view why CRE beats variance in characterizing diffusion anisotropy. Let X be a random variable, $Var(X)$ be its variance. According to proof in [24], $E(|X - E(X)|) \leq 2CRE(X)$. In our case, X is e^{-bd} whose magnitude is multiple of $10^{-2} < 1$, so we have $Var(X) = E(|X - E(X)|^2) \leq E(|X - E(X)|) \leq 2CRE(X)$. Our experiment results show that magnitude of CRE is almost 10 times of that of $Var(X)$. Higher magnitude of CRE makes it less sensitive to rounding errors. One more result from [24] is $CRE(X) \leq \sqrt{Var(X)}$, thus $Var(X) \leq 2CRE(X) \leq 2\sqrt{Var(X)}$, which implies CRE has smaller range than variance does. This is verified by Fig.3(c) where the graph of variance is way below that of CRE. Moreover, in Fig.4(d), which representing the the variance of e^{-bd}, the Genu/Splenium of corpus callosum is so bright that regions besides it are not clearly visualized, so CRE is much better than variance visually.

Fig.5(a) shows a partition of isotropic,one-fiber and two-fiber diffusion based on ADC calculated from 55 measurements. The black, gray, white voxels are identified as isotropic, one-fiber and two-fiber diffusion, respectively. The characterization is consistent with the known fiber anatomy. Fig.5(b) represents the characterization result based

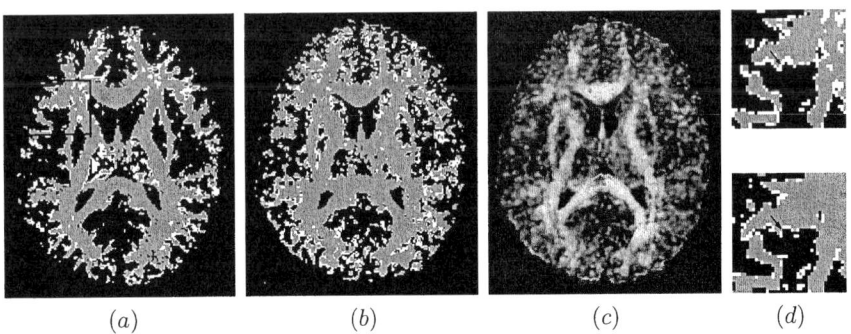

Fig. 5. (a)-(b). Characterization: black, gray, and white regions represent the voxels with isotropic, one-fiber, and two-fiber diffusion, respectively.(a) using 55 measurements, (b) using 12 carefully selected measurements. (c) Image of CRE calculated from 12 measurements. (d) Characterization results of the region inside the black box in (a) using CRE (top) and variance (bottom) based on 55 measurements

on the ADC estimated from 12 measurements. It is very close to that from 55 measurements. CRE based on ADC estimated from 12 measurements (Fig.5(c)) is also comparable to that from 55 measurements (Fig.4(c)). Thus our characterization is not sensitive to number of measurements. Fig.5(d) illustrates a two-fiber diffusion voxel(pointed by black arrow) that is incorrectly characterized as one-fiber diffusion using variance (bottom image) but characterized as two-fiber correctly using CRE (top image). This further verify superiority of CRE over variance in characterizing diffusion anisotropy.

4 Summary

In this paper, we present a novel variational framework for simultaneous smoothing and estimation of ADC profiles depicted by two diffusion tensors. To our knowledge this is the first attempt to use the least amount of measurement to detect two-fiber diffusion from human brain HARD MRI data. We also demonstrated our algorithm for using CRE of e^{-bd} to characterize the diffusion anisotropy.

Our experiments on two sets of human brain HARD MRI data showed the effectiveness and robustness of the proposed model in the estimation of ADC profiles and the enhancement of the characterization of diffusion anisotropy. The characterization of diffusion from the proposed method is consistent with the known neuroanatomy.

In this article, we have not included the work for determination of fiber directions and the method for automated fiber tracking. The study addressing these problems will be reported in separate papers.

Acknowledgment

We thank Dr. Guojun He from the Brain Institute, University of Florida for his technical help in data collecting.

References

1. C. Beaulieu, "The basis of anisotropic water diffusion in the nervous system - a technical review," *NMR Biomed.*, vol. 15, pp. 435–455, 2002.
2. P. J. Basser, "Inferring microstructural features and the physiological state of tissues from diffusion-weighted images," *NMR Biomd.*, vol. 8, pp. 333–344, 1995.
3. P. J. Basser, J. Mattiello, and D. Lebihan, "Estimation of the effective self-diffusion tensor from the NMR," *Spin Echo. J. Magn. Reson.*, vol. series B 103, pp. 247–254, 1994.
4. D. S. Tuch, R. M. Weisskoff, J. W. Belliveau, and V. J. Wedeen, "High angular resolution diffusion imaging of the human brain," in *Proc. of the 7th ISMRM*, Philadelphia, 1999, p. 321.
5. V. J Wedeen, T. G. Reese, Tuchand D. S., M. R. Weigel, J. G. Dou, R. M. Weisskoffand, and D. Chesler, "Mapping fiber orientation spectra in cerebral white matter with fourier transform diffusion MRI.," in *Proc. of the 8th ISMRM*, Denver, 2000, p. 82.
6. T. L. Chenevert, J. A. Brunberg, and J. G. Pipe, "Anisotropic diffusion in human white matter: Demonstration with MR techniques in vivo," *Radiology*, vol. 177, pp. 401–405, 1990.

7. R Deriche, D Tschumperlé, and C Lenglet, "DT-MRI estimation, regularization and fiber tractography," in *Proc. of the 2nd ISBI*, Washington D.C, 2004, pp. 9–12.
8. C. Feddern, J. Weickert, and B. Burgeth, "Level-set methods for tensor-valued images," in *Proc. of the 9th Annual Meeting of ISMRM*, Nice, 2003, pp. 65–72.
9. G. J. M. Parker, J. A. Schnabel, M. R. Symms, D. J. Werring, and G. J. Baker, "Nonlinear smoothing for reduction of systematic and random errors in diffusion tensor imaging," *Magn. Reson. Med.*, vol. 11, pp. 702–710, 2000.
10. C. Poupon, J. F. Mangin, C. A. Clark, V. Frouin, J. Regis, D. LeBihan, and I. Block, "Towards inference of human brain connectivity from MR diffusion tensor data," *Med. Image Anal.*, vol. 5, pp. 1–15, 2001.
11. B. C. Vemuri, Y. Chen, M. Rao, and T. H. Mareci, "Automatic fiber tractograph from dti and its validation," in *Proc. of the 1st IEEE ISBI*, 2002, pp. 505–508.
12. Z. Wang, B.C. Vemuri, Y. Chen, and T.H. Mareci, "A constrained variational principle for direct estimation and smoothing of the tensor field from complex DWI," *IEEE Tran. Med. Imag.*, vol. 23, pp. 930–940, 2004.
13. P. J. Basser, J. Mattiello, and D. LeBihan, "MR diffusion tensor spectroscopy and imaging," *Biophys*, vol. 66:259, pp. 267, 1994.
14. A. L. Alexander, K. M. Hasan, M. Lazar, J.S. Tsuruda, and D. L. Parker, "Analysis of partial volume effects in diffusion-tensor MRI," *Magn. Reson. Med.*, vol. 45, pp. 770–780, 2001.
15. L. Frank, "Anisotropy in high angular resolution diffusion-weighted MRI," *Magn Reson Med*, vol. 45, pp. 935–939, 2001.
16. L. Frank, "Characterization of anisotropy in high angular resolution diffusion weighted MRI," *Magn Reson Med*, vol. 47, pp. 1083–1099, 2002.
17. G. J. M. Parker and D. C. Alexander, "Probabilistic monte carlo based mapping of cerebral connections utilising whole-brain crossing fiber information," in *Information Processing in Medical Imaging*, Ambleside UK, 2003, pp. 684–696.
18. D. S. Tuch, T. G. Reese, M. R. Wiegell, N. Makris, J. W. Belliveau, and V. J. Wedeen, "High angular resolution diffusion imaging reveals intravoxel white matter fiber heterogeneity," *Magn. Reson. Med.*, vol. 48, pp. 577–582, 2002.
19. Y. Chen, W. Guo, Q. Zeng, G. He, B. C. Vemuri, and Y. Liu, "Recovery of intra-voxel structure from hard MRI," in *IEEE International Symposium on Biomedical Imaging*, Arlington, Virginia, 2004, pp. 1028–1031.
20. E. Özarslan and T. H. Mareci, "Generalized diffusion tensor imaging and analytical relationships between diffusion tensor imaging and high angular resolution diffusion imaging," *Magn. Reson. Med.*, vol. 50, pp. 955–965, 2003.
21. D. C. Alexander, G. J. Barker, and S. R. Arridge, "Detection and modeling of non-gaussian apparent diffusion coefficient profiles in human brain data," *Magn. Reson. Med.*, vol. 48, pp. 331–340, 2002.
22. Y. Chen, W. Guo, Q. Zeng, X. Yan, F. Huang, H. Zhang, G. He, B. C. Vemuri, and Y. Liu, "Estimation, smoothing, and characterization of apparent diffusion coefficient profiles from high angular resolution DWI," in *IEEE Int. Conf. in Computer Vision and Pattern Recognition (CVPR)*, Washington, D.C., 2004, pp. 588–593.
23. M. Rao, Y. Chen, B. C. Vemuri, and F. Wang, "Cumulative residual entropy: A new measure of information," *IEEE Trans. on Info. Theory*, vol. 50, pp. 1220–1228, 2004.
24. M. Rao, "More on a new concept of entropy and information," *Journal of Theoretical Probability*, to appear.

Linearization of Mammograms Using Parameters Derived from Noise Characteristics

Nico Karssemeijer, Peter R. Snoeren, and Wei Zhang

Department of Radiology, Radboud University Nijmegen Medical Centre,
PO Box 9101, 6500HB Nijmegen, The Netherlands
n.karssemeijer@rad.umcn.nl

Abstract. A method is proposed for converting digitized mammograms to a normalized representation, in which pixel values are linearly related to the logarithm of x-ray exposure. This method is based on a signal dependent noise model. By exploiting this model unknown parameters of the non-linear response of the film-screen system can be estimated from signal dependence of the image noise. The method was applied to a series of 1372 mammograms acquired over a period of 8 years. Sudden changes in estimated parameters corresponded well with the introduction of new film-screen systems.

1 Introduction

Quantitative analysis of mammograms requires reliable knowledge of acquisition parameters. If these are available mammograms can be converted to a normalized representation, from which tissue properties can be extracted more reliably. The use of such representations may increase robustness of computer aided detection (CAD) systems, and may allow more accurate estimation of clinically relevant features like breast density. Methods for normalized representation of mammograms have been proposed in the literature. Most notably, a physics based method was developed by Highnam and Brady [1, 2], which assumes that the breast is composed of two classes of tissue, fat and a mixture of dense tissue types. This method converts mammograms to a representation of dense tissue thickness. Other investigators have used linearization methods when dealing with digitized mammograms, to correct for the non-linear reponse of the film/screen system. or used a representation in which image noise is equalized.

In this paper we focus on linearization, which is defined as a process in which mammograms are converted to a space in which pixel values are linearly related to the logarithm of the exposure E. For quantitative analysis this is a naturale scale, as in first approximation there is a linear relation between $\log E$ and the average x-ray attenuation μd of the tissue mapping on a pixel, with μ the average linear attenuation coefficient and d the tissue thickness. On this scale, local measures of contrast, gradients, and other derivatives only depend on physical properties of the projected anatomical structures and not on the pixel value itself. Without taking into account the non-linear response of the acquisition system contrast related measurements cannot be made accurately.

With modern full field digital mammography (FFDM) systems images can be archived in a raw format, in which pixel values are proportional to exposure. For computer aided detection methods this is an important advantage. However, it will take a long time before annotated databases with FFDM cases are sufficiently large to develop CAD systems that are trained exclusively with FFDM. For the near future the use of digitized mammograms will be necessary, and if adequate normalization methods are available continued use of large databases of digitzed mammograms will be advantageous. After all, the size and quality of databases will be one of the key elements in future development of CAD systems.

When dealing with digitized films it is difficult to retrieve acquisition parameters, in particular those related to the nonlinear response of the screen-film system. In a previous paper, we explored the use of temporal matching of mammograms to retrieve the relation between pixel values in digitized films and exposure. In this paper we investigate a method to estimate parameters for linearisation from the image itself. The method is based on analysis of high frequency components in the image noise.

2 Screen-Film Noise in Digitized Mammograms

2.1 Theory

Radiographic mottle in screen-film mammography systems has been investigated by by Barnes [3]). There are three independent random processes involved, film granularity, quantum mottle and screen structure mottle. The resulting density fluctuations due to these processes can be described as

$$\sigma^2(D) = \sigma_g^2(D) + \sigma_q^2(D) + \sigma_s^2(D) \quad (1)$$

with D the optical density. According to Barnes, in mammography the latter component is very small, which is confirmed by more recent studies [4]. Here it will be neglected. Noise due to film granularity can be described in first approximation by

$$\sigma_g(D) \propto \sqrt{D} \quad (2)$$

Quantum noise fluctuations in the x-ray exposure at the detector are proportional to $\sqrt{E}$. In the optical density domain they can be written in the form of

$$\sigma_q(D) \propto \frac{G}{\sqrt{n}} \quad (3)$$

with n the average x-ray photon fluence absorbed in the screen and $G(D)$ the slope of the characteristic curve of the screen-film system at density D. The inverse relation is due to the fact that characteristic curves are defined as a function of $\log E$. Film noise dominates quantum noise at high spatial frequencies, very low exposures, or very high exposures [4].

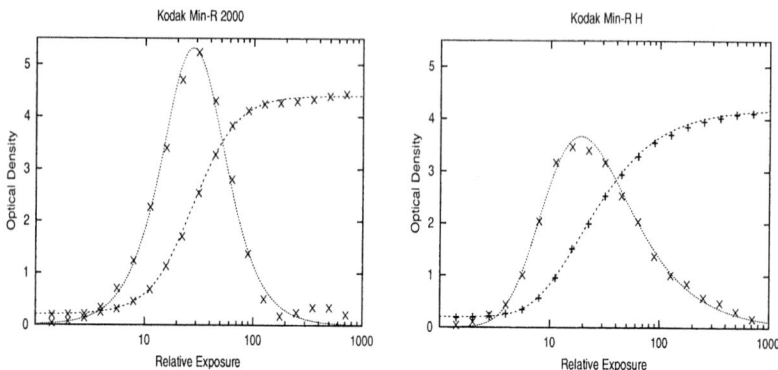

Fig. 1. Characteristic curves and gradients of a Kodak Min-R 2000 film and a Kodak Min-R H film. The plotted curves are model fits

2.2 Characteristic Curves

Over the last decades mammographic film-screen systems have gradually increased contrast. By increasing the film gradient the peripheral zone of the breast and the skin line are imaged at high optical densities, often rendering them invisible under normal viewing conditions. To improve this, some companies developed dual-emulsion films in which the gradient is high at low densities but smaller in the mid and high density ranges.

It was found experimentally that the screen-film response can well be modeled by

$$D(E) = D_{bf} + D_{max} \left[\frac{1}{1 + e^{-g \cdot (\ln E - s)}} \right]^q$$
$$= D_{bf} + D_{max} \left[1 + (E/s)^{-g} \right]^{-q} \quad (4)$$

with x-ray exposure denoted by E, with $D(E)$ the optical density, D_{bf} the base plus fog optical density of the unexposed film, and D_{max} the optical density of the fully exposed film. The parameters g and s represent the gradient and speed of the film, respectively. The parameter q can be used to model an asymmetric shape of the curve. An example of a symmetric model ($q = 1$) fitted to the characteristic curve of a Kodak Min-R 2000 film is shown in figure 1. To model the Kodak Min-R H response an asymmetric model was used (figure 1). It is noted that characteristic curves of screen-film systems vary over time due to changes in developer conditions.

For medical x-ray films it is common to measure the average gradient G_{av} between the optical densities of 0.25 and 2.00 above base plus fog, using

$$G_{av} = \frac{2.0 - 0.25}{\log E1 - \log E2} \quad (5)$$

where $E1$ and $E2$ are the relative exposure values at densities 0.25 and 2.0 above base plus fog, respectively.

2.3 Quantum Noise

Quantum noise fluctuations are transfered through the imaging system and give rise to pixel value fluctuations in digitized mammograms. To analyze this process the screen-film and digitizer transfer functions are modeled. We assume that the digitizer response is linear with optical density:

$$y(E) = y_0 - c_d D(E)$$

with y the pixel value and y_0 the pixel value at density $D = 0$.

At a given image intensity the fluctuation of pixel values $\sigma_y(y)$ due to quantum noise can be written as a function of variation in exposure $\sigma_E(y)$

$$\sigma_y(y) = \left| \frac{\partial y(E)}{\partial D} \frac{\partial D}{\partial E} \right|_y b \sigma_E(y)$$

with b a constant that takes blurring in the imaging system into account at the scale of the filter used to measure fluctuations. We assume that this constant is independent of E. Using the square root model for quantum noise

$$\sigma_E(y) = p\sqrt{E(y)}$$

it can be derived from using the characteristic curve model in 4 that,

$$\sigma_y(y) = c_q\, c_d\, g\, q\, D_{max} \frac{1}{\sqrt{E(y)}} \left[1 + (E(y)/s)^{-g}\right]^{-q-1} (E(y)/s)^{-g} \qquad (6)$$

with $E(y)$ the exposure corresponding with pixel value y, and $c_q = bp$ a constant that we will refer to as the quantum noise factor. The $1/\sqrt{E}$ factor is in accordance with (3).

Taking the inverse of the film curve exposure can be expressed as

$$E(y) = s \left[\left(\frac{D_{max}}{D(y) - D_{bf}} \right)^{\frac{1}{q}} - 1 \right]^{\frac{1}{g}}$$

$$= s\, t(y)^{-\frac{1}{g}} \qquad (7)$$

with

$$t(y) = \left(\frac{D_{max}}{D(y) - D_{bf}} \right)^{\frac{1}{q}} - 1 \qquad (8)$$

$$= (E(y)/s)^{-g}$$

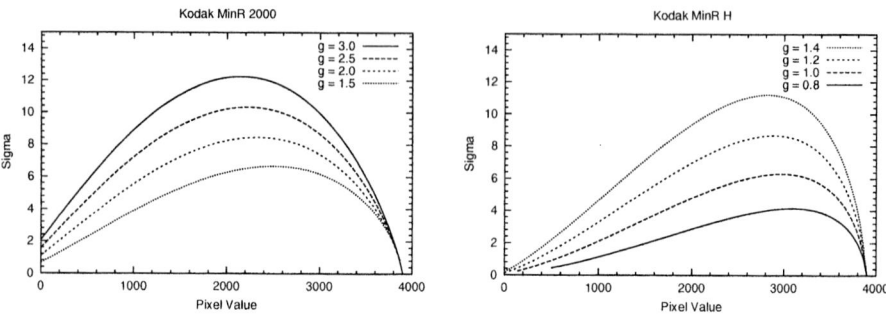

Fig. 2. Changes of quantum noise due to variation of the gradient g of the characteristic curve for two types of film

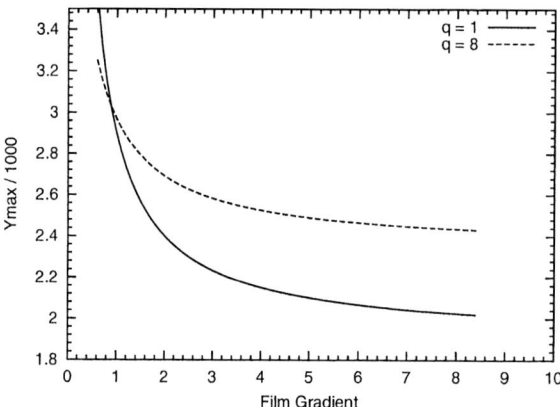

Fig. 3. Pixel value at which the quantum noise maximum occurs as a function of film gradient for two values of q

By substitution of $t(y)$ in equation (6) we can derive

$$\sigma_y(y) = c_q\, c_d\, g\, q\, D_{max} \frac{1}{\sqrt{s}} t(y)^{1+1/2g}(1+t(y))^{-q-1} \qquad (9)$$

In figure 2 it is shown how the quantum noise component modeled by relation 6 behaves when the gradient of the film is varied. Changes of the film speed did not affect the location of the maximum. An analytical expression for the maximum can be found by differentiation of (9). The optical density D_M at which this maximum occurs is given by

$$D_M = D_{bf} + D_{max}\left(1 + \left[\frac{2g+1}{2gq-1}\right]\right)^{-q} \qquad (10)$$

Figure 3 shows a graph of the maximum location as a function of the film gradient.

The fact that the quantum noise maximum D_M shifts when the film gradient is varied provides an opportunity for estimating the film gradient from the noise characteristics in a digitized film. The speed of the film cannot be retrieved in this way. It is noted that the noise maximum strongly depends on digitizer calibration and film curve parameters q, D_{max}, D_{bf}.

2.4 Film Granularity

As mentioned before, noise due to film granularity cannot be neglected. In a paper by Bunch [4] the relative contribution of film granularity to the noise power spectrum was determined for a number of mammographic film-screen systems from Kodak. At 5 lp/mm, which corresponds with a 100 micron pixel size, the relative contribution of film noise is fairly constant at a level of 40 % at low optical densities. It increases for densities higher than 1.2. At an optical density of 2.0 the relative contribution is 80 %.

3 Noise Measurements

To measure noise a high pass filter was applied to compute local contrast fluctuations. The filtered image was obtained by subtracting a smoothed image from the original. We used a Gaussian kernel for smoothing with $\sigma = 100$ micron. All experiments were done with images that were averaged down to 100 micron resolution. To compute image noise as a function of pixel value the gray-scale was divided in non-overlapping bins of fixed size N. Local contrast distributions were computed for each bin and the standard deviations $s(y_n)$ of these distributions were estimated, with y_n the weighted mean pixel value in bin n. In all experiments a fixed bin-size of $N = 20000$ pixels was used.

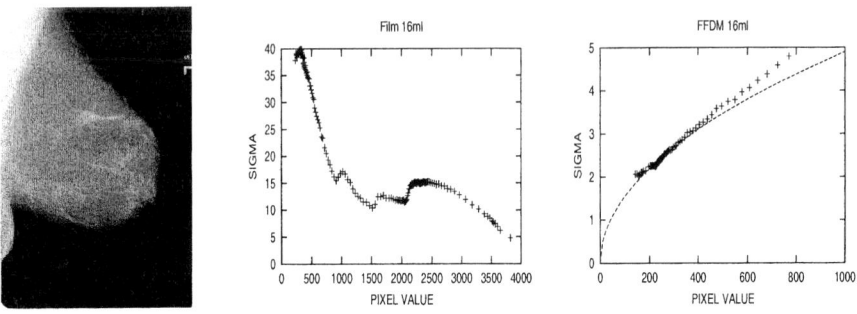

Fig. 4. Example of a mammograms for which both a film-screen (Min-R 2000) and a FFDM image was available. The middle figure shows noise measured in the film-screen images. Noise determined in the FFDM image is shown right

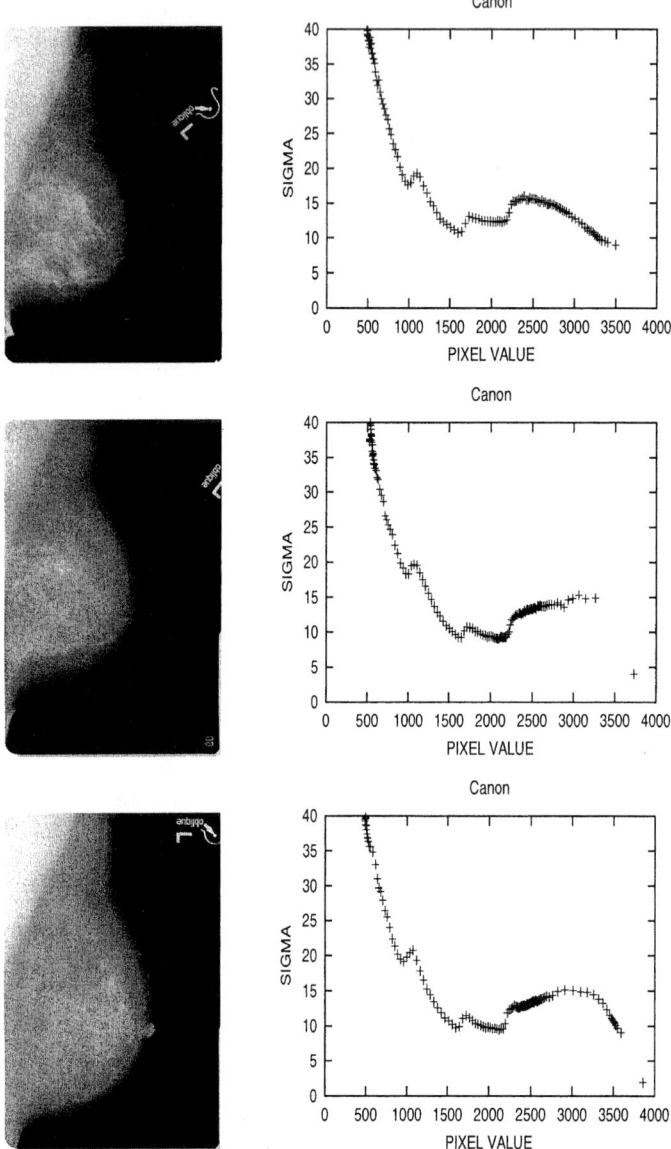

Fig. 5. Examples of noise measured in three mammograms. The top row shows an image recorded with a Kodak Min-R 2000 film. The other examples are Min-R films. The images on the first and second row are from the same woman. The example demonstrates how the film type affects the shape of the curves

A typical example is shown in figure 4. A case was chosen for which both a conventional mammogram and a digital mammogram were available. The time between the two acquisitions was less than two weeks. In the noise plot of the

FFDM image a square root model for quantum noise is indicated by a dashed line. This appears to fit well to the data up to some point. Experimentally it was found that the model fit was good in the area where the breast is fully compressed. In the uncompressed tissue part there is an additional noise component, which appeared to be due to skin surface roughness. The noise plot of the digitized film shows the expected gradual decrease at higher pixel values (see figure 2). For low pixel values the scanner noise is dominant. Other examples are shown in figure 5. The image in the upper row was made with a Kodak Min-R 2000 film, whereas the other images were older Kodak films with a lower gradient. In this example the expected shift of the maximum to the right for lower film-gradients can be observed.

It appeared that there were three distinct discontinuities in the noise characteristics of digitized film which were at the same grey level for all images. This was due to the digitizer we used. To reduce scanner noise an increasing amount of smoothing was applied in the scanner at lower pixel values.

4 Film Curve Parameter Estimation

4.1 Method

In section 2 it has been shown how the shape of the film curve is reflected in the relation between optical density and high frequency noise. We investigate if this relation allows retrieval of film curve parameters from a digitized mammogram.

It should be noted that it is not be possible to determine film speed from the image noise, because the effect on σ_D of a shift of the film curve along the $\log E$ axis might as well be caused by a combined change of unknown variables as exposure time, the constants p and b representing quantum noise contribution, and the modulation transfer function (see equations 2.3 and 2.3). Therefore, we use a fixed relative speed in our parameter estimation process. According to ANSI specifications, X-ray film speed is defined as the exposure required for the film to reach net optical density 1. We arbitrarily chose a value of $logE = 1.2$ to correspond with $D + D_{bf} = 1.0$. It is noted that in our film curve model the parameters s and g are not defined in the same way as the relative film speed defined above and the average film gradient G_{av} used in practice (eq 5).

Inaccuracy of the digitization process limits applicability of the aproach. The results in the previous section show that digitizer noise is dominant at higher optical densities and, moreover, that image noise may be affected by noise reduction processes in the digitizer. For the digitizer used in the study it was determined that up to a optical density of about 1.8 ($y > 2300$) noise measurements are accurate. For higher optical densities the noise reduction scheme activated in the scanner causes problems. This makes estimation of the film curve at higher optical densities problematic. It does not prohibit, however, estimation of the film curve in the mid and low optical density range. As most of the relevant structures in mammograms are imaged at lower optical densities this may not be a problem. In our experiments scanner calibration was fixed and known. We used $c_d = 1000$ and $y0 = 4000$.

To estimate the film curve parameters from the measured noise characteristics using relation (6) we have to take the film noise component σ_f into account. The digitizer noise is neglected in the range of interest. For the noise at pixel value y_i we assume

$$\sigma_{model}(y_i)^2 = \sigma_q(y_i)^2 + c_f D \qquad (11)$$

where film noise variance is assumed to be proportional to optical density (equation 2) and c_f is a constant. We were not able to develop a stable procedure to estimate this parameter together with the film curve parameters. Therefore, we used a fixed value of c_f chosen as such that thee mean contribution of film noise relative to the total noise was 0.4 at optical density 1.5. This choice was motivated by data found in the literature ([4]).

Given the fixed relative speed of the film, the model we use has five unknown parameters parameters, representing the average gradient G_{av}, asymmetry q, the quantum noise factor c, maximum density D_{max} and base plus fog density density D_{bf}. For the latter we use a fixed value $D_{bf} = 0.20$. The other four parameters were estimated. To increase the robustness of the esimation method, prior information about the expected parameter values was used in two ways. Firstly, the range of variation of the three film curve parameters was limited to realistic intervals. Secondly, the expected value and variance of the parameters D_{max} and G_{av} were used to penalize unrealistic film curve models. Ranges, means and variances were determined from various sets of characteristic curves obtained from quality assurance procedures in recent years.

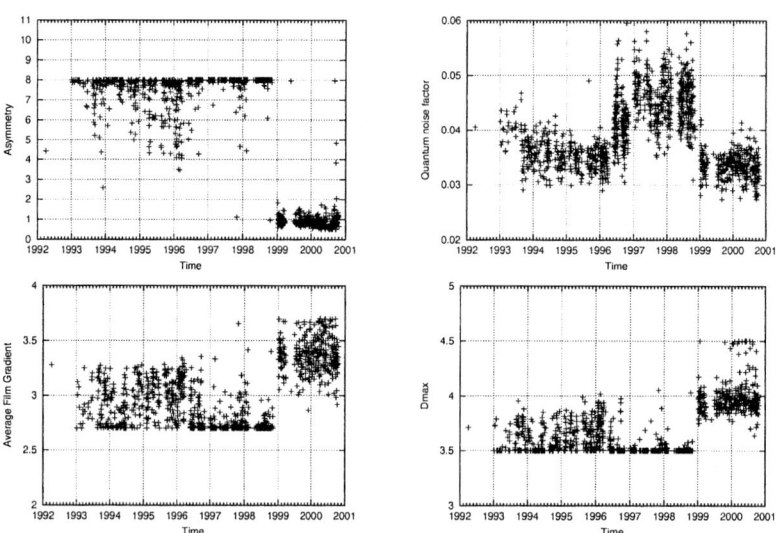

Fig. 6. Film curve parameter estimation for a series of 1372 case (left MLO images). Prior distributions for the average gradient and maximum density were used ($w = 0.02$)

For parameter estimation we used a regularized least squares fit. Minimization was performed with the simplex method. The function that was minimized is given by

$$J(\mathbf{r}) = \frac{1}{N}\sum_{i=0}^{i=N}(\sigma(y_i) - \sigma_{model}(y_i))^2 + w\left[\left(\frac{(G_{av} - \mathrm{E}(\mathrm{G_{av}}))^2}{\mathrm{var}(\mathrm{G_{av}})} + \frac{(D_{max} - \mathrm{E}(\mathrm{D_{max}}))^2}{\mathrm{var}(\mathrm{D_{max}})}\right)\right] \quad (12)$$

with the parameter vector $\mathbf{r} = (q, D_{max}, G_{av}, p)$. The weight of the regularization term was determined experimentally.

4.2 Results

A series of 1372 cases was used to evaluate the method. Only left MLO images were processed. Results are shown in figure 6. Transitions from Kodak MinRH to MinR2000 in January 1999 and from an older film/screen type in 1996 are

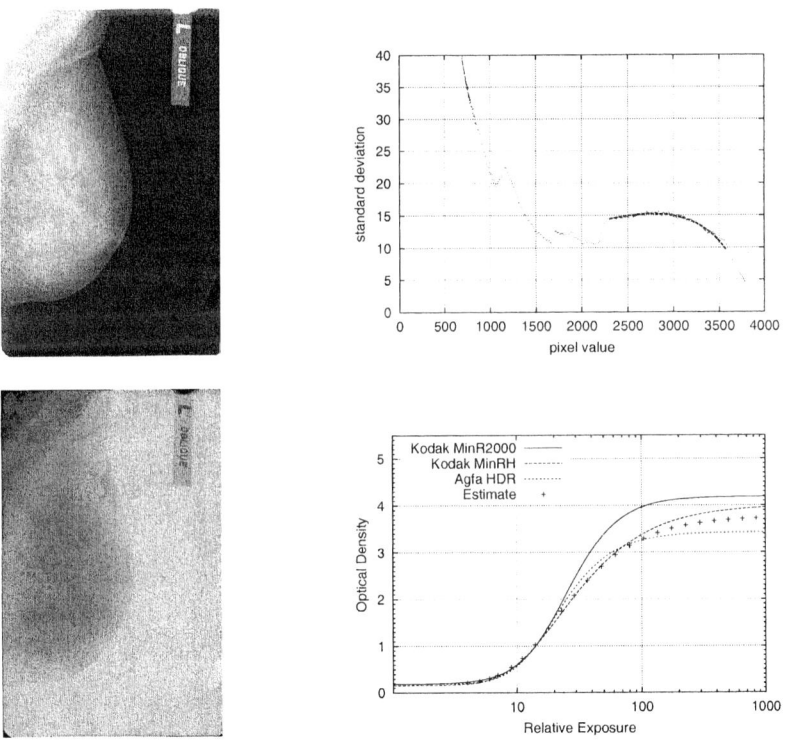

Fig. 7. Example of film curve estimation in a mammogram (a Kodak film from 1993). The linearized mammogram is shown on the bottom. For comparison, typical film curves of Kodak MinRH, MinR2000 and Agfa HDR are also shown

clearly marked. In particular the difference between the asymmetry parameter value of the new MinR2000 film and the older ones is very distinct and estimates of asymmetry appear to be very consistent.

5 Conversion to Linear Mammogram Representation

When the film curve and calibration parameters are known mammograms can be converted to a linearized representation in which pixel values are linear with $\log E$. This is attractive because in first order approximation that scale is also linear with the X-ray attenuation of the imaged dense tissue thickness:

$$\begin{aligned}
\log E &= \log\left[E_0 \, e^{-\mu_d t_d - \mu_f t_f}\right] \\
&= -\mu_d t_d - \mu_f t_f + \log E_0 \\
&= -\mu_d t_d - \mu_f (T - t_d) + \log E_0 \\
&= t_d (\mu_f - \mu_d) + constant
\end{aligned} \tag{13}$$

with t_d and t_f the thickness of dense and fatty tissue, μ_d and μ_f the attenuation coefficients and T the breast thickness.

To map the pixel values to the log E domain a value of the constant in the equation above must be chosen. Mapping the fatty tissue in the compressed region of the breast to a fixed value seems to be a natural choice. It can be determined in a digitized mammogram after segmentation by taking the minimum pixel value in the interior part of the compressed breast region. Perhaps, correction for scatter might be useful as well, this would also make the relation to dense tissue thickness more accurate. For very dense breasts, determination of the fatty tissue background may require another method.

6 Discussion

Estimation of film curve parameters from the pixel value to noise relation is possible, but some assumptions have to be made to make estimation robust. Speed of the film cannot be retrieved. However, as speed does not influence contrast (changes of $\log E$) this may not be a problem in most applications. Given the parameters of the film curve and the digitizer calibration mammograms can be converted to a linear mammogram representation (LMR) in which pixel values are linear with $\log E$. As this scale is also linear with the imaged dense tissue thickness, in first approximation, it seems to be a good choice for quantitative image processing.

One application of film curve estimation is temporal mammogram analysis. However, when the last mammogram is digital a very different approach is possible, because then we have the linear FFDM recording available as a reference. By registration of the FFDM case with the digitized film a pixel to pixel match can be obtained which allows computation of a 2D probability density function of the Gray values on both images. Actually this pdf is already computed when a method like mutual information is used for registration. The pdf allows estimation of the film curve parameters.

When a mammogram only has a limited dynamic range there may not be enough information to determine filmcurve parameters. In particular for CC images of fatty breast cases this may be a problem. Because images of the same case will have the same filmcurve parameters the best approach would be to extract the pixel value to noise relation simultaneously from all images of the case. Alternatively, the filmcurve derived the first image that is processed can be used for all. It should be avoided to process images from the same case with different curves, because inaccuracy of the estimation might then hamper CC/MLO and left/right comparisons.

References

1. R P Highnam, J M Brady, and B J Shepstone. A representation for mammographic image processing. *Med Imag Analysis*, 1:1–18, 3 1996.
2. R Highnam and M Brady. *Mammographic image analysis*. Kluwer Academic Publishers, P.O. Box 17, 3300 AA Dordrecht, The Netherlands, 1 edition, 1999.
3. G T Barnes and D P Chakraborty. Radiographic mottle and patient exposure in mammography. *Radiology*, 145:815–821, 1982.
4. Bunch P C. Objective imaging characteristics of mammographic screen-film systems. *SPIE Medical Imaging 1996*, 2708:241–271, 1996.

Knowledge-Driven Automated Detection of Pleural Plaques and Thickening in High Resolution CT of the Lung

Mamatha Rudrapatna[1], Van Mai[1], Arcot Sowmya[1], and Peter Wilson[2]

[1] School of Computer Science and Engineering, University of New South Wales,
Sydney, NSW 2052, Australia
[2] I-MED / MIA Network, Sydney, NSW 2000, Australia
{mamathar, vmma518, sowmya}@cse.unsw.edu.au
pcwilson2@bigpond.com

Abstract. Consistent efforts are being made to build Computer-Aided Detection and Diagnosis systems for radiological images. Such systems depend on automated detection of various disease patterns, which are then combined together to obtain differential diagnosis. For diffuse lung diseases, over 12 disease patterns are of interest in High Resolution Computed Tomography (HRCT) scans of the lung. In this paper, we present an automated detection method for two such patterns, namely Pleural Plaque and Diffuse Pleural Thickening. These are characteristic features of asbestos-related benign pleural disease. The attributes used for detection are derived from anatomical knowledge and the heuristics normally used by radiologists, and are computed automatically for each scan. A probabilistic model built on the attributes using naïve Bayes classifier is applied to recognise the features in new scans, and preliminary results are presented. The technique is tested on 140 images from 13 studies and validated by an experienced radiologist.

1 Introduction

Digital technology has revolutionised the acquisition, processing and storage of medical images. The next step is the automation of disease pattern detection and diagnosis. Current imaging modalities are producing ever more images with increasing detail. Even though their availability have increased the diagnostic sensitivity, the burden on radiologists is also increasing due to the large volume of data produced. The need for automated techniques is self-evident, as fatigue and oversight are major contributors to diagnostic error [1]. In addition, errors due to inexperience and inter- and intra observer variations are not uncommon. Computer-aided detection systems are being developed to help alleviate these problems and make the diagnostic process more objective. Inevitably, such systems are built in a bottom-up manner since images must be processed, segmented and analysed before a diagnosis can be made. Subsequently, diagnosis systems can be built on top of the detection systems.

High Resolution Computer Tomography (HRCT) is considered to be the best tool available for detection of diffuse lung diseases [2]. HRCT has proven to be more sensitive than chest X-Rays and CT scans. HRCT refers to scans with very thin collimation of 1 to 1.5 mm. Even though the images are normally obtained with up to 20 mm gap between consecutive slices, the increased resolution and limited artefacts compensates for any deficiency arising from non-contiguous sampling. This protocol on average produces 25 images per patient, however the latest volumetric multi-detector row scanners can produce up to 300 contiguous thin-section scans per patient.

Our focus is on asbestos related diseases. Even though the mining of asbestos has been terminated in many countries, the exposure to asbestos continues due to its ubiquitous usage in building products till the 1970's. As the latency period between asbestos exposure and the development of pleural diseases is anywhere from 20 to 30 years, the incidence of asbestos related diseases is peaking now in some countries and yet to peak in others. Asbestos related diseases can be broadly classified into three categories: asbestos-related benign pleural disease, asbestosis and malignant pleural mesothelioma (MPM). We present an automated detection technique for two characteristic features of benign pleural disease, namely pleural plaque and diffuse pleural thickening. Pleural plaques are often the first signs of asbestos exposure, since the pleura appears to be more sensitive to the effects of asbestos infiltration than the lung parenchyma. Bilateral plaques (appearing in both the lungs) and calcification of plaques are distinctive characteristics of asbestos exposure. The incidence of pleural plaque in non-asbestos exposed population is very low [3], and therefore pleural plaques and thickening are considered as prime indicator of asbestos-related diseases; consequently they are very significant disease features to detect and monitor.

To the best of our knowledge, no automated technique for detection of pleural plaques has been reported to date. Other diffuse lung disease pattern detection has been automated. Lung nodule detection has attracted a bigger share of attention [4 - 7], while automated techniques are also being developed for detection of patterns such as Emphysema [8], Ground-Glass Opacity [9] and other interstitial [10] and airway abnormalities [11]. Recently, we have reported on other characteristic features of asbestosis such as Parenchymal bands and end stage Honeycombing [12, 13].

In the next section, some background information on pleural plaques is discussed. Section 3 presents our automated technique for detection of pleural plaque and diffuse pleural thickening. Preliminary results are presented in section four and section five concludes with a summary and future directions.

2 Background

The lung may be visualised as a pair of sacs, as illustrated in Fig 1. The inner visceral layer covers the lung, while the outer parietal layer lines the chest cavity and the upper surface of the diaphragm. The lung region where the trachea bifurcates into main bronchi and enters the lungs is known as the hilum. The hilum is an important landmark since it helps to divides the lung roughly into apical, middle and basal regions. Many diseases show predominance in one or more of these regions.

Pleural plaques are defined as discrete elevated areas of hyaline fibrosis arising from the parietal pleura. On HRCT, they appear as smooth, sharply defined regions especially underneath visible rib segments. Diffuse pleural thickening occurs when

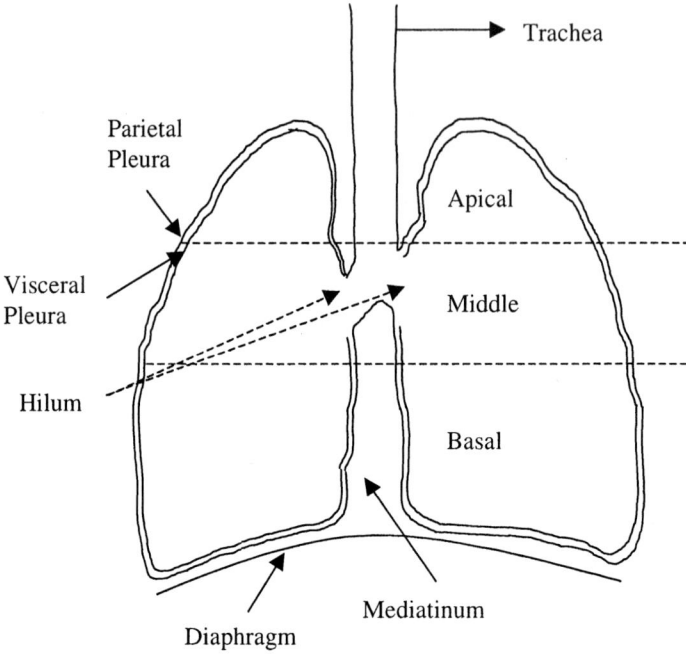

Fig. 1. Lung Anatomy

thickened visceral pleura fuses with the parietal pleura over a wide area [3]. For the purpose of detection, we may classify pleural plaques into three distinct types based on location, namely diaphragmatic plaques, paravertebral plaques and costal plaques. Examples of these types and other anatomical details are shown in Fig 2.

Even though there are no reports on automated detection techniques for pleural plaques, their visual appearance on CT / HRCT scans has been well studied. It is known that pleural plaques are not commonly seen in the apical region of the lungs, whereas diffuse pleural thickening is observable there. Even though the size and number of plaques vary vastly, they are rarely solitary. Pleural plaques are commonly seen indenting the lung parenchyma to form "pleural bumps". Diffuse pleural thickening, on the other hand, is often smooth.

Costal plaques are by far the easiest to detect when located internal to the rib segments. This is because only the pleura and extrapleural fat normally lie internal to the ribs, and in normal patients, are too thin to be resolved on the HRCT scans. Even though the intercostal muscles have visual characteristics very similar to those of plaques, they pass in between, and not internal to the rib segments. In many cases however, the pleural plaque region may appear to merge or extend into the intercostal muscle and surrounding soft tissues, since the extrapleural fat layer that separates them may be very thin and invisible. This makes the segmentation task very challenging. In the case of diffuse pleural thickening, the region of interest extends in between and internal to the rib segments and again, this region often appears merged with the surrounding soft tissue.

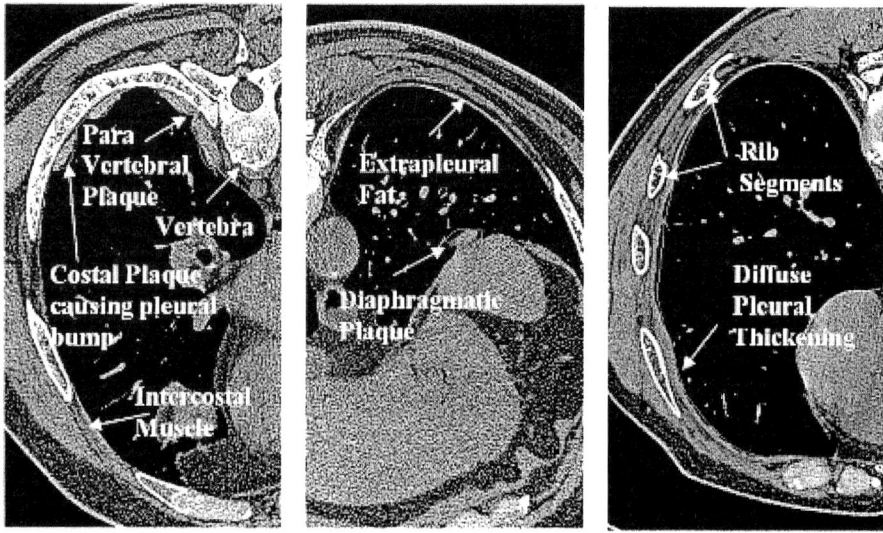

Fig. 2. Costal plaque, Diaphragmatic Plaque and Diffuse Pleural Thickening

Normal anatomy near the vertebral region can mimic the appearance of a plaque since the intercostal vessels make the soft tissue appear thicker, thereby resulting in false positive detection of pleural plaque. It has been suggested that the detection of plaques in this region should be considered at multiple levels. Diaphragmatic plaques are by far the most difficult to detect, since they are not well delineated and show only a marginal variation of curvature in the plane of scan. However, it is suggested that if these regions show calcification, they are more likely to be plaques.

3 Method

In this section we describe the image features specially designed to capture the anatomical and morphological knowledge discussed above. Also, the image processing techniques employed to extract such features and relevant anatomical structures are explained.

3.1 Feature Design

The domain knowledge acquired from expert radiologists was used in image feature design and are summarized in Table 1. The diagnosis of pleural plaques depends heavily on their location. They are easiest to identify when they are located internal to the rib segments. The feature "CanReachRibs" encodes this knowledge. Since the confidence near the paravertebral region is somewhat lower, the spinal bones are treated differently and the feature "CanReachSpine" is extracted.

Focal pleural plaques often appear to be indented into the lung parenchyma causing small "bumps" along the lung boundary. This serves as another strong indicator of plaques and the feature "IsOnBump" reflects this knowledge. Sometimes when a layer of extrapleural fat is visible, it can used to distinguish plaques especially from the intercostal muscles and other soft tissues. The feature "CanReachFat" is used for this purpose.

Unlike pleural plaques, diffuse pleural thickening has a very smooth appearance and does not form an undulating bumpy interface with the lung parenchyma. Further, as the fat layer is usually not visible and parts of the thickened region might merge with the surrounding soft tissues, we require other features to help group confident regions and not-so-confident regions. For such cases, we look at whether any other portions of the candidate region are internal to the ribs and / or fat layer and whether the region is considerably long, in order to arrive at a decision. The features with percentage measures are used for this purpose. In addition, it was found that the thickness of the candidate region helps to minimise false positives.

Table 1. Features used for classification

Feature	Explanation	Comments
CanReachRibs	Pixel lies internal to rib segment	Very good predictor of plaque
CanReachSpine	Pixel lies internal to Vertebra	Confidence is somewhat low due, as intercostal tissues in paravertebral region may appear thick and mimic plaque
CanReachFat	Pixel lies internal to fat layer	Not very reliable since in many cases the layer is too thin to be visible
IsOnBump	Pixel lies on pleural bump	Good predictor of plaque, however accurate assessment using simple image processing techniques is difficult
PctBump	% pixels on pleural bump for the region	These features help identify whether a plaque region is made up of pixels that show characteristics such as internal to ribs, fat etc. If a major portion displays such characteristics, then the other portions may be included with confidence. Helps in detection of diffuse pleural thickening
PctIntRibs	% pixels internal to ribs for the region	
PctIntFat	% pixels internal to fat layer for the region	
PctIntSpine	% pixels internal to vertebra for the region	
Thickness	Thickness of the region	Helps eliminate pleural regions that may appear thick due to imaging artifacts
Length	Length of the region	Useful for recognition of diffuse pleural thickening

Since diaphragmatic plaques are not well demarcated, a different approach is needed. The features described above are not sufficient to recognise diaphragmatic plaques and may cause large number of false positives. Therefore, we decided to exclude regions detected near the diaphragm at this stage.

For every slice in the HRCT study, and for every candidate plaque pixel, the features in Table 1 are extracted. Knowledge of anatomy is used in this process. Classification and post-processing steps are carried out to arrive at the final output. The block diagram in Fig 3 outlines the sequence. Techniques used for parameter tuning and model building are also included.

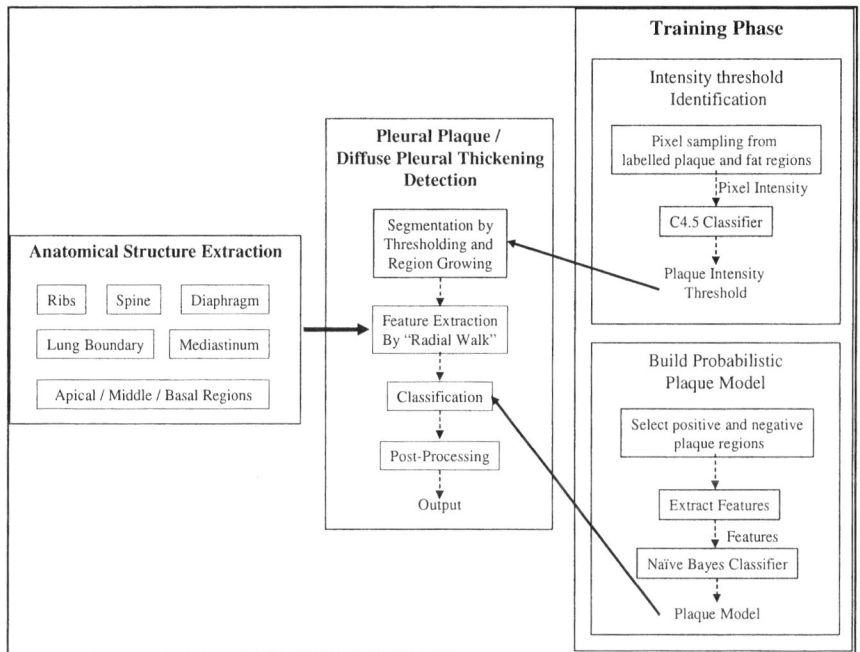

Fig. 3. System Architecture

3.2 Extraction of Anatomical Details

Some anatomical structures found to be useful in localising and improving the detection outcome are extracted from the images. There are not sufficient landmarks within the lungs to create reference atlases. However, knowledge of certain anatomical structures can be exploited in the detection of pleural plaques. Since pleural plaques can be easily discriminated from adjacent ribs and vertebral regions, extraction of relevant anatomical these structures helps to localise the plaques. Since pleural plaques are constrained on the inner side by lung parenchyma, good extraction of the lung boundary is also necessary. In the following sections, the HRCT images are blurred to highlight the regions of interest, which are **cross-hatched** for better visibility.

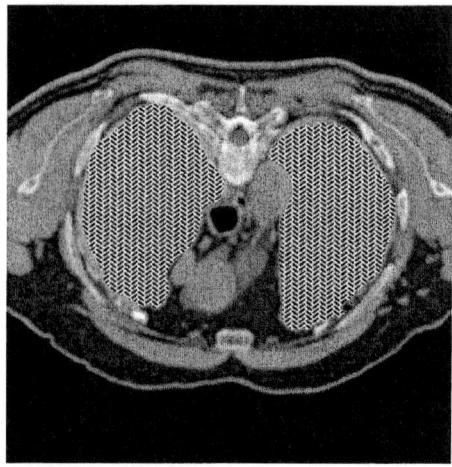

Fig. 4. Lung Boundary

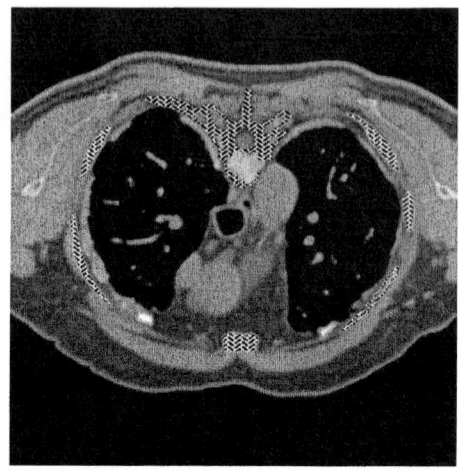

Fig. 5. Segmented ribs and vertebra

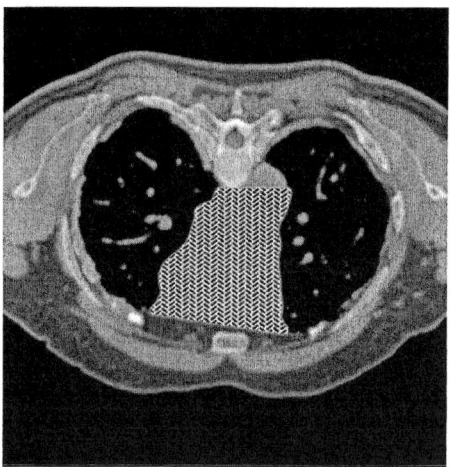

Fig. 6. Mediastinum Mask

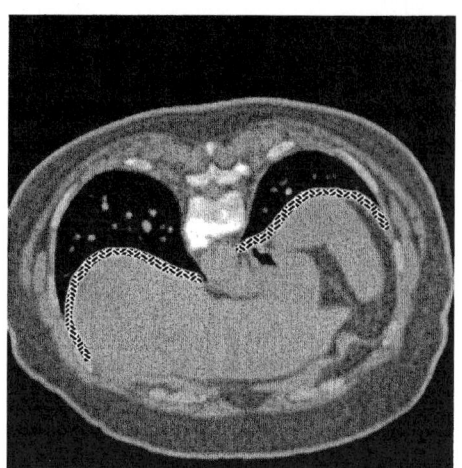

Fig. 7. Diaphragm Surface

The lung boundary is extracted by applying simple image processing techniques. A threshold level of -700 HU (Hounsfield Unit) is selected for segmentation from the surrounding soft tissues, as the lungs are mostly filled with air. Morphological operators, which alter the contours of regions using small structuring elements, are applied to obtain a smooth boundary as shown in Fig. 4.

Ribs have the highest pixel intensity in the image and hence are easily segmented. They are contrasted best when viewed in the soft tissue window of 50/350 HU. The pixel values are adjusted for this window and thresholded at an intensity level of 250. The segmented regions, however, contain calcified plaque regions as well, which must then be separated. Calcified plaques are solid in appearance compared to ribs and vertebrae, as they enclose the soft tissue of bone marrow and spine respectively. In the segmented binary image these appear as black holes surrounded by white bone.

Euler number of a region, which represents the number of holes in the region, can be easily calculated using the component labelling technique. Component labelling is an algorithm that assigns a unique label to each segmented region. For each bone sub-image, black regions are labelled. If one or more black regions larger than a certain area are detected, such bone regions are deemed to be ribs or vertebrae. The vertebra (interchangeably referred to as spine at times) is identified as the largest bone region in the top half of the image (after it is flipped if the scan is taken in a supine position). Segmented ribs and spine are highlighted in Fig. 5 and clearly calcified plaque regions are omitted.

Another useful anatomical region is the mediastinum, the structure between the lungs containing the heart, the large arteries and the veins. Pleural plaques along the mediastinum are rare and hence any region detected here is likely to be a false positive. With a mediastinum mask, all such regions can be easily excluded. A convex hull of the two lung regions is obtained from which the lungs are subtracted. From this, only the region below the level of the spine is retained, which gives the desired mediastinum mask as shown in Fig. 6.

Since detection of plaques along the diaphragm is difficult and the designed features work better for other types of plaques, a large number of false positives are detected along this surface. Hence we exclude all such regions with a diaphragm mask. The diaphragm surface is visible only in the last few slices of the basal region and anatomically the lung shape is wider here compared to its height. The aspect ratio can be a good predictor given the lung region. Hence, we first identify the lung region for each slice using our earlier work on hilum detection [14]. The bounding rectangle for each lung provides the length and width measurements to calculate aspect ratio. We extracted these attributes for nearly 450 lungs (left and right) from around 350 slices belonging to 15 studies. A decision tree learner (C4.5 in Weka [15]) was used to obtain classification rules. Once a slice is identified to contain the diaphragm, we divide each lung vertically (sagittal section) into two halves. The local minima of the lung boundary in these two halves give the starting and ending points of the diaphragm. Tracing the lung boundary between these two points provides the diaphragm surface as seen on HRCT slices. The result is as shown in Fig. 7.

The detection techniques for rib segments, spine, mediastinum mask and diaphragm were tested on the same 13 patient studies that are later used for testing pleural plaque detection. The region-based accuracy of these detection methods is shown in Table 2. It should be noted that the detection accuracy of the spine heavily influences accuracy of the mediastinum and an improvement in the former will automatically improve the latter.

Table 2. Performance measures for anatomical region detection

Module	Accuracy
Rib Segments	74%
Spine	64%
Mediastinum	69%
Diaphragm	80%

3.3 Pre-processing and Segmentation

Thresholding is usually the first operation used in any segmentation and the threshold level may be determined either empirically or statistically. We used a simple decision tree learner to determine the appropriate pixel intensity of the plaque pixels. On HRCT scans, the plaques are separated from the ribs and the extrapleural soft tissue by a thin layer of fat. Since the plaques are best contrasted when viewed in soft tissue window of 50/350 HU, the pixels are first adjusted to the soft tissue window (i.e. pixels in the range −125HU and +225HU with centre at 50HU are mapped linearly to 256 grey-scale levels and pixels below and above this range are set to zero and 255 respectively). A total of 20 images from 5 studies labelled by radiologists were used. Pixels sampled from the plaque and extra-pleural fat regions were fed into a decision tree learner (C4.5 in Weka) to obtain the threshold level.

Region growing techniques are normally used to group pixels belonging to one class to form a region. However, a seed point is needed to start the region growing process. Also, a stopping condition is required, which is normally based on the pixel intensity of the neighbouring pixels. Using anatomical knowledge, a simpler method of region growing was implemented to segment the candidate plaque regions. Since the pleural plaques are constrained by the lung parenchyma, lung boundary pixels provide a good starting point. The stopping condition based on pixel intensity was deemed unsuitable, as in many cases the fat layer that separates the plaques from extrapleural soft tissue is very thin and therefore unresolved on HRCT scans.

The lung masks are first dilated by one pixel. All pixels that lie within the dilated masks and having pixel intensity greater than the threshold learned above are marked. The lung mask is then dilated by one more pixel. Now every pixel located within the expanded band with pixel intensity greater than the threshold and also in the neighbourhood of the previously marked is included. The neighbourhood policy is enforced to terminate the growth at the fat layer when it is visible, and not grow into intercostal muscle region. These steps are repeated a number of times (determined empirically to be 7), which captures the average thickness of the plaques and gives a satisfactory result. While the focus was on capturing the percentage involvement of the pleura, further tuning of the parameters will be required while targeting, say, the pleural thickening seen on patients with mesothelioma. This process is very close to a constrained region growing technique. The candidate regions extracted from this step may include intercostal muscles and other false positives. Various feature values, extracted using anatomical knowledge help minimise such false positives.

3.4 Feature Extraction and Classification

Anatomical and pathological knowledge acquired from expert radiologists was used in feature design. Features are extracted for each pixel in the candidate region using what we call a "Radial Walk" technique. The pixels on the lung boundary internal to the candidate plaque region are extracted from the intersection of the lung boundary and the dilated candidate plaque region (see Fig 8). Pixels lying on the extrapolated line joining the lung centroid and each of the short-listed boundary pixels are labelled as belonging to candidate plaque, fat or rib regions, based on the pixel intensity and location on various anatomical masks explained above. If two or more rib pixels are encountered, then the feature "CanReachRib" is assigned to true for all plaque pixels lying on the extrapolated line. Instead, if a vertebral mask is detected, the feature "CanReachSpine" is assigned to true. Similarly, if one or more fat pixels are encountered immediately after the plaque pixels, then the feature "CanReachFat" is assigned to true. No features are extracted for pixels that are missed between the extrapolated lines. We deal with such pixels in the post-processing phase.

The pleural bumps are extracted by subtracting the lung boundary from its convex hull. Since the convex hull joins the outer most points with a line, only a portion of the bumpy region is extracted. For all candidate pixels that lie on the bumpy region, the feature "IsOnBump" is set to true.

These features were extracted for around 30,000 pixels belonging to plaque and non-plaque regions (mainly intercostal muscles) from 14 labelled images in two studies. We used a simple naïve Bayes classifier (implemented in Weka [15]) to deduce the probabilities for each feature class. This supervised learner is based on the Bayes rule for calculating posterior probabilities from prior probabilities. It is well known that even though the naïve Bayes classifier assumes conditional independence among features given the class label, it works remarkably well even when this assumption is not valid [16]. Clearly some of the features we extract are not independent. We calculate the probabilities of a pixel belonging to plaque or non-plaque class and the pixel is assigned to the class with the highest probability. Fig 9 and 10 show the candidate regions and the regions after classification.

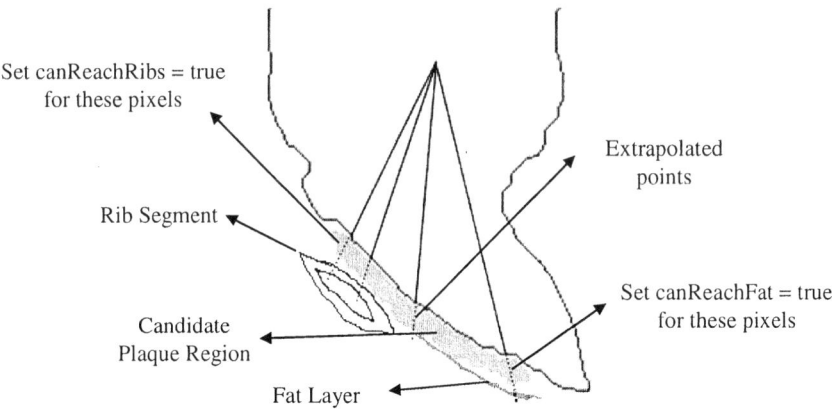

Fig. 8. Feature extraction using "Radial Walk", dotted lines depict extrapolated points (not to scale)

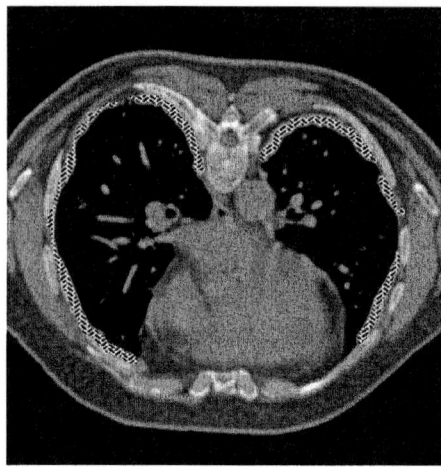 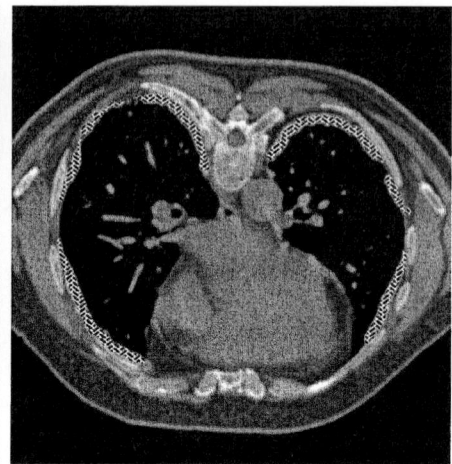

Fig. 9. Candidate regions **Fig. 10.** Classification output

3.5 Post-processing

When we extract features with the "radial walk", some pixels fall between the radial lines, therefore no features are extracted and no class label is assigned to these pixels. For such pixels we assign the majority class label in the 3 x 3 neighbourhood. Since the class labels are based on the probabilities, some portions of the candidate regions may be classified as plaque and others as non-plaque. Regions with fewer that 20% plaque pixels are ignored.

4 Results

The methods were developed and tested using 1 mm collimation scans with 15 mm inter-slice gap. The algorithm was run on 13 studies from 13 different patients, which were different from the studies used in the training set. We divided the studies into two groups. The first group contained 10 studies. After removing the first and last few slices, where the lungs were either not visible or very small, a total of 130 images was presented to a senior radiologist along with the output from the automated detection technique. This group included one case of pleural plaque and two cases of diffuse pleural thickening, forming the positive test set, and seven other studies with non-pleural diseases formed the control or negative set in the group. Of these, two predominantly had emphysema, one had predominant honeycombing, two had ground-glass opacity, one had large nodules and masses and the last one was mostly normal with one or two small lung nodules.

Since the percentage involvement of the pleural surface is clinically important, we computed our performance measures using the total number of pleural pixels involved vs. the number of pixels on the lung boundary. A radiologist was asked to mark the start and end of the pleural boundary where the plaques were wrongly detected (false positive) and where the technique missed detection (false negative). From this feedback we are able to determine the true positive (TP), false positive (FP), true negative (TN) and false negative (FN) numbers, explained below.

- TP: Number of pleural pixels labelled by radiologist as plaque and recognised as such by our method.
- FP: Number of pleural pixels identified as plaque by our method, but not labelled so by radiologist.
- TN: Number of pleural pixels labelled by radiologist as NOT plaque and recognised as such by our method.
- FN: Number of pleural pixels labelled by radiologist as plaque, but NOT recognised as such by our method.

The following performance measures were calculated.

Sensitivity = TP / (TP + FN) (1)

Specificity = TN / (TN + FP) (2)

Precision = TP / (TP + FP) (3)

Accuracy = TP + TN / (TP + FP + TN + FN) (4)

The performance results are shown in Table 3.

Table 3. Performance measures on the first test group

Measure	Positive + Control Set	Positive Set alone
Sensitivity	81 %	81%
Specificity	95%	95%
Precision	53%	83%
Accuracy	94%	91%

The precision in the positive plus control group is low compared to positive set alone since no positive example were found in the control set (TP = 0, FN = 0) and only FP were found. However, the performance on the studies in the control set with extensive pulmonary fibrosis (honeycombing) and ground-glass opacity proved satisfactory.

The second group comprised 11 images from three studies and they contained pleural plaques. They were pre-labelled by two radiologists without having seen the computerised output. However, not all occurrence of plaque was labelled on these images and hence we cannot deduce true positives and true negatives. The proportion of plaque pleural pixels detected by our technique over the plaque region labelled by radiologists yielded 60.5 %.

5 Discussion

The technique performs well on images with pleural plaque / diffuse pleural thickening, missing relatively a few regions. However on non-plaque images, many false positives are reported. These tend to be mostly in the paravertebral region (around 49%) where normal anatomy mimics the appearance of plaques. Another point of failure occurs where the rib segments are very slender and containing very little bone marrow, resulting in inadequate segmentation of ribs. The paravertebral region can be improved by taking into consideration the slices above and below. To improve bone detection, more rigorous methods such as template matching may be required, or extraction of more features than just the Euler number currently used.

It is clear from Table 1 that not all features contribute equally to the detection of pleural plaques. Feature such as "CanReachRibs" is highly reliable where as features "CanReachFat" and "IsOnBump" are not so reliable. The latter two are not reliable for very different reasons. In the case of "CanReachFat", it is due to the fact that the fat layer may or may not be visible whereas for "IsOnBump", even though it is always visible, a more sophisticated extraction method is needed.

In a trial, we accumulated confidence levels for each pixel based on the features, where each feature was weighted differently. We assigned an initial value of 1 to every candidate pixel. If fat layer could be reached, we added 1. If spine could be reached a value of 2 was added, and 3 was added if ribs could be reached. We mapped these numbers into different colours from red to green, red being the lowest and any value above 5 being green (possible values were 1 to 7). One such colour-coded image is show in Fig. 11. We are currently working on more formal methods for assigning priorities to different features. More results are presented in Fig.12.

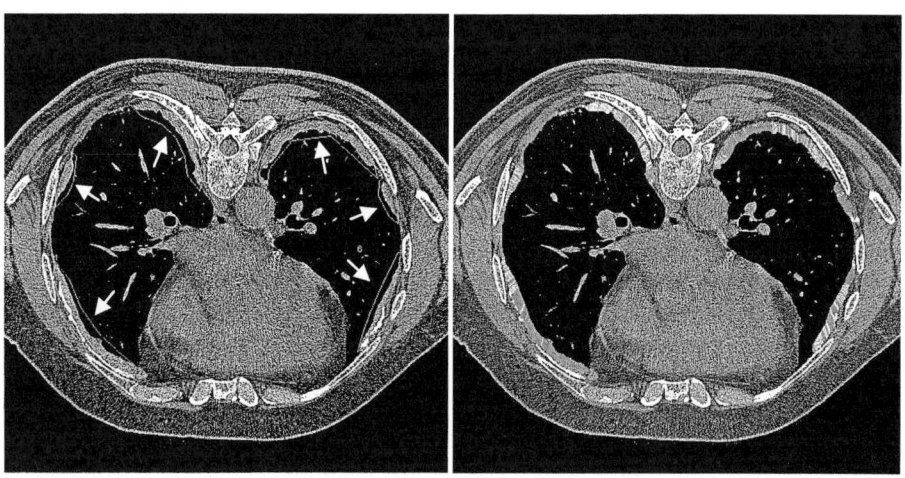

Fig. 11. Left: Original image marked by radiologist (outlined regions with arrows pointing), Right: Result with confidence levels assigned to pixels based on features. Colors range from red, yellow, blue, cyan and green; red being the lowest (darker shade represents red)

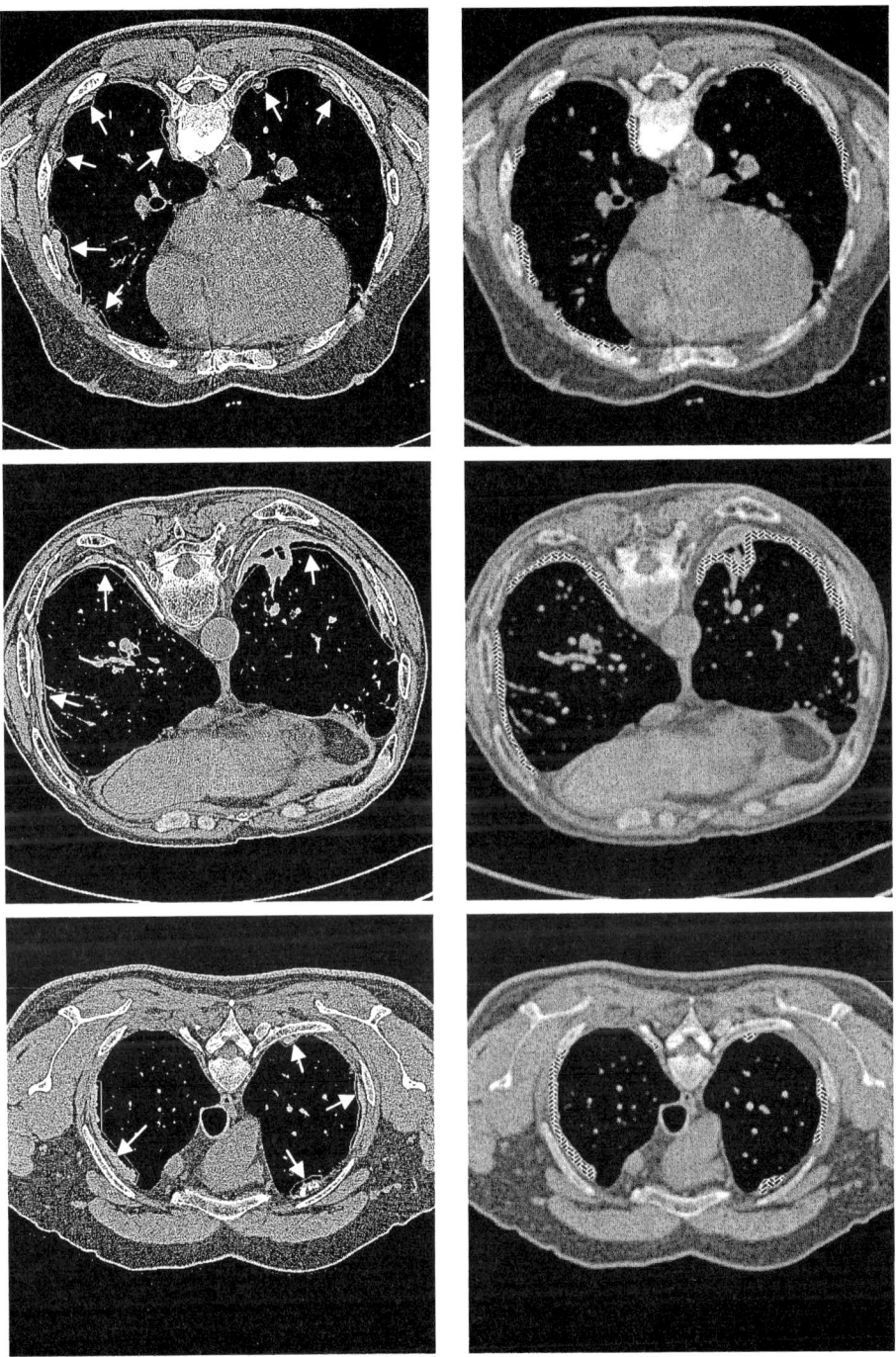

Fig. 12. Left: Original images marked by radiologist (outlined regions with arrows pointing), Right: Results of automated technique on right

Acknowledgement

This research was partially supported by the Australian Research Council through a Linkage grant (2002 – 2004), with Medical Imaging Australasia as clinical and Philips Medical Systems as industrial partners. We thank Thienco Bui for his assistance in testing some of the anatomy modules.

Reference

[1] CS White, BM Romney, AC Mason, JH Austin, BH Miller, and Z Protopapas, "Primary carcinoma of the lung overlooked at CT: analysis of findings in 14 patients", *Radiology*, Radiological Society of North America, **199**, 109 – 115, 1996.
[2] W.R. Webb, N.L. Muller, D.P. Naidich, "High-Resolution CT of the Lung, Third Edition", Lippincott Williams & Wilkins, 2001.
[3] C. Peacock, S.J. Copley, D.M. Hansell, "Asbestos-Related Benign Pleural Disease", *Clinical Radiology*, The Royal College of Radiologists, **55**, 422 – 432, 2000.
[4] Michael F. McNitt-Gray, Eric M. Hart, Nathaniel Wyckoff, James W. Sayre, Jonathan G. Goldin, and Denise R. Aberle, "A pattern classification approach to characterizing solitary pulmonary nodules imaged on high resolution CT: Preliminary results", *Medical Physics*, American Association of Physicists in Medicine, **26**, 880 – 888, 1999.
[5] Y. Matsuki, K. Nakamura, H. Watanabe, T. Aoki, H. Nakata, S. Katsuragawa, K. Doi, "Usefulness of an artificial neural network for differentiating benign from malignant pulmonary nodules on high-resolution CT: Evaluation with receiver operating characteristics analysis", *American Journal of Roentgenology*, American Roentgen Ray Society, **178**, 657 – 663, 2002.
[6] S.G. Armato III, M.L Giger, H. MacMahon, "Automated detection of lung nodules in CT scans: Preliminary results", *Medical Physics*, American Association of Physicists in Medicine, **28**(8), 1552 – 1561, 2001.
[7] K. Kanazawa, Y. Kawata, N.Niki, H.Satoh, H.Ohmatsu, R. Kakinuma, M.Kaneko, N. Moriyama, K. Eguchi, "Computer-aided diagnosis for pulmonary nodules based on helical CT images", *Computerized Medical Imaging and Graphics*, Elsevier Science Ltd, **22**, 157 – 167, 1998.
[8] R. Uppaluri, E.A. Hoffman, M. Sonka, P.G. Hartley, G.W. Hunninghake, G. McLennan, "Computer recognition of regional lung disease patterns", *American Journal of Respiratory and Critical Care Medicine*, The American Thoracic Society, **160**, 648 – 654, 1999.
[9] H.U. Kauczor, K. Heitmann, C.P. Heussel, D. Marwede, T. Uthmann, M. Thelen, "Automatic Detection and quantification of ground-glass opacities on high-resolution CT using multiple neural networks: Comparison with a density mask", *American Journal of Roentgenology*, American Roentgen Ray Society, **175**, 1329 – 1334, 2000.
[10] S.Delorme, M.A.K. Reichenbecher, I.Zuna, W.Schlegel, G.K. Gerhard, "Usual Interstitial Pneumonia: Quantitative assessment of high-resolution computed tomography findings by computer-assisted texture-based image analysis", *Investigative Radiology*, Lippincott-Raven Publishers, **32**(9), 566 – 574, 1997.
[11] François Chabat, Xiao-Peng Hu, David M. Hansell, and Guang-Zhong Yang, "ERS Transform for the Automated Detection of Bronchial Abnormalities on CT of the Lungs", *IEEE Transactions On Medical Imaging*, **20** (9), 2001.

[12] M. Rudrapatna, A. Sowmya, P. Wilson, "Automatic Detection of Hilum and Parenchymal Bands on HRCT Lung Images", proceedings of *IEEE Conference on Cybernetics and Intelligent Systems*, 768 – 773, 2004.
[13] C. Wang, M. Rudrapatna, A. Sowmya, "Lung Disease Detection Using Frequency Spectrum Analysis", proceedings of *Fourth Indian Conference on Computer Vision, Graphics and Image Processing*, 485 – 490, 2004.
[14] A. Misra, M. Rudrapatna, A. Sowmya, "Automatic Lung Segmentation: A Comparison of Anatomical and Machine Learning Approaches" proceedings of *International Conference on Intelligent Sensors, Sensor Networks and Information Processing*, 451 – 456, 2004.
[15] Ian H. Witten, Eibe Frank, "Data Mining: Practical machine learning tools with Java implementations", Morgan Kaufmann, 2000.
[16] Pedro Domingos and Michael Pazzani, "On the Optimality of the Simple Bayesian Classifier under Zero-One Loss", *Machine Learning*, Kluwer Academic Publishers, **29**, 103 – 130, 1997.

Fundamental Limits in 3D Landmark Localization

Karl Rohr

University of Heidelberg, IPMB, DKFZ Heidelberg,
Dept. Intelligent Bioinformatics Systems, Biomedical Computer Vision Group,
Im Neuenheimer Feld 580, D-69120 Heidelberg, Germany
k.rohr@dkfz.de

Abstract. This work analyses the accuracy of estimating the location of 3D landmarks and characteristic image structures. Based on nonlinear estimation theory we study the minimal stochastic errors of the position estimate caused by noisy data. Given analytic models of the image intensities we derive closed-form expressions for the Cramér-Rao bound for different 3D structures such as 3D edges, 3D ridges, 3D lines, and 3D blobs. It turns out, that the precision of localization depends on the noise level, the size of the region-of-interest, the width of the intensity transitions, as well as on other parameters describing the considered image structure. The derived lower bounds can serve as benchmarks and the performance of existing algorithms can be compared with them. To give an impression of the achievable accuracy numeric examples are presented. Moreover, by experimental investigations we demonstrate that the derived lower bounds can be achieved by fitting parametric intensity models directly to the image data.

1 Motivation

Performance characterization in biomedical image analysis is gaining increased importance as more and more approaches for the same or similar tasks are developed. On the one hand, performance characterization serves a clear practical need, e.g., when we have to select an algorithm for a certain application. On the other hand, validation and evaluation studies are a major step towards a sound description of algorithms as well as the foundation of the field.

This work is concerned with characterizing the performance of *3D landmark localization*. Landmarks are preferred features for a variety of image analysis tasks, e.g., multi-modality image registration, motion analysis, as well as object measurement, and the performance in these tasks directly depends on the quality of extracting these features from images. However, work on performance evaluation of 3D landmark extraction is rare. For an experimental study on 3D differential approaches for point landmark extraction in 3D tomographic images of the human brain see [3]. Here, we describe an *analytic study* on 3D landmark localization. We take the statistical point of view to analyze the localization errors caused by noisy data. We consider a continuous image model that represents the blur as well as noise introduced by an imaging system. For this model we derive analytic results stating lower bounds for the localization uncertainty (highest possible precision). The lower bounds are evaluated for explicitly given feature models. We show that the precision of localization in general depends on the noise level, the size of the region-of-interest, the width of the intensity transitions, as well as on other parameters describing the systematic intensity variations.

Our study on the positional random errors is based on nonlinear estimation theory and the Cramér-Rao bound (CRB). As explicitly given models of image features we investigate 3D edges, 3D ridges, 3D lines, and 3D blobs. This generalizes the work in [4] on 2D step edges and that in [6] on 2D edges and corners. Note, that the derivation of analytic results for 3D image features is much more extensive in comparison to the 2D case. For use of Cramér-Rao bounds in the case of prior edge extraction and 2D curve fitting we refer to [2],[5].

We derive closed-form expressions and also provide numeric examples which represent the highest possible precision for localizing the considered landmarks. This means, we can use the formulas and numeric values as *benchmarks* and compare them with the performance of existing algorithms for 3D landmark localization. Note, that here we derive uncertainty lower bounds for the location. Therefore, we may assume that all model parameters except the ones for the location are known. On the other hand, if the other parameters are also unknown and thus have to be estimated then the resulting bound can only increase. Therefore, the bounds derived here are indeed *fundamental limits*. In addition, as a comparison, we perform an experimental study where we apply the model fitting approach in [9] for localizing 3D landmarks in 3D tomographic images. It turns out that the theoretical lower bounds can actually be achieved.

2 Nonlinear Estimation Theory and Cramér-Rao Lower Bound

Our aim is to derive *analytic* results for the highest possible precision (minimal uncertainty) in localizing landmarks in images. To this end we model landmarks by their systematic intensity variations which are disturbed by an additive noise process. Our observations $g(\mathbf{x})$ are continuous functions extended over certain intervals. Signal measurements are available within finite regions of an image (regions-of-interest). We deal with space-dependent random variables, i.e. random processes. The model $g_M(\mathbf{x}, \mathbf{p})$ describing the systematic intensity variations depends on the parameter vector $\mathbf{p} = (p_1, ..., p_n)^T$ and, in general, is nonlinear. Therefore, nonlinear estimation theory (e.g., van Trees [8]) is the suitable framework.

Depending on the image dimension (2D or 3D) and the type of landmark (0D, 1D, or 2D image feature) the number of location parameters to be estimated differs. In the case of 2D images, for example, point landmarks such as blobs require two parameters while for (straight) lines and edges only one parameter determines their location (the position in orthogonal direction is not uniquely defined). In the case of 3D images we have to estimate the following number of location parameters: Three for point landmarks (0D feature), two for lines and ridges (1D feature), and one for edges (2D feature).

The image noise $n(\mathbf{x})$ will be assumed to be a sample function from an additive zero-mean white Gaussian noise process that is independent of the signal and has a spectral power density $L_n(\mathbf{u}) = \sigma_n^2$. Our image model then reads

$$g(\mathbf{x}) = g_M(\mathbf{x}, \mathbf{p}) + n(\mathbf{x}), \quad \mathbf{x}_1 \leq \mathbf{x} \leq \mathbf{x}_2. \tag{1}$$

Note that by choosing a particular space point $\mathbf{x} = \mathbf{x}_i$ a random variable $n(\mathbf{x}_i)$ with variance σ_n^2 is defined. Note also that the assumed noise model is an approximation to the error statistics of biomedical images. While the assumption of the Gaussian noise model often holds, it has been argued that for large signal-to-noise ratios the dependence of the noise on the signal should be taken into account [1]. However, here we assume that this dependence can be neglected.

In the following we suppose to have no statistical a priori knowledge about $\mathbf{p}$ and therefore treat $\mathbf{p}$ as a non-random variable. In general, we have to deal with the case of multiple parameter estimation. The uncertainties of the estimated parameter vector $\hat{\mathbf{p}} = (\hat{p}_1, ..., \hat{p}_n)^T$ are represented by the covariance matrix

$$\boldsymbol{\Sigma} = cov\{\hat{\mathbf{p}}\} = E\{(\hat{\mathbf{p}} - \mathbf{p})(\hat{\mathbf{p}} - \mathbf{p})^T\} = \begin{pmatrix} \sigma_{\hat{p}_1}^2 & \cdots & \sigma_{\hat{p}_1 \hat{p}_n} \\ \vdots & \ddots & \vdots \\ \sigma_{\hat{p}_n \hat{p}_1} & \cdots & \sigma_{\hat{p}_n}^2 \end{pmatrix}.$$

Lower bounds for the elements of this matrix are determined by the *Fisher information matrix*. In the case of 3D images this matrix can be stated as

$$\mathbf{F} = \frac{1}{\sigma_n^2} \int_{x_1}^{x_2} \int_{y_1}^{y_2} \int_{z_1}^{z_2} \frac{\partial g_M(\mathbf{x}, \mathbf{p})}{\partial \mathbf{p}} \cdot \left(\frac{\partial g_M(\mathbf{x}, \mathbf{p})}{\partial \mathbf{p}} \right)^T d\mathbf{x}. \tag{2}$$

If $\hat{\mathbf{p}}$ is an unbiased estimate of $\mathbf{p}$ then the errors are bounded by

$$\boldsymbol{\Sigma} \geq \mathbf{F}^{-1}, \tag{3}$$

which means that the symmetric matrix $\boldsymbol{\Sigma} - \mathbf{F}^{-1}$ is positive semidefinite. Since the diagonal elements of positive semidefinite matrices are larger or equal to zero, the uncertainty of an element of $\hat{\mathbf{p}}$ is bounded by

$$\sigma_{\hat{p}_i}^2 \geq (\mathbf{F}^{-1})_{ii}, \tag{4}$$

where $(\mathbf{F}^{-1})_{ii}$ is the ii-th element of $\mathbf{F}^{-1}$. This inequality is usually referred to as *Cramér-Rao bound (CRB)*. The lower bound can be compared with the actual variance of a certain estimation scheme. For an efficient estimate, (4) is satisfied with equality. However, this is only the case if g_M depends linearly on $\mathbf{p}$. Then, the maximum-likelihood estimate is the estimate with minimum variance. It is possible that the variance in the nonlinear case approaches this bound (see below).

For general 3D image features the location is defined by three parameters $\mathbf{p} = (x_0, y_0, z_0)^T$ and we have a symmetric 3×3 matrix

$$\mathbf{F} = \begin{pmatrix} F_{11} & F_{12} & F_{13} \\ F_{21} & F_{22} & F_{23} \\ F_{31} & F_{32} & F_{33} \end{pmatrix}, \quad (5)$$

where $F_{21} = F_{12}, F_{31} = F_{13}$, and $F_{23} = F_{32}$. With

$$det\mathbf{F} = F_{11}(F_{22}F_{33} - F_{23}^2) - F_{12}(F_{12}F_{33} - F_{23}F_{13}) + F_{13}(F_{12}F_{23} - F_{22}F_{13})$$

we thus have for the positional parameters the following bounds:

$$\sigma_{\hat{x}_0}^2 \geq CRB_{\hat{x}_0} = \frac{F_{22}F_{33} - F_{23}^2}{det\mathbf{F}} \quad (6)$$

$$\sigma_{\hat{y}_0}^2 \geq CRB_{\hat{y}_0} = \frac{F_{11}F_{33} - F_{13}^2}{det\mathbf{F}} \quad (7)$$

$$\sigma_{\hat{z}_0}^2 \geq CRB_{\hat{z}_0} = \frac{F_{11}F_{22} - F_{12}^2}{det\mathbf{F}}. \quad (8)$$

Regions-of-interest (observation windows) are specified by the half-widths $w_x, w_y,$ and w_z around the landmark position $(x_0, y_0, z_0)^T$.

3 Cramér-Rao Bounds for 3D Landmark Localization

The framework described above is now applied to derive closed-form expressions for the Cramér-Rao bound for different 3D image structures. We consider 3D edges, 3D ridges, 3D lines, and 3D blobs. The investigated structures are examples for 0D, 1D, and 2D features. Note, that the derivation of analytic results for 3D image features is much more extensive in comparison to the 2D case. On the one hand, the Fisher information matrix in (2) and (5) contains nine elements in comparison to four elements, and, on the other hand, the integrals that have to be calculated are much more complex. For reasons of space restriction we concentrate on the main steps and results.

We also note, that the models under consideration depend on several parameters, however, here we are only interested in deriving uncertainty lower bounds for the location. Therefore, in the following, we may assume that all model parameters except the ones for the location are known. On the other hand, if all parameters are unknown and thus have to be estimated then the resulting bound can only increase (see Scharf [7]). Therefore, the bounds derived here are indeed lower bounds (fundamental limits).

3.1 3D Edges

First, we consider a Gaussian smoothed 3D step edge with contrast a and transition width σ. We arbitrarily assume that the edge has intensity variations only

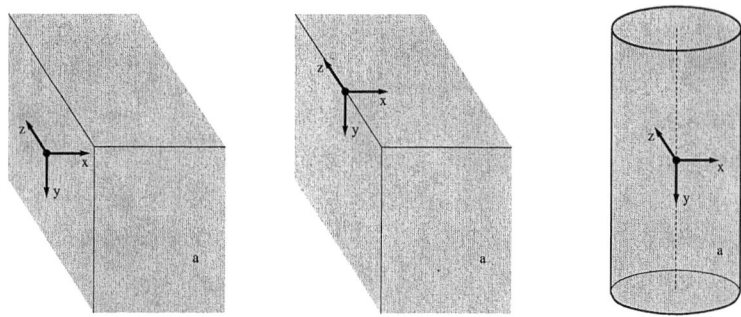

Fig. 1. Models of a 3D edge (left), 3D ridge (middle), and 3D line (right)

along the x-axis and denote its location by x_0 (see Fig. 1, left). To simplify the calculations we choose the coordinate system in such a way that $x_0 = 0$. The region-of-interest (ROI) defined by the half-widths w_x, w_y, and w_z is placed symmetrically around x_0 and some position $y_0 = 0$ and $z_0 = 0$ in y- and z-direction. The model function of this image feature is given by

$$Edge3D(x,y,z) = a\phi(\frac{x}{\sigma}), \tag{9}$$

with the Gaussian error function $\phi(x) = \int_{-\infty}^{x} G(\xi)d\xi$. For this model there is one uniquely defined location parameter and the Cramér-Rao bound calculates to

$$\sigma^2_{\hat{x}_0, Edge3D} \geq CRB_{\hat{x}_0, Edge3D} = \frac{\sqrt{\pi}\sigma}{2a^2 \text{erf}(\frac{w_x}{\sigma})} \cdot \frac{\sigma_n^2}{w_y w_z}, \tag{10}$$

where $\text{erf}(x) = 2\phi(\sqrt{2}x) - 1$. To easier interpret the formula we can derive an approximation by assuming that the width w_x is much larger than the width σ of the Gaussian, i.e. $w_x \gg \sigma$ (this means that the significant intensity variations essentially lie within the ROI, which is typically the case). Then we obtain

$$CRB_{\hat{x}_0, Edge3D} \approx \frac{\sqrt{\pi}\sigma}{2a^2} \cdot \frac{\sigma_n^2}{w_y w_z}. \tag{11}$$

We see that the bound is proportional to the ratio $\sigma_n^2/(w_y w_z)$ of the noise level and the width of the ROI in y- and z-direction. The contrast a has a large influence on the precision since it appears (inverse) quadratically. The approximate bound depends linearly on the edge width σ. We also see that if the structural intensity variations are essentially captured in x-direction then the precision cannot be improved by increasing w_x. On the other hand, we can improve the localization precision by extending the ROI in y- or z-direction (enlarging w_y or w_z). The relation to an analogous 2D edge model is $CRB_{\hat{x}_0, Edge3D} = 1/(2w_z) \cdot CRB_{\hat{x}_0, Edge2D}$.

3.2 3D Ridges

Next we consider a model of a 3D ridge structure. This structure is a 1D feature and its extremal points define a line in 3D images. Actually, such a structure can be modeled by extending a Gaussian smoothed 2D L-corner model to 3D. We use an L-corner with an aperture angle of 90° and assume that we have no variation in z-direction (Fig. 1, middle):

$$Ridge3D(x,y,z) = a\phi(\frac{x}{\sigma})\phi(\frac{y}{\sigma}). \tag{12}$$

Assuming that $w_x, w_y \gg \sigma$, the analytic lower bounds for the two positional parameters compute to

$$CRB_{\hat{x}_0, Ridge3D} \approx \frac{\sqrt{\pi}\sigma}{a^2} \cdot \frac{\sigma_n^2}{w_y w_z} \tag{13}$$

$$CRB_{\hat{y}_0, Ridge3D} \approx \frac{\sqrt{\pi}\sigma}{a^2} \cdot \frac{\sigma_n^2}{w_x w_z}. \tag{14}$$

3.3 3D Lines

3D lines are 1D features in 3D images. We analyze a 3D Gaussian line model with elliptic cross-section and extended in y-direction (Fig. 1, right). Such a model is often used for representing 3D vessels and can be written as

$$Line3D(x,y,z) = a\, e^{-\frac{x^2}{2\sigma_x^2}} e^{-\frac{z^2}{2\sigma_z^2}}. \tag{15}$$

For the lower bounds we obtain

$$\sigma^2_{\hat{x}_0, Line3D} \geq \frac{\sigma_x}{\pi a^2 \sigma_z \left(-2\sqrt{2}\frac{w_x}{\sigma_x}G(\frac{\sqrt{2}w_x}{\sigma_x}) + \text{erf}(\frac{w_x}{\sigma_x})\right)\text{erf}(\frac{w_z}{\sigma_z})} \cdot \frac{\sigma_n^2}{w_y} \tag{16}$$

$$\sigma^2_{\hat{z}_0, Line3D} \geq \frac{\sigma_z}{\pi a^2 \sigma_x \text{erf}(\frac{w_x}{\sigma_x})\left(-2\sqrt{2}\frac{w_z}{\sigma_z}G(\frac{\sqrt{2}w_z}{\sigma_z}) + \text{erf}(\frac{w_x}{\sigma_x})\right)} \cdot \frac{\sigma_n^2}{w_y}. \tag{17}$$

Assuming $w_x \gg \sigma_x$ and $w_z \gg \sigma_z$ we have

$$CRB_{\hat{x}_0, Line3D} \approx \frac{\sigma_x}{\pi a^2 \sigma_z} \cdot \frac{\sigma_n^2}{w_y} \tag{18}$$

$$CRB_{\hat{z}_0, Line3D} \approx \frac{\sigma_z}{\pi a^2 \sigma_x} \cdot \frac{\sigma_n^2}{w_y}. \tag{19}$$

In comparison to an analogous 2D Gaussian line model, the result depends on the ratio between σ_x and σ_z. Assuming $\sigma_x = \sigma_z = \sigma = 1$ the uncertainty for the 3D Gaussian line is a factor of $\sqrt{\pi}$ smaller compared to the 2D Gaussian line.

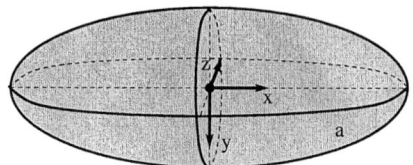

Fig. 2. Model of a 3D blob

3.4 3D Blobs

Finally, we consider 3D anisotropic blobs as point landmarks in 3D images (Fig. 2). Such a model can be used, for example, to represent artificial markers, parts of bone structures, the human eye, or the ventricular horns in human brain images (if we take one half of the model, cf. [9]). We define the centerpoint as the point we want to localize and model such structures by a trivariate Gaussian

$$Blob3D(x,y,z) = a\, e^{-\frac{x^2}{2\sigma_x^2}}\, e^{-\frac{y^2}{2\sigma_y^2}}\, e^{-\frac{z^2}{2\sigma_z^2}}. \quad (20)$$

The localization uncertainty for this structure computes to

$$\sigma_{\hat{x}_0,Blob3D}^2 \geq \frac{2\sigma_x \sigma_n^2}{\pi^{\frac{3}{2}} a^2 \sigma_y \sigma_z \left(-2\sqrt{2}\frac{w_x}{\sigma_x} G(\frac{\sqrt{2}w_x}{\sigma_x}) + \mathrm{erf}(\frac{w_x}{\sigma_x})\right) \mathrm{erf}(\frac{w_y}{\sigma_y}) \mathrm{erf}(\frac{w_z}{\sigma_z})} \quad (21)$$

$$\sigma_{\hat{y}_0,Blob3D}^2 \geq \frac{2\sigma_y \sigma_n^2}{\pi^{\frac{3}{2}} a^2 \sigma_x \sigma_z \,\mathrm{erf}(\frac{w_x}{\sigma_x}) \left(-2\sqrt{2}\frac{w_y}{\sigma_y} G(\frac{\sqrt{2}w_y}{\sigma_y}) + \mathrm{erf}(\frac{w_y}{\sigma_y})\right) \mathrm{erf}(\frac{w_z}{\sigma_z})} \quad (22)$$

$$\sigma_{\hat{z}_0,Blob3D}^2 \geq \frac{2\sigma_z \sigma_n^2}{\pi^{\frac{3}{2}} a^2 \sigma_x \sigma_y \,\mathrm{erf}(\frac{w_x}{\sigma_x}) \mathrm{erf}(\frac{w_y}{\sigma_y}) \left(-2\sqrt{2}\frac{w_z}{\sigma_z} G(\frac{\sqrt{2}w_z}{\sigma_z}) + \mathrm{erf}(\frac{w_z}{\sigma_z})\right)} \quad (23)$$

Assuming $w_x \gg \sigma_x, w_y \gg \sigma_y, w_z \gg \sigma_z$, we obtain the relatively simple formulas

$$CRB_{\hat{x}_0,Blob3D} \approx \frac{2\sigma_x \sigma_n^2}{\pi^{\frac{3}{2}} a^2 \sigma_y \sigma_z} \quad (24)$$

$$CRB_{\hat{y}_0,Blob3D} \approx \frac{2\sigma_y \sigma_n^2}{\pi^{\frac{3}{2}} a^2 \sigma_x \sigma_z} \quad (25)$$

$$CRB_{\hat{z}_0,Blob3D} \approx \frac{2\sigma_z \sigma_n^2}{\pi^{\frac{3}{2}} a^2 \sigma_x \sigma_y}. \quad (26)$$

For x_0 the precision depends on the ratio $\sigma_x/(\sigma_y \sigma_z)$. The result for y_0 and z_0 is analogous. In the case of an isotropic blob ($\sigma_x = \sigma_y = \sigma_z = \sigma$) we have

$$CRB_{\hat{x}_0,Blob3D} = CRB_{\hat{y}_0,Blob3D} = CRB_{\hat{z}_0,Blob3D} \approx \frac{2\sigma_n^2}{\pi^{\frac{3}{2}} a^2 \sigma}. \quad (27)$$

In contrast to an analogously defined 2D blob the result depends on the width σ. The relation between isotropic 2D and 3D blobs can be stated as $CRB_{\hat{x}_0,Blob3D} =$

$1/(\sqrt{\pi}\sigma) \cdot CRB_{\hat{x}_0, Blob2D}$. Thus, for $\sigma = 1$, for example, the localization uncertainty for a 3D blob is a factor of 0.56 lower in comparison to a 2D blob, while for $\sigma = 0.1$ the localization uncertainty is a factor of 5.64 higher.

4 Numeric Examples and Experimental Investigations

In this section, we present numeric examples of the achievable precision for the above studied landmark models as well as describe results of experimental investigations. The resulting precision will be presented in terms of the image grid by identifying the units of the space coordinates with pixel or voxel positions. The pixel or voxel spacing will be denoted by *pix* or *vox*, respectively, and the intensity values will be characterized by the dimension *gr*.

4.1 Numeric Examples

We state numeric results for the following landmark models: 2D and 3D step edges, 2D and 3D lines, as well as 2D and 3D blobs. To ease a comparison we use the same parameter values for all examples below. We use ROIs of size 25×25 pixels (2D) or $25 \times 25 \times 25$ voxels (3D), which means that $w_x = w_y = 12pix$ or $w_x = w_y = w_z = 12vox$. Furthermore, for the intensity contrast we choose $a = 100gr$ and for the noise level we assume $\sigma_n^2 = (5gr)^2$. Note, that we present the numeric values of the uncertainties in terms of the standard deviation (square root of the variance) in order to be better comparable with the space coordinates.

We first consider a 2D step edge with transition width $\sigma = 1pix$. Note, that we can use the same model as in the 3D case in (9). Applying the approximation of the Cramér-Rao bound, which is valid since $w_x = 12pix \gg \sigma = 1pix$, the localization precision computes to $\sigma_{\hat{x}_0, Edge2D} \approx 0.0192pix$. For the 3D step edge $Edge3D(\mathbf{x})$ with the same parameter setting and applying (11) we obtain $\sigma_{\hat{x}_0, Edge3D} \approx 0.0039vox$. Thus, the precision is about five times better than in the 2D case. It should be noted that this (subvoxel) precision can only be achieved if a and σ (and the orientation of the edge) are determined correctly and surely only if the model is valid. However, the obtained precision which is better than $1/100vox$ is amazing.

Next we consider a 2D Gaussian line model. The model is analogous to the 3D case in (15) except that the term including the z-coordinate is omitted. Using the same parameter values as above and $\sigma_x = 1pix$ we yield $\sigma_{\hat{x}_0, Line2D} \approx 0.0108pix$. In the 3D case, for the model $Line3D(\mathbf{x})$ applying (18),(19) with $\sigma_x = \sigma_z = 1vox$ we obtain $\sigma_{\hat{x}_0, Line3D} = \sigma_{\hat{z}_0, Line3D} \approx 0.0081vox$. It can be seen that the precision in the 3D case is somewhat better than in the 2D case.

Finally, we present numeric results for 2D and 3D blob structures. For the 2D Gaussian blob model (analogous to the 3D case) with $\sigma_x = \sigma_y = 1pix$ the localization precision calculates to $\sigma_{\hat{x}_0, Blob2D} = \sigma_{\hat{y}_0, Blob2D} \approx 0.0399pix$. For the 3D Gaussian blob model $Blob3D(\mathbf{x})$ in (20) with $\sigma_x = \sigma_y = \sigma_z = 1vox$ we obtain $\sigma_{\hat{x}_0, Blob3D} = \sigma_{\hat{y}_0, Blob3D} = \sigma_{\hat{z}_0, Blob3D} \approx 0.0300vox$. Also in this case the precision in 3D is better than in 2D.

4.2 Experimental Investigations

The numeric values stated above are theoretical values and represent the highest possible precision for localizing the considered landmarks. This means, we can use these values as benchmarks and compare them with the performance of existing algorithms for landmark localization. Here, as a comparison, we apply a model fitting approach which has been introduced in [9] for localizing 3D landmarks in 3D tomographic images. With this approach parametric intensity models are directly fit to the image data using least-squares minimization to determine estimates of the model parameters including the position.

Our study is based on 2D and 3D images which have been generated using the intensity models introduced above with additive white Gaussian noise of different levels. For each image we randomly varied (using a uniform distribution) the correct (subvoxel) position of the landmark within an interval of $[-1,1]vox$ in each coordinate. In addition, to initialize the model fitting approach we randomly varied (again using a uniform distribution) the model parameters around the correct values within certain intervals. We varied the intensity levels of the background and structure a_0, a_1 within $[-10,10]gr$, each coordinate of the position x_0, y_0, z_0 within $[-1,1]vox$, and the blurring (width) parameters $\sigma_x, \sigma_y, \sigma_z$ within $[-0.2, 0.2]vox$. In total, for each noise level, we carried out 1000 experiments, i.e., using 1000 different images and 1000 different initializations of the model fitting approach. The precision of the position estimate is then computed as the standard deviation, for example, in case of the x-coordinate as

$$\sigma_{\hat{x}_0} = \sqrt{\frac{1}{N-1} \sum_{i=1}^{N} (x_{0,i} - \overline{x}_0)^2}, \qquad (28)$$

where $\overline{x}_0$ denotes the mean and N the number of experiments ($N = 1000$ in our case). In all our experiments we used ROIs of sizes 25×25 pixels or $25 \times 25 \times 25$ voxels, respectively, i.e. $w_x = w_y = w_z = 12vox$.

In the experiments, the noise level is specified by the standard deviation σ_n as in the formulas above. In addition, we also state the corresponding signal-to-noise ratio (SNR), which is computed as the ratio between the variance of the signal and that of the noise by

$$SNR = \frac{\sigma_g^2}{\sigma_n^2} = \frac{1}{m\,\sigma_n^2} \sum_{i=1}^{m} (g(\mathbf{x}_i) - \overline{g})^2, \qquad (29)$$

where $\overline{g}$ is the mean intensity over all intensities $g(\mathbf{x}_i)$ within the ROI consisting of m pixels (voxels).

We first study the localization of line (vessel) structures in 2D images using the Gaussian line model. The landmark position is the center point of the line along a cross-section within a symmetric ROI. As parameter values for the intensity levels of the background and the structure we choose $a_0 = 50gr$ and $a_1 = 150gr$, i.e., the contrast is $a = 100gr$. For the width of the line we choose $\sigma = 3pix$. From the experiment it turned out that the position es-

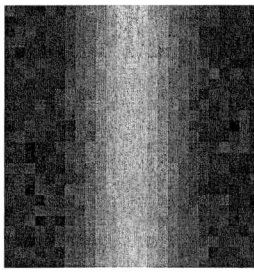 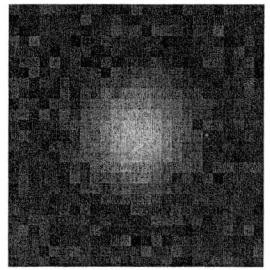 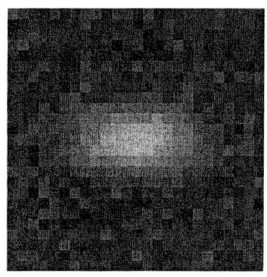

Fig. 3. 3D example images with noise. Isotropic 3D Gaussian line: Longitudinal (left) and axial cross-section (middle) ($a_0 = 50gr, a_1 = 150gr, \sigma_x = \sigma_y = 3vox, \sigma_n = 5gr$), and anisotropic 3D blob: xz−cross-section (right) ($\sigma_x = 4vox, \sigma_y = 3vox, \sigma_z = 2vox$)

timate is unbiased, i.e., the systematic error is zero. The result for the precision of the position estimate as a function of the noise level σ_n when applying the model-fitting approach has been summarized in Tab. 1. We chose values of $\sigma_n = 1, 3, 5, 10, 50gr$ which correspond to signal-to-noise ratios of $SNR = 1222.22, 135.80, 48.89, 12.22, 0.49$, respectively. In addition, we carried out experiments without noise ($\sigma_n = 0gr$), where we obtained a precision of ca. $10^{-8}vox$, i.e., the uncertainty can be considered to be zero. In comparison, in Tab. 1 we have also listed the theoretically derived values based on the Cramér-Rao bound. It can be seen that the agreement between the theoretical and the experimental values is very good. The agreement is even more remarkable since the analytic derivation does not consider discretization effects due to sampling and quantization, while in the experiments naturally discrete images have to used. Moreover, in the experiments we also estimated the model parameters a_0, a_1, and σ in addition to the positional parameters.

We have also analyzed the 3D Gaussian line model $Line3D(\mathbf{x})$ in (15). We have used the same parameter values as in the 2D case and assumed a circular cross-section of the line of width $\sigma_x = \sigma_z = 3vox$. The noise levels $\sigma_n = 1, 3, 5, 10, 50gr$ correspond to SNR levels $SNR = 370.54, 41.17, 14.82, 3.71, 0.15$. As an example, we show in Fig. 3 (left, middle) images of longitudinal and axial cross-sections of the 3D Gaussian line model with added noise of $\sigma_n = 5gr$. Tab. 2 reveals that the agreement between the theoretical and experimental values is very good. The accuracy in the 3D case is about a factor of two better than in the 2D case.

Next we study the localization of blobs in 2D images consisting of a bivariate anisotropic Gaussian function. The landmark position is the center point of the blob. As above we choose an intensity contrast of $a = 100gr$ ($a_0 = 50gr$, $a_1 = 150gr$). We first consider an isotropic blob ($\sigma_x = \sigma_y = \sigma$) with $\sigma = 3pix$. Again, from the experiment it turned out that the position estimate is unbiased. The result for the precision of the position estimate as a function of the noise level σ_n for the model-fitting approach has been summarized in Tab. 3. We chose values of $\sigma_n = 1, 3, 5, 10, 50gr$ which correspond to signal-to-noise ratios of $SNR = 370.54, 41.17, 14.82, 3.71, 0.15$. In comparison, in Tab. 3 we have also listed the theoretically derived values based on the Cramér-Rao bound. It can be seen that the agreement between the theoretical and the experimental values is very good.

The result for an anisotropic 2D blob with $\sigma_x = 4pix$ and $\sigma_y = 2pix$ has been listed in Tab. 4. Here the accuracy in $y-$direction is a factor of two better than in $x-$direction.

Finally, we consider the localization of a blob in 3D images using the 3D blob model $Blob3D(\mathbf{x})$ in (20) consisting of a trivariate Gaussian function. The landmark position is the center point of the 3D blob. We choose the same parameter values for the intensity levels as above and first investigated an isotropic

Table 1. Localization of a 2D Gaussian line with $\sigma_x = 3pix$: Standard deviation of the precision as a function of the standard deviation σ_n of the noise

$\sigma_n [gr]$	1	3	5	10	50
Theory, $\sigma_{\hat{x}_0}$ [pix]	0.0038	0.0113	0.0188	0.0376	0.1878
Experiment, $\sigma_{\hat{x}_0}$ [pix]	0.0037	0.0111	0.0182	0.0367	0.1798

Table 2. Localization of a 3D Gaussian line with $\sigma_x = \sigma_z = 3vox$: Standard deviation of the precision as a function of the standard deviation σ_n of the noise

σ_n [gr]	1	3	5	10	50
Theory, $\sigma_{\hat{x}_0}$ [vox]	0.0016	0.0049	0.0081	0.0163	0.0814
Experiment, $\sigma_{\hat{x}_0}$ [vox]	0.0016	0.0049	0.0082	0.0162	0.0831

Table 3. Localization of an isotropic 2D blob with $\sigma_x = \sigma_y = 3pix$: Standard deviation of the precision as a function of the standard deviation σ_n of the noise

σ_n [gr]	1	3	5	10	50
Theory, $\sigma_{\hat{x}_0}$ [pix]	0.0080	0.0239	0.0399	0.0798	0.3989
Experiment, $\sigma_{\hat{x}_0}$ [pix]	0.0081	0.0236	0.0399	0.0800	0.3944

Table 4. Localization of an anisotropic 2D blob with $\sigma_x = 4pix$, $\sigma_y = 2pix$: Standard deviation of the precision in $x-$ and $y-$direction as a function of the standard deviation σ_n of the noise

σ_n [gr]	1	3	5	10	50
Theory, $\sigma_{\hat{x}_0}$ [pix]	0.0113	0.0339	0.0564	0.1128	0.5642
Experiment, $\sigma_{\hat{x}_0}$ [pix]	0.0112	0.0337	0.0558	0.1168	0.5937
Theory, $\sigma_{\hat{y}_0}$ [pix]	0.0056	0.0169	0.0282	0.0564	0.2821
Experiment, $\sigma_{\hat{y}_0}$ [pix]	0.0055	0.0175	0.0281	0.0565	0.2909

Table 5. Localization of an isotropic 3D blob with $\sigma_x = \sigma_y = \sigma_z = 3vox$: Standard deviation of the precision as a function of the standard deviation σ_n of the noise

σ_n [gr]	1	3	5	10	50
Theory, $\sigma_{\hat{x}_0}$ [vox]	0.0035	0.0104	0.0173	0.0346	0.1730
Experiment, $\sigma_{\hat{x}_0}$ [vox]	0.0035	0.0105	0.0176	0.0342	0.1832

Table 6. Localization of an anisotropic 3D blob with $\sigma_x = 4vox$, $\sigma_y = 3vox$, and $\sigma_z = 2vox$: Standard deviation of the precision in $x-$, $y-$, and $z-$direction as a function of the standard deviation σ_n of the noise

σ_n [gr]	1	3	5	10	50
Theory, $\sigma_{\hat{x}_0}$ [vox]	0.0049	0.0147	0.0245	0.0489	0.2447
Experiment, $\sigma_{\hat{x}_0}$ [vox]	0.0049	0.0145	0.0238	0.0485	0.2537
Theory, $\sigma_{\hat{y}_0}$ [vox]	0.0037	0.0110	0.0184	0.0367	0.1835
Experiment, $\sigma_{\hat{y}_0}$ [vox]	0.0036	0.0111	0.0183	0.0364	0.1830
Theory, $\sigma_{\hat{z}_0}$ [vox]	0.0024	0.0073	0.0122	0.0245	0.1223
Experiment, $\sigma_{\hat{z}_0}$ [vox]	0.0025	0.0073	0.0123	0.0239	0.1224

3D blob of $\sigma_x = \sigma_y = \sigma_z = \sigma = 3vox$. Tab. 5 shows that the agreement between theory and experiment is again very good, and that the accuracy is about a factor of two better in comparison to the 2D case (cf. Tab. 3). The noise levels $\sigma_n = 1, 3, 5, 10, 50gr$ correspond to $SNR = 88.82, 9.87, 3.55, 0.89, 0.04$. The result for an anisotropic 3D blob ($\sigma_x = 4vox$, $\sigma_y = 3vox$, $\sigma_z = 2vox$) can be seen in Tab. 6. For an example of a cross-section image see Fig. 3 (right). Again we observe a remarkable agreement between theory and experiment.

Acknowledgement

I thank Stefan Wörz for carrying out the experiments as well as for discussions.

References

1. C.K. Abbey, E. Clarkson, H.H. Barrett, S.P. Müller, and F.J. Rybicki, "A method for approximating the density of maximum-likelihood and maximum *a posteriori* estimates under a Gaussian noise model", *Med. Image Analysis* 2:4 (1998) 395-403
2. Y.T. Chang and S.M. Thomas, "Cramer-Rao Lower Bounds for Estimation of a Circular Arc Center and Its Radius", *Graphical Models and Image Processing* 57:6 (1995) 527-532
3. T. Hartkens, K. Rohr, and H.S. Stiehl, "Evaluation of 3D Operators for the Detection of Anatomical Point Landmarks in MR and CT Images", *Computer Vision and Image Understanding* 86:2 (2002) 118-136
4. R. Kakarala and A.O. Hero, "On Achievable Accuracy in Edge Localization", *IEEE Trans. on Pattern Anal. and Machine Intell.* 14:7 (1992) 777-781

5. K. Kanatani, "Cramer-Rao Lower Bounds for Curve Fitting", *Graphical Models and Image Processing* 60:2 (1998) 93-99
6. K. Rohr, "On the Precision in Estimating the Location of Edges and Corners", *J. of Mathematical Imaging and Vision* 7:1 (1997) 7-22
7. L.L. Scharf, *Statistical Signal Processing: Detection, Estimation, and Time Series Analysis*, Addison-Wesley Reading/Massachusetts 1991
8. H.L. van Trees, *Detection, Estimation, and Modulation Theory*, Part I, John Wiley and Sons, New York London 1968
9. S. Wörz and K. Rohr, "Localization of Anatomical Point Landmarks in 3D Medical Images by Fitting 3D Parametric Intensity Models", *Proc. 18th Internat. Conf. on Information Processing in Medical Imaging (IPMI'03)*, Ambleside, UK, July 20-25, 2003, In *Lecture Notes in Computer Science* 2732, C. Taylor and J.A. Noble (Eds.), Springer-Verlag Berlin Heidelberg 2003, 76-88

Computational Elastography from Standard Ultrasound Image Sequences by Global Trust Region Optimization

Jan Kybic[1] and Daniel Smutek[2]

[1] Center for Machine Perception, Czech Technical University, Prague, Czech Republic
kybic@fel.cvut.cz
http://cmp.felk.cvut.cz/~kybic
[2] Faculty of Medicine I, Charles University, Prague, Czech Republic

Abstract. A new approach is proposed to estimate the spatial distribution of shear modulus of tissues in-vivo. An image sequence is acquired using a standard medical ultrasound scanner while varying the force applied to the handle. The elastic properties are then recovered simultaneously with the inter-frame displacement fields using a computational procedure based on finite element modeling and trust region constrained optimization. No assumption about boundary conditions is needed. The optimization procedure is global, taking advantage of all available images. The algorithm was tested on phantom, as well as on real clinical images.

1 Introduction

Elastography, or elasticity imaging [1,2], aims at noninvasive measurement of elastic properties of tissues and their spatial distributions. Knowing elastic parameters can be very useful for biomedical modeling as well as for diagnostics. As an example, many carcinoma are harder than the surrounding healthy tissue [3–5], as are some lesions. It has been established that several diseases of breast, kidney, prostate, blood vessels and other organs are also accompanied by a change of elastic properties of tissues. After all, palpation, a precursor to elastography, has been used for medical diagnosis since perhaps several thousand years.

Many kinds of elastographic procedures have been proposed in recent years [6–10]. In most cases, a small force is applied to the tissue and the resulting displacement is measured. Typically, the induced displacement is extremely small and a special device is needed to measure it. In ultrasound based elastography, we often need to resolve displacements significantly smaller than the wavelength. A special ultrasound scanner is used, allowing the sampling of the received signal (RF signal) at very high frequency [11–13], so that it can be correlated with the emitted pulse.

However, such specialized devices are not yet readily available in clinical practice. Therefore, we attempt to develop an elastography approach using only a standard ultrasound machine, without any special hardware. The tissue is deformed by varying the force applied by the operator on a standard ultrasound hand-held transducer while acquiring the image sequence. A specialized reconstruction algorithm is used, simultaneously estimating the shear modulus distribution and the displacement fields between a chosen reference frame and the rest of the images in the sequence.

We have already confirmed the feasibility of reconstructing elastic properties of tissues from standard ultrasound images in our previous work [14], where we have used a pair of images for the reconstruction. Like all similar methods described in the literature [8–10, 15], we were forced to provide stress (force) boundary conditions for the elasticity problem even on the virtual internal boundaries of the imaged region, where no measurement is available. Using displacement-only boundary conditions leads to an inherently ill-posed and unstable inverse problem, even if additional boundary conditions for the elastic modulus μ are imposed [16]. In practical terms it means that there are many different modulus distributions consistent with the two acquired images within measurement accuracy.

The new reconstruction algorithm described here can find a shear modulus distribution μ consistent with a whole set of images, allowing us to choose a trade-off between the robustness and accuracy of the estimation and the time and memory requirements. The applied force does no longer have to be strictly perpendicular to the sensor array, maintaining the same image plane is enough. Moreover, no assumptions are needed about the boundary forces any more. By virtue of using more images, the problem is better posed. It has been shown recently [17] that the elastic modulus can be reconstructed almost uniquely (up to 4 constants) from two displacement fields, i.e. 3 images in our case, and up to 1 constant from 4 displacement fields (5 images). To the best of our knowledge, this is the first algorithm described in the literature that combines information from several images (or equivalently, from several displacement fields), to reconstruct elasticity parameters.

2 Method

2.1 Data Acquisition

An ultrasound probe (transducer) of a Philips Envisor scanner is placed on a skin above the zone of interest, such as the thyroid gland, breast, or liver. An image sequence of about 10 s at 5 ∼ 10 frames per second is acquired while the operator slowly varies the pressure applied on the handle. The operator is instructed to keep the same image plane as closely as possible. Out of this sequence, a smaller number of approximately equidistant images (in time) are selected for further processing, ideally with no motion and other artifacts. The selected 2D images will be denoted f_t for $-n_1 \leq t \leq n_2$. Image f_0 will be called a reference image. The images of an area denoted Ω are taken in a moving coordinate system attached to the sensor (Figure 1).

2.2 Elasticity Equations

Let us consider the tissue movement between two adjacent images f_{t_-}, and f_t, where $t_- = t - \operatorname{sign} t$. In other words, f_{t_-} is the image preceding f_t towards the

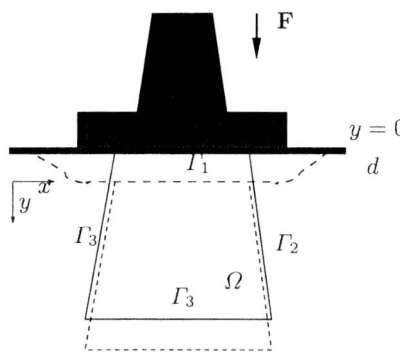

Fig. 1. The tissue is deformed by varying the pressure on the ultrasound probe (black). Dashed lines show the position of the skin and the sensed region after the probe is shifted (in this case downward by a distance d)

reference image f_0. Since we do not have any information about the movement of the tissue outside the imaging plane, we will make the standard assumption of a *plane strain*, i.e. that all the out-of-plane strains (displacements) are zero. Let us denote $\mathbf{v}_t$ the displacement field between f_{t_-} and f_t

$$\mathbf{v}_t\bigl(\mathbf{u}_{t_-}(\mathbf{x})\bigr) = \mathbf{u}_t(\mathbf{x}) - \mathbf{u}_{t_-}(\mathbf{x}) \tag{1}$$

where $t \mapsto \mathbf{u}_t(\mathbf{x})$ is the trajectory of a tissue point that is at coordinates $\mathbf{x}$ in frame f_0; $\mathbf{u}_0(\mathbf{x}) = \mathbf{x}$. Note that $\mathbf{v}_t$ is expressed in the coordinate system of f_{t_-}. We shall assume that the displacement is small and that the tissue is isotropic and incompressible. Then, the displacement field satisfies the standard elasticity equations [1, 10] governed by a Lamé parameter $\mu(\mathbf{x}) > 0$, the shear modulus:

$$\left.\begin{array}{r}-\nabla p_t + \nabla \cdot \bigl(2\mu \nabla^s \mathbf{v}_t\bigr) = \mathbf{0} \\ -\nabla \cdot \mathbf{v}_t = 0\end{array}\right\} \text{ in } \Omega \tag{2}$$

where p_t is a pressure, positive for compression, and $\varepsilon_t = \nabla^s \mathbf{v}_t = \frac{1}{2}(\nabla \mathbf{v}_t + \nabla \mathbf{v}_t^T)$ is a symmetric strain tensor. Note that there are $n = n_1 + n_2$ independent displacements $\mathbf{v}_t$ and pressures p_t, one for each image f_t, $t \neq 0$, while there is only one field μ, defined in the reference coordinate system, common to all images. All equations (2) must be satisfied simultaneously, for all images t, $-n_1 \leq t \leq n_2$, $t \neq 0$. The only boundary condition we impose is

$$\mathbf{u}_t = \mathbf{v}_t = \mathbf{0} \quad \text{on } \Gamma_1 \tag{3}$$

It comes from the assumption that the ultrasound sensor is always in touch with the upper edge Γ_1 of the imaged region Ω (the skin).

2.3 Weak Formulation

We convert the strong formulation (2) into an equivalent weak one [10]. We say that fields $\mu \in L_\infty^+(\Omega)$, $\{\mathbf{v}_t\} \in H_1(\Omega)^n$, $\{p_t\} \in L_2(\Omega)^n$, are consistent with the elasticity constraints, iff (3) holds and

$$0 = A\bigl(\mu; \{\mathbf{v}_t\}, \{p_t\}, \{\mathbf{w}_t\}, \{q_t\}\bigr) \stackrel{\text{def}}{=} \sum_{t \neq 0} A_t(\mu; \mathbf{v}_t, p_t, \mathbf{w}_t, q_t)$$

$$A_t(\mu; \mathbf{v}_t, p_t, \mathbf{w}_t, q_t) = \int_\Omega 2\mu_t \nabla^s \mathbf{v}_t : \nabla^s \mathbf{w}_t - (\nabla \cdot \mathbf{w}_t) p_t - (\nabla \cdot \mathbf{v}_t) q_t \, d\Omega \quad (4)$$

for all sufficiently regular and integrable test functions $\mathbf{w}_t \in H^1(\Omega)$ and $q_t \in L_2(\Omega)$ such that $\mathbf{w}_t = \mathbf{0}$ on $\partial\Omega$. We write

$$\boldsymbol{\xi} \stackrel{\text{def}}{=} \bigl(\mu, \{\mathbf{v}_t\}, \{p_t\}\bigr) \in \mathcal{C} \iff \forall \mathbf{w}_t, q_t;\; A\bigl(\mu; \{\mathbf{v}_t\}, \{p_t\}, \{\mathbf{w}_t\}, \{q_t\}\bigr) = 0 \quad (5)$$

where $\mathcal{C}$ is a manifold representing all consistent modulus, displacement, and pressure fields. Note that no boundary conditions are imposed apart from (3).

2.4 Finite Element Method

We convert the continuous formulation (4) to a corresponding linear system of equations using the Galerkin method [18]. The domain Ω is triangulated to form a mesh with a maximum edge size h. The mesh topology is the same for all frames, while the mesh nodes follow the tissue, i.e. the trajectory of a node with an initial position $\mathbf{x}$ (corresponding to the reference frame) is $\mathbf{u}_t(\mathbf{x})$. We shall denote N_v the total number of vertices in the mesh, N_u the number of vertices except the top, non-moving edge, and N_i the number of internal vertices, not lying on any edge.

The modulus μ, the displacement fields $\mathbf{v}_t$ and the test functions $\mathbf{w}_t$ are discretized with P1 basis functions φ_i (equal to 1 at vertex i, 0 on other vertices, and piecewise linear on each triangle). The pressure p_t and test functions q_t are discretized with P0 basis functions ψ_i (piecewise constant):

$$\mu^h = \sum_i \mathrm{m}_i \varphi_j \qquad \mathbf{v}^h = \sum_i \begin{bmatrix} \mathrm{v}_{2i} \\ \mathrm{v}_{2i+1} \end{bmatrix} \varphi_i = \sum_j \mathbf{v}_j \varphi_j \quad (6)$$

$$p^h = \sum_j \mathrm{p}_j \psi_j \quad (7)$$

(and similarly for $\mathbf{w}^h$ and q^h) where the superscript h denotes the discretized version. To relax the incompressibility condition in order to avoid mesh locking, the support of functions ψ_i is chosen to be triangles adjacent to vertex i, where ψ_i is 1, and zero elsewhere. Consequently, we have $2N_u$ degrees of freedom for each $\mathbf{v}_t$, N_v degrees of freedom for μ and each p_t and q_t, and N_i degrees of freedom for each $\mathbf{w}_t$. Note also that with this discretization, the bilinear form A (4) can be integrated exactly.

The discretized state $\boldsymbol{\xi}^h$ of the modulus and displacement reconstruction problem is completely described by a finite-dimensional state vector $\boldsymbol{\Xi}$ with $N_x = n(2N_u + N_v) + N_v$ degrees of freedom.

$$\boldsymbol{\xi}^h \stackrel{\text{def}}{=} \bigl(\mu^h, \{\mathbf{v}_t^h\}, \{p_t^h\}\bigr) \longleftrightarrow \boldsymbol{\Xi} = \bigl(\{\mathrm{m}_i\}, \{\mathrm{v}_{j,t}\}, \{\mathrm{p}_{k,t}\}\bigr) \in \mathbb{R}^{N_x} \qquad t \neq 0$$

The corresponding discretized version of the manifold (5) of consistent solutions is

$$\mathcal{C}^h = \left\{ \boldsymbol{\xi}^h = \left(\mu^h, \{\mathbf{v}_t^h\}, \{p_t^h\}\right); \mu^h > 0, \mathbf{c}(\boldsymbol{\xi}^h) = \mathbf{0} \right\}$$

with a vector of constraints

$$\mathbf{c}(\boldsymbol{\xi}^h) = D_\lambda A^h(\boldsymbol{\xi}^h, \mathbf{w}^h, q^H) \quad \text{and} \quad \begin{bmatrix} \mathbf{w}^h \\ q^h \end{bmatrix} = \boldsymbol{\Phi}\boldsymbol{\lambda}$$

where $\boldsymbol{\lambda} = (\{w_{i,t}\}, \{q_{j,t}\})$ is a vector expressing the test functions $\mathbf{w}^h$ and q^h using P1 and P0 basis functions (6),(7). As A^h is linear in $\boldsymbol{\lambda}$, we have $\forall \boldsymbol{\lambda}; A^h(\boldsymbol{\xi}^h, \boldsymbol{\lambda}) = 0$ iff $\mathbf{c}(\boldsymbol{\xi}^h) = D_\lambda A^h(\boldsymbol{\xi}^h, \boldsymbol{\lambda}) = \mathbf{0}$. To simplify the notation, we will from now on drop the superscript h even if the resulting algorithm must obviously represent the continuous quantities in the appropriate finite dimensional bases.

2.5 Image Similarity Criterion

A solution $\boldsymbol{\xi} = (\mu, \{\mathbf{v}_t\}, \{p_t\})$, besides satisfying the elasticity constraints, must also be consistent with the image sequence $\{f_t\}$. The displacements $\mathbf{v}_t^h$ must correspond to the observed movement in the image sequence. The similarity between a pair of images f, g is measured by a normalized version of the SSD criterion

$$J_s(f,g) = \frac{1}{2} \frac{\sum_{\mathbf{i} \in I} m_g(\mathbf{i})\, m_f(\mathbf{i}) \left(g(\mathbf{i}) - f(\mathbf{i})\right)^2}{\sum_{\mathbf{i} \in I} m_g(\mathbf{i})\, g(\mathbf{i})^2 + m_f(\mathbf{i}) f(\mathbf{i})^2}$$

where I is the set of pixel coordinates in the images and m_f and m_g are masks, determining the region of interest. There is one mask m_t associated with each image f_t. This criterion is fast to calculate, invariant to image intensity scale changes and largely insensitive to changes of overlap. This is important in our application where the imaged region is changing from frame to frame. We chose to evaluate the similarity between the reference image f_0 and deformed images $(T_{\mathbf{u}_t} f_t)(\mathbf{x}) = f_t(\mathbf{u}_t(\mathbf{x}))$, where $\mathbf{u}_t$ and $\mathbf{v}_t$ are recursively related by (1)

$$\mathbf{u}_t(\mathbf{x}) = \mathbf{u}_{t_-}(\mathbf{x}) + \mathbf{v}_t\bigl(\mathbf{u}_{t_-}(\mathbf{x})\bigr) \quad \text{and} \quad \mathbf{u}_0(\mathbf{x}) = \mathbf{x}$$

In our experience [19, 20] comparing each image with a reference is more accurate than evaluating the similarity between adjacent images. Bilinear interpolation and zero boundary conditions are used to evaluate the warped image $T_{\mathbf{u}_t} f_t$ and the corresponding warped mask $T_{\mathbf{u}_t} m_t$. The global similarity criterion over the whole sequence is:

$$J(\boldsymbol{\xi}) = J(\{\mathbf{v}_t\}) = \sum_{t \neq 0} J_s(f_0, T_{\mathbf{u}_t} f_t)$$

2.6 Problem Definition

Given the definitions above our problem of simultaneous reconstruction of elastic properties of the tissue and the displacements consistent with the elasticity equations and the acquired image sequence can be described as a constrained optimization:

$$\boldsymbol{\xi}^* = \arg\min_{\boldsymbol{\xi}} J(\boldsymbol{\xi}) \quad \text{for} \quad \boldsymbol{\xi} \in \mathcal{C} \tag{8}$$

The difficulty lies in the complicated nonlinear structure of the manifold $\mathcal{C}$, coming from the $\mu \nabla^s \mathbf{v}_t$ products (4) and the the displacement accumulation $\{\mathbf{v}_t\} \mapsto \{\mathbf{u}_t\}$. In other words, the PDE (2) is solved in a curved space, the local curvature of which is influenced by the deformation in preceding frames. The problem (8) may have several local minima. Therefore, finding a good starting point $\boldsymbol{\xi}_0$ is important. Usually, we use $\mathbf{v}_t = \mathbf{0}$, $p_t = 0$, and $\mu = 1$, or multiresolution (Section 2.8).

According to our tests, most higher-order approximations used by standard optimization methods are only useful in a close vicinity of the solution point. We therefore chose a modified trust region optimization method [21], described in the following section, as it was the only method tested providing the required robustness.

2.7 Trust Region Optimization

In contrast to the classical trust region approach that uses linearized constraints and quadratic approximation to the criterion, we found that a linear approximation of the criterion is adequate, while the constraints have to be take into account exactly in each step, otherwise the convergence is not ensured.

Major Iterations. Starting from an initial (feasible) estimate $\boldsymbol{\xi}_0$, the trust region optimizer attempts to find a sequence of estimates $\boldsymbol{\xi}_0, \boldsymbol{\xi}_1, \boldsymbol{\xi}_2, \ldots$ on the manifold $\mathcal{C}$, (i.e., such that $\mathbf{c}(\boldsymbol{\xi}_i) = \mathbf{0}$ for all i), and so that further the sequence of criterion values $J(\boldsymbol{\xi}_0), J(\boldsymbol{\xi}_1), J(\boldsymbol{\xi}_2), \ldots$ is decreasing. Each step $\boldsymbol{\xi}_i \to \boldsymbol{\xi}_{i+1}$ is termed a major iteration. Major iterations terminate if the decrease of J is below an a priori chosen relative or absolute threshold (we normally use a relative threshold of 10^{-3}) or if the process stagnates (no improvement can be found).

Within each major iteration i, we linearize the criterion around $\boldsymbol{\xi}_i$

$$\tilde{J}(\boldsymbol{\xi}_i + \mathbf{z}) = J(\boldsymbol{\xi}) + D_{\boldsymbol{\xi}} J(\boldsymbol{\xi}_i) \mathbf{z} = J_i + \mathbf{a}^T \mathbf{z} \tag{9}$$

and solve the reduced problem

$$\mathbf{z}^* = \arg\min \tilde{J}(\boldsymbol{\xi}_i + \mathbf{z}) = \arg\min \mathbf{a}^T \mathbf{z} \quad \text{for} \quad \mathbf{z} + \boldsymbol{\xi}_i \in \mathcal{C}, \ \|\mathbf{z}\| < \varrho_i \tag{10}$$

where ϱ_i is the trust region radius. We start with $\varrho_0 = 0.3$ (units of ϱ partly correspond to pixels). If the problem (10) is successfully solved and $J(\boldsymbol{\xi}_i + \mathbf{z}^*) < J(\boldsymbol{\xi}_i)$ (the linear approximation is valid), we accept the step by setting $\boldsymbol{\xi}_{i+1} = \boldsymbol{\xi}_i + \mathbf{z}^*$ and increase $\varrho_{i+1} = 1.5\varrho_i$. Otherwise, we try to solve (10) again with $\varrho_i \leftarrow 0.1\varrho_i$.

The problem (10) is equivalent to

$$\mathbf{z}^* = \arg\min \mathbf{a}^T \mathbf{z} + \frac{\alpha}{2}\|\mathbf{z}\|^2 \quad \text{for} \quad \mathbf{z} + \boldsymbol{\xi}_i \in \mathcal{C} \tag{11}$$

for some Lagrange multiplier α. The appropriate α is found by a binary search, stopping if $0.1\varrho \leq \|\mathbf{z}\| \leq \varrho$ and using the last value of α as a first guess. If no such α can be found, the major iteration is declared to fail.

Minor Iterations. The problem (11) is again solved iteratively, producing a sequence $\mathbf{z}_0, \mathbf{z}_1, \ldots$. Each step is called a minor iteration. The first of them, $\mathbf{z}_0$ is chosen to minimize (9) in the trust region, regardless of the constraints

$$\mathbf{z}_0 = \arg\min \mathbf{a}^T \mathbf{z} \quad \text{for} \quad \|\mathbf{z}\| \leq \varrho \tag{12}$$

The solution (except degenerate cases) is $\mathbf{z}_0 = -\varrho \mathbf{a}/\|\mathbf{a}\|$. Then, for each minor iteration estimate $\mathbf{z}_j$ we find the next estimate $\mathbf{z}_{j+1}$ as a solution to the constrained optimization problem (11) with linearized constraints

$$\mathbf{z}_{j+1} = \arg\min_{\mathbf{z}} \mathbf{a}^T \mathbf{z} + \frac{\alpha}{2}\|\mathbf{z}\|^2$$
$$\text{with} \quad 0 = \mathbf{d} + \mathsf{B}(\mathbf{z} - \mathbf{z}_j)$$
$$\text{where} \quad \mathbf{d} + \mathsf{B}(\mathbf{z} - \mathbf{z}_j) = \mathbf{c}(\boldsymbol{\xi}_i + \mathbf{z}_j) + \left(D_{\boldsymbol{\xi}}\, \mathbf{c}(\boldsymbol{\xi}_i + \mathbf{z}_j)\right)(\mathbf{z} - \mathbf{z}_j) \approx \mathbf{c}(\boldsymbol{\xi}_i + \mathbf{z})$$

We form the Lagrangian

$$\mathscr{L} = \mathbf{a}^T \mathbf{z} + \frac{\alpha}{2}\|\mathbf{z}\|^2 + \mathbf{y}^T \left(\mathbf{d} + \mathsf{B}(\mathbf{z} - \mathbf{z}_j)\right)$$

and find its first order optimality conditions for $\delta \mathbf{z} = \mathbf{z}_{j+1} - \mathbf{z}_j$:

$$\begin{aligned} \alpha\,\delta\mathbf{z} + \mathsf{B}^T \mathbf{y} &= -\mathbf{a} - \alpha \mathbf{z}_j \\ \mathsf{B}\,\delta\mathbf{z} &= -\mathbf{d} \end{aligned} \tag{13}$$

The sparse symmetric linear system of equations (13) is solved using the (iterative) MINRES method [22].

We monitor the constraint fulfillment $\|\mathbf{c}(\boldsymbol{\xi}_i + \mathbf{z}_j)\|$ during minor iterations. Normally only a few iterations ($3 \sim 5$) are needed to ensure that the dicrepancy is sufficiently small ($\|\mathbf{c}(\boldsymbol{\xi}_i + \mathbf{z}_j)\| < 10^{-4}$). If divergence is detected (the discrepancy $\|\mathbf{c}(\cdot)\|$ increases), the minor iterations are declared to fail. Consequently, in the next major iteration, smaller ϱ will be used and so the linear approximation of the constraints will be more accurate and the major iterations thus less likely to diverge.

Summary of the Trust Region Optimization. The trust region algorithm consists of four cascaded iteration loops. The outermost, major iterations, finds a sequence of feasible solutions $\boldsymbol{\xi}_i$ with decreasing criterion values. The second level attempts to find a suitable value α such that the step $\mathbf{z}^*$ of (11) has a correct amplitude $\|\mathbf{z}^*\| \leq \varrho$. The third level (minor iterations) iteratively solves (11). Finally, the innermost, fourth level, iteratively solves a linear system of equation (13) within each minor iteration.

Unfeasible Starting Points. If only an infeasible (not belonging to $\mathcal{C}$) starting point $\boldsymbol{\xi}_0'$ is available, we project it to $\mathcal{C}$ by minimizing

$$\boldsymbol{\xi}_0 = \arg\min_{\boldsymbol{\xi}} \|\boldsymbol{\xi} - \boldsymbol{\xi}_0'\|_W^2 \quad \text{for} \quad \boldsymbol{\xi} \in \mathcal{C} \tag{14}$$

where $\|(\mu, \{\mathbf{v}_t\}, \{p_t\})\|_W^2 = 10^3 \|\mu\|^2 + \|\{\mathbf{v}_t\}\|^2 + \|\{p_t\}\|^2$ is a weighted Euclidean norm which gives more weight to the μ components of $\boldsymbol{\xi}$, expressing our a priori estimate of the precision of the various components. The minimization problem (14) is solved by repeated projections to the linearized constraint subspace with respect to $\|\cdot\|_W$, until convergence is reached, similarly to the minor iterations described above (13). Infeasible starting point may arise for example when interpolating a coarse solution in a multiresolution framework (Section 2.8). Normally, however, the distance from the constraint space is small, just due to numerical errors, so only a few iterations are needed and the choice of the projection norm is not crucial.

Maintaining Feasibility. We had to add two additional rules to the evaluation of the success of each major iteration, preventing the algorithm from running astray. First, we require that μ is everywhere positive. If not, we project the proposed μ to the allowed space by selectively setting the offending components to small positive numbers (10^{-6}). Second, we require that the change of all accumulated displacements $\mathbf{u}_t$ be less than 0.5 pixels in magnitude everywhere. Both rules could be implemented within the trust region approach albeit with a slightly higher computational cost. We opted for this hybrid approach since both rules only affect the optimization during a few initial steps.

2.8 Multiresolution

To improve speed and robustness of the optimizer, a multiresolution approach was used with respect to both mesh and image size. We start with a coarse mesh and coarse versions of the images — normally a mesh with 3×3 nodes and images of about 64×64 pixels are used. Once the coarse problem is solved (which is fast), its solution is used as a starting point for a finer one. In the outer loop we progressively refine the mesh by subdivision. In the inner loop, we increase the image resolution, so that the problem is solved at optimum level — as a rule of thumb, we attempt to have image size $5l \sim 10l$ pixels, where l is the maximum edge length for the mesh. We continue until the desired mesh and image resolution is reached. The image pyramid is built by convolution with a 3×3 smoothing filter and down-sampling by a factor of 2.

When the mesh or image resolution is changed, the status vector $\boldsymbol{\xi}$ must be updated accordingly. This involves multiplying $\mathbf{v}_t$ by 2 (for image size change) or taking the mean of the parent node values (for mesh expansion). The interpolated state vector has to be projected to $\mathcal{C}$ (see (14)).

3 Experiments

First experiment is based on data acquired on a Gammex 429 Ultrasound Biopsy Phantom[1] that mimics normal breast tissue and contains eleven test objects filled with low or high density gel, simulating lesions (Figure 2). Two of the acquired images with different views of different lesions are shown, each representing a whole sequence. Corresponding reconstructions using 3 images are shown; using 2 images did not converge to an acceptable solution, using more than 3 images did not improve the results significantly.

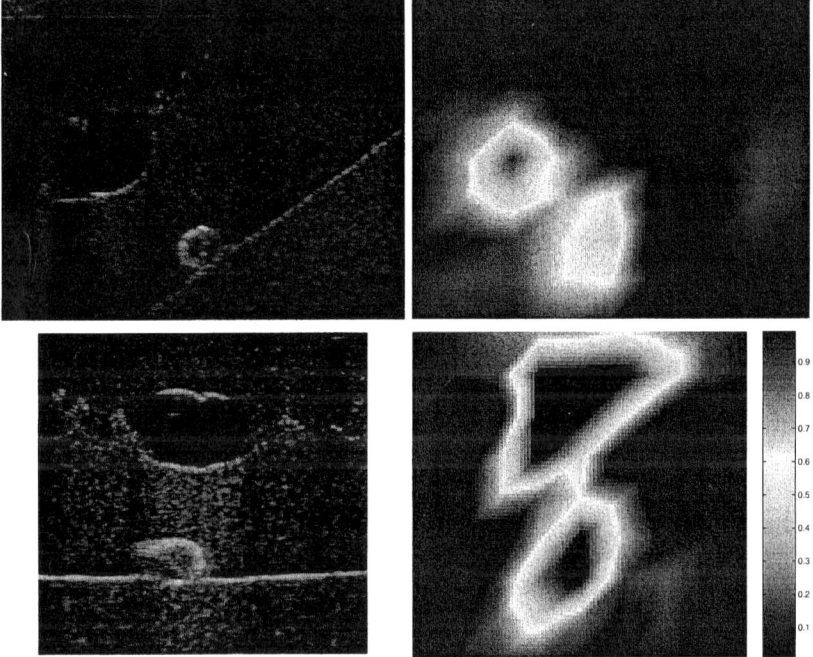

Fig. 2. Phantom images (left column) and corresponding reconstruction of the relative modulus μ from sets of 3 images with a 10 × 10 node mesh (right column). The same color scale is used in both images

Figure 3 (top) shows a reconstruction based on a real thyroid gland ultrasound sequence of a normal subject using 3 images. Finally, for illustration, the bottom image shows a reconstruction from thyroid gland sequence taken from a subject with acute thyroiditis, [2] reconstructed using a twice finer mesh and 5 images.

---

[1] www.gamex.com
[2] We suspect there might be a difference in the elastic properties however it probably is not discernible at the current resolution level of the elastograms.

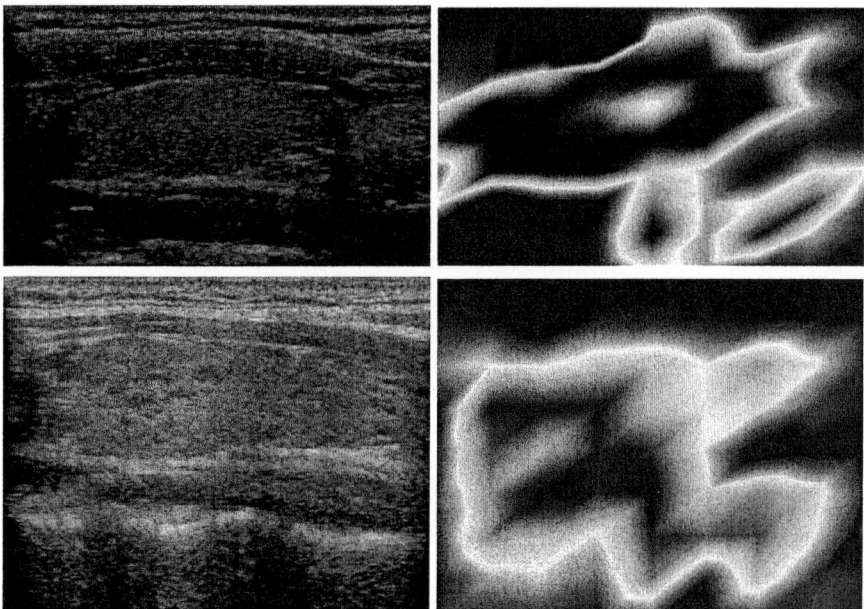

Fig. 3. Normal thyroid gland image (top left) and the reconstructed elastogram from a 3 image set (top right). Acute thyroiditis subject image (bottom left) and the corresponding elastogram reconstructed using a finer mesh and 5 images (bottom right). The same color scale is used as in Fig. 2

4 Timings and Resolution

Most reconstructions shown above used 3 images of about 500×500 pixels and moderate density meshes with about 10×10 nodes. Such reconstruction takes 10 min $\sim$ 1 h on a standard PC (1.4 GHz Pentium). The time increases significantly with both mesh density and number of images. As an illustration, the thyroiditis reconstruction above with 20×20 nodes and 5 images took over 5 h.

5 Conclusions

We have presented an algorithm for simultaneous estimation of displacement field and shear modulus distribution from a series of standard ultrasound images. The novelty of the method is in its ability of combining information from several images in a global manner. It is based on the theoretical observation that while reconstructing a shear modulus from a pair of images is bound to lead to an ill-defined problem [17], the situation is improved if several deformation fields are available. This way we avoid inventing essentially unmeasurable boundary data for the direct elasticity problem. The reconstruction task is formulated as a constrained optimization method. Unfortunately, since we no longer have a uniquely solvable direct problem, the feasible subspace that needs to be searched is a highly convoluted manifold of all solutions consistent with linear elasticity equations. Therefore, the computation time is rather long. Also, since our data is relatively noisy and low resolution, we suspect there might not even be enough information to obtain more details of the shear modulus distribution. In any case, the new method gives better results than the previous algorithm [14], based on only two images.

Acknowledgements

The first author was sponsored by the Czech Ministry of Education, grant MSM6840770012, the second author by the Grant Agency of the Czech Academy of Sciences, grant 1ET101050403.

References

1. Ophir, J., Kallel, F., Varghese, T., Konofagou, E., Alam, S.K., Garra, B., Krouskop, T., Righetti, R.: Elastography: Optical and acoustic imaging of acoustic media. C. R. Acad. Sci. Paris **2** (2001) 1193–1212 serie IV.
2. Insana, M.F., Cook, L.T., P., C.: Analytical study of bioelasticity ultrasound systems. In A., K., M., S., A., T.P., eds.: Information Processing in Medical Imaging (IPMI), Berlin (1999)
3. Liu, H.T., Sun, L.Z.: Analytic modeling of breast elastography. Medical Physics **30** (2003) 2340–2349
4. Yeh, W.C., Li, P.C., Jeng, Y.M., Hsu, H.C., Kuo, P.L., Li, M.L., Yang, P.M., Lee, P.H.: Elastic modulus measurements of human liver and correlation with pathology. Ultrasound in Medicine & Biology **28** (2002) 467–474
5. Yin, Sun, Wang, Vannier, M.: Modeling of elastic modulus evolution of cirrhotic human liver. IEEE Trans. Biomed Eng. **51** (2004) 1854–1856
6. Lin, J., McLaughlin, J.: Recovery of the Lamé parameter μ in biological tissues. Inverse Problems (2004) 1–24
7. McLaughlin, J.R., J.-R., Y.: Unique identifiability of elastic parameters from time-dependent interior displacement measurement. Inverse Problems (2004) 24–45
8. Bishop, J., Samani, A., Sciaretta, J., B., P.D.: Two-dimensional MR elastography with linear inversion reconstruction: methodology and noise analysis. Phys. Med. Biol. (2000) 2081–2091
9. Liu, H., Shi, P.: Robust identification of object elasticity. In Šonka, M., Kakadiaris, A.I., Kybic, J., eds.: Computer Vision and Mathematical Methods in Medical and Biomedical Image Analysis (CVAMIA+MMBIA). Number 3117 in Lecture Notes in Computer Science. Springer, Heidelberg (2004) 423–435
10. Oberai, A., Gokhale, N., Feijóo, G.: Solution of inverse problems in elasticity imaging using the adjoint method. Inverse Problems (2003) 297–313
11. Srinivasan, S., Ophir, J.: A zero-crossing strain estimator for elastography. Ultrasound in Medicine and Biology **29** (2003) 227–238
12. Brusseau, E., Fromageau, J., Rognin, N., Delacharte, P., Vray, D.: Local estimation of RF ultrasound signal compression for axial strain imaging: theoretical developments and experimental design. IEEE Engineering in Medicine and Biology Magazine **21** (2002) 86–94

13. Barbone, P., Gokhale, N., Richards, M., Oberai, A., Doyley, M.: Simultaneous elastic image registration and elastic modulus reconstruction. In: Proceedings of the 2004 IEEE International Symposium on Biomedical Imaging: From Nano to Macro, Arlington, VA, USA, 15-18 April 2004, IEEE (2004) 543–546
14. Kybic, J., Smutek, D.: Estimating elastic properties of tissues from standard 2d ultrasound images. In: Proceedings of the SPIE Conference on Medical Imaging, SPIE (2005)
15. Washington, C.W., Miga, M.I.: Modality independent elastography (MIE): A new approach to elasticity imaging. IEEE Transactions on Medical Imaging (2004) 1117–1126
16. Barbone, P.E., Bamber, J.C.: Quantitative elasticity imaging: what can and cannot be inferred from strain images. Phys. Med. Biol. (2002) 2147–2164
17. Barbone, P.E., Gokhale, N.H.: Elastic modulus imaging: on the uniqueness and nonuniqueness of the elastography inverse problem in two dimensions. Inverse Problems (2004) 283–296
18. Nečas, J., Hlaváček, I.: Mathematical Theory of Elastic and Elasto-Plastic Bodies. Elsevier, Amsterdam (1981)
19. Ledesmay-Carbayo, M.J., Kybic, J., Desco, M., Santos, A., Unser, M.: Cardiac motion analysis from ultrasound sequences using non-rigid registration. In Niessen, W.J., Viergever, M.A., eds.: Proceedings of MICCAI, Springer-Verlag (2001) 889–896
20. Ledesma-Carbayo, M.J., Kybic, J., Sühling, M., Hunziger, P., Desco, M., Santos, A., Unser, M.: Cardiac ultrasound motion detection by elastic registration exploiting temporal coherence. In: Proceedings of the First 2002 IEEE International Symposium on Biomedical Imaging: Macro to Nano (ISBI'02), 445 Hoes Lane, Piscataway, NJ, U.S.A., IEEE (2002) 585 – 588
21. Moré, J., Sorensen, D.: Computing a trust region step. SIAM Journal on Scientific and Statistical Computing (1983) 553–572
22. Barret, R., Berry, M., Chan, T.F., Demmel, J., Donato, J., Dongarra, J., Eijkhout, V., Pozo, R., Romine, C., van der Vonst, H.: Templates for the Solution of Linear Systems: Building Blocks for Iterative Methods. SIAM, Philadelphia (1994) Available from netlib.

Representing Diffusion MRI in 5D for Segmentation of White Matter Tracts with a Level Set Method

Lisa Jonasson[1], Patric Hagmann[1,2], Xavier Bresson[1], Jean-Philippe Thiran[1], and Van J. Wedeen[3]

[1] Signal Processing Institute (ITS),
Swiss Federal Institute of Technology (EPFL), CH-1015 Lausanne, Switzerland
[2] Department of Diagnostic and Interventional Radiology,
Lausanne University Hospital (CHUV), CH-1011 Lausanne, Switzerland
[3] Athinoula A. Martinos Center for Biomedical Imaging,
Massachusetts General Hospital and the Harvard Medical School,
Boston, MA, United States

Abstract. We present a method for segmenting white matter tracts from high angular resolution diffusion MR images by representing the data in a 5 dimensional space of position and orientation. Whereas crossing fiber tracts cannot be separated in 3D position space, they clearly disentangle in 5D position-orientation space. The segmentation is done using a 5D level set method applied to hyper-surfaces evolving in 5D position-orientation space.

In this paper we present a methodology for constructing the position-orientation space. We then show how to implement the standard level set method in such a non-Euclidean high dimensional space. The level set theory is basically defined for N-dimensions but there are several practical implementation details to consider, such as mean curvature.

Finally, we will show results from a synthetic model and a few preliminary results on real data of a human brain acquired by high angular resolution diffusion MRI.

1 Introduction

Diffusion Weighted Magnetic Resonance Imaging is a modality that permits non-invasive quantification of the water diffusion in living tissues. The tissue structure will affect the Brownian motion of the water molecules which will lead to an anisotropic diffusion. Today, a diffusion tensor (DT) model is the most frequently used method to map the structural anisotropy. The tensor model, which basically only contains information about anisotropy and principal diffusion, has limited possibilities of resolving complex brain white matter architectures, particularly in regions with fiber crossings.

A recent approach first presented by Wedeen et al. in [1] is the Diffusion Spectrum Imaging (DSI) that provides a full 3D probability density function (PDF) of the diffusion at each location. This PDF provides a detailed description of the diffusion and manages to resolve highly complex cytoarchitecture such as fiber crossings. For simplicity the PDF is normally reduced to an orientation density function (ODF) which is the radial projection of the PDF. Other approaches such as q-ball imaging [2] and persistent angular structure (PAS) [3] aim at directly obtaining the ODF without first measuring the PDF. All these methods are commonly referred to as high angular resolution diffusion (HARD) MRI. Currently, the HARD data is used to map cerebral connectivity through fiber tractography [4].

Jonasson et al. [5] presented a 3D geometric flow algorithm designed for segmenting fiber tracts from DT-MRI. The method was based on the assumption that adjacent voxels in a tract have similar properties of diffusion and we defined similarity measures between tensors to propagate the surface. Various problems can benefit from fiber tract segmentation, like quantitative investigation of the diffusion inside the chosen fiber tracts, white matter registration and surgical planning.

By diagonalizing the DT several practical representations can be computed such as direction of principal diffusion, anisotropy and comparisons between different compartments of diffusion. These simplifications are less straightforward for the ODF. Frank et al. [6] presented a way of determining the anisotropy from HARD data but only anisotropy is not sufficient for segmentation of white matter tracts and the problem of crossing fibers remain unsolved. By augmenting the dimensionality of our data many of these problems can be solved simultaneously. Instead of considering a 3D map of ODFs, we define a 5D position-orientation space (POS) as a combination of a spherical space of orientation and an Euclidean space of position. Two fiber tracts with different directions of diffusion that are crossing each other in the same voxel become separated in this 5D space and can be segmented separately without interference from one another. Another positive aspect of this 5D space is that it consists of only scalar values which allow us to adapt classical segmentation methods for grayscale images.

Firstly we will explain the underlying principles of POS and show how to define it from a 3D map of ODF. We will then show that it is possible to segment white matter structures from HARDI MRI data by propagating a hyper-surface in this non-Euclidean 5D space. The evolution of the interface is implemented using the level set method proposed by Osher and Sethian [7,8,9]. The level set formalism is defined for N-dimensions and we will show how to practically apply it in 5D, with an emphasis on the computation of mean curvature in 5D.

2 Background Theory

2.1 Position Orientation Space

A HARDI experiment provides a 3D map of ODFs. Thus, for every position vector $\mathbf{x} = (x, y, z)$, in Euclidean 3D space, $\mathbb{R}^3$, there is an ODF measuring the intensity of diffusion in any direction, $\mathbf{u} = (\varphi, \theta)$ where $\mathbf{u}$ is a vector restricted

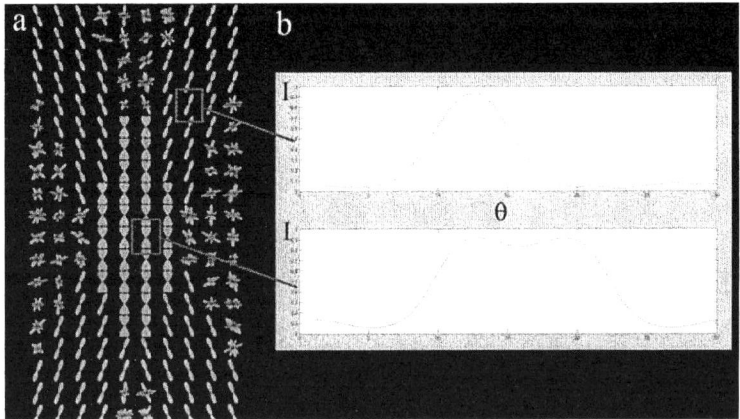

Fig. 1. Example of POS for a 2D slice of a volume of ODFs. The intensity is plotted for each angle

to the unit sphere, S^2, with $(0 \leq \theta < 2\pi, 0 \leq \varphi \leq \pi)$. The cartesian product of $\mathbb{R}^3$ and S^2 forms POS that we note Ω:

$$(\mathbf{x}, \mathbf{u}) \in \Omega = \mathbb{R}^3 \times S^2. \quad (1)$$

And its implied metric tensor allows us to determine the gradient operator as:

$$\nabla = \hat{\mathbf{x}}\frac{\partial}{\partial x} + \hat{\mathbf{y}}\frac{\partial}{\partial y} + \hat{\mathbf{z}}\frac{\partial}{\partial z} + \hat{\varphi}\frac{\partial}{\partial \varphi} + \frac{1}{\sin(\varphi)}\hat{\theta}\frac{\partial}{\partial \theta}. \quad (2)$$

To get some intuition about what POS is and why it is useful for fiber tract segmentation is it instructive to consider the case of a 2D map of ODF restricted to a plane. In Fig. 1a a 2D slice of ODFs is shown. The slice shows a crossing between two fiber tracts. The ODFs in the figure are restricted to the plane and can therefore be described through only one angle, θ. The intensity of the ODF varies with the angle. In the case where we only have one fiber there will be a peak in the intensity for the angle that corresponds to the direction of the fiber. In positions where two fiber tracts cross there will be two intensity peaks, one for the direction of each fiber. These two cases are illustrated in Fig.1b.

The third dimension represents the orientation of diffusion, hence the 2D ODF map is mapped as a 3D scalar field. This means that even though the two fiber tracts cross over in 2D, they will be separated in 3D and can therefore easily be segmented. Fig. 2 shows how the two fibers are segmented in 3D and then projected back to 2D.

2.2 Level Set Evolution of N-Dimensional Interfaces

Since the level set method was first introduced by Osher and Sethian [7, 8, 9] it is becoming a more and more popular numerical tool within image processing, fluid

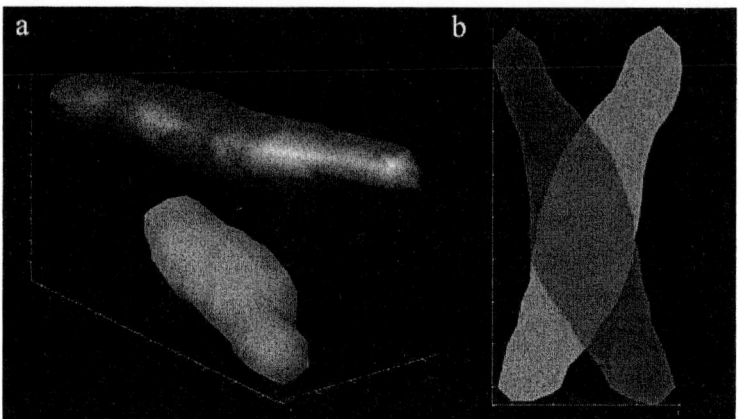

Fig. 2. Example of POS for a 2D slice of a volume of ODFs

mechanics, graphics, computer vision etc. It is basically used for tracking moving fronts by considering the front as the zero level set of an embedding function, called the level set function, of the moving front. In image processing the level set method is most frequently used as a segmentation tool through propagation of a contour by using the properties of the image as well as properties of the contour itself, such as the mean curvature. It was originally used to detect edges in an image [10], but more recent applications detect textures, shapes, colors etc. The level set theory was initially used for two dimensional images but its general formulation makes it possible to use for N-dimensional images. The theoretical extension to three dimensions is commonly used and even though some of the properties of the 2D curves, such as the property of shrinking to a point under curvature flow, do not hold in the 3D case, the main part of the theory remains valid and works well for segmentation of 3D objects [11]. The extension to even higher dimensions is straightforward.

Let the level set, $\phi(\mathbf{x}, t)$, be a smooth function where $\mathbf{x} \in \text{POS}$ and $t \in \mathbb{R}^+$. Then the hyper-surface in 5-dimensions is represented by the level set defined by $\{\mathbf{x} = (x, y, z, \varphi, \theta) \in POS : \phi(\mathbf{x}, t = 0)$.

The evolution of the hyper-surface embedded in the level set function is generally described through this equation:

$$\frac{\partial \phi}{\partial t} = F \mid \nabla \phi \mid, \tag{3}$$

where F is a speed function. For the particular case

$$F = -\nabla \cdot \left(\frac{\nabla \phi}{\mid \nabla \phi \mid} \right), \tag{4}$$

F is the mean curvature of level sets of ϕ and (3) becomes the 5-D mean curvature flow.

Chan and Vese presented in [12] a method for segmenting images without edge detection by using the weak formulation of the Mumford-Shah functional [13]. The resulting equation for the interface evolution becomes [12]:

$$\begin{cases} \frac{\partial \phi}{\partial t} = \delta_\epsilon(\phi) \left[\mu \nabla \cdot \left(\frac{\nabla \phi}{|\nabla \phi|} \right) - (u_0 - c_1)^2 + (u_0 - c_2)^2 \right] & \text{in } \Omega \\ \frac{\delta_\epsilon(\phi)}{|\nabla \phi|} \frac{\partial \phi}{\partial \vec{n}} = 0 & \text{on } \partial \Omega \end{cases} \quad (5)$$

where Ω is the image domain, in our case POS, and $\partial \Omega$ is the boundary of Ω. $\delta_\epsilon(\phi)$ is the ϵ-regularized Delta function [12] and $\mu > 0$ is a fixed parameter. u_0 is a given image which in our case is the ODF map represented as a scalar volume of intensity values in POS and c_1 and c_2 are defined as:

$$\begin{cases} c_1 = \frac{\int_\Omega H_\epsilon(\phi) u_0 dx}{\int_\Omega H_\epsilon(\phi)} \\ c_2 = \frac{\int_\Omega (1 - H_\epsilon(\phi)) u_0 dx}{\int_\Omega (1 - H_\epsilon(\phi))} \end{cases} \quad (6)$$

Here we have that $H_\epsilon(\phi)$ is the ϵ-regularized version of the Heaviside function and c_1 and c_2 are respectively the averages of the image u_0 on the region $\{\phi \geq 0\}$ and $\{\phi < 0\}$.

3 Method and Implementation

3.1 Creating POS

We have constructed the 5D POS from a 3D map of ODF. The values of the ODF are placed on a 2D grid. Due to the symmetry of the diffusion data only a hemisphere is sampled so we have that:

$$(\varphi, \theta) \in \{0, \frac{\pi}{n}, ..., \pi - \frac{\pi}{n}\} \times \{0, \frac{\pi}{n}, ..., \pi\}, \quad (7)$$

where n is the sampling step.

Due to the spherical geometry of the space there is a periodicity in the data. The two extremities along the θ-axis are neighbors. Due to the symmetry of the diffusion data this periodicity is also present along the φ-axis. If, due to the same symmetry, only a hemisphere is considered, the periodicity along the φ-axis can be disregarded. To cope with the periodicity of the data an exchange between the two ends of the level set along the θ-axis is made after every iteration.

3.2 Evolution of the Hyper-Surface

The hyper-surface is evolved according to (5). Once the POS is defined we have a scalar image not too different from a classical gray scale image. The specific considerations except for the high number of dimensions are the periodicity and the computation of the gradients, see (2). Implementing a level set function in 5D is theoretically straightforward but practically difficult. One of the main problem is handling the storage of the huge amount of data that is treated. Optimizing

Fig. 3. A hyper-cube evolving under 5D mean curvature flow. a) x-z-plane, b) y-θ-plane

the computation of the level set function and its re-initialization is crucial. There is however one important issue to consider theoretically: the computation of the curvature.

For evolving curves in 2D and surfaces in 3D the expression in (4) is already complicated. In the 2D case the expression of the mean curvature becomes:

$$\nabla \cdot \left(\frac{\nabla \phi}{|\nabla \phi|} \right) = \frac{\phi_{xx}\phi_y^2 - 2\phi_x\phi_y\phi_{xy} + \phi_{yy}\phi_y^2}{(\phi_x^2 + \phi_y^2)^{1/2}}. \tag{8}$$

Computing this equation for 5D, Mathematica gives a several pages long answer which is not satisfactory from a numerical point of view.

A lot of work has already been done for N-D mean curvature flows [14, 15]. Hence, we propose to use the theory developed by Ambrosio and Soner [14] to determine the mean curvature in a 5D space.

Differential geometry decomposes the mean curvature, Γ, into its principal curvatures, κ_n, such as:

$$\Gamma = \frac{\kappa_1 + ... + \kappa_N}{N}. \tag{9}$$

The principal curvatures of a hyper-surface embedded in a level set function, ϕ, of codimension one are then given by the eigenvalues of the following $N \times N$ matrix:

$$\frac{1}{|\nabla \phi(x)|^2} P_{\nabla \phi(x)} \nabla^2 \phi(x) P_{\nabla \phi(x)}, \tag{10}$$

where P_p is a projection operator onto the space normal to the nonzero vector p:

$$P_p = I - \frac{p \otimes p}{|p|^2}, \tag{11}$$

where I is the identity matrix.

To test these theories we have evolved a 5D hyper-cube through a mean curvature flow and seen how it first turns into a hyper sphere and then finally shrink to a point, see Fig 3.

The level set function is re-initialized at every iteration using the fast marching method [16]:
$$|\nabla \phi| = 1 \quad (12)$$

4 Results

4.1 Synthetic Data

To test the method we constructed a 3D volume of ODFs modelling two crossing fiber tracts, see left figure in Fig. 4. The ODFs are normalized by removing the minimum from each ODF. One surface was initialized by placing a small surface of a few voxels in each fiber tract. The hyper surface was evolved until convergence and then projected back into 3D Euclidean space. The result can be seen in Fig. 4. We see how each fiber tract is segmented completely without influence from the other crossing fiber.

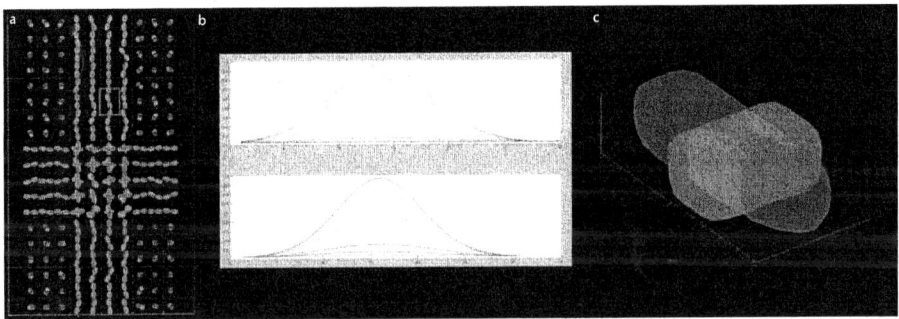

Fig. 4. a) Slice of the synthetic 3D volume of ODFs. b) The intensity of the different angles plotted against each other. c) The 3D projection of the 5D result

4.2 Real Data

Material. The diffusion images were obtained on a healthy volunteer with a 3T Philipps Intera scanner. We used a diffusion weighted single shot EPI sequence with timing parameters: TR/TE/Δ/ δ =3000/154/47.6/35 ms, bmax = 12000mm2/s and a spatial resolution of 2x2x3mm3. The data were acquired by sampling q-space on a 3D grid with 515 diffusion encoded directions restricted to the interior of a sphere of radius 5. From this acquisition the ODF map is reconstructed according a standard DSI scheme [17].

Informed consent was obtained in accordance with institutional guidelines for all of the volunteers.

Results. The ODFs are normalized by removing the minimum from each ODF. The small initial surfaces were placed inside brain region known to contain well

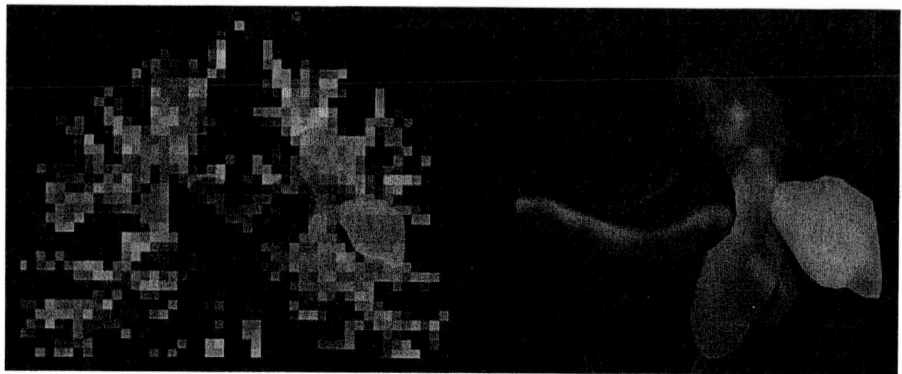

Fig. 5. Results from application on HARD MRI from a human brain. The red surface is a part of the cortico spinal tract. The blue surface is a segment of the corpus callosum and the green is the arcuate fasciculus

known fiber tracts. The result are shown in Fig. 5 and display the core of important fiber tracts such as the corpus callosum (blue), the cortico spinal tract (red) and the arcuate fasciculus in green. These are early results but show proof of principle. The current problem is the handling of data storage and only smaller volumes can be treated at the moment.

5 Discussion and Conclusion

We have shown how extending the dimensionality of the segmentation space from 3D to 5D disentangles originally overlapping structures. We have seen from the result on synthetic data, that crossing fiber tracts in 3D are represented in 5D POS as separate objects characterized by intense diffusion. The results shown for brain HARD MRI data are the early results. Due to the huge 5D matrices only parts of the structures have been segmented. However, they clearly show the potential of this approach to clearly delimit structures of coherent diffusion. The problem of data handling will be solved with better computer power and a more efficient implementation and data storage.

Further, we have shown that it is possible to implement the level set method for evolving a hyper-surface in a non-Euclidean 5D space. To solve the problem of the implementation of the mean-curvature flow we have proposed to use the theory developed by Ambrosio and Soner [14].

Segmenting regions in HARD MRI is a new approach for interpreting data with a different objective than classical fiber tractography. Fiber tractography provides a map of the cerebral connectivity and aims at visualizing fiber tracts as a set of lines. Our approach treats one fiber tract as one single object characterized by intense and coherent diffusion. This representation gives a different view of the brain architecture that can be more appropriate for applications such quantitative investigation of the diffusion as well as for surgical planning and white matter registration.

Acknowledgements

This work is supported by NIH 1R01-MH64044 grant and the Swiss National Science Foundation grant number 2153-066943.01.

References

[1] V.J. Wedeen, T.G. Reese, D.S. Tuch, M. R. Wiegell, T.G. Weisskoff, and D. Chessler, "Mapping fiber orientation spectra in cerebral white matter with fourier-transform diffusion mri," in *Proceedings of 8th Annual Meeting ISMRM*, Denver, 2000, p. 82.

[2] DS Tuch, TG Reese, MR Wiegell, and VJ Wedeen, "Diffusion mri of complex neural architecture.," *Neuron*, vol. 40, no. 5, pp. 885–895, 2003.

[3] K.M. Jansons and D.S. Alexander, "Persistent angular structure: new insights from diffusion mri data.," *Inverse problems*, vol. In Press, 2003.

[4] P. Hagmann, T. Reese, W. Tseng, R. Meuli, JP. Thiran, and Wedeen V, "Diffusion spectrum imaging tractography in complex cerebral white matter: An investigation of the centrum semiovale," in *ISMRM 12'th scientific meeting*, May 2004, vol. 12, p. 623.

[5] L. Jonasson, X. Bresson, P. Hagmann, R. Meuli, O. Cuisenaire, and J.-Ph. Thiran, "White matter fiber tract segmentation in dt-mri using geometric flows.," *Medical Image Analysis*, vol. In Press, 2004.

[6] L.R. Frank, "Anisotropy in high angular resolution diffusion-weighted mri," *Magn Reson Med*, vol. 45, no. 6, pp. 935–9, 2001.

[7] S. Osher and J.A. Sethian, "Fronts propagating with curvature-dependent speed: Algorithms based on Hamilton-Jacobi formulations," *Journal of Computational Physics*, vol. 79, pp. 12–49, 1988.

[8] S. Osher and N. Paragios, *Geometric Level Set Methods in Imaging, Vision, and Graphics*, 2003.

[9] JA. Sethian, *Level set methods and fast marching methods: Evolving interfaces in computational geometry, fluid mechanics, computer vision, and materials science*, 1999.

[10] V. Caselles, R. Kimmel, and G. Sapiro, "Geodesic active contours," *International Journal of Computer Vision*, vol. 22, pp. 61–79, 1997.

[11] V. Caselles, R. Kimmel, G. Sapiro, and C. Sbert, "Minimal surfaces: A three dimensional segmentation approach," *Numerische Mathematik*, vol. 77, no. 4, pp. 423–451, 1997.

[12] T.F. Chan and Vese L. A., "Active contours without edges.," *IEEE Tansactions on Image Processing*, vol. 10, no. 2, pp. 266–277, 2001.

[13] D. Mumford and J. Shah, "Optimal approximation by piecewise smooth functions and associated variational problems.," *Commun. Pure Appl. Math.*, vol. 42, pp. 577–685, 1989.

[14] L. Ambrosio and H.M. Soner, "Level set approach to mean curvature flow in arbitrary codimension," *Journal of Differential Geometry*, vol. 43, pp. 693–737, 1996.

[15] Y.G. Chen, Y. Giga, and S. Goto, "Uniqueness and existence of viscosity solutions of generalized mean curvature flow equations," *Journal of Differential Geometry*, vol. 33, pp. 749–786, 1991.

[16] D. Adalsteinsson and J.A. Sethian, "A fast level set method for propagating interfaces," *Journal of Computational Physics*, vol. 118, pp. 269–277, 1995.

[17] V.J. Wedeen, P. Hagmann, WYI. Tseng, and T.G. Reese, T.G.and Weisskoff, "Mapping complex tissue architecture with diffusion spectrum magnetic resonance imaging," *Accepted Magn Res Med*, 2005.

Automatic Prediction of Myocardial Contractility Improvement in Stress MRI Using Shape Morphometrics with Independent Component Analysis*

A. Suinesiaputra[1], A.F. Frangi[2], H.J. Lamb[1], J.H.C. Reiber[1], and B.P.F. Lelieveldt[1]

[1] Department of Radiology, Leiden University Medical Center,
Leiden, the Netherlands
[2] Computational Imaging Lab, Dept. of Technology,
Pompeu Fabra University, Barcelona, Spain

Abstract. An important assessment in patients with ischemic heart disease is whether myocardial contractility may improve after treatment. The prediction of myocardial contractility improvement is generally performed under physical or pharmalogical stress conditions. In this paper, we present a technique to build a statistical model of healthy myocardial contraction using independent component analysis. The model is used to detect regions with abnormal contraction in patients both during rest and stress.

1 Introduction

Ischemic heart disease is a major heart disease in the western world. Non-invasive diagnosis of ischemia has been developed in recent years (see [1] for the survey of different imaging techniques). Among others, Magnetic Resonance Imaging (MRI) has attracted many clinicians due to its excellent spatial and temporal resolution, high-contrast of soft tissue, accurate and reproducible global and regional ventricular function, flow and perfusion during rest and pharmacological stress, and the possibility of using paramagnetic contrast agent to enhance the intensity of myocardial infarction areas [2, 3].

One crucial assessment in ischemic heart disease is to determine whether hibernating or stunning myocardium occurs. This is viable but dysfunctional myocardium, which may improve its function after treatment [1]. The prediction

---

* This work is supported by the Dutch Science Foundation (NWO), under an innovational research incentive grant, vernieuwingsimpuls 2001. This work was also supported in part by a grant from Fundación MAPFRE Medicina and grants TIC2002-04495-C02 from the MEyC, and FIS-PI040676 and G03/185 from ISCIII. The work of A.F. Frangi was supported in part by a Ramon y Cajal Research Fellowship from the Spanish MEyC.

of improvement of myocardial contraction is only possible during physical or pharmacological stress [4]. Thus, the identification of dysfunctional myocardium that improves under stress is an important factor in the treatment of ischemic heart disease.

Low-dose dobutamine stress MRI can be used to evaluate improvement of myocardial contraction in infarct patients [1,5]. In this procedure, a low dose of dobutamine is administered to stimulate dysfunctional, but potentially viable myocardium. Usually, visual comparison between the rest and stress cine images is used to perform visual wall motion scoring. However, this visual assessment is very difficult and subjective to perform, because differences between rest and stress motion may be very subtle.

The goal of this work is to develop a method to automatically detect subtle changes in cardiac contraction between rest and stress. In this paper, we further expand previously described work on modeling the myocardial contraction of healthy hearts [6]. A statistical contraction model is trained from myocardial contours in rest condition using Independent Component Analysis (ICA) to construct a set of locally selective basis functions. Analysis is performed by projecting patient shapes onto this basis, and in [6], this model is used to automatically detect and localize abnormal cardiac contraction in rest. The main novelty of this work is twofold:

- We improve upon the ICA modeling framework by adopting a principled way of selecting the optimal number of components, and introducing kernel density estimation to describe the model parameter distributions for normal contraction.
- We apply the framework to the rest-stress comparison problem. By comparing the projection parameters in rest and stress conditions, one can assess which regions of myocardium show contractility improvement under stress, and therefore may be viable.

This paper is organized as follows. Section 2 describes the statistical modeling of normal contraction by using ICA. In Section 3, we present the qualitative prediction results of myocardial viability in stress condition, followed by a discussion in Section 4.

2 Methodology

ICA is originally used for finding source signals from a mixture of unknown signals without prior knowledge other than the number of sources [7]. There have been some studies to use ICA in machine learning for feature extraction [8], face recognition [9] and classification [10]. Previously, we have reported a statistical model to detect regional abnormalities from infarct patients using ICA [6]. The advantage of using ICA over other decompositions is the fact that ICA yields locally independent detectors that can be used to determine regional shape abnormalities, whereas PCA yields global shape variations that influence the entire shape.

ICA is a linear generative model, where every training shape can be approximated by a linear combination of its components. Let $x = (x_1, y_1, \ldots, x_m, y_m)^T$ be a shape vector, consisting of m pairs of (x, y) coordinates of landmark points. The linear generative model is formulated as follows:

$$x \approx \bar{x} + \Phi b .\tag{1}$$

The matrix $\Phi \in \mathbb{R}^{2m \times p}$ defines the independent components (ICs) and $b \in \mathbb{R}^p$ is the weight coefficient vector. The mean shape, $\bar{x}$, is defined by

$$\bar{x} = \frac{1}{n} \sum_{i=1}^{n} x_i .\tag{2}$$

where n is the number of shapes and p is the number of retained components.

The goal of ICA is to find a matrix, Ψ, such that

$$b = \Psi (x - \bar{x}) \tag{3}$$

with a constraint that columns of Ψ correspond to statistically independent directions. Thus the independent components are given by $\Phi = \Psi^{-1}$. The matrix Ψ is estimated by a suitable optimisation algorithm (see [11] for survey of ICA).

2.1 Modeling Contraction of Healthy Myocardium

In this paper, the observed shapes are taken from LV epi- and endocardial contours from short-axis MR images. To model the contractility pattern, contours for each subject are combined serially into one shape vector in the following order: endocardium contour at *end-diastole* (ED), epicardium contour at ED, endocardium contour at *end-systole* (ES) and epicardium contour at ES.

Prior to shape modeling, Procrustes shape alignment on the 4 contours at once was performed as a pre-processing step to eliminate global differences in pose and scale between the samples [12]. Mean shape of the training shapes after the alignment is shown in Fig. 1.

Since we want to determine the improvement of motion contraction from rest to stress, *centerline* points, i.e. points in the the middle between epi- and

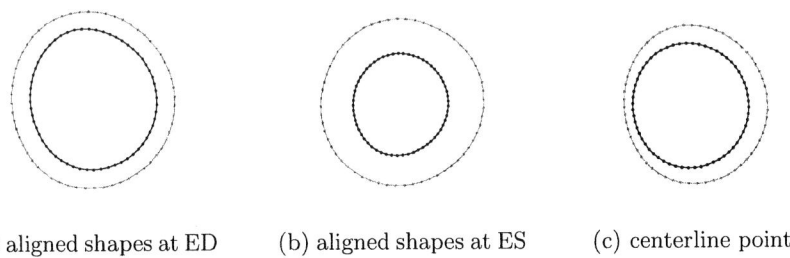

(a) aligned shapes at ED   (b) aligned shapes at ES   (c) centerline points

Fig. 1. Mean shape of the aligned training shapes

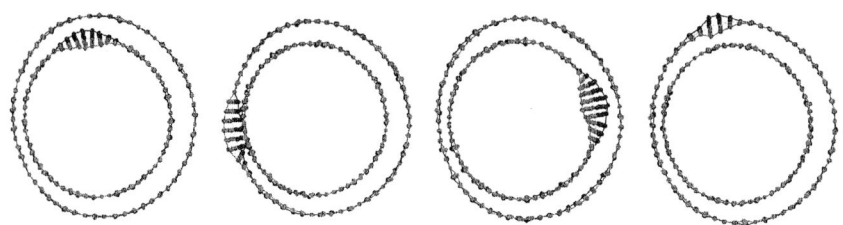

Fig. 2. Four examples of independent components from model. Dots are shape variations, where the maximum is $\pm 3\sigma$ (standard deviation). The inner and outer contours are ES and ED centerline points, respectively

endocardial contours, were used in ICA. The centerline method has already been used in the rest and stress studies to diagnose coronary artery disease [13]. Figure 1(c) shows the centerline points from the mean shapes.

Four examples of independent components are shown in Fig. 2. The independent components (ICs) show an interesting and important property where shape variations are local. In the diagnosis, these shape variations are used as detectors to determine local shape abnormalities, i.e. regions with abnormal contraction.

2.2 Determining the Number of Independent Components

If the number of source signals in ICA is not known a priori, the number of components needs to be determined. Many methods have been proposed to estimate this parameter, for instance, by using mutual information [14], neural networks [15], a Bayesian approach [16], and clustering techniques [17]. Though these approaches are different, the basic idea is to determine which are "weak" and "strong" independent components. Strong ICs represents reliable components.

In this paper, we adopted the clustering technique, proposed by Himberg et. al. [17][1]. In this approach, reliable ICs are determined from a number of different realizations of ICs with different initialization and by subsequently performing clustering on the resulting ICs. This approach was selected because of stochastic nature of computing ICs with the FastICA [7], the most popular and robust ICA algorithm that we used in this study.

After each trial, each IC is represented as a single point in a source space. The reliability of the estimated ICs can be analyzed by looking at the spread of the obtained ICs. The ICs form clusters in the source space, and the more compact and isolated the cluster of an IC, the more reliable is the IC (see Fig. 3(b)). To measure the reliability, an agglomerative hierarchical clustering is performed. A quality index of an IC, I_q, that reflects the compactness and isolating of a cluster, is defined as

$$I_q(C_m) = \frac{1}{|C_m|^2} \sum_{i,j \in C_m} \sigma_{ij} - \frac{1}{|C_m||C_{-m}|} \sum_{i \in C_m} \sum_{j \in C_{-m}} \sigma_{ij} \qquad (4)$$

---

[1] The implementation is known as the Icasso package [17].

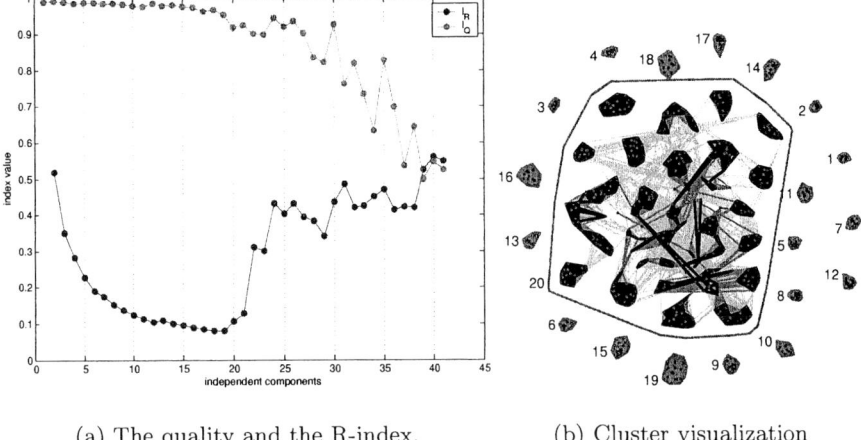

(a) The quality and the R-index. (b) Cluster visualization

Fig. 3. I_q and I_R plot and the visualization of the estimated ICs in the cluster space. In the right figure, clusters are indicated by red convex hulls. Grey lines connect estimates whose similarity is larger than a threshold, the darker the line the stronger the similarity. Labels correspond to independent components. Notice that reliable components are compact and isolated

where C_m and C_{-m} are the set of indices that belong and do not belong to the m-cluster, respectively. The σ_{ij} is a similarity measurement between i-th and j-th IC using their mutual correlation coefficient r_{ij}, i.e.

$$\sigma_{ij} = |r_{ij}| \ . \tag{5}$$

The value of I_q increases when C_m becomes more compact and isolated.

Another measurement to indicate reliable ICs in the clustering technique is the R-index, I_R.

$$I_R = \frac{1}{L} \sum_{m=1}^{L} \frac{S_m^{\text{in}}}{S_m^{\text{ex}}} \tag{6}$$

where

$$S_m^{\text{in}} = \frac{1}{|C_m|^2} \sum_{i,j \in C_m} d_{ij}$$

$$S_m^{\text{ex}} = \min_{m' \neq m} \frac{1}{|C_m||C_{m'}|} \sum_{i \in C_m} \sum_{j \in C_{m'}} d_{ij} \ .$$

d_{ij} is a dissimilarity measurement, defined as $d_{ij} = 1 - \sigma_{ij}$. The R-index is basically a ratio between the *within-cluster* and *between-cluster* ratio.

The R-index and the quality index indicate improved clustering in opposite directions. The optimal value for the number of computed ICs is when I_q is large and I_R is small. The plot of I_q and I_R for our study is shown in Fig. 3(a).

The estimated ICs can be visualized in the cluster space (see Fig. 3(b)). Each estimated IC is represented as a single point in the cluster space. Reliable ICs form compact and isolated clusters. In Fig. 3(b), ICs number 1 until 19 are reliable, whereas the remaining ICs are not reliable (they are glued together as one cluster number 20). The gray lines in Fig. 3(b) denote dependencies at some threshold values between clusters.

2.3 Density Estimation of Coefficient Values from the ICA Model

In Eq. 1, the b vector represents, the projection of a shape X onto the IC basis, Φ. The b vector contains coefficient values for the model that are needed to approximate the shape X from the IC basis. If X is similarly shaped to the shapes that construct the IC basis, then the coefficient values are within the distribution of the b vector of the model. On the contrary, if X is not similar to the shapes of the model, then the coefficient values are outside of the distribution. Hence, the detection of abnormal shapes becomes a problem of estimating the probability density function of the model coefficient values.

Since the ICA model is built from n training shapes, Eq. 1 can be simply reformulated in matrix form as:

$$X = \bar{x} \cdot \mathbf{1}^T + \Phi B \ . \tag{7}$$

We want to estimate the probability density of each column in matrix B. Figure 4 shows the distribution of each coefficient value from the healthy heart contraction for each IC (column of B), with an example of a projected patient shape.

In ICA, components are sought to be statistically independent. This is achieved by finding the direction of components that maximizes the nongaussianity [7].

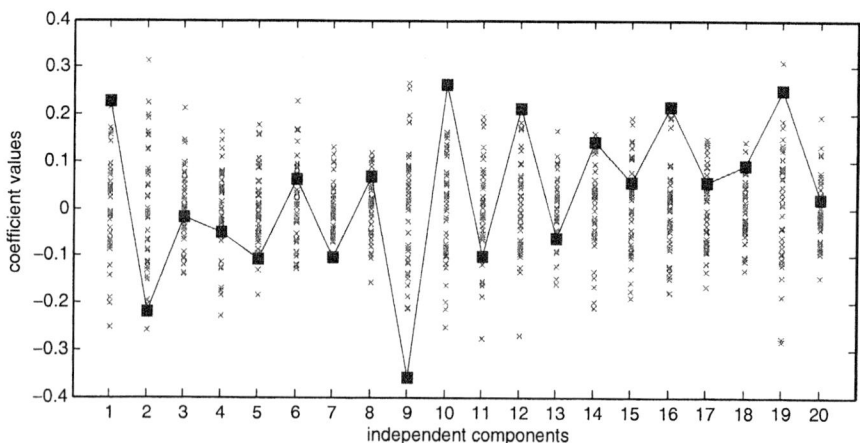

Fig. 4. Distribution of coefficient values of healthy heart contraction (crosses) with an example of coefficient values from the projected shape of a patient (solid lines)

The result is an independent basis which is non-orthogonal. The components have non-gaussian distribution, or at most only one with a gaussian distribution. Thus we cannot use an assumption of normal distribution to estimate the probability density function of the matrix $\boldsymbol{B}$.

However there is one important advantage of using ICA. A multivariate density estimation of the matrix $\boldsymbol{B}$ can be simplified into univariate density estimation, because of the independency. This cannot be done in other linear representation, such as PCA [18]. Thus we can estimate the probability density function on each of IC separately.

Based on those ICA properties, we used the non-parametric kernel density estimation [19] on each of the independent component separately. The kernel density estimation for the j-th component is defined by

$$\hat{f}_j(x) = \frac{1}{nh} \sum_{i=1}^{n} K\left(\frac{x - \boldsymbol{B}_{i,j}}{h}\right) \qquad (8)$$

where $\boldsymbol{B}_{i,j}$ is the coefficient values in the matrix $\boldsymbol{B}$ in Eq. 7 at j-th independent component. The bandwidth h and the kernel function $K(u)$ are the two parameters of the kernel density estimation method.

We choose the Gaussian function:

$$K(u) = \frac{1}{\sqrt{2\pi}} \exp\left(-\frac{u^2}{2}\right) \qquad (9)$$

as the kernel function. Note that the choice of kernel function is not really critical for the kernel density estimation, but rather for the choice of bandwidth [19].

The bandwidth h controls the amount of smoothing. A small difference in setting h can yield a big difference in the probability function. We use the Sheather-Jones solve-the-plugin method level 2 to estimate the optimal bandwidth [20]. The solve-the-plugin method solves an unknown functional parameter in the optimal bandwidth equation (see the equation in [20]) directly from the sample distribution.

After estimating the probability density function $\hat{f}_j(x)$ for each IC, the quantification of abnormalities is straightforward. We define a probability map of being abnormal for each IC as

$$\hat{p}_j(x) = 1 - \hat{f}_j(x) \ . \qquad (10)$$

A threshold value ρ is defined to determine the abnormality. Coefficient values that fall below that threshold are considered to be normal.

3 Experimental Results

3.1 Model Construction

An ICA model of healthy myocardial heart contraction was built by selecting epicardial and endocardial borders at ED and ES phases from 42 healthy volunteers. The mid-ventricular level from short-axis MRI was taken from each

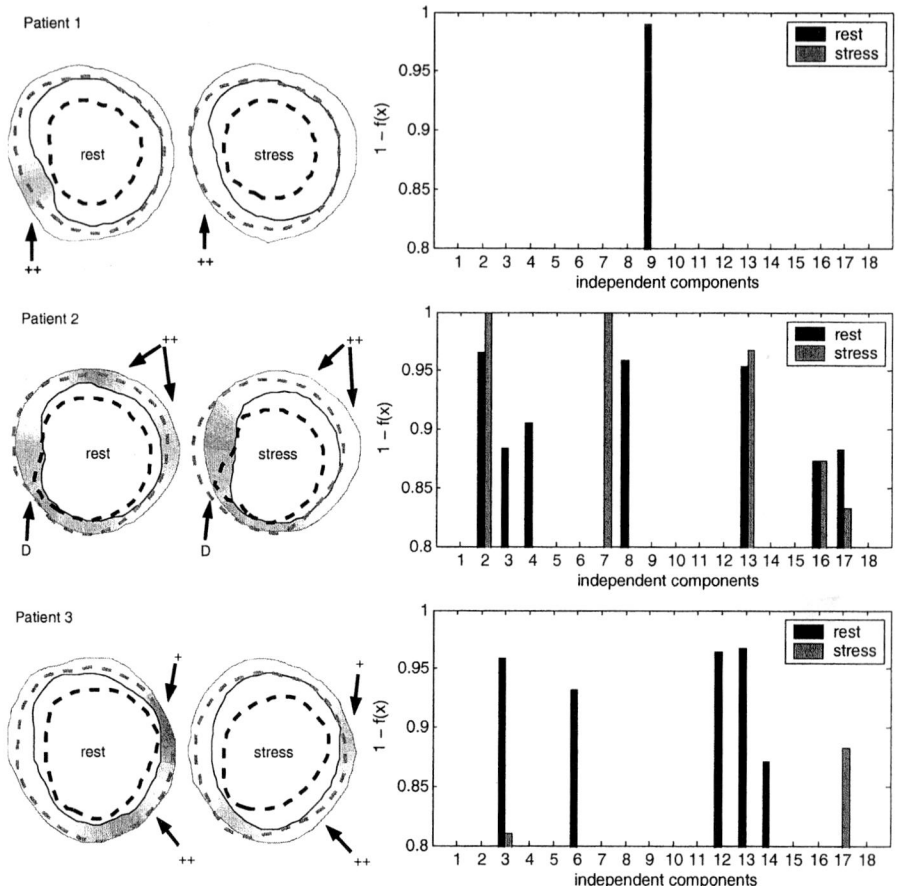

Fig. 5. Qualitative prediction results of myocardial contractility improvement from Patients 1, 2, and 3. The leftmost and middle figures are quantification of abnormal regions from rest and stress respectively. ED and ES contours are drawn in solid and dashed lines respectively, to visualize contraction of the heart. The right most figure shows the abnormal independent components

subject. Contours were drawn manually and used 60 landmark points per contour, defined by equi-angular sampling from the center of the myocardium. To ensure point correspondence between shapes, a fixed reference point was defined at the the intersection between the left and the right ventricle.

ICA was performed using the FastICA algorithm [7], implemented in Matlab. FastICA uses an optimization algorithm to maximize the *non-Gaussianity* of each component's direction to ensure that components are statistically independent between each other. The nonlinearity objective function used in the optimization process is $g(y) = 3y^2$ (or *pow*) and with symmetric orthogonalization. The number of independent components was determined following Himbergs approach [17], as has been described in Sec. 2.2. The number of trials was set to 20. The plot of the quality index and the R-index of the estimated ICs is shown in Fig. 3(a), yields 19 ICs.

3.2 Qualitative Prediction Results of Contractility Improvement

To qualitatively evaluate the prediction of myocardial contractility improvement under stress, MR data of 6 representative patients with acute myocardial infarction were selected. The threshold value, ρ, separating abnormal from normal coefficient values, is empirically defined as 0.8. Figure 5 and 6 show the visualization of abnormal regions in rest and stress for those 6 patients.

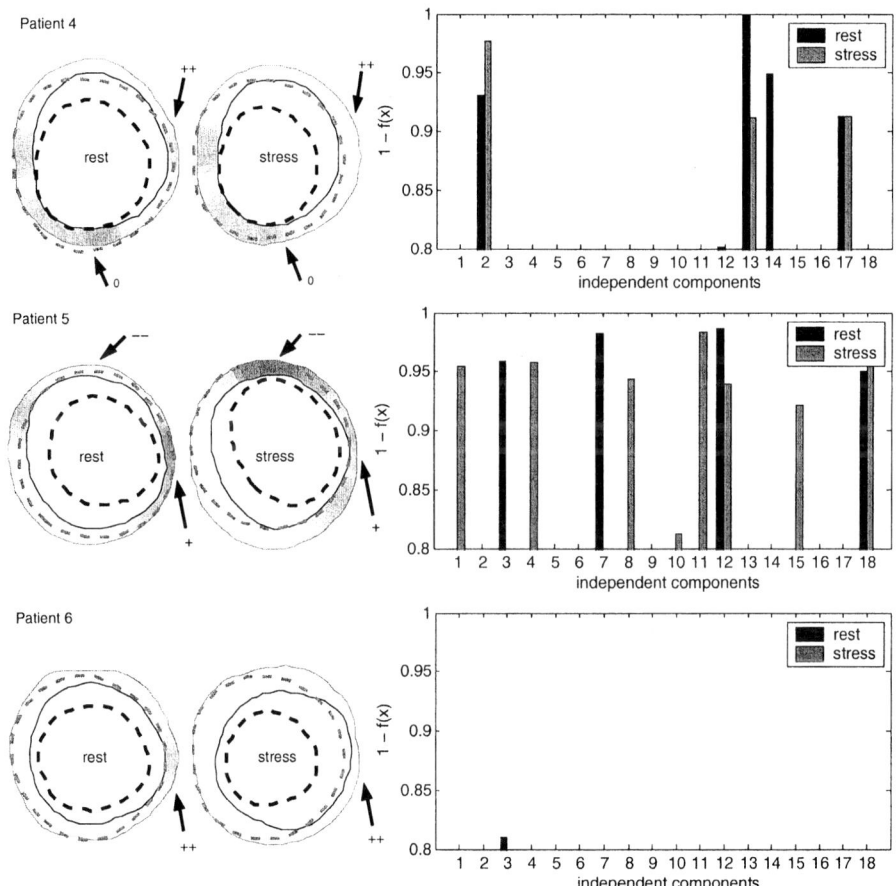

Fig. 6. Qualitative prediction results of myocardial contractility improvement from Patients 4, 5, and 6. The leftmost and middle figures are quantification of abnormal regions from rest and stress respectively. ED and ES contours are drawn in solid and dashed lines respectively, to visualize contraction of the heart. The right most figure shows the abnormal independent components

The left and middle figures are the quantification of abnormal contraction regions from our method in rest and stress, respectively. Regions with abnormal contraction are shown with dark colors inside of the myocardium. The darker the color, the more abnormal the regional motion. Thus regions with contractility improvement are visible by the decreasing amount of darkness from rest to stress in the corresponding regions.

Each of the abnormal regions has a corresponding abnormal independent component that is shown as bar plot at the right figure, given as the probability value of being abnormal. Contractility improvement of an IC is shown as a decreasing amount of the probability value from rest to stress.

Contraction motion is visualized with the ED (solid lines) & ES (dashed lines) contours that are plotted together. It can be seen from Fig. 5 and 6 that regions with abnormal contraction motion correspond visually with the dark areas.

Arrows in Fig. 5 and 6 point to some interesting regions in each patient. If contraction in a region is improved, then the arrow is marked with '+' sign (Patient 3 and 5). Regions with a lot of contractility improvement, where they are detected as normal in stress, are marked with '++' sign. These are seen at Patient 1, 2, 3, 4 and 6.

There is a case where an abnormal region does not improve its contractility in stress (Patient 4 with '0' sign) or even the contraction is getting worse in stress (Patient 5 with '−' sign). Another interesting case appears in Patient 2, where there is a region that has a small contraction in rest (see the arrow with 'D' sign), an improved contraction in stress, but abnormal motion in stress. This is detected by the model as an abnormal region.

4 Discussion

This paper explores the potential of using ICA to model contraction of healthy hearts. The model is used to detect myocardial regions with abnormal contraction, both in rest and stress. Comparing the detection between rest and stress gives an indication of areas that may improve after treatment.

In Fig. 5 and 6, we show 6 examples of the prediction results using the ICA model. These examples show that the method is capable to perform comparative morphometrics between rest and stress. Abnormal myocardial regions in rest with decreasing probability value in stress are identified as viable but dysfunctional myocardium. These are regions that may gain improvement after treatment.

The detected abnormal regions both in rest and stress correspond visually with the lack of contractility on those regions (see Fig. 5 and 6). The method can also detect an abnormal motion in stress, even with increased contraction. This is possible, because the model is statistically trained from normal cardiac contraction, all deviations from normal contraction or motion are labeled as abnormal.

Currently, we are working on validating the method with clinical visual wall motion scores to provide a quantitative evaluation of the method. The gold standard for the assessment of ischemic heart disease is post-treatment data when it comes to the question whether myocardium improves or not after treatment. This validation is performed on a larger patient group.

To gain more accurate prediction of contractility improvement for the whole heart, extending the ICA model into a semi 3D model is necessary to detect abnormal myocardial segments for the 3 major coronary arteries [21]. This involves inclusion of three levels of short-axis MRI (apical, middle and basal) and one segment from vertical long axis.

References

[1] Underwood, S.R., Bax, J.J., et. al.: Imaging techniques for the assessment of myocardial hibernation. European Heart Journal **25** (2004) 815–836
[2] van der Wall, E.E., Vliegen, H.W., et. al.: Magnetic Resonance Imaging in Coronary Artery Disease. Circulation **92** (1995) 2723–2739
[3] van der Geest, R.J., Reiber, J.H.: Quantification in Cardiac MRI. Journal of Magnetic Resonance Imaging **10** (1999) 602–608
[4] Nagel, E., Fleck, E.: Functional MRI in Ischemic Heart Disease Based on Detection of Contraction Abnormalities. Journal of Magnetic Resonance Imaging **10** (1999) 411–417
[5] Baer, F., Voth, E., et. al.: Gradient-echo magnetic resonance imaging during incremental dobutamine infusion for the localization of coronary artery stenoses. European Heart Journal **15** (1994) 218–225
[6] Suinesiaputra, A., Üzümcü, M., Frangi, A., Reiber, J., Lelieveldt, B.: Detecting Regional Abnormal Cardiac Contraction in Short-Axis MR Images Using Independent Component Analysis. In Barillot, C., Haynor, D.R., Hellier, P., eds.: 7th MICCAI Conf., LNCS 3216, Springer-Verlag (2004) 737–744
[7] Hyvärinen, A., Karhunen, J., Oja, E.: Independent Component Analysis. John Wiley & Sons, Inc. (2001)
[8] Akaho, S.: Conditionally Independent Component Analysis for Supervised Feature Extraction. Neurocomputing **49** (2002) 139–150
[9] Bartlett, M.S., Movellan, J.R., Sejnowski, T.J.: Face Recognition by Independent Component Analysis. IEEE Trans. on Neural Network **13** (2002) 1450–1464
[10] Lee, T.W., Lewicki, M.S.: Unsupervised Image Classification, Segmentation, and Enhancement Using ICA Mixture Models. IEEE Trans. on Image Processing **11** (2002) 270–279
[11] Hyvärinen, A.: Survey on Independent Component Analysis. Neural Computing Surveys **2** (1999) 94–128
[12] Dryden, I.L., Mardia, K.V.: Statistical Shape Analysis. John Wiley & Sons (2002)
[13] van Rugge, F.P., van der Wall, E.E., et. al.: Magnetic Resonance Imaging During Dobutamine Stress for Detection and Localization of Coronary Artery Disease. Circulation **90** (1994) 127–138
[14] Stögbauer, H., Andrzejak, R.G., et. al.: Reliability of ICA Estimates with Mutual Information. In Puntonet, C., Prieto, A., eds.: ICA 2004, LNCS 3195, Granada, Spain, Springer-Verlag (2004) 209–216
[15] Cichocki, A., Karhunen, J., et. al.: Neural Networks for Blind Separation with Unknown Number of Sources. Neurocomputing **24** (1999) 55–93

[16] Roberts, S.J.: Independent Component Analysis: Source Assessment & Separation, a Bayesian Approach. IEEE Proceedings - Vision, Image & Signal Processing **3** (1998) 149–154
[17] Himberg, J., Hyvärinen, A., Esposito, F.: Validating the Independent Components of Neuroimaging Time-Series via Clustering and Visualization. NeuroImage **22** (2004) 1214–1222
[18] Bressan, M., Vitrià, J.: Independent Modes of Variation in Point Distribution Models. In Arcelli, C., Cordella, L., di Baja, G.S., eds.: 4th Int. Workshop on Visual Form, IWVF4, LNCS 2059, Springer-Verlag (2001) 123–134
[19] Silverman, B.: Density Estimation for Statistics and Data Analysis. Monographs on Statistics and Applied Probability. Chapman and Hall, London (1986)
[20] Wand, M., Jones, M.C.: Kernel Smoothing. Chapman and Hall (1995)
[21] Cerqueira, M.D., Weissman, N.J., et. al.: Standardized Myocardial Segmentation and Nomenclature for Tomographic Imaging of the Heart: A Statement for Healthcare Professionals From the Cardiac Imaging Committee of the Council on Clinical Cardiology of the American Heart Association. Circulation **105** (2002) 539–542

Brain Segmentation with Competitive Level Sets and Fuzzy Control

Cybèle Ciofolo and Christian Barillot

IRISA / CNRS - Team Visages,
35042 Rennes Cedex, France
{Cybele.Ciofolo, Christian.Barillot}@irisa.fr
http://www.irisa.fr/visages/visages-eng.html

Abstract. We propose to segment 3D structures with competitive level sets driven by fuzzy control. To this end, several contours evolve simultaneously toward previously defined anatomical targets. A fuzzy decision system combines the a priori knowledge provided by an anatomical atlas with the intensity distribution of the image and the relative position of the contours. This combination automatically determines the directional term of the evolution equation of each level set. This leads to a local expansion or contraction of the contours, in order to match the borders of their respective targets. Two applications are presented: the segmentation of the brain hemispheres and the cerebellum, and the segmentation of deep internal structures. Experimental results on real MR images are presented, quantitatively assessed and discussed.

1 Introduction

Segmentation of anatomical structures is a critical task in medical image processing, with a large range of applications going from visualization to diagnosis. For example, to delineate structures in the mid-sagittal plane of the brain in the context of a pre-operative planning, an accurate segmentation of the hemispheres, and especially of their internal faces, is needed. In such a task, the main difficulties are the non-homogeneous intensities within the same class of tissue, and the high complexity of anatomical structures such as white and gray matter, as well as their large variability.

Various methods using deformable models have been proposed for image segmentation. Parametric methods [1], including the first active contours, showed limited abilities to deal with topological changes and complex, highly convoluted shapes, both being frequent in 3D medical images. The non-parametric approaches, including gradient-based methods [2, 3], region-based methods [4, 5, 6], or both [7, 8], proved a better adaptability to medical applications. The level set formalism [9] provides an efficient implementation for these approaches, with the following advantages: (i) efficient numerical schemes are available, (ii) topological changes are allowed, and (iii) extension of the method to higher dimensions is easy. The evolution force of a level set depends on internal properties of the corresponding contour, such as the local curvature, on external parameters and on additional propagation terms. The role of these additional terms is to drive the contour to dedicated areas, depending on the target application. To this end, both image data such as the gray levels and prior knowledge are critical to get accurate results in the context of medical image segmentation. Thus, our goal is to take advantage of as much information as possible in the level set evolution.

Recent approaches [6, 7] generally use energy minimization techniques to define the additional terms of the force. However, in medical imaging, the structures of interest are often very small compared to the image resolution and may have complex shapes. This makes it difficult to define energy constraints that remain both general and adapted to specific structures and pathologies.

Another approach consists in translating the available information into decision rules that are directly used to drive the level set evolution. To do so, a strong theoretical background and effective tools are provided by fuzzy logic [10]. In particular, the use of fuzzy sets is appropriate to describe data that belong to ill-defined categories, where neither arbitrary classes nor fixed borders are defined, such as the voxels corresponding to partial volumes on cerebral MRI data. Consequently, the fuzzy sets theory has already been used in medical image segmentation. Some authors [12] use an adaptative fuzzy c-means algorithm that is combined with an isosurface algorithm and a deformable surface model to reconstruct the brain cortex. Automatic segmentation methods for brain internal structures are also proposed [13], where the segmentation is based on a symbolic spatial description of the structures and finally refined with a deformable model.

Our approach differs from these ones. As we wish to process larger structures and more complex shapes, we propose to introduce a regularization constraint as soon as the segmentation begins. To do so, we use a level set algorithm, whose evolution parameters are automatically tuned by a specific type of fuzzy decision system: a fuzzy controller [15]. In particular, this decision system takes advantage of the structure labels provided by an atlas, the anatomical description brought by experts and the intensities of the processed volumes. Following previous work [16, 17], we focus on the competition between several level sets to segment structures that cannot be distinguished with only their intensities. As a first example, we apply our method to the segmentation of the brain hemispheres and the cerebellum, with the objective to get a fine segmentation of the hemispheres internal faces. We also use our algorithm to segment the basal ganglia and thalami, which correspond to a critical target area for electrical stimulation in Parkinson's disease treatment. The method can also be used in many other contexts where the target regions cannot be segmented with only the statistics of the image.

This paper is organized as follows. The segmentation method is described in Section 2 with a focus on the level set formulation. Section 3 presents the tuning of the expansion-contraction term of the level set equation with a fuzzy controller and the application to the label competition. Our results on real MRI volumes are then presented and discussed in Section 4.

2 Level Set Segmentation Driven by Fuzzy Control

2.1 General Formulation of the Level Set Evolution

The design of our level set is based on the region-based evolution force proposed in [18]:

$$F = g(P_T)(\rho\kappa - \nu), \qquad (1)$$

where ν is a constant module force, whose sign leads the current contour toward the desired border; κ is the local curvature of the contour; ρ is the weight on curvature; g is a decreasing function; and P_T is the probability of transition between the inside and the outside of the structure to be segmented. Thus the role of the term $g(P_T)$ is to stop the evolution of the contour at the desired location.

The ν and P_T terms are computed according to a preliminary classification of tissues before the beginning of the level set evolution. The image intensities are viewed as samples of a Gaussian Mixture Model (GMM), whose parameters are estimated according to a Maximum A Posteriori principle, with a SEM algorithm [14]. The classes that are mainly represented inside the initialization volume are automatically detected and determine the reduced GMM corresponding to the inside of the object to segment. For further details concerning the computation of these terms, see [18].

The advantages of the evolution force described in Eq. (1) is that it is very simple and directly derived from the original geometric active contour formulation [2]. It assigns a precise role to each term, while preserving the ability to modify each term according to geometrical constraints corresponding to visual requirements.

2.2 Adding Dedicated Geometrical Constraints with Fuzzy Control

Our goal is to take advantage of the strong background presented in Section 2.1, and to improve it while meeting the requirements of real medical problems. These requirements are difficult to model with a robust mathematical formulation. In particular, the energy minimization methods are often too global to lead to a fine segmentation of thin structures, and when they give satisfactory results, they generally use weighting parameters that need to be manually tuned.

To avoid this, our approach is to extract as much information as possible from the intensities of the MRI volume and to combine it with the knowledge brought by an atlas and the anatomical descriptions provided by some experts. Finally, the result is directly used in the level set evolution law. This implies to perform the fusion between numerical data (coming from both the MRI volume and the atlas) and symbolic data (the spatial description of the brain structures), which is the typical field of application of the theory of fuzzy sets [10].

However, let us stress that we want to preserve the precision of the data coming from the MRI volume. For this reason, the use of a fuzzification process, which would blur the data, does not seem appropriate, and we prefer to work in a context where precise measurements are directly applicable as inputs of the fuzzy decision system. This requirement leads us to focus on a particular application of the theory of fuzzy sets : fuzzy control [15].

The fuzzy controller is a fuzzy decision system that efficiently translates evolution rules, which are formulated by sentences in natural language, into constraints that are introduced in the level set equation. In previous works, we showed how to combine the gradient and region information to improve the stopping criterion $g(P_T)$ in Eq. (1) [16], and how to use fuzzy labels to automatically tune the weighting parameter on curvature ρ in Eq. (1) so that the white matter is accurately segmented, or to have the level set evolve to a selected area, for example the left hemisphere of the brain [17].

In this paper, we focus on the competitive evolution of several level sets, according to various constraints. The advantage of competition between level sets is that, under certain conditions, it can be considered as a shape constraint when there is no statistical information to distinguish between several regions of the MRI volume. For example, the left and right hemispheres of the brain are similar with respect to their image intensities and the contour curvature. However, using their spatial localization, their identification is easy.

Consequently, for each level set, our method takes into account both the distance of the corresponding contour to the fuzzy map associated to the structure to segment and the distance to the other contours, as well as the gray levels of the MRI volume. Inputs for the fuzzy decision system are then defined from these sources of data. As we aim at defining a privileged propagation direction for the contour, the output of the fuzzy controller is the value of the ν parameter in Eq. (1). In other words, for each voxel, the local value of ν will be assigned so as to favor contraction or expansion of the contour, as shown in Section 3.

3 Tuning of the Expansion-Contraction Term ν

This section presents in detail the fuzzy decision system that assigns the value of ν for each voxel of the processed volume, at each iteration step of the level set algorithm.

3.1 Principle of the Fuzzy Decision System

In [18], the proposed computation of ν is:

$$\nu = \text{Sign}(P(\lambda \in \Lambda_i | \mathbf{x}) - P(\lambda \in \Lambda_e | \mathbf{x})), \qquad (2)$$

where $\mathbf{x}$ is the current voxel, λ is the class of the current voxel estimated from the volume histogram, and Λ_i and Λ_e are the reduced GMM representing respectively the inside and the outside of the structure to be segmented. We aim at replacing this equation by a law constituted of three constraints:

1. Several contours that evolve in competition must not intersect even if each of them can split in several components;
2. Each contour must stay in the vicinity of the fuzzy label describing its segmentation target;
3. Eq. (2) is valid under Conditions 1 and 2.

Condition 1 corresponds to the idea of competition between the evolving contours. Some methods have been developed to solve this problem, such as region competition algorithms [6]. However this approach is applicable if the regions can be distinguished by their statistics. In the case of regions presenting similar gray levels, such as the brain hemispheres, one must use other features, like labels coming from an atlas, to guarantee that the different contours will not intersect. Another repulsive constraint has also been proposed in [19]: if a pixel is covered by another contour than the current one, the current contour is pushed away. The advantage of this condition is its simplicity, both for implementation and introduction into an energetical model. But this requires to have well-defined classes, which does not correspond to the segmentation of brain MRI volumes. Consequently, we choose to take advantage of this idea and adapt it to our application in order to fulfill the above three conditions. The role of the fuzzy decision system, more specifically the fuzzy controller, is thus to translate this repulsive constraint in a fuzzy environment. Let us note that even if there is a distinct equation evolution for each contour, all of them have to match the same general constraints, consequently only one fuzzy controller is needed and used successively for all the level sets.

A fuzzy controller is characterized by three main elements: the inputs, the outputs and the decision rules. The inputs and outputs are fuzzy variables that are characterized by several states modeled by fuzzy sets. The decision rules are expressed in natural language and determine the fusion of the inputs in order to compute the value of the outputs.

3.2 Inputs of the Fuzzy Controller

Three fuzzy variables are used as inputs of the fuzzy controller, each one corresponding to one of the conditions listed in Section 3.1.

1. Dc represents the distance from the current contour to the other ones.
2. $Dlab$ represents the signed distance from the current contour to the label corresponding to its segmentation target. An example of distance map, or fuzzy label map of the left brain hemisphere is shown on Fig. 1.
3. Dp represents the difference of probability presented in Eq. (2).

Dc and $Dlab$ are five-state variables. Each state is represented by a fuzzy set with a trapezoidal or triangular membership function. Dp is a simpler variable, since only the sign of the difference of probability in Eq. (2) was shown to have a real influence on the contour evolution [18]. Consequently, Dp is characterized by two states only, which also have trapezoidal membership functions.

Let us note that we also used Gaussian-like functions to represent the states of the variables. However, as reported in [15, 11], we did not observe any significant modification of the segmentation results.

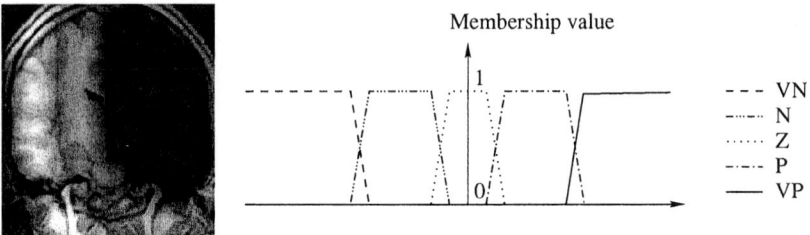

Fig. 1. Left: example of distance map from the left hemisphere. Right: the five fuzzy states of the *Dlab* variable: very negative (VN), negative (N), around zero (Z), positive (P) and very positive (VP)

3.3 Outputs of the Fuzzy Controller

The unique output of the fuzzy controller is the variable ν, which has two states: P and N, which respectively mean *positive* and *negative*. We choose this representation in relation with Eq. (1) and Eq. (2), where ν is a constant module force.

3.4 Decision Rules of the Fuzzy Controller

The fuzzy decision rules are the translation of the conditions described in Section 3.1. They are formulated as "IF ... THEN..." expressions. An example of these rules is:

"IF (*Dlab* is P) AND (*Dp* is P) AND ((*Dc* is F) OR (*Dc* is RC) OR (*Dc* is C) OR (*Dc* is TC)) THEN (ν is P)"

The conjunction operator AND was implemented with the t-norm *min* and the disjunction operator OR with the t-conorm *max*. The results are defuzzified to obtain the final value of ν with the centroid method. Let us note that, as reported in [10, 11], these choices are very common, but not critical, in the context of fuzzy control.

The fuzzy decision rules that were set up in this work are summarized in Table 1. In order to meet Condition 1, which avoid overlapping between contours corresponding to different level sets, the ν output of the fuzzy set is tuned to act as a repulsion or contraction force (ν=N), when a contour is too close to another one (*Dc*=N). This corresponds to the first line of the table.

Condition 2, which is related to the distance maps, is translated by a majority of P states in the right part of the table and N states in the left part. This means that if the processed voxel of the contour is far outside its label (*Dlab*=N or VN), it needs to contract (ν=N). On the contrary, if it is inside the label (*Dlab*=P or VP), it needs to expand (ν=P).

Condition 3 is mainly visible in the central part of the table (*Dlab*=Z and *Dc*=TC to F). This corresponds to the case where the contour is within the vicinity of its label and not too close to another one. Then the state of ν depends on the intensities of the volume only, as explained in Eq.(2).

Table 1. Fuzzy decision rules for the output variable ν. The states of the variable $Dlab$ are very negative (VN), negative (N), around zero (Z), positive (P), and very positive (VP). The states of the variable Dc are null (N), too close (TC), close (C), rather close (RC) and far (F). The states of the variables Dp and ν are negative (N) and positive (P)

	$Dlab$=VN		$Dlab$=N		$Dlab$=Z		$Dlab$=P		$Dlab$=VP	
	Dp=N	Dp=P	Dp=N	Dp=P	Dp=N	Dp=P	Dp=N	Dp=P	Dp=N	Dp=P
Dc=N	N	N	N	N	N	N	N	N	N	N
Dc=TC	N	N	N	N	N	P	N	P	P	P
Dc=C	N	N	N	N	N	P	N	P	P	P
Dc=RC	N	N	N	N	N	P	N	P	P	P
Dc=F	N	N	N	N	N	P	N	P	P	P

4 Experiments and Results

We focus on two applications to illustrate our method. First, we use three level sets in competition to segment simultaneously the left and right hemispheres of the brain and the cerebellum. The goal of this experiment is to obtain an accurate segmentation of the internal faces of the hemispheres, in order to later on delineate structures on these faces, like the calcarine sulci. Another interesting issue in pre-operative planning is the segmentation of internal structures such as the thalami and parts of the basal ganglia. These structures correspond to target areas for electrical stimulation in the context of Parkinson's disease treatment for example. For this application, we use four level sets, one for each of these structures: thalami, caudate nuclei, pallida and putamens.

4.1 Data

We test our method on a database provided on the Internet Brain Segmentation Repository (IBSR), and available at the Center for Morphometric Analysis, Massachusetts General Hospital (http://www.cma.mgh.harvard.edu/ibsr).

This database, which will be called the IBSR dataset in this document, contains 18 real T1-weighted MR scans and the corresponding manual segmentation of 43 structures, performed by a trained expert. We consider this manual segmentation as the ground truth to assess our results. The MR scans are 256x256x128 volumes, with slices of thickness 1.5mm, and pixel dimension going from 0.84mm to 1mm on each slice.

We also use another database of 18 real T1-weighted volumes without ground truth to qualitatively assess the robustness of the segmentation of the brain hemispheres and the cerebellum. This set of volumes is called the GIS dataset, and each MR scan (GE, 1.5T) is 256x256xN, where N is the number of 1mm slices (typically between 150 and 190), with isotropic voxels.

4.2 A Fully Automatic Processing

In order to achieve the segmentation of brain structures of interest in MRI volumes coming from any acquisition system, we include the segmentation algorithm in a fully automatic succession of operations. These operations are the same for each processed MRI volume.

First, one subject is randomly selected among the IBSR dataset. It is isolated as the reference subject for this set of volumes and its manual segmentation is considered as the atlas for all the experiments that are run on the 17 remaining subjects. Concerning the GIS database, we use the BrainWeb dataset [20] as the reference atlas.

A brain mask and fuzzy label maps (or distance maps) are then created from the atlas for each of the processed subjects. Afterwards, the segmentation is performed with a level set algorithm including the fuzzy decision module described in the previous sections.

Creation of a Brain Mask. To create an adjusted brain mask for the processed volume from the atlas, we use an affine registration algorithm (12 parameters that maximize the mutual information are computed). The gray matter, white matter and internal CSF volumes of the reference subject were previously combined to obtain a reference brain segmentation. We then use a morphological dilation on the registration result to get a mask including the whole brain of the processed volume.

Creation of the Fuzzy Label Maps. As for the brain mask, the labels corresponding to the target structures (hemispheres and cerebellum or internal structures) are extracted from the manual segmentation of the reference subject and registered with a non-linear algorithm towards the processed volume. For each structure to segment, the signed distance to the corresponding registered label border is then computed and normalized to be used as the D_{lab} input of the fuzzy decision system.

4.3 Segmentation of the Hemispheres and the Cerebellum

These experiments are run both on the IBSR dataset and the GIS dataset. The three level sets are initialized with boxes located respectively in the left and right hemispheres and in the cerebellum.

Fig. 2 shows the segmentation results on both datasets, with the same set of parameters. The boxes are deformed in order to correctly match the complex shapes of the three structures. The mean computation time is around 30 minutes on a 2.6GHz PC Linux. The visual quality of the segmentation results on the internal faces of the hemispheres is good. Note that these results show the robustness of the method, since the contours are initialized far from their targets and the intensity distribution strongly varies from one dataset to the other one, and inside the IBSR dataset itself.

In order to quantitatively assess our results on the IBSR dataset, we compute the mean distance M_d between our results and the ground truth provided by

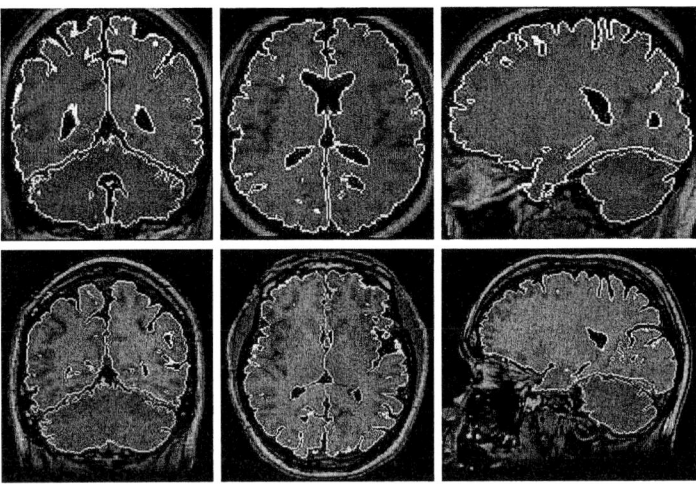

Fig. 2. Segmentation with labels of the left hemisphere, right hemisphere and cerebellum. Top row: IBSR dataset, bottom row: GIS dataset

Table 2. Mean values of the similarity indexes for the segmentation (Seg.) and the registration (Reg.) of the hemispheres (LH and RH) and the cerebellum (C) on the IBSR dataset

Index	LH Seg.	LH Reg.	RH Seg.	RH Reg.	C Seg.	C Reg.
Spatial accuracy index S	0.95	0.89	0.95	0.89	0.92	0.80
Mean distance M_d (mm)	1.5	2.0	1.6	2.1	2.1	2.6

the manual segmentation. We also use the spatial accuracy index S, which is a similarity index based on the overlapping rate between the result and the truth [21]:

$$S = 2 \cdot \frac{\text{Card}(R \cap T)}{\text{Card}(R) + \text{Card}(T)} \qquad M_d = \frac{\sum_{r \in R} \min_{t \in T} d(r,t)}{\text{Card}(R)},$$

where R is the segmentation result and T is the ground truth. Our results are summarized in Table 2. This table also contains the index values corresponding to the similarity between the non-linear registration result of the atlas structures and the ground truth. This shows that the segmented volumes are clearly closer to the ground truth than the ones that were obtained with a registration algorithm only.

4.4 Segmentation Results of Internal Structures

The objective of these experiments is to show another application of the competitive level set algorithm. The segmentation of internal structures of the brain gray matter is peculiarly difficult since they are located in partial volume areas

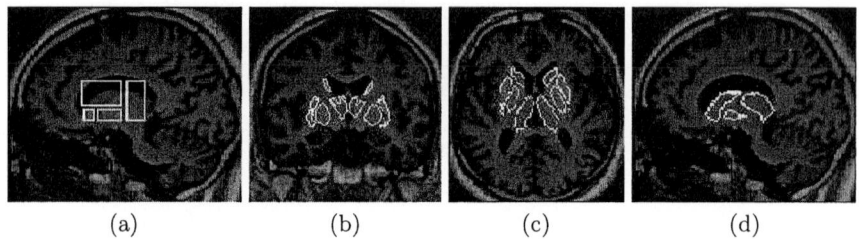

Fig. 3. (a): Initialization of the level set with boxes. (b), (c), (d): Segmentation with labels of the thalami, caudate nuclei, pallida and putamens

and their borders are largely blurred. In this section, we present promising preliminary results that should be improved by future refinement of the method.

As no ground truth is available for the GIS dataset, these experiments are run on the IBSR dataset. We wish to take into account the a priori knowledge provided by the registered labels of each target region: thalami, caudate nuclei, pallida and putamens. Consequently the level sets are initialized with seed regions obtained by morphological erosion of the labels. The mean computation time is 8 minutes. Let us note that, as for the previous experiments, the segmentation is done with exactly the same set of parameters for all the volumes in the dataset.

An example of the segmentation results is shown on Fig. 3. The visual quality of the segmented structures is globally good on 14 subjects of the dataset. For 3 cases, the results are too small or too large compared to the ground truth. This is due to the location of the target structures, which corresponds to partial volume areas on the MR scans. Due to the small range of the histogram of these 3 cases, the preliminary classification process (see Section 2.1 and 3.1) does not succeed in accurately classifying the partial volumes. Consequently, the role of the Dp input of the fuzzy controller is not completely adapted to the desired evolution of the level sets. We believe that this should be improved with a better adaptation of the classification process to the range of the histogram. Another solution would be to introduce a priori spatial relations between the internal structures as inputs of the fuzzy decision system, as suggested in [13]. This should help the contours to jointly evolve toward their respective targets.

The left part of Fig. 3 shows an illustration of the level sets topological flexibility. They are initialized with a box roughly located in the area of the target structures, and split in four boxes, one for each level set. Each box evolves toward its specific target and the segmentation results are similar to the ones with registered seed regions.

The quantitative evaluation of the results is shown in Table 3. The spatial accuracy index is good for the thalami. For the caudate nuclei, pallida and putamens, the lower values can be explained by the small size of the corresponding structures. Consequently, even a small difference between the result and the ground truth leads to a large variation in the spatial accuracy index. As an example, let us consider the result of a morphological erosion on the ground truth of one of these structures with a structuring element of size 1. The mean S value

Table 3. Similarity indexes values for the segmentation (Seg.) and the registration (Reg.) of the thalami (Th), caudate nuclei (CN), pallida (GP) and putamens (Pu)

Index	Th. Seg.	Th. Reg.	CN Seg.	CN Reg.	GP Seg.	GP Reg.	Pu. Seg.	Pu. Reg.
S	0.77	0.75	0.65	0.59	0.58	0.62	0.70	0.72
M_d (mm)	1.70	1.79	1.71	1.81	1.51	1.69	1.46	1.59

computed between the ground truth and the erosion result is only 0.77. For this reason, the index values obtained between the non-linearly registered labels and the ground truth were included in the table. They show that the segmentation improves the registration results for both thalami and caudate nuclei. On the contrary, for the smallest structures, pallida and putamens, the similarity slightly decrease with the segmentation process. However, the mean distances between the result and the ground truth remain very low even for these structures, which shows that the competitive level set segmentations can be considered as promising premilinary results for internal structures. Moreover, note that we used a manual segmentation as the ground truth, without taking into account the intra and inter-observer variability that is generally observed on manual results, and should be included in the computation of similarity indexes.

5 Conclusion and Future Work

We presented an automatic method for the simultaneous segmentation of several regions with competitive level sets driven by fuzzy control. The level set evolution depends on the intensity distribution of the image, the distance to other evolving contours, and the distance to a target label registered from an atlas. This method was applied in two contexts: the segmentation of the brain hemispheres and the cerebellum, and the segmentation of internal structures of the brain.

Experimental results show that the competitive level sets can adapt to several datasets and precisely segment complex shapes such as the internal faces of the brain hemispheres, even if they are initialized far from the desired result. However, the method still needs improvement on internal structures because of the partial volumes and the small size of the structures.

This leads to introduce new a priori knowledge in the fuzzy decision system, such as the spatial relations between the target structures. A variety of medical applications could thus take advantage of this technique to assess the evolution of anatomical structures, such as lesions.

Acknowledgements

We thank the Center for Morphometric Analysis at Massachusetts General Hospital (http://www.cma.mgh.harvard.edu/ibsr/) for providing the MR brain data sets and their manual segmentations.

This work was supported by the CNRS and the Region Bretagne Council.

References

1. Kass, M., Witkin, A., Terzopoulo, D.: Snakes: Active contour models. Int. Journal of Computer Vision, Vol 1 **1** (1988) 321–331
2. Malladi, R., Sethian, J. A., Vemuri, C.: Shape modeling with front propagation: a level set approach. IEEE Trans. PAMI Vol 17 **2** (1995) 158–175
3. Caselles, V., Kimmel, R., Sapiro, G.: Geodesic Active Contours. Int. Journal of Computer Vision, Vol 22 **1** (1997) 61–79
4. Yezzi Jr., A., Tsai, A., Willsky, A.: A Statistical Approach to Snakes for Bimodal and Trimodal Imagery. Proceedings of ICCV'99, (1999) 898–903
5. Chan, T. F., Vese, L. A.: Active contours without edges. IEEE Trans. Image Processing, Vol 10 **2** (2001) 266–277
6. Vese, L. A., Chan, T. F.: A Multiphase Level Set Framework for Image Segmentation using the Mumford and Shah Model. Int. Journal of Computer Vision, Vol 50, **3** (2002)
7. Paragios, N.: A Variational Approach for the Segmentation of the Left Ventricle: Int. Journal of Computer Vision, Vol 50 **3** (2002) 345–362
8. Sifakis, E., Garcia, C., Tziritas, G.: Bayesian Level Sets for Image Segmentation. Journal of Visual Communication and Image Representation, Vol 13 (2002) 44–64
9. Osher, S., Sethian, J. A.: Fronts Propagating with Curvature Dependant Speed: Algorithms Based on Hamilton-Jacobi Formulation. Journal of Computational Physics, Vol 79 (1988) 12–49
10. Bouchon-Meunier, B., Marsala, C.: Logique floue, principes, aide à la décision. Hermès Science Publications (2003)
11. Logique floue Observatoire Français des Techniques Avancées (1994)
12. Xu, C., Pham, L., Rettmann, M. E., Yu, D. N., Prince, J. L.: Reconstruction of the Human Cerebral Cortex from Magnetic Resonance Images. IEEE Trans. Medical Imaging, Vol 18 **6** (1999) 467–480
13. Colliot, O., Camara, O., Dewynter, R., Bloch, I.: Description of brain internal structures by means of spatial relations for MR image segmentation Proceedings of SPIE'2004 Medical Imaging, (2004) 444-455
14. Celeux, G., and Diebolt, J.: L'algorithme SEM : un algorithme d'apprentissage probabiliste pour la reconnaissance de mélanges de densités. Revue de statistiques appliquées, Vol 34 **2** (1986) 35–51
15. Bouchon-Meunier, B., Marsala, C.: Traitement de données complexes et commande en logique floue. Hermès Science Publications (2003)
16. Ciofolo, C., Barillot, C., Hellier, P.: Combining fuzzy logic and level set methods for 3D MRI brain segmentation Proceedings of ISBI'2004, (2004) 161–164
17. Ciofolo, C.: Atlas-based segmentation using level sets and fuzzy labels Proceedings of MICCAI'2004 (2004) 310–317
18. Baillard, C., Hellier, P., Barillot, C.: Segmentation of brain 3D MR images using level sets and dense registration, Medical Image Analysis, Vol 5 **3** (2001) 185–194
19. Zhang, B., Zimmer, C., Olivo-Marin, J.-C.: Tracking fluorescent cells with coupled geometric active contours. Proceedings of ISBI'2004, (2004) 476–479
20. Collins, D. L., Zijdenbos, A. P., Kollokian, V., Sled, J. G., Kabani, N. J., Holmes, C. J., Evans, A. C.: Design and construction of a realistic digital brain phantom. IEEE Trans. Medical Imaging, Vol 17 **3** (1998) 463–468
21. Zijdenbos, A. P., Dawant, B. M., Margolin, R. A., Palmer, A. C.: Morphometric Analysis of White Matter Lesions in MR Images: Method and Validation. IEEE Trans. Medical Imaging, Vol 13 **4** (1994), 716–724

Coupled Shape Distribution-Based Segmentation of Multiple Objects*

Andrew Litvin and William C. Karl

Boston University, Boston, Massachusetts
{litvin, wckarl}@bu.edu

Abstract. In this paper we develop a multi-object prior shape model for use in curve evolution-based image segmentation. Our prior shape model is constructed from a family of shape distributions (cumulative distribution functions) of features related to the shape. Shape distribution-based object representations possess several desired properties, such as robustness, invariance, and good discriminative and generalizing properties. Further, our prior can capture information about the interaction between multiple objects. We incorporate this prior in a curve evolution formulation for shape estimation. We apply this methodology to problems in medical image segmentation.

1 Introduction

The use of prior information about shape is essential when image intensity alone does not provide enough information to correctly segment objects in a scene. Such cases arise due to the presence of clutter, occlusion, noise, etc. In this work we concentrate on curve evolution-based image segmentation approaches [1] and prior shape models matched to this framework. In a typical curve evolution scheme, the regions of interest in the image (i.e. the shapes or objects) are represented by non-self-intersecting closed contours. Curve evolution methods allow convenient handling of object topology, efficient implementation, and possess variational and associated probabilistic interpretations. In a typical curve evolution implementation, the shape-capturing curve is evolved under the combined action of two classes of forces: those dependent on the observed image data (data-dependent forces) and those reflecting prior knowledge about the segmented shape or boundary (regularizing forces). This work is focused on the development of shape models suitable for such prior shape force terms in curve evolution.

---

* This work was partially supported by AFOSR grant F49620-03-1-0257, National Institutes of Health under Grant NINDS 1 R01 NS34189, Engineering research centers program of the NSF under award EEC-9986821. The MR brain data sets and their manual segmentations were provided by the Center for Morphometric Analysis at Massachusetts General Hospital and are available at http://www.cma.mgh.harvard.edu/ibsr/.

Desirable qualities in a shape-based prior include invariance with respect to transformations such as scale, translation, and rotation, independence from knowledge of correspondence, robustness of the resulting solution to initialization, the ability to generate the prior model from training data, and subsequent robustness to small training set size. Shape distributions have been used in the computer graphics community [14] to characterize shapes and, more recently, have been successfully applied to shape classification problems. They were shown to possess the desired properties of robustness, invariance, and flexibility. To date, however, shape distributions have not been used in an estimation context.

In this work we develop a novel multi-object prior based on such shape distributions for use in estimation. We then present a method to use this prior in curve evolution-based segmentation problems. Finally, we suggest the promise of this prior for challenging medical image segmentation tasks through an example. In our formulation, the shape prior is constructed by designing a shape similarity measure penalizing the difference between shape distributions extracted from boundary curves under comparison.

In Section 2 we give an overview of existing shape modeling approaches and the motivations behind our technique. In Section 3 we review the curve evolution framework and introduce the shape distribution concept. Section 4 presents our experimental results and Section 5 concludes this paper.

2 Prior Work

Different approaches have been proposed for the inclusion of prior information in deformable curve-based image segmentation. The most common regularization method for curve evolution penalizes a quantity such as total curve length or object area [1, 10]. Such "generic" penalties are stationary along the curve, in that every point on the boundary experiences the same effect. Such priors can remove object protrusions and smooth salient object detail when the boundary location is not well supported by the observed data, since they seek objects with short boundaries or small area.

Deformable template approaches construct prior models based on allowable deformations of a template shape. Some approaches are based on representing and modeling shape as a set of landmarks (see [5, 4] and references therein). Other approaches use principal component analysis based on parameterized boundary coordinates or level-set functions to obtain a set of shape expansion functions [20, 22] that describe the subspace of allowable shapes. Still other approaches construct more complex parametric shape representations, such as the MREP approach in [16], or deformable atlas based approach in [3]. These methods are effective when the space of possible curves is well covered by the modeled template deformations as obtained through training data, but may not generalize well to shapes unseen in the training set.

Motivated by such limitations in existing approaches and by the representational richness of the ideas in [24, 14], we propose construction of a shape prior based on an energy which penalizes the difference between a set of feature *distributions* of a given curve and those of a prior reference set. Such prior shape distributions capture the existence of certain visual features of a shape regardless of the location of these features. Shape distributions have been successfully applied to shape classification tasks (e.g. [8, 14] and references therein), and these results indicate that shape distributions are robust, invariant, flexible shape representations with good discriminative properties. In this work, we apply such shape distribution-based models to problems of boundary estimation in medical imaging, suggesting their potential.

Simultaneous multiple object segmentation is an important direction of research in medical imaging. The positions of segmented parts are often highly correlated and can be used to further constrain the resulting boundary estimation. In [23, 18] the authors extend the PCA shape model to constrain multiple object locations. In [6], a PDM model was extended to model multiple shapes. In [7, 15] the authors mutually constrained shapes by penalizing quantities such as area of overlap between different objects. These approaches do not include shape specific information regarding the different objects. Our approach shares a common idea with [13], where the concept of a force histogram was used to characterize shapes. In [13] histogram-based descriptors were used solely in discrimination while our focus is to use similar descriptors in estimation problems.

In [11], the authors present preliminary results on constructing shape distribution-based shape models for single objects. This paper improves upon and extends this technique to the multiple object case. In contrast to existing approaches, this model attempts to directly encode properties of a class of shapes (versus simply penalizing points of high curvature), yet does not depend on the specific embedding of a shape, and thus generalizes well to unseen objects. As another major contribution, analytical expressions for energy minimizing gradient curve flows are derived, providing useful insights as well as efficient curve evolution implementation. Our approach seems to provide an interesting alternative shape prior, well matched to curve evolution approaches, with promise for challenging segmentation problems.

3 General Formulation and Shape Distribution Prior

3.1 Segmentation by Energy Minimization Based on Curve Evolution

First, we review the overall approach of segmentation in a curve evolution framework based on energy minimization. We assume that each object (shape) in the image is defined by a separate closed curve. An energy functional is defined for each object (in contrast to the multi-phase approach in [21]) and each boundary is evolved to minimize the overall energy. For a single object, then, the solution curve C^* is sought as:

$$C^* = \underset{C}{\operatorname{argmin}}\ E(C) \qquad (1)$$

The energy $E(C)$ consists of a data term and a shape prior term:

$$E(C) = E_{data}(C) + \alpha E_{prior}(C) \qquad (2)$$

The data term E_{data} favors the fidelity of the solution to the image data. This term is sensor and application specific. In this paper we use two definitions of E_{data}: the bimodal image energy in [2] and the information theoretic energy in [9]. Our contribution is focused on the shape prior term E_{prior}, which we base on the concept of shape-distributions, discussed in Sec. 3.2. The positive scalar α is a regularization parameter that balances the strength of the prior and data.

The gradient curve flow minimizing (2) can be found using variational approaches or shape-gradient approaches. In this work we utilize variational approaches. The curve is then evolved according to the gradient curve flow $dC/dt = -\nabla E(C)$, were t is an artificial time parameter. We implement the curve evolution via the level-set framework [17]. This framework is very general, and our prior term can be coupled with many existing data terms (ex. [2,9]). In the multi-object case the simultaneous evolution of multiple boundaries effectively minimizes an energy which is a sum of terms (2) corresponding to the individual objects.

3.2 The Shape Distribution Concept

Distributions of features measured over shapes in a uniform way, are called shape distributions [14]. As shown by recent shape classification experiments [14], such shape distributions can capture the intuitive similarity of shapes in a flexible way while being robust to a small sample size and invariant to object transformation.

In a continuous formulation, shape distributions are defined as sets of cumulative distribution functions (CDFs) of feature values (one distribution per collection of feature values of the same kind) measured along the shape boundary or across the shape area. Joint CDFs of multiple features can also be considered, although in this work we only consider one-dimensional distributions. An illustrative example of the shape distribution idea is shown in Figure 1, using boundary curvature as the feature. We define the shape distribution for a class or set of shapes as an average of the cumulative distribution functions corresponding to the individual shapes in the group. This approach is equivalent to combining feature value representations (continuous functions or discrete sets of values) measured on individual shapes into a single set and then defining the overall CDF of the resulting set.

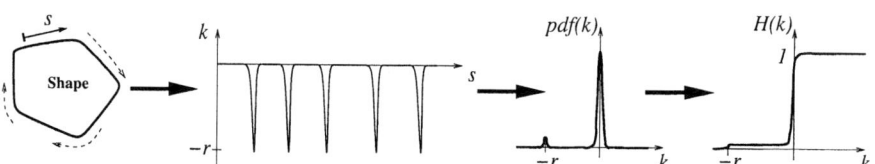

Fig. 1. An example of constructing a shape distribution for a curve (left) based on curvature $\kappa(s)$ measured along the boundary (second graph). Third and fourth graphs show the sketches of $pdf(\kappa)$ and cumulative distribution function $H(\kappa)$ of curvature respectively. Note the invariance of $H(\kappa)$ with respect to the choice of the initial point of arc-length parameterization

We will call a set of feature values extracted from a shape a "feature class". In the example of Figure 1 the feature class is boundary curvature. Separate feature classes capturing different characteristics of shapes can be combined in a single framework, creating a more versatile prior. We distinguish two types of feature classes. For the first type of feature, which we term autonomous, the values for a particular curve are computed with reference only to the curve itself. For the second type of feature, which we term directed, the feature values are computed with reference to the curves of other objects. By incorporating directed feature classes into our shape models we provide a mechanism for modeling the relationships between different objects in a scene and, thus, create a framework for multi-object segmentation.

3.3 A Prior Energy Based on Shape Distributions

We now introduce our formulation of the shape prior in the continuous domain. Let $\Phi \in \Omega$ be a continuously defined feature (e.g. curvature along the length of a curve), and let λ be a variable spanning the range of values Λ of the feature. Let $H(\lambda)$ be the CDF of Φ:

$$H(\lambda) = \frac{\int_\Omega h\{\Phi(\Omega) < \lambda\} \, d\omega}{\int_\Omega d\omega} \quad (3)$$

where $h(x)$ is the indicator function, which is 1 when the equality is satisfied and 0 otherwise.

We define the prior energy $E_{prior}(C)$ for the boundary curve C in (2) based on this shape distribution as:

$$E_{prior}(C) = \sum_{i=1}^{M} w_i \int_\Lambda \left[H_i^*(\lambda) - H_i(C, \lambda) \right]^2 d\lambda \quad (4)$$

where M is the number of different distributions (i.e. feature classes) being used to represent the object, $H_i(C, \lambda)$ is the distribution function of the ith feature class for the curve C, and the non-negative scalar weights w_i balance the relative contribution of the different feature distributions. Prior knowledge of object behavior is captured in the set of target distributions $H_i^*(\lambda)$. These target distributions H_i^* can correspond to a single prior shape, an average derived from a group of training shapes, or can be specified by prior knowledge (e.g. the analytic form for a primitive, such as a square). In practice, we compute the feature values, the corresponding shape distributions, and evolution forces dC/dt by discretizing curves and their properties through uniform sampling.

We use three specific feature classes in our experiments in this work, which we define below and illustrate in Figure 2.

- **Feature class # 1.** Inter-node Distances (Autonomous feature type). The feature value set $\{F\}$ consists of the normalized distances between nodes of the discrete curve.

$$\{F\} = \frac{\{d_{ij} \mid (i,j) \in S\}}{\text{mean}\left(\{d_{ij} \mid (i,j) \in S\}\right)} \quad (5)$$

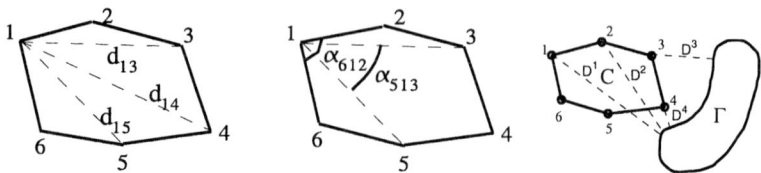

Fig. 2. Feature value sets used in this work illustrated for a curve C discretized using 6 nodes. Feature class #1 (left): interpoint distances $\{d_{13}..d_{15}\}$. Feature class #2 (center): interpoint angles $\{\alpha_{-1,1,2}..\alpha_{-n,1,n}\}$ ($n = 2$) are shown. Feature class #3 (right): feature set values for curve C are defined as shortest signed distances from the curve Γ to nodes of the curve C

The set S defines the subset of internodal distances used in the feature. For $(a, b) \in [0, 1]$, $S_{(a,b)}$ defines such subset of nodes in a multi-scale way: $\{(i, j) \mid (j - i) * ds/L \in [a, b]\}$, where a and b are the lower and upper bounds of the interval respectively; ds is the distance between neighboring boundary nodes and L is the total boundary length. In the experiments presented in this paper we used 4 different, non-overlapping intervals. Note that the features defined above are invariant to shape translation, rotation and scale.

- **Feature class # 2.** Multiscale curvature (Autonomous feature type).
  The feature value set $\{F\}$ consists of the collection of angles between nodes of the discrete curve.

$$\{F\} = \{\angle_{i-j,i,i+j} \quad (i, j) \in S\} \tag{6}$$

where $\angle(ijk)$ is the angle between nodes i, j, and k. Again, the set S defines the subset of internodal angles used in the feature and again we used S in a multi-scale way, as described in Feature class #1. Similar invariance properties hold for this feature class by construction.

- **Feature class # 3.** Relative inter-object distances. (Directed feature type)
  The set $\{F\}$ consists of the collection of shortest signed distances between each node of C and the boundary of object Γ (negative for nodes of C inside Γ). These distances are normalized by the average radius of Γ with respect to its center of mass. This feature class encodes the relative position of C with respect to Γ. Note that the prior defined using this feature class provides a descriptor richer than those in penalty based approaches in [7, 15], while being less restrictive than a PCA based prior. Again, this feature is invariant to translation, rotation and scale applied to the pair of shapes C and Γ.

3.4 Gradient Flow Computation

In order to use the energy in (4) as a prior in a curve evolution context we must be able to compute the curve flow that minimizes it. For simplicity, we consider here an energy defined on just a single feature class. Since (4) is additive in the different feature classes, minimizing flows for single individual feature classes can be added with the corresponding weights to obtain the overall minimizing flow. The energy for a single feature class is given by:

$$E(C) = \int \left[H^*(\lambda) - H(C,\lambda)\right]^2 d\lambda \qquad (7)$$

Because the energy depends on the whole curve in non-additive way, the minimizing flow at any location on the curve also depends on the whole curve, and not just the local curve properties.

The minimizing flow and its computation will, of course, depend on the specifics of the feature classes chosen. In [11], a numerical scheme was proposed to estimate the flow. Such a scheme can be employed for any definition of the feature class; although, it is computationally expensive. Here we introduce an efficient approach to analytically compute the minimizing flows for the feature classes presented previously using a variational framework. The resulting flows guarantee reduction of the energy functionals (7).

Due to the space constraints we only briefly outline the steps required to derive the flows and present final results for our specific feature classes.

1. Find the Gâteaux semi-derivative of the energy in (7) with respect to a perturbation β. Using the definition of the Gâteaux semi-derivative, the linearity of integration, and the chain rule we obtain

$$\mathcal{G}(E,\beta) = 2\int \left[H^*(\lambda) - H(\Gamma,\lambda)\right] \mathcal{G}\left[H(\gamma,\lambda),\beta\right] d\lambda \qquad (8)$$

2. If the Gâteaux semi-derivative of a linear functional f exists, then according to the Rietz representation theorem, it can be represented as

$$\mathcal{G}(f,\beta) = <\nabla f, \beta> \qquad (9)$$

were ∇f is the gradient flow minimizing the functional f. Therefore, we must find the boundary functional representation $\nabla H(\Gamma, \lambda)$ for the feature such that $\mathcal{G}\left[H(\Gamma,\lambda),\beta\right] = <\nabla H(\Gamma,\lambda),\beta>$.

3. The overall flow minimizing (7) is then given by

$$\nabla E = 2\int \left[H^*(\lambda) - H(\Gamma,\lambda)\right] \nabla H(\Gamma,\lambda) d\lambda \qquad (10)$$

A detailed derivation of the gradient flows for the three features used in this work can be found in the technical report [12]. We simply summarize those results here. For feature class #1 the minimizing flow is given by:

$$\nabla E(\Gamma)(s) = 2\int_{t \in S} \boldsymbol{n}(s) \cdot \frac{\boldsymbol{\Gamma}(s,t)}{|\boldsymbol{\Gamma}(s,t)|} \left[H^*(|\boldsymbol{\Gamma}(s,t)|) - H(\Gamma,|\boldsymbol{\Gamma}(s,t)|)\right] dt \qquad (11)$$

where Γ is the parameterized curve as a function of arc length $\{X(s), Y(s)\}$ with $s \in \{0,1\}$, $\boldsymbol{\Gamma}(s,t)$ is a vector with coordinates $\{X(t) - X(s), Y(t) - Y(s)\}$, and

$n(s)$ is the outward normal at $\{X(s), Y(s)\}$. The flow at each s is an integral over the curve, indicating the non-local dependence of the flow. The expression under the integral can be interpreted as a force acting on a particular pair of locations on the curve, projected on the normal direction at s.

For feature class #2, the minimizing flow is given by

$$\nabla E(\Gamma)(s) = -\int_{t \in S} \left[\left\{ \begin{array}{ll} \frac{\cos(\beta)\cos(n(s),\Gamma^+) + \cos(\gamma)\cos(n(s),\Gamma^-)}{\sin \alpha} & \text{if } \alpha \neq \pi \\ \sin(n(s), \Gamma^-)) & \text{otherwise} \end{array} \right\} \times \frac{a \cdot r^{(s,t)}}{bc} - f^{(s-t)} \frac{\sqrt{1 - \left(n(s-t) \cdot \frac{\Gamma^-}{|\Gamma^-|}\right)^2}}{|\Gamma^-|} - f^{(s+t)} \frac{\sqrt{1 - \left(n(s+t) \cdot \frac{\Gamma^+}{|\Gamma^+|}\right)^2}}{|\Gamma^+|} \right] \times \left[H^*(\alpha(s,t)) - H(\Gamma, \alpha(s,t)) \right] dt \quad (12)$$

where $r^{(s,t)}$ and $f^{(s+t)}$ take values -1 and 1 and indicate the sign of change of the angle $\alpha(s,t) = \angle(\Gamma^-, \Gamma^+)$ with respect to along-the-normal perturbation of the point $\Gamma(s)$ and $\Gamma(s+t)$ respectively, $\Gamma^+ = \Gamma(s, s+t)$; $\Gamma^- = \Gamma(s, s-t)$; $a = |\Gamma^+ - \Gamma^-|$; $b = |\Gamma^-|$; $c = |\Gamma^+|$; $\beta = \angle(-\Gamma^+, \Gamma^- - \Gamma^+)$; $\gamma = \angle(-\Gamma^-, \Gamma^+ - \Gamma^-)$.

Finally, for feature class #3, relating the curve Γ to another object Ω, the gradient flow is given by:

$$\nabla E(\Gamma)(s) = n(s) \cdot \nabla D_\Omega(s) \left[H^* \left(\frac{D_\Omega(s)}{R(\Omega)} \right) - H \left(\Gamma, \frac{D_\Omega(s)}{R(\Omega)} \right) \right] \quad (13)$$

where $D_\Omega(s)$ is value of signed distance function generated by curve Ω at the point on the curve Γ given by $\{X(s), Y(s)\}$, and $R(\Omega)$ is the mean radius of the shape Ω relative to its center of mass.

4 Results

In this section we apply our shape distribution based prior to both a synthetic and a real example. The real data example arises in segmentation of brain MRI. We compare both single object and multi-object priors. The benefit of using a multi-object prior is expected to be greater when the object boundary is not well supported by the observed image intensity gradient or when initialization is far from the true boundary.

In the first experiment we apply our prior to a synthetic 2-object segmentation problem with very low SNR, simulating two closely positioned organs, shown in Figure 3, panel (a). Both objects in the ground truth image have the same known intensity. The background intensity is also known as in the model

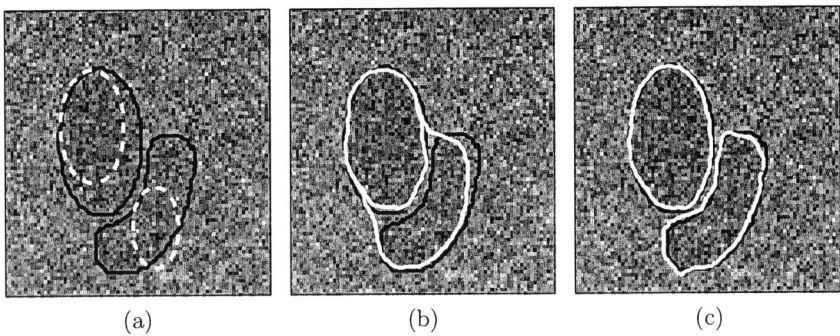

Fig. 3. Synthetic 2 shape example: (a) Noisy image; Solid black line shows the true objects boundaries; dashed white lines - initial boundary position; (b) Segmentation with curve length prior; (c) - Segmentation with new multiobject shape distribution prior including all three feature classes. Solid black line shows the true objects boundaries; solid white lines - final boundary

Table 1. Symmetric difference (area based) segmentation error. For each object the error measure is computed as a symmetric difference between final segmented region and true segmented region. The values in the table are computed as a sum of error measures for individual objects

	Curve length	PCA method	Our method
Experiment I	1092		146
Experiment II	1090	1437	758

[2]. Gaussian IID noise (SNR= -18dB) was added to this bimodal image to form the noisy observed image. The data term E_{data} in (2) and the corresponding data-term gradient curve flow are formed according the data model in [2].

In Figure 3 we show the results obtained by segmenting this image using energy minimizing curve evolution based on two different shape priors: (b) shows the results with a curve length penalty; (c) shows the results with our multi-object shape distribution prior including all 3 feature classes. The prior target distributions for case (c) were constructed using the true objects in (a). The regularization parameter was chosen in each case to yield the subjectively best result. The curve length prior result in (b) yields an incorrect segmentation for one of the objects or leads to a collapse of one of the contours. With the directed feature class included in the segmentation functional (c), both objects can be correctly segmented since the energy term corresponding to feature class #3 effectively prevents intersection of boundaries. Segmentation errors (area based) are summarized in Table 1.

In our second example we apply our techniques to 2D MRI brain data segmentation. A data set consisting of 12 normal adult subjects was used. Manual expert segmentations of the subjects was provided and those of 11 of these subjects was used as training data to construct our shape prior. The prior was then

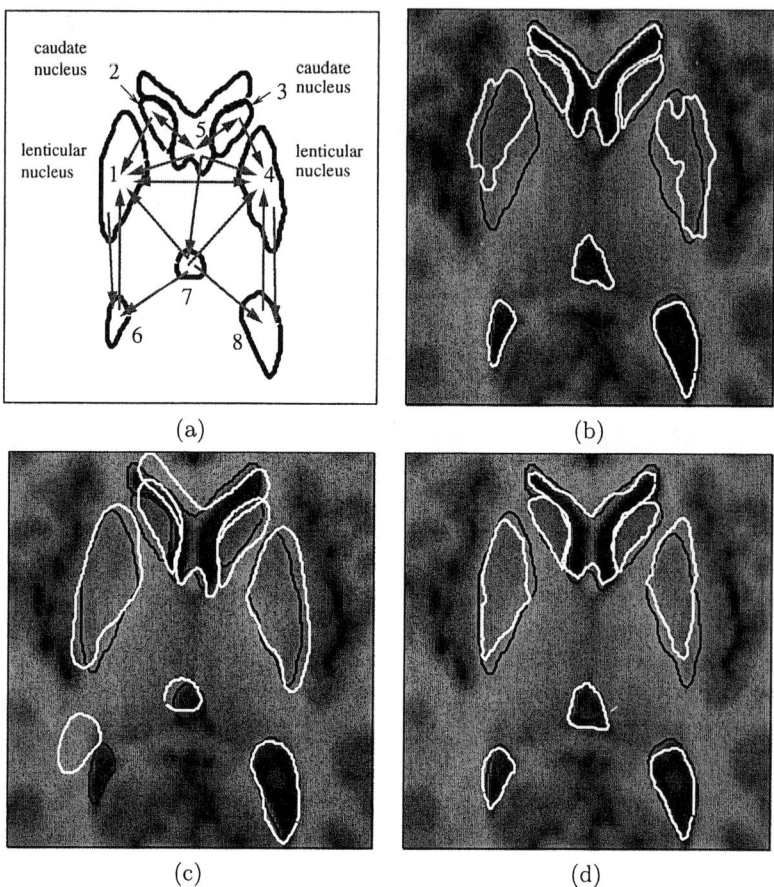

Fig. 4. Brain MRI segmentation: (a) Multiple structures and interactions used for feature class #3; (b) Segmentation with independent object curve length prior. (c) Segmentation using multiobject PCA technique in [19] (d) Segmentation with new multiobject shape distribution prior. Solid black line shows the true objects boundaries; solid white line - final segmentation boundary

applied to segment the data of the omitted subject. The eight numbered structures shown in Figure 4, panel (a) were simultaneously segmented. For the data dependent energy term E_{data}, we used the information theoretic approach of [9] by maximizing the mutual information between image pixel intensities and region labels (inside or outside), therefore favoring segmented regions with intensity distributions that were different from the background intensity distribution.

In Figure 4 we present our results. Panel (b) gives the segmentation with a standard curve length prior applied independently to each object. One can see that Structures 1 and 4 are poorly segmented, due to their weak image boundaries. In panel (c) we present the result given by the multi-shape PCA technique in [19] using 5 principle components defining the subspace of allowable shapes. The segmentation is sought as the shape in this subspace, optimizing the same information-theoretic criteria [9] as used with our shape prior. The usage of the same data term simplifies the comparison with our approach since only the shape model components of the method are different. One can see that structures 2,5,6, and 7 are not segmented properly due to the poor generalization by the PCA prior. Expanding the subspace by choosing 10 PCA components did not improve the result given by this method. Finally, our result is shown in panel (d). We obtain satisfactory segmentation for the structures for which PCA method failed (2,5,6,7), while performing equally well for structures 1,3,4 and 8. The choice of initialization did not significantly influence our results. Segmentation errors given in Table 1 qualitatively confirm the superior performance attained using our prior.

5 Conclusions

In this paper we present a shape distribution-based object prior for use in curve evolution image segmentation. This prior allows encoding of multi-object information. We apply a variational approach to analytically compute the energy minimizing curve flows for three feature classes. We investigate the application of our shape distribution prior to medical image segmentation involving multiple object boundaries. In our experiments we achieved the performance superior to that obtained using the traditional curve length minimization methods and a multi-shape PCA shape prior reported in the literature.

References

1. V. Caselles, R. Kimmel, and G. Sapiro, "Geodesic active contours," *International journal of computer vision*, vol. 22(1), pp. 61–79, 1997.
2. T. Chan and L. Vese, "Active contours without edges," *IEEE trans. on Image Processing*, vol. 10, no. 2, pp. 266–277, February 2001.
3. G. Christensen, "Deformable shape models for anatomy," Ph.D. dissertation, Washington University, St. Louis, US, 1994.
4. T. Cootes, C. Taylor, D. Cooper, and J. Graham, "Active shape models – their training and application," *Computer Vision and Image Understanding*, vol. 61, no. 1, pp. 38–59, 1995.
5. I. Dryden and K. Mardia, *Statistical shape analysis*. John Wiley & Sons, 1998.
6. N. Duta and M. Sonka, "Segmentation and interpretation of mr brain images: an improved active shape model," *IEEE trans. on Med. Im.*, vol. 17, no. 7, pp. 1049–1062, 1998.
7. G. Ho and P. Shi, "Domain partitioning level set surface for topology constrained multi-object segmentation," in *Proc. IEEE Intl. Symp. Biomedical Imaging*, Washington DC, US, 2004.
8. C. Y. Ip, D. Lapadat, L. Sieger, and W. Regli, "Using shape distributions to compare solid models," in *SMA '02: Proceedings of the seventh ACM symposium on Solid modeling and applications*. Saarbrcken, Germany: ACM Press, 2002, pp. 273–280.

9. J. Kim, J. W. Fisher, A. Yezzi, M. Cetin, and A. S. Willsky, "Nonparametric methods for image segmentation using information theory curve evolution," in *Proc. ICIP*, Rochester, USA, September 2002.
10. M. E. Leventon, W. E. L. Grimson, O. Faugeras, and W. M. W. III, "Level set based segmentation with intensity and curvature priors," *IEEE Workshop on Mathematical Methods in Biomedical Image Analysis Proceedings (MMBIA'00)*, pp. 4–11, 2000.
11. A. Litvin and W. C. Karl, "Using shape distributions as priors in a curve evolution framework," in *Proceedings of 2004 IEEE International Conference on Acoustic Speech and Signal Processing (ICASSP)*, Montreal, Canada, 2004.
12. ———, "Coupled shape distribution-based segmentation of multiple objects," Boston University, Boston, USA, Tech. Rep. ECE-2005-01, March 2005.
13. P. Matsakis, J. M. Keller, O. Sjahputera, and J. Marjamaa, "The use of force histograms for affine-invariant relative position description," *IEEE trans. on PAMI*, vol. 26, no. 1, pp. 1–18, 2004.
14. R. Osada, T. Funkhouser, B. Chazelle, and D. Dobkin, "Shape distributions," *ACM transactions on graphics*, vol. 21(4), pp. 807–832, 2002.
15. N. Paragios and R. Deriche, "Coupled geodesic active regions for image segmentation: A level set approach," in *European Conference in Computer Vision*, Dublin, Ireland, 2000.
16. S. M. Pizer, D. S. Fritsch, P. A. Yushkevich, V. E. Johnson, and E. L. Chaney, "Segmentation, registration, and measurement of shape variation via image object shape," *IEEE Transactions on Medical Imaging*, vol. 18(10), pp. 851–865, 1996.
17. J. Sethian, *Level set methods and fast marching methods*. Cambridge University Press, 1999.
18. A. Tsai, W. Wells, C. Tempany, G. E., and A. Willsky, "Coupled multi-shape model and mutual information for medical image segmentation," in *Proc. IPMI (Information Processing in Medical Imaging)*, Ambleside, UK, July 2003, pp. 185–197.
19. A. Tsai, W. Wells, C. Tempany, E. Grimson, and A. Willsky, "Mutual information in coupled multi-shape model for medical image segmentation," *Medical Image Analysis*, vol. 8, no. 4, pp. 429–445, 2004.
20. A. Tsai, A. Yezzi, W. Wells, C. Tempany, D. Tucker, A. Fan, W. Grimson, and A. Willsky, "Model-based curve evolution technique for image segmentation," *IEEE Conference on Computer Vision and Pattern Recognition (CVPR'01)*, 2001.
21. L. Vese and T. Chan, "A multiphase level set framework for image segmentation using the Mumford and Shah model," *International Journal of Computer Vision*, vol. 50, no. 3, pp. 271–293, 2002.
22. Y. Wang and L. Staib, "Boundary finding with prior shape and smoothness models," *IEEE Trans. on Pattern Analysis and Machine Intelligence (PAMI)*, vol. 22, no. 7, pp. 738–743, 2000.
23. J. Yang, L. H. Staib, and J. S. Duncan, "Neighbor-constrained segmentation with 3d deformable models," in *Proc. IPMI (Information Processing in Medical Imaging)*, Ambleside, UK, July 2003, pp. 198–209.
24. S. Zhu, "Embedding gestault laws in markov random fields," *IEEE trans. on PAMI*, vol. 21, no. 11, 1999.

Partition-Based Extraction of Cerebral Arteries from CT Angiography with Emphasis on Adaptive Tracking

Hackjoon Shim[1], Il Dong Yun[2], Kyoung Mu Lee[1], and Sang Uk Lee[1]

[1] School of Electrical Engineering and Computer Science,
Seoul National University, Seoul, 151-742, Korea
hjshim@diehard.snu.ac.kr, kmlee@ee.snu.ac.kr, sanguk@ipl.snu.ac.kr
[2] School of Electronics and Information Engineering,
Hankuk University of Foreign Studies, Yongin, 449-791, Korea
yun@hufs.ac.kr

Abstract. In this paper a method to extract cerebral arteries from computed tomographic angiography (CTA) is proposed. Since CTA shows both bone and vessels, the examination of vessels is a difficult task. In the upper part of the brain, the arteries of main interest are not close to bone and can be well segmented out by thresholding and simple connected-component analysis. However in the lower part the separation is challenging due to the spatial closeness of bone and vessels and their overlapping intensity distributions. In this paper a CTA volume is partitioned into two sub-volumes according to the spatial relationship between bone and vessels. In the lower sub-volume, the concerning arteries are extracted by tracking the center line and detecting the border on each cross-section. The proposed tracking method can be characterized by the adaptive properties to the case of cerebral arteries in CTA. These properties improve the tracking continuity with less user-interaction.

1 Introduction

The wall of a cerebral artery may become weak and have a bulging spot like a thin balloon. This is an aneurysm inside which the flowing blood can rupture the weakened wall and result in a subarachnoid hemorrhage (SAH). However, most people with unruptured aneurysms have no symptoms. The overall annual risk of rupture of an intact intracranial aneurysms is 1.9%[1]. Therefore, periodical screening by medical images is considerably required for potential patients.

As the imaging technology develops, the resolution becomes higher, but at the same time, the amount of data becomes enormous increasing the burdens of the experts examining vessels and the associated pathologies. For prognosis of SAH it is crucial to examine the vascular structure exactly not hindered by bone or vein. If only the vascular structure can be segmented out in CTA, it will be very helpful for prognosis or surgery planning.

The most basic method for segmentation is the combination of thresholding and connected-component analysis (CCA)[2]. However, being applied to the segmentation of cerebral arteries from bone or vein in CTA, it has some problems mainly due to the following two facts. One is the overlapping intensity distributions of bone and vessels making thresholding not effective. The other is the close contact between arteries and bone or vein resulting in the infeasibility of CCA. Bone usually has higher intensity values than arteries. However the partial volume effect (PVE)[3] causes in-between voxels to have in-between intensity values so that the intensity distributions of bone and arteries overlap with each other. Veins have only a little lower intensity values than arteries and are very close to arteries.

To settle these problems it is required to make use of some prior information or anatomic knowledge about arteries like follows:

- Vessels are smoothly varying structures with nearly circular or elliptical cross-sections.
- In the cranial cavity the arteries of main interest flow apart from bone. However below the floor of the cranial cavity the arteries often pass through bone.

Until now a number of papers have been published on the vessel extraction in magnetic resonance angiography (MRA) [4, 5, 6]. MRA does not show bone which makes vessel extraction more easily than CTA. As for CTA only a few researches have been performed.

Suryanarayanan et. al [8] took account of the profiles of bone and sinus (cavity) and partitioned the head volume into three sub-volumes. Each sub-volume has a consistent spatial relationship between bone and vessels enabling separate segmentation algorithm to be applied. This work is not on segmentation itself but on the proper partitioning of volumes for segmentation.

Wink et. al [9] extracted the abdominal aorta based on tracking of the center line. The abdominal aorta is thick and mostly straight, consequently much simpler to extract than cerebral arteries. Their method is very similar to the proposed method in this paper. However, in being applied to the case of cerebral arteries in CTA, consideration of obscure boundary of arteries, especially to bone or vein was not sufficiently. The proposed method adds some adaptive properties to the extraction of cerebral arteries in CTA. Its better performance in tracking will be confirmed by some experiments in section 3.

Hong et. al [10] eliminated bone in brain with two CT volumes scanned before and after the injection of contrast dye, respectively. They performed rigid registration between the two CT volumes and subtracted the pre-contrast volume from the post-contrast volume. This work belongs to a digital subtraction angiography (DSA) and can make a perfect extraction theoretically. The drawback of this approach is that it requires twice of scanning which doubles the burden and cost for patients.

The outline of this paper is as follows. In section 2 the overall workflow of the proposed method will be explained. In section 3 the experimental results and the analysis will be provided. And finally we will conclude with section 4.

2 Description of the Overall Workflow

This paper proposes a method to extract cerebral arteries from CTA. The overall workflow is composed of the following five sub-sections. First, a CT data is acquired, re-sampled and pre-processed. Then the head CT volume is partitioned into two sections each of which has a consistent spatial relationship between bone and vessels. To each sub-volume a separate segmentation algorithm is applied. Therefore the next two sub-sections describe these two algorithms, repectively. Finally, to remove the discontinuities between the sub-volumes, the inter-partition tracking is devised and will be explained in the last sub-section.

2.1 Data Acquisition and Pre-processing

A CT data is sampled in an anisotropic space, where the resolution in each of x-, y-, and z-directions is not equal. For further processing of volume data, we interpolated the intensity value on each grid in the z-direction by trilinear interpolation. To suppress the effects of noise and artifacts, the isotropically resampled volume is pre-processed by the convolution with a Gaussian kernel.

2.2 Partitioning of a Head CT Volume

In the cranium, the arteries of main interest are called as the Circle of Willis and aneurysms usually happen on the Circle of Willis located on the floor of the cranial cavity. The cranial cavity corresponds to the upper part of the head CT volume data, and has the concerned arteries separated far away from bone. In the while, below the floor of the cranial cavity, the arteries often pass through bone and run closely to vein. As mentioned earlier, these circumstances produce obscure boundaries of the arteries which require special treatment of the lower sub-volume.

If we consider the profile of bone, in the upper sub-volume, bone forms an outer boundary as in Fig. 1 (a). As we go down, bone approaches closer to the inner arteries and consequently constitutes a complex structure as seen in Fig. 1 (b). We assume a square region on each slice as in Fig. 1 (c). From the top of the head the ratio r_{bone} of the number of bone voxels in the square to the total number of voxels in the square is computed on each slice. At first no bone voxels can be found, but as we go down, the number of bone voxels increases and the slice where it exceeds a threshold t_{bone} is the partitioning slice. Empirically t_{bone} is set to 0.002.

2.3 Extraction in the Upper Sub-volume (Threshold-Morphological Method)

As bone and vessels are not adjacent to each other in the upper sub-volume, they can be well separated mostly by intensity thresholds and CCA. On the contrary as stated in the introduction, the PVE produces voxels of in-between intensity values on the boundary of the bone structure. These voxels are what should have

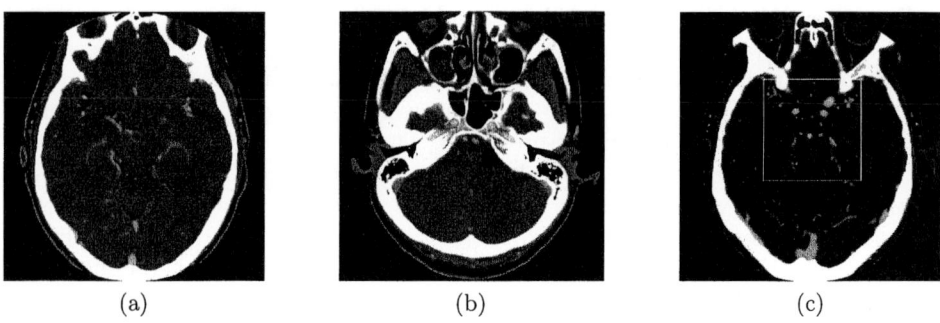

Fig. 1. Bone voxel distributions in : (a) A slice of the upper sub-volume, (b) a slice of the lower sub-volume, (c) The partitioning slice

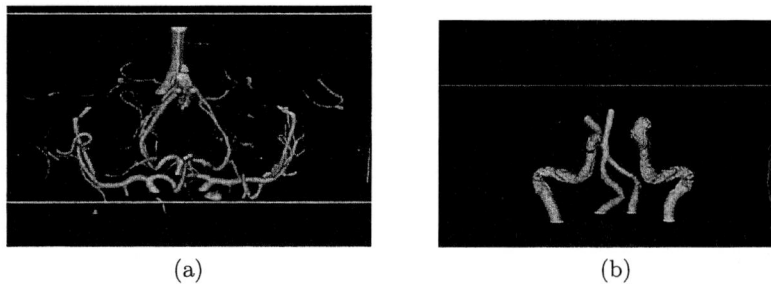

Fig. 2. Vessels extracted: (a) In the upper sub-volume, (b) In the lower sub-volume

been removed together with bone structure. Thus, we applied morphological dilation operation with the ball-shaped structuring element to add these voxels to the bone structure. Next, after the application of CCA, only the components which satisfies the size and the shape criteria remain as vessel segments. The size criterion is that the size of a component should be larger than a threshold t_{size} and the shape one is that the component has a saturation value less than another threshold t_{sat}. Saturation is a compactness measure being the ratio of the number of voxels in the component to the number of voxels in the bounding box of the component. Empirically, t_{size} t_{sat} are 100 and 0.1, respectively.

Fig. 2 (a) shows the vessels extracted by the method in the upper sub-volume. The upper part of the Circle of Willis can be examined clearly with the bone structure removed. Some veins are visualized together, but they can be removed by a simple post-processing using some anatomical knowledge.

2.4 Extraction in Lower Partition (Adaptive Tracking Method)

In the lower sub-volume, as the arteries are often adjacent to bone or veins, they could not be segmented out only by intensity information. In this paper, the main arteries are extracted by tracking the central axes and detecting the border

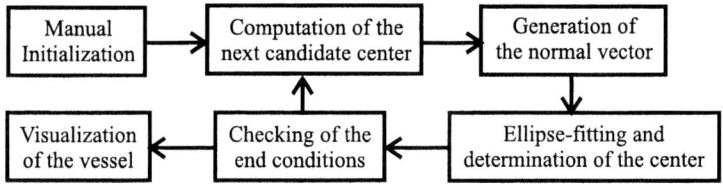

Fig. 3. The block diagram of the segmentation in the lower sub-volume

points on each cross-section. The tracking method in the lower sub-volume is composed of several step as shown in Fig. 3. The most important steps are the ones of "Generation of the normal vector" and "Ellipse-fitting and determination of the center".

Manual Initialization and Computation of the Next Candidate Center: The tracking is initialized by the user designating a center point and a normal vector. The arteries of main interest are left-right internal carotid arteries (ICA) and left-right vertebral arteries (VA), consequently four pairs of an initial center and an initial normal vector are required.

The candidate center for the next cross-section C_{cand} is computed by adding the step vector b to the previous center C_{last}. The step vector b is in the same orientation of the normal vector computed for the last cross-section.

Generation of the Normal Vector: As seen in Fig. 4, vessels are assumed to be cylinders, and the direction of vessel axis and the area of its perpendicular cross-section are denoted by n_0 and S_0, respectively at the center O. Then, an arbitrary cross-section with the angle of ϕ has its area S of (1). Consequently the perpendicular cross-section is determined by minimizing S which means that $\phi = 0$.

$$S = \frac{S_0}{\cos \phi}, \qquad 0 \leq \phi \leq \frac{\pi}{2}. \tag{1}$$

However the real vessel is generally not a cylinder. Therefore to minimize the cross-section area, both of θ and ϕ of the spherical coordinate system should

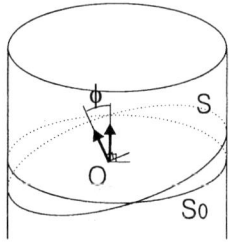

Fig. 4. Cross-sections and their normal vectors

be sampled in uniform intervals as (2) and (3). θ is the azymuthal angle in the xy-plane from the x-axis with $0 \leq \theta \leq 2\pi$ and ϕ is the zenith angle from the z-axis with $0 \leq \phi \leq \frac{\pi}{2}$ [11].

$$\Theta = \{\theta_i \mid \theta_i = 2\pi \frac{i}{M}, \quad i = 0, \ldots, M-1\}. \tag{2}$$

$$\Phi = \{\phi_j \mid \phi_j = \frac{\pi}{2} \frac{j}{N}, \quad j = 0, \ldots, N\}. \tag{3}$$

The normal vector, **n** is computed as (4) at the pair of (θ, ϕ).

$$\mathbf{n}(\theta, \phi) = (\cos\theta \sin\phi, \sin\theta \sin\phi, \cos\phi). \tag{4}$$

When we denote as $\mathbf{n}_{ij} = \mathbf{n}(\theta_i, \phi_j)$, the correct normal vector of the cross-section, $\mathbf{n}_{min} = \mathbf{n}(\theta_{i_{min}}, \phi_{j_{min}})$ is defined from (5).

$$(i_{min}, j_{min}) = \arg \min_{\substack{i \in \{0,\ldots,M-1\} \\ j \in \{0,\ldots,N\}}} S_{ij}, \tag{5}$$

where $S_{ij} = $ Area of the cross-section determined by (θ_i, ϕ_j).

However S_{ij} can be calculated only after the border of the cross-section is correctly obtained over all the possible pair of (θ_i, ϕ_j). It is worth to note that if the detected border points are scattered sparsely, S_{ij} will be large and vice versa. Therefore we determine the normal vector by minimizing the variance of the positions of the border points instead of the area of the cross-section.

Ellipse-Fitting and Determination of the Center: At the cross-section perpendicular to the previous normal vector, the border points of the artery are detected and fitted to an ellipse. From the candidate center of the cross-section, rays are cast along the directions equally sampled around the candidate center as in Fig. 5 (d). The radial component of the gradient along each ray is plotted as in Fig. 6. Fig. 5 (a) and (d) show the usual case where the artery is surrounded only by normal tissues. The contrast-enhanced artery has higher intensity value than the surrounding tissues, so the border point along the ray is detected as the first negative extremum below some negative threshold t_-.

Fig. 5 (b) and (e) show the case where the artery passes through bone. Since bone has much higher intensity values that the artery, the plot of the radial gradient component shows large positive values. For this reason, we invert the sign of the negative threshold t_- into some positive value t_+ and detect the border point as the first positive extremum above t_+.

Finally Fig. 5 (c) and (f) are the case where the artery is adjacent to vein. As veins have similar intensity values to arteries resulting in a plain plot of the radial gradient component, we reduce the magnitude of t_-. With this smaller t_- the border point is detected.

Fig.5 (e) and (f) show the detected border points in these special cases. Although there are some outliers, the modified thresholds generally produce proper border points. These outliers should be removed in the ellipse-fitting

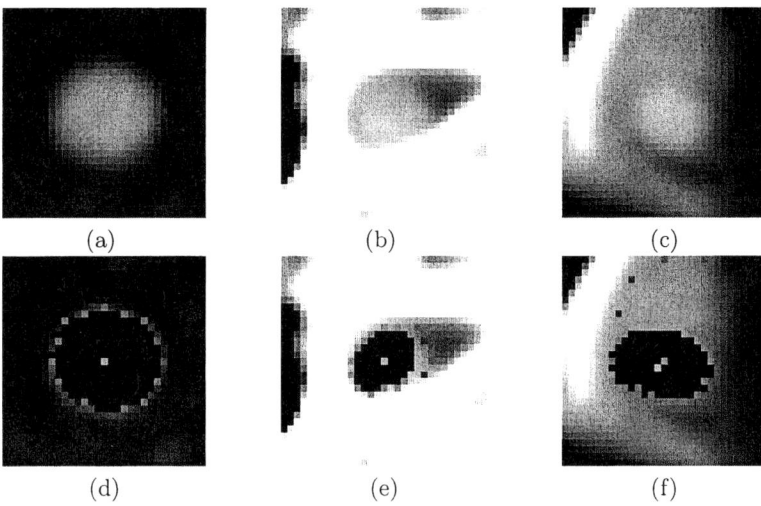

Fig. 5. Artery cross-sections : (a) Surrounded by only normal tissues, (b) Surrounded by bone structure, (c) Adjacent to vein, (d) (e) (f) The detected border points, the outliers, and the fitted ellipse of (a), (b), and (c), respectively

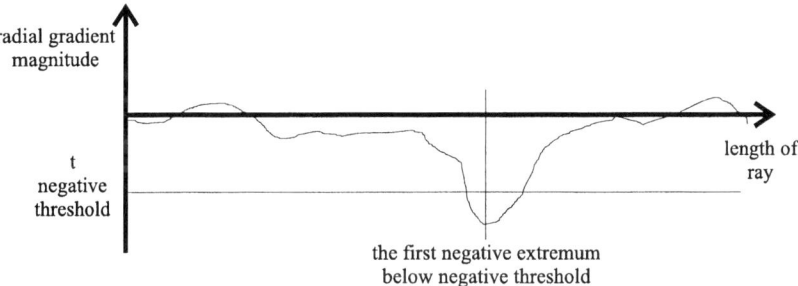

Fig. 6. The radial component of the gradient along a ray

which can be certified by the blue ellipse not effected by the outliers in Fig. 5 (e) and (f). The ellipse-fitting was implemented by the use of Intel OpenCV library[12].

The removal of outliers are performed by two separate processes. The first process is illustrated in Fig. 7 (a). E is the ellipse fitted in the previous cross-section and E_t is the translation of E by the amount of the step vector b. Since arteries have smoothly varying structure as stated in the introduction, if the length of b is sufficiently small, the new boundary in the current cross-section will not be much different from E_t. Therefore, the border points which are the most distant from E_t are removed and are named as the absolute outliers denoted by 'o' in Fig. 7 (a). If n_{total} and n_{ao} denote the number of all the

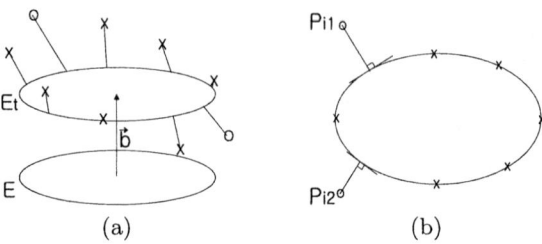

Fig. 7. Removal of outliers: (a) Absolute outliers, (b) Relative outliers

detected border points in a cross-section and the absolute outliers, respectively, the ratio $r_{ao} = n_{ao}/n_{total}$ can be adjusted according to the obscureness of the boundary. Next the relative outliers are removed among the remained border points as in Fig. 7 (b). If the number of the relative outliers is denoted by n_{ro}, the number of all the possible n_{ro}-tuples each of which is composed of n_{ro} points is $n_{tuple} = \binom{n_{total}-n_{ao}}{n_{ro}}$.

For each n_{ro}-tuple $T_i = \{P_{i1}, \ldots P_{in_{ro}}\}$, $i = 1, \ldots, n_{tuple}$, an ellipse E_i is approximated using the rest border points except the points of T_i. If the 3D distance from a point P to the boundary of an ellipse E is denoted by $d(E, P)$, the sum of distances d_i of (6) measures how much each T_i will be taken as the relative outliers. ω_j is the weight for P_{ij} and empirically is set to 1 if P_{ij} is exterior to the ellipse E_i and set to 0.2 otherwise. This is for the purpose of weighting the exterior outliers more than the interior ones, because they produce larger errors in ellipse-fitting. Afterwards the points of T_i minimizing d_i are removed as the relative outliers.

$$d_i = \sum_{j=1}^{n_{ro}} \omega_j d(E_i, P_{ij}). \tag{6}$$

Checking of the End Conditions and Visualization of the Vessel: The possible end conditions can be the maximum length of the artery, the z-coordinate of the center point, or whether being out of the artery boundary. If the end condition is not satisfied, the workflow goes back to the stage of "To compute the next candidate center" of Fig. 3. Otherwise, the workflow terminates and the accumulated cross-sections will be visualized. Fig. 2 (b) shows left-right ICA's and left- right VA's. In spite of the varying diameter of the arteries and the overlapping intensity distributions, the proposed tracking scheme has extracted the main arteries effectively.

2.5 Inter-partition Tracking

The proposed method applies a separate segmentation algorithm to each sub-volume. This inevitably causes discontinuities on the partitioning slice between the two sub-volumes as in Fig. 8 (a). We perform the inter-partition tracking to

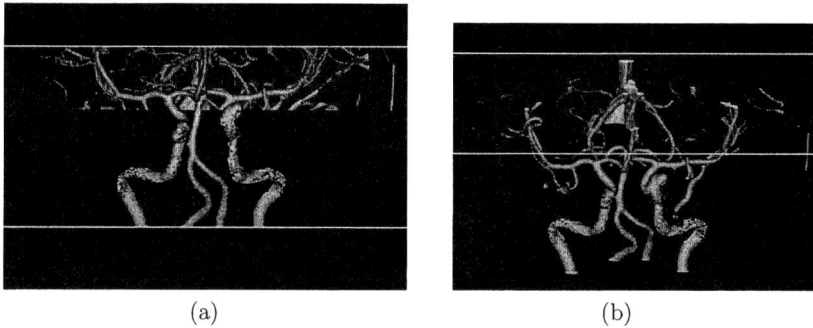

Fig. 8. Inter-partition tracking to eliminate the discontinuities on the partitioning slice: (a) Before, (b) After

eliminate these discontinuities. First, 2-D CCA is executed on the partitioning slice. Among the connected components, only those that are large enough and in the region of interest are selected as the seeds for tracking. The central mean of each seed is the initial center point and the initial normal vector is downward to the lower sub-volume. From each seed the tracking is initiated to connect the discontinuities. Fig. 8 (b) is the result after the inter-partition tracking and shows that most of the discontinuities are eliminated.

3 Results and Discussion

We performed experiments with 24 data sets which were provided by a company and a hospital (not-specified due to anonymous reviewing). Three of them are the double-scanned data sets composed of before-injection, after-injection, and their DSA result. Let us call them as DS (double-scaned) data sets of from DS01 to DS03. The rest are the single-scanned volumes scanned after the injection and are named as from SS01 to SS21. Mainly concerned about the tracking in the lower sub-volume, we defined some subjective evaluation criterion. It designates a result as a success when at most one of the arteries of main interest is missed or cut with no re-initialization. According to this criterion 17 out 24 data sets marked as the success and the subjective success rate can be 70.83% = 17/24.

3.1 Adaptiveness of the Proposed Tracking

To evaluate the proposed tracking method more objectively, we performed experiments with the left ICA of DS03 data set. The most important measure about the tracking performance can be the ability to continue tracking without getting astray or making turnovers which requires user's re-initialization. We counted the number of requirements for re-initialization (in short, NRR) as the sum of the number of getting astray (NGA) and the number of turnovers (NTO). For tracking to get astray means that the new center point is out of

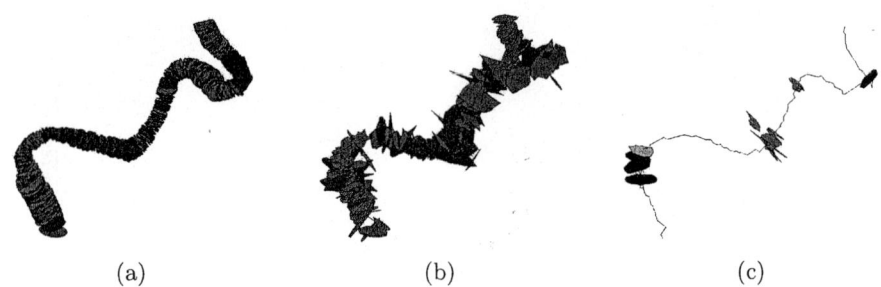

Fig. 9. Left ICA : (a) The cross-sections tracked by the proposed method, (b) The cross-sections tracked by a conventional method[9], (c) The cross-sections re-initialized by the user in the conventional method[9] with the green ones owing to getting astray and the blue ones owing to turnovers, repectively

the true artery boundary. Fig. 9 (a) shows the tracking result of the proposed method by the accumulated cross-sections. It required no re-initialization, i.e. $NRR = NGA + NTO = 0$.

On the contrary, Fig. 9 (b) is the cross-sections by the tracking method[9] using the center-likelihood (CL) measure for determining the new center point on a cross-section This method[9] was targeted for the abdominal aorta which is simpler to extract than the cerebral arteries. It used the difference between the last two center points for the generation of the step vector and provided not enough consideration to deal with outliers. Hence it is not appropriate for the extraction of the cerebral arteries as shown in Fig. 9 (b). When the left ICA passes through bone or is adjacent to veins, the border points are not exactly detected making the cross-sections irregular. Besides, in Fig. 9 (c), the green cross-sections are the re-initialized ones owing to getting astray and the blue ones indicate the re-initialization owing to turnovers. In this case, $NGA = 8$ and $NTO = 4$.

This comparison illustrates the adaptiveness of the proposed tracking which is due to the following facts.

- The normal vector at each cross-section is determined by minimizing all the cross-sections computed by the sampled pairs of (θ, ϕ).
- The gradient threshold is modified in the case where the artery is adjacent to veins.
- The outliers in detecting border points on a cross-sections are removed by two separate processes.

3.2 Visual Comparison to DSA Results

Each of the DS data sets has three volumes. We call them, as Before-volume, After-volume, and DSA-volume[10], respectively. The vascular structure including arteries can be seen clearly in Fig. 10 (a), (c), and (e). However this result

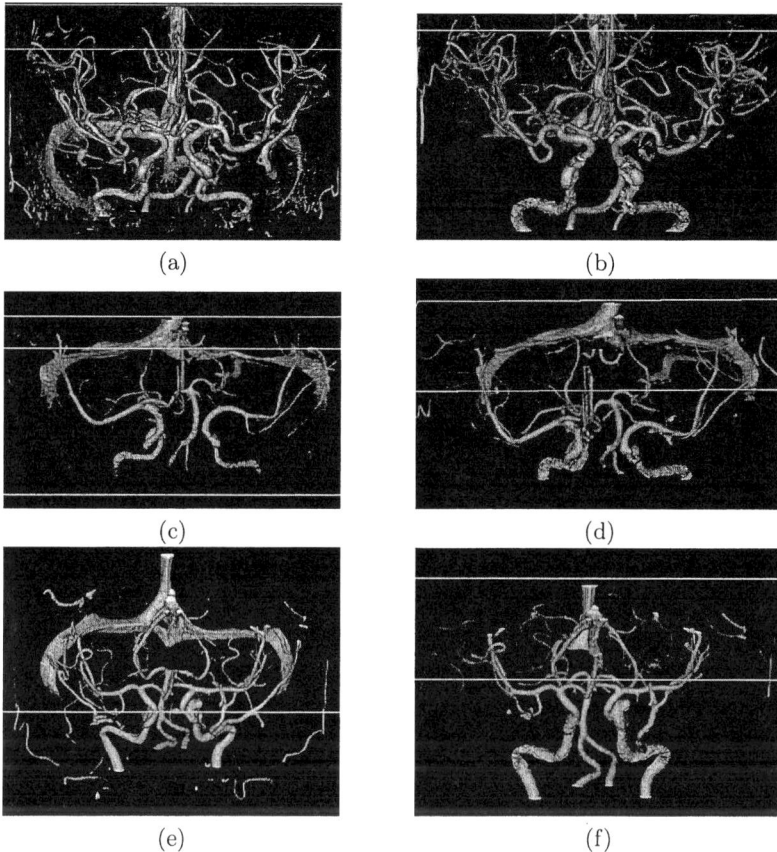

Fig. 10. Visual comparison to DSA results[10] : (a) (c) (e) The DSA results of DS01, DS02, and DS03, respectively, (b) (d) (f) The results of the proposed method of DS01, DS02, and DS03, repectively

requires double-scanning. The results of the proposed method are shown in Fig. 10 (b), (d), and (f) and are comparable to (a), (c), and (e).

The results of the proposed method show that where the arteries pass through bone, their surfaces are mixed with the colors of bone and vessel. This is inevitable when the segmentation result is being displayed using a bit-mask operation. Due to the PVE the voxel at the artery boundary adjacent to bone has higher intensity value than the normal artery surface voxel.

4 Conclusion

In this paper we proposed a method for the extraction of cerebral arteries in CTA. CTA also shows bone structure which hinders arteries to be seen. When veins are adjacent to the arteries of interest, their spatial closeness and small intensity difference make the segmentation of arteries more difficult. The proposed method partitioned the CT volume into two sub-volumes and applied a separate segmentation algorithm to each segment. Specially, in the lower sub-volume, we added some adaptive properties to the simple tracking and they enhances the continuity of tracking in spite of the above difficulties. The experimental results confirmed that the proposed method had produced considerable amount of results which are subjectively satisfying and had enhanced the continuity of the tracking. The visual comparison to the DSA result illustrated that the proposed method is comparable to the result with double-scanned volumes which means a high applicability to the practical clinical use.

Acknowledgements. This research was supported by INFINITT Co. which also provided the data sets[13].

References

1. Rinkel, G.J.E., Djibuti, M. , Algra, A., Gijn, J.V., Prevalence and risk of rupture of intracranial aneurysms: a systematic review, Stroke, Vol. 29(1998), 251-256
2. Higgins, W.E., Spyra, W.J.T., Ritman, Automatic extraction of the arterial tree from 3-d angiograms, IEEE Conf. Eng. in Medicine and Bio., Vol. 2(1989) 563-564
3. Sonka, M., Fitzpatrick, J.M., Handbook of Medical Imaging, SPIE Press (2000)
4. Flasque, N., Desvignes, M., Constans, J., Revenu, M., Acquisition, segmentation, and tracking of the cerebral vascular tree on 3D magnetic resonance angiography images, Medical Image Analysis, Vol. 5(2001), 173-183
5. Sabry, M., Sites, C.B1., Farag, A.A., Hushek, S., A Fast Automatic Method for 3D Volume Segmentation of the Human Cerebrovascular, CARS (2002)
6. Wilson, D.L., Noble, J.A., An Adaptive Segmentation Algorithm for Time-of-flight MRA Dat, IEEE Trans. on Medical Imaging, Vol. 18(1999) 938-945
7. Chapman, B.E., Stapelton, J.O., Parker, D.L., Intracranial vessel segmentation from time-of-flight MRA using pre-processing of the MIP Z-buffer: accuracy of the ZBS algorithm, Medical Image Analysis, Vol. 8(2004) 113-126
8. Suryanarayanan, S., Mullick, R., Mallya, Y., Kamath, v., Automatic Partitioning of Head CTA for enabling Segmentation, SPIE Proceedings of Medical Imaging (2004)
9. Wink, O., Niessen, W.J., Viergever, M.A., Fast Delineation and Visualization of Vessels in 3-D Angiographic Images, IEEE Trans. on Medical Imaging, Vol. 19(2000) 337-346
10. Hong, H., Lee, H., Shin, Y.G., Seong, Y.H., Three-Dimensional Brain CT-DSA using Rigid Registration and Bone Masking for Early Diagnosis and Treatment Planning, Lecture Note on Artificial Intelligence 3378 (2004)
11. Zwillinger, D. (Ed.). Spherical Coordinates in Space, 4.9.9 in CRC Standard Mathematical Tables and Formulae, Boca Raton, FL: CRC Press (1995) 297-298
12. Open Source Computer Vision Library: Reference Manual, Intel Co. (2000)
13. http://www.infinitt.com/English/default.html

Regional Whole Body Fat Quantification in Mice

Xenophon Papademetris[1,2], Pavel Shkarin[2], Lawrence H. Staib[1,2], and Kevin L. Behar[3]

[1] Departments of Biomedical Engineering,
[2] Diag. Radiology
[3] Psychiatry, Yale University New Haven, CT 06520-8042
xenophon.papademetris@yale.edu

Abstract. Obesity has risen to epidemic levels in the United States and around the world. Global indices of obesity such as the body mass index (BMI) have been known to be inaccurate predictors of risk of diabetes, and it is commonly recognized that the distribution of fat in the body is a key measure. In this work, we describe the early development of image analysis methods to quantify regional body fat distribution in groups of both male and female wildtype mice using magnetic resonance images. In particular, we present a new formulation which extends the expectation-maximization formalism commonly applied in brain segmentation to multi-exponential data and applies it to the problem of regional whole body fat quantification. Previous segmentation approaches for multispectral data typically perform the classification on fitted parameters, such as the density and the relaxation times. In contrast, our method directly computes a likelihood term from the raw data and hence explicitly accounts for errors in the fitting process, while still using the fitted parameters to model the variation in the appearance of each tissue class. Early validation results, using magnetic resonance spectroscopic imaging as a gold standard, are encouraging. We also present results demonstrating differences in fat distribution between male and female mice.

1 Introduction

Obesity is rapidly becoming an epidemic in the United States and around the world. This was particularly highlighted in a series of recent NIH workshops [5]. The relation of obesity to insulin resistance and impaired glucose tolerance leading to type 2 diabetes is well established [22, 7]. Body fat distribution in humans has also been linked to ischemic heart disease [13, 15] and cancer [2]. Further, it has been known for decades that global indices of obesity, such as the body mass index (B.M.I.), are often not an accurate predictor of the risk of diabetes and heart disease. For example, the amount of visceral abdominal fat (i.e. fat inside the abdominal cavity) seems to correlate more highly with risk for diabetes. As stated in lay language in a recent New York Times article [9], "People who are shaped like apples, carrying excess weight in the abdomen, are more likely to have diabetes and heart disease than are those built like pears, who deposit fat in their hips, thighs and backsides." This was even further emphasized by a recent study by Klein et al [11] that demonstrated an absence of effect of liposuction on insulin resistance. This was attributed to the fact that liposuction primarily removes subcutaneous fat (i.e. fat just under the skin and outside the abdominal cavity), whose presence appears less correlated with insulin resistance.

Transgenic mouse models of obesity offer the unique ability to study the effect of factors such as age, gender, diet and therapeutic agents on disease progression, in statistically significant numbers of subjects in a tightly controlled environment. There are currently, however, no effective automated methods for the non-invasive measurement of fat distribution in rodents. While such measurements can be made invasively (via dissection [21]), non-invasive techniques will enable longitudinal studies of the same group of animals, and the development of automated image analysis techniques will facilitate large scale studies.

Multi-echo magnetic resonance imaging offers a unique non-invasive technique for quantifying soft tissue structural differences between wildtype mice and transgenic mouse models of obesity and for regional quantification of fat in a whole body image. The parameters that can be estimated from such images, namely the T1-weighted proton density and the relaxation rate r_2, offer jointly a high contrast marker for the detection of fat as well as optimal soft tissue contrast for image registration. Accurate image registration is necessary for bringing information from different mice into a common space for the purpose of statistically comparing fat distributions and morphometric differences in different groups.

In this paper, we present preliminary work aimed at the effective quantification of such images. In particular, we present a method for image classification for the purpose of determining tissue composition in terms of fat, lean muscle (non-fatty soft tissue) and bone/air. The main mathematical contribution of this work is the development of a probabilistic model for the modeling of multi-exponential data in the presence of noise for optimal tissue classification.

Our work is related to previous work in voxel based image classification and segmentation which has been extensively studied in the literature. Many of the methods in this area rely on the formalism of Markov random fields as originally presented by Geman and Geman [8]. The major application of such techniques in medical imaging has been in the voxel-based classification of brain images into gray matter, white matter and cerebro-spinal fluid. Our work is close in spirit to the approach of Wells et al. and others [24, 25], where an Expectation-Maximization strategy is used to simultaneously estimate tissue classes (gray, white, CSF) while simultaneously estimating additional parameters (in this case the bias field) which aid in the classification. Cline et al. [4] use multispectral voxel classification in conjunction with connectivity to segment the brain into tissue types. Material mixture models [12] have also been used. There has also been additional work explicitly aiming at fuzzy classification where each voxel, instead of being classified as exclusively belonging to a specific class, is given partial memberships into multiple classes e.g. [14, 19, 17]. Our proposed whole body classification is particularly close to the work of Pham et al [17] which aims to fuzzily classify multi-spectral acquisitions using a fuzzy c-means method, and exponential fits to estimate tissue properties.

Simple thresholding techniques have been used by many investigators in more clinically focused studies to determine fat volumes (e.g. the work of Weiss et al [23].) Threshold selection, however, is often performed in an arbitrary manner and the measurements produced using such methods are highly sensitive to the exact threshold settings. There has been some work in automated fat quantification from MRI (e.g. [3, 10]) which either utilize simplified thresholding based algorithms, and/or very specific acquisition methods, which are not suitable for whole body fat quantification.

The rest of this paper reads as follows. In, Section 2, we provide details for both the conventional imaging and spectroscopic imaging (CSI) methods used to obtain both the images and the CSI data used as a gold standard. Next, in Section 3, we describe the mathematical formulation of our classification method. Validation results are presented in Section 4, and results illustrating differences in fat distribution between groups of male and female mice are presented in Section 5. Conclusions and plans for future work are discussed in Section 6.

2 Imaging and Spectroscopy Methods

Our imaging/spectroscopy methods were developed on a Bruker 4T small-animal imager with an inner diameter of 16 cm. Three-dimensional images were acquired with a resolution of approximately $0.15 \times 0.20 \times 0.15 mm$, and an imaging matrix of $128 \times 512 \times 128$, using a 3D multi-echo multi-spin (MSME) sequence with 6 echos $TE = 15, 30, 45, 60, 75, 90 ms$ and $TR = 300 ms$. This yielded six images of different contrast which in turn enable the fitting of a mono-exponential model to each voxel for the purpose of computing tissue parameters such as the relaxation rate r_2 and the T1-weighted density d. Because the dimensions of our current imaging coil were not long enough to image the full length of some male mice, in these cases mice were imaged twice with repositioning between the acquisitions and the resulting images were joined together to form the whole body image. Example images, as well as fitted mono-exponential parameters d and r_2, are shown in Figure 1.

Chemical shift spectroscopic imaging (CSI) acquisition was used as a *gold standard data* of tissue composition for a small portion of the mouse. The CSI data were acquired with a resolution of $0.4 \times 0.4 \times 1 mm^3$, dimensions $64 \times 64 \times 12$, and a spectral width of $4006 Hz$ resulting in good water and fat separation. Fat was quantified by integrating the resulting spectra for each voxel around the fat peak, as was done in the images shown in Figure 2 (on page 375). Although the acquisition time required for CSI is prohibitively long for routine work (more than two hours for a small section of the mouse), these data provide a gold standard for the validation of faster acquisitions (such as our multi-echo data) combined with more rigorous image analysis techniques.

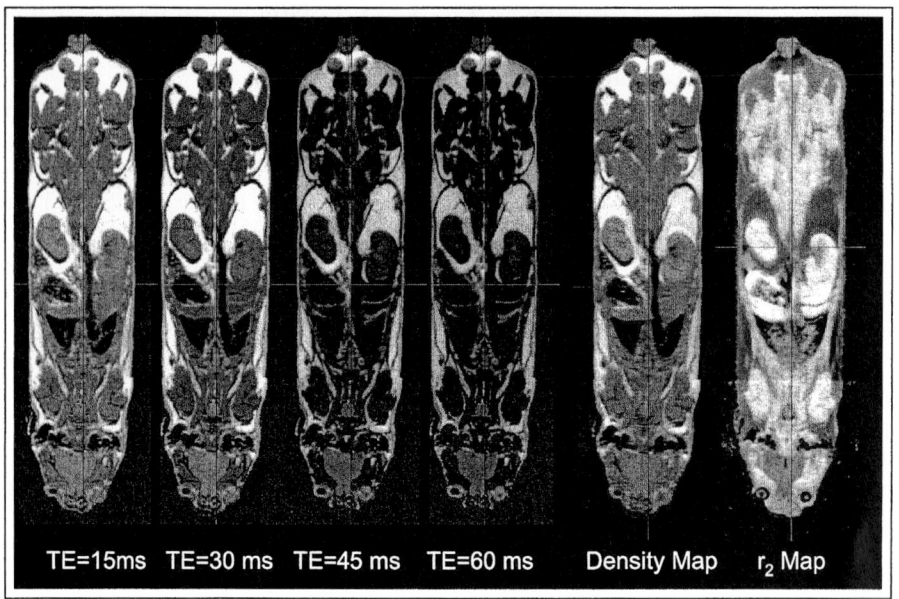

Fig. 1. Example images from multi-echo acquisitions. *Leftmost four columns:* Four different contrasts obtained using a multi-echo sequence. Rightmost two columns: Exponential fit of T1-weighted density and relaxation rate r_2

3 Tissue Classification

In this section, we describe our methodology for tissue classification from MRI. Our method for classification extends the EM-like classification methods of Wells et al and Zhang et al [24, 25], to properly apply to the vector-valued imaged data that are available to us.

Image Model: We acquire a number $N_e = 6$ of images at multiple echo times $T_e = [15, 30, 45, 60, 75, 90]$ ms, and we model the image intensity at image location $\mathbf{x}$ for a given T_e using a mono-exponential model:

$$I(\mathbf{x}, T_e) = d(\mathbf{x})e^{-T_e r_2(\mathbf{x})} + e_f(\mathbf{x}) \tag{1}$$

where T_e is the echo-time for the acquisition, $d(\mathbf{x})$ and $r_2(\mathbf{x})$ are the T1-weighted proton density and the relaxation rate at location $\mathbf{x}$ ($r_2 = 1/t_2$, where t_2 is the relaxation time), and e_f is the noise term, which we assume to be normally distributed.

For the purpose of the classification, we assume that any given voxel belongs to one of three classes $c = [$ 1=bone/air, 2=lean muscle, 3=fat $]$, and that the density d and relaxation rate r_2 for each class can be described as independent normally distributed random variables with means m_d, m_{r2} and standard deviations s_d, s_{r2}. We group the parameters for each class $i \in [1, 2, 3]$ into a parameter vector $\theta_i = [m_d^i, m_{r2}^i, s_d^i, s_{r2}^i]$, and further concatenate the three parameter vectors θ_i into a global parameter vector Θ. In addition, we define the labeling function $M(\mathbf{x})$ which determines the class value for each voxel. $M(\mathbf{x})$ can take values [1, 2, 3]. At each image location $\mathbf{x}$ (we will drop the explicit dependence on $\mathbf{x}$ from here on), we estimate the optimal values of d and r_2. This is accomplished by minimizing a standard least squares merit function of the form:

$$\chi^2 = \sum_{j=1}^{N_e} \frac{\left(I(\mathbf{x}, T_e(j)) - de^{-T_e(j)r_2}\right)^2}{\sigma_n^2} = \sum_{j=1}^{N_e} \frac{e_f(j)^2}{\sigma_n^2} \qquad (2)$$

We label the optimal estimates at location $\mathbf{x}$ as $\hat{d}$ and $\hat{r}_2$, and σ_n is an estimate of the image noise at this location. We model the fitting errors $e_f(i)$ as independent and normally distributed with zero mean. The quality of the fit can be modeled using the Student's t distribution with $N_e - 2$ degrees of freedom [17]. Hence, we can compute at each voxel a probability of fit $q(\mathbf{x})$[18], given the optimal residual error χ^2. Further, we can estimate the variance of the fitting error e_f, s_e^2 which will be useful in the classification process. In summary, the application of this procedure at each voxel results in the computation of optimal tissue parameters $(\hat{d}, \hat{r}_2)$, the likelihood that the model is applicable q, and the variance of the fitting error s_e^2.

Classification Algorithm: The goal of our classification strategy can then be expressed as estimating the optimal segmentation M and parameter vector Θ given the input image vector $\mathbf{I}$. We express this mathematically as:

$$\hat{M}, \hat{\Theta} = \underset{M, \Theta}{\arg\max}\, p(M, \Theta | \mathbf{I}) \qquad (3)$$

As is commonly done, this can be solved iteratively (where k labels the iteration) in the same spirit as the EM-framework as:

$$\textbf{E-Step:}\ \Theta^k = \underset{\Theta}{\arg\max}\, p(\Theta | \mathbf{I}, M^{k-1}), \quad \textbf{M-Step:}\ M^k = \underset{M}{\arg\max}\, p(M | \mathbf{I}, \Theta^k) \qquad (4)$$

where at iteration k, in the E-Step we estimate a new set of parameters Θ^k given the current classification M^{k-1} and then, in the M-Step, using the newly estimated Θ^k we estimate a new classification M^k.

E-Step: This is straightforward. For each class i we estimate the mean and standard deviation of d and r_2 by a weighted sum of the $\hat{d}$ and $\hat{r}_2$ of all the voxels where $M = i$, using the quality of fit terms q as the weights. This ensures that parameter estimates from better fits are weighted more heavily in the estimation process [17].

M-Step: This takes the form of a Bayesian a-posterior maximization. First we express

$$\hat{M} = \underset{M}{\arg\max}\, \log p(M | \mathbf{I}, \Theta^k) = k_1 + \log p(\mathbf{I}, \Theta^k | M) + \log p(M) \qquad (5)$$

where k_1 is a constant. This equation is easily maximized by a greedy search strategy as M can only take values of $1, 2, 3$. The prior term on the classification, $p(M)$, can be defined by modeling M as a Markov random field resulting in a Gibbs distribution for M of the form: $P(M) = e^{-k_m U(M(\mathbf{x}))}$ [25], which ensures local smoothness of the classification (k_m is a normalization constant.) We express the likelihood (or data-adherence) term for each possible value of $M = i$ as:

$$p(\mathbf{I}, \Theta^k | M = i) = p(\mathbf{I}|\Theta^k, M = i) P(\Theta_k | M = i) \propto \Pi_{j=1}^{N_e} p(I(T_e^j)|\theta^i) \quad (6)$$

The term $p(I(T_e^j)|\theta^i)$ can be derived using the imaging model (Equation 1). First we linearize this using a Taylor series expression as:

$$I(T_e^j) \approx m_d^i e^{-T_e^j m_{r2}^i} + (d - m_d^i) e^{-T_e^j m_{r2}^i} + (r_2 - m_{r2}^i) T_e^j m_d^i e^{-T_e^j m_{r2}^i} + e_f \quad (7)$$

By assuming that d, r_2 and e_f are normally distributed random variables, we can conclude that the conditional density $p(I(T_e^j)|\theta^i)$ is also a normal distribution, as $I(T_e^j)$ is effectively a weighted sum of three normal random variables. Further we can derive the mean and standard deviation of this distribution as:

$$\text{Mean}(p(I(T_e^j)|\theta^i)) = \mu(M, T_e^j) = m_d^i e^{-T_e^j m_{r2}^i}, M = i \quad (8)$$

$$\text{Variance}(p(I(T_e^j)|\theta^i)) = \sigma^2(M, T_e^j) = (T_e^j m_{r2}^i)^2 (s_d^2 + (m_d^i)^2 T_e^2 s_{r2}^2), M = i \quad (9)$$

Based on this derivation, we can express Equation 5 in its final form as:

$$\hat{M} = \underset{M}{\arg\min} \underbrace{\sum_{j=1}^{N_e} \frac{(I(T_e^j) - \mu(M, T_e^j))^2}{2\sigma(M, T_e^j)^2} - \log \sigma(M, T_e^j)}_{\text{Vector Data Adherence Term}} - \underbrace{k^m U(M)}_{\text{Smoothness}} \quad (10)$$

This formulation is superior to the more standard approach where the classification is performed directly on fitted tissue parameters (e.g. in this case the T1-weighted density d and the relaxation rate r_2) because it takes into account directly the fact that such parameter fitting is an approximation to the real data. In cases where the local parameter fit is inaccurate (i.e. the residual error in the fitting of d and r_2, which is not uncommon in motion-corrupted data) a standard classification based on these estimates can yield erroneous results, whereas by performing the classification using the original image data such errors can be avoided. Consider, for example, the case where a mono-exponential model badly approximates the data at a given voxel. If the fitted parameters are used, the data adherence term will push for the voxel to be classified in one of the given classes regardless. In our method, the values for the (vector) data adherence term will be high for all classes, hence allowing the local classification to be driven by the smoothness term as is appropriate in cases of uncertain data.

Initialization: The algorithm is initialized using a k-means clustering procedure [6, 17], which initially forms clusters based on the fitted density measurements $\hat{d}$. Then, using the output as a starting point, the algorithm performs a joint clustering on the pair $[\hat{d}, \hat{r}_2]$.

4 Validation of Segmentation Using CSI

We performed preliminary validation of the MRI-based fat quantification algorithm by comparing its output to a direct measure of fat using chemical shift spectroscopic imaging (CSI). While CSI provides high quality measurements, the imaging time is *prohibitive for in-vivo* whole body imaging. We acquired both whole body MR images and also CSI data covering a small portion of the abdomen (typically 2.5x2.5x2 cm^3) of 12 wildtype C57BL6 mice (6 male, 6 female, average age 11 weeks), using the methods described in Section 2.

CSI Processing. The CSI data were first corrected to align the water peaks in the spectra of the individual voxels (as shown in Figure 2 (top right)). Next we

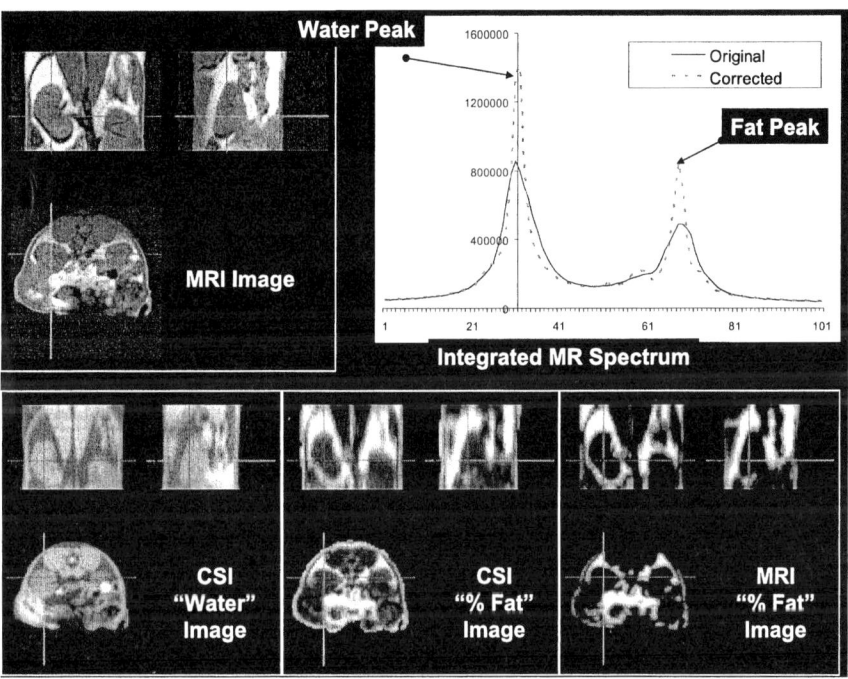

Fig. 2. Preliminary validation of the MRI-based fat measurements using spectroscopic (CSI) imaging. (Top Left) Section of the MRI image for which CSI data was acquired. (Top Right) Integrated MRS Spectrum from all CSI voxels illustrating the effect of correcting for local field inhomogeneities by shifting the individual CSI-voxel water peaks to the center of the spectrum. Note that both the water and the fat peaks become higher and narrower as a result of the correction. (Bottom Left) Spectroscopic-"water" image showing contrast that is similar to that obtained using MRI – without the fat . (Bottom Middle) Spectroscopic "% fat" image (Bottom Right) Fat probability map generated by the classification algorithm and MRI, at the same resolution as the CSI data. The correlation between the two fat maps was 0.78. When the small signal dropout region near the mouse's back is excluded the correlation rises to 0.82

Table 1. Quantitative validation of the MRI-based fat measurements with CSI. The total amount of fat in the imaged region from CSI (CSIFAT) is compared with MRI derived measurements (MRIFAT) as estimated by our algorithm (using three different smoothness parameters 0.1,0.5,1.0). The *voxelwise* correlation between the CSI percentage fat map and the algorithm output is given in the rightmost three columns. (The mouse identifier begins with 'F' for female mice and 'M' for male mice.)

Mouse	CSI FAT	MRI FAT			Correlation		
		0.1	0.5	1	0.1	0.5	1
F1	269271	279303	275568	271401	0.574	0.570	0.565
F2	295106	215768	210516	205431	0.520	0.517	0.512
F3	305127	178272	174510	170722	0.506	0.502	0.498
F4	286950	342248	338066	335099	0.542	0.537	0.530
F5	245584	170922	165038	158983	0.413	0.407	0.401
F6	363370	299371	294440	289295	0.608	0.605	0.602
M1	648171	700656	694753	686846	0.656	0.654	0.653
M2	1043136	659980	661060	659450	0.744	0.744	0.744
M3	451314	300178	296097	291818	0.744	0.743	0.742
M4	1123495	824133	820210	814955	0.779	0.778	0.777
M5	1972404	1687532	1686527	1685327	0.854	0.854	0.854
M6	512522	310780	307982	303555	0.790	0.789	0.789
Overall	7516450	5969141.1	5924766.5	5872883	0.748	0.748	0.747

computed a water signal and a fat signal for each voxel by integrating over the appropriate portions of the spectrum around the water and fat peaks respectively. A water image is shown in Figure 2 (bottom left), and a percentage fat image is shown in Figure 2 (bottom middle).

MRI-based Fat Quantification. Our algorithm was used to quantify fat in the MRI data and a corresponding MRI percentage fat image was computed, by first rigidly registering the MRI image to the MRS 'water image' using the method by Studholme et al. based on normalized mutual information[20] (top left, and bottom left of Figure 2 respectively) and computing the percentage of MRI voxels in the space occupied by a single CSI voxel labeled as fat by the algorithm. The results are tabulated in Table 1, and the overall trend is encouraging. The overall correlation (obtained by concatenating the fat maps from all the mice and computing a single correlation) was approximately 0.75 and the algorithm's total fat estimate was approximately 80% of the CSI total fat estimate. Further the output of the algorithm was fairly insensitive to the setting of the smoothness parameter as shown in the table.

For the male mice, the CSI slices were acquired in the kidney region where fat content is generally higher, whereas for the female mice CSI slices were through the liver where the fat is more dispersed inside the organ. The lower correlations for the female mice were expected. The error for the male mice is less as the fat around the kidney is easier to quantify from MRI (and see visually). This may be due to our hard classification strategy which does not allow for partial voxel labeling. Also, in general our approach under-estimated the total amount of fat possibly due to the inability of the mono-exponential model to accurately quantify fat dispersed in tissue.

5 Quantification of Group Differences

5.1 Fat Quantification in Male and Female Mice via ROI Analysis

To illustrate the potential applications of our methodology in the evaluation of groups of mice, we performed regional fat quantification for two groups of mice, a group of $N = 5$ male mice and a group of $N = 5$ female mice. The two groups were approximately age matched (average age 10.6 vs 10 weeks). They are a subset of the mice used for evaluation of our tissue classification algorithm presented in Section 4, in particular two mice were omitted from the original $N = 12$ mice of Table 1 for the purpose of this analysis to make the groups approximately age matched.

Our tissue classification strategy described in Section 3 was used to classify the images. Using this classification, we computed the following measures which are tabulated in Table 2: (a) Total mouse volume, (b) Total body fat volume, (c) Abdominal fat volume – this was defined as the total volume of fat inside the abdomen. A region of interest (ROI) inside the abdomen was defined by the semi-automatically extracted abdominal surfaces in each mouse. (d) Subcutaneous Fat Volume – defined as the total amount of fat outside the abdomen, (e) % abdominal fat, defined as the ratio of abdominal fat to total fat and (f) % body fat, defined as the ratio of total fat volume to total mouse volume.

The results tabulated in Table 2, demonstrate that in these two (admittedly small) groups, male mice tend to be bigger and have proportionally more fat than female mice, Further, we illustrate our ability to quantify regional fat measures such as abdominal fat, as opposed to simply whole body fat. We additionally note that the computed % body fat numbers are in the same range as those reported in the literature[1] using a whole body MR-spectrometer on similar mice.

Table 2. Quantification of key parameters using our tissue classification algorithm (*Top:* M = Males $N = 5$. *Bottom:* F = Females $N = 5$). Mice were approximately age-matched (10.6 vs 10 weeks old)

	M1	M2	M3	M4	M5	Average
Age (weeks)	9	10	10	12	12	10.6
Volume (mm^3)	15265	20267	15467	21497	21433	18785.8
Total Fat (mm^3)	2219	3272	2338	5371	6223	3884.6
Abd. Fat (mm^3)	1002	1678	1090	2489	2731	1798.0
Sub. Fat (mm^3)	1217	1594	1248	2882	3492	2086.6
% Abd Fat	45%	51%	47%	46%	44%	47%
% Body Fat	15%	16%	15%	25%	29%	20%

	F1	F2	F3	F4	F5	Average
Age (weeks)	8	8	11	11	12	10.0
Volume (mm^3)	11070	11780	14507	13583	14530	13094.0
Total Fat (mm^3)	1787	1519	2247	1823	2097	1894.6
Abd. Fat (mm^3)	640	743	1001	805	864	810.6
Sub. Fat (mm^3)	1147	776	1246	1018	1233	1084.0
% Abd. Fat	36%	49%	45%	44%	41%	43%
% Body Fat	16%	13%	15%	13%	14%	14%

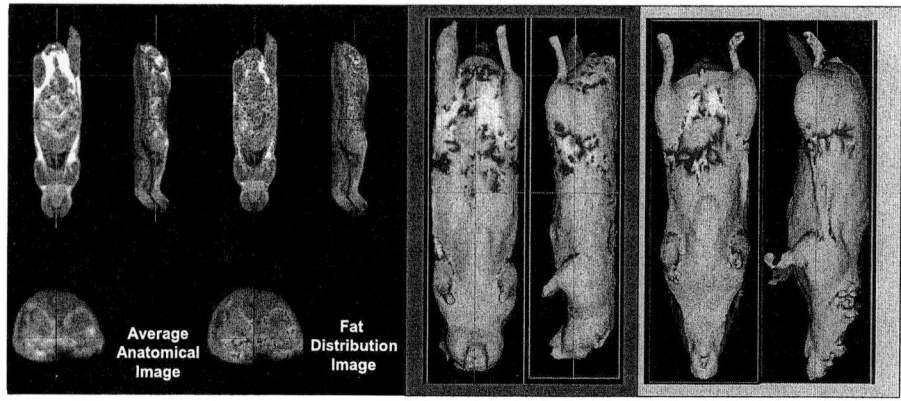

Fig. 3. Left: Average anatomical image (left) and fat distribution image (right) from $N = 5$ male mice, computed using non-rigid registration. The fat distribution is overlaid on the average anatomical image (right) where the color scale is such that voxels shown in red were classified as fat in at least half the mice, with progressively brighter shades of yellow indicating that those areas were classified as fat in more mice. **Middle & Right:** Fat distributions of $N = 5$ male (middle) and $N = 5$ female (right) projected onto the outer skin surface of the reference male and female mice respectively. At each point in the surface we plot the average value of the fat distribution on a line segment of length 7 mm parallel to the local surface normal

5.2 Fat Distributions in Male and Female Mice

For the same $N = 5$ male and $N = 5$ female mice used in the previous section we computed fat distribution maps by (a) registering the individual male and female mice into a common space using our integrated registration method [16] – that used both image intensities and points sampled from pre-segmented surfaces (an example is shown in Figure 4), and (b) averaging the warped individual fat maps to generate average fat distribution maps for each group. The fat distribution maps are shown in Figure 3. Visually it is again obvious that in this case the male mice had substantially more fat, especially in the area around the reproductive organs (between the rear two legs). Such fat distributions generated by the registration of individual mouse tissue classification maps to a common space afford a direct look of what the typical fat distribution is in a group of mice.

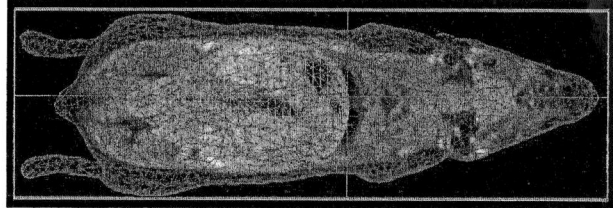

Fig. 4. Example of a point-set used for registration – from a female mouse. Red: outer skin surface, orange: abdominal surface, green and yellow: right and left kidney surfaces respectively

6 Conclusions and Future Work

With the segmentation and quantification method described in this paper it has been possible to estimate regional body fat which overcomes a number of inadequacies in previous studies. The current method achieves an accurate quantification of subcutaneous fat pads, however the accuracy of the method to detect intra-organ fat (e.g. in the liver) which is dispersed in normal tissue is limited by its reliance on binary classification and mono-exponential tissue modeling. To address these limitations, it should be possible to use a larger number of non-uniformly spaced echos to enable the robust estimation of multi-exponential tissue models, which in turn will enable the use of fuzzy classification techniques. Additional ongoing work aims to optimize whole body mouse non-rigid registration to address the issue of forming composite fat maps and eliminating the need for the manual ROI analysis, which was used in the results presented in Section 5.1. The classification methods presented in this paper are also applicable in both human and rodent neuroimaging in cases where multi-echo data is available.

References

1. DE Berryman, EO List, KT Coschigano, K Behar, JK Kim, and JJ Kopchick. Comparing adiposity profiles in three mouse models with altered GH signaling. *Growth Hormone & IGF Research*, 14:309–18, Aug 2004.
2. E. E. Calle and R. Kaak. Overweight, obesity and cancer: Epidemiological evidence and proposed mechanisms. *Nature Reviews Cancer*, 4:579–591, 2004.
3. K. K. Changani, A. Nicholson, A. White, J.K. Latcham, D.G. Reid, and J. C. Clapham. A longitudinal magnetic resonance imaging (MRI) study of differences in abdominal fat distribution between normal mice and lean overexpressors of mitochondrial uncoupling protein-3 (UPC-3). *Diabetes, Obesity and Metabolism*, 5:99–105, 2003.
4. H. E. Cline, W. E. Lorensen, R. Kikinis, and F. Jolesz. Three-dimensional segmentation of MR images of the head using probability and connectivity. *Journal of Computer Assisted Tomography*, 14(6):1037–1045, Nov./Dec. 1990.
5. NIH Obesity-Related Scientific Meetings Conferences and Workshops. http://obesityresearch.nih.gov/news/meetings-archive.htm.
6. R. Duda and P. Hart. *Pattern Classification and Scene Analysis*. John Wiley and Sons, N.Y., 1973.
7. DJ Evans, RG Hoffmann, RK Kalkhoff, and AH Kissebah. Relationship of body fat topography to insulin sensitivity and metabolic profiles in premenopausal women. *Metabolism*, 33(1):68–75, Jan 1984.
8. D. Geman and S. Geman. Stochastic relaxation, Gibbs distribution and the Bayesian restoration of images. *IEEE Trans. Pattern Analysis and Machine Intelligence*, 6(6):721–741, November 1984.
9. Denise Grady. The secret life of a potent cell. *The New York Times*, F::1, July, 6th 2003.
10. S. A. Gronemeyer, R. G. Steen, W. M. Kauffman, W. E. Reddick, and J. O Glass. Fast adipose tissue (FAT) assesment by MRI. *Magnetic Resonance Imaging*, 18:815–818, 2000.

11. S Klein, L. Fontana, V. Young, Leroy. C., R. Andrew, C. Kilo, B. W. Patterson, and B. S. Mohammed. Absence of an effect of liposuction on insulin action and risk factors for coronary heart disease. *New England Journal of Medicine*, 350(25):2549–2557, June, 17th 2004.
12. Z. Liang, R. F. Jaszczak, and R. E. Coleman. Parameter estimation of finite mixtures using the EM algorithm and information criteria with application to medical image processing. *IEEE Trans. Nucl. Sci.*, 39(4):1126–1133, 1992.
13. JE Manson, GA Colditz, MJ Stampfer, WC Willett, B Rosner, RR Monson, FE Speizer, and CH Hennekens. A prospective study of obesity and risk of coronary heart disease in women. *N Engl J Med.*, 322(13):882–9, Mar 1990.
14. A. Noe and J. C. Gee. Partial volume segmentation of cerebral MRI scans with mixture model clustering. In *Information Processing in Medical Imaging (IPMI)*, pages 423–430, 2001.
15. LO Ohlson, B Larsson, K Svardsudd, L Welin, H Eriksson, L Wilhelmsen, P Bjorntorp, and G. Tibblin. The influence of body fat distribution on the incidence of diabetes mellitus. 13.5 years of follow-up of the participants in the study of men born in 1913. *Diabetes*, 34(10):1055–8, Oct 1985.
16. X. Papademetris, A. Jackowski, R. T. Schultz, L. H. Staib, and J. S. Duncan. Integrated intensity and point-feature nonrigid registration. In *Medical Image Computing and Computer Aided Intervention (MICCAI)*, 2004.
17. D. L. Pham and J. L. Prince. Adaptive fuzzy segmentation of magnetic resonance images. *IEEE Transactions on Medical Imaging*, 18(9):737–752, September 1999.
18. W. H. Press, S. A. Teukolsky, W. T. Vetterling, and B. P. Flannery. *Numerical Recipes in C: The Art of Scientific Computing*. Cambridge University Press, Cambridge, U. K., 1994, Second Edition.
19. D.W. Shattuck, S. R. Sandor-Leahy, K.A. Schaper, D.A. Rottenberg, and R.M. Leahy. Magnetic resonance image tissue classification using a partial volume model. *NeuroImage*, 13(5):856–876, May 2001.
20. C. Studholme, D. Hill, and D. Hawkes. Automated three-dimensional registration of magnetic resonance and positron emission tomography brain images by multiresolution optimisation of voxel similarity measures. *Medical Physics*, 24(1):25–35, 1997.
21. Y-S. Tsai, H-J Kim, N. Takahashi, H-S. Kim, J. Hagaman, J. K. Kim, and N. Maeda. Hypertension and abnormal fat distribution but not insulin resistance in mice with p465l pparγ. *J. Clin. Invest.*, 114:240–249, 2004.
22. R. Weiss, S. Dufour, S. Taksali, W. V. Tambolrane, K. F. Petersen, R. C. Bonadonna, L. Boselli, G. Barbetta, K Allen, F. Rife, M. Savoye, J. Dziura, R. Sherwin, G. I. Shulman, and S. Caprio. Prediabetes in obese youth: a syndrome of impaired glucose tolerance, severe insulin resistance and altered myocellular and abdominal fat partitioning. *Lancet*, 362:951–7, 2003.
23. R. Weiss, S.E. Taksali, S. Dufour, C.W. Yeckel, X. Papademetris, G. Kline, W.V. Tamborlane, J. Dziura, G.I. Shulman, and S. Caprio. The "Obese Insulin Sensitive adolescent" – importance of adiponectin and lipid partitioning. *J. Clin Endocrinol. Metab.*, March 2005.
24. W.M. Wells, R. Kikinis, W.E.L Grimson, and F. Jolesz. Adaptive segmentation of MRI data. *IEEE Transactions on Medical Imaging*, 15:429–442, 1996.
25. Y. Zhang, M. Brady, and S. Smith. Segmentation of brain MR images through a hidden markov random field model and the expectation maximization algorithm. *IEEE Transactions on Medical Imaging*, 20(1):45–57, 2001.

Surface Matching via Currents

Marc Vaillant[1] and Joan Glaunès[2]

[1] CIS, Johns Hopkins University, Baltimore, MD
marc@jhu.edu
[2] LAGA, Université Paris 13, Villetaneuse, France
glaunes@math.univ-paris13.fr

Abstract. We present a new method for computing an optimal deformation between two arbitrary surfaces embedded in Euclidean 3-dimensional space. Our main contribution is in building a norm on the space of surfaces via representation by currents of geometric measure theory. Currents are an appropriate choice for representations because they inherit natural transformation properties from differential forms. We impose a Hilbert space structure on currents, whose norm gives a convenient and practical way to define a matching functional. Using this Hilbert space norm, we also derive and implement a surface matching algorithm under the large deformation framework, guaranteeing that the optimal solution is a one-to-one regular map of the entire ambient space. We detail an implementation of this algorithm for triangular meshes and present results on 3D face and medical image data.

1 Introduction

Surfaces embedded in 3D are important geometric models for many objects of interest in image analysis. They are often the appropriate abstractions for studying gross shape, either because the structure of interest is inherently 2D (e.g. the outer cortex of the human brain, human face, etc.), or because its shape can be efficiently and completely captured by its bounding surface (e.g. planes, animals, or anatomical structures of the human body, etc.). A fundamental task in image analysis applications is to perform a non rigid matching (deformation) between two occurrences of the same structure. For example, it has been recognized as early as 1917 by D'Arcy Thompson [1], that given representations of a particular anatomic structure in two subjects, an appropriate methodology for comparing their gross morphological differences is to study a *transformation*–uniquely characterized by a natural optimality property–from one structure into the other.

Surface matching is usually achieved via semi-automated procedures in which a small number of substructures, such as landmark points or curves, are identified by hand and then used to guide the transformation of the entire surface [2, 3, 4, 5, 6]. One interpretation of the problem is to consider surface matching as a "point correspondence" task: for each point on the discretized template surface find its corresponding point on the target. Fully automated approaches to this problem have been developed in [7]. However, a fundamental issue with this point of view is that, due to discretization, a point on one surface need not have a homologous point on the other. This problem is handled in [7] by simultaneously identifying and rejecting points with no corresponding pair as "outliers". A second issue is that geometric information is necessarily discarded when reducing surfaces–inherently 2D objects–to 0-dimensional point sets. Another related approach is the work of Wang et. al. [8]. This approach does use local geometric constraints by including surface curvature in their matching criterion. Its advantage is that both triangulation and correspondence is established simultaneously. Another elegant approach includes the work of Davies et. al. [9] in which the correspondence problem is tackled by building the "best" model via a set of optimality criteria.

We develop a surface matching approach in which the two issues mentioned above are overcome naturally in the fundamental theoretical framework. Our approach follows most closely the work of [10], but differs in that we represent surfaces as the generalized distributions of deRham called **currents** [11], instead of the classical distributions of Schwartz. As in [10], distribution representations allow us to get away from a strict pointwise representation of surfaces and therefore enable us to treat the problem as true surface matching without the point correspondence issue. Furthermore, representation via currents captures the geometry of the structure because it is sensitive to both location and to the first order local geometric structure. We are therefore able to overcome the two issues above via the natural choice of current representation. In this paper we provide a detailed theoretical development of a norm on surfaces which can be used as a matching criterion for finding an optimal transformation from one surface into another. We present one such variational optimization problem under the large deformation diffeomorphism framework. Finally, we derive a discretized version of this variation problem, detail its implementation, and provide results on 3D face and medical image data.

2 Surfaces as Currents

In order to build a surface matching algorithm, we need a criterion that measures how "close" or similar one surface is to another. Our strategy is to represent surfaces as objects in a linear space and then to equip this space with a computable norm. The generalized distributions from geometric measure theory, called currents, will serve as the representers. In this section we set the notation and introduce currents as representations of surfaces. The main power, and hence motivation, for using these representations will become clear in Section 2.2 where we see that they are preserved under coordinate transformations.

2.1 2-Forms and Currents

The paradigm of the approach is built from mathematical objects called differential m-forms. Although the theory is more general than presented here, we restrict the discussion to the setting of interest: surfaces embedded in $\mathbb{R}^3$. In this setting, we need only introduce differential 2-forms. A differential **2-form** on $\mathbb{R}^3$ is a differential mapping $x \mapsto \omega(x)$ such that for each $x \in \mathbb{R}^3$, $\omega(x)$ is a skew-symmetric bilinear function on $\mathbb{R}^3$. A 2-form is a natural object to be integrated over an oriented smooth surface S because, as we will see, it automatically transforms correctly under a change of coordinates. For each $x \in S$, let u_x^1, u_x^2 be an orthonormal basis of the tangent plane at x. Abusing notation slightly, we then associate to S the function

$$S(\omega) = \int_S \omega(x)(u_x^1, u_x^2) d\sigma(x), \tag{1}$$

where $d\sigma$ is the element of surface area. Thus, the surface S is seen as a linear functional on the space of 2-forms via (1). More generally, the space of 2-dimensional **currents** is defined as the dual space to C^∞ 2-forms with compact support. It is equipped with the correct topology as in the classical theory of distributions of Schwartz. This definition extends to more singular geometric objects, such as triangular meshes, by replacing the surface measure with 2-dimensional Hausdorff measure. In fact a wide class of geometric subsets of $\mathbb{R}^3$, called rectifiable sets, can be viewed as currents [12].

In the sequel, we continue to abuse notation by using the same letter to denote both a surface as well as its associated representation as a current.

2.2 Push Forward of a Current

The fundamental property ultimately motivating the representation of surfaces by currents is that it is possible to define an action of diffeomorphisms $\phi : \mathbb{R}^3 \to \mathbb{R}^3$ on currents which coincides with the natural action of ϕ on surfaces (i.e. $S \mapsto \phi(S)$).

First define the **pull back** of a 2-form ω by: $\phi^\sharp \omega(x)(\eta, \nu) = \omega(\phi(x))\left((d_x\phi)\eta, (d_x\phi)\nu\right)$. The **push forward** $\phi_\sharp S$ of a current S is $\phi_\sharp S(\omega) = S(\phi^\sharp \omega)$. The change of coordinates for integration of differential forms [13] states

$$S(\phi^\sharp \omega) = \phi(S)(\omega). \tag{2}$$

That is, $\phi_\sharp S$ is indeed the current associated with $\phi(S)$, which is exactly the natural property we would like our representations to have.

2.3 Vectorial Representation

It will be convenient to use a vectorial representation of skew-symmetric bilinear functions on $\mathbb{R}^3$. If B is such a function, its representer $\overline{B} \in \mathbb{R}^3$ satisfies $B(\eta, \nu) = \overline{B} \cdot (\eta \times \nu)$, where $\cdot$ and $\times$ are the euclidean dot and cross products respectively. Therefore a 2-form, $\omega(x)$, will be represented by the vector field $\overline{\omega}(x)$ via this association. Formally, the association between 2-forms and vectors is given by the hodge star operator and duality (see [13]).

2.4 Hilbert Space of Currents

Recall that the motivation for introducing representations is as a vehicle for constructing a norm on the space of hypersurfaces of $\mathbb{R}^3$. In practice, this norm must be computable. We see in this section that the currents of interest, i.e. those associated with hypersurfaces of $\mathbb{R}^3$ via (1), can be equipped with a Hilbert space structure having an easily computable norm. The machinery of Reproducing kernel Hilbert space (r.k.h.s.) theory is fundamental in this construction (see [14]). Background in the somewhat uncommon setting of differential forms is given next, together with the derivation of the norm.

Let $(W, \langle \cdot, \cdot \rangle_W)$ be a Hibert space of differential 2-forms. The dual space (space of continuous linear functionals) of W is denoted W^*. By the Riesz-Frechet theorem, each $S \in W^*$ has a representer $K_W S \in W$ such that for every $\omega \in W$, $S(\omega) = \langle K_W S, \omega \rangle_W$. K_W is in fact an isometry between W^* and W. We say that W is a r.k.h.s. if for every $x, \xi \in \mathbb{R}^3$, the associated linear **evaluation functional**, δ_x^ξ, defined by $\delta_x^\xi(\omega) = \overline{\omega}(x) \cdot \xi$ belongs to W^*. If W^* is a r.k.h.s., we define the **reproducing kernel** operator k_W by

$$k_W(x,y)\xi = \overline{K_W \delta_x^\xi(y)}.$$

Thus it is in fact the reproducing kernel of $\overline{W}$, the space of vector fields corresponding to W. From this definition follows the formula:

$$\langle \delta_x^\xi, \delta_y^\eta \rangle_{W^*} = k_W(x,y)\xi \cdot \eta \tag{3}$$

We impose a slightly stronger constraint than continuity of the evaluation functionals: W is constructed so that it is continuously embedded in the space of continuous bounded 2-forms. That is, there exists some constant c such that $|\omega|_\infty \leq c|\omega|_W$ for all $\omega \in W$. This immediately implies continuity of the evaluation functionals, and furthermore, if S is a surface, we have

$$|S(\omega)| \leq \int_S |\delta_x^{u_x^1 \times u_x^2}(\omega(x))| d\sigma(x) \leq \sigma(S) \, c |\omega|_W.$$

Hence $S \in W^*$, and we are now able to compare submanifolds via the dual space norm on W^*.

3 Surface Matching

Equipped with an appropriate representative space W^*, as described in the previous section, we can now state an optimization problem for mapping one surface into another. We have chosen the well established "large deformation" setting which provides a solution that is a diffeomorphism of the ambient space. This framework is founded in the paradigm of Grenander's group action approach for modeling objects. Abstractly, an appropriate group of transformations, $\mathcal{G}$, is defined together with a group action, which act on a set of objects or structures of interest, $\mathcal{M}$. The idea is to study two elements S_1 and S_2 of $\mathcal{M}$ through an "optimal" transformation $\phi \in \mathcal{G}$ that registers these objects (i.e. $\phi S_1 = S_2$). This approach shifts the focus of the modeling effort onto the study of transformations, as envisioned by D'Arcy Thompson.

In the large deformation setting, $\mathcal{G}$ is a subgroup of diffeomorphisms and the structures of interest in this paper, $\mathcal{M}$, are hypersurfaces of $\mathbb{R}^3$. Optimality is realized by considering all curves $\phi_t \in \mathcal{G}, t \in [0,1]$ connecting two elements in $\mathcal{G}$ via the group action. The optimal transformation is given by ϕ_1, for the curve which minimizes the accumulated infinitesimal variations in $\mathcal{G}$ through a riemannian structure. We next detail the construction of the group $\mathcal{G}$ and define formally the optimization problem.

3.1 Large Deformation Framework

The fundamental object of construction is a Hilbert space V, with inner product $\langle \cdot, \cdot \rangle_V$, of smooth vector fields (at least C^1) defined on the background space $\mathbb{R}^3$. For all time dependent families of elements of V, written $v_t \in V$ for $t \in [0, 1]$, such that $\int_0^1 |v_t|_V dt < \infty$, the solution ϕ_t at time $t = 1$, of

$$\frac{\partial \phi}{\partial t} = v_t \circ \phi_t, \qquad (4)$$

with $\phi_0(x) = x$, is a unique diffeomorphism (see [15, 16]). The collection of all such solutions defines our subgroup of diffeomorphisms $\mathcal{G}_V$, and the inner product $\langle \cdot, \cdot \rangle_V$ equips it with a Riemannian structure. We will sometimes denote ϕ^v for an element of $\mathcal{G}$, explicitly characterizing it by its associated vector field v. The geodesics of $\mathcal{G}$ provide the transformations which match objects in the orbit, and are characterized by extremals of the kinetic energy $\frac{1}{2} \int_0^1 |v_t|_V^2 dt$. In fact, $\mathcal{G}$ can be equipped with a natural right-invariant geodesic distance

$$d_V(\phi, \phi') = \inf \left\{ \left(\int_0^1 |v_t|_V^2 dt \right)^{1/2}, \phi_1^v \circ \phi = \phi' \right\}.$$

3.2 Variational Formulation

We define the optimal matching, ϕ_* between two currents S and T as a minimizer of $J_{S,T}(\phi) \doteq d_V(Id, \phi)^2 + |\phi_\sharp S - T|_{W^*}^2 / \sigma_R^2$, where σ_R^2 is a trade-off parameter. Equivalently we have $\phi_* = \phi_1^{v_*}$ where v_* is a minimizer of

$$J_{S,T}(v) = \int_0^1 |v_t|_V^2 dt + \frac{1}{\sigma_R^2} |(\phi_1^v)_\sharp S - T|_{W^*}^2 \qquad (5)$$

The first term of this energy is referred to as the regularizing term, and the second is referred to as the matching, or data attachment term.

In practice, a surface is approximated by a triangular mesh, which also has a current representation. Our strategy is to approximate triangle mesh associated currents in order to derive a computable gradient of the energy (5). We next detail the approximation and gradient derivation.

Let S be a triangular mesh in $\mathbb{R}^3$. Given a face f of S, let f^1, f^2, f^3 denote its vertices, $e^1 = f^2 - f^3, e^2 = f^3 - f^1, e^3 = f^1 - f^2$ its edges, $c(f) = \frac{1}{3}(f^1 + f^2 + f^3)$ its center, and $N(f) = \frac{1}{2}(e^2 \times e^3)$ its normal vector with length equal to its area. We will also denote by S_t the triangular mesh at time t, with faces f_t having vertices $f_t^i = \phi_t(f^i)$, $i = 1, 2, 3$.

The mesh S is represented as a current in the following way

$$S(\omega) = \sum_f \int_f \overline{\omega}(x) \cdot (u_x^1 \times u_x^2) d\sigma_f(x),$$

where σ_f is the surface measure on f. Now, we approximate ω over a face by its value at the center. Thus, we have the approximation $S(\omega) \approx \sum_f \overline{\omega}(c(f)) \cdot N(f)$, so in fact, the approximation is a sum of linear evaluation functionals $\mathcal{C}(S) = \sum_f \delta_{c(f)}^{N(f)}$, and the matching error can be easily computed using the reproducing kernel as in (3).

From the identity $\phi_\sharp S = \phi(S)$ we can infer two possible approximations to $\phi(S)$:

1. compute the approximation $\mathcal{C}(S)$ and then apply the push forward formula $(\phi_1)_\sharp \mathcal{C}(S)$:

$$\phi_\sharp \delta_x^\xi = \delta_{\phi(x)}^{\det(d_x \phi)(d_x \phi^*)^{-1}\xi} \tag{6}$$

2. first compute S_1 and then compute the approximation $\mathcal{C}(S_1)$.

We have implemented the second approximation. The advantage is that it does not involve the derivatives of ϕ_1, which simplifies the computation of the gradient (cf 3.3). Note, however, that in this case an additional approximation is made since $S_1 \neq \phi_1(S)$. Given either approximation, we can compute explicitly the metric between two surfaces S and T. Let f, g index the faces of S and q, r index the faces of T, the metric $\mathcal{E} = |\mathcal{C}(S) - \mathcal{C}(T)|_{W^*}^2$ between these two surfaces under the second approximation becomes

$$\mathcal{E} = \sum_{f,g} N(f)^t k_W(c(g), c(f)) N(g) - 2 \sum_{f,q} N(f)^t k_W(c(q), c(f)) N(q)$$
$$+ \sum_{q,r} N(q)^t k_W(c(q), c(r)) N(r).$$

After a considerable amount of theoretical work, we have arrived at a fairly simple formula which we can analyze intuitively. The first and last terms enforce structural integrity of the two surfaces, while the middle term penalizes geometric and spatial mismatch. Using this approximation we now turn to the computation of the gradient with respect to v_t.

3.3 Gradient of J in $L^2([0, 1], V)$

Let x^j index the vertices of S. Like all point-based matching problems in the large deformation setting, it can be shown that the optimal vector fields v_t are of the form

$$v_t(x) = \sum_j k_V(x_j, x) \alpha_t^j, \tag{7}$$

where k_V denotes the reproducing kernel *of the deformation space V* (see [4, 5]). The vectors α_t^j are referred to as **momentum vectors** do to the connection of the large deformation setting to Hamiltonian mechanics (see [17, 18]). It follows from the flow equation that the matching functional (5) is a function only of the trajectories x_t^j.

Gradient of the Data Attachment Term. The gradient of the data attachment term, $\mathcal{E}$, in the space $L^2([0,1], V)$ of vector fields is of the form $\nabla \mathcal{E}_t(x) = \sum_j k_V(x_t^j, x) d_{x_t^j} \phi_{t1}^*$ $\nabla_{x_t^j} \mathcal{E}$. Indeed, for a variation $v_{t,\epsilon} = v_t + \epsilon \tilde{v}_t$ of the vector field v_t, the corresponding variation of $x_1^j = \phi_1(x^j)$ is (see [19])

$$\tilde{x}_1^j = \partial_\epsilon x_1^j|_{\epsilon=0} = \int_0^1 d_{x_t^j} \phi_{t1} \tilde{v}_t(x_t^j) dt,$$

and thus the variation of $\mathcal{E}$ is

$$\partial_\epsilon \mathcal{E}|_{\epsilon=0} = \sum_j \partial_{x_t^j} \mathcal{E} \widetilde{x_1^j} = \int_0^1 \partial_{x_t^j} \mathcal{E} d_{x_t^j} \phi_{t1} \widetilde{v}_t(x_t^j) dt$$

$$= \int_0^1 \langle k_V(x_t^j, \cdot) d_{x_t^j} \phi_{t1}^* \nabla_{x_t^j} \mathcal{E}, \widetilde{v}_t \rangle_V dt$$

We have reduced the computation to the derivative of $|\mathcal{C}(S_1) - \mathcal{C}(T)|^2_{W^*}$ with respect to the vertices of S_1. Let $\partial_{f_1^i} \mathcal{E}$ denote the contribution of a face f_1 to its vertex f_1^i. We have $\partial_{f_1^i} \mathcal{E}\, \eta = 2[\partial_{f_1^i} \mathcal{C}(S_1)\, \eta](\omega)$, where $\omega = K_W(\mathcal{C}(S_1) - \mathcal{C}(T))$ and $\mathcal{C}(S_1)(\omega) = \sum_f \delta^{N(f_1)}_{c(f_1)}(\omega) = \sum_f N(f_1) \cdot \overline{\omega}(c(f_1))$. Thus,

$$\partial_{f_1^i} \mathcal{E}\, \eta = 2\partial_{f_1^i} N(f_1)\, \eta \cdot \overline{\omega}(c(f_1)) + N(f_1) \cdot d\overline{\omega}(c(f_1)) \partial_{f_1^i} c(f_1)\, \eta,$$

$$= (\eta \times e_1^i) \cdot \overline{\omega}(c(f_1)) + \frac{2}{3} N(f_1) \cdot d\overline{\omega}(c(f_1))\, \eta,$$

so that $\nabla_{f_1^i} \mathcal{E} = (e_1^i \times \overline{\omega}(c(f_1))) + \frac{2}{3} d\overline{\omega}(c(f_1))^* N(f_1)$. It is left to compute $d_{x_t^i} \phi_{t1}$. It follows from properties of the differential that $\frac{d}{dt}(d_{x_t^i} \phi_{t1}) = -d_{x_t^i} \phi_{t1} d_{x_t^i} v_t$ (see [10]). Therefore we have the ordinary differential equation

$$\frac{d}{dt} \nabla_{x_t^i} \mathcal{E} = -(d_{x_t^i} v_t)^* \nabla_{x_t^i} \mathcal{E}, \tag{8}$$

which can be solved by integrating backward from time $t = 1$, since we can compute $d_{x_t^i} v_t$ using (7). Finally, we obtain $\nabla_{x_1^i} \mathcal{E}$ by summing $\nabla_{f_1^i} \mathcal{E}$ over all faces which share x_1^i as a vertex.

Gradient of J. By a direct computation, the gradient of the regularization term, $\int_0^1 |v_t|^2_V$, is simply $2v_t$ so that the gradient of the functional J becomes

$$\nabla J_t(x) = 2 \sum_j k_V(x_t^j, x)(d_{x_t^j} \phi_{t1}^* \nabla_{x_t^j} \mathcal{E} + \alpha_t^j) \tag{9}$$

3.4 Description of the Algorithm

On the basis of remarks made in 3.3, we compute the functional and gradient as functions of the momentum variables α_t^j. The trajectories $x_t^j = \phi_t(x^j)$ being computed by solving the flow equation, written $\partial_t x_t^j = \sum_k k_V(x_t^k, x_t^j) \alpha_t^k$. Therefore the dimension of the parameter space is $3 * nt * nf$ where nt is the number of time steps and nf the number of faces of S. Equipped with equations (8) and (9), we implement a simple steepest descent algorithm.

4 Experiments

4.1 Experiments with Faces Dataset

In this experiment we used 10 segmented surfaces from the USF HumanID database [20] together with manually selected landmarks. The landmarks are used only for validation purposes. The first face was chosen as the template S to be matched to the

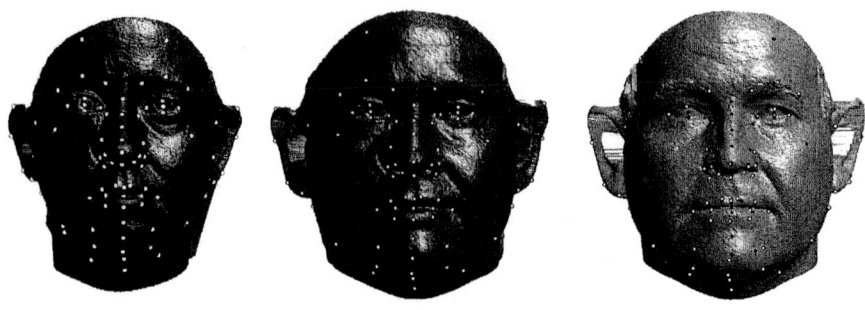

Fig. 1. Left: template, right: target, center: mapped template

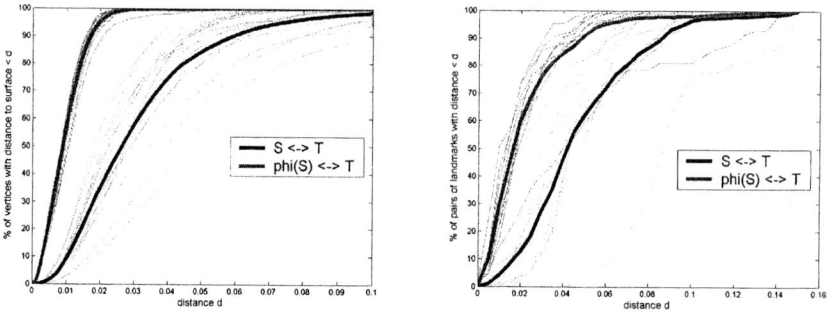

Fig. 2. Face experiments: distance graphs for vertices (left) and landmarks (right). Mean distance is given by the bold curves

other 9 surfaces. For each experiment we downsampled the original surfaces from 60 thousands triangles to 5 thousands triangles and we computed the optimal deformation between the downsampled meshes. Figure 1-left shows the image of the *original* template surface with its landmarks overlayed. Figure 1-right shows a target surface with its landmarks as well as the landmarks of the mapped surface. The mapped template is shown in the center panel. Figure 2-left shows distance error graphs, before and after the matching process (i.e. between S and T and between $\phi(S)$ and T). The left graph plots the percentage of vertices whose distance to the other surface is less than d, as a function of distance d. On the right we plot the distance graphs for the sets of landmarks, i.e. the percentage of landmarks on target T such that the distance to their corresponding landmarks on S (resp. $\phi(S)$) is less than d. Note that the matching is visually satisfying, which is confirmed by the surface distance graph. However, success in matching some of the landmarks such as those along the chin, neck and jaw was not achieved. In fact, this may reflect the somewhat unreliable choice of these landmark points, which do not necessarily correspond to clearly defined features that can be reliably identified.

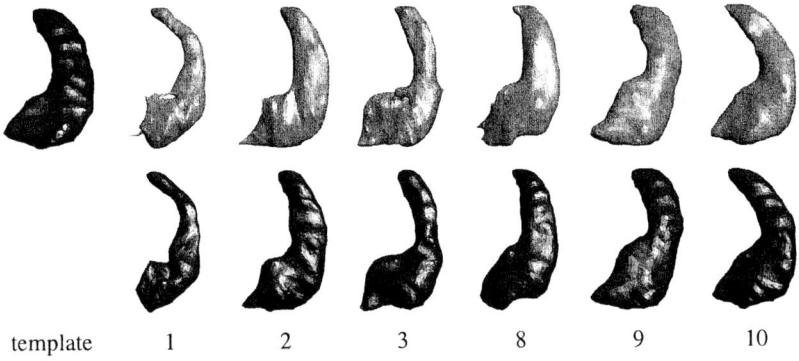

Fig. 3. up: 7 left hippocampi segmented surfaces (1,2 and 3 are of Alzheimer type). bottom: deformations of template through the action of the optimal diffeomorphisms.

4.2 Experiments on Hippocampus Data

Next we applied the matching algorithm to 15 left hippocampi segmented surfaces (see [21] for the method used); the first 7 belong to patients with Alzheimer disease and the others belong to normal subjects. In this experiment, the surfaces were down-sampled to 500 triangles.

Figure 3 displays the deformations of the template surface from the matching process. Figure 4 shows the distance graph for this set of experiments. Note that for almost all vertices the distance is lower than 2mm. Also notice the small variance for these experiments.

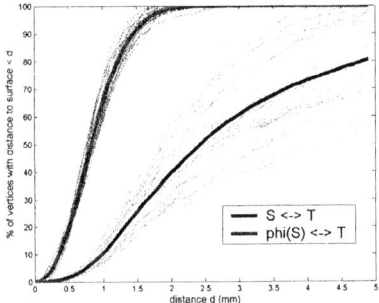

Fig. 4. Distance graph for the hippocampi experiments

4.3 Experiments on Planum Temporale Segmented Surfaces

As a final experiment, we applied the surface matching algorithm to segmentations of left and right planum temporales (PT) from 17 different subjects with 8 having auditory disorders. There is a high variability in sizes and shapes for this part of the brain, even between normal subjects, and also between left and right PTs of the same subject.

We chose to run two types of experiments on this set of data. In the first experiment we fixed one PT surface as the template and then registered it to the other 16 PTs with our current matching algorithm. This was done for both left and right sets of data. Bilateral PT asymmetry studies are an active area of research, so in the second experiment we mapped each PT to its symmetric pair of the same subject. I.e. for each left PT we used its corresponding right PT as the template, and conversely for each right PT we used its corresponding left PT as the template. Figure 5 shows the distance graphs obtained for the left PT data of the first experiment, and for the left to right symmetry matchings.

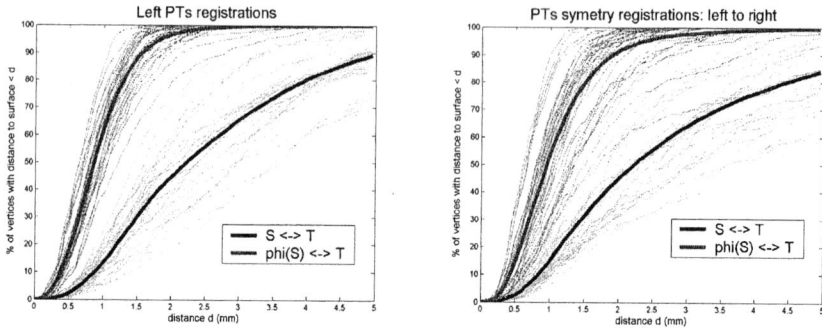

Fig. 5. Distance graphs for the planum temporale experiments

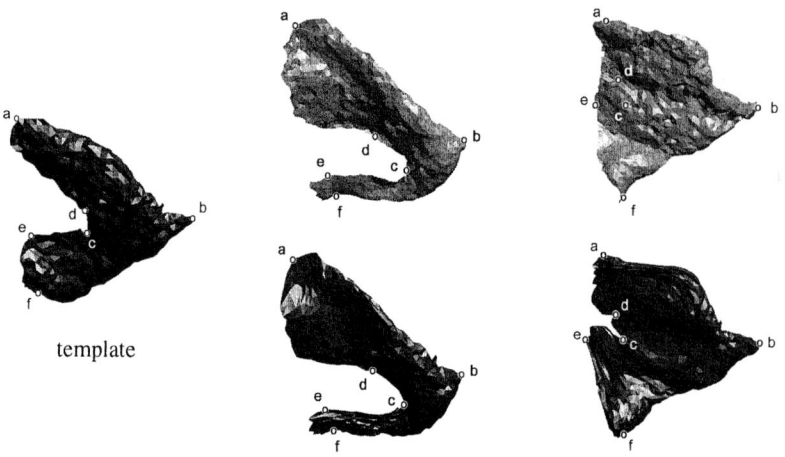

Fig. 6. Planum temporale experiments: correspondences of landmarks selected on template

The mean performance for this data was quite good, and similar to the performance for the hypocampus. Note, however the high variance of the distance measures in the graphs. This may be explained by the fact that the boundaries of the mapped template and target need not match if the geometries near the boundary are quite different from one another. For example, in Figure 6 we show a template on the left and two targets in the top row. In the bottom row are the mapped templates corresponding to the target of the same column. Overlayed on the template are manually defined landmarks which are also flowed under the mapping and overlayed on the mapped template. The landmarks shown on the target were estimated from the mapped template by choosing the closest point on the target for each landmark on the mapped template. In the first case (left) the algorithm gives correspondences which are consistent with what one may select by hand, whereas in the second case it gives correspondences for c and d landmarks which are not on the boundary. Indeed here there are no obvious corresponding landmarks on the target since its shape is globally different from template.

5 Conclusion

We have presented a novel matching criterion for surfaces based on a sound theoretical framework. We integrated this criterion into a large deformation based variational problem, derived a discrete version and an algorithm for implementing its optimization via gradient descent. Finally we demonstrated its performance on different types of data. The main contribution was in recognizing currents as an appropriate mathematical modeling object for surfaces. Given the recent active developments in exterior calculus [22] and current based approaches to curvature estimation [23], we expect the representations to become more sophisticated (perhaps incorporating second order geometric information), and that discretization will continue to get better.

A promising and exciting immediate application of the diffeomorphic matching in this paper is in statistical inference of shape via momentum representation of flow, as described in [18]. It has been shown in [17] that the image of the template S under the flow ϕ_t is completely determined by the momentum (α^i) at time $t = 0$. Hence, the momenta encode the non-linear transformation from one structure into another, and furthermore, they live in a linear space which lends itself to linear statistical analysis.

Acknowledgements

Hippocampus surfaces were provided by M. Chupin, Cognitive Neuroscience and Brain Imaging Laboratory, CNRS, Paris and B. Dubois, Neurology Unit, Hopital de La Salpetriere, Paris. This research was partially supported by NIH grants 5R01MH064838-02, 5P41RR015241-04 and 2P01AG003991-21.

References

1. D'Arcy W. Thompson. *On Growth and Forms*. Cambridge University Press, Cambridge, England, 1917.
2. L Bookstein, F. *Morphometric tools for landmark data; geometry and biology*. Cambridge University press, 1991.
3. C. Davatzikos. Spatial transformation and registration of brain images using elastically deformable models. *Comp. Vision and Image Understanding*, 66(2):207–222, May 1997.
4. S. C. Joshi and M. I. Miller. Landmark matching via large deformation diffeomorphisms. *IEEE Trans. Image Processing*, 9(8):1357–1370, 2000.
5. V. Camion and L. Younes. Geodesic interpolating splines. *EMMCVPR*, pages 513–527, 2001.
6. J. Glaunès, M. Vaillant, and M. I. Miller. Landmark matching via large deformation diffeomorphisms on the sphere. *Journal of Mathematical Imaging and Vision, MIA 2002 special issue*, 20, 2004.
7. H. Chui and A. Rangarajan. A new point matching algorithm for non-rigid registration. *Computer Vision and Image Understanding*, 89:114–141, 2003.
8. Yongmei Wang, Bradley S. Peterson, and Lawrence H. Staib. 3d brain surface matching based on geodesics and local geometry. *Computer Vision and Image Understanding*, 89:252–271, 2003.

9. R. H. Davies, T. F. Cootes, and C. J. Taylor. 3d statistical shape models using direct optimisation of description length. In *ECCV*, 2002.
10. J. Glaunès, A. Trouvé, and L. Younes. Diffeomorphic matching of distributions: A new approach for unlabelled point-sets and sub-manifolds matching. In *CVPR*, pages 712–718. IEEE Computer Society, 2004.
11. G. deRham. Variétés différentiables, formes, courants, formes harmoniques. *Act. Sci. Indust.*, 1222, 1955.
12. F. Morgan. *Geometric measure theory, 2nd ed.* Acad. Press, INC., 1995.
13. M.P. do Carmo. *Differential Forms and Applications.* Springer-Verlag, 1994.
14. G. Wahba. *Spline Models for Observational Data.* CBMS-NSF Regional conference series. SIAM, 1990.
15. A. Trouvé. An infinite dimensional group approach for physics based models. Technical report (electronically available at http://www.cis.jhu.edu), 1995.
16. P. Dupuis, U. Grenander, and M. I. Miller. Variational problems on flows of diffeomorphisms for image matching. *Quaterly of Applied Math.*, 56:587–600, 1998.
17. M. I. Miller, A. Trouvé, and L. Younes. Geodesic shooting in computational anatomy. Technical report, Center for Imaging Science, Johns Hopkins University, 2003.
18. M. Vaillant, M. I. Miller, L. Younes, and A. Trouvé. Statistics on diffeomorphisms via tangent space representations. *NeuroImage*, 23:161–169, 2004.
19. M. I. Miller, A. Trouvé, and L. Younes. On the metrics and Euler-Lagrange equations of computational anatomy. *Annual Review of Biomedical Engineering*, 4:375–405, 2002.
20. USF HumanID 3D faces database, courtesy of Professor Sudeep Sarkar, University of South Florida, Tampa FL. Http://marthon.csee.usf.edu/HumanID/.
21. M. Chupin, D. Hasboun, S.Baillet, S. Kinkingnhun, B.Dubois, and L. Garnero. Competitive segmentation of the hippocampus and the volumetry in alzheimer's disease. In *10th Annual Meeting of the Organization for Human Brain Mapping*, June 13-17,2004.
22. A.N. Hirani. *Discrete exterior calculus.* PhD thesis, California Institute of Technology, 2003.
23. David Cohen-Steiner and Jean-Marie Morvan. Restricted delaunay triangulations and normal cycle. In *SCG '03: Proceedings of the nineteenth annual symposium on Computational geometry*, pages 312–321. ACM Press, 2003.

A Genetic Algorithm for the Topology Correction of Cortical Surfaces

Florent Ségonne[1,2], Eric Grimson[1], and Bruce Fischl[1,2]

[1]MIT C.S.A.I.L.
[2]Athinoula A. Martinos Center - MGH/NMR Center

Abstract. We propose a technique to accurately correct the spherical topology of cortical surfaces. We construct a mapping from the original surface onto the sphere to detect topological defects as minimal non-homeomorphic regions. A genetic algorithm corrects each defect by finding the maximum-a-posteriori retessellation in a Bayesian framework. During the genetic search, incorrect vertices are iteratively identified and eliminated, while the optimal retessellation is constructed. Applied to synthetic and real data, our method generates optimal topological corrections with only a few iterations.

1 Introduction

The human cerebral cortex is a highly folded ribbon of gray matter that lies inside the cerebrospinal fluid and outside the white matter of the brain. Locally, its intrinsic "unfolded" structure is that of a two-dimensional (2-D) sheet, which is several millimeter thick. The analysis of cortical data is greatly facilitated by the use of accurate 2-D models of the cortical sheet [1, 5], which alleviates most drawbacks of the three-dimensional embedding space (such as the underestimation of true cortical distances or the overestimation of cortical thicknesses). In the absence of pathology, each cortical hemisphere is a simply-connected 2-D sheet of neurons that carries the simple topology of a sphere. There has been extensive research dedicated to the extraction of accurate and topologically-correct models of the brain surface that allows for the establishment of a global 2-D coordinate system onto the cortical brain surface. However, because of its highly convoluted nature that results in most of its surface being buried within folds, noise, imaging artifacts, partial voluming effects and intensity inhomogeneities, the automatic extraction of accurate and topologically correct cortical surfaces is still a challenging problem.

Methods for producing topologically correct cortical models can be divided into two categories. Several approaches directly incorporate topological constraints into the segmentation process. A model, carrying the desired topology, is iteratively deformed onto the cortical surface while preserving its topology. To this end, active contours [3, 4, 2, 9, 19] and digital models [12, 15] have shown to be extremely useful. Unfortunately, the energy functionals driving the deformation are highly non-convex and the achievement of the desired final surface most often requires an initialization of the model that is close to its final configuration. In addition, local topological constraints can easily lead to large geometric inaccuracies in the final cortical representation, which are difficult to correct.

Recently, new approaches have been developed to retrospectively correct the topology of an already segmented image. These techniques, which do not enforce any topological constraints into the segmentation process, can focus on more accurate models. Many segmentation techniques, using local intensity, prior probabilities, and/or geometric information without regard to topology, will be able to generate accurate cortical surfaces, with few topological inconsistencies.

Most methods assume that the topological defects in the segmentation are located at the thinnest parts of the volume and aim at correcting the topology by minimally modifying the volume or tessellation [17, 8, 18]. While these methods can be effective, most of them do not use any geometric or statistical information. Although they will often lead to accurate results, due to the accuracy of initial segmentations, topological corrections may not be optimal: additional information, such as the expected local curvature or the local intensity distribution, may lead to different corrections, i.e. hopefully comparable to the ones a trained operator would make.

Only a few techniques have been proposed to integrate additional information into the topology correction process. Using a digital framework, Kriegeskorte and Goeble [11] developed a technique that corrects each topological defect, located at the thinnest parts of the volume, by maximizing an empirical fitness function. More recently, another method to correct the topology of sub-cortical structures has been proposed but has not yet been applied to the reconstruction of cortical surfaces [16]. Unfortunately, digital approaches fail to integrate geometric information into the topology correction process.

In previous work, Fischl et al. [7] proposed an automated procedure to locate topological defects by homeomorphically mapping the initial triangulation onto a sphere. Topological defects are identified as regions in which the homeomorphic mapping is broken and a greedy algorithm is used to retessellate incorrect patches, constraining the topology on the sphere S while preserving geometric accuracy by a maximum likelihood optimization. In this approach, all possible edges in a defective region are ordered using some measure, then each edge is sequentially added to the existing tessellation if and only if it does not intersect any of the existing or previously added edges.

Although this approach can result in reasonable surfaces in many cases, it is worth noting that the information necessary to evaluate the "goodness" of an edge does not exist in isolation, but only as a function of the tessellation of which the edge is a part. This is a critical point, as it implies that a greedy algorithm cannot in general achieve geometrically accurate surfaces, as the necessary information does not exist at the time that the edge ordering is constructed. Another subtle point to be noted is that every vertex in the original defect, even those present due to segmentation inaccuracies, will be present in the final retessellation, resulting in extremely jagged patches that only a strong smoothing could correct. As a consequence, the final configuration will approximately correspond to an average of all vertex positions in the original configuration. Finally, we note that, even though the final intrinsic topology will be the correct one (the one of a sphere, corresponding to an Euler number $\mathcal{X} = 2$ [1]), the proposed method does not guarantee that the final surface will not self-intersect.

In this paper, we propose a technique that directly extends the approach taken by Fischl et al. in [7], addressing most of its limitations. We focus on the retessellation problem and introduce a genetic algorithm to explore the space of possible surface retessellations and to select an optimal configuration. During the search, incorrect vertices are iteratively identified and eliminated from the tessellation.

2 Methods

In order to extend the greedy retessellation developed in [7], we propose to take a somewhat different approach, and evaluate the goodness of fit of the entire retessellation, not of individual edges.

Our method proceeds as follow:

1) Generate a mapping from the original cortical surface onto the sphere that is maximally homeomorphic. Each topological defect is identified as a set of overlapping triangles.
2) Discard the tessellation in each defect and generate an optimal retessellation using a genetic algorithm to search the space of potential retessellations.

2.1 Identification of Topological Defects

The first step is identical to the approach developed by Fischl et al. in [7]. Briefly, the identification of topological defects begins with the inflation and projection of the cortical surface $\mathcal{C}$ onto a sphere $\mathcal{S}$. Next, we generate a maximally homeomorphic mapping $\mathcal{M} : \mathcal{C} \to \mathcal{S}$ by minimizing an energy functional that directly penalizes regions in which the determinant of the Jacobian matrix of $\mathcal{M}$ becomes zero or negative (non-homeomorphic regions). More specifically, noting that the Jacobian yields a measure of the deformation of an oriented area element under $\mathcal{M}$, the energy functional $E_\mathcal{M}$ limits the penalization of compression primarily to negative semi-definite regions. If the initial area on the folded surface of the ith face is A_i^0, and the area on the spherical surface $\mathcal{S}$ at time t of the numerical integration is A_i^t, then the energy functional is given by:

$$E_\mathcal{M} = \sum_{i=0}^{F} \log(\frac{1+e^{kR_i}}{k}) - R_i \ , \ R_i = \frac{A_i^t}{A_i^0}.$$

---

[1] The Euler number of a surface is a topological invariant. For a tessellation, it can be easily computed as: $\mathcal{X} = \#vertices - \#edges + \#faces$. The Euler number of a sphere is $\mathcal{X} = 2$.

The resulting mapping - from the initial tessellation to the sphere - is maximally homeomorphic. Multivalued regions, containing overlapping triangles, constitute topological defects where the homeomorphic mapping is broken. $\mathcal{M}$ associates at each vertex v of the initial cortical surface $\mathcal{C}$ a vertex $v_\mathcal{S} = \mathcal{M}(v)$ on the sphere $\mathcal{S}$. Vertices with spherical coordinates that intersect a set of overlapping triangles are marked as defective and topological defects are identified as connected sets of defective vertices (we refer to [7] for more details).

2.2 Definition of the Retessellation Problem

Once a topological defect has been identified, its tessellation is discarded. The retessellation problem can then be stated as follows.

> *Given a set of defective vertices, each of which has been assigned a spherical location by the quasi-homeomorphic mapping $\mathcal{M}$, find the vertices that should be kept in the defect and the set of edges connecting them, so that an energy functional, measuring the goodness of the retessellation, is maximized.*

Topological inconsistencies, which are resulting from mislabeled voxels in the segmentation process, generate tessellations that include incorrect vertices. These vertices should be identified and discarded from the final solution. A potential topological correction of the defect corresponds to the generation of a new tessellation such that no edge intersection occurs in the spherical surface. Many such tessellations exist [2], and one would like to select an optimal solution that maximizes the goodness of fit of the retessellation.

We evaluate the fitness of a corrected region with the maximum-a-posteriori estimate of the retessellation, given geometric information about the observed surface, and the underlying MRI values. The numerical technique we propose to explore in the maximization of the fitness function is a genetic algorithm or GA (for a good introduction see [14]). The GA is an appropriate choice for this type of problem as the space to be searched is potentially quite large (the defects can contain upwards of 300,000 candidate edges), and there is no easy way to compute gradient information. More importantly, we define a set of genetic operations used to propagate information from one generation to the next that correspond to 'relevant' surface operations.

2.3 A Genetic Algorithm for the Surface Retessellation

Genetic Algorithms were developed by John Holland in the 1960s as a means of importing the mechanisms of natural adaptation into computer algorithms and numerical optimization [10]. In genetic algorithms, a candidate solution to a problem is typically called a chromosome, and the evolutionary viability of each chromosome is given by a fitness function. Typically, genetic algorithms are defined by different operators: Selection, Crossover and Mutation.

---

[2] For a defect composed of n vertices, the number of potential edges is $N = n(n-1)/2$, leading to a space of size $O(2^N)$.

In the next paragraphs, we explain the role of these operators in detail and specify how their definition is meaningfully tailored to the current problem.

A - Representation and Retessellation: perhaps the most important decision in the construction of a GA is the choice of representation for the underlying problem. Here we have a number of constraints that must be satisfied that lead to the representation we use. These essentially amount to the requirement that every potential edge be represented exactly once in an ordering for the retessellation. This guarantees that the retessellation will result in the proper topology [7]. Thus the representation we choose is an edge ordering, represented by a permutation of N integers. The retessellation procedure then simply involves adding edges in the order specified by the permutation.

Such a procedure will generate retessellated patches that include all vertices present in the defect, resulting in irregular jagged surfaces. In order to alleviate this problem, we directly encode the vertex selection into the representation. Given an edge ordering, we construct the corresponding tessellation and assign to each vertex an arrival number based on the order in which they were added. Next, we discard all the vertices that were added after all of its neighbors, i.e. vertices with lower arrival numbers. This way, edges added first in the retessellation will force their bordering vertices to be included in the final retessellation. The edges added last, which most often generate the surface irregularities, will consequently be discarded.

B - Selection of the Initial Population: the selection of the initial population is particularly significant for the considered problem. The space to be searched is potentially quite large and the selection of a "good" initial population can drastically improve convergence of the algorithm. Topological defects are constituted of sets of overlapping triangles. The intersecting edges on the sphere $\mathcal{S}$ correspond to different topological paths in the original cortical surface $\mathcal{C}$. In order to generate an initial population with a large variance, i.e. composed of individuals with large *shape* differences, we first group the non-overlapping edges into different clusters. Using the spherical quasi-homeomorphic mapping M, intersecting edges are iteratively segmented into different clusters. Next, these clusters are used to select the initial population of chromosomes. We say that a chromosome is generated from a cluster C_i, if the first edges (in the ordering) constituting this chromosome comes from C_i. Consequently, chromosomes generated from different clusters will have different shapes, hopefully leading to an initial population with a large variance. Figure 1 provides a few examples of initially selected chromosomes in the case of a simple topological defect.

C - Mutation and Crossover: the two most important operations used in GAs are mutation and crossover. Mutation involves the random modification of a part of the code of an "individual" in the population and crossover the exchange of a part of the code of an "individual" with another one in the population. We define these operations in order to accommodate the nature of the current problem. Intersecting edges represent choice between different surface configurations. In the following section, we note I_i the set of edges intersecting the edge e_i: $I_i =$

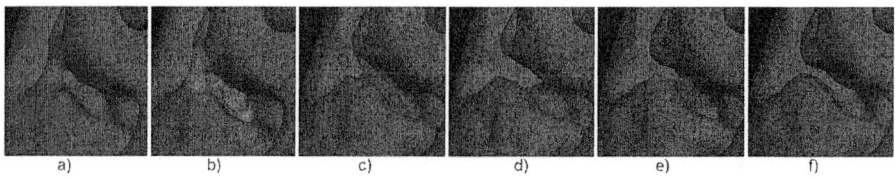

Fig. 1. a) Example of a topological defect containing 2 handles and constituted of 183 defective vertices. b) Result of the clustering of the non-intersecting edges into 5 segments. c-e) These candidate retessellations represent different configurations of the initial population generated using the edge clustering. f) The optimal solution generated by our genetic approach in 15 generations after 4 mutations and 8 crossovers

$\{e_j | \text{int}(e_i, e_j) = 1\}$, where $\text{int}(e_i, e_j)$ is the intersection operator, and returns 1 if edge e_i intersects edge e_j, and 0 otherwise.

For mutation, we perform the following operation for each possible edge in the tessellation:

1) Draw a random number r from $U_\mathbb{R}(0,1)$, the uniform distribution on the real numbers between 0 and 1.
2) If $r > p_{mut}$ then continue with the next edge.
3) Draw a random number k from $U_\mathbb{N}(1, \#I_i)$, the uniform distribution on the natural numbers between 1 and $\#I_i$.
4) Exchange the positions of e_i and e_j, where e_j is the kth entry in the set I_i.

This procedure will allow the selective exploration of the different retessellations represented by different members of I_i, thus reducing the size of the effective search space.

The crossover operator we define is the random combination of permutations. Some care must be taken here to insure that every edge is represented exactly one time. Towards that end, the crossover operator will add a random number of edges from each parent retessellation, only if that edge has not been added. The crossover operator will randomly select one of the permutations to draw from first, then copy a random number of edges from it to the "offspring" retessellation. For each edge, we draw a random number r from $U_\mathbb{R}(0,1)$, and stop copying edges if $r < 1/2$. Next, a random number of edges will be copied from the second parent, if they are not already represented in the offspring. This procedure will continue until every edge is represented.

It is important to note that the previously defined genetic operations carry meaningful geometric operations. Mutation, which randomly swaps the ordering of intersecting edges, corresponds to local jumps from one configuration to another one. The crossover operation naturally combines different parts of the code from the two candidate tessellations, generating a configuration that often expresses distinct local surface properties of both parents. In addition, since the edge ordering naturally encodes which vertices are discarded (the vertices included last being discarded), the crossover operation, which iteratively combines two edge orderings, most often generates offspring chromosomes that preserve the best geometric characteristics of the parents (most likely, the same vertices will be discarded).

D - Fitness and Likelihood Functions: we use some prior knowledge about the cortex to define the fitness function. A cortical surface is a smooth manifold $\mathcal{C}$ that partitions the embedding space into an inside part, composed of white matter, and an outside part, composed of gray matter. We characterize the goodness of a retessellation by measuring two of its properties:

(1) The smoothness of the resulting surface,
(2) the MRI values I inside and outside the surface.

Formally, the posterior probability of the ith retessellation T_i is given by:

$$p(T_i|\mathcal{C}, I) \propto p(I|\mathcal{C}, T_i) p(T_i|\mathcal{C}).$$

The likelihood term $p(I|\mathcal{C}, T_i)$ encodes information about the MRI intensities inside and outside the surface. Each retessellated patch, being topologically correct, separates the underlying MRI volume into two distinct components [3], an inside part $\mathcal{C}^-$ and an outside part $\mathcal{C}^+$. An acceptable candidate solution should generates a space partition with most of its inside and outside voxels corresponding to white and gray matter voxels respectively. In order to estimate the likelihood $p(I|\mathcal{C}, T_i)$, we assume that the noise is spatially independent. This probability can be rewritten:

$$p(I|\mathcal{C}, T_i) = \underbrace{\prod_{x \in \mathcal{C}^-} p_w(I(x)|\mathcal{C}, T_i) \prod_{x \in \mathcal{C}^+} p_g(I(x)|\mathcal{C}, T_i)}_{\text{volume-based information}} \underbrace{\prod_{v=1}^{V_i} p(g_i(v), w_i(v)|\mathcal{C}, T_i)}_{\text{surface-based information}},$$

$p_w(I(x)|\mathcal{C}, T_i)$ and $p_g(I(x)|\mathcal{C}, T_i)$ are the likelihood of intensity values at location x in the volume inside and outside the tessellation respectively, $p(g_i(v), w_i(v)|\mathcal{C}, T_i)$ is the joint likelihood of intensity values inside and outside the tessellation at vertex v in tessellation T_i.

Geometric information can be incorporated via $p(T_i|\mathcal{C})$, which represents priors on the possible retessellation. For example, $p(T_i|\mathcal{C})$ could have the form:

$$p(T_i|\mathcal{C}) = \prod_{v=1}^{V_i} p(\kappa_1(v), \kappa_2(v)|\mathcal{C}),$$

where κ_1 and κ_2 are the two principal curvatures of the surface, computed at vertex v.

Given that the vast majority of the surface is in general not defective, we fortunately have ample amounts of data with which to estimate the correct forms

---

[3] We use the angle weighted pseudo-normal algorithm to compute the signed distance of the tessellation. The voxel grid is partitioned into inside negative values and outside positive values

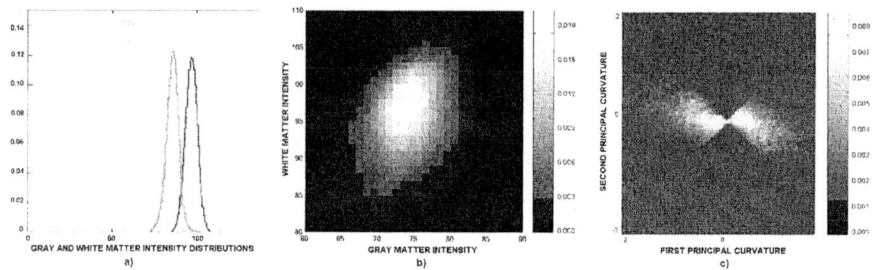

Fig. 2. a) Example of the gray and white matter distributions estimated locally from a given a topological defect. b) Joint distribution of gray and white matter given the surface computed using the non-defective portion of the gray/white boundary representation of a single subject. The gray and white matter intensity are two correlated variables, as indicated by the diagonal structure of the joint distribution. c) Joint distribution of two principal curvatures of the surface

of the distributions $p(T_i|\mathcal{C})$, $p_g(I(x)|\mathcal{C}, T_i)$, $p_w(I(x)|\mathcal{C}, T_i)$ and $p(g_i, w_i|\mathcal{C}, T_i)$. In particular, the single tissue distributions $p_g(I(x)|\mathcal{C}, T_i)$ and $p_w(I(x)|\mathcal{C}, T_i)$ are locally estimated around each topological defect in a region that excludes the defect itself (we exclude all voxels that intersect one of the N potential edges). This makes the resulting procedure completely adaptive and self-contained, in the sense that no assumptions need to be made about the contrast of the underlying MRI image(s), and no training or parametric forms are required for $p(T_i|\mathcal{C})$. An example of the estimation of $p(g_i, w_i|\mathcal{C}, T_i)$ and $p(T_i|\mathcal{C})$ is given in Fig. 2. Image b) shows the joint distribution of gray and white matter given the surface computed using the non-defective portion of the gray/white boundary representation of a single subject. Note the diagonal character of the distribution, indicating that the intensities are mutually dependent - brighter white matter typically means brighter gray matter due to factors such as bias fields induced by RF inhomogeneities and coil sensitivity profiles, as well as intrinsic tissue variability. One possible form of the priors on the tessellation is given in Fig. 2c, which shows the joint distribution of the two principal curvatures κ_1 (green) and κ_2 (red) computed over the non defective portion of a single surface. It is important to note in this context that all these distributions can only be applied after a candidate retessellation has been completed, as the gray/white joint density requires surface normals, gray and white intensity distributions necessitate the underlying MRI volume to be partitioned in two separate components and the principal curvatures require the calculation of the second fundamental form, all of which are properties of the surface, not of individual edges.

E - Iterative Elimination of Vertices: During the genetic search, some vertices will be consistently discarded from the best patches. These vertices, which are the ones that were erroneously kept in the initial cortical tessellation, should be identified and eliminated from the final tessellation. To this end, we introduce in our genetic search, an elimination operator, which selectively eliminates the worst vertices from the defect. The elimination step operates as follow: after every few iterations, we eliminate the vertices that were consistently discarded from the best candidate patches.

The proposed approach is implemented with the following parameters. The initial population size is chosen depending on the number of defective vertices. The retessellation process is quadratic in the number of vertices contained within the convex hull of each defect. Typical defect contains on the order of 100 vertices for a population size of 20 candidate retessellations. At each step of the genetic search, a new population is generated from selected chromosomes based on their fitness. Given a population of individuals, the top one third is selected to form the elite group. These chromosomes are kept for the next generations. The worst individuals, corresponding to the bottom one third, are replaced with mutated copies of the best. Finally, the remaining ones are generated from crossover operations from parents iteratively chosen from the elite population. The mutation rate p_{mut} is experimentally chosen to be 10%. The algorithm stops when no new best candidate has been found for the past 10 generations. For a typical topological defect of size 100 vertices, the algorithm usually converges in less than 50 generations, which corresponds to a computational time of approximately 10 minutes on a 1-G-Hz Pentium IV. An optimal configuration is usually the result of approximately 30 genetic operations, 80% of which are crossovers and 20% mutations. The elimination operator is applied every 5 generations. The number of discarded vertices depends on the topological defect. In some cases, more than 40% will be eliminated.

3 Results and Discussion

Before reporting results of the proposed approach on synthetic and real datasets, we measure the goodness of our method relatively to a random search algorithm. This is to verify that our approach actually improves the speed of convergence and that the genetic operations allow the generation of superior candidate retessellations.

Genetic versus Random Search: we compared our approach with a random search algorithm, in which random permutations of the edge ordering were iteratively generated. The graphs in Fig. 3 illustrate the strength of our approach on a real data example. The topological defect is shown in Fig. 1a. For each method, the first candidate tessellation corresponded to the solution generated by the greedy approach proposed in [7] with its vertices added last being discarded (see sect 2.3.A). Compared to a random search, the genetic search converges much faster (at least, second order magnitude). The genetic algorithm boosts the overall fitness of the population by keeping the best representations at each generation and producing new candidates using the elite population. In a few generations composed of a small number of chromosomes (20 chromosomes per generation in this example), the genetic search is able to produce new optimal retessellations (see Fig. 1f).

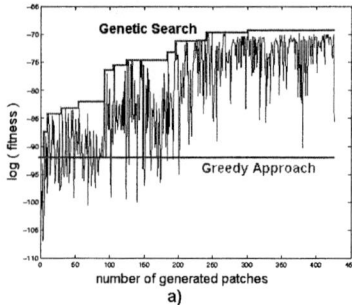 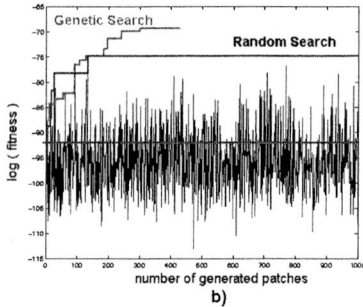

Fig. 3. a) Evolution of the log of the fitness function during the genetic search. b) Evolution of the log fitness function during a random search. Note how the genetic search iteratively improves the average fitness of each generated chromosome, which, as a consequence, will be able to generate new optimal chromosomes. On the other hand, random retessellation rarely generates new optimal patches. In this defect, which was constituted of 183 vertices, even after 50000 random draw, the fitness function of the best randomly generated chromosome was still 5 order of magnitude below the best GA chromosome (generated as the 300th offspring during the 15th generation)

Application to Synthetic Data and Real Data: in order to validate the proposed method, we first generated surfaces containing simple topological defects (handles, holes). These data were used to explore the performance of the algorithm relatively to typical topological defects. The underlying MRI volumes were generated by adding white noise to the expected tissue intensities : gray and white intensity values were drawn from Gaussian distributions $G(\mu_g = 90, \sigma_g = 5.0)$ and $G(\mu_w = 110, \sigma_w = 5.0)$ respectively. Figure 4, top row, illustrates the behavior of the algorithm relatively to different MRI volumes, when the same topological defect has to be corrected (left: a simple handle). We note that traditional active contour models could not have generated the same results due to the amount of noise in the images and the presence of large local minima in the energy functional.

We have applied our proposed approach on 35 real images. The dataset was composed of MRI volumes of different qualities, from different populations. Results were evaluated by an expert to assess the correctness of the final corrections. The algorithm was able to generate correct solutions that the initial greedy approach [7] failed to produce. Methods that do not integrate statistical and geometric information will often fail to produce solutions comparable to the ones a trained operator would make. This is illustrated in Fig. 4, bottom, where valid solutions do not always correspond to minimal corrections (i.e. cutting the handle in the two examples of Fig. 4). Only general approaches that integrate additional information can lead to correct solutions. An average cortical surface contains on the order of 50 topological defects, most of which are relatively small. A full brain is corrected in approximately 2 hours on a 1GHz PII machine. The average Hausdorff distance computed for each defect in between automatically and manually corrected surfaces is less than $0.2mm$.

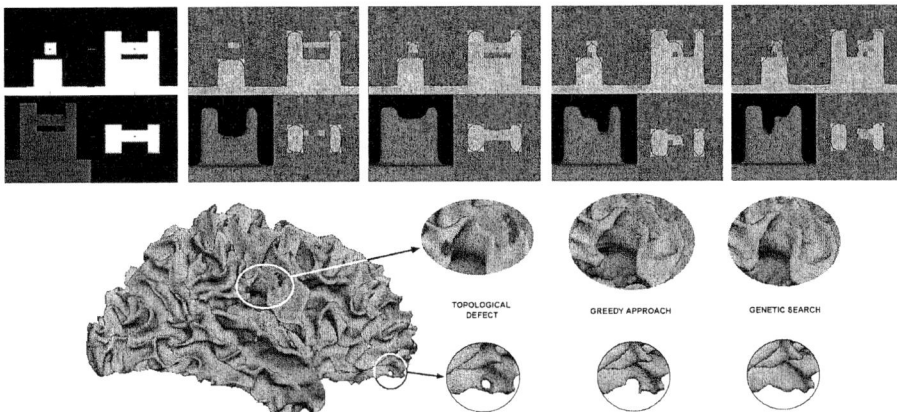

Fig. 4. Top row) Results of our proposed approach on different phantom examples. The same topological defect (left: a small handle constituted of about 100 vertices) is corrected using different underlying MRI volumes. In each case, our approach generated an optimal configuration corresponding to the expected solution. Bottom row) Topology correction of a cortical representation. The initial surface was constituted of 30 defects (Euler number $\mathcal{X} = -58$). Compared to the greedy approach of Fischl et al. [7], which failed to find the correct solutions in many defects, our approach was able to generate valid solutions. This is illustrated on two examples, in which valid topological solutions do not correspond to minimal corrections

We note that the proposed method does not directly prevent the final surface from self-intersecting. Self-intersecting configurations typically have low fitness values and are naturally discarded during the genetic search. The self-intersecting constraint could be directly integrated into the retessellation process, but would drastically slow down the proposed approach. In our experience, final corrected representations rarely intersect (less than one in ten thousand faces, which corresponds to approximately 1 defect per brain). In order to ensure that the solution generates a valid manifold, we retrospectively check that the final retessellation does not self-intersect. In the case of self-intersection, we re-apply the genetic algorithm with the additional constraint of only generating valid candidate patches. Self-intersecting patches are identified and discarded from the population.

4 Conclusion and Future Work

We have proposed an automated method to accurately correct the topology of cortical representations. Our approach integrates statistical and geometric information to select the optimal correction for each defect. In particular, we have developed a genetic algorithm that is specifically adapted to the retessellation problem. Iterative genetic operations generate candidate tessellations that are selected for reproduction based on their goodness of fit. The fitness of a retessellation is measured by the smoothness of the resulting surface and the local MRI intensity profile inside and outside the surface. The resulting procedure is completely adaptative and self-contained. During the search, defective vertices are identified and discarded while the optimal retessellation is constructed.

Given a quasi-homeomorphic mapping from the initial cortical surface onto the sphere, our method will be able to generate optimal solutions. For each defect, the space to be searched (i.e. the edge ordering) is dependent on the spherical location of the defective vertices. Some configurations of the quasi-homeomorphic mapping could lead to optimal but incorrect retessellations. In future work, we plan to address this limitation by directly integrating the generation of the homeomorphic mapping into the correction process.

References

1. A. M. Dale and M. Sereno, "Improved localization of cortical activity by combining EEG and MEG with MRI cortical surface reconstruction: A linear approach," J. Cogn. Neurosci., vol. 5, no.2, pp.162-176, 1993.
2. A. M. Dale, B. Fischl, and M. I. Sereno, "Cortical surface-based analysis I: Segmentation and surface reconstruction," NeuroImage, vol.9, pp. 179-294, 1999.
3. C. Davatzikos, and R.N. Bryan, "Using a Deformable Surface Model to Obtain a Shape Representation of the Cortex". IEEE T.M.I., 1996. 15: p. 785-795.
4. D. MacDonald, N. Kabani, D. Avis, and A. C. Evens, "Automated 3D extraction of inner and outer surfaces of cerebral cortex from MRI," NeuroImage, vol.12, pp. 340-356, 2000.
5. D. C. van Essen, and H. Drury, "Structural and functional analyses of human cerebral cortex using a surface-based atlas," Journal of Neuroscience, vol.17, no.18, pp7079-7102, 1997.
6. B. Fischl, and M. I. Sereno, and A. M. Dale, "Cortical surface-based analysis II: Inflation, flattening, and a surface-based coordinate system," NeuroImage, vol.9, pp. 195-207, 1999.
7. B. Fischl, A. Liu, and A. M. Dale, "Automated manifold surgery: Constructing geometrically accurate and topologically correct models of the human cerebral cortex," IEEE T.M.I., vol. 20, pp. 70-80, 2001.
8. X. Han, C. Xu, U. Braga-Neto, and J. L. Prince, "Topology correction in brain cortex segmentation using a multiscale, graph-based approach," IEEE T.M.I., vol. 21(2): 109–121, 2002.
9. X. Han, C. Xu, D. Tosun, and J. L. Prince, "Cortical Surface Reconstruction Using a Topology Preserving Geometric Deformable Model," MMBIA, Kauai, Hawaii, Dec. 2001, pp. 213-220.
10. Holland, J.H., "Adaptation in Natural and Artificial Systems," 1975, Ann Arbor: University of Michigan Press.
11. N. Kriegeskorte and R. Goeble, "An efficient algorithm for topologically segmentation of the cortical sheet in anatomical mr volumes. NeuroImage, vol. 14, pp. 329-346, 2001.
12. J.-F. Mangin, V. Frouin, I. Bloch, J. Regis, and J. Lopez-Krahe, "From 3D magnetic resonance images to structural representations of the cortex topography using topology preserving deformations," Journal of Mathematical Imaging and Vision, vol. 5, pp.297-318, 1995.

13. T. McInerney and D. Terzopoulos, "Deformable models in medical image analysis: A survey," Medical Image Analysis, vol.1, no.2, pp.91-108,1996.
14. M. Mitchell, "An introduction to genetic algorithms," MIT Press.
15. F. Poupon and J.-F. Mangin and D. Hasboun and C. Poupon and I. Magnin and V. Frouin, "Multi-object Deformable Templates Dedicated to the Segmentation of Brain Deep Structures", LNCS 1496, pp. 1134-1143, 1998.
16. F. Ségonne, B. Fischl, and E. Grimson, "Topology correction of Subcortical Structures," MICCAI 2003, LNCS 2879, pp.695-702.
17. D. W. Shattuck and R. Leahy, "Automated Graph-Based Analysis and Correction of Cortical Volume Topology," NeuroImage, vol. 14, pp. 329-346, 2001.
18. I. Guskov and Z. Wood, "Topological noise removal," GI 2001 proceedings, pp. 19-26, 2001.
19. X. Zeng, L. H. Staib, R. T. Schultz, and J. S. Duncan, "Segmentation and measurement of the cortex from 3D MR images using coupled surfaces propagation," IEEE T.M.I., vol. 18, pp. 100-111, 1999.

Simultaneous Segmentation of Multiple Closed Surfaces Using Optimal Graph Searching

Kang Li[1], Steven Millington[2], Xiaodong Wu[3],
Danny Z. Chen[4], and Milan Sonka[3]

[1] Dept. of Electrical and Computer Engineering, Carnegie Mellon University,
5000 Forbes Ave, Pittsburgh, PA 15213, USA
kangl@cmu.edu
[2] Frank Stronach Institute, Infeldgasse 21B/II, A8010 Graz, Austria
steven.millington@tugraz.at
[3] Dept. of Electrical and Computer Engineering, The University of Iowa,
4016 Seamans Center, Iowa City, IA 52242-1595, USA
{xiaodong-wu, milan-sonka}@uiowa.edu
[4] Dept. of Computer Science and Engineering, The University of Notre Dame
Notre Dame, IN 46556, USA
dchen@cse.nd.edu

Abstract. This paper presents a general graph-theoretic technique for simultaneously segmenting multiple closed surfaces in volumetric images, which employs a novel graph-construction scheme based on triangulated surface meshes obtained from a topological presegmentation. The method utilizes an efficient graph-cut algorithm that guarantees global optimality of the solution under given cost functions and geometric constraints. The method's applicability to difficult biomedical image analysis problems was demonstrated in a case study of co-segmenting the bone and cartilage surfaces in 3-D magnetic resonance (MR) images of human ankles. The results of our automated segmentation were validated against manual tracings in 55 randomly selected image slices. Highly accurate segmentation results were obtained, with signed surface positioning errors for the bone and cartilage surfaces being 0.02±0.11mm and 0.17 ± 0.12mm, respectively.

1 Introduction

Optimal segmentation of surfaces representing object boundaries in volumetric datasets is important and challenging for many medical image analysis applications. Recently, we proposed an efficient algorithm for d-D ($d \geq 3$) optimal hyper-surface detection with hard smoothness constraints, making globally optimal surface segmentation in volumetric images practical [1,2]. By modeling the problem with a *geometric graph*, the method transforms the segmentation problem into computing the minimum s-t graph cut that is well-studied in graph theory, and makes the problem solvable in a low-order polynomial time. The solution is guaranteed to be globally optimal in the considered region by theoretical

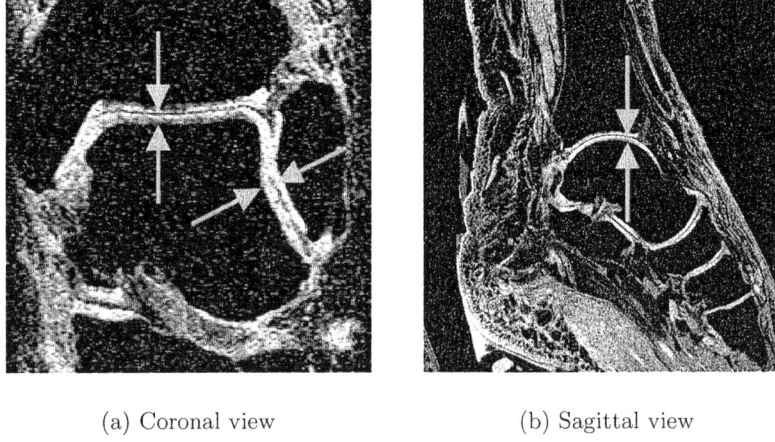

(a) Coronal view (b) Sagittal view

Fig. 1. Two sample slices of a 3-D MR image of human ankle

proofs [1]. We have also developed a multi-surface segmentation algorithm [3]. However, these methods were both limited to segmenting height-field or cylindrical surfaces in regular grids.

In this paper, we present a non-trivial extension of our previous work. We focus on the problem of segmenting *optimal multiple closed* surfaces in 3-D. The new method for multiple surfaces segmentation is motivated by the need to accurately segment cartilage layers in diseased joints. In this application, the articular cartilage and corresponding subchondral bone surfaces can be imaged by 3-D high-resolution MRI (Fig. 1). However, no segmentation method exists that would allow a rapid, accurate, and reproducible segmentation for quantitative evaluation of articular cartilage.

The main contribution of our work is that it extends the optimal graph-searching techniques to closed surfaces, while the backbone of our approach – graph-cuts – is radically different from traditional graph searching. Consequently, many existing problems that were tackled using graph-searching in a slice-by-slice manner can be migrated to our new framework with little or no change to the underlying objective function formulation.

2 Methods

The proposed method allows segmenting multiple inter-related surfaces in volumetric images and facilitates subsequent quantitative analysis. We will utilize the bone–cartilage segmentation task to help make the method description intuitively clear. The general strategy of our method is to achieve the final segmentation in two stages. The initial stage provides approximate segmentation of the three-dimensional object (in our case, of the bone), and the final segmentation is achieved by accurate and simultaneous segmentation of its multiple surfaces of interest. The outputs of the algorithm are triangulated meshes that are ready for visualization and quantitative measurement.

The method consists of the following three main steps:

1. *Bone surface presegmentation.* A level set based algorithm is used. Starting from several seed-spheres, the method uses the image-derived edge and regional information to evolve a smooth surface toward the bone boundary. The presegmented surface serves as an initialization to the subsequent segmentation.
2. *Mesh generation and optimization.* The presegmentation results in an implicit surface that is the zero level set of a 4-D function embedded in a volumetric digital grid. An isosurfacing algorithm (e.g., marching cubes) is used to convert the implicit surface into an explicit triangulated mesh. The mesh is optimized by removing or merging isolated and redundant triangles. The resolution of the mesh can be increased or decreased using progressive level of detail approaches when necessary.
3. *Co-segmentation of the cartilage and bone surfaces.* The mesh generated by the second step is used to initialize a graph in a narrow-band around the presegmented bone surface. A novel multi-surfaces graph search algorithm is used to simultaneously obtain the precise positions of the bone and cartilage surfaces based on two cost functions separately designed for the two surfaces while considering specific geometric constraints.

Since the mesh manipulation step involves largely standard techniques in graphics, only the first and third steps are described in detail.

2.1 Bone Surface Presegmentation

The presegmentation algorithm is based on the *MetaMorphs* deformable shape and texture model presented in [4]. The method provides a unified gradient-descent framework for modeling both the boundary and texture information in an image, and is relatively efficient in computation.

Let Ω denote the image domain, and $\partial\Omega$ be the surface represented by the model, which is the zero level set of a signed distance function ϕ. ϕ is positive in the model interior, denoted Ω^+. Instead of directly evolving the function ϕ, the deformation of the surface is controlled by a set of uniformly-spaced control points artificially embedded in the image domain. The motion of the control points is computed using image-derived information. The deformation at any voxel location can then be derived using the cubic B-spline based Free Form Deformation (FFD). As such, the level set function ϕ can be updated using a geometric transformation of itself at each descent step. The motion of the control points is determined by minimizing the weighted combination of two edge-based cost terms and two region-based cost terms. For more detail of the cost terms and the model evolution, we refer to reader to [4].

Particularly, in [4], the authors suggested a Gaussian kernel-based nonparametric approach for modeling image pixel (voxel) intensity distributions. This approach, however, is computationally expensive in 3-D. Considering our application domain and taking advantage of the physical properties of the MR images, voxel intensities in the bone region are approximated by a Rayleigh distribution:

$$P(I|b) = \frac{Ie^{-I^2/2b^2}}{b^2}, \quad I \geq 0, \; b > 0 \tag{1}$$

with I being the pixel intensity. This distribution has only one free parameter b, which is estimated using the sample mean μ of voxel intensities inside the initializing spheres, as:

$$b = \mu\sqrt{\frac{2}{\pi}} \tag{2}$$

2.2 Simultaneous Segmentation of Cartilage and Bone Surfaces

After the bone surface is presegmented and converted into a triangulated mesh, a novel graph-based algorithm is applied to co-optimize the cartilage and bone surfaces. Note that anatomically, the cartilage only covers certain parts of the bone surface. To simplify the problem, we assume the cartilage extends the full surface area of the bone. However, in some areas the "cartilage" surface merges with the bone, so that the cartilage thickness is effectively zero in those areas.

Preliminaries. A triangulated mesh consists of a set of *vertices* connected by *edges*. We use $\mathcal{M}(\mathcal{V}, \mathcal{E})$ to denote a mesh with vertex set $\mathcal{V}$ and edge set $\mathcal{E}$. Two vertices are said to be *adjacent* if they are connected by an edge. Each vertex has an associated surface *normal*, which is perpendicular to the surface that the mesh represents at the vertex.

A graph $\mathcal{G}(\mathcal{N}, \mathcal{A})$ is a structure that consists of a set of *nodes* $\mathcal{N}$ and a set of *arcs* $\mathcal{A}$. The arc connecting two nodes n_1 and n_2 is denoted by $\langle n_1, n_2 \rangle$. For *undirected* arcs, the notations $\langle n_1, n_2 \rangle$ and $\langle n_2, n_1 \rangle$ are considered equivalent. For a *directed* arc, they are considered distinct. The former one denotes the arc from n_1 to n_2, and the latter one from n_2 to n_1. In addition, a *geometric* graph is a graph whose nodes have certain geometric positions in space.

Graph Construction. Since the bone and cartilage surfaces are to be segmented simultaneously, two spatially-coincident *columns* of equidistant nodes are constructed along the normal at each vertex of the triangular mesh obtained from the presegmentation (Fig. 2). The number of nodes in each column is determined by the required resolution, and the extent of each column depends on the width of the region where the cartilage and bone surfaces are expected – a narrow-band around the presegmented surface. A set of arcs is carefully constructed between the nodes to ensure the geometric constraints, including the *smoothness constraint*, which controls the stiffness of the output surfaces, and the surface *separation constraint*, which defines the relative positioning and the distance range of the two surfaces.

Suppose there are N vertices on the mesh, and let v_i be one of them ($i \in \{0, \ldots, N-1\}$). The two columns of nodes constructed along the normal at v_i are denoted by $\mathcal{K}_0(v_i) \equiv \{n_{0i}^0, \ldots, n_{0i}^{K-1}\}$ and $\mathcal{K}_1(v_i) \equiv \{n_{1i}^0, \ldots, n_{1i}^{K-1}\}$,

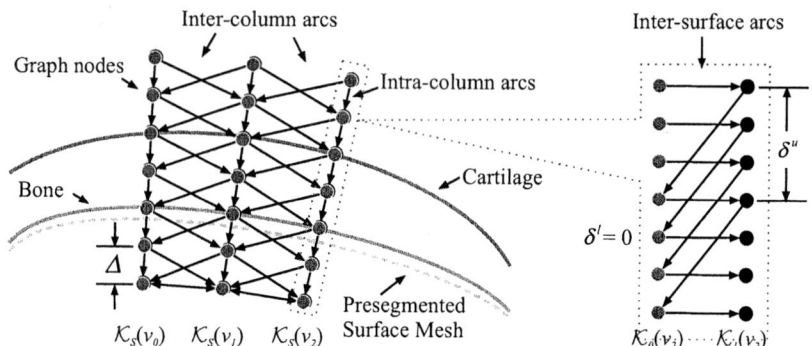

Fig. 2. Graph construction

respectively, where K is the number of nodes in each column. The collection of columns $\bigcup \mathcal{K}_s(v_i)$ with $s = 0, 1$ and $i = 1, \ldots, N-1$ constitutes the node set $\mathcal{N}$.

Next, assuming that each column $\mathcal{K}_0(v_i)$ intersects with the bone surface at exactly one node, denoted n^*_{0i}, and each column $\mathcal{K}_1(v_i)$ intersects with the cartilage surface at exactly one node n^*_{1i}, the collections of nodes $\mathcal{N}^*_0 \equiv \{n^*_{0i} : i = 0, \ldots, N-1\}$ and $\mathcal{N}^*_1 \equiv \{n^*_{1i} : i = 0, \ldots, N-1\}$ will represent discretizations of the bone surface and the cartilage surface, respectively. In this way, the segmentation problem is converted to a graph search problem, in which the node sets $\mathcal{N}^*_0$ and $\mathcal{N}^1_1$ are to be identified.

Apparently, the choices of $\mathcal{N}^*_0$ and $\mathcal{N}^*_1$ are not arbitrary. Cost values are assigned to the graph nodes according to two cost functions constructed specifically for the bone and cartilage surfaces. $\mathcal{N}^*_0$ and $\mathcal{N}^*_1$ will correspond to the set of nodes with the minimum total cost in the graph. Furthermore, several constraints are imposed on the geometric relations of the nodes in $\mathcal{N}^*_0$ and $\mathcal{N}^*_1$. These constraints are enforced by the graph arcs, constructed as follow.

- *Intra-column arcs* $\mathcal{A}^a$: Along each column $\mathcal{K}_s(v_i)$, every node n^k_{si} has a directed arc to the node n^{k-1}_{si}, i.e.,

$$\mathcal{A}^a = \{\langle n^k_{si}, n^{k-1}_{si} \rangle : k = 1, \ldots, K-1; \forall i, s\} \quad (3)$$

- *Inter-column arcs* $\mathcal{A}^r$: The inter-column arcs encode the smoothness constraint, which is imposed between each pair of adjacent columns. Two columns $\mathcal{K}_s(v_i)$ and $\mathcal{K}_s(v_j)$ ($s \in \{0, 1\}$, $i \neq j$) are said to be adjacent if the two vertices v_i and v_j are adjacent on the mesh. Suppose one of the sought surfaces intersects with two adjacent columns $\mathcal{K}_s(v_i)$ and $\mathcal{K}_s(v_j)$ at nodes $n^{k_i}_{si}$ and $n^{k_j}_{sj}$, respectively. If the surface is smooth, k_i and k_j should not differ too much. The smoothness constraint Δ defines the maximum allowed difference between k_i and k_j, i.e., $\Delta = \max |k_i - k_j|$. Smaller Δ forces the surface to be smoother. To encode the smoothness constraint in the graph, the following directed arcs are constructed:

$$\mathcal{A}^r = \{\langle n^k_{si}, n^{\max(0, k-\Delta)}_{sj} \rangle : \forall s, k; \ v_i, v_j \text{ adjacent}\} \quad (4)$$

- *Inter-surface arcs* $\mathcal{A}^s$: These arcs model the separation constraint between the two surfaces. Suppose the bone and cartilage surfaces intersect $\mathcal{K}_0(v_i)$ and $\mathcal{K}_1(v_i)$ at nodes $n_{0i}^{k_0}$ and $n_{1i}^{k_1}$, respectively. Because the thickness of the cartilage is within some known range, $n_{0i}^{k_0}$ and $n_{1i}^{k_1}$ are at least δ^l, and at most δ^u nodes apart, i.e., $\delta^l \leq k_1 - k_0 \leq \delta^u$. The inter-surface arcs are constructed between columns $\mathcal{K}_0(v_i)$ and $\mathcal{K}_1(v_i)$ for all $v_i \in \mathcal{V}$ as:

$$\mathcal{A}^s = \{\langle n_{1i}^k, n_{0i}^{\max(0, k-\delta^u)}\rangle, \langle n_{0i}^k, n_{1i}^{\min(K-1, k+\delta^l)}\rangle : \forall i, k\} \tag{5}$$

For more than two surfaces, the separation constraint is specified pairwisely.

Cost Functions. The cost functions are crucial for accurate surface localization. For this pilot study, relatively simple cost functions are used. Specifically, the cost function for the bone surface, C_{bone}, is the negated gradient magnitude of the Gaussian-smoothed image G,

$$C_{bone} = -|\nabla G| \equiv -\sqrt{G_x^2 + G_y^2 + G_z^2} \tag{6}$$

where $G_x \equiv \frac{\partial}{\partial x} G$, $G_y \equiv \frac{\partial}{\partial y} G$ and $G_z \equiv \frac{\partial}{\partial z} G$ are partial derivatives of the image. The cost function for the cartilage surface is computed as a weighted combination of the response of a 3-D "sheet filter" [5] and the directional image gradients. The sheet filter is formulated using the Hessian matrix $\nabla^2 G$ of the image intensity. Let the eigenvalues of $\nabla^2 G$ be λ_0, λ_1 and λ_2, ($\lambda_0 \geq \lambda_1 \geq \lambda_2$). The sheet filter is defined as:

$$F_{sheet}(G) = \begin{cases} |\lambda_2| \cdot \omega(\lambda_1, \lambda_2) \cdot \omega(\lambda_0, \lambda_2), & \lambda_2 < 0, \\ 0, & \text{otherwise.} \end{cases} \tag{7}$$

The function ω is given by:

$$\omega(\lambda_a, \lambda_b) = \begin{cases} (1 + \frac{\lambda_a}{|\lambda_b|})^\gamma, & \lambda_b \leq \lambda_a \leq 0, \\ (1 - \alpha \frac{\lambda_a}{|\lambda_b|})^\gamma, & \frac{|\lambda_b|}{\alpha} > \lambda_a > 0, \\ 0, & \text{otherwise,} \end{cases} \tag{8}$$

where α, γ are parameters. In our experiments, we chose $\alpha = 0.25$ and $\gamma = 0.5$. In summary, the cost function for cartilage surface is computed as:

$$C_{cartilage} = \begin{cases} -F_{sheet}(-G) - \tau_x G_x, & \text{if } G_x > 0, \\ -F_{sheet}(-G) & \text{otherwise,} \end{cases} \tag{9}$$

where the value of τ_x is chosen to be 1.0 in our experiments.

The above cost functions are computed in the image domain. The node costs are assigned using spatial interpolation based on the positions of the nodes. Specifically, the costs of nodes n_{0i}^k are assigned according to C_{bone}, and the costs of nodes n_{1i}^k are computed from $C_{cartilage}$.

Optimization. Once the graph is constructed and the node costs assigned, we can use the same technique described in [3] to transform the graph into an s-t graph $\mathcal{G}_{st}$ that has a source node s and a sink node t, and apply a minimum s-t cut algorithm to compute the optimal surfaces. The final surfaces will correspond to the upper envelope of the set of nodes that can be reached from s in $\mathcal{G}_{st}$, i.e., the source set of $\mathcal{G}_{st}$.

3 Case Study

Osteoarthritis and articular cartilage injuries are very common – one in six people in the USA is affected by some form of arthritis. The socio-economic impact of degenerative joint diseases is massive, with an estimated annual cost of \$65 billion in the USA during the 1990's. As such, there is a huge research interest in the field of chondro-protective and chondro-restorative treatments.

The proposed method allows segmenting the articular cartilage surface and the corresponding subchondral bone surface in volumetric MRI images that facilitates subsequent quantitative analysis. The segmentation is initiated by a few (normally 3 or less) roughly-placed seed points in the bone region, but is otherwise fully automated.

Data. The method was tested in 8 high-resolution 3-D MR data sets of human ankles. The images were acquired using a 1.5T MR scanner, with in plane resolution 0.3×0.3 mm^2 and slice thickness 0.3 mm. The acquisition time was 17 minutes and 14 seconds. Overall, each MR image data set consisted of approximately $512 \times 512 \times 150$ voxels.

Independent Standard. In the 8 MR images, 55 coronal or sagittal slices were randomly selected to be manually traced by an expert observer (orthopedic surgeon) and formed the independent standard. The selection of coronal as well as sagittal slices allows assessing the performance of the inherently 3-D segmentation method using 2-D manual tracings.

Comparisons with the Independent Standard. Computer segmentation of the talus bone and the cartilage surfaces was performed in 3-D. Consequently, the segmented surfaces were available for the entire closed 3-D object. The automated segmentation method locally failed in 5 of the 55 image slices for which independent standard was available due to local pre-segmentation errors. The segmentation accuracy was assessed in the 50 image slices by computing signed, unsigned, and RMS surface positioning errors. The positioning errors were defined as the shortest distances between the manually traced borders and the computer-determined surfaces in the coronal and sagittal MR slices for which the independent standard was available. The errors are reported on a per-slice basis as mean $\pm$ standard deviation.

Reproducibility. To assess the reproducibility of cartilage segmentation, the method was independently initialized 5 times and the mean and maximum car-

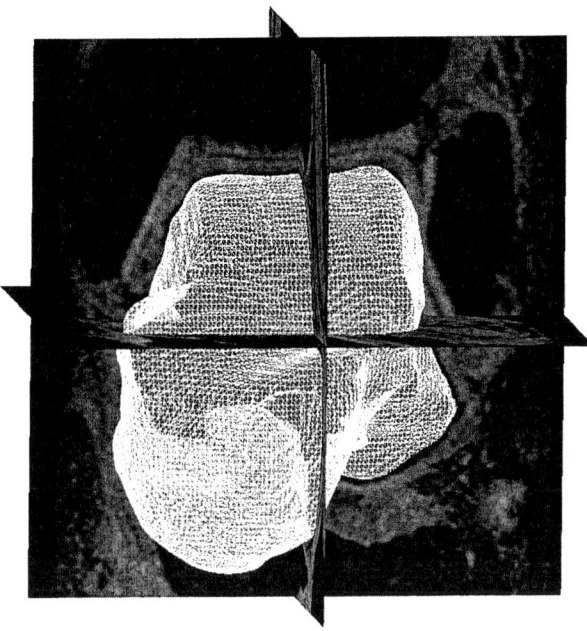

(a) Presegmented talus surface

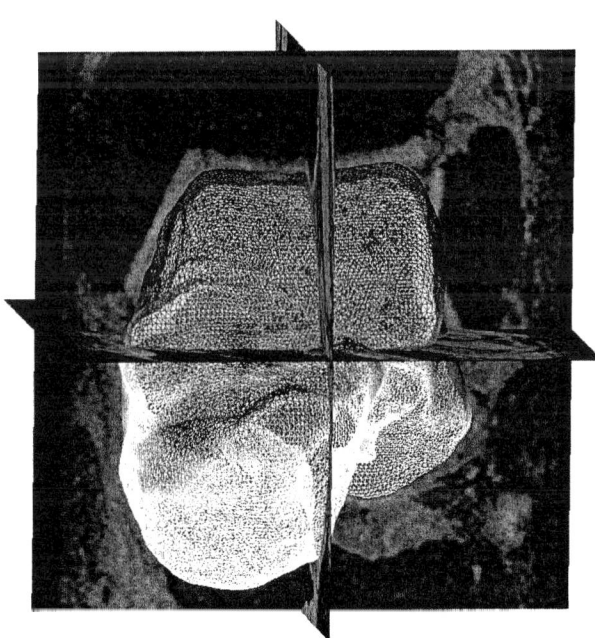

(b) Segmented talus and cartilage

Fig. 3. Presegmentation and segmentation. Cartilage surfaces are color-coded, with darker shadings depicting thicker cartilage

tilage thicknesses were determined for each of the 8 talus cartilages. The reproducibility was assessed by calculating mean ± standard deviation of differences between the average values obtained in the 5 reproducibility runs and the individual results.

Results. All experiments were performed on a workstation with dual 3.0GHz processors and 4GB of RAM. For each data set, we used 3 seed-spheres inside the

Table 1. Overall surface positioning accuracy

	Signed Error (mm)	Unsigned Error (mm)	RMS Error (mm)
Bone	0.02 ± 0.11	0.25 ± 0.08	0.03 ± 0.01
Cartilage	0.17 ± 0.12	0.39 ± 0.09	0.04 ± 0.01

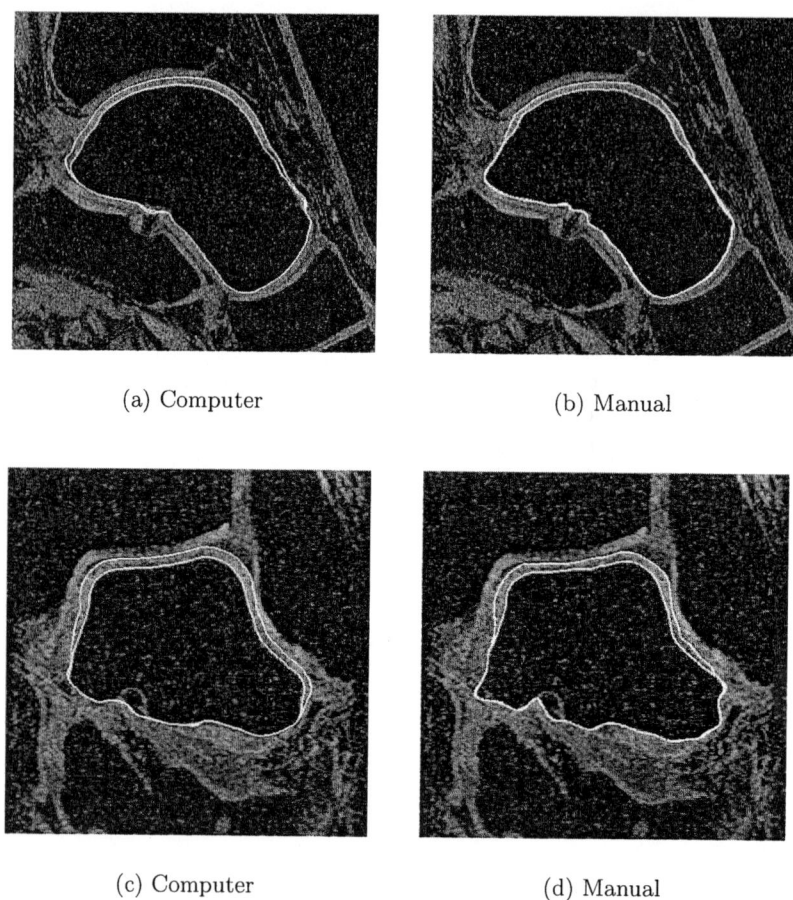

(a) Computer (b) Manual

(c) Computer (d) Manual

Fig. 4. Comparison of computer and manual segmentations

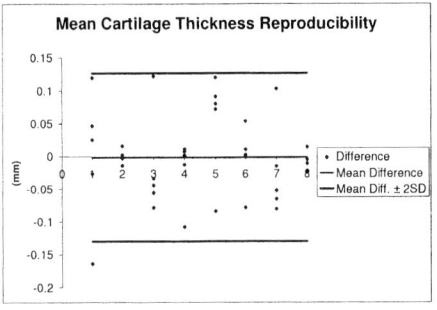 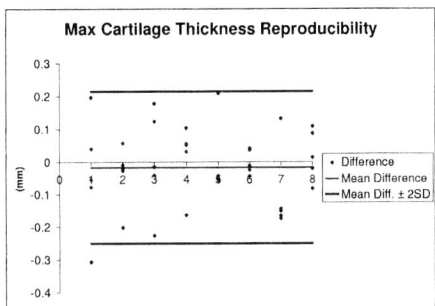

(a) Mean cartilage thickness (b) Max cartilage thickness

Fig. 5. Bland-Altman plots of cartilage thickness reproducibility

bone region to initialize the presegmentation. To reduce running time, the regions containing the talus bones were cropped from the original MR images to form smaller images of approximately 250×250×150 voxels each. The presegmentation was performed on 2-times downsampled copies of the cropped images, while the final segmentation was performed on the original full-resolution images.

The parameters used for final segmentations were $K = 30$, $\delta^l = 0$, $\delta^u = 12$ and $\Delta = 1$. For each data set, the average execution times of the presegmentation and segmentation stages were about 200 seconds and 70 seconds, respectively. The overall surface positioning errors of the computer-segmented talus bone and its cartilage surfaces are shown in Table 1. Examples of computer-segmented and manually-traced bone and cartilage contours are shown in Fig. 4.

The mean cartilage thickness measurements achieved a signed error of 0.08 ± 0.07mm, and an unsigned error of 0.09 ± 0.06mm. The corresponding measurements of maximum cartilage thicknesses have signed and unsigned errors of 0.01 ± 0.19mm and 0.16 ± 0.10mm, respectively. All border positioning errors show subvoxel accuracy (voxel size $0.3 \times 0.3 \times 0.3$ mm^3).

In the reproducibility experiment, the initializing spheres were modified from the original settings by adding up to 10% of random perturbations to their radii and 2 to 5 voxels of random translations to each coordinate of their positions. The Bland-Altman plots of the signed differences between each individual measurement and the average measurements are shown in Fig. 5 demonstrating that repeated measurement of cartilage thickness is unbiased and reproducible.

4 Discussion and Conclusion

Traditional techniques such as manual segmentation and gradient based edge detection are not suitable for automated, accurate, reproducible detection of the cartilage and subchondral bone surfaces in thin congruent cartilage layers. The objective of this study was to provide a proof of concept that the cartilage and subchondral bone surfaces can be accurately detected simultaneously in 3-D, using a novel segmentation method, and perform its pilot validation in comparison with an independent standard.

Properties of the Method. The graph-based segmentations utilized hard geometric constraints, which are intuitive and easily controllable. The definition of the smoothness constraint, however, requires that the edges in the surface mesh be as equidistant as possible. This could be achieved by using sophisticated mesh optimization algorithms. An alternative and simpler way is to make the smoothness constraint vary between graph columns by modulating it according to the corresponding edge length. When the mesh is dense enough, however, the effect of unequal edge length could be ignored for our application. Therefore, neither approach was used in the reported experiments. A drawback of the presented graph-search approach is its dependence on presegmentation, which is crucial for obtaining good final results. However, a one-shot approach using either numerical or discrete mathematical tools alone could be difficult to design, computationally inefficient and may not yield a satisfactory outcome. In addition, its reliance on surface normals makes the method suffer from surface self-intersections. However, this problem is avoidable by detecting spatially intersecting node columns and pruning the affected nodes during the graph-construction.

The employed presegmentation method uses free form deformation, with which one can use large step size for surface evolution. Moreover, in practice, the number of control points required for the FFD is usually much fewer than the number of image voxels. These make the method computationally efficient.

Overall, the method was shown to be highly reproducible in our experiments. However, the initialization of the presegmentation is quite strategic. As a rule of thumb, the seed-spheres should be roughly centered at the maxima of the "shape image" in the bone interior. Automatic initialization methods can be designed following this strategy.

Cartilage Segmentation. A variety of 2-D image segmentation techniques have been utilized on articular cartilage images in the past, including manual segmentation, seed point and region growing algorithms, fully automated 2-D shape recognition, interpolated B-splines, B-spline snakes, and directional gradient vector flow snakes [6,7,8]. All of these techniques have limitations as they require an accurate initialization. Manual surface segmentation is both labor intensive and prone to error and is influenced by subjective judgment of the operator leading to inter-observer variability. Moreover, the accuracy and reproducibility of existing fully automated and semi-automated algorithms in noisy images of cartilage layers are often suboptimal. This poses particular problems in thin highly congruent, curved cartilage layers, which require subvoxel measurement accuracy. Previous studies utilizing computer-assisted techniques suffer from measurement errors of up to 100% or exclude large areas of the joint surface. As a result there has been a return to manual segmentation techniques with the focus being on the development of time saving devices such as touch screen interactive segmentation. The reported 3-D approach addresses a number of the existing challenges and carries a substantial promise for the future utility of automated quantitative analysis of cartilage in 3-D.

Conclusion. A novel method for simultaneously segmenting multiple closed surfaces was demonstrated. The method utilizes an efficient graph-based algorithm that produces optimal solutions according to certain cost functions and geometric constraints. The proposed method achieved highly accurate results in segmenting cartilage and bone surfaces in MR images of human ankles. Although this paper concentrated on closed surfaces, the presented method can segment surfaces of other topologies according to different initializing meshes.

References

1. X. Wu and D. Z. Chen, "Optimal net surface problems with applications," in *Proc. of the 29th International Colloquium on Automata, Languages and Programming (ICALP)*, July 2002, pp. 1029–1042.
2. K. Li, X. Wu, D. Z. Chen, and M. Sonka, "Efficient optimal surface detection: Theory, implementation and experimental validation," in *Proc. SPIE International Symposium on Medical Imaging: Image Processing*, vol. 5370, May 2004, pp. 620–627.
3. ——, "Globally optimal segmentation of interacting surfaces with geometric constraints," in *Proc. IEEE Computer Society Conference on Computer Vision and Pattern Recognition (CVPR)*, vol. I, June 2004, pp. 394–399.
4. X. Huang, D. Metaxas, and T. Chen, "Metamorphs: Deformable shape and texture models," in *Proc. IEEE Computer Society Conference on Computer Vision and Pattern Recognition (CVPR)*, vol. I, June 2004, pp. 496–503.
5. Y. Sato, C.-F. Westin, A. Bhalerao, S. Nakajima, N. Shiraga, S. Tamura, and R. Kikinis, "Tissue classification based on 3D local intensity structure for volume rendering," *IEEE Trans on Visualization and Computer Graphics*, vol. 6, no. 2, pp. 160–180, 2000.
6. C. G. Peterfy, C. F. van Dijke, D. L. Janzen, C. C. Gluer, R. Namba, S. Majumdar, P. Lang, and H. K. Genant, "Quantification of articular cartilage in the knee with pulsed saturation transfer subtraction and fat-suppressed MR imaging: optimization and validation," *Radiology*, vol. 192, pp. 485–491, 1994.
7. A. Stammberger, F. Eckstein, M. Michaelis, K. H. Englmeier, and M. Reiser, "Interobserver reproducibility of quantitative cartilage measurement: comparison between B-spline snakes and manual segmentation," *Magnetic Resonance Imaging*, vol. 17, pp. 1033–1042, 1999.
8. J. Tang, S. Millington, S. Acton, J. Crandall, and S. Hurwitz, "Cartilage surface tracking using directional gradient vector flow snakes," in *IEEE Int. Conf. on Image Processing*, Singapore, 2004.

A Generalized Level Set Formulation of the Mumford-Shah Functional for Brain MR Image Segmentation

Lishui Cheng[1], Jie Yang[1], Xian Fan[1], and Yuemin Zhu[2]

[1] Institute of Image Processing and Pattern Recognition, Shanghai Jiao Tong University (SJTU), Shanghai, 200030, P.R.China
{lishuicheng, jieyang, Yivanne}@sjtu.edu.cn
[2] CREATIS, CNRS UMR 5515 & INSERM Unit 630, 69621 Villeurbanne cedex,France
Yue-Min.Zhu@creatis.insa-lyon.fr

Abstract. Brain MR image segmentation is an important research topic in medical image analysis area. In this paper, we propose an active contour model for brain MR image segmentation, based on a generalized level set formulation of the Mumford-Shah functional. The model embeds explicitly gradient information into the Mumford-Shah functional, and incorporates in a generic framework both regional and gradient information into segmentation process simultaneously. The proposed method has been evaluated on real brain MR images and the obtained results have shown the desirable segmentation performance.

1 Introduction

Segmentation of anatomical structures is of utmost significance both for clinical diagnosis and visualization purposes. Because of the huge amount of data and the complexity of these organs and structures, manual segmentation is extremely tedious and often unfeasible. Computer-based automatic segmentation methods are required to fully exploit medical data.

Active contour model, since it was first proposed in [1], has been extensively studied and used in the field of image segmentation. The central idea behind active contour model is to evolve a curve or surface based on energy minimization method under the influence of image dependent forces, regularity constraints and certain user-specified constraints. Originally, active contour models are parameterized curves or surfaces which iteratively evolve toward the desired locations according to the energy minimization criterion. The limitations of such kind of contour models are well known. For example, they are sensitive to initial conditions and should be placed usually near to the boundary of objects of interest. Besides, due to the explicit parameterization of the model, they can not cope with significant protrusions and topological changes.

Level set method provides an alternative solution to energy minimization-based image segmentation problem. The main idea behind level set method, which was first introduced by Osher and Sethian [2], consists of regarding the evolution curve as a higher dimension function which evolves under certain forces. It provides efficient numerical techniques for tracking and analyzing curve evolution problems. Moreover, level set-based contours are parametric independent and thus particularly appropriate for segmenting complex anatomical shapes. The evolution contour can change its topology naturally and the result is less dependent on initialization than parametric active contour models.

Many approaches have been proposed to address medical image segmentation problems with level set method. Geodesic active contour, which was proposed in [3], has been developed and extended to medical imagery in [4] and [5]. However, geodesic deformable contours are usually dependent on local features of an image, such as gradient, which makes them sensitive to noise. In [6], Zeng et al. derived a method for segmenting three-dimensional (3-D) brain cortex using coupled level set surface propagation based on certain geometric constraints of cortex thickness. The evolving surfaces are driven to boundaries of anatomical objects by forces derived from a specific designed local image information operator. On the other hand, there has been a great interest in region based active contours. In [7], Chan and Vese proposed a region-based active contour which was derived from the Mumford-Shah functional [8]. This model can detect interior contours automatically and the initial curve can be placed anywhere in the image. Methods for magnetic resonance (MR) brain image segmentation based on Chan-Vese model have been developed and implemented in [9] and [10]. Recently, Yang et al. [11] proposed a neighbor-constrained segmentation method for 3-D MR image analysis based on a combination of level set shape representation and Chan-Vese model. We notice that Tsai et al. in [12] also did similar work in this period.

Region-based active contours can provide a global criterion for image segmentation and are usually more robust to noise than boundary-based active contours. However, edge information of an image has more strength in the localization of boundaries. Moreover, because boundary finding usually relies on changes in the gray level, rather than their actual values, it is less sensitive to changes in the gray level distributions. Based on these observations, a number of researchers have tried to integrate region and boundary information in image segmentation. Chakraborty et al. [13] proposed a deformable model for medical images by integrating gradient and region information. In [14], Zhu and Yuille proposed a statistical variational approach which combines the geometrical features of a snake/balloon model and the statistical region growing techniques. Paragios also introduced a geodesic active region model which was implemented in level set method [15]. Note that the authors of [16] and [17] have done similar work in an attempt to combine gradient vector flow (GVF) [18] with geodesic active contour [3].

In this paper, a new variational active contour model for brain MR image segmentation is proposed. The model is based on the generalized level set formulation of the Mumford-Shah functional. It embeds explicitly gradient information into the Mumford-Shah functional, and incorporates in a general framework both regional and gradient information in segmentation process. Region-based forces make our method less sensitive to noise, while the gradient information allows for a better spatial localization. Furthermore, the method is very general, and does not require external information (such as an atlas) nor makes extra anatomy assumptions for brain MR image segmentation.

The rest of the paper is organized as follows. Section 2 briefly introduces the Mumford-Shah image segmentation problem. In section 3, the basic formulation of the proposed model is described in detail. In section 4, we depict the use of the basic model for multiphase brain MR image segmentation. Experimental results and conclusion are given in sections 5 and 6, respectively.

2 Background

In the variational framework, an image I_0 is usually considered as a real-valued bounded function defined on $\overline{\Omega}$, where Ω is a bounded and open subset of R^2 (in two dimension case) with $\partial\Omega$ its boundary.

Let I be a differentiable function on Ω, Γ is a set of discontinuities (i.e. contours). In [8], Mumford and Shah proposed the following functional to segment an image into homogeneous objects:

$$E^{MS}(I,\Gamma) = \mu \int_{\Omega} (I - I_0)^2 dxdy + \int_{\Omega-\Gamma} \|\nabla I\|^2 dxdy + \nu |\Gamma| \quad (1)$$

where $|\Gamma|$ stands for the total length of the arcs making up Γ, μ and ν are fixed parameters. The first term asks I is a good approximation of I_0, the second term asks that I is smooth and the third term ensures the boundaries that accomplish this be as short as possible. The smaller E is, the better (I,Γ) segments I_0.

A reduced form of this segmentation problem is simply the restriction of I to piecewise constant functions, i.e. I =constant c_i on each connected component Ω_i. Under this circumstance, the image segmentation problem, which is now called "minimal partition problem", is solved through minimizing the following functional:

$$E_0^{MS}(I,\Gamma) = \sum_i \mu_i \int_{\Omega_i} (I_0 - c_i)^2 dxdy + \nu \times Length(\Gamma) \quad (2)$$

where μ_i and ν are scaling parameters.

Traditionally, Mumford-Shah functional provides a region based method for image segmentation. In [7], Chan and Vese formulated this functional in terms of the level set formalism. Later, they generalized this method to treat multiple regions [19], and applied it to medical imaging [9]. The similar work was also proposed by Tsai et al. [20]. However, their method did not consider the gradient information of an image in segmentation process. Furthermore, as pointed out by F. Gibou and R. Fedkiw [21], under suitable assumptions, Chan-Vese model [7] simply reduces to the k-means algorithm [22].

3 Description of the Model

In this section, we present the generalized level set formulation of the Mumford-Shah functional in bimodal case. According to level set theory originally proposed by Osher and Sethian in [2], a geometric active contour can be represented by the zero level set of a real-valued Lipschitz function $\phi: \Omega \subset R^2 \to R$ which evolves in an image I_0 according to a variational flow in order to segment the object from the background. Since it was proposed, level set theory has received increasing interest in medical image analysis community [23]. Some of the biggest advantages of level set method are as follows. Firstly, unlike traditional parametric active contour models [1], level set based active contours are parametric-independent and hence can deal with topological changes naturally. Secondly, level set contours can be extended to three and higher dimensions, which is needed in many medical image processing and analysis applications. Thirdly, level set method usually has mature numerical implementation and is convenient to compute some geometry properties, such as curvature and normal [2].

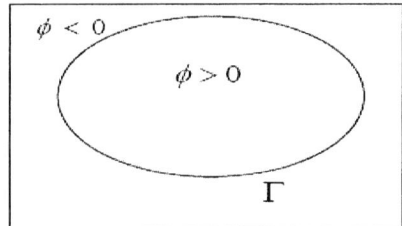

Fig. 1. The domain Ω divided into two regions by the curve Γ on which $\phi = 0$

The boundary curve Γ in Mumford-Shah model can be represented by the zero level set of the function ϕ, as depicted in Fig.1 for bimodal case. As in [7], the first term of Eq. (2) can be represented as follows:

$$\mu_1 \int_\Omega (I_0 - c_1)^2 H(\phi) dxdy + \mu_2 \int_\Omega (I_0 - c_2)^2 (1 - H(\phi)) dxdy \tag{3}$$

where c_1 and c_2 are the mean intensities inside and outside the active contour Γ (Fig. 1), respectively, and $H(\phi)$ is the Heaviside function defined as:

$$H(\phi) = \begin{cases} 1, \phi > 0 \\ 0, else \end{cases} \tag{4}$$

Now let us consider the length term of the Mumford-Shah functional. In [24], the line (surface) integral of a function $f(\vec{x})$ in $R^2(R^3)$ is defined as the following formula :

$$\int_\Omega f(\vec{x})\delta(\vec{x})d\vec{x} \qquad (5)$$

where the region of integration is all of Ω, and $\delta(\vec{x})$ the Delta function defined as follows:

$$\delta(\vec{x}) = \begin{cases} 1, \vec{x}=0 \\ 0, else \end{cases} \qquad (6)$$

Because the Delta function prunes out everything except the boundary $\partial\Omega$ automatically, the one-dimensional Delta function can be used to rewrite the line integral in level set framework as (for more details, see [24]):

$$\int_\Omega f(\vec{x})\delta(\phi)|\nabla\phi|d\vec{x} \qquad (7)$$

Based on this definition of line integral, the length term in the Mumford-Shah functional can be represented by a weighted length as follows:

$$\int_\Omega g(\vec{x})\delta(\phi)|\nabla\phi|d\vec{x} \qquad (8)$$

where $g(\vec{x})$ is a positive and decreasing function, indicating the boundary features of an image. Usually, $g(\vec{x})$ can be defined as (in 2 dimension):

$$g(\vec{x}) = g(x,y) = \frac{1}{1+|\nabla G_\sigma(x,y) * I_0(x,y)|^p}, p \geq 1 \qquad (9)$$

where $G_\sigma * I_0$, a smoother version of I_0, is the convolution of the image I_0 with the Gaussian $G_\sigma(x,y) = \sigma^{-1/2}e^{-|x^2+y^2|/4\sigma}$. The function $g(\vec{x})$ is supposed to be positive in homogeneous regions and zero in edges. In fact, similar to geodesic active contour model in [3], the corresponding curve that can minimize (8) is a geodesic curve. So here we are seeking to use a geodesic length which can stand for the length term in the Mumford-Shah functional.

Taking into account Eq. (3) and (8), the Mumford-Shah functional defined by Eq.(2) can be, using level set theory, reformulated as the following form that unifies both region and boundary features of an image:

$$E(\phi) = \mu_1 \int_\Omega (I_0 - c_1)^2 H(\phi)dxdy + \mu_2 \int_\Omega (I_0 - c_2)^2 (1 - H(\phi))dxdy$$
$$+ \nu \int_\Omega g(x,y)\delta(\phi)|\nabla\phi|dxdy \qquad (10)$$

where μ_1, μ_2 and ν are positive parameters, which have a scaling role. The first two terms encode the region statistics of the image while the last term carries the gradient information of the image. By adjusting the values of μ_1, μ_2 and v, we can choose different weights of region and gradient information.

Using the fundamental lemma of calculus of variations, minimizing E with respect to ϕ leads to the following Euler-Lagrange equation:

$$E_\phi = \delta(\phi)[\mu_1(I_0 - c_1)^2 - \mu_2(I_0 - c_2)^2 - v\nabla \bullet (g\frac{\nabla \phi}{|\nabla \phi|})] \tag{11}$$

Then, using the steepest descent method, we obtain the evolution equation as follows (see Appendix):

$$\phi_t = \delta(\phi)[\mu_2(I_0 - c_2)^2 - \mu_1(I_0 - c_1)^2 + v\frac{\nabla g \bullet \nabla \phi}{|\nabla \phi|} + vg\nabla \bullet (\frac{\nabla \phi}{|\nabla \phi|})] \tag{12}$$

Eq. (12) constitutes the basic formulation of our new active contour model. The first two terms describe the attraction of region homogeneity forces, the third term prevents curves from crossing over edges, and the last term is the part of force that depends on the intrinsic geometry, especially the curvature of the contour. Furthermore, both the last two terms are also dependent on gradient information of the image, which drives the contour to the boundaries of objects. Therefore, our active contour model provides a generic framework that unifies the region and boundary features of an image for segmentation problems.

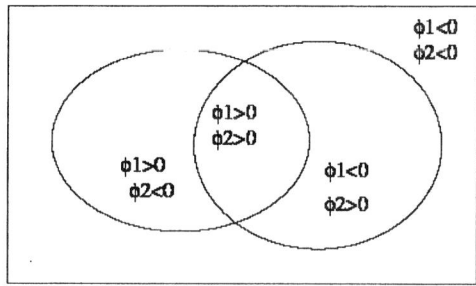

Fig. 2. Four regions separated using two level set functions (ϕ_1, ϕ_2)

4 MR Image Segmentation Scheme

In brain MR image segmentation problems, an image is often to be segmented into four regions: white matter (WM), grey matter (GM), cerebro-spinal fluid (CSF) and the background. So, in order to segment more than two objects using the active contour model described in the preceding section, it is necessary to extend the model to multimodal or multiphase case. This can readily be achieved by following the same idea as that in [19]. For simplicity, we give below the energy functional only for four phases (Fig. 2):

$$E(\phi_1,\phi_2) = \mu_{11}\int_\Omega (I_0-c_{11})^2 H(\phi_1)H(\phi_2)dxdy$$
$$+\mu_{10}\int_\Omega (I_0-c_{10})^2 H(\phi_1)(1-H(\phi_2))dxdy$$
$$+\mu_{01}\int_\Omega (I_0-c_{01})^2 (1-H(\phi_1))H(\phi_2)dxdy \qquad (13)$$
$$+\mu_{00}\int_\Omega (I_0-c_{00})^2 (1-H(\phi_1))(1-H(\phi_2))dxdy$$
$$+v_1\int_\Omega g(x,y)\delta(\phi_1)|\nabla\phi_1|dxdy + v_2\int_\Omega g(x,y)\delta(\phi_2)|\nabla\phi_2|dxdy$$

where $\mu_{11},\mu_{10},\mu_{01},\mu_{00},v_1$, and v_2 are scaling parameters, ϕ_1 and ϕ_2 are two level set functions, c_{11},c_{10},c_{01} and c_{00} are the mean values of the four regions, defined as follows:

$$c_{11} = mean(I_0) \text{ in } \{(x,y):\phi_1(x,y)>0,\phi_2(x,y)>0\}$$
$$c_{10} = mean(I_0) \text{ in } \{(x,y):\phi_1(x,y)>0,\phi_2(x,y)<0\}$$
$$c_{01} = mean(I_0) \text{ in } \{(x,y):\phi_1(x,y)<0,\phi_2(x,y)>0\}$$
$$c_{00} = mean(I_0) \text{ in } \{(x,y):\phi_1(x,y)<0,\phi_2(x,y)<0\}$$

Following the same idea as in section 3, we can obtain the corresponding evolution equations for the two level set functions:

$$\phi_{1_t} = \delta(\phi_1)\{v_1[\frac{\nabla g \bullet \nabla \phi_1}{|\nabla \phi_1|} + g\nabla\bullet(\frac{\nabla \phi_1}{|\nabla \phi_1|})] - [(\mu_{11}(I_0-c_{11})^2 - \mu_{01}(I_0-c_{01})^2)H(\phi_2)$$
$$+(\mu_{10}(I_0-c_{10})^2 - \mu_{00}(I_0-c_{00})^2)(1-H(\phi_2))]\} \qquad (14)$$

and

$$\phi_{2_t} = \delta(\phi_2)\{v_2[\frac{\nabla g \bullet \nabla \phi_2}{|\nabla \phi_2|} + g\nabla\bullet(\frac{\nabla \phi_2}{|\nabla \phi_2|})] - [(\mu_{11}(I_0-c_{11})^2 - \mu_{10}(I_0-c_{10})^2)H(\phi_1)$$
$$+(\mu_{01}(I_0-c_{01})^2 - \mu_{00}(I_0-c_{00})^2)(1-H(\phi_1))]\} \qquad (15)$$

Thus, we evolve two level sets simultaneously in order to segment a brain MR image into four regions, WM, GM, CSF and background.

In the numerical implementation, $H(\phi)$ is the regularized Heaviside function defined as:

$$H_\varepsilon(z) = \frac{1}{2}(1+\frac{2}{\pi}\arctan(\frac{z}{\varepsilon})) \qquad (16)$$

Likewise, $\delta(\phi)$ is the regularized version of Delta function defined as:

$$\delta_\varepsilon(z) = \frac{1}{\pi} \bullet \frac{\varepsilon}{\varepsilon^2 + z^2} \qquad (17)$$

Note that when $\varepsilon \to 0$, both regularized versions converge to standard Heaviside function and Delta function [7]. $\nabla g \bullet \nabla \phi$ and $|\nabla \phi|$ are discretized using upwind difference scheme [2]. The discretization of $\nabla \bullet \frac{\nabla \phi}{|\nabla \phi|}$ is with central difference scheme and the temporal derivative with a forward difference scheme.

In practice, the segmentation process is initialized with two level set functions defined as the distance function from initial surfaces. In order to accelerate the convergence of the algorithm, we adopted seeded initialization which was used in [15] and [19] as a common level set implementation technique. To be specific, these initial surfaces are defined as a number of cylinders centered at regularly spaced locations across the entire data volume. The number of cylinders is set according to the volume size. After convergence, we use a simple 3-D connectivity algorithm to correct for spurious isolated pixels in the three regions, WM, GM, and CSF. Finally, by checking the sign of the two level set functions, we can obtain the four segmented regions as the result of combination of inside and outside areas (Fig.2).When necessary, the data is filtered by anisotropic diffusion [25] before being fed into the segmentation algorithm.

5 Experimental Results and Discussion

In our experiments, we fixed $\mu_{00} = \mu_{01} = \mu_{10} = \mu_{11} = \mu, v_1 = v_2 = v$. This leaves us only two free parameters (μ and v) to balance the influence of two forces, the region homogeneity and the gradient-based forces.

To evaluate the performance of our method, we used a quantitative criterion, the Dice Similarity Coefficient (DSC), which has been adopted for voxel-by-voxel classification agreement [26]. For any type T, assuming that V_m denotes the set of pixels assigned for it by manual segmentation and V_a denotes the set of pixels assigned for it by the automatic segmentation algorithm, DSC is defined as follows:

$$DSC = 2 \bullet \frac{|V_m \cap V_a|}{|V_m| + |V_a|} \qquad (18)$$

It can be considered as a special case of the widely used Kappa coefficient [27]. Since manual segmentations are not "ground truth", DSC provides a reasonable way to evaluate automated segmentation methods.

5.1 Validation on Real Brain MR Data

We applied our method on 12 real brain MR data sets, which were acquired with a 1.5 T MR imaging system (GE, Signa) with the resolution 0.94 x 1.25 x 1.5 mm (256 x

192 x 124 voxels). These data sets have been previously labeled through a labor-intensive (usually 50 hours per brain) manual method by an expert. Since in this paper our main focus is on the cortical structures, the subcortical structures and non-brain tissues were removed by using manually labeled data sets as binary masks. We first applied our method on these data sets and then compared with expert results. The obtained results are shown in Fig. 3 and Table 1. Furthermore, we also compared our algorithm with Chan-Vese model [19] using the same data sets. The experiments indicated that our method usually got a DSC 2%-6% higher than that of Chan-Vese model.

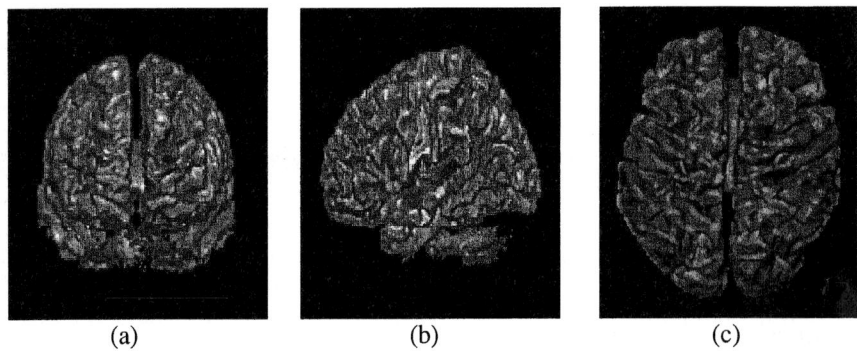

(a) (b) (c)

Fig. 3. Three views of the interface between GM/WM for case 7. (a) Coronal view. (b) Sagittal view. (c) Axial view

Table 1. Comparison of our method with manual segmentation using DSC (%)

Tissue	Case1	2	3	4	5	6	7	8	9	10	11	12
WM	87	86	84	86	84	85	89	84	80	87	88	79
GM	77	76	70	74	72	78	80	74	72	79	79	71
Average	82	81	77	80	78	82	85	79	76	83	84	75

5.2 Discussion

According to Zijdenbos's statement [26] that DSC>0.7 indicates excellent segmentation, the results shown in Table.1 indicate that our method has achieved desirable performance in MR brain image segmentation.

Because of the varieties of the real data sets, the average DSC of our method ranges from 75% to 85% in the experiment. The performance of WM segmentation is relatively better than that of GM segmentation. One reason for this is that GM is usually much more convoluted than WM, and the evolving surfaces have difficulty in moving into extremely narrow sulcus (1-2 pixels wide). Another reason is that GM usually has a much smaller area than WM, and misclassification of only one pixel has a much greater influence on GM segmentation than WM segmentation. Finally, labeling of MR data can also bear some error because accurate localization of anatomical structures is difficult even for an expert.

Although our method is specifically designed to be valid for brain MR image segmentation, it remains versatile. Unlike other specific techniques, for example [6], our technique does not need any geometric constraints; nor does it make use of priori shape information [11]. So, our segmentation method can be used for a wide variety of structures and modalities.

6 Conclusion and Future Work

Starting from the original Mumford-Shah functional, we have reformulated the latter using level set theory. In particular, we have introduced a weighted length term in the Mumford-Shah functional, thus allowing for incorporating gradient information in the Mumford-Shah model. The proposed active contour model is particularly suitable for brain MR image segmentation problems, and bears all the advantages of a parametric independent active contour. By driving two level set functions through the use of both region and boundary information, we have achieved a good segmentation of brain MR volumes into four regions, white matter, grey matter, cerebro-spinal fluid and the background.

In order to keep the consistency of mathematical formulation with the original Mumford-Shah functional, we did not include some possible modifications which may improve the performance of the proposed method. For example, in [28], the variance is considered in order to fit the Gaussian intensity distribution. In [29], the authors introduced a multiplicative gain field to Mumford-Shah functional which is adaptive to intensity inhomogeneities. These may be also incorporated in our method and are the subjects of future research.

Acknowledgements. The first author Lishui Cheng would like to particularly thank for the many helpful and stimulating discussions with Dr. Chenyang Xu on medical image segmentation. The first author also thanks Professor Vicent Caselles providing his paper and Mr. Yun Zhu for the very beneficial discussion about level set method .The first and third authors thank Dr. L. Yao, Dr. Y. Zhou, Ms. S. Ding, Mr. Y. Zheng, X. Li, K. Xie, H.Qin, G. Sun, Z. Zhang, S.Wu and other members of PAMI lab of SJTU for the friendship. The authors thank Ms. Hongxia Yang of Beijing Tumor Hospital and Ms. Yulei Jiang of Qingdao Women and Children's Hospital, for providing the data and useful medical expertise. The authors would also like to thank the anonymous reviewers whose valuable comments have greatly improved the presentation of this paper. The work is partially supported by the Natural Science Foundation of China (NSFC) under grant number 30170274.

References

1. M. Kass, A.Witkin, and D.Terzopoulos, "Snakes: Active contour models," International Journal of Computer Vision, vol. 1, pp. 321-331, 1988
2. S. Osher, and J. A. Sethian, "Fronts propagating with curvature dependent speed: algorithms based on Harmilton-Jacobi formulations," Journal of Computational Physics, vol. 79, pp. 12-49, 1988

3. V. Caselles, R. Kimmel, and G. Sapiro, "On geodesic active contours," International Journal of Computer Vision, vol. 22, no. 1, pp. 61-79,1997
4. A. Yezzi, Jr., S. Kichenassamy, P. Olver, A. Kumar and A. Tannenbaum, "A Geometric Snake Model for Segmentation of Medical Imagery," IEEE Transactions on Medical Imaging, vol. 16, no.2, pp. 199-209, 1997
5. W. J. Niessen, B. M. ter Haar Romeny, and M. A. Viergever, "Geodesic Deformable Model for Medical Image Analysis," IEEE Transactions on Medical Imaging, vol. 17, no.4, PPpp. 634-641,1998
6. X. Zeng, L. H. Staib, R. T. Schultz, and J. S. Duncan, "Segmentation and Measurement of the Cortex from 3-D MR Images Using Coupled-surfaces," IEEE Transactions on Medical Imaging, vol. 18, pp. 927-937,1997
7. T.F. Chan, and L.A. Vese, "Active contours without edges," IEEE Transactions on Image Processing, vol. 10, no. 2, pp. 266-277,2001
8. D. Mumford, and J. Shah, "Optimal approximations by piecewise smooth functions and associated variational problems," Communication on Pure and Applied Mathematics, vol. 42, pp. 577-684, 1989
9. T.F. Chan, and L.A. Vese, "Active Contours and Segmentation Models Using Geometric PDE's for Medical Imaging," University of California, Los Angeles, CA, USA,CAM Report 00-41, 2000
10. E. D. Angelini, T. Song, B. D. Mensh, and A. Laine, "Multi-phase Three-Dimensional Level Set Segmentation of Brain MRI," MICCAI 2004, LNCS 3216,pp.318-326,2004
11. J. Yang , L. H. Staib and J. S. Duncan, " Neighbor-Constrained Segmentation With Level Set Based 3-D Deformable Models," IEEE Transactions on Medical Imaging, vol. 23, no. 8, pp. 940-948,2004
12. A. Tsai, A. Yezzi, Jr., W. Wells, C. Tempany, D. Tucker, A. Fan and A. Willsky, "A Shape-Based Approach to the Segmentation of Medical Imagery Using Level Sets," IEEE Transactions on Medical Imaging, vol. 22, no. 2, pp. 137-153,2003
13. A. Chakraborty, L. H. Staib and J. S. Duncan, "Deformable Boundary Finding in Medical Images by Integrating Gradient and Region Information," IEEE Transactions on Medical Imaging, vol. 15, no. 6, pp. 859-870, 1996
14. 14.S.Zhu,and A. Yuille, "Region competition: unifying snakes, region growing and bayes/MDL for multiband image segmentation," IEEE Transactions on Pattern Analysis and Machine Intelligence, vol. 18, no. 9, pp. 884-900,1996
15. N. Paragios, and R. Deriche, "Geodesic active regions: a new paradigm to deal with frame partition problems in computer vision," Journal of Visual Communication and Image Representation, vol. 13, pp. 249-268, 2002
16. X. Xie, and M. Mirmehdi, "RAGS: region-aided geometric snake," IEEE Transactions on Image Processing, vol. 13, no. 5, pp. 640-652, 2004
17. N. Paragios, O. Mellina-Gottardo and V. Ramesh, "Gradient Vector Flow Fast Geodesic Active Contours," International Conference in Computer Vision (ICCV), pp. I: 67-73, 2001
18. C. Xu and J. L. Prince, "Snakes, Shapes, and Gradient Vector Flow," IEEE Transactions on Image Processing, vol.7, no. 3, pp. 359-369, 1998
19. L. A. Vese and T. F. Chan, "A Multiphase Level Set Framework for Image Segmentation Using the Mumford and Shah Model," International Journal of Computer Vision, vol.50, no.3, pp. 271-293, 2002
20. A. Tsai, A. Yezzi, A. Willsky, "Curve evolution implementation of the Mumford-Shah functional for image segmentation, denoising, interpolation, and magnification," IEEE Transactions on Image Processing, vol. 10, no. 8, pp. 1169-1186, 2001

21. F. Gibou and R. Fedkiw, "A fast level set based algorithm for segmentation," 4th Annual Hawaii International Conference on Statistics and Mathematics, pp.281-291, 2005
22. J. C. Dunn, "A fuzzy relative of the isodata process and its use in detecting compact well-separated clusters," Journal of Cybernetics, vol. 3(3), pp. 32-57, 1973
23. J. S. Suri, K.Liu, S. Singh , S. N. Laxminarayan, L. Reden and X. Zeng, "Shape Recovery Using Level Sets in 2-D/3-D Medical Imagery: A State-of-the-Art Review," IEEE Transactions on Information Technology in Biomedcine,vol.6, no. 1,pp.8-28,2002
24. S. Osher and R. Fedkiw, "Level Set Methods and Dynamic Implicit Surface," Springer-Verlag, pp. 13-15, ISBN: 0387954821, 2002
25. P. Perona and J. Malik, "Scale-space and edge detection using anisotropic diffusion," IEEE Transactions on Pattern Analysis Machine Intelligence, vol. (12), no.7, pp.:629–639, 1990
26. A. P. Zijdenbos, B.M. Dawant, R. A. Margolin, A.C. Palmer, "Morphometric analysis of white matter lesions in MR images: Method and validation," IEEE Transactions on Medical Imaging, vol. 13, no. 4, pp. 716-724, 1994
27. L. Hubert, "Kappa Revisited," Psycholog. Bullet. , vol. 84, no.2, pp. 289-297, 1977
28. N. Lin, W. Yu, J.S. Duncan, "Combinative Multi-Scale Level Set Framework for Echocardiographic Image Segmentation," Medical Image Analysis, vol.7, no.4, pp. 529-537, 2003
29. Fei Liu, Yupin Luo and Dongcheng Hu, "Adaptive level set image segmentation using the Mumford and Shah functional, " SPIE, Optical Engineering, 41(12):3002-3003, 2002

Appendix

We show our demonstration for bimodal case. The problem is: for the following functional (A.1), the evolution equation is given by Eq. (12).

$$E(\phi) = \mu_1 \int_\Omega (I_0 - c_1)^2 H(\phi) dxdy + \mu_2 \int_\Omega (I_0 - c_2)^2 (1 - H(\phi)) dxdy \\ + \nu \int_\Omega g(x,y) \delta(\phi) |\nabla \phi| dxdy \quad (A.1)$$

Proof:
The Frechet derivative of $E(\phi)$ with respect to $\phi(x,y)$ in the direction $\varphi(x,y)$, which is denoted by $dE(\phi, \varphi)$, can be computed as:

$$dE(\phi, \varphi) = \int_\Omega \{\delta(\phi)[\mu_1 (I_0 - c_1)^2 - \mu_2 (I_0 - c_2)^2]\varphi \\ + \nu[\delta'(\phi)|\nabla \phi| g\varphi + \delta(\phi) g \frac{\nabla \phi}{|\nabla \phi|} \bullet \nabla \varphi)]\} dxdy \quad (A.2)$$

where $\delta'(\phi)$ denotes the first derivative of the Delta function.

Applying Green's theorem to (A.2),

$$dE(\phi,\varphi) = \int_\Omega \delta(\phi)[\mu_1(I_0-c_1)^2 - \mu_2(I_0-c_2)^2]\varphi dxdy$$

$$+v\int_\Omega \delta'(\phi)|\nabla\phi|g\varphi dxdy + v\oint_{\partial\Omega}\frac{\delta(\phi)}{|\nabla\phi|}\frac{\partial\phi}{\partial \vec{n}}g\varphi dS - v\int_\Omega \nabla\bullet(\delta(\phi)g\frac{\nabla\phi}{|\nabla\phi|})\varphi dxdy$$

$$= \int_\Omega \delta(\phi)[\mu_1(I_0-c_1)^2 - \mu_2(I_0-c_2)^2]\varphi dxdy + v\oint_{\partial\Omega}\frac{\delta(\phi)}{|\nabla\phi|}\frac{\partial\phi}{\partial \vec{n}}g\varphi dS \qquad (A.3)$$

$$+v\int_\Omega \delta'(\phi)|\nabla\phi|g\varphi dxdy - v\int_\Omega [\delta'(\phi)|\nabla\phi|g\varphi + \delta(\phi)\nabla\bullet(g\frac{\nabla\phi}{|\nabla\phi|})\varphi]dxdy$$

$$= \int_\Omega \delta(\phi)[\mu_1(I_0-c_1)^2 - \mu_2(I_0-c_2)^2 - v\nabla\bullet(g\frac{\nabla\phi}{|\nabla\phi|})]\varphi dxdy$$

under the natural boundary condition. $\frac{\partial \phi}{\partial \vec{n}} = 0$.

So from Schwartz inequality, it is obvious that the direction that reduces the energy functional most rapidly is given by:

$$\varphi_s = \delta(\phi)[\mu_2(I_0-c_2)^2 - \mu_1(I_0-c_1)^2 + v\nabla\bullet(g\frac{\nabla\phi}{|\nabla\phi|})] \qquad (A.4)$$

Introducing an artificial time t, we get:

$$\phi_t = \varphi_s = \delta(\phi)[\mu_2(I_0-c_2)^2 - \mu_1(I_0-c_1)^2 + v\frac{\nabla g\bullet\nabla\phi}{|\nabla\phi|} + vg\nabla\bullet(\frac{\nabla\phi}{|\nabla\phi|})] \qquad (A.5)$$

which is the same as Eq.(12).

Integrable Pressure Gradients via Harmonics-Based Orthogonal Projection

Yuehuan Wang and Amir A. Amini

CVIA Laboratory, Campus Box 8086, 660 S. Euclid Ave.,
Washington University School of Medicine,
St. Louis, MO 63110, USA

Abstract. In the past, several methods based on iterative solution of pressure-Poisson equation have been developed for measurement of pressure from phase-contrast magnetic resonance (PC-MR) data. In this paper, a non-iterative harmonics-based orthogonal projection method is discussed which can keep the pressures measured based on the Navier-Stokes equation independent of the path of integration.

The gradient of pressure calculated with Navier-Stokes equation is expanded with a series of orthogonal basis functions, and is subsequently projected onto an integrable subspace. Before the projection step however, a scheme is devised to eliminate the discontinuity at the vessel boundaries.

The approach was applied to velocities obtained from computational fluid dynamics (CFD) simulations of stenotic flow and compared with pressures independently obtained by CFD. Additionally, MR velocity data measured in in-vitro phantom models with different degree of stenoses and different flow rates were used to test the algorithm and results were compared with CFD simulations. The pressure results obtained from the new method were also compared with pressures calculated by an iterative solution to the pressure-Poisson equation. Experiments have shown that the proposed approach is faster and is less sensitive to noise.

1 Introduction

Phase-Contrast (PC) MR methods are widely used for measurement of blood flow velocities [1]. PC MR imaging relies on the phase changes of moving spins when subjected to a magnetic field gradient. In the absence of acceleration and higher order terms, it can be shown that the accumulated phase offset is directly proportional to the spin velocities, and all three orthogonal components of the velocity vector for points within a prescribed image slice may be determined. The velocity field can then be used to obtain flow patterns, wall shear stress, vascular compliance, and blood pressure.

Previously, Urchuk et al. [2] developed a method to determine the pressure wave from time-resolved PC MRI data. Yang et al. [3] developed a technique for pressure calculation, which performs iterative integration of pressure gradients data in two-dimensions. The method was extended by Tyszka et al. [4]

to three-dimensions. Both of the techniques in [3] and [4] are similar in spirit to a method developed earlier by Song et al. [5], who proposed a solution to the pressure-Poisson equation for derivation of intraventricular blood pressures, from ultra-fast X-ray CT. More recently, Ebbers [6] has developed a technique to integrate pressure gradients along specific flow streamlines computed from PC MR data, and Thompson [7] has proposed a single slice method to measurement of intra-cardiac pressures. In previous work, we developed an iterative solution to the pressure-Poisson equation in axisymmetric geometries for pressure measurements [8]. In this paper, we propose a novel non-iterative approach to pressure calculations which offers significant advantages over previously proposed methods.

The idea is based on a method originally proposed by Frankot and Chellappa [9] for solving the shape from shading problem in computer vision. In this paper, Frankot and Chellappa's method is extended and adapted to blood pressure measurement from MR velocity fields. The approach was applied to CFD simulated velocity fields of stenotic flow as well as in-vitro MR velocity data. The results were compared with the pressure generated by CFD and the iterative solution to pressure-Poisson equation, in terms of accuracy and speed.

2 Method

2.1 Calculation of Pressure Gradient

The law of "Conservation of Momentum" [10], described by the Navier-Stokes equations, governs the fluid motion. If the dynamic viscosity μ can be considered a constant (a good approximation for an incompressible Newtonian Fluid), the Navier-Stokes equations take the following form:

$$\nabla \mathbf{P} = -\rho \frac{\partial \mathbf{u}}{\partial t} - \rho(\mathbf{u}.\nabla)\mathbf{u} + \mu \nabla^2 \mathbf{u} + \rho \mathbf{f}, \quad (1)$$

where $\mathbf{u}$ is the fluid velocity, $\mathbf{P}$ is the pressure, ρ is the density of fluid, and $\mathbf{f}$ is the body force such as gravity which is generally ignored.

This vector equation completely describes the dynamics of Newtonian fluids such as water and air. In axi-symmetric coordinates, one can obtain the gradient for steady flow as

$$\begin{cases} \hat{P}_r = \frac{\partial \mathbf{P}}{\partial r} = -\rho \left(u \frac{\partial u}{\partial r} + w \frac{\partial u}{\partial z} \right) + \mu \left(\frac{1}{r} \frac{\partial}{\partial r} \left(r \frac{\partial u}{\partial r} \right) + \frac{\partial^2 u}{\partial z^2} - \frac{u}{r^2} \right), \\ \hat{P}_z = \frac{\partial \mathbf{P}}{\partial z} = -\rho \left(u \frac{\partial w}{\partial r} + w \frac{\partial w}{\partial z} \right) + \mu \left(\frac{1}{r} \frac{\partial}{\partial r} \left(r \frac{\partial w}{\partial r} \right) + \frac{\partial^2 w}{\partial z^2} \right) \end{cases} \quad (2)$$

where u is the radial component and w is the axial component of PC velocities and $\hat{P}_r$ and $\hat{P}_z$ denote the r and z components, respectively, of the gradient of pressure as calculated from the PC data.

Due to noise, the vector field $(\hat{P}_r, \hat{P}_z)$ is not curl-free, and therefore by definition it can not be the true gradient of the scalar pressure field.

2.2 Non-iterative Harmonics-Based Orthogonal Projection

For the vector field $(\hat{P}_r, \hat{P}_z)$ to be integrable, it needs to be the gradient of a scalar function (i.e., integral is path-independent) and therefore,

$$\frac{\partial \hat{P}_r}{\partial z} = \frac{\partial \hat{P}_z}{\partial r} \tag{3}$$

The projection of $\widehat{\nabla \mathbf{P}}(r,z) = (\hat{P}_r, \hat{P}_z)$ onto an integrable subspace involves minimizing the following energy function:

$$D = \iint_\Omega \left| \tilde{P}_r - \hat{P}_r \right|^2 + \left| \tilde{P}_z - \hat{P}_z \right|^2 r \, dr \, dz \tag{4}$$

where $(\tilde{P}_r, \tilde{P}_z)$ is the projection onto the integrable subspace, that is, it minimizes D in equation (4).

Provided a series of orthogonal integrable basis function $\phi(r, z, \underline{\omega})$, with $\underline{\omega}$ as the vector (ω_r, ω_z) of spatial frequencies, the pressure $\tilde{\mathbf{P}}$ can be expanded as:

$$\tilde{\mathbf{P}} = \sum \tilde{C}(\underline{\omega}) \phi(r, z, \underline{\omega}) \tag{5}$$

and its gradient will have:

$$\tilde{P}_r = \sum \tilde{C}(\underline{\omega}) \phi_r(r, z, \underline{\omega}), \tag{6}$$

$$\tilde{P}_z = \sum \tilde{C}(\underline{\omega}) \phi_z(r, z, \underline{\omega}). \tag{7}$$

where $\phi_r = \frac{\partial \phi}{\partial r}$ and $\phi_z = \frac{\partial \phi}{\partial z}$

The measured gradient can also be expanded as:

$$\hat{P}_r = \sum \hat{C}_1(\underline{\omega}) \phi_r(r, z, \underline{\omega}), \tag{8}$$

$$\hat{P}_z = \sum \hat{C}_2(\underline{\omega}) \phi_z(r, z, \underline{\omega}). \tag{9}$$

Following Frankot and Chellappa [9], the coefficient of expanssion of the projected pressure $\tilde{\mathbf{P}}$ in the integrable subspace, is related to $\hat{C}_1$ and $\hat{C}_2$ by:

$$\tilde{C} = \frac{\hat{C}_1 T_r + \hat{C}_2 T_z}{T_r + T_z} \tag{10}$$

where $T_r = \int_{\Re^3} |\phi_r|^2 r \, dr \, dz$ and $T_z = \int_{\Re^3} |\phi_z|^2 r \, dr \, dz$.

Then $\tilde{P}$ can be retrieved with inverse projection of $\tilde{C}$. Herein, Fourier basis functions are adopted for $\phi(\underline{\omega})$ for convenience of computations using the fast implementation of the Discrete Fourier Transform.

3 Effect of Discontinuities at Boundaries

The projection can not work in presence of pressure discontinuity. As an example, Fig. 1 shows the pressure profile along the center of a rigid tube under steady

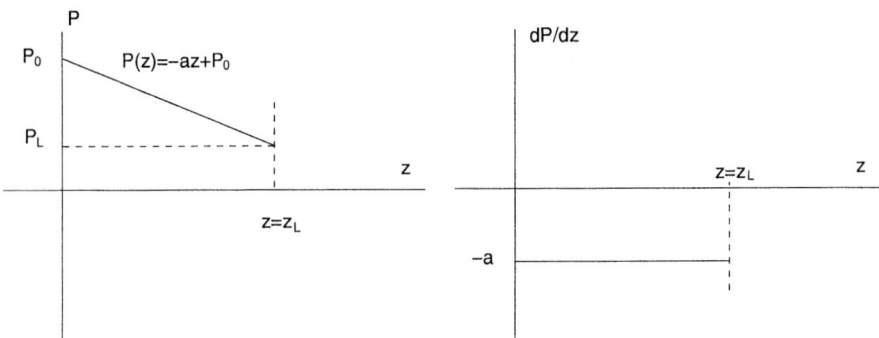

Fig. 1. A pressure profile and its gradient

flow (linear pressure drop along z) with the in-flow boundary being at $z = 0$ and out-flow boundary being at $z = z_L$.

Now consider Fourier expansion of $\mathbf{P}(z) = \sum C(\omega_z) e^{j\omega_z z}$ and derivative of $\mathbf{P}(z)$: $\sum j\omega_z C(\omega_z) e^{j\omega_z z}$. One can show that because of the discontinuity at $z = 0$ and $z = z_L$, Fourier expansion of $\frac{d\mathbf{P}}{dz}$:

$$\frac{d\mathbf{P}}{dz} = \sum C_d(\omega_z) e^{j\omega_z z} \tag{11}$$

will not yield $C_d(\omega_z) = j\omega_z C(\omega_z)$

There are two kinds of discontinuities that affect the harmonics-based orthogonal projection. First, because of the non-rectangular geometry, both the area inside and outside of the vessel will be included in the data to be projected. Therefore, a discontinuity exists at the boundaries of blood vessel $\{(r,z)|r = r_b(z)\}$ ($r_b(z)$ is the radial coordinate of the boundary point at z; see Figure 2). Another discontinuity exists at locations $r = 0$, $r = r_L$, $z = 0$, and $z = z_L$ (Figure 2) since the Discrete Fourier Transform assumes that the data is periodic.

For the discontinuities across the vascular boundary, the gradient components were set as follows:

$$\hat{P}_r(r,z) = \begin{cases} \hat{P}_r(r_b, z) & \text{if } r_b(z) < r \leq r_L \\ \hat{P}_r(r,z) & \text{if } r \leq r_b(z) \end{cases} \tag{12}$$

$$\hat{P}_z(r,z) = \begin{cases} \hat{P}_z(r_b, z) & \text{if } r_b(z) < r \leq r_L \\ \hat{P}_z(r,z) & \text{if } r \leq r_b(z) \end{cases} \tag{13}$$

To keep continuity in the periodic extension, a symmetric extension of pressure can be adopted:

$$\hat{\mathbf{P}}(r,z) = \hat{\mathbf{P}}(r,-z) = \hat{\mathbf{P}}(-r,z) = \hat{\mathbf{P}}(-r,-z)$$

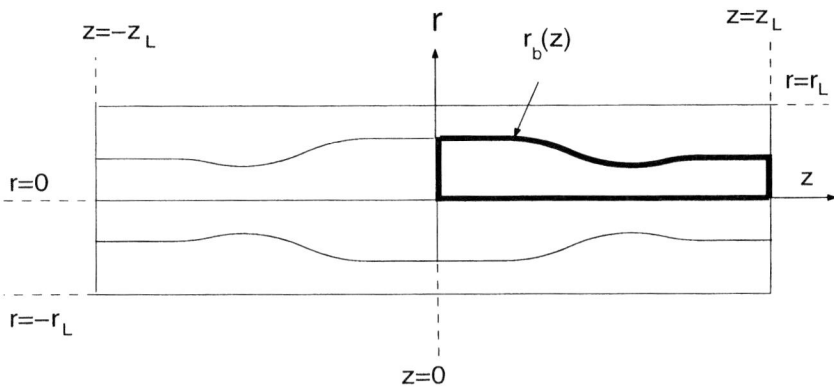

Fig. 2. Illustration of stenotic flow in axisymmetric coordinate system and solution to the discontinuity problem at boundaries. The figure in bold illustrates a physical axi-symmetric vessel phantom with $0 \leq r \leq r_b(z)$ and $0 \leq z \leq z_L$

which means that the gradient components adhere to:
$$\hat{P}_r(r,z) = \hat{P}_r(r,-z) = -\hat{P}_r(-r,z) = -\hat{P}_r(-r,-z),$$
$$\hat{P}_z(r,z) = -\hat{P}_r(r,-z) = \hat{P}_z(-r,z) = -\hat{P}_z(-r,-z)$$

for all $r \in [0, r_L], z \in [0, z_L]$

The process of harmonics-based orthogonal projection is then applied to $\widehat{\nabla \mathbf{P}}(r,z), r \in [-r_L, r_L], z \in [-z_L, z_L]$, as shown in Fig. 2.

4 Experiments

4.1 Flow Phantom

In order to study the pressure changes in blood flow across stenoses, we have studied flow patterns in in-vitro models. Three axi-symmetric models, which mimic 50, 75 and 90 percent area stenoses in larger vessels, were manufactured in house and were used to acquire velocity information using magnetic resonance (MR) imaging techniques.

This vascular pathology was modeled as a symmetric spindle-shaped narrowing in a rigid pipe with straight entrance and exit tubes. A 1.5 m long straight rigid acrylic tube was placed upstream of the test section to ensure a fully developed laminar flow (Poiseuille flow) at the entrance of the model.

Figure 3 shows a schematic diagram of the flow apparatus including the stenosis test section. The dimensions L_0, L_1, H, and R_S, in Fig. 3 are 150 cm, 20 cm, 8 cm, and 0.95 cm respectively.

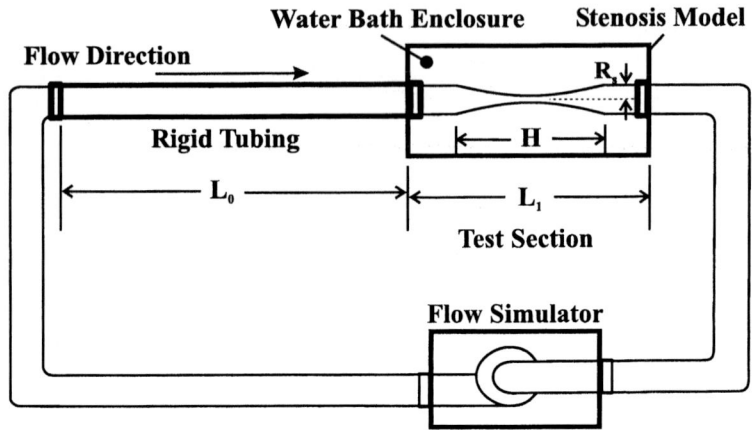

Fig. 3. Schematic diagram of the flow apparatus, including the test section, with major features of the flow loop used in the in vitro MR experiments. The flow simulator is a positive displacement pump with a computer-controlled system that can produce steady and pulsatile flows. Rigid tubing is placed upstream of the test section to ensure an undisturbed flow at the entrance of model. The water bath enclosure is a cylindrical reservoir that holds the model inside, and is used to satisfy the minimum load requirement of the scanner. The water bath enclosure sits inside a head coil during the MRI experiment. The replaceble concentric stenosis models are made from clear acrylic with different dimensions

4.2 MRI

After purging the system of air bubbles from the flow circuit shown in Fig. 3, a constant flow rate was driven through the flow system by a computer controlled UHDC flow simulator (Shelley Medical Imaging Technologies, London, Ontario, Canada). The working fluid employed was the Shelley blood mimicking fluid, which mimics the MR relaxation properties of the blood ($T_1 = 1300$ ms and $T_2 = 185$ ms at 1.5 Tesla). It has a viscosity of 0.00255 kg/(m.s) (2.55 centi-poise), slightly lower than the normal blood.

The test section was placed in a head coil inside a 1.5T MR imaging system (Magnetom Symphony, Siemens Medical Systems, Erlangen, Germany). Imaging parameters were as follows: slice orientation = coronal, number of slices = 1, slice thickness = 2.0 mm, in-plane pixel size = 0.1172 cm, flip angle = 20 degree, 7.1 ms < TE < 8.5 ms, TR = 40 ms, field of view = 300 mm, and number of signal averages = 32. V_{enc} was set to different values in the axial and radial directions. Its value depended upon the specific phantom and flow rate which is given in Table 1. Some typical images are shown in Fig. 4.

4.3 Experimental Results

Comparison with CFD To validate the pressures calculated with the non-iterative harmonics-based orthogonal projection method, the CFD code FLU-

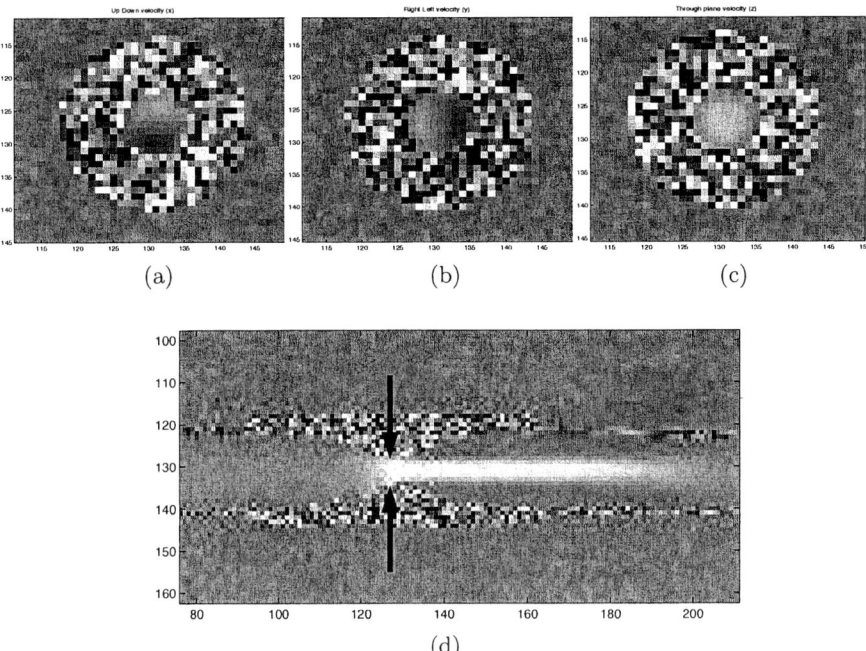

Fig. 4. Typical axial images of the three velocity components in the 90% area stenosis model. (a) u (right-left) encoded. (b) v (anterior-posterior) encoded. (c) w (superior-inferior) encoded. (d) Coronal image containing the axis of symmetry for the same model, displaying w (superior-inferior) encoded velocities. The axial images were acquired at the center of the stenosis

Table 1. In the in-vitro phantom experiments, V_{enc} (cm/s) was set to different values in the axial and the radial directions

Stenosis models	flow rate = 10ml/s		flow rate = 15ml/s		flow rate = 20ml/s	
	Radial	Axial	Radial	Axial	Radial	Axial
50%	4	12	4	18	5	22
75%	5	22	5	30	7	40
90%	7	50	11	70	16	90

ENT 6 (Fluent Inc., Lebanon, NH) was used to perform simulation for laminar, steady flow of a blood mimicking fluid (density 1.03 g/cm^3 and viscosity 2.5 centi-poise), in axisymmetric phantom geometries employed in PC-MRI experiments. FLUENT's output included velocity components as well as pressure maps. To validate PC-MRI based pressure calculations, the velocity field produced by FLUENT was used independently by our program to calculate pressure, $\tilde{\mathbf{P}}$, which was then compared with the pressure obtained from FLUENT, $\mathbf{P}_f$.

Table 2. RError of the AC component of pressure calculated with non-iterative harmonics-based orthogonal projection, $\tilde{\mathbf{P}}$, based on velocities simulated using FLUENT, when compared with pressure independently generated by FLUENT, $\mathbf{P}_f$

stenosis models	flow rate = 10ml/s	flow rate = 15ml/s	flow rate = 20ml/s
50%	3.24%	5.10%	6.31%
75%	4.12%	5.26%	5.95%
90%	6.79%	7.26%	7.53%

Table 3. CPU Time (in seconds) of the non-iterative harmonics-based orthogonal projection method when applied to the FLUENT simulated velocities, running on a SUN Ultra SPARC 10 workstation

stenosis models	flow rate = 10ml/s	flow rate = 15ml/s	flow rate = 20ml/s
50%	3.30	3.23	3.23
75%	4.25	4.23	3.25
90%	3.25	3.27	3.26

Table 4. RError of the AC component pressure calculated with iterative solution to Pressure-Poisson equation, based on the same velocities simulated by FLUENT, when compared with $\mathbf{P}_f$

stenosis models	flow rate = 10ml/s	flow rate = 15ml/s	flow rate = 20ml/s
50%	7.13%	4.29%	3.71%
75%	10.68%	10.60%	9.60%
90%	5.11%	7.55%	8.92%

To estimate error, a normalized error measure was adopted:

$$RError = \sqrt{\frac{\int_\Omega (\tilde{\mathbf{P}} - \mathbf{P}_f)^2 r dr dz}{\int_\Omega \mathbf{P}_f^2 r dr dz}} \tag{14}$$

The results are given in Table 2 and 3.

For comparison, the relative RMS error of pressures calculated with the iterative solution to pressure-Poisson equation discussed in [8] using the same input velocities is presented in Table 4. The CPU times for arriving at solutions are given in Table 5.

In these two tests, as well as in the following tests, the RErrors were measured between the AC component of the calculated pressures and the AC component of pressures independently generated by FLUENT; all DC components were omitted. The results are for the flow region from $z = $ -4 cm to $z = $ 18 cm ($z = 0$ is the center of the stenosis). The results indicate that on average, some gains in accuracy are obtained; however, computational times are dramatically reduced when using the proposed non-iterative harmonics-based orthogonal projection method.

Table 5. CPU Time (in seconds) of the iterative solution to pressure-Poisson equation when applied to the velocity data simulated with FLUENT, and running on the same workstation

stenosis models	flow rate = 10ml/s	flow rate = 15ml/s	flow rate = 20ml/s
50%	7.91	10.81	13.87
75%	7.18	5.93	5.82
90%	154.3	154.5	154.3

Table 6. Comparison of RErrors when using the non-iterative and iterative approach to pressure calculation from CFD velocity data corrupted by additive Gaussian noise for the case of 90% stenosis and flow rate = 20ml/s. For results in this table, a pre-filter was first applied to the velocity data before pressure calculation

σ_φ	RError of non-iterative method	RError of iterative method
0.02	15.41%	16.93%
0.04	15.29%	17.88%
0.06	15.84%	19.95%
0.08	17.01%	22.98%

Table 7. Comparison of RErrors when using the non-iterative and iterative approach to pressure calculation from CFD velocity data corrupted by additive Gaussian noise for the case of 90% stenosis and flow rate = 20ml/s. For results in this table, no filtering was performed before pressure calculation. N/A (Not Available) = the program did not converge

σ_φ	RError of non-iterative method	RError of iterative method
0.02	28.53%	119.98%
0.04	49.47%	299.72%
0.06	71.42%	N/A
0.08	95.15%	N/A

Effect of Noise. Since the pressure is computed based on Eq. (2), a nonlinear differential equation in velocity components, the noise on velocity plays an important role in accurate pressure computation.

In PC-MRI, velocity **u** is proportional to phase φ. According to [11], if both components of the acquired MR signal are Gaussian-distributed with variance σ^2, and SNR (signal to noise ratio) of the magnitude R is relatively large, noise on the phase φ can be well simulated by a Gaussian distribution with variance σ_φ^2. Then the noise on PC velocities is also Gaussian and its standard deviation is:

$$\sigma_v = \frac{V_{enc}}{\pi}\sigma_\varphi \quad (15)$$

Different values of σ_φ were used to add noise to the velocity field produced by FLUENT. In the first test, a pre-filter was adopted, and in the second test no filtering was performed. The tests were carried out on all nine combinations of the three models (50%, 75%, 90% stenosis) and three flow rates (10ml/s, 15ml/s, 20ml/s). In Tables 6 and 7 the results for 90% stenosis and flow rate at 20ml/s are given.

The results demonstrate that with weak noise, even without a pre-filter, the proposed non-iterative harmonics-based orthogonal projection method can still work, while the iterative solution to pressure-Poisson equation completely fails. In reality, we have observed that in most cases where there is significant noise, the iterative method will not even converge without a pre-filter.

It should be noted that the filter used here was not optimized. However, since the same filter was applied to velocities, the comparisons are valid.

In vitro Results. The pressure fields calculated from in-vitro PC-MR velocity data were compared with $\mathbf{P}_f$ independently obtained by FLUENT. The

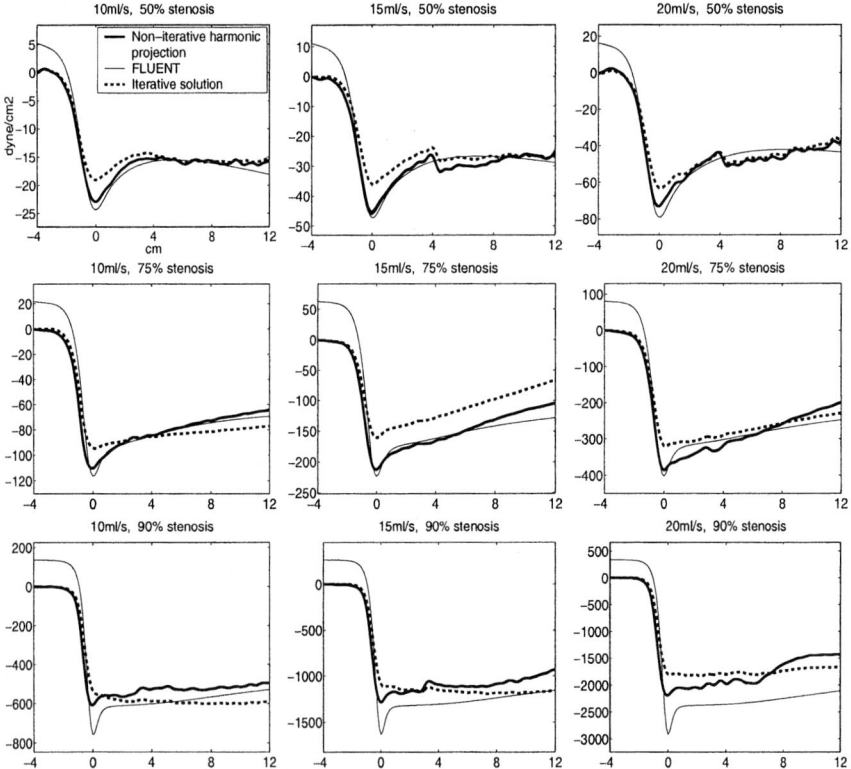

Fig. 5. Comparison of FLUENT generated pressures (thin lines) with those calculated with non-iterative harmonics-based orthogonal projection using PC-MR velocity data (thick lines) and iterative solution to Pressure-Poisson equation (dashed lines) also from the same PC-MR velocity data

Table 8. CPU Time (in seconds) of the non-iterative harmonics-based orthogonal projection method when applied to in-vitro PC-MR velocity data

stenosis models	flow rate = 10ml/s	flow rate = 15ml/s	flow rate = 20ml/s
50%	2.89	2.88	2.93
75%	2.62	2.64	2.67
90%	2.66	2.69	2.66

Table 9. CPU Time (in seconds) of the iterative solution to pressure-Poisson equation when applied to the same PC-MR velocity data

stenosis models	flow rate = 10ml/s	flow rate = 15ml/s	flow rate = 20ml/s
50%	40.21	76.97	26.94
75%	46.45	79.27	63.67
90%	60.63	155.65	95.92

comparisons of pressure along axis of symmetry are plotted in Fig. 5, and the CPU time for the computations are listed in Tables 8 and 9. For these tests, no filtering was performed before pressure calculations.

4.4 Discussion

If one compares the in-vitro results and the CFD validations, one concludes that the CPU time for the iterative solution to the pressure-Poisson equation is significantly higher than the proposed method. In fact, in the case of 90% stenosis phantom, the convergence rate of the iterative solution is far slower than in the other cases. The CPU time of the non-iterative harmonics-based orthogonal projection method is almost directly proportional to the size of the input data, whereas that of the iterative approach is determined primarily by noise level.

5 Conclusion

In this paper, a non-iterative harmonics-based orthogonal projection approach was proposed for pressure measurement from PC-MR velocity data in 3-D axisymmetric geometries. With validations performed on CFD simulated velocity data and PC-MRI velocity data, the method shows slight gain in accuracy in comparison to the iterative solution to pressure-Poisson equation. At the same time, it is much faster and is far less sensitive to noise (when using no pre-filter). It is expected that the gains in accuracy and compute time will be more substantial when dealing with 3-D geometries and pulsatile flows. This is the topic for current research.

Acknowledgements

We gratefully acknowledge Geoffrey Behrens who performed the FLUENT CFD simulations used in this paper. Chinese Scholarship Foundation (No. 2003842104) has funded Yuehuan Wang's visit to the CVIA lab. Support for the project was provided by BJH foundation and NSF grant IRI-9796207.

References

1. NJ Pelc, FG Sommer, KCP Li, TJ Brosnan, and DR Enzmann. Quantitative magnetic resonance flow imaging. *Magnetic Resonance Quarterly*, 10:125–147, 1994.
2. SN Urchuk, SE Fremes, and DB Plewes. In-vivo validations of MR pulse pressure measurement in an aortic flow model: preliminary results. *Magn. Res Med.*, 38:215–223, 1997.
3. GZ Yang, PJ Kilner, NB Wood, and SR Underwood. Computation of flow pressure fields from MR velocity mapping. *Magn Res Med*, 36:520–526, 1996.
4. JM Tyszka, DH Laidlaw, JW Asa, and JM Silverman. Three-dimensional time-resolved (4D) relative pressure mapping using MRI. *JMRI*, 12:321–329, 2000.
5. SM Song, RM Leahy, DP Boyd, BH Brundage, and S. Napel. Determining cardiac velocity fields and intraventricular pressure distribution from a sequence of ultrafast CT cardiac images. *IEEE Trans. on Medical Imaging*, 13:386–397, 1994.
6. T. Ebbers, L. Wigstrom, A. Bolger, J. Engvall, and M. Karlsson. Estimation of relative cardiovascular pressures using time-resolved three-dimensional phase-contrast MRI. *Magn Res Med.*, 45:872–879, 2001.
7. R. Thompson and E. McVeigh. Fast measurement of intracardiac pressure differences with 2D breath-hold PC MRI. *Magn Res Med.*, 49:1056–1066, 2003.
8. A.N. Moghaddam, G. Behrens, N. Fatouraee, R. Agarwal, E.T. Choi, and A.A. Amini. Factors affecting the accuracy of pressure measurements in vascular stenoses from phase-contrast MRI. *Magn Res Med.*, 52:300–309, 2004.
9. R. Frankot and R. Chellappa. A method for enforcing integrability in shape from shading algorithms. *IEEE Trans. on Pattern Analysis and Machine Intelligence*, 10(4):439–451, July 1988.
10. I. Currie. *Fundamental Mechanics of Fluids*. McGraw-Hill, New York, 1993.
11. H. Gudbjartsson and S. Paltz. The Rician distribution of noisy MRI data. *Magnetic Resonance in Medicine*, 34:910–914, June 1995.

Design of Robust Vascular Tree Matching: Validation on Liver

Arnaud Charnoz[1,3], Vincent Agnus[1], Grégoire Malandain[2], Stéphane Nicolau[1], Mohamed Tajine[3], and Luc Soler[1]

[1] IRCAD R&D, Strasbourg, France
[2] Epidaure Research group, INRIA, Sophia Antipolis, France
[3] LSIIT, CNRS/ULP, Strasbourg, France

Abstract. In this paper, we propose an original and efficient tree matching algorithm for intra-patient hepatic vascular system registration. Vascular systems are segmented from CT-scan images acquired at different times, and then modeled as trees. The goal of this algorithm is to find common bifurcations (nodes) and vessels (edges) in both trees.
   Starting from the tree root, edges and nodes are iteratively matched. The algorithm works on a set of match solutions that are updated to keep the best matches thanks to a quality criterion. It is robust against topological modifications due to segmentation failures and against strong deformations.
   Finally, this algorithm is validated on a large synthetic database containing cases with various deformation and segmentation problems.

1 Introduction

Motivations: Liver Tumors Follow-Up. The main purpose of our work is to make an intra-patient follow-up of tumors (see our previous work [3]). This approach is motivated by the fact that the liver is a highly deformable organ and that tumors evolution study needs the determination of this volumic deformation. Now it is well-known that the most reliable landmarks to estimate deformations sustained by the liver are provided by its vascular network [2, 6, 12, 7, 10].

Previous Works. Related works propose algorithms to match and/or register vascular systems (brain, liver and, in a similar manner, lung airways). Generally, veins are modeled as graphs computed from segmented images and skeletons [11]. Some authors use some tree structure notions in their algorithms to register a tree with an image [2] or two trees [6]. Other approaches really match structures (nodes and vessels), but use general graph matching methods [12, 7, 8] or specific methods like subtree isomorphism [10] which do not take segmentation problems into account.
   The oriented tree matching problem is more specific than graph matching because the structure is oriented and the path that connects two nodes is unique. Moreover, it cannot be considered as a oriented subtree isomorphism problem

because of segmentation problems. Indeed, the segmentation process can miss some vessels (edges). This implies a (virtual) pruning on both trees (for example an edge in a tree could be represented by several successive edges on the other tree) and thus the tree topology differs between acquisitions.

In our previous work [3], vascular systems are modeled as a tree and then tree vertices are matched together without taking possible segmentation errors into account. The previous algorithm works well on most branches but suffers from a lack of robustness in complex (but real) cases, especially on small branches where segmentation problems are important.

Proposal. The new algorithm proposed in this paper does not to focus on the best solution (given two edge sets to match) like in our previous algorithm but on the most likely solutions which are updated along the process. The remainder of this paper is organized as follows. The first part presents our iterative oriented tree matching. We describe how we generate solutions at each step of the tree according to local criteria, and how we select the most likely ones with a global quality criterion.

In the second part, an evaluation of our algorithm on large database shows that in standard cases (20% of pruning or less), our algorithm matches 90% of nodes and that even in worst, cases 75% of matches are correct.

2 A New Iterative Tree Matching Technique

Skeletons computed from segmented vascular systems can be represented as an oriented tree. Thus, the proposed algorithm is a tree matching. The orientation symbolizes blood circulation flow. Nodes represent bifurcations and edges correspond to vessels between two bifurcations. And in our algorithm, some geometric vessel attributes are used (3D positions, radius, vessel path).

Vascular trees segmented for a patient follow-up represent the same vascular system; our goal is to find common bifurcations and registering them. However, their topology and 3D positions may differ due to segmentation errors and deformations applied on them. The main challenge consists in using tree topology to detect deformations, and in parallel, geometric informations to detect topology problems. In the following, we assume that we work on standard patient case, thus that tree roots are known (detection of vascular system entrance) and that tree deformations are small.

In next sections, we explain our tree matching. Firstly, we focus on a global view of the algorithm framework. Then, we detail the solution creations and the quality criteria that select at each step the most likely solutions.

2.1 Notations

In this paper, we use the notions of oriented tree [1]. We work on a tree noted $T = (V, E, r)$ where V represents the set of vertices, $E \subset V \times V$ the set of edges and r the root. We note $\|T\|$ the number of vertices of T. For a node u in a tree T, $T(u)$ denotes the subtree of T induced from u. For a vertex v, $sons(v)$ denotes the set of their child vertices, $father(v)$ its father vertex, $out(v)$ the set of out-edges of v, and $in(v)$ its in-edge. For an oriented edge $e = (v, u)$, we define $src(e) = v$ and $tgt(e) = u$. For two vertices $v, w \in V$, $P(v, w)$ is the unique path in T linking v to w. Let e be an edge and v its target vertex, $DV_L(e) = \{u/u \in$ vertices of $T(v), \|P(v,u)\| \leq L\}$ denotes the descendant vertex set composed of L-first depth level vertices in subtree induced from e. For a vertex v, $T_+(v)$ denote the subtree $T(v)$ to which $father(v)$ is added to the vertex set and $in(v)$ to the edge set. More generally, A being a finite set, A^i is the ith element of A, and $|A| = card(A)$. So $A = \{A^i : 1 \leq i \leq |A|\}$. We introduce also some notations on functions. $\mathcal{B}_{A,B}^k$ is the set of bijections from subset of k elements of A to subset of k elements of B. For $f \in \mathcal{B}_{A,B}^k$, $D_f(A)$ (resp. $I_f(B)$) is the domain (resp. the image) of f. So $f(D_f(A)) = I_f(B)$ and $|D_f(A))| = |I_f(B)| = k$

2.2 Framework of the Algorithm

Our algorithm searches for the best tree matching between $T_1 = (V_1, E_1, r_1)$ and $T_2 = (V_2, E_2, r_2)$ starting from roots (r_1 match with r_2). Since possibilities are high, we propose to generate and select the most likely solutions. The algorithm starts by studying the root match and updates selected solutions when it explores and finds other possible matches in both trees. This means that some solutions selected at a process step can be eliminated later if they become unlikely. The likelihood of solutions is evaluated at each tree depth step with quality match criteria.

Our algorithm studies simultaneously N likely solutions $(S_i^0 \ldots S_i^N)$, i being the depth step. S_i^0 contains a set of matched vertices which descendant vertices are not studied yet. To continue building the final solution (all nodes analysed in both trees), the algorithm have to explore, one by one, these vertex matches. The exploration of one of them generates new solutions more complete noted S_{i+1}^j. Our algorithm progresses in solution exploration from S_i to S_{i+1}^j when a vertex match is analysed. Solutions are studied and developed simultaneously to be able to compare themselves.

In particular, the figure 1 shows the creation of the most likely solution S_1^i of the first tree depth step of process by exploring the root vertex match of the initial solution S_0. This figure details the constuction of match solutions from an initial vertex in S_0 (root match between r_1 and r_2). The first process step (1.a) consists in generating all out-edge match set hypotheses, noted HE^i (two hypotheses are shown among all: HE^A and HE^B). However, the number of solution is too high to be explored and a local quality criterion ($cost(HE^i)$) is computed to keep only the n best hypotheses (1.b). Then, we study each hypothesis to find next vertex match associated with an out-edge match. The figure shows the vertex match research of one out-edge match set $((a_1, a_2), (b_1, b_2))$ corresponding to the hypothesis HE^A.

The second process step (2.a) consists in generating path match hypotheses, noted $^nHP^i$, from the nth out-edge match (for instance, two hypotheses are shown, $^1HP^1$ and $^1HP^2$ corresponding to the first out-edge match (a_1, a_2)).

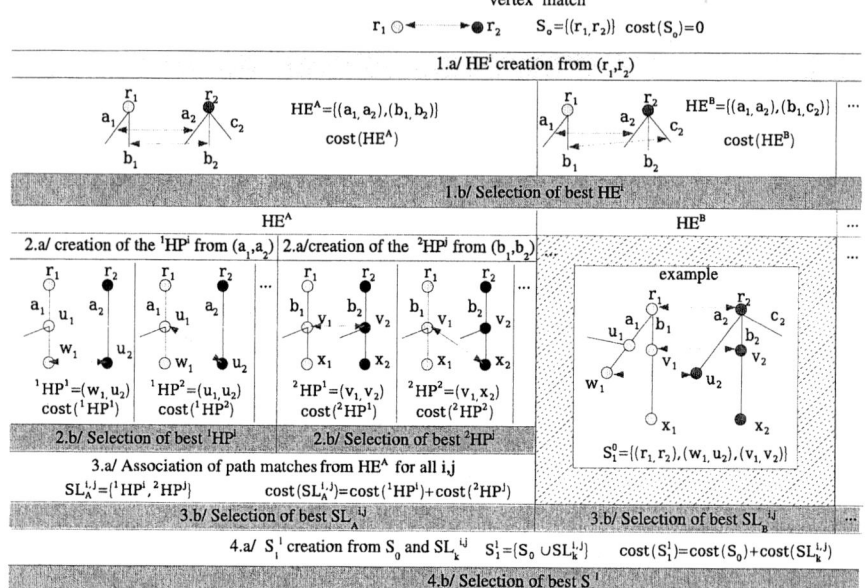

Fig. 1. This figure details the constuction of solutions on a tree depth step

Once again, the number of solution is too high to be explored and a local quality criterion ($cost(^1HP^i)$) is computed to keep only the m best hypotheses (2.b). When the algorithm finishes to compute all best path match hypotheses for each out-edge match, we test all possible permutations and reassemble them (3.a) in local solutions noted $SL_k^{i,j}$ where k is the kth out-edge match set hypothesis, i and j the path match chosen for the first out-edge matches. Once again, only the best of them are selected (3.b). In (4.a) and (4.b), we build and select all best solutions resulting of different out-edge matches set hypotheses and path match hypotheses. A global solution example possible is shown on the right in the figure and is noted S_1^0. The algorithm restart this process from one of vertex matches included in different solutions S_1^l.

In next subsections, we detail how we generate out-edge match set hypotheses and path match hypotheses and how we select the best most likely one using either local or global quality criterion.

2.3 Hypothesis Generation

Step I: Out-Edge Match Set Hypothesis. This step consists in generating out-edge match possibilities from a vertex match, noted (v_1, v_2), to continue the match of $T_1(v_1)$ and $T_2(v_2)$. Two possiblilities are shown on figure 2. Let $O_1 = out(v_1)$ and $O_2 = out(v_2)$. An out-edge match set hypothesis is noted $\mathcal{HE}(v_1, v_2)$. An hypothesis $\mathcal{HE}^i(v_1, v_2)$ is represented by an out-edge match set $\mathcal{E}_f(v_1, v_2)$ which characterizes a match between k elements of O_1 with k elements

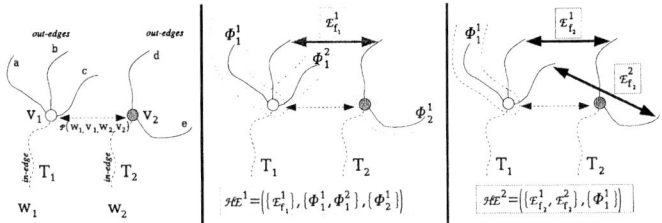

Fig. 2. Illllustration of a creation of out-edge match set hypotheses from a vertex match. The left figure resumes the vertices match between v_1 and v_2. The others show two possible solutions, in which an out-edge match set is chosen for each solution ($\{\mathcal{E}_{f_1}^1\}$ for $\mathcal{H}E^1$ and $\{\mathcal{E}_{f_2}^1, \mathcal{E}_{f_2}^2\}$ for $\mathcal{H}E^2$). Hypotheses suppose that some out-edges do not have their equivalent in other trees and thus that the corresponding subtree is not matched ($\{\phi_1^1, \phi_1^2, \phi_2^1\}$ for $\mathcal{H}E^1$ and $\{\phi_1^1\}$ for $\mathcal{H}E^2$)

of O_2. $\mathcal{E}_f(v_1, v_2) = \{(e, f(e))/e \in D_f(O_1), f \in \mathcal{B}_{O_1,O_2}^k\}$. This out-edge match set assumes implicitly that some out-edges of O_1 (respectively O_2) noted $D_f(O_1)^c$ (respectively $I_f(O_2)^c$) have no association. Thus, some subtrees have no match in the other tree. A cost will be attributed to them to be able to compare hypotheses with or without lost subtrees. Thus these lost subtrees must be retained in the solution (this was deliberately omitted in the figure 1 explications for clarity reason). Let $\phi(v, OE) = \{T_+(u)/\forall(v,u) \in OE\}$ be the subtree induced by a vertex and a subset OE of its out-edges. We note $O_{min} = min(|O_1|, |O_2|)$, then possible hypotheses are given by:

$$\mathcal{H}E(v_1, v_2) = \bigcup_{k=0\ldots O_{min}} \bigcup_{f \in \mathcal{B}_{O_1,O_2}^k} \{(\mathcal{E}_f(v_1, v_2), \phi(v_1, D_f(O_1)^c), \phi(v_2, I_f(O_2)^c)\}$$

Step II: Path Match Hypothesis. This step consists in generating path match possiblilities from an out-edge match, noted (e_1, e_2). Tree possiblilities are shown on figure 3. We assume that an edge $e_1 \in O_1$ and an edge $e_2 \in O_2$ match (representing the same starting vessel). the algorithm must find the next common bifurcation in subtrees $T_1(tgt(e_1))$ and $T_2(tgt(e_2))$ closest to v_1 and v_2. Due to segmentation defects, $tgt(e_1)$ and $tgt(e_2)$ do not necessarily represent the same bifurcation (this case happens frequently when branches are small). We search a vertex match in subtrees and not only between $tgt(e_1)$ and $tgt(e_2)$ (Fig. 3).

The research of next vertex match is restricted on the L first level of subtrees $T_1(tgt(e_1))$ and $T_2(tgt(e_2))$. Thus, we search the best vertex match between $DV_L(e_1)$ and $DV_L(e_2)$. In our algorithm, L is empirically choosen and is generally fixed 3.

Now, let (w_1, w_2) be a vertex match with $w_1 \in DV_L(e_1)$ and $w_2 \in DV_L(e_2)$. w_1 does not necessarily equal $tgt(e_1)$ and this vertex match defines a path match $\mathcal{P}(v_1, w_1, v_2, w_2) = (P(v_1, w_1), P(v_2, w_2))$. This match of pathes implies that some subtrees starting from them are not matched. We note this forest of no

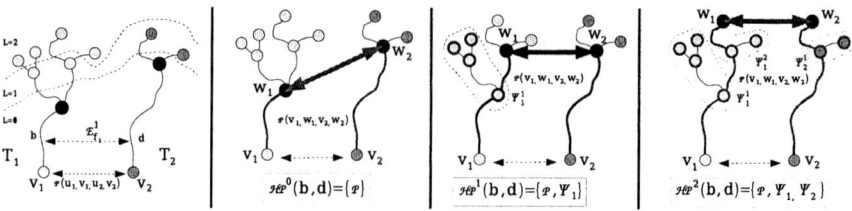

Fig. 3. Figures show the creation of path match hypotheses from an out-edge match. The different depths L are shown on the left figure and three solutions are illustrated

match subtrees $\psi(v,w) = \{T_+(u), u \in sons(k), k \in V_P, T_+(u) \cap P(v,w) = \{k\}\}$ where $V_P = \{\text{vertices of } P(v,w)\}\setminus\{v,w\}$. if we note $v_1 = src(e_1)$ and $v_2 = src(e_2)$, the set of possible path matches is defined as:

$$\mathcal{HP}(e_1, e_2) = \bigcup_{w_1 \in DV_L(e_1)} \bigcup_{w_2 \in DV_L(e_2)} \{\mathcal{P}(v_1, w_1, v_2, w_2), \psi(v_1, w_1), \psi(v_2, w_2)\}$$

2.4 Hypotheses Selection

In the previous section, we have seen how to generate all out-edge match set hypotheses and path match hypotheses. matches. However, all possible tree matching solutions cannot be explored due to huge combinatorial possibilities: Selections must be made.

Therefore some cost functions are computed to determine the quality of matches. In our algorithm, two types of cost are computed: a global cost to determine the solution quality $S_i(cost(S_i))$, and two local costs to determine the quality of each out-edge match set hypothesis $\mathcal{HE}^i$ and each path match hypotheses $\mathcal{HP}^i$ (Fig. 1). We give here general expression of the cost functions. Each term of these cost functions are detailed in the next paragraph.

We define the two following local costs that select the most likely $\mathcal{HE}^i$ and the most likely $\mathcal{HP}^i$.

$$cost(\mathcal{HE}^i(v_1, v_2)) = \sum_{j=1}^{N_1} cost(\mathcal{E}_f^j(v_1, v_2)) + \sum_{j=1}^{N_2} cost(\phi^j(v_1, D_f(O_1)^c))$$
$$+ \sum_{j=1}^{N_3} cost(\phi^j(v_2, I_f(O_2)^c))$$
$$cost(\mathcal{HP}^i(e_1, e_2)) = cost(\mathcal{P}(v_1, w_1, v_2, , w_2)) + \sum_{j=1}^{N_4} cost(\psi^j(v_1, w_1))$$
$$+ \sum_{j=1}^{N_5} cost(\psi^j(v_2, w_2))$$

The global cost expression selects the most likely solutions S_i. If algorithm explores a vertex match (v_1, v_2) of a current solution S_i, we obtain new solutions S_{i+1}^l (for example $S_{i+1}^l = S_i \bigcup_{e \in D_f(O_1)} \mathcal{HP}^T(e, f(e))$ where T is different for each out-edge match). S_{i+1}^l is caracterised by an out-edge match set from v_1 and v_2 and a path match for each out-edge match. The value of solution cost is given by:

$$\text{cost}(S^l_{i+1}) = \sum_{e \in D_f(O_1)} \text{cost}(\mathcal{H}P^T(e, f(e)) + \sum_{j=1}^{N_2} \text{cost}(\phi^j(v_1, D_f(O_1)^c))$$
$$+ \sum_{j=1}^{N_3} \text{cost}(\phi^j(v_2, I_f(O_2)^c)) + \text{cost}(S_i)$$

In these equations, N_i represents the different set cardinals. Note that there are three kinds of costs: a cost between two out-edges, a cost between two paths and a cost for subtrees which have no correspondence in the other tree.

Physical Cost Used: We define here the basic functions that allow to compare the geometric properties of match solutions (vertex or edge). The cost C_E represents the distance between extremity edges, C_R represents the radius difference along edges (vessels), C_{OE} represents the difference between the out-edges number from each extremity edge, C_S represents the scale between edges and C_A represents the angle between edges. These costs are normalized thanks to a truncated quadratic robust estimator ρ and its empirically chosen parameter α [5]. The perfect match is symbolised by a zero cost.

We remind that an edge e represents a vessel between two bifurcations. In the following cost formulas, $e(t)$ is the 3D parametric curve representation of the vessel, $r(t)$ represents the vessel's radius along the curve and l is the curve's length. Thus by default, $e(t)$ (respectively $r(t)$) is defined between $t \in [0, l]$ where $e(0)$ and $e(l)$ represent the vessel extremities. We note $\mathbf{e}$ the vector between two points $e(0)$ and $e(l)$. For each cost comparison between e_1 and e_2, we supposed that $e_1(0) = e_2(0)$.

$$C_E(e_1, e_2) = \rho(\|e_1(l_1) - e_2(l_2)\|, \alpha_E)$$

$$C_R(e_1, e_2) = \rho\left(\int_0^1 \|r_1(s \times l_1) - r_2(s \times l_2)\| ds, \alpha_R\right)$$

$$C_S(e_1, e_2) = \rho\left(1 - \frac{l_1}{l_2}, \alpha_S\right), \quad \text{if } l_1 < l_2$$

$$C_A(e_1, e_2) = \rho\left(1 - \frac{\|\mathbf{e_1} \cdot \mathbf{e_2}\|}{\|\mathbf{e_1}\| \|\mathbf{e_2}\|}, \alpha_A\right)$$

$$\rho(v, \alpha) = \begin{cases} \left(\frac{v}{\alpha}\right)^2 & \text{if } |v| < |\alpha| \\ 1 \end{cases}$$

Out Edge Match Cost: $\text{cost}(\mathcal{E}^i_f(v_1, v_2))$ compare edge orientation and radius.

$$\text{cost}(\mathcal{E}^i_f(v_1, v_2)) = \frac{1}{\gamma_1 + \gamma_2}(\gamma_1 C_A(e'_1, e'_2) + \gamma_2 C_R(e'_1, e'_2))$$

with $e'_1(t)$ (respectively $e'_2(t)$) is $e_1(t)$ ($e_2(t)$) defined on $[0, \min(l_1, l_2)]$ and where γ_1 and γ_2 are weights used to favor robust characteristics in the algorithm.

Path Match Cost: In $cost(\mathcal{P}(v_1, w_1, v_2, w_2))$, weights are added to favor path matches with same small length, same orientation and same vessel radius and vessel extremities.

$$cost(\mathcal{P}(v_1, v_2, w_1, w_2)) = \frac{1}{\beta_1 + \ldots + \beta_4}(\beta_1 C_A(e_1, e_2) + \beta_2 C_R(e_1, e_2) + \beta_3 C_S(e_1, e_2) + \beta_4 C_E(e_1, e_2)) + \min_i cost(\mathcal{H}E^i(w_1, w_2))$$

with $e_1 = P(v_1, w_1)$ and $e_2 = P(v_2, w_2)$. This cost is composed of a local cost representing the current edge comparison and the cost of the next best out-edge matches from current extremity edges. This last term allows the algorithm to be more efficient and robust because an information is added on the vessel extremity similarity.

No Match Tree Cost: We have previously considered a cost for no inclusion subtrees in the match solution represented by $\phi^i(u, E)$ and $\psi^j(u, w)$. Each subtree $T_+(v)$ is defined by a vertex v. Cost computation is the same in both cases and is noted $costLost(v)$. We highlight that choosing the weight of this cost is difficult and depends on other match costs. If this cost is too high, then all nodes are matched (we forbid a subtree lost and then the algorithm is not robust against segmentation problem). Conversely, if it is too low, the algorithm does not select matches (the algorithm looses all branches). Hence a minimum cost $cost_{min}$ is introduced.

$$costLost(v) = R'(v) + \sum_{w_k \in sons(v)} costLost(w_k)$$

with: $R(v) = \frac{1}{\mu_1 + \mu_2}(\mu_1 \frac{\|T(v)\|}{\|T\|} + \mu_2 \int_0^1 \|r(s) - R_{min}\| ds)$
$R'(v) = \max(R(v), cost_{min})$

the constant R_{min} corresponds to minimum radius to detect vessels in images. This cost is composed of two terms, the first one give us an information on the subtree surface to avoid loosing big subtree, the second one is an information on vesssel radius to avoid loosing large vessel (vessels with large radius are not concerned by segmentation problem and thus can be found in the other tree)

3 Experiments and Validation

3.1 Virtual Patient Creations

To test and validate our algorithm, we have worked on a liver and its hepatic vascular system. To work on a complex vascular system (380 nodes), the Visible Man (cf. The Visible Human Project of NLM) has been segmented. The matching is harder (more bifurcations) than for a real patient case. This leads to better tests to evaluate the algorithm robustness.

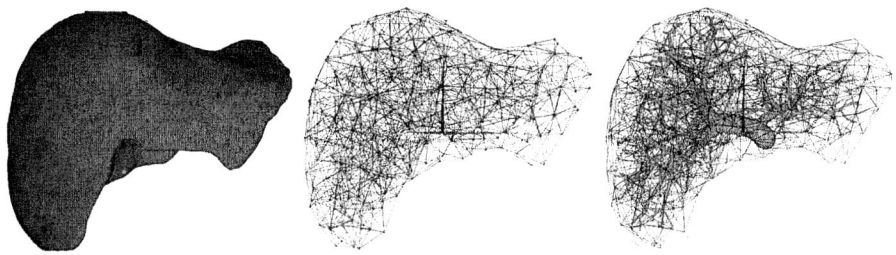

Fig. 4. The surgery simulator prototype is used to simulate liver and vascular system deformations thanks to a volumic model. [**Left**] Surfacic model [**Center**] Volumic model [**Right**] Volumic model and portal vascular system

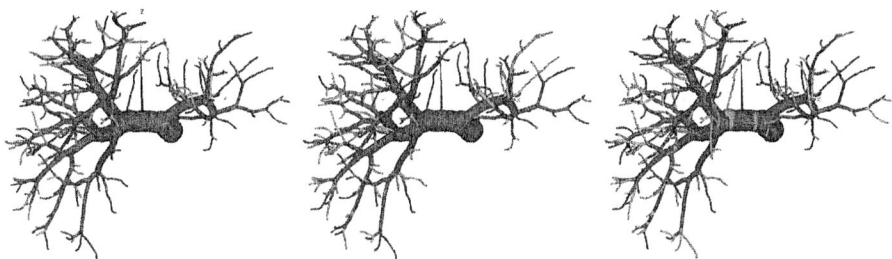

Fig. 5. The visible Man's portal vascular system is randomly pruned to loose approximately 20%, 30% and 40% of length in both trees. Lost branches appear in green

To simulate deformations, we have used the minimally invasive hepatic surgery simulator prototype developed at INRIA [9]. The goal of this simulator is to provide a realistic training framework to learn laparoscopic gestures. For this paper, we used it only to simulate deformations of the liver and its vascular system (Fig. 4). This simulator uses complex biomechanical models, based on linear elasticity and finite element theory, which include anisotropic deformations.

To simulate segmentation errors on our phantom, we have pruned random tree branches. The probability to loose small vessels is greater than to loose large ones (Fig. 5).

To test the algorithm, a database of 600 patient follow-up cases has been generated from 2 types of deformations : a small (mean distance between commun points = 9 mm) and a strong (30mm) and 5 pruning steps (0,10,20,30,40 %) with on each step, 20 randomly generated prunings (Tab. 1 and 2).

3.2 Results on a Virtual Patient

Algorithm parameters have been chosen and fixed empirically to work more efficiently on all these cases. These paramater choices and their different consequences on the algorithm process (error, robustness, procesus time) are not detailed here but in a future journal paper.

Table 1. Matching results with a small deformation: Each line represents a pruning configuration with 20 randomly computed cases. Each column shows the mean result of these 20 cases with their magnitude. Three results are shown : the number of common nodes (match number in the reference solution) between both pruned trees, the sensitivity which is the number of correct found matches among the number of solutions matches and the efficiency which is the number of correct found matches among the number of found matches (correct and uncorrect)

% T_1 pruning	% T_2 pruning	common nodes	% sensitivity	% efficiency
0	0	380 ± 0	100 ± 0	100 ± 0
0	10	314 ± 7	98,7 ± 0,8	98,9 ± 0,7
0	20	242 ± 8	96,2 ± 3,1	97,5 ± 0,7
0	30	189 ± 7	92,1 ± 5,2	94,9 ± 1,5
0	40	144 ± 3	84,0 ± 5,8	90,9 ± 2,5
10	10	260 ± 9	98,5 ± 0,7	97,8 ± 1,1
10	20	203 ± 7	97,4 ± 1,0	94,7 ± 1,3
10	30	164 ± 6	94,9 ± 2,5	93,0 ± 1,5
10	40	128 ± 6	90,5 ± 6,4	89,7 ± 4,9
20	20	169 ± 8	96,2 ± 1,8	92,8 ± 1,0
20	30	135 ± 10	96,2 ± 1,7	89,9 ± 1,6
20	40	108 ± 6	90,3 ± 6,9	85,4 ± 3,3
30	30	115 ± 7	94,3 ± 3,6	87,0 ± 2,6
30	40	90 ± 6	90,8 ± 6,5	82,6 ± 3,5
40	40	71 ± 6	93,5 ± 3,2	79,5 ± 3,8

The process is fast (about 10 minutes to register 380 nodes on 1GHz PC). Two process results are shown (Fig. 6) for a small and a strong deformation and pruned to loose approximately 20% of surface branches in both trees. Tab. 1 and 2 show that on small deformations the algorithm is very robust (practically all possible matches with a small standard deviation were found in the different cases) even with large pruning. With strong deformations and large pruning, the process is less robust (around 80%).

Results are reported in terms only of node identification. In fact, the consequences of performing an incorrect connection may be much larger in a proximal branch than peripherally. However, we noticed that most of the match errors (incorrect node correspondences and lost branches) are localized on terminal edges. On these nodes, the algorithm suffers from a lack of information (no subtree, dense node concentrations, small vessels). This makes the matching task harder.

To conclude, deformations and prunings (20% or less) used for these tests correspond with standard observed real cases. For this values, experts consider our algorithm efficient (sensitivity and similarity greater than 90%) to find a good approximation of the 3D liver deformation.

Table 2. Matching results with a strong deformation: see description Tab. 1. The standart deviation of cases (0-30%) and (0-40%) is very high. Our algorithm attains its limits when we have a great difference between pruning (topology of trees become very different) associated with a strong deformation. These configuration cases occurre infrequently

% T_1 pruning	% T_2 pruning	common nodes	% sensitivity	% efficiency
0	0	380 ± 0	100 ± 0	100 ± 0
0	10	311 ± 9	97,7 ± 1,0	98,7 ± 0,6
0	20	246 ± 6	94,4 ± 0,8	95,8 ± 0,8
0	30	195 ± 10	75,1 ± 37,3	76,9 ± 35,1
0	40	147 ± 6	69,6 ± 34,5	72,3 ± 32,7
10	10	257 ± 6	95,7 ± 1,8	96,0 ± 1,3
10	20	206 ± 5	93,0 ± 2,7	92,5 ± 1,3
10	30	162 ± 7	92,9 ± 2,2	91,4 ± 1,7
10	40	128 ± 7	88,2 ± 4,5	86,5 ± 3,0
20	20	169 ± 7	92,9 ± 4,2	91,3 ± 1,1
20	30	138 ± 7	90,3 ± 4,8	87,6 ± 2,6
20	40	109 ± 6	88,9 ± 5,4	85,6 ± 2,6
30	30	114 ± 7	90,0 ± 7,3	85,6 ± 2,0
30	40	93 ± 6	91,6 ± 2,5	82,9 ± 3,6
40	40	73 ± 4	87,7 ± 5,8	78,0 ± 4,4

4 Conclusion

The purpose of this paper was to present the design of our original new robust method to match liver vascular systems between two CT/NRI acquisitions. This method is well adapted, fast and robust on a complex vascular system. Thanks to the virtual database generated by the INRIA simulator, we have tested numerous configurations.

Currently, we are working on the second step of tumor follow-up: the estimation of liver deformation computed from the vascular system matching. In parallel, we have started first tests on a real patient database with very encouraging results (Fig. 7). These results will be detailed in a future paper.

Then, we will validate our works with surgeons on a real patient database with the collaboration of the Strasbourg hospital and also propose a new tool for automatic diagnosis of tumor evolution in the liver.

Acknowledgments. We thank the Strasbourg hospital and their surgeons for providing images as well as their advice on "standard" deformations applied on the liver. This work has benefited from the segmentation program of the vascular system developed by the IRCAD R&D team. The realistic liver deformations are provided by the INRIA simulator from the Epidaure project. Many thanks to Clément Forest [4] for his assistance during the use of the simulator.

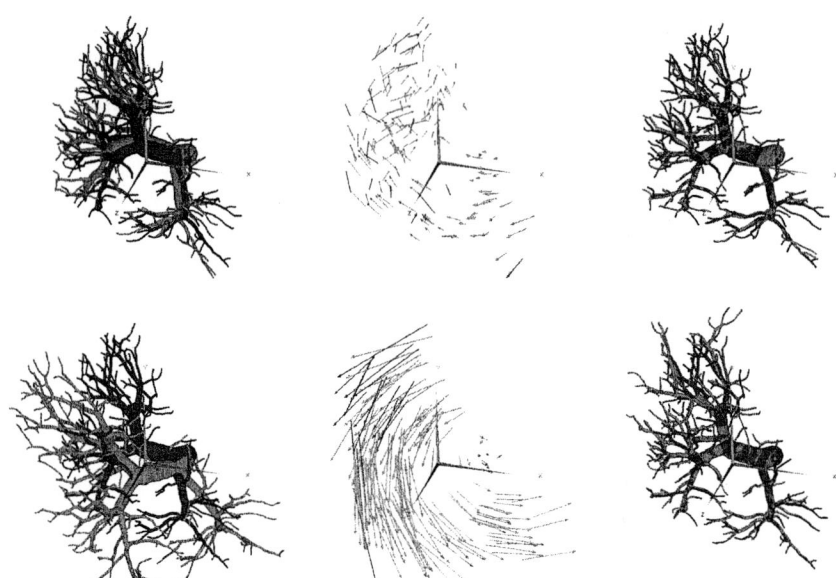

Fig. 6. [**Top**] On the left, small deformation case is pruned at 20%. The center figure shows the result of our oriented tree matching, good matches are represented by green arrows and represent 95% of all nodes and wrong matches by red arrows. The right figure shows the tree registration after the process. [**Bottom**] A strong deformation with an equivalent pruning where the algorithm find 91% of all nodes

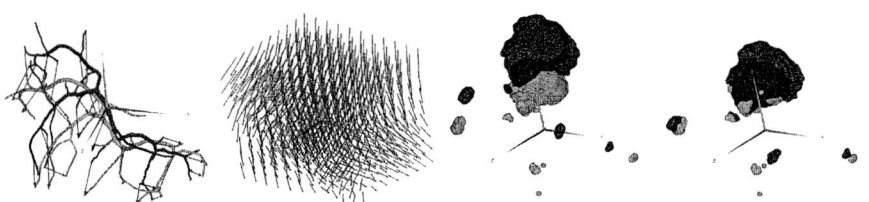

Fig. 7. [a]Real patient where the vascular system has been matched where vertex matches are shown in red. [b]Deformation field computed from matches. [c,d]Tumors before and after registration

References

1. *The Design and Analysis of Computer Algorithms.* Addison-Wesley, 1974.
2. S.R. Aylward, J. Jomier, S. Weeks, and E. Bullitt. Registration and analysis of vascular images. *IJCV*, 55(2-3):123–138, 2003.
3. A. Charnoz, V. Agnus, and L. Soler. Portal vein registration for the follow-up of hepatic tumours. In *MICCAI*, volume 3217 of *LNCS*, pages 878–886, Saint-Malo, France, September 2004. Springer Verlag.

4. C. Forest, H. Delingette, and N. Ayache. Surface contact and reaction force models for laparoscopic simulation. In *International Symposium on Medical Simulation*, June 2004.
5. F. R. Hampel, E. M. Ronchetti, P. J. Rousseeuw, and W. A. Stahel. Robust statistics. In *John Wiley and Sons*, New York, 1986.
6. T. Lange, S. Eulenstein, M. Hunerbein, H. Lamecker, and P.-M Schlag. Augmenting intraoperative 3d ultrasound with preoperative models for navigation in liver surgery. In *MICCAI*, volume 3217 of *LNCS*, pages 534–541, Saint-Malo, France, September 2004. Springer Verlag.
7. Y. Park. *Registration of linear structures in 3-D medical images*. PhD thesis, Osaka University, Japan. Departement of informatics and Mathematical Science, 2002.
8. M. Pelillo, K. Siddiqi, and S.W. Zucker. Matching hierarchical structures using association graphs. *PAMI*, 21:1105–1120, November 1999.
9. G. Picinbono, J-C. Lombardo, H. Delingette, and N. Ayache. Improving realism of a surgery simulator: linear anisotropic elasticity, complex interactions and force extrapolation. *JVCA*, 13(3):147–167, jully 2002.
10. C. Pisupati, L. Wolff, W. Mitzner, and E. Zerhouni. Tracking 3-d pulmonary tree structures. In *MMBIA*, page 160. IEEE Computer Society, 1996.
11. L. Soler, H. Delingette, G. Malandain, J. Montagnat, N. Ayache, J.-M. Clément, C. Koehl, O. Dourthe, D. Mutter, and J. Marescaux. A fully automatic anatomical, pathological and fonctionnal segmentation from CT-scans for hepatic surgery. In *Medical Imaging*, SPIE proceedings, pages 246–255, San Diego, February 2000.
12. J. Tschirren, K. Palágyi, J.M. Reinhardt, E.A. Hoffman, and M. Sonka. Segmentation, Skeletonization, and Branchpoint Matching - A Fully Automated Quantitative Evaluation of Human Intrathoracic Airway Trees. In *MICCAI*, volume 2489 of *LNCS*, pages 12–19. Springer-Verlag, 25 September 2002.

A Novel Parametric Method for Non-rigid Image Registration

Anne Cuzol, Pierre Hellier, and Etienne Mémin

IRISA, Université de Rennes 1 - INRIA,
Campus de Beaulieu,
35 042 Rennes Cedex, France
{acuzol, phellier, memin}@irisa.fr

Abstract. This paper presents a novel non-rigid registration method. The main contribution of the method is the modeling of the vorticity (respectively divergence) of the deformation field using vortex (respectively sink and source) particles. Two parameters are associated with a particle: the vorticity (or divergence) strength and the influence domain. This leads to a very compact representation of vorticity and divergence fields. In addition, the optimal position of these particles is determined using a mean shift process. $2D$ experiments of this method are presented and demonstrate its ability to recover evolving phenomena (MS lesions) so as to register images from 20 patients.

1 Introduction

Non-rigid image registration is the process of estimating a non-linear geometric transformation that puts two images into correspondence. Beyond rigid transformations, non-rigid registration is needed when deformable phenomena are observed. Application field of non-rigid registration are numerous: motion computation of beating organs (heart), estimation of inter-subject anatomical variability (construction of anatomical atlases), monitoring of changes over time (evolving lesions in multiple sclerosis disease), *etc.*

This is a very active field of research and numerous methods have been proposed so far. We refer the reader for comprehensive surveys on this area [5, 7, 10, 11].

Non-rigid registration methods based on image luminance can usually be classified according to the image similarity and the deformation field regularization. Most often, methods tend to regularize deformation fields using a Gaussian regularization (demon's), a first-order or second-order regularization (penalization of the deformation discontinuities) or a intrinsically regularized deformation model (B-splines deformation fields for instance). These regularizations amount to zeroing the vorticity and divergence of the deformation field. These two variables are related to the first-order derivatives of the deformation field indeed.

However, matter apparition or dissipation lead to a divergent field, therefore we think that this information needs to be accurately estimated in case of monitoring anatomical changes over time. This paper presents an original $2D$ registration method that overcomes this difficulty. We rely on vortex and source particles to model the deformation field.

2 Definitions and Properties of Vector Fields

In this section, we present first known analytic results on planar vector fields. We shall rely on them to develop an original method for fluid motion estimation.

A two-dimensional vector field w is a $\mathbb{R}^2$-valued map defined on a bounded set Ω of $\mathbb{R}^2$. We denote it $\mathbf{w}(\mathbf{x}) = (u(\mathbf{x}), v(\mathbf{x}))^T$, where $\mathbf{x} = (x, y)$ and x and y are the spatial coordinates. Each component of the vector field will be supposed twice continuously differentiable: $u, v \in C^2(\Omega, \mathbb{R})$.

Noting $\nabla = (\frac{\partial}{\partial x}, \frac{\partial}{\partial y})$ the operator whose components are the partial derivatives with respect to the coordinates x and y, we define the *divergence*: div $\mathbf{w} = \frac{\partial u}{\partial x} + \frac{\partial v}{\partial y} = \nabla.\mathbf{w}$ and the scalar *vorticity* of the vector field: curl $\mathbf{w} = \frac{\partial u}{\partial y} - \frac{\partial v}{\partial x} = \nabla.\mathbf{w}^\perp$, where $\mathbf{w}^\perp = (-v, u)$ is the orthogonal counterpart of w.

The vorticity accounts for the presence of a rotating motion, while the divergence is related to the presence of *sinks* or *sources* in the flow. A vector field whose divergence is null at every point is called *solenoidal*. Similarly, a field with zero vorticity will be called *irrotational*. It is well known that for irrotational fields there exists a scalar function ϕ, called the *velocity potential*, such that $\mathbf{w} = \nabla \phi$. Similarly, for solenoidal fields there exists a scalar function ψ called the *stream function* such that $\mathbf{w}^\perp = \nabla \psi$.

Any continuous vector field that vanishes at infinity can be decomposed into a sum of an irrotational component with null vorticity and a solenoidal component with null divergence. This is called the *Helmholtz Decomposition*. When the null border condition can not be imposed, an additional component, named the *laminar* component, which is both irrotational and solenoidal, has to be included. The decomposition reads then: $\mathbf{w} = \mathbf{w}_{irr} + \mathbf{w}_{sol} + \mathbf{w}_{lam}$. In practice, an affine registration (by maximization of mutual information [6]) is performed first, so that we can assume a null border condition at infinity.

Substituting the two components $\mathbf{w}_{irr}$ and $\mathbf{w}_{sol}$ by their expressions in terms of potential functions and considering the divergence and the curl of the motion field enables to write the potential function as solution of two Poisson equations:

$$\Delta \phi = \text{div} \mathbf{w}_{irr} \quad \text{and} \quad \Delta \psi = -\text{curl} \mathbf{w}_{sol}, \qquad (1)$$

where Δ denotes the Laplacian operator. These solutions may be expressed as convolution products:

$$\phi = \int G(\mathbf{x} - \mathbf{u}) \text{div } \mathbf{w}_{irr}(\mathbf{u}) d\mathbf{u} = G \otimes \text{div } \mathbf{w}_{irr}, \qquad (2)$$

$$\psi = -\int G(\mathbf{x} - \mathbf{u}) \text{curl } \mathbf{w}_{sol}(\mathbf{u}) d\mathbf{u} = -G \otimes \text{curl } \mathbf{w}_{sol}, \qquad (3)$$

where G is the Green's function associated to the two-dimensional Laplacian:

$$G(\mathbf{x}) = \frac{1}{2\pi} \ln(|\mathbf{x}|). \qquad (4)$$

As the vector fields $\mathbf{w}_{irr}$ and $\mathbf{w}_{sol}$ are respectively the gradient and the orthogonal gradient of the potential functions ϕ and ψ, equation (2-3) may be rewritten as:

$$\mathbf{w}_{irr} = K \otimes \text{div } \mathbf{w}_{irr} \text{ and } \mathbf{w}_{sol} = -K^\perp \otimes \text{curl } \mathbf{w}_{sol}, \qquad (5)$$

where K denotes the gradient of the Green kernel. The second equation of (5) is known as the *Bio-Savart* integral. These two equations state that the solenoidal and the irrotational components (and consequently the whole vector field) may be recovered through a convolution product knowing the divergence and the vorticity of the velocity field.

3 Vortex Particles

The idea of vortex particles methods [1,4] consists in approximating the vorticity of a field w by a discrete sum of delta functions located at *point vortices* z_i:

$$\text{curl } \mathbf{w}(\mathbf{x}) \approx \sum_{i=0}^{n} \gamma_i \delta(\mathbf{x} - \mathbf{z}_i), \tag{6}$$

with δ denotes the Dirac measure.

This discretization of the vorticity into a limited number of elements enables to evaluate the velocity field directly from the Bio-Savart integral (equ. 5). Due to the singularity of the Green kernel gradient, K, the induced field develops $\frac{1}{r}$-type singularities, where r is the distance to the point vortices.

These singularities can be removed by smoothing the Dirac measure with a *cutt-off* or *blob* function, leading to a smoothed version of K. Let f_ϵ be such a blob function scaled by a parameter ϵ: $f_\epsilon(\mathbf{x}) = \frac{1}{\epsilon^2} f(\frac{\mathbf{x}}{\epsilon})$. The smoothed kernel is defined as $K_\epsilon = K \otimes f_\epsilon$. The amount of smoothing is determined by the value of ϵ. If $\epsilon \to 0$, f_ϵ tends to the Dirac function and $K_\epsilon \to K$.

In the same way, for the divergence map a *source* particles representation reads then:

$$\text{div } \mathbf{w}(\mathbf{x}) \approx \sum_{i=0}^{n} \gamma_i f_{\epsilon_i}(\mathbf{x} - \mathbf{z}_i), \tag{7}$$

where z_i denotes the center of each basis function f_{ϵ_i}, the coefficient γ_i is the strength associated to the particle i, and ϵ_i represents its influence domain. These parameters are free to vary from a function to another.

4 Registration Method Using Vortex Particles

In this section we present how a vortex and source particles representation may be used in conjunction with an appropriate cost function to design the registration method.

4.1 Deformation Modeling

As we mentioned above, the discretization of the vorticity map with vortex particles, along with a Gaussian smoothing of the Dirac measure leads through Bio-Savart integral to the following representation of the solenoidal component of the motion field:

$$\mathbf{w}_{sol}(\mathbf{x}) \approx \sum_{i=0}^{n^{sol}} \gamma_i^{sol} K^\perp \otimes f_{\epsilon_i^{sol}}(\mathbf{z}_i^{sol} - \mathbf{x}) = \sum_{i=0}^{n^{sol}} \gamma_i^{sol} K^\perp_{\epsilon_i^{sol}}(\mathbf{z}_i^{sol} - \mathbf{x}), \tag{8}$$

where $K_{\epsilon_i}^\perp$ is a new kernel function obtained by convolving the orthogonal gradient of the Green kernel with the blob function. Obviously, a similar representation of the irrotational component can be obtained using source particles.

As a result, we exhibit an approximation of the complete motion field as weighted sums of *basis functions* defined by their centers location and their respective spatial influence. A Gaussian smoothing allows to derive analytically the associated smoothed kernel K_ϵ. Thus, the final expressions of the motion field components are:

$$\mathbf{w}_{sol}(\mathbf{x}) = \sum_{i=0}^{n^{sol}} \gamma_i^{sol} \frac{(\mathbf{z}_i^{sol} - \mathbf{x})^\perp}{2\pi|\mathbf{x} - \mathbf{z}_i^{sol}|^2}(1 - e^{-\frac{|\mathbf{x}-\mathbf{z}_i^{sol}|^2}{\epsilon_i^{sol2}}}), \tag{9}$$

and

$$\mathbf{w}_{irr}(\mathbf{x}) = \sum_{i=0}^{n^{irr}} \gamma_i^{irr} \frac{\mathbf{x} - \mathbf{z}_i^{irr}}{2\pi|\mathbf{x} - \mathbf{z}_i^{irr}|^2}(1 - e^{-\frac{|\mathbf{x}-\mathbf{z}_i^{irr}|^2}{\epsilon_i^{irr2}}}). \tag{10}$$

This representation will be incorporated within a spatio-temporal variation model of the luminance function in order to perform the registration.

4.2 Brightness Variation Model

The linearized version of the usual brightness consistency equation ($\frac{dI}{dt} = 0$) is used. This data model reads:

$$\nabla I(\mathbf{x}, t)^T . \mathbf{w}(\mathbf{x}) + I_t(\mathbf{x}, t) = 0, \tag{11}$$

where $\nabla I(\mathbf{x}, t)$ is the spatial gradient of the luminance function I and $I_t(\mathbf{x}, t)$ the temporal gradient.

Because of the linearization, this optical flow constraint is not valid in cases of large displacements. The use of a multiresolution scheme will insure the validity of the equation.

Considering this constraint holds almost everywhere on the whole image plane leads to seek a motion field $\mathbf{w}(\mathbf{x})$ minimizing the following cost function:

$$\mathcal{F}(I, \mathbf{w}) = \int_\Omega \left[\nabla I(\mathbf{x}, t)^T . \mathbf{w}(\mathbf{x}) + I_t(\mathbf{x}, t)\right]^2 d\mathbf{x}. \tag{12}$$

We have chosen to embed the vortex deformation model into the brightness constancy assumption. However, this is not restrictive and the deformation model could be used with more general measures such as mutual information for instance. However, the minimization scheme that is presented below would need to be adapted since the partial derivatives of mutual information cannot be readily computed (a Powell optimization scheme would be required for instance).

4.3 General Minimization Problem

Considering such a cost function for an unknown motion field approximated through vortex and source particles representations comes down to solve the following minimization problem:

$$\hat{\beta} = \arg\min_{\beta} \mathcal{F}(I, \mathbf{w}(\beta)), \tag{13}$$

with $\beta = (\{\mathbf{z}_i^{sol}, \gamma_i^{sol}, \epsilon_i^{sol}\}_{i=1:n^{sol}}, \{\mathbf{z}_i^{irr}, \gamma_i^{irr}, \epsilon_i^{irr}\}_{i=1:n^{irr}})$.

One seeks therefore the minimizer of the cost function $\mathcal{F}$ in terms of particles location, strength coefficients and influence domains. Due to the peculiar form of the field components (9) and (10) this minimization is a difficult problem, which is highly non linear with respect to some of the unknowns. To face the problem we have chosen to rely on a least square process embedded in a multi-resolution framework and associated to a generalized conjugated gradient optimization known as *Fletcher-Reeves* method.

We present more precisely in the next section how this difficult global optimization issue is handled.

5 Estimation

In order to cope with large displacements, the minimization is performed in a classical incremental multiresolution framework. At the coarsest level, the linearized version of the consistency equation can be used. At the finest levels, an incremental field is estimated.

5.1 Incremental Estimation Scheme

We assume first that a previous estimate of the set of unknowns is available. All these unknowns combine in the deformation modeling to form a deformation field $\widetilde{\mathbf{w}}$. Dropping the time indices of the intensity function for sake of clarity we end up with the following functional to be minimized according to $\mathbf{h}$, an unknown correction motion field:

$$\mathcal{F}(\mathbf{h}) = \int_{\Omega} \left[\boldsymbol{\nabla}\tilde{I}(\mathbf{x})^T . \mathbf{h}(\mathbf{x}) + \tilde{I}_t(\mathbf{x}) \right]^2 d\mathbf{x}. \tag{14}$$

In this equation we have introduced a compact notation $\tilde{I}(\mathbf{x})$ for the backward registered image $I(\boldsymbol{x} + \widetilde{\mathbf{w}}(\mathbf{x}), t+1)$. The correction field $\mathbf{h}$ is a combination of a solenoidal component $\mathbf{h}_{sol}$ and of an irrotational component $\mathbf{h}_{irr}$ according to the Helmholtz decomposition. Like the field $\widetilde{\mathbf{w}}$, this correction field is parameterized on the basis of a set of vortex and source particles. In practice, this kind of scheme is embedded into a pyramidal multiresolution data representation scheme. Such a representation is obtained through low-pass filtering and sub-sampling. At a given level, the known motion estimate $\widetilde{\mathbf{w}}$ is fixed to be the projected estimate obtained at the previous level. At the first level, the field is a null field.

5.2 Resulting Minimization Problem

The incremental estimation scheme transforms the original optimization problem (13) into a succession of minimization problems with respect to three kinds of unknowns. The derivatives with respect to the different variables are explicit and given by:

$$\frac{\partial \mathcal{F}(\mathbf{h})}{\partial \gamma_i} = \int_\Omega \frac{r_i(\mathbf{x})}{\pi |r_i(\mathbf{x})|^2}(1 - e^{-\frac{|r_i(\mathbf{x})|^2}{\epsilon_i^2}})\nabla \tilde{I}(\mathbf{x})[\nabla \tilde{I}(\mathbf{x})^T.\mathbf{h}(\mathbf{x},\gamma_i) + \tilde{I}_t(\mathbf{x})]d\mathbf{x}, \quad (15)$$

$$\frac{\partial \mathcal{F}(\mathbf{h})}{\partial \beta_i}\bigg|_{\beta_i = \frac{1}{\epsilon_i}} = \int_\Omega \frac{2\gamma_i}{\pi \epsilon_i} \frac{r_i(\mathbf{x})}{|r_i(\mathbf{x})|^2} e^{-\frac{|r_i(\mathbf{x})|^2}{\epsilon_i^2}} \nabla \tilde{I}(\mathbf{x})[\nabla \tilde{I}(\mathbf{x})^T.\mathbf{h}(\mathbf{x},\epsilon_i) + \tilde{I}_t(\mathbf{x})]d\mathbf{x},$$

(16)

$$\nabla_{\mathbf{z}_i} \mathcal{F}(\mathbf{h}) = \begin{pmatrix} \frac{\partial \mathcal{F}(\mathbf{h})}{\partial x_i} \\ \frac{\partial \mathcal{F}(\mathbf{h})}{\partial y_i} \end{pmatrix}, \quad (17)$$

where:
$$\frac{\partial \mathcal{F}(\mathbf{h})}{\partial x_i} = \int_\Omega -\frac{\frac{2}{\epsilon_i^2}|r_i(\mathbf{x})|^2 r_i^2(x) + (|r_i(\mathbf{x})|^2 + r_i^2(x))(1 - e^{-\frac{|r_i(\mathbf{x})|^2}{\epsilon_i^2}})}{\pi |r_i(\mathbf{x})|^4} \quad (18)$$

$$\nabla \tilde{I}(\mathbf{x})[\nabla \tilde{I}(\mathbf{x})^T.\mathbf{h}(\mathbf{x},x_i) + \tilde{I}_t(\mathbf{x})]d\mathbf{x},$$
$$r_i(\mathbf{x}) = (r_i(x), r_i(y))^T = \mathbf{x} - \mathbf{z}_i(\text{irr. part}) \text{ or } (\mathbf{z}_i - \mathbf{x})^\perp (\text{sol. part}). \quad (19)$$

Equations (15,16 and 17) lead to three different kinds of systems. The first one, in terms of coefficient strength is linear, the second one in terms of particles influence domain is non linear. No constrained minimization is required for both of them. A gradient descent process can be devised for this set of unknowns. For the third one an additional constraint to keep the particles into the image plane must be added. Such a constrained minimization problem, combined with the kind of non linearity, leads to a very tough minimization problem. Besides, if we do not make assumptions about the initial particles location, we must devise a method allowing eventual long range moves of the particles coordinates.

Thus, we have decoupled the estimation of the three unknowns. The two first (the strength coefficients and the influence domains of the particles) will be solved with a generalized conjugated gradient process presented in section 5.3 while the particles locations are frozen. The particles location will be in turn updated through a mean shift process presented in section 5.4.

5.3 Fletcher-Reeves Optimization

Fletcher-Reeves optimization consists in a non linear extension of conjugate gradient algorithms. Given an iterate $\Theta_k = \{\gamma_k^{sol}, \epsilon_k^{sol}, \gamma_k^{irr}, \epsilon_k^{irr}\}$ and a direction $\mathbf{d}_k$, a line search (w.r.t. α_k) is performed along $\mathbf{d}_k$ to produce $\Theta_{k+1} = \Theta_k + \alpha_k \mathbf{d}_k$. The Fletcher-Reeves variant of the nonlinear conjugate algorithm generates $\mathbf{d}_{k+1}$ from the recursion:

$$\mathbf{d}_{k+1} = \beta_k \mathbf{d}_k - \nabla \mathcal{F}(\Theta_{k+1}) \text{ with } \beta_k = \left(\frac{\|\nabla \mathcal{F}(\Theta_{k+1})\|_2}{\|\nabla \mathcal{F}(\Theta_k)\|_2}\right)^2.$$

Let us note that for the linear part of our system the method comes to a standard conjugated gradients. During this optimization, the particle locations are fixed. We initialize the domain of influence in an adaptive way. Their values are fixed to the value of the distance to the nearest particles. At convergence, we obtain a representation of the unknown correction field for fixed particle locations. Let us now describe how we propose to adjust these locations.

5.4 Estimation of Optimal Particle Positions

Definition of the Error Function. Considering that estimates of the strength coefficients and influence domains are available for both irrotational and solenoidal components we consider two different error surfaces. For each component, the surface is the registration discrepancy, considering the other orthogonal component fixed. For the solenoidal component the error surface is defined at each point of the image domain as:

$$\mathcal{D}^{sol}(\mathbf{x}) = I_{t+1}(\mathbf{x} + \tilde{\mathbf{w}}(\mathbf{x}) + \tilde{\mathbf{h}}^{irr}(\mathbf{x})) - I_t(\mathbf{x}), \tag{20}$$

where $\tilde{\mathbf{h}}^{irr}$ is a first estimate of the irrotational increment, with a set of fixed initial positions for the source particles. This error surface gathers all the reconstruction errors due to the solenoidal component. Similarly the error surface corresponding to the irrotational component is defined as:

$$\mathcal{D}^{irr}(\mathbf{x}) = I_{t+1}(\mathbf{x} + \tilde{\mathbf{w}}(\mathbf{x}) + \tilde{\mathbf{h}}^{sol}(\mathbf{x})) - I_t(\mathbf{x}). \tag{21}$$

Extension to a Characteristic Surface. The quality of the modelization we consider depends on the accuracy of the discrete approximation of the divergence and curl map. To achieve the best approximation as possible with a limited number of particles we should try to have a great number of particles to describe areas with strong divergence or vorticity and only few of them for the rest of the image. The surface error as defined by (20) or (21) can help to guide a particle towards a new location in accordance with its nature (vortex or source). However, it can guide a particle to an unappropriate location if the initial estimation of the components is not informative, because $\mathcal{D}^{sol}$ could highlight an error associated to the irrotational component, and vice versa.

To overcome this problem we choose to add a term to each error surface, based on the amount of vorticity or divergence estimated by the particles method. Particles could therefore be encouraged to go toward locations of high error magnitude associated to high concentration of vorticity or divergence. We end up with two surfaces, for the solenoidal and the irrotational part:

$$\mathcal{S}^{sol}(\mathbf{x}) = \frac{(\mathcal{D}^{sol}(\mathbf{x}))^2}{\int_\Omega (\mathcal{D}^{sol}(\mathbf{x}))^2 d\mathbf{x}} + \frac{(\operatorname{curl}\tilde{\mathbf{h}}(\mathbf{x}))^2}{\int_\Omega (\operatorname{curl}\tilde{\mathbf{h}}(\mathbf{x}))^2 d\mathbf{x}}, \tag{22}$$

and

$$\mathcal{S}^{irr}(\mathbf{x}) = \frac{(\mathcal{D}^{irr}(\mathbf{x}))^2}{\int_\Omega (\mathcal{D}^{irr}(\mathbf{x}))^2 d\mathbf{x}} + \frac{(\operatorname{div}\tilde{\mathbf{h}}(\mathbf{x}))^2}{\int_\Omega (\operatorname{div}\tilde{\mathbf{h}}(\mathbf{x}))^2 d\mathbf{x}}. \tag{23}$$

Finally, in order to restrict the displacements of the different particles to localized areas we combine these functions with an *a priori* prior on the particles location.

A Priori Probability Distribution for Particles Location. Considering $\mathbf{z}_i^k$ the random vector denoting the location of particle i at step k, we propose to fix a distribution of $\mathbf{z}_i^{k+1}$, knowing $\mathbf{z}_{1:n}^k$, where $\mathbf{z}_{1:n}^k$ represents the set of the n vectors $(\mathbf{z}_1^k, ..., \mathbf{z}_n^k)$ at step k.

We assume this probability distribution is Gaussian, defined as $\mathbf{z}_i^{k+1}|\mathbf{z}_{1:n}^k \sim \mathcal{N}(\mathbf{z}_i^k, \sigma_i^k)$, The standard deviation σ_i^k is set to the half of the distance between $\mathbf{z}_i^k$ and the closest center among $\{\mathbf{z}_j^k\}_{j=1,\ldots,n, j\neq i}$. The distribution takes into account the previous location of the particles through a Gaussian prior of mean $\mathbf{z}_i^k$ but also the dependency between $\mathbf{z}_i^{k+1}$ and all the other particles through the expression of σ_i^k.

Conditional Version of the Probability Distribution. Combining the *a priori* distribution $p_{\mathbf{z}_i^{k+1}|\mathbf{z}_{1:n}^k}$ defined above with the surface described before, denoted $\mathcal{S}_{\mathbf{z}_{1:n}^k}$ and characterized by (22) or (23), we can define a conditional probability distribution function of a particle $\mathbf{z}_i^{k+1}$ given the others:

$$p_{\mathbf{z}_i^{k+1}|\mathbf{z}_{1:n}^k, \mathcal{S}_{\mathbf{z}_{1:n}^k}}(\mathbf{x}) \propto \mathcal{S}_{\mathbf{z}_{1:n}^k}(\mathbf{x}) \cdot p_{\mathbf{z}_i^{k+1}|\mathbf{z}_{1:n}^k}(\mathbf{x}). \tag{24}$$

This pdf balances an *a priori* for the location of one given particle (whose role is to confine the particle to stay in a certain area between two iterates) and the information brought by the characteristic surface (associated to all the particles locations) in the neighborhood of this position. Once known this distribution for each particle we propose to shift $\mathbf{z}_i^k$ towards the pdf local mode in order to adjust optimally the location of the particles set.

Shifting the Particles Towards the Pdf Modes. From the sample $\{\mathcal{S}_{\mathbf{z}_{1:n}^k}(\mathbf{s})\}_{\mathbf{s}\in\mathcal{S}}$ evaluated at pixel coordinates $\mathbf{s}$, and the probability distribution $p_{\mathbf{z}_i^{k+1}|\mathbf{z}_{1:n}^k}$, a statistical non parametric estimate of the conditional probability distribution $p_{\mathbf{z}_i^{k+1}|\mathbf{z}_{1:n}^k, \mathcal{S}_{\mathbf{z}_{1:n}^k}}$ may be obtained [9] as

$$\hat{p}_{\mathbf{z}_i^{k+1}|\mathbf{z}_{1:n}^k, \mathcal{S}_{\mathbf{z}_{1:n}^k}}(\mathbf{x}) \propto \frac{\sum_{\mathbf{s}\in\mathcal{S}} \mathcal{S}_{\mathbf{z}_{1:n}^k}(\mathbf{s}) p_{\mathbf{z}_i^{k+1}|\mathbf{z}_{1:n}^k}(\mathbf{s}) K(\frac{\mathbf{x}-\mathbf{s}}{h})}{\sum_{\mathbf{s}\in\mathcal{S}} K(\frac{\mathbf{x}-\mathbf{s}}{h})}, \tag{25}$$

where K is a kernel and h is its corresponding window size.

The continuous pdf $\hat{p}_{\mathbf{z}_i^{k+1}|\mathbf{z}_{1:n}^k, \mathcal{S}_{\mathbf{z}_{1:n}^k}}(\mathbf{x})$ is thus expressed as a linear combination of basis functions with weighted coefficients given by $w(\mathbf{s}) = \mathcal{S}_{\mathbf{z}_{1:n}^k}(\mathbf{s}) p_{\mathbf{z}_i^{k+1}|\mathbf{z}_{1:n}^k}(\mathbf{s})$.

To shift a center $\mathbf{z}_i^k$ towards the nearest mode of $\hat{p}_{\mathbf{z}_i^{k+1}|\mathbf{z}_{1:n}^k, \mathcal{S}_{\mathbf{z}_{1:n}^k}}$ we rely on the *mean shift* estimate of the gradient of a density function [2, 3]. This estimate called the *mean shift vector* reads:

$$M_{h,G}(\mathbf{x}) = \frac{\sum_{\mathbf{s}\in\mathcal{S}} w(\mathbf{s}) \mathbf{s} G(\frac{\mathbf{x}-\mathbf{s}}{h})}{\sum_{\mathbf{s}\in\mathcal{S}} w(\mathbf{s}) G(\frac{\mathbf{x}-\mathbf{s}}{h})} - \mathbf{x}, \tag{26}$$

where G is the kernel obtained by derivation of the kernel K. This vector gives at each point the direction of the maximum increase of the density function estimated through the weights $w(\mathbf{s})$ and the kernel K. Different choices can be done for this kernel. Usual choices are the Epanechnikov kernel or a Gaussian kernel. The gradient of the Epanechnikov kernel is a box function kernel whereas G remains Gaussian for a Gaussian kernel K.

Given this estimate of the pdf gradient, an iterative convergent [2] process called mean shift naturally arises. This process consists in moving iteratively the kernel center $\mathbf{x}$ following $M_{h,G}(\mathbf{x})$ until a stationary point (i.e., zero gradient) of the underlying density is found.

In our case, the mean shift procedure is applied to the $n^{sol} + n^{irr}$ centers of the basis functions (or particles) involved in our motion field modeling. Each particle is shifted towards the nearest mode of the conditional density $\hat{p}_{\mathbf{z}_i^{k+1}|\mathbf{z}_{1:n}^k, S_{\mathbf{z}_{1:n}^k}}$. We have chosen to use the Epanechnikov kernel. Besides, the choice of the window size is crucial. Different choices can be made. In our case we have settled adaptive window sizes. They are fixed to the distance of the nearest particles. Such a choice make sense in our case. As a matter of fact, for distant particles only a rough and smooth estimate of the pdf function is needed whereas for close particles an accurate estimate of the density is at the opposite required to approximate at best the vorticity and divergence maps.

5.5 Overall Estimation Scheme

The overall estimation scheme consists in an alternate updating of the different unknowns. It is composed by the following two steps, repeated in turn until convergence:

1. For a given set of particles at fixed locations, the strength coefficients and the influence domains attached to the particles blob function are estimated through the generalized conjugated gradient optimization described in section 5.3.
2. The vortex and source particles locations are shifted toward the nearest local mode of the corresponding pdf. This shift is realized applying the mean shift procedure described in section 5.4.

The whole process is stopped when the divergence and vorticity reach a certain stability. This criterion is expressed as:

$$\left(\frac{\|\operatorname{div} \tilde{\mathbf{h}}^{k+1} - \operatorname{div} \tilde{\mathbf{h}}^k\|_2}{\|\operatorname{div} \tilde{\mathbf{h}}^k\|_2} \right)^2 + \left(\frac{\|\operatorname{curl} \tilde{\mathbf{h}}^{k+1} - \operatorname{curl} \tilde{\mathbf{h}}^k\|_2}{\|\operatorname{curl} \tilde{\mathbf{h}}^k\|_2} \right)^2$$

6 Results

In this section we illustrate our method with two real examples. The first one shows the evolution of a multiple sclerosis (MS) lesion for the same patient between two different times. Two $3D$ T2 (among other modalities) were acquired within 6 months and rigidly registered [6]. The MR volumes were registered with a $3D$ rigid transformation and an axial $2D$ slice extracted to experiment the non-rigid registration method. The lesion appears as a white stain in the left part of the brain at t_0 and has grown at t_0+6 months (see fig. 1).

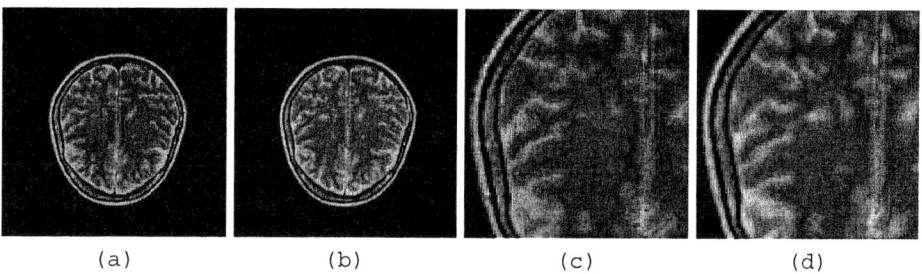

Fig. 1. (a) T2-MR slice at time t_0; (b) T2-MR corresponding slice at time t_0+6 months; (c)-(d) Zoom centered on the lesion

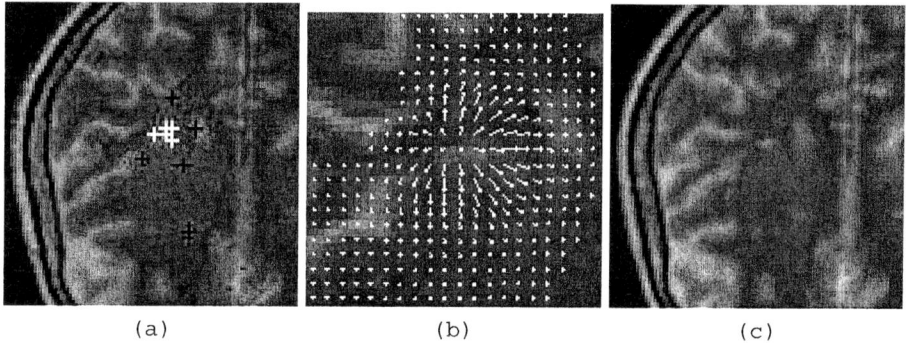

Fig. 2. (a) Automatic shifting of the source particles towards the region of interest. The black points represents the initial positions of the source particles (manual initialization), the white points the final optimal positions after the mean shift process; (b) Zoom on the resulting divergent field, centered in the lesion. The deformation field ; (c) Registered image (image at time t_0+6 months registered toward image at time t_0)

The source particles are initialized manually near the lesion. The user can fix the positions of the particles without precision because the estimation method allows to guide the particles towards the region of interest (fig. 2 (a)). An accurate deformation field is estimated (fig. 2 (b)), corresponding to a divergent motion centered in the lesion. The corresponding registered image is represented in fig. 2 (c). The difference image between the original and the deformed image (fig.3 (a)) can be compared with the difference image after registration (fig.3 (b)). The error due to the lesion has been removed by the estimation method. The remaining error , mainly around sulci, is due to rigid registration error and interpolation artifacts.

The second example illustrates the application of our method to a basis of 20 subjects. For each subject, a T1 $3D$ MR was acquired and the brain was extracted using the Brain Extraction Tool [8]. All the IRM images have been first registered rigidly toward a reference subject (a $3D$ transformation was estimated and a $2D$ slice was extracted for each subject after registration). The goal is here to estimate the non rigid deformation between all the rigidly registered images and the reference one. The deformations are

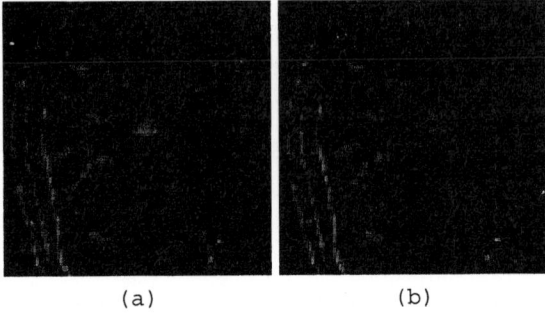

Fig. 3. (a) Difference between the two images after rigid registration; (b) Difference after non rigid registration. The image discrepancy has decreased significantly on the lesion. The image discrepancy on the sulci is not due to a misalignment, but to a luminance variation because of the interpolation artifact

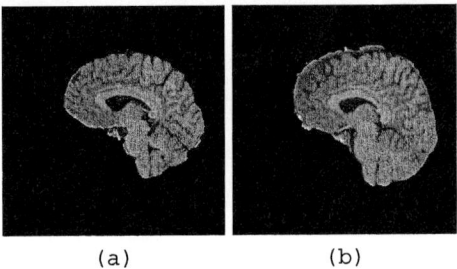

Fig. 4. (a) Reference subject; (b) Rigidly registered image for another subject of the database

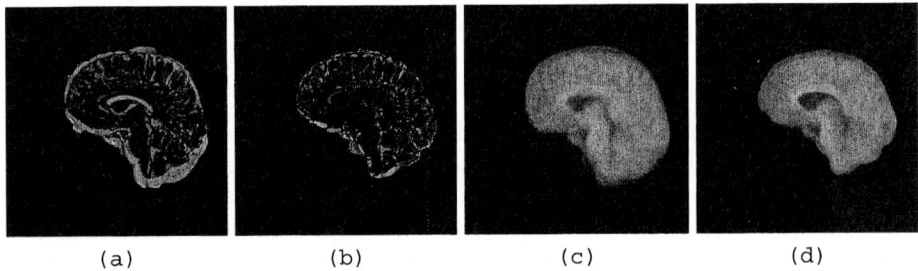

Fig. 5. (a) Original difference image between one given subject and the reference one, after rigid registration; (b) Difference image after non rigid registration for this subject; (c) Average image after rigid registration over the 20 subjects; (d) Average image after non rigid registration over the 20 subjects

here much more complicated than for the first example. To obtain an accurate result, we choose to fix a dense grid of source and vortex particles, recovering the brain region. We present an example of registration for one given subject (fig.4 (b)) with respect to the reference one (fig.4 (a)). The corresponding difference images before and after non rigid registration are shown in fig.5 (a-b). The estimation method brings a significant reduction of the important regions of error. Finally, fig.5 (c-d) shows the average image after rigid registration and the average image after non-rigid registration.

7 Conclusion

In this paper, a parametric method for non-rigid image registration was presented. The deformation field is described by two sets of so-called vortex and source particles, leading to a compact representation. The deformation parameters (for each particle, the vorticity or divergence, and the influence domain) are computed using a generalized conjugate gradient descent. The optimal positions of the particles are also estimated using a mean shift process.

This method was implemented for $2D$ images and experimented on various real data. It is shown that this method is capable of recovering efficiently divergent fields, and show its ability to register a set of 20 images (T1-MR sagittal images of different subjects).

Future work will focus on the $3D$ extension of this registration modeling. Concerning the divergent component, the $3D$ extension is straightforward since divergence is still a scalar variable. However, the $3D$ extension of the vorticity component will be more problematic since vorticity is no longer a scalar but a vector: vorticity cannot be bound to a particle but to a manifold such as a line or a surface.

References

1. A. Chorin. Numerical study of slightly viscous flow. *J. Fluid Mech.*, 57:785–796, 1973.
2. D. Comaniciu and P. Meer. Mean shift: A robust approach toward feature space analysis. *IEEE PAMI*, 24(5):603–619, 2002.
3. K. Fukanaga and L.D. Hostetler. The estimation of the gradient of a density function, with applications in pattern recognition. *IEEE Trans. on Info. Theory*, 21(1):32–40, 1975.
4. A. Leonard. Vortex methods for flow simulation. *J. Comp. Phys.*, 37, 1980.
5. H. Lester and S. Arridge. A survey of hierarchical non-linear medical image registration. *Pattern Recognition*, 32:129–149, 1999.
6. F. Maes, A. Collignon, D. Vandermeulen, G. Marchal, and P. Suetens. Multimodality image registration by maximisation of mutual information. *IEEE TMI*, 16(2):187–198, 1997.
7. J. Maintz and MA. Viergever. A survey of medical image registration. *MedIA*, 2(1):1–36, 1998.
8. S.M. Smith. Fast robust automated brain extraction. *HBM*, 17(3):143–155, 2002.
9. R.A. Thisted. *Elements of statistical computing*. Chapman and Hall, 1988.
10. A. Toga and P. Thompson. The role of image registration in brain mapping. *Image and Vision Computing*, 19:3–24, 2001.
11. B. Zitova and J. Flusser. Image registration methods: a survey. *Image and Vision Computing*, 21:977–1000, 2003.

Transitive Inverse-Consistent Manifold Registration

Xiujuan Geng, Dinesh Kumar, and Gary E. Christensen

Department of Electrical and Computer Engineering,
The University of Iowa, Iowa City, IA, 52242
{xiujuan-geng, dinesh-kumar, gary-christensen}@uiowa.edu

Abstract. This paper presents a new registration method called Transitive Inverse-Consistent Manifold Registration (TICMR). The TICMR method jointly estimates correspondence maps between groups of three manifolds embedded in a higher dimensional image space while minimizing inverse consistency and transitivity errors. Registering three manifolds at once provides a means for minimizing the transitivity error which is not possible when registering only two manifolds. TICMR is an iterative method that uses the closest point projection operator to define correspondences between manifolds as they are non-rigidly registered. Examples of the TICMR method are presented for matching groups of three contours and groups of three surfaces. The contour registration is regularized by minimizing the change in bending energy of the curves while the surface registration is regularized by minimizing the change in elastic energy of the surfaces. The notions of inverse consistency error (ICE) and transitivity error (TE) are extended from volume registration to manifold registration by using a closest point projection operator. For the experiments in this paper, the TICMR method reduces the average ICE by 200 times (contour)/ 6 times (surface) and the average TE by 40 times (contour)/ 2-4 times (surface) compared to registering with a curvature constraint alone. Furthermore, the TICMR is shown to avoid some local minimum that are not avoided when registering with a curvature constraint alone.

1 Introduction

This paper introduces a new registration approach called Transitive Inverse Consistent Manifold Registration (TICMR). The novelty of this approach is that it jointly registers three manifolds together instead of two allowing both the inverse consistency error [1] and the transitivity error [2] to be minimized. TICMR is a general approach that has applications for many types of manifolds. In this paper we present two registration algorithms based on the TICMR framework: one for registering contours and one for registering surfaces.

Fig. 1 defines the notation used throughout the paper. Transformation $h_{ij} : x \to y$ defines a pointwise correspondence mapping between all points x on manifold j and their corresponding projections y on or near manifold i. The closest point operator [3] is used to map points $y = h_{ij}(x)$ onto manifold i if necessary. All six pictured transformations are jointly estimated using the TICMR approach to find the correspondences between the three manifolds.

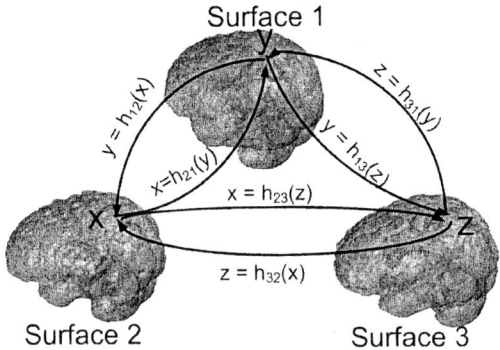

Fig. 1. The transformations $h_{12}, h_{21}, h_{13}, h_{31}, h_{23}$, and h_{32} satisfy the transitivity property if $h_{ij}(x) = h_{ik}(h_{kj}(x))$ for every x on surface i and $i \neq j \neq k$. These transformations are inverse consistent if $h_{ij}(x) = h_{ji}^{-1}(x)$ for every x on surface j and $i \neq j$

The goal of this work is to identify important sources of registration error and develop a registration algorithm to minimize those errors. This type of approach is needed since there is no "gold standard" for evaluating non-rigid image registration performance. Thus, the best we can do is to identify necessary conditions/properties that the registration algorithms should satisfy—such as zero to near zero inverse consistency error and transitivity error—and try to achieve them.

Parameterized contours and surfaces play an important role in medical image analysis because surfaces are relatively easy to define and are a rich source of shape information. The geometric properties of curves and surfaces are conserved between individual images, making them useful landmarks for morphometric comparisons and provide important boundary conditions [4] for image registration constrained by regions of interest. Surface-based mapping can offer advantages over volume based mapping in some medical imaging registration applications such as brain mapping. For example, 3D registration accuracy based on matching intensity values of brain images does not ensure the alignment of sulcal and gyral pattens of the individual cortical surfaces [5].

2 The TICMR Registration Method

Let C_{SIM} represent a similarity cost function that defines the correspondences between the three manifolds to be registered. Let C_{REG} represent a constraint for regularizing the estimation procedure. Finally, let C_{ICC} and C_{TRANS} correspond to the inverse consistency constraint and the transitivity constraint, respectively. The TICMR problem statement is to jointly estimate a set of six transformations $h_{12}, h_{21}, h_{13}, h_{31}, h_{23}$, and h_{32} that satisfy

$$h_{ij} = \arg\min_{h_{ij}} \sigma C_{SIM} + \rho C_{REG} + \chi C_{ICC} + \gamma C_{TRANS} \tag{1}$$

where σ, ρ, χ, and γ are weighting factors.

In this paper, we present two registration algorithms based on solving Eq. 1; the first is contour-based and the second is surface-based. Contours are assumed to be represented by a linked list of node points connected with straight lines. Surfaces is assumed to be represented by a triangulated surface mesh. The parameters for contour registration are the displacement vectors from each node on the template contour to the target contour. Likewise, the parameters for surface registration are displacement vectors from each vertex in the template surface to the corresponding point on the target surface.

2.1 Similarity Cost Function

We used the closest point similarity cost function [3] to define the correspondences for the contour-to-contour and surface-to-surface TICMR algorithms. The closest point similarity cost function is a convenient method for defining correspondences between manifolds when exact correspondences are unknown. The cost function we used is given by

$$C_{SIM} = \sum_{i=1}^{3} \sum_{\substack{j=1 \\ j \neq i}}^{3} \int_{S_j} ||D_{S_i}(h_{ij}(x))||^2 dx \qquad (2)$$

where D_{S_i} corresponds to the distance map of S_i. That is, $D_{S_i}(x)$ gives the closest distance from point x to S_i. The manifold S_i represents a contour for contour-to-contour matching or a surface for surface-to-surface matching. The distance maps were computed using Voronoi Feature Transform (VFT) presented in Maurer et. al [6].

The six terms in Eq. 2 correspond to the unidirectional similarity cost functions required to match each manifold to the other two manifolds (see Fig. 1). Although the cost function in Eq. 2 is simple and effective, it can be replaced by more complicated similarity functions if desired. For example, feature vectors can be used to define correspondence as in the HAMMER registration algorithm[7].

2.2 Regularization Constraint

Correspondences defined solely by the similarity cost in Eq. 2 are independent of the neighborhood structure of S_i and will produce poor correspondences if not regularized. Regularization is used to constrain the estimation procedure to produce correspondence maps or transformations that are smooth spatially. Different regularizing constraints for contour and surface matching are needed due to the differences in topology of contours and surfaces.

The regularization cost used to constrain the contour-to-contour registration is given by

$$C_{REG} = \sum_{i=1}^{3} \sum_{\substack{j=1 \\ j \neq i}}^{3} \int_{S_j} ||\frac{dh_{ij}(x(s))}{ds} - \frac{dx(s)}{ds}||^2 ds \qquad (3)$$

where s is arc length of the curve. The registration of curves S_1, S_2, and S_3 is regularized by penalizing the change of the tangent vector along the deforming curve. Notice that this cost function is similar to that used to regularize snake active contour models [8] except that Eq. 3 is defined in a Eulerian coordinate system instead of a Lagrangian coordinate system. The consequence of this is that the curves do not deform in our formulation, but their projections do.

The regularization used for surface matching is different than that used for contour matching since points on a contour are ordered while the points on a surface are not. Following Hsu et. al [9], the elastic energy $E(S)$ of a surface S can be defined by $E(S) = \int_S (a + bH^2 + cG)dA$ where H and G are mean and Gaussian curvatures of S, respectively; A is the surface area of S; b and c are "bending" energies, and a is a surface tension or "stretching" energy. Setting a equal to zero makes $E(S)$ scale invariant. To regularize the transformation so there is no penalty for the original shape of the surface, we replace H with $H - H_S$, where H_S is the mean curvature of the original surface S and plays a role as boundary condition. The third term in $E(S)$ is a constant because $\int_S GdA = 2\pi\chi(S)$ where $\chi(S)$ is a constant for surfaces with the same topology. Combining these observations produces the elastic energy function

$$C_{REG} = \sum_{i=1}^{3} \sum_{\substack{j=1 \\ j \neq i}}^{3} \int_{S_j} (H(h_{ij}(x)) - H_{S_j}(x))^2 a(h_{ij}(x)) dx \qquad (4)$$

where $a(x)$ is the area around point x and $\sum_x a_x$ is the total surface area. Moving the surface vertex at x in the direction of the gradient of the area a_x (i.e., the same direction of the normal vector at this point) decreases the energy. Making the assumption that the mean curvature at x is a constant, we can simplify the the derivative of the regularization cost as $H(h_{ij}(x)) - H_{S_j})N(h_{ij}(x)a(h_{ij}(x))$, where $N(x)$ is the normalized normal vector at point x.

2.3 Inverse Consistency Constraint and Projection Error

The contribution of each transformation $h_{i,j}$ in the similarity cost function C_{SIM} and the regularization constraint C_{REG} is independent. Therefore minimizing the similarity cost and regularization constraint produces 6 uni-directional registration problems and are not sufficient to guarantee that h_{ij} and h_{ji} are inverse consistent. In this paper, we define an inverse consistency constraint (ICC) to minimize inverse consistency error for manifold registration in a similar manner to the work in [1] for registering volumetric images.

We begin by defining the inverse consistency error (ICE) and projection error (PE) of the forward and reverse transformations between two manifolds as shown in Fig. 2. This figure illustrates that the forward transformation h_{12} does not have to project from manifold 1 to manifold 2 and vice versa for the reverse transformation h_{21}. The difference between the projection of a point from one manifold to the closest point on the other manifold is defined as the PE.

Fig. 2 shows two ways to define the inverse consistency error (ICE). Panel a defines the ICE as the difference between the identity map and the concatenation of h_{21} and h_{12}. This method can be used to evaluate the inverse consistency error between the forward and reverse transformations. Panel b defines the ICE as the difference between the projection of x through h_{12} and x' through h_{21}^{-1} where x' is the closest point to x that is in the range space of h_{21}^{-1}. The method in panel b is the one we use to minimize the inverse consistency error.

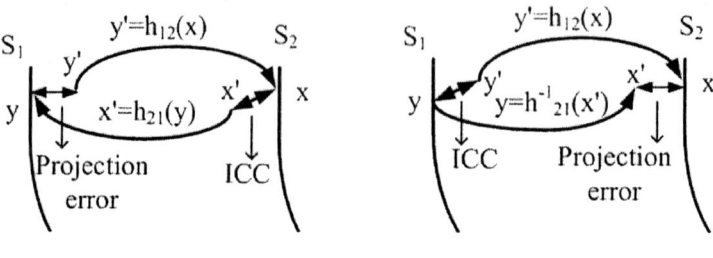

(a) Projection error and Inverse Consistency error

(b) Compute Inverse Consistency error

Fig. 2. Illustration of the projection error and the two ways to calculate the inverse consistency error

The inverse consistency constraint for the six transformations between three manifolds (see Fig. 1) is defined as

$$C_{ICC} = \sum_{i=1}^{3} \sum_{\substack{j=1 \\ j \neq i}}^{3} \int_{S_j} ||h_{ij}(x) - f_{ij}(x)||^2 dx \qquad (5)$$

where $f_{ij}(x) = \arg\min_{y \in S_i} ||h_{ji}(y) - x||^2$.

2.4 Transitivity Constraint

One of the most important points of this paper is that both the inverse consistent error and the joint transitivity error can be minimized together. Based on the transitivity relationships illustrated in Figure 1, we define the transitivity constraint as

$$C_{TRANS} = \sum_{i=1}^{3} \sum_{\substack{j=1 \\ j \neq i}}^{3} \sum_{\substack{k=1 \\ k \neq i \neq j}}^{3} \int_{S_j} ||h_{ik}(h_{kj}(x)) - h_{ij}(x)||^2 dx. \qquad (6)$$

To minimize the transitivity cost, we assume that h_{ij} is independent of h_{kj} and h_{ik} for $k \neq i \neq j$. Therefore, for each partial cost in Eq. 6, we fix the term $(h_{ik}(h_{kj}(x))$ to estimate the parameters of $h_{ij}(x)$. Making this assumption simplifies the estimation procedure by making it linear in the parameters of h_{ij} rather than nonlinear in the parameters of h_{kj} due to the concatenation with the transformation h_{ik}.

3 Results

3.1 Contour-Based Registration Results

The contour-based registration algorithm was tested using contours extracted from 2D CT images of human lungs. Fifteen lung contours were extracted from 15 different data

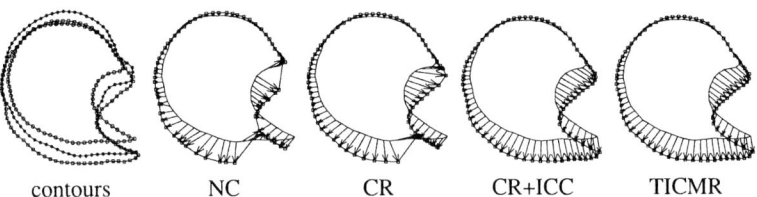

Fig. 3. Typical contour-to-contour registration results. Arrows show the displacement vectors starting at points on contour 2 mapped through the estimated transformation h_{12}. Every tenth displacement vector is visualized. The bases and points of adjacent vectors have been connected by lines to visualize contour 2 and the estimated shape of contour 1. The panels from left to right show the three contours super-imposed used to generate the results, registration with no constraints (NC), registration with curvature regularization (CR), registration with CR + inverse consistency constraints (CR+ICC), and registration with CR+ICC+transitivity constraints (TICMR)

sets using a boundary finding algorithm after segmenting the CT images. The number of points making up the lung boundary contours varied from 700 to 1000 points depending on the size of the lung cross sectional area. The 15 data sets were divided in to five groups of three contours each. Each group of three contours were registered using 100 iterations, the similarity weight ($\sigma = 1$) and

1. No constraints (NC) ($\rho = \chi = \gamma = 0$),
2. Curvature regularization (CR) only ($\rho = 1, \chi = \gamma = 0$),
3. CR+inverse consistency constraints (CR+ICC) ($\rho = \chi = 1, \gamma = 0$), and
4. CR+ICC+transitivity constraints (TICMR) ($\rho = \chi = 1.0; \gamma = 0.1$).

The results for one transformation estimated using the four constraint sets are illustrated in Fig. 3. The left panel shows the three contours used to produce the registrations shown in the other panels. The arrows show every tenth estimated displacement vector from contour 2 to contour 1. The displacement vectors at each contour node were initialized to zero and converged to the target contour within 100 iterations. All the displacement vectors were estimated independently of each other for the unconstrained (NC) registration result. The arrows show that displacement field is not uniform/smooth, there are many-to-one mappings, and poor correspondence at places. The CR registration produced uniform/smooth displacements, but still had many-to-one mappings and poor correspondence in places. The CR+ICC registration produced a uniform/smooth displacement field, a one-to-one mapping from one contour to the other, and a good correspondence from one contour to the other. The TICMR registration is very similar to the CR+ICC result although there are slight differences.

The images in Fig. 4 show how the inverse consistency error is typically affected by the four sets of constraints. The boxed region in each image is zoomed to help show differences. This figure shows the trajectories of points from contour $2 \to 1 \to 2$ using the estimated transformations h_{12} and h_{21}. The final position of the trajectories should match the starting location if the forward and reverse transformations are inverse consistent. We see that the inverse consistency for the NC and CR registrations are not good and could be expected from the results shown in Fig. 3. However, the CR+ICC

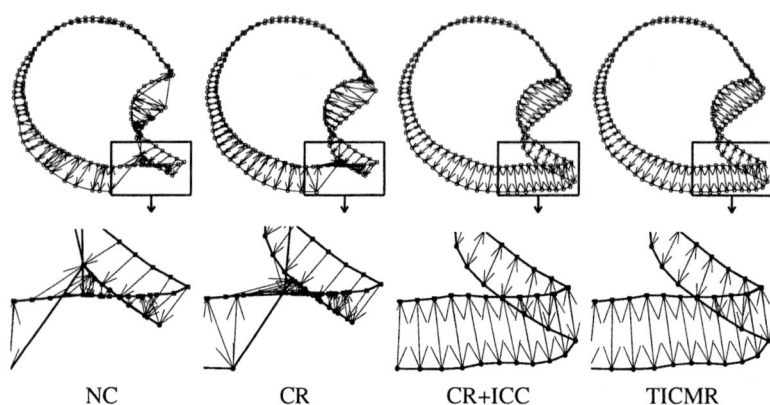

Fig. 4. Typical inverse consistency errors for contour-based registration. Arrows show the trajectories of points starting on contour 2, mapped through transformation h_{12}, projected onto closest point on contour 1, and then mapped through transformation h_{21}. The distance between the starting and final positions is defined as the inverse consistency error. Arrows are shown for every tenth displacement vector estimated along contour 2. The panels from left to right correspond to registrations with no constraints (NC), curvature regularization (CR), CR+inverse consistent constraint (CR+ ICC), and CR+ICC+transitive constraint (TICMR). The bottom row shows a zoomed version of the boxed region in the top row

and the TICMR registrations are essentially inverse consistent over the whole contour and there is very little noticeable difference between them.

The results in Fig. 5 illustrate typical transitivity errors for the four constraint sets. In this figure, the arrows show the trajectories of points from contour $2 \to 1 \to 3 \to 2$. The final position of the trajectories should point to the start location if the transformations have the transitivity property. Again the NC and CR registration results show large transitivity error. However, unlike the two previous cases, we can now see a difference between CR+ICC and TICMR registrations. The TICMR registration produced essentially transitive transformation, while the CR+ICC did not do so well.

Figure 6 shows the summary statistics for the five groups of three lung contours with respect to the average similarity error (ASE), average regularization error (ARE), average inverse consistency error (AICE) and average transitivity error (ATE) for the four sets of constraints. The ASE is the average distance from the estimated displacement vectors to the target curve. The ASE is lowest for unconstrained registration and highest when using curvature regularization alone. Adding inverse consistency and transitivity constraints the curvature regularization reduces the ASE slightly. The median ASE is less than 0.1 pixels for h_{12} but close to 1.0 pixel for the h_{31} and h_{23} transformations.

The ARE is a measure of the smoothness of the estimated displacement vectors. It is defined as the cost C_{REG} in Eq. 3 normalized by the number of nodes in the discrete contour. This measure can only be used to access the relative smoothness of a transformation since it depends on the shape of the template and target contours. In all three cases shown, the ARE is high for the unconstrained registration and is essentially the same for the three results that include the curvature regularization.

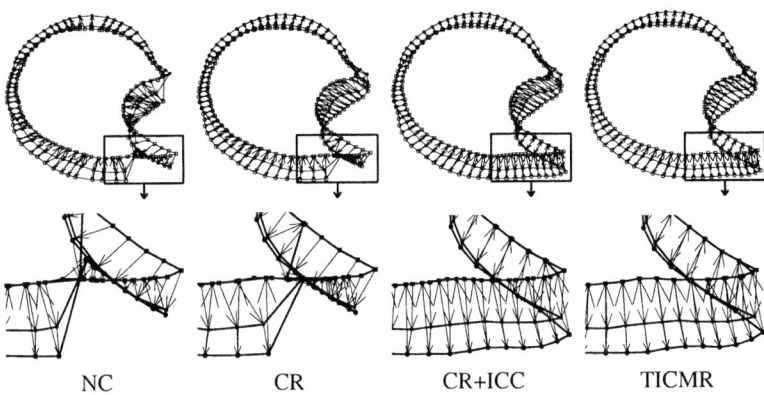

Fig. 5. Typical transitivity errors for contour-based registration. Arrows show the trajectories of points starting on contour 2, mapped through h_{12}, projected onto closest point on contour 1, mapped through h_{31}, projected onto closest point on contour 3, and mapped through h_{23}. The distance between the starting and final positions is defined as the transitivity error. Arrows are shown for every tenth displacement vector estimated along contour 2. The panels from left to right correspond to registrations with no constraints (NC), curvature regularization (CR), CR+inverse consistent constraint (CR+ ICC), and CR+ICC+transitive constraint (TICMR). The bottom row shows a zoomed version of the boxed region in the top row

The Average Inverse Consistency Error (AICE) is defined as C_{ICC} in Eq. 5 normalized by the number of nodes in the discrete contour. The AICE is much larger for the NC and CR registration results than for the the CR+ICC and TICMR results. These findings are to be expected since the CR+ICC and the TICMR results were generated by specifically minimizing the the AICE. It is important to note that the AICE was reduce to less than 0.11 pixels on average for the CR+ICC and TICMR results giving a 200 times improvement over only using CR.

The Average Transitivity Error (ATE) is defined as C_{TRANS} in Eq. 6 normalized by the number of nodes in the discrete contour. Again the ATE is much larger for the NC and CR registration results than for the the CR+ICC and TICMR results. However, the ATE is much smaller for the TICMR result compared to the CR+ICC result demonstrating the importance of the transitivity constraint. The TICMR results reduced the median ATE by approximately 40 times compared to CR registration and approximately 2 times compared to CR+ICC registration.

Fig.7 shows the effect of varying χ and γ on the similarity, inverse consistency and transitivity errors. The left column shows that varying the inverse consistency constraint weight χ without the transitivity constraint ($\gamma = 0$) has little effect on the average similarity error (ASE), but has a large effect on the average inverse consistency error (AICE) and on the average transitivity error (ATE). The right column shows that varying the transitivity constraint weight γ while keeping $\chi = 1$ has little effect on the ASE and AICE, but does have a substantial effect on lowering the ATE. Similar results were found for the 3D experiments discussed in the next section.

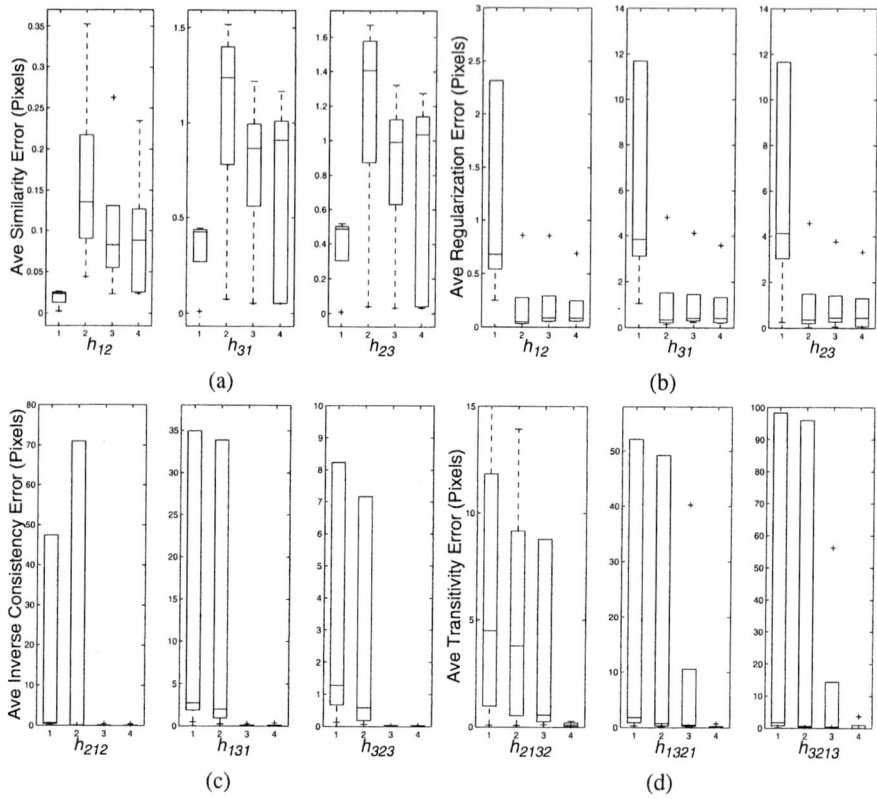

Fig. 6. Summary box plots for the 5 groups of 3 contour-based registration experiments. Only 3 of 6 plots for each error measure are shown to save space. The boxes stretch from the 25th percentile (bottom) to the 25th percentile (top). The median is shown as the line across the box. Some of the maximum values are out side of the range of the scale shown. The boxes in each plot are numbered from 1 to 4 and correspond to NC, CR, CR+ICC, and TICMR, respectively, at the 100th iteration. Notation: h_{iji} means $h_{ij}(h_{ji})$ and h_{ijki} means $h_{ij}(h_{jk}(h_{ki}))$

3.2 Surface-Based Registration Results

The surfaced-based TICMR algorithm was tested using surfaces generated from 3D phantom images (12 images in total) and the brain surfaces extracted from MRI image volumes (6 images in total). Two groups of three torus-shaped phantom surfaces and 2 groups of three ellipsoid-shaped phantom surfaces were generated from $64 \times 64 \times 64$ voxel volumes. The 6 surfaces of the human brain were generated from $128 \times 160 \times 128$ voxel MRI image volumes. All triangulated surfaces were generated from binarized 3D image data using the regularized marching tetrahedra technique [10]. The surfaces had approximately 3500 vertices and 7500-9500 faces for the torus phantoms, 2600-4400 vertices and 4800-5100 faces for the ellipsoid phantoms, and approximately 7500-8400 vertices and 15,000-16,700 faces for the brain surfaces. Down-sampling the original

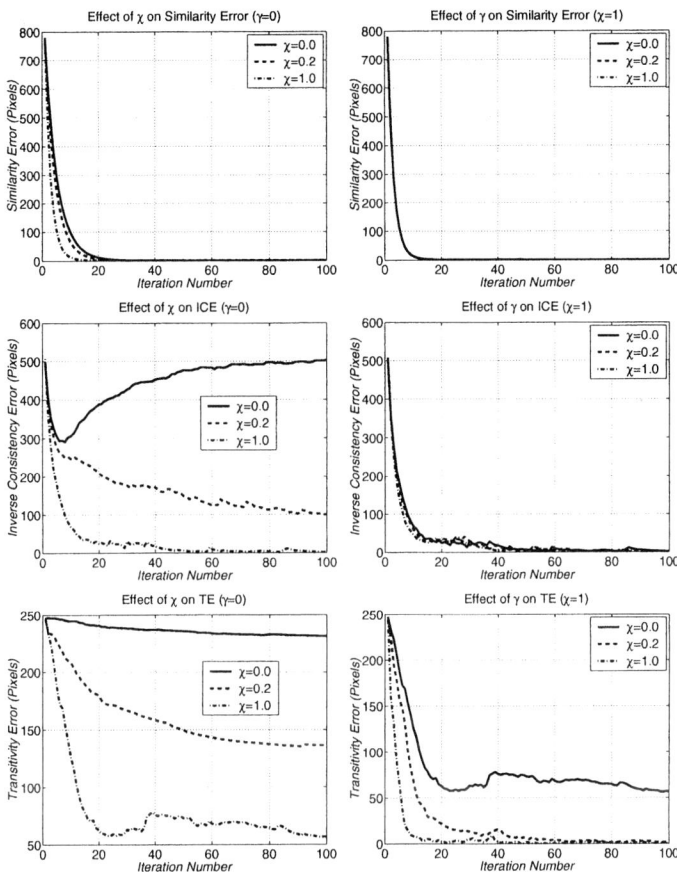

Fig. 7. Typical convergence rates for the contour-based registration experiments. χ is the inverse consistency constraint (ICC) weight, and γ is the transitivity constraint (TC) weight. In the left column, χ varies while keeping $\gamma = 0$; in the right column, γ varies while keeping $\chi = 1$

image volumes before generating the surfaces was used to reduce the number of vertices and faces for the triangulated surfaces so no further decimation of the surface meshes was required. The normal vector at vertex v on the surface was computed by averaging normals of its adjacent faces weighted by the area of each face. The mean curvature at a vertex v was computed using the method of Joshi et al. [11]. In this method, the surface at v is approximated by fitting a quadratic surface patch to the neighboring vertices of v using least squares estimation. The principal curvatures are extracted from the quadratic surface patch and averaged.

The parameters estimated for surface registration were displacement vectors at each node in the template surface to the corresponding point on the target surface. The surfaces were approximated with triangular surface patches between vertices for the closest point computations. The closest point computations were computed efficiently using the 3D distance maps generated using the method described in Maurer et. al[6]. Surfaces and their displacement vectors were visualized using the Matlab^{TM} software (see Fig. 8).

For the torus and ellipsoid experiments, the TICMR method reduced the average inverse consistency error (AICE) by 6 times and the average transitivity error (ATE) by 4 times compared to curvature regularized (CR) registration. For the brain surface registration, the TICMR approach reduced the AICE by 10 times compared to the CR registration. Fig. 8 shows a 3D visualization of the transitivity error for the brain surface

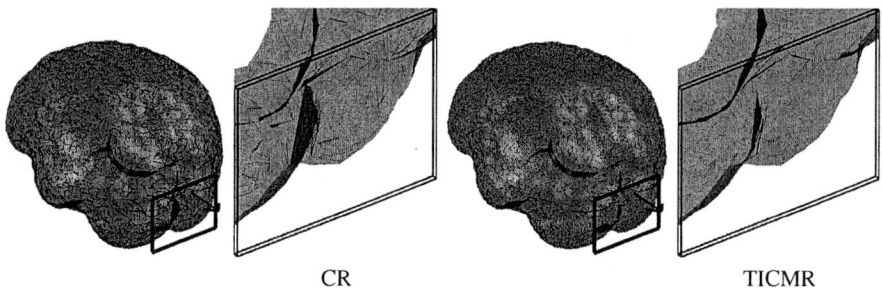

Fig. 8. Visualization of transitivity error (TE) for uni-directional surface registration with curvature regularization (left) and TICMR surface registration (right). The short lines on the surface show the transitivity error of the composite transformation h_{2132} that maps points from surface 2 to 3 to 1 to 2. Not all transitivity error vectors are shown

registration results. The short lines on the surface represent transitivity error of the composite transformation $h_{2132}(x) = h_{21}(h_{13}(h_{32}(x)))$. The average transitivity error (ATE) was reduced by a factor of 2 for the TICMR brain surface registration compared to the uni-directional curvature regularized registration.

The contour and surface-based TICMR algorithms were implemented in C++ and run on a dual processor 2GHz AMD Athlon computer with 3.5 GB of RAM. The computation time for the contour-based TICMR algorithm was less than 5 minutes for 100 iterations. The surface-based TICMR registrations took approximately 20 minutes for the torus and ellipsoid surfaces and approximately 70 minutes for the brain surfaces for 100 iterations. In contour case, approximately 90% of time is used for computing the inverse transformations and interpolating the closest contour points. In surface case, 85% of time was used for compute inverse transformations (20%) and interpolating points on the surfaces (65%).

4 Discussion and Conclusions

This paper presented a new registration method for jointly registering groups of three manifolds called the transitive inverse consistent manifold registration (TICMR). Example TICMR registration algorithms were given for curve-based and surface-based registration. The curve-based and surface-based TICMR algorithms gave much better correspondences than non-rigid, uni-directional, closest-point curve and surface-based registration with curvature regularization.

Acknowledgments

This work was supported in part by the NIH grants EB004126, CA096679 and HL64368.

References

1. G.E. Christensen and H.J. Johnson, "Consistent image registration," vol. 20, no. 7, pp. 568–582, July 2001.
2. G.E. Christensen and H.J. Johnson, "Invertibility and transitivity analysis for nonrigid image registration," *Journal of Electronic Imaging*, vol. 12, no. 1, pp. 106–117, Jan. 2003.
3. P.J. Besl and N.D. McKay, "A method for registration of 3-d shapes," vol. 14, no. 2, 1992.
4. G.E. Christensen, "Inverse consistent registration with object boundary constraints," in *Proceedings of the 2004 IEEE International Symposium on Biomedical Imaging: From Nano to Macro*, Arlington, VA, USA, April 2004, IEEE.
5. B. Fischl, M.I. Sereno, R.B.H. Tootell, and A.M. Dale, "High-resolution inter-subject averaging and a coordinate system for the cortical surface," *Human Brain Mapping*, vol. 8, no. 4, pp. 272–284, 1999.
6. C.R. Maurer, R. Qi, and V. Raghavan, "A Linear Time Algorithm for Computing Exact Euclidean Distance Transforms of Binary Images in Arbitrary Dimensions," vol. 25, no. 2, pp. 265–270, Feb. 2003.
7. D. Shen and C. Davatzikos, "Hammer: hierarchical attribute matching mechanism for elastic registration," *IEEE Trans. on Medical Imaging*, vol. 21, no. 11, pp. 1421–1439, Dec 2002.
8. M. Kass, A. Witkin, and D. Terzopoulos, "Snakes: Active contour models," *International Journal of Computer Vision*, vol. 4, pp. 609–331, 1988.
9. L. Hsu, R. Kusner, and J. Sullivan, "Minimizing the squared mean curvature integral for surfaces in space forms," *Experiment. Math.*, vol. 1, no. 3, pp. 191–207, 1992.
10. G.M. Treece, R.W. Prager, and A.H. Gee, "Regularised marching tetrahedra: improved iso-surface extraction," Cambridge university engineering department technical report, Sept. 1998.
11. Sarang C. Joshi, Jing Wang, Michael I. Miller, David Van Essen, and Ulf Grenander, "Differential geometry of the cortical surface," in *Vision Geometry IV*, R.A. Melter, A.Y. Wu, F.L. Bookstein, and W.D. Green, Eds., 1995, Proceedings of SPIE Vol. 2573, pp. 304–311.

Cortical Surface Alignment Using Geometry Driven Multispectral Optical Flow

Duygu Tosun and Jerry L. Prince

Electrical and Computer Engineering, Johns Hopkins University,
Baltimore, MD, 21218, USA
{dtosun, prince}@jhu.edu
http://iacl.ece.jhu.edu/index.html

Abstract. Spatial normalization is frequently used to map data to a standard coordinate system by removing inter-subject morphological differences, thereby allowing for group analysis to be carried out. In this paper, we analyze the geometry of the cortical surface using two shape measures that are the key to distinguish sulcal and gyral regions from each other. Then a multispectral optical flow (OF) warping procedure that aims to align the shape measure maps of an atlas and a subject brain's normalized maps is described. The variational problem to estimate the OF field is solved using a Euclidean framework. After warping one brain given the OF result, we obtain a better structural and functional alignment across multiple brains.[1]

1 Introduction

Developments in medical imaging techniques, particularly magnetic resonance imaging (MRI), have allowed for imaging studies concerning the structure of the human cerebral cortex and its function with large number of subjects. A major challenge has been the development of automated spatial normalization methods that allow analysis of data from multiple subjects in a standard coordinate system, designed to remove intersubject morphological differences.

Traditionally, scaled volumetric transformations are utilized to warp each brain into a standard (reference) coordinate system [1, 2, 3]. The simplest approaches rely on affine transformations only [1], and complex warping algorithms with large number of degrees of freedom improve the spatial normalization [2,3]. Comparison of local intensity and density of cortical tissues is a common key element of such voxel-based normalization approaches, which ignore geometric properties intrinsic to the cortex.

Recent advances in reconstruction of cortical surfaces from three-dimensional (3-D) MR brain image volumes have made surface-based visualization and detailed analyses on the cortical surface through surface warping possible [4, 5].

---

[1] This work was supported by the NIH/NINDS under grant R01NS37747. See http://iacl.ece.jhu.edu/duygu/research/Pubs.html for color version of figures.

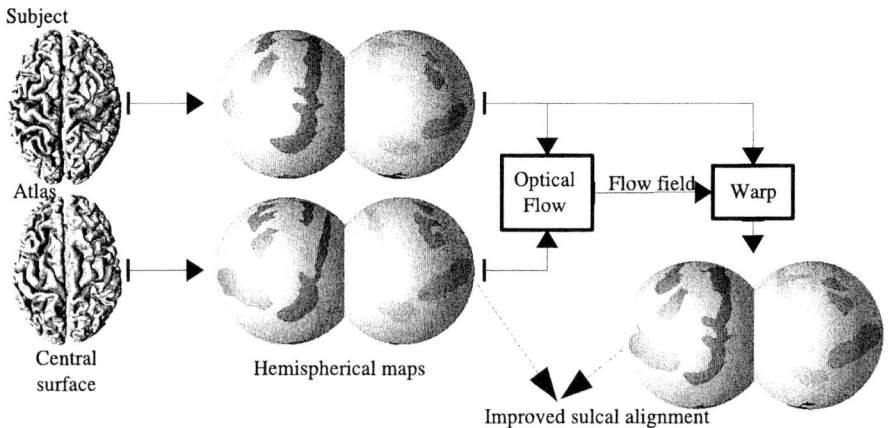

Fig. 1. Main goal: Anatomical feature matching by optical flow warping (displaying sulcal segmentation)

Visualization and analyses on the cortical surface, however, is difficult because of the extensive sulcal and gyral convolutions and their variability among individuals. Cortical unfolding procedures have been developed to address these problems. These procedures expose the buried folds of cortical gray matter, to reveal the entire structure of part or all of the cortex on a flat, convex, or radial surface [6, 7, 8, 9, 10, 11, 12, 13, 14, 15]. Preservation of the metric details — i.e., creation of approximately isometric maps — of the 3D surface has been a major goal in flattening [6, 11, 12, 13]. Several mapping approaches choose to map cortical surface onto a shape whose intrinsic properties are similar to cortex or introduce "cuts" in the surface, which are generally made manually, to control the distortion.

In order to carry out analyses on normalized cortical surfaces, it is desirable to create maps that are in a "standardized" coordinate system, in the sense that they put known anatomical features at the same coordinates in the mapped space [7, 8, 11, 14, 15]. It is believed that many major sulci are linked to the underlying cytoarchitectonic and functional organization of the cortex [16]. Hence, the main anatomical features of interest are the primary sulci common among individuals. Some methods enforce manually identified corresponding features to correspond on the computed maps [8, 14]. Others derive correspondence by maintaining strict point correspondences between parametric models that are initialized and deformed in similar fashion throughout the surface estimation process [11, 4].

In this work, we develop an automated procedure to align the key anatomical features from the individual brains in the normalized cortical coordinate system as outlined in Fig. 1. Because of the large variability of cortical geometry, a challenge is to reliably identify key anatomical features and map them to the same location on the normalized cortical coordinate system. Instead of identifying the anatomical features of interest explicitly, we analyze the geometry of the cortical surface by using two shape measures that distinguish sulcal and gyral regions from each other. This approach gives an implicit representation of the features. In order to align the dominant anatomical features of the two brains, an optical flow (OF) field is computed using both shape features as input, and the resulting deformation is used to warp the subject brain into correspondence with the template brain (atlas).

As shown in Fig. 1, the variational problem to estimate the OF field is defined on the normalized cortical surface. This variational problem can be solved on the surface via finite element approximation; however, such approaches can be time consuming and numerically unstable. To avoid these problems, we adopt the Euclidean framework described in [17] and modify it for our purpose. The basic idea of this approach is to embed the surface-based variational problem in the 3-D Euclidean space, and use Cartesian coordinate based differential operators.

The proposed feature matching procedure, when applied to multiple brains, gives a good alignment of major sulcal regions. In addition to testing for alignment of anatomical features, we also look at the alignment of functional data before and after the feature matching procedure and quantify the improvement in functional data alignment by estimating the mutual information between atlas and subject brains.

2 Preliminaries

Cortical Surface Reconstruction. In this paper, we start with a triangle mesh representation of the human brain cortex. We use *Cortical Reconstruction Using Implicit Surface Evolution* (CRUISE) [5] to find the central surface that lies at the geometric center of the gray matter tissue. CRUISE is a data-driven method combining a robust fuzzy segmentation method, an efficient topology correction algorithm, and a geometric deformable surface model. The cortical surface extraction starts with a 3-D T1-weighted SPGR volumetric axial MR data set obtained from the Baltimore Longitudinal Study of Aging (BLSA) [18]. Each reconstructed central surface is a triangle mesh comprising approximately 300,000 vertices.

Cortical Normalization. The feature matching procedure described in this paper assumes that the cortical surface extracted from the 3-D MR image volume is normalized onto a common manifold. We used the cortical normalization technique presented in [15] to map each cortical hemisphere onto its own unit sphere (i.e., hemispherical maps). The key components of the cortical normalization technique are parametric surface relaxation, iterated closest point registration, and conformal mapping. The cortical normalization automatically produces spherical coordinates on each cortical hemisphere separately. (A hemispherical map is the map of a single cortical hemisphere onto the entire unit sphere surface). The key anatomical landmarks — e.g., major sulci — are mapped to approximately the same location on the hemispherical maps and represents a good starting point for the geometry-based surface alignment that we describe herein.

3 Anatomical Feature Matching by Optical Flow Warping

A general warping procedure can be stated as following: Given two manifolds — an atlas A and a subject S — and a similarity measure, find the best coordinate system transformation that associates any point of S to a corresponding point at A while maximizing the similarity measure between the warped manifold S and the atlas manifold A. In our setting, the manifolds A and S are the hemispherical map pairs of the atlas and subject brains on the unit sphere surface, respectively. Therefore, we are looking for a warping procedure that warps a unit sphere into another unit sphere with the feature matching constraints. Each cortical hemisphere is warped separately on its own hemispherical map sphere. In this paper, we use an optical flow (OF) technique for this purpose.

Incorporating the key anatomical features such as sulcal and gyral landmarks into the warping procedure [8,3] is the key to obtaining the desired match on the hemispherical maps. Unlike the methods described in [8,14], our goal is to derive a warping procedure that does not require manually identified landmarks and does not require strict point correspondences throughout the estimation process. The primary focus of the warping procedure is to match prominent features such as the major sulci that are common across multiple brains. This creates the challenge of automated extraction of features to drive the warping procedure.

In order to force a focus on the prominent features, we use the geometry of a partially flattened surface (PFS) representation of the cortex. A PFS representation of the cortex is generated by smoothing the triangle mesh representation of the central surface using a relaxation operator [6,12]. There are two reasons behind our use of PFS representation instead of the central surface representation. First, the PFS is a smoother surface having smaller curvatures than the original central surface. The degree of detailed folding can be easily controlled by the surface relaxation algorithm's stopping criterion. In particular, we stop when the L_2 norm of the mean curvature function H defined on the surface, $\|H\|_2$, reaches a pre-selected value (see [15]). $\|H\|_2$ is a global measure that quantifies the global shape of the surface, allowing meaningful comparison between PFSs from different individuals. Second, the surface relaxation operator used to generate our PFS allows the preservation of the most prominent anatomical details representing the major sulci while smoothing out the cortical folds highly variable among individuals.

In this section, we first introduce the shape measures that we use to automatically identify the key surface features. Then, an OF warping procedure with multispectral constraints based on these shape measures is proposed to warp the subject brain's hemispherical map to the atlas brain's hemispherical map in order to match their shape measure maps.

3.1 Shape Measures

The two principal curvatures κ_1 and κ_2, where $\kappa_1 \leq \kappa_2$, have the necessary information to fully describe the local shape of the surface. However, curvature based analysis of the folding pattern requires individual measures that possess a coordinate independent *geometrical* meaning such that the *shape* of the surface can be specified independent of the *size*. The widely used Gaussian and mean curvature measures, by themselves, fail to capture the intuitive notion of local shape very well. In particular, the Gaussian curvature vanishes both at planar points (i.e., $\kappa_1 = \kappa_2 = 0$), and at parabolic points (i.e., $\kappa_1 \neq 0$ and $\kappa_2 = 0$), thereby failing to distinguish these two shapes.

In [19], *shape index* and *curvedness* measures were introduced as a pair of local shape indicator measures. The shape index, SI, and the curvedness, C, are defined as

$$\text{SI} = \frac{2}{\pi} \arctan \frac{\kappa_2 + \kappa_1}{\kappa_2 - \kappa_1} \quad \text{and} \quad C = \sqrt{\frac{\kappa_1^2 + \kappa_2^2}{2}}. \quad (1)$$

The shape index specifies the local surface geometry up to a scaling factor (i.e., similarity), and takes values in $[-1, +1]$. The extreme values of the shape index represents local shapes look like either the inside (SI $= -1$) or the outside (SI $= 1$) of a spherical surface, and intermediate values correspond to the local surface shapes observed when these shapes smoothly morphed one to other.

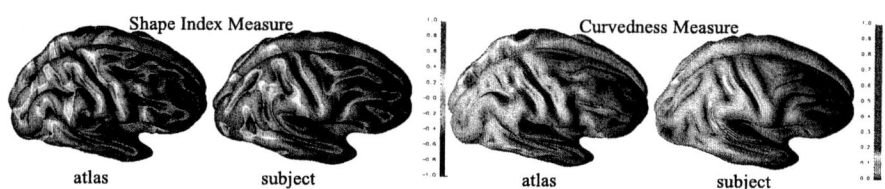

Fig. 2. Shape measures of two example partially flattened surfaces (PFSs)

As a scale-independent measure, the shape index does not specify the magnitude of the local shape. In contrast, the curvedness measure is inversely proportional with the *size* of the surface patch independent of the coordinate. Unlike the Gaussian and mean curvature measures, the shape index and curvedness measures complement each other in defining the local surface *shape* and the *size*.

Fig. 2 shows the shape index and curvedness measure maps of two example PFSs. It is observed that the shape index measure successfully distinguishes the sulci and gyri on the PFSs. One can also see that the curvedness measures of the subject and atlas brains' PFSs are comparable in magnitude and similar in overall pattern.

3.2 Optical Flow with Multispectral Constraints

We now describe an optical flow (OF) technique defined on the unit sphere to warp the atlas and subject brains' hemispherical maps to match their key anatomical features on the hemispherical map coordinate system. Let $\mathbf{I}(\mathbf{V}(t)) = [w_{SI}I_{SI}(\mathbf{V}(t)), w_C I_C(\mathbf{V}(t))]$ be the shape measure vector extracted from the PFS representation, where $\mathbf{V} \in \Re^3$ is the surface mesh node on the hemispherical map of the atlas brain when $t = 0$, and of the subject brain when $t = 1$. I_{SI} and I_C are the shape index and curvedness measure maps with scalar weights w_{SI} and w_C, respectively.

Hemispherical maps are 2-D manifolds embedded in the 3-D Euclidean space. Let $\mathbf{I}(\mathbf{x}) = [w_{SI}I_{SI}(\mathbf{x}), w_C I_C(\mathbf{x})]$ denote the shape measure vector in $\Re^3$ where $\mathbf{x} = \mathbf{x}(t) = [x_1(t), x_2(t), x_3(t)] \in \Re^3$, but restricted to the unit sphere surface — i.e., $S^2 \subset \Re^3$ — where the hemispherical maps are defined. Starting with the constant intensity constraint of OF, $\frac{d\mathbf{I}(\mathbf{x})}{dt} = \mathbf{0}$, and using the chain rule of differentiation, the left hand side of this equation can be expressed as

$$w_j \left(\langle \nabla_{S^2} I_j(\mathbf{x}), \mathbf{u} \rangle + \frac{dI_j(\mathbf{x})}{dt} \right) = 0 \quad \text{for } j = \text{SI, C} \tag{2}$$

where $\mathbf{u} = \mathbf{u}(\mathbf{x}(t)) = [u_1(\mathbf{x}(t)), u_2(\mathbf{x}(t)), u_3(\mathbf{x}(t))] = d\mathbf{x}(t)/dt$ represents the flow field vector at $\mathbf{x}$, and ∇_{S^2} is the the spatial gradient operator defined on S^2.

To estimate a smooth flow field $\mathbf{u}$ with the multispectral OF constraint given in (2) and the incompressibility (divergence-free) constraint [20,21], we pose the following optimization problem:

$$\operatorname*{argmin}_{\mathbf{u} \in \mathcal{F}} \int_{S^2} \left(\sum_{i=1}^{3} \rho(\|\nabla_{S^2} u_i\|, \mu) \right) dx_1 dx_2 dx_3$$

$$\text{s.t. } w_j \left(\langle \nabla_{S^2} I_j(\mathbf{x}), \mathbf{u} \rangle + \frac{dI_j(\mathbf{x})}{dt} \right) = 0 \text{ for } j = \text{SI, C and } \nabla_{S^2} \cdot \mathbf{u} = 0, \tag{3}$$

where $\rho(\epsilon, \mu) = \log(1 + \frac{1}{2}(\frac{\epsilon}{\mu})^2)$ is a robust Lorentzian error measure [22] introduced to handle discontinuities and outliers, and $\mathcal{F}$ is the set of flow fields. The set of flow fields is defined as $\mathcal{F} = \{\mathbf{u} \in W^{1,2}(S^2 \subset \Re^3) \text{ s.t. } \|\mathbf{u} + \mathbf{x}\| = \|\mathbf{x}\|\}$, where $W^{1,2}(S^2, \Re^3)$ denotes the Sobolev space of functions, so that every point on a sphere of a given radius is mapped back onto the same sphere surface.

Rather than solving the optimization problem given in (3) directly, we solve the problem of unconstrained minimization of the energy function for given α and β parameters

$$E(\mathbf{u}) = \int_{S^2} \rho \left(\sqrt{\sum_{j-\text{SI,C}} w_j^2 \left(\langle \nabla_{S^2} I_j(\mathbf{x}), \mathbf{u} \rangle + \frac{dI_j(\mathbf{x})}{dt} \right)^2}, \mu \right) dx_1 dx_2 dx_3$$

$$+ \alpha \int_{S^2} \left(\sum_{i=1}^{3} \rho(\|\nabla_{S^2} u_i\|, \mu) \right) dx_1 dx_2 dx_3 + \beta \int_{S^2} \rho \left(\|\nabla_{S^2} \cdot \mathbf{u}\|, \mu \right) dx_1 dx_2 dx_3. \tag{4}$$

To derive the Euler-Lagrange equation of this variational problem, we need to compute the gradient descent of (4). Let $\phi = \phi(\mathbf{x}) \in C_0^\infty(S^2, \Re^3)$, the space of smooth functions in S^2 vanishing outside a compact subset of S^2. The flow field function should satisfy $\|\mathbf{u} + \mathbf{x}\| = \|\mathbf{x}\|$; thus, for a small enough perturbation s, the admissible function is defined as $\mathbf{u}(s) = [(\mathbf{u} + s\phi + \mathbf{x})\frac{\|\mathbf{x}\|}{\|\mathbf{u}+s\phi+\mathbf{x}\|} - \mathbf{x}] \in W^{1,2}(S^2, \Re^3)$. Computing $\frac{d}{ds}E(\mathbf{u}(s))|_{s=0}$ gives the following Euler-Lagrange equation.

$$0 = \frac{\sum_{j=\text{SI,C}} \left[w_j^2 \left(\langle \nabla_{S^2} I_j, \mathbf{u}(s)\rangle + \frac{dI_j}{dt}\right)\left(\frac{\partial}{\partial x_k}I_j - \langle \nabla_{S^2} I_j, \mathbf{y}\rangle y_k\right)\right]}{\mu^2 + \frac{1}{2}\sum_{j=\text{SI,C}} w_j^2 \left(\langle \nabla_{S^2} I_j, \mathbf{u}(s)\rangle + \frac{dI_j}{dt}\right)^2}$$

$$+ \alpha\left[y_k \sum_{i=1}^{3} \left(\frac{y_i \Delta_{S^2} u_i + 2\langle \nabla_{S^2} u_i, \mathbf{x}\rangle \frac{y_i}{\|\mathbf{u}+\mathbf{x}\|^2}}{\mu^2 + \frac{1}{2}\|\nabla_{S^2} u_i\|^2}\right) - \alpha \frac{\Delta_{S^2} u_k}{\mu^2 + \frac{1}{2}\|\nabla_{S^2} u_k\|^2}\right]$$

$$+ \beta\left[\frac{\frac{(2\nabla_{S^2}\cdot\mathbf{u})\langle \mathbf{y},\mathbf{x}\rangle}{\|\mathbf{u}+\mathbf{x}\|^2} + y_k\langle \nabla_{S^2}(\nabla_{S^2}\cdot\mathbf{u}), \mathbf{y}\rangle - y_k\frac{\partial}{\partial x_k}(\nabla_{S^2}\cdot\mathbf{u})}{\mu^2 + \frac{1}{2}\|\nabla_{S^2}\cdot\mathbf{u}\|^2}\right] \qquad (5)$$

for $k = 1, 2, 3$, where $\mathbf{y} = \frac{\mathbf{u}+\mathbf{x}}{\|\mathbf{u}+\mathbf{x}\|} = [y_1, y_2, y_3]$, and Δ_{S^2} is the Laplace-Beltrami operator on the S^2 surface.

Numerical Implementation. The shape measures are defined on the triangle mesh representation of the hemispherical maps. Therefore, in order to compute the solution to (5), the differential operators must be discretize on the triangulated surface. This involves a finite element approximation of the differential operators defined on S^2. Such approaches can be not only tedious and time consuming, but also unstable if the surface triangulation is not regularized. In [17], a new concept was introduced that allows us to transform the variational problem defined on the surface into a variational problem embedded in the entire 3-D Euclidean space ($\Re^3$).

In order to utilize this Eulerian framework to solve the PDE given in (5), we first need to transfer the given explicit surface representation of S^2 into an implicit surface representation, and then extend the shape measure maps defined on the surface to maps defined for the entire $\Re^3$. Although the triangle mesh representation of the unit sphere has thousands of mesh nodes, its implicit representation in $\Re^3$ occupies only a cubic region of size $2 \times 2 \times 2$. The unit sphere surface needs to be resized to a sphere of size $R \gg 1$ to properly transfer the surface data into the entire 3-D Euclidean space with enough details. Its implicit surface representation is given as the zero level set of the signed distance function $\phi: \Re^3 \to \Re, \phi(\mathbf{x}) = \|\mathbf{x}\| - R$. The shape measure maps on S^2 are then extended to the entire 3-D Euclidean space in such a way that the maps are constant in the surface normal directions — i.e., $\langle \nabla \mathbf{I}, \nabla \phi\rangle = 0$ [17], where ∇ is the spatial gradient operator in the 3-D Cartesian coordinates.

This transformation allows us to calculate the spatial gradient and Laplace-Beltrami operators, intrinsic to the surface, by using the simple differential operators defined in the 3-D Cartesian coordinates. Hence, $\nabla_{S^2} f = P_{\nabla\phi} \nabla f$ and $\Delta_{S^2} f = \nabla \cdot (P_{\nabla\phi} \nabla f)$, where $P_{\nabla\phi}$ is the operator that projects a 3-D vector onto the plane orthogonal to $\nabla\phi$ (see [17]). Eqn. (5) is discretized by using the classical scheme of forward differences in time, and combination of forward and backward differences in space, thereby making the numerical implementation straightforward and faster compared to that of a finite element approximation on the triangulated surface. From various possible combinations of the forward and backward differences, upwinding scheme in the direction of $\nabla\phi$ is used in computing the projected gradient, and upwinding scheme in the direction of $-\nabla\phi$ is used in computing the divergence.

Iterative Procedure. First the shape measure maps extended to the 3-D space are regularized using the intrinsic isotropic diffusion operator in 3-D Cartesian coordinates — i.e., $\nabla \cdot (P_{\nabla\phi} \nabla I_{SI}) = 0$ and $\nabla \cdot (P_{\nabla\phi} \nabla I_C) = 0$ — to stabilize the OF field estimation. To speed up the iterative procedure, we solve the variational problem only at the narrow-band points that satisfies $\|\phi(\mathbf{x})\| < h$ for a given constant h. Finally, to address the large deformation problem, a multiscale scheme is utilized as outlined in the following pseudo-code.

Algorithm 1 (Multiscale Scheme for Optical Flow Warping)
1. Initialize the parameters w_{SI}, w_C, R, h, μ, α, and β.
2. Resize the hemispherical maps to a sphere of size $R \gg 1$.
3. Extend the shape measure maps to the 3-D Euclidean space.
4. Regularize the shape measure maps via intrinsic isotropic diffusion operator in 3-D Cartesian coordinate.
5. Set $\mathbf{u} = \mathbf{0}$ at all 3-D Cartesian grip points.
6. Use the Euler-Lagrange equation given in (5) to solve for $\mathbf{u}$ at narrow-band points using a iterative procedure.
7. Map $\mathbf{u}$ onto the hemispherical map of subject brain and deform the hemispherical map accordingly.
8. Increase R and decrease α and β parameters.
9. Repeat the above steps until $\|\mathbf{u}\| < \epsilon$ almost everywhere for a small ϵ.

4 Experimental Results and Discussion

Hemispherical maps of 32 subject brains were warped to the atlas brain's hemispherical map using the multiscale OF warping procedure described in Sect. 3. The algorithm parameters at the last iteration of the multiscale scheme were $w_{SI} = w_C = 1$, $R = 50$, $h = 5$, $\mu = 2$, $\alpha = 5$, and $\beta = 1$. Choosing $R = 50$ makes each hemispherical map's surface area comparable to the actual cortical surface area. We want to note that since the proposed OF warping does not have a built in diffeomorphism criterion, a large α algorithm parameter was chosen to obtain a smooth flow field. The multiscale scheme convergences after 10–20 iterations, and each iteration takes 30–60 seconds depending on the size of R.

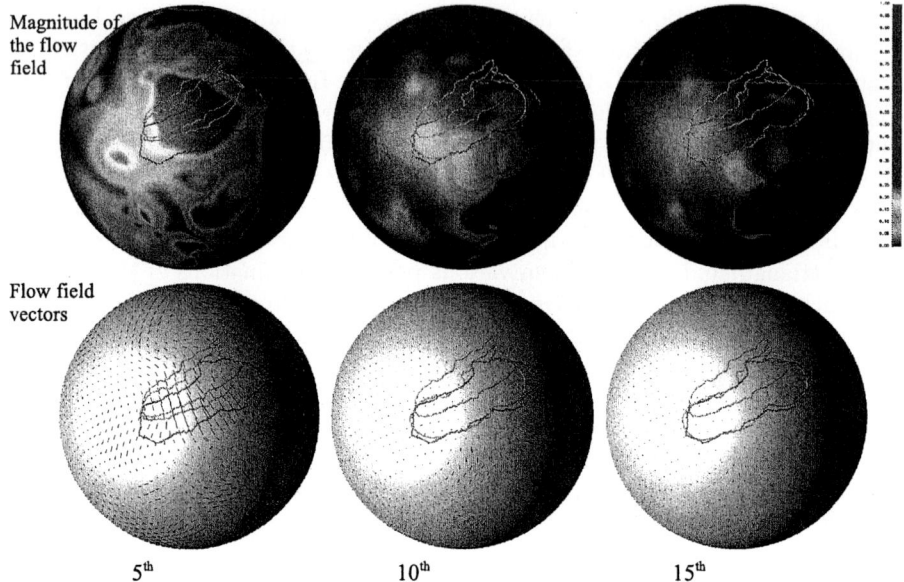

Fig. 3. Optical flow field after 5th, 10th and 15th iterations of the multiscale scheme. Top row: magnitude of the field vectors; Bottom row: direction of the field vectors. Contours: The boundary of the central sulcus region of the atlas brain (in magenta) and of the subject brain initially and after the OF warping after these iterations (in yellow and cyan, respectively)

Fig. 3 shows an example. The magnitude of the resulting flow field (top row) and the field vectors (bottom row) on the warped hemispherical map are shown after 5th, 10th and 15th iterations of the multiscale scheme. The field vectors are downsampled for display purposes. The boundary of the central sulcus region of the atlas brain (in magenta) and of the subject brain initially and after the OF warping after these iterations (in yellow and cyan, respectively) are also shown in Fig. 3. (Note that sulcal boundary information was not used in the OF process.)

In order to evaluate how well common anatomical features map to similar locations on the sphere using the proposed OF warping procedure, we analyzed the locations to which four primary sulci are mapped in 33 individual brains (one atlas brain and 32 subject brains). Four sulcal regions — the central sulcus (cs), superior frontal (sf), cingulate sulcus (cn) and parieto-occipital sulcus (po) on both the left and right cortical hemispheres — were automatically segmented [23] and manually labeled on all 33 brains.

To see where the four sulci map on the hemispherical map of the atlas brain, we generated probabilistic maps comprising an estimated conditional probability of the location of a sulcal region for each of four sulcal regions. Fig. 4 shows the probabilistic maps of the sulcal regions on the left cortical hemisphere before and after the OF warping. The maximum values of the probabilistic maps, and the surface area of the regions on the atlas brain's hemispherical map where

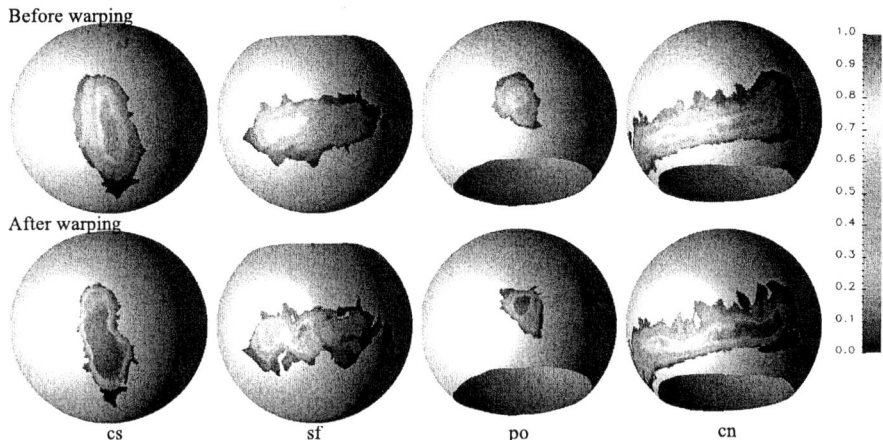

Fig. 4. Probabilistic maps of the four sulcal regions on the left cortical hemisphere before and after the optical flow warping

Table 1. Alignment of the major sulcal regions

	lcs	lsf	lpo	lcn	rcs	rsf	rpo	rcn
average sulcal area	0.29	0.21	0.08	0.46	0.28	0.18	0.08	0.48
max before OF	1.00	0.93*	0.94	1.00	0.94	0.88	0.88	1.00*
area(Prob > 0.5) before OF	0.28	0.15	0.07	0.45	0.23	0.07	0.07	0.44
max after OF	1.00	1.00*	1.00	1.00	1.00	1.00	1.00	1.00*
area(Prob > 0.5) after OF	0.32	0.24	0.06	0.42	0.33	0.14	0.06	0.41

*Only 31 subjects data were used because of missing labels in 2 subjects.

Prob > 0.5 are given in Table 1 along with the average surface area of each sulcal region. Improvements in both of these measures, and the visual inspection of the results shown in Figs. 3 and 4 show that by geometry driven OF warping we achieve a significantly better sulcal alignment, close to perfect alignment in fact.

In order to demonstrate a potential use of the proposed OF warping technique in neuroscience applications, we utilize the warped hemispherical maps in cross-sectional analysis of functional images of cerebral blood flow using positron emission tomography (PET-CBF) from older adults in the neuroimaging substudy of the BLSA [18]. For each neuroimaging session, three PET scans were performed during: Rest, and Verbal and Figural Recognition Memory. For each scan, 75mCi of [^{15}O] water were injected as a bolus, and scans were acquired on a GE 4096+ scanner (resolution = 6 mm FWHM), and the activation intensity range is [0,511]. Each subject's PET-CBF data was preprocessed and aligned with its structural MRI data by following the processing steps described in [24], and then the PET-CBF data values were mapped onto the central surface mesh nodes by integrating the PET-CBF data over a curvilinear line bounded by the

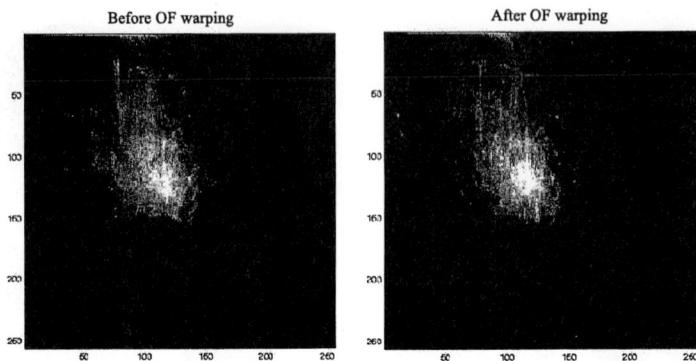

Fig. 5. Joint probability distribution of PET-CBF activation before and after the OF warping

GM tissue thickness at this point. The CBF data on the surface was regularized using the intrinsic isotropic diffusion operator.

The OF warping approach presented in this paper aims to improve alignment of the anatomical features, which should also improve the alignment of function for gross tasks involving vision and speech in the major sulci. To quantify any such improvement in functional data alignment, we estimated the mutual information before and after OF warping, which is widely used in the medical image registration techniques [25]. The PET-CBF activation values mapped onto the surfaces are quantized into 256 levels. The probability that the activation level x occurs in brain X, $p_X(x)$, is estimated as $N(x)/\sum_i N(i)$, where $N(i)$ is the total surface area on the given hemispherical map with activation level $i \in [0, 255]$. The joint probabilities are estimated in a similar fashion.

The joint probability distribution of atlas and subject brains' PET-CBF activations before and after the OF warping are shown in Fig. 5. We observe a subtle decrease in the spread of the joint probability distribution, and the peak values are larger after the OF warping as well. Averaged over 32 subjects, we observe a 45% increase in the mutual information metric of PET-CBF activation during rest once the normalized cortical maps are matched using the proposed method. The improvement on the mutual information metric is 50% for PET-CBF activation during both verbal and figural memory tasks.

Conclusion. We have presented a feature matching technique based on two shape measures and optical flow warping with multispectral constraints. The shape measure vector, **I**, can be extended to a $n \times 1$ vector by incorporating additional features inherent to that specific application such as features extracted from functional data, or information regarding the relative location of structures of interest. The mathematical derivations presented in this paper can be generalized to optical flow warping of any manifolds with n constraints, which gives the opportunity of utilizing the proposed method in a wide variety of image processing and analysis research where alignment of data on a surface is desired.

References

1. J. Talairach and P. Tournoux. *Co-Planar Stereotaxic Atlas of the Human Brain. 3-Dimensional Proportional System: An Approach to Cerebral Imaging.* Thieme Medical Publisher, Inc., Stuttgart, New York, 1988.
2. K. Friston, J. Ahburner, J. Poline, C. Frith, J. Heather, and R. Frackowiak. Spatial realignment and normalization of images. In *Human Brain Mapping*, 1995.
3. L. Collins and A. C. Evans. ANIMAL: Automatic nonlinear image matching and anatomical labeling. In *Brain warping*. Academic Press, 1999.
4. D. MacDonald, N. Kabani, D. Avis, and A. Evans. Automated 3D extraction of inner and outer surfaces of cerebral cortex from MRI. *NeuroImage*, 12(3), 2000.
5. X. Han, D. L.Pham, D. Tosun, M. E. Rettmann, C. Xu, and J. L. Prince. CRUISE: Cortical reconstruction using implicit surface evolution. *NeuroImage*, 23(3), 2004.
6. H. A. Drury, D. C. V. Essen, C. H. Anderson, W. C. Lee, T. A. Coogan, and J. W. Lewis. Computerized mapping of the cerebral cortex: A multiresolution flattening method and a surface-based coordinate system. *J. Cogn. Neuro.*, 8(1), 1996.
7. J. I. Sereno, A. M. Dale, A. Liu, and R. B. H. Tootell. A surface-based coordinate system for a canonical cortex. *Proc. 2nd Int. Conf. Hum. Brain Mapping, NeuroImage*, 3(3).
8. P. M. Thompson and A. W. Toga. A surface-based technique for warping three-dimensional images of the brain. *TMI*, 15, 1996.
9. M. K. Hurdal, P. L. Bowers, K. Stephenson, D. W. L. Sumners, K. Rehm, K. Schaper, and D. A. Rottenberg. Quasi-conformally flat mapping the human cerebellum. In Berlin Springer, editor, *Lecture Notes in Computer Science*.
10. S. Angenent, S. Haker, A. Tannenbaum, and R. Kikinis. On the Laplace-Beltrami operator and brain surface flattening. *IEEE Trans. Med. Imag.*, 18(8), 1999.
11. B. Fischl, M. I. Sereno, and A. M. Dale. Cortical surface-based analysis II: Inflation, flattening, and a surface-based coordinate system. *NeuroImage*, 9(2), Feb. 1999.
12. B. Timsari and R. Leahy. Optimization method for creating semi-isometric flat maps of the cerebral cortex. In *Proc. SPIE Conf. Med. Imag.*, 2000.
13. Ruth Grossmann, Nahum Kiryati, and Ron Kimmel. Computational surface flattening: A voxel-based approach. *Lecture Notes in Computer Science*, 2059.
14. X. Gu, Y. Wang, T. F. Chan, P. M. Thompson, and S. T. Yau. Genus zero surface conformal mapping and its application to brain surface mapping. In *Information Processing in Medical Imaging*, Ambleside, UK, July 2003.
15. D. Tosun, M. E. Rettmann, and J. L. Prince. Mapping techniques for aligning sulci across multiple brains. *Medical Image Analysis - Special issue: Medical Image Computing and Computer-Assisted Intervention - MICCAI 2003 - Edited by R. Ellis and T. Petters*, 8(3), 2004.
16. W. I. Welker. The significance of foliation and fissuration of cerebellar cortex. The cerebellar folium as a fundamental unit of sensorimotor integration. *Arch. Italienned de Biologie*, 128, 1990.
17. M. Bertalmio, L. T. Cheng, S. Osher, and G. Sapiro. Variational problems and partial differential equations on implicit surfaces: The framework and examples in image processing and pattern formation. *J. Comput. Physics*, 174(2), 2001.
18. S. M. Resnick, A. F. Goldszal, C. Davatzikos, S. Golski, M. A. Kraut, E. J. Metter, R. N. Bryan, and A. B. Zonderman. One-year age changes in MRI brain volumes in older adults. *Cerebral Cortex*, 10(5), 2000.
19. J. J. Koenderink and A. J. van Doorn. Surface shape and curvature scales. *Image and Vision Computing*, 10(8), 1992.

20. B. K. P. Horn and B. G. Schunck. Determining optical flow. *Artificial Intelligence*, 17, 1981.
21. S. M. Song and R. M. Leahy. Computation of 3-D velocity fields from 3-D cine CT images of a human heart. *IEEE Trans. Med. Imag.*, 10(3), 1991.
22. M. J. Black, G. Sapiro, D. H. Marimont, and D. Heeger. Robust anisotropic diffusion. *IEEE Trans. Imag. Proc.*, 7(3), 1998.
23. M. E. Rettmann, X. Han, C. Xu, and J. L. Prince. Automated sulcal segmentation using watersheds on the cortical surface. *NeuroImage*, 15, 2002.
24. L. L. Beason-Held, S. Golski, M. A. Kraut, G. Esposito, and S. M. Resnick. Brain activation during encoding and recognition of verbal and figural information in older adults. *Neurobiol. Aging*, 26(2), 2005.
25. C. Studholme, D. L. G. Hill, and D. J. Hawkes. An overlap invariant entropy measure of 3d medical image alignment. *Pattern Recog.*, 32, 1999.

Inverse Consistent Mapping in 3D Deformable Image Registration: Its Construction and Statistical Properties

Alex Leow[1], Sung-Cheng Huang[2], Alex Geng[1], James Becker[3], Simon Davis[3], Arthur Toga[1], and Paul Thompson[1]

[1] Rm. 4238, 710 Westwood Plaza, LONI, UCLA School of Medicine
[2] Dept. of Molecular and Medical Pharmacology, UCLA School of Medicine
[3] Dept. of Neurology, Psychiatry, and Psychology, Univ. of Pittsburgh
aliao@loni.ucla.edu

Abstract. This paper presents a new approach to inverse consistent image registration. A uni-directional algorithm is developed using symmetric cost functionals and regularizers. Instead of enforcing inverse consistency using an additional penalty that penalizes inconsistency error, the new algorithm directly models the backward mapping by inverting the forward mapping. The resulting minimization problem can then be solved uni-directionally involving only the forward mapping, without optimizing in the backward direction. Lastly, we evaluated the algorithm by applying it to the serial MRI scans of a clinical case of semantic dementia. The statistical distributions of the local volume change (Jacobian) maps were examined by considering the Kullback-Liebler distances on the material density functions. Contrary to common belief, the values of any non-trivial Jacobian map do not follow a log-normal distribution with zero mean. Statistically significant differences were detected between consistent versus inconsistent matching when permutation tests were performed on the resulting deformation maps

1 Introduction

Non-linear image registration is a well-established field in medical imaging with many applications in functional and anatomic brain mapping, image guided surgery, and multimodality image fusion [1-3]. The goal of image registration is to align, or spatially normalize, one image to another. In multisubject studies, registration reduces subject-specific anatomic differences by deforming individual images onto a population average brain template. Using a similar procedure, maps visualizing structural brain change over time can be generated by deforming baseline scans onto subsequent scans of the same subject, and using the deformation map to quantify local changes.

To formulate the image registration problem mathematically, we denote the two images to be registered as T and S (both defined on an image domain Ω). We seek to estimate a transformation h so that $S(h(x))$ is "closest" to $T(x)$ in terms of certain matching criteria. Ideally, this transformation mapping h should be smooth, one-to-one, and differentiable (i.e., a diffeomorphism). Conventionally, researchers in the field of non-linear image registration use the notation $u=(u_x, u_y, u_z)$, the displacement vector field away from the identity map, to represent the transformation h (i.e.,

$h(x) = x - u(x)$). The inverse map h^{-1} of h (i.e., $h^{-1}(h(x))=x$ for all x) thus maps the target to the source image. We will also use the notation u^{-1} to denote the displacement field of the inverse map h^{-1}.

To make the transformation smooth, one-to-one, and differentiable, a regularizing constraint on the displacement field is needed. Thus, the problem of image registration is often cast as a minimization problem with a total cost functional E expressed in general as $E = E_M(S,T) + R(h)$, where E_M is the matching criterion cost function, and $R(h)$ is the regularizing constraint on the transformation.

Intuitively, the problem of image registration is symmetric, i.e., the correspondences established between the two images should not depend on the order we use to compare the two images. However, early approaches for non-linear image registration were not symmetric and various terms (e.g., source, target, template, study, and reference) have been used to describe the direction of this comparison. In this paper, we will adopt the term *source* or S to describe the floating/deforming image and the term *target* or T to describe the image that the source image is deformed to match. This dependence on the direction of comparison not only complicates the notation but also has serious disadvantages. Firstly, the deformation field depends on which image is assigned the source and which image the target. This dependence can be termed *inverse inconsistency* as inconsistency arises if we switch the order of source and target. Secondly, as pointed out in [4], these inversely inconsistent approaches penalize the expansion of image regions more than the shrinkage of image regions. This imbalance in the penalty was also noticed and discussed in another paper [5] by the same group in which shrinking brain lesions were found to be easier to detect than expanding ones using inversely inconsistent methods. Thus, conventional inverse-inconsistent non-linear registration techniques may be problematic in applications where the Jacobian of the transformation h is interpreted as measuring tissue loss or expansion, a step commonly performed in computational neuroanatomy (e.g., in tensor-based morphometry).

One of the first approaches for inverse consistent registration [6] symmetrized not only the matching cost functional, but also the regularization of the displacement. Using the sum of squared differences of the intensities as the matching cost functional, the following total cost function E was proposed:

$$E(T,S) = \underbrace{\int_\Omega |S(h(x)) - T(x)|^2 dx + \lambda R(h)}_{E_1} + \underbrace{\int_\Omega |T(h^{-1}(x)) - S(x)|^2 dx + \lambda R(h^{-1})}_{E_2} \quad (1)$$

Here λ is a positive scalar weighting of the regularizers applied to the forward and inverse mappings. The above cost function is symmetric and does not depend on the order of T and S, i.e., $E(T,S) = E(S,T)$. To solve (1) numerically, [6] solved for h and g separately as follows and additional inverse consistency constraints were added so that g numerically realized h^{-1}.

$$E_h(T,S) = \int_\Omega |S(h(x)) - T(x)|^2 dx + \lambda R(h) + \rho \int_\Omega \left\| h - (g)^{-1} \right\|^2 dx; \quad (2)$$

$$E_g(T,S) = \int_\Omega |T(g(x)) - S(x)|^2 dx + \lambda R(g) + \rho \int_\Omega \left\| g - (h)^{-1} \right\|^2 dx.$$

Iterative gradient descent methods can be employed and the numerical algorithm for minimizing eq. (2) can be summarized as follows. At initialization, both h and g are set to be the identity map. At each time step, the gradient descent of E_h is computed to update h while fixing the map g, and similarly Eg is used to update g while fixing the map h. This avoids the highly nonlinear nature of the original minimization problem eq. (1) in which both the forward and backward mappings are involved and need to be optimized while maintaining the inverse relation between them.

Although the alternative formulation eq. (2) was extensively tested, with good experimental results, it has some disadvantages compared to the original formulation in eq. (1). Firstly, the algorithm proposed to solve eq. (2) is essentially a two step strategy and creates a lagging-behind situation in estimating h and g. Either h and g has to be alternately fixed (i.e., the two maps are not estimated simultaneously). Moreover, an extra weighting parameter for the inverse consistency constraints has to be considered and was tuned case-by-case in [6].

2 Method

2.1 Inverting Gradient Descent Direction

We seek to solve the original symmetric formulation for non-linear registration in eq. (1) instead of the modified formulation in eq. (2). To this end, we propose to directly couple the backward and forward mappings, allowing all driving body forces to be combined in the forward direction. As a result, the corresponding minimization problem can be optimized in a unidirectional fashion, i.e. by considering the forward mapping only. Thus, the proposed algorithm can be thought of as a unidirectional procedure with embedded inverse consistency.

To simplify the derivation of this procedure, we will illustrate it using the sum of squared difference (SSD) as the matching cost functional. This can easily be extended to other intensity/feature-based cost functionals. As mentioned before, we will convert the gradient descent direction involving the backward mapping (E_2 in eq. (1)) to a corresponding gradient descent direction in the forward direction. More precisely, we wish to update h and h^{-1} by perturbing the mappings from the previous time step in a descent direction with respect to the total cost functional E.

$$h \to h + \varepsilon\eta_1 + \varepsilon\eta_2; \; h^{-1} \to h^{-1} + \varepsilon\xi_1 + \varepsilon\xi_2. \tag{3}$$

Here, ε is an infinitesimally small positive number and η_1 and ξ_1 are vector fields that represent the gradient descent direction of E_1 in eq. (1) in the forward and backward direction respectively, with η_2 and ξ_2 similarly defined for the term E_2. Notice that the terms η_1 and ξ_2 can be computed using standard calculus. Formally, we can write η_1 and ξ_2 as follows

$$\eta_1(x) = \big(S(h(x)) - T(x)\big)\nabla S(h(x)) + \lambda\nabla R(h); \tag{4}$$

$$\xi_2(x) = \big(T(h^{-1}(x)) - S(x)\big)\nabla T(h^{-1}(x)) + \lambda\nabla R(h^{-1}).$$

Here the gradient operator applied to the regularizer denotes the gradient descent direction of the regularizer (or a regularized/smoothed body force). In order to numerically compute (3), we need to solve for η_2 and ξ_1 using eqs. (3) and (4). To this end, we first utilize the inverse relationship given in eq. (3)

$$\left(h^{-1} + \varepsilon\xi_1 + \varepsilon\xi_2\right) \circ \left(h + \varepsilon\eta_1 + \varepsilon\eta_2\right) = id. \tag{5}$$

where id is the identity mapping. By expanding (5) using Taylor's expansion and collecting up to first order terms of ε, we obtain

$$Dh^{-1}(h(x))\{\eta_1(x) + \eta_2(x)\} = -\xi_1(h(x)) - \xi_2(h(x)). \tag{6}$$

Here D denotes the Jacobian matrix operator. Using the relationship: $\left(D(h(x))\right)^{-1} = Dh^{-1}(h(x))$, derived by differentiating the identity relation $h^{-1}(h) = id$, we obtain the following alternative form to (6)

$$\eta_1(x) + \eta_2(x) = -D(h(x))\{\xi_1(h(x)) + \xi_2(h(x))\}. \tag{7}$$

With (7), we can now express η_2 and ξ_1 using the known quantities ξ_2 and η_1

$$\eta_2(x) = -D(h(x))\xi_2(h(x)); \tag{8}$$

$$\xi_1(x) = -D(h^{-1}(x))\eta_1(h^{-1}(x))$$

With all the quantities known, we now have a recipe for minimizing the symmetric forward-backward problem (1) using an iterative approach with the updating formulae (3). Moreover, as the two updating formulae in (3) are designed to be consistent with each other, we can simply update in the forward direction (first formula) without using the backward updating formulae at all. Notice that with eq. (8), the inversion of a body force from the backward direction to the forward direction can be carried out using only the forward mapping h (without involving h^{-1}). This property is desirable due to the unavoidable numerical errors incurred when inverting between h and h^{-1}.

Thus, at each time step of the gradient descent method, we sum up the total forward body force by combining the forward body force and the inverted backward body force obtained by applying (8). To evaluate (8) numerically, interpolations are necessary and we use a bi-linear or tri-linear technique to interpolate the backward body force in the non-grid point position $h(x)$.

In this paper, the linear elastic operator is chosen as in [6] for the regularizer

$$R(u) = \int \left\| -\alpha\Delta u - \beta\nabla(\nabla \cdot u)\right\|^2 dx. \tag{9}$$

where Δ is the Laplacian and α and β are the Lamé constants (both set to be 1.0). The Fast Fourier transform technique (FFT) is applied to parameterize the displacement field. A multi-resolution minimization scheme can then be implemented in the frequency domain.

2.2 Statistical Properties of Deformation Maps

In this section, we discuss the statistical properties of the deformation maps arising from non-linear image registration. In tensor-based morphometry, the Jacobian determinants of deformation maps are used to index local volume compressions or dilations and their distribution is typically assumed to be log-normal [7]. However, we now show that the determinant of the Jacobian operator applied to any bijective (one-to-one and onto) globally volume-preserving mapping h cannot have a log-normal distribution with zero mean. To this end, let us denote the Jacobian matrix of a transformation h as Dh (with the (i,j)-th element $\partial h_j / \partial x_i$), and the local volume loss/expansion map (Jacobian map) can thus be defined as $J(x) = |Dh(x)|$. Notice that J encodes the local volume change of the source with respect to the target image, and may be considered to reside on the target reference frame. Since h is a diffeomorphic and bijective mapping from Ω to itself, we obtain the following using a change of variable

$$\frac{1}{|\Omega|} \int_\Omega |Dh(x)| dx \stackrel{y=h(x)}{=} \frac{1}{|\Omega|} \int_\Omega dy = 1. \tag{10}$$

Here, the first integral should be evaluated with respect to the target domain and the second integral with respect to the source domain, and $|\Omega|$ is the total volume of Ω. Given eq. (10), we can define a probability density function (PDF) P on Ω as $P(x) = |Dh(x)|/|\Omega|$ as it integrates to 1. Let us also use $Q(x) = 1/|\Omega|$ to denote the PDF of the uniform distribution on Ω. Then, using the relation $\log(1/a) = -\log(a)$, we can compute the mean of $\log(J)$ in the target reference frame on Ω as follows

$$\frac{1}{|\Omega|} \int_\Omega \log|Dh(x)| dx = -\int_\Omega \frac{1}{|\Omega|} \log\left(\frac{1/|\Omega|}{|Dh(x)|/|\Omega|}\right) dx \tag{11}$$

$$= -\int_\Omega Q \log \frac{Q}{P} dx = -KL(Q,P).$$

Here KL, the non-negative asymmetric Kullback-Leibler (K-L) distance, between two PDF's X and Y is defined as

$$KL(X,Y) = E_X\left[\frac{X}{Y}\right] = \int_\Omega X \log \frac{X}{Y} dx \geq 0; \tag{12}$$

$$KL(X,Y) \neq KL(Y,X); \; KL(X,Y) = 0 \; \text{iff} \; X \equiv Y.$$

Eq. (12) suggests that calculating the mean of a log-transformed volume change map is the same as computing the negative K-L distance between Q and P, and is *always non-positive* (zero only when J equals 1 everywhere, i.e., when the flow is incompressible). By contrast, let us also show that the log transform of $J \circ h^{-1} = J(h^{-1}(x))$, the volume change map pulled back onto the source reference frame, has a mean larger than zero, unless the flow is incompressible. Thus, the pulled-back Jacobian map does not have a log-normal distribution with zero mean either.

$$\frac{1}{|\Omega|}\int_\Omega \log J\left(h^{-1}(y)\right)dy \stackrel{y=h(x)}{=} \frac{1}{|\Omega|}\int_\Omega (\log J(x))|Dh|dx$$

$$=\frac{1}{|\Omega|}\int_\Omega (\log|Dh(x)|)|Dh|dx = \int_\Omega \frac{|Dh|}{|\Omega|}\log\left(\frac{|Dh(x)|/|\Omega|}{1/|\Omega|}\right)dx \quad (13)$$

$$=\int_\Omega P\log\frac{P}{Q}dx = KL(P,Q).$$

Similarly, calculating the mean of the pulled-back logged volume change map is equivalent to computing the *K-L* distance between P, and Q, and is always non-negative. Conventional log-normal modeling of the Jacobian distributions may therefore be less appropriate than non-parametric estimation, as illustrated in the Results.

3 Results

3D T1-weighted magnetic resonance images (MRI) of a 57 year-old male patient diagnosed with semantic dementia were obtained using a gradient echo acquisition (TR 25ms, TE 5ms, slice thickness 1.5mm, FOV 24x18cm, flip angle 40 degrees, no gaps). A total of four serial scans were obtained (baseline scan in 02/1993; follow-up scans in 10/1994, 02/1996, and 08/1999). The baseline (target) and the final follow-up (source) scans were used to evaluate the proposed approach. The two scans were first rigidly aligned and re-sliced to an isotropic volume of size 180×180×180 (a voxel = 1mm^3). The proposed inverse consistent registration algorithm was used to deform the source back to the target by maximizing the mutual information (MI) [8] between the deforming source and target images. This spatial normalization of scans over time allowed local tissue change to be estimated as mentioned in previous sections. A multi-resolution scheme starting from the 32×32×32 FFT resolution was used (λ=1e-4; time step=3e-6), and numerical convergence was checked every 20 iterations (convergence criteria was met when the MI failed to increase by 0.001 after one iteration). 40 iterations were computed in each FFT resolution before the resolution was increased by a factor of 2 (with the time step decreased to one-tenth) in each dimension. The top panel of Fig. 1 plots the target image (baseline scan) from an angle showing temporal lobes bilaterally, the second panel the source image from the same angle. The MRI scans show existing left temporal lobe atrophy (LT) with relative preservation of the right temporal lobe (RT). However, closer inspection of the Jacobian map (Fig. 2) shows active atrophy in the right temporal lobe, as well as bilateral caudate (RC, LC), putamen (RP, LP), and thalamus (RT, LT) tissue loss, while no active atrophy was detected in the left temporal lobe during the same time period (not shown here). Fig. 3 plots the values of MI and regularizer versus iterations in the forward and backward direction using (1) the proposed inverse consistent approach, and (2) an inconsistent approach (minimizing only the term E_1 in eq. (1)). The proposed consistent algorithm achieved not only higher MI values, but also lower regularizer values.

In order to validate the inverse consistency property of the proposed algorithm, we compared the deformation with that obtained by switching the source/target. Ideally, the deformation should not depend on this order, and thus inverse consistency can be assessed by looking at the difference (Table 1) between the deformation pair. For comparison, the corresponding errors using the inconsistent algorithm are also reported. Notice that the proposed algorithm yielded smaller errors in all aspects, and on average decreased the mean error to about one-seventh compared to the inconsistent algorithm.

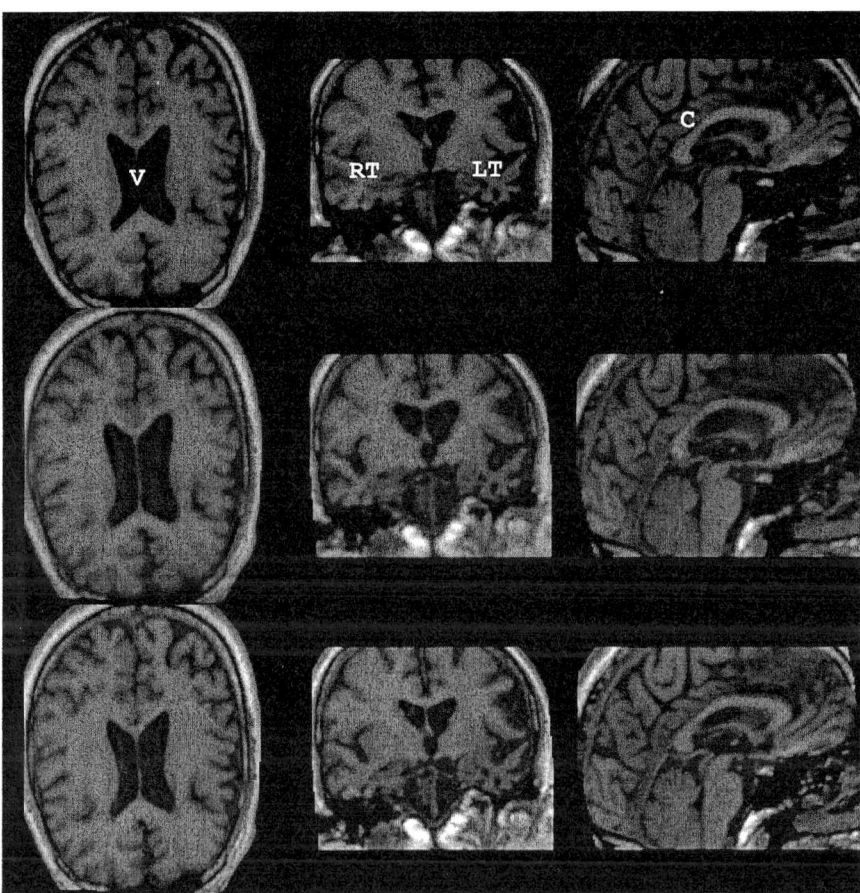

Fig. 1. The first row shows the baseline MRI scan of a patient diagnosed with semantic dementia. The second row shows the follow-up MRI scan of the same patient in which ventricle (V) dilation and copus callosum (C) shape change can be observed. The third row shows the follow-up MRI scan deformed to match the baseline scan using the proposed inverse consistency algorithm with maximization of mutual information (see text)

We then examined the statistical properties of the log(J) values. The left panel in the first row of Fig. 4 shows the histogram of the log(J) values under the proposed inverse consistent mapping (mean −0.0011; skewness −0.01657), and the right panel the corresponding histogram using inconsistent matching (mean −0.0017; skewness − 0.648). Notice the slight visual difference in these two histograms. We first tested if

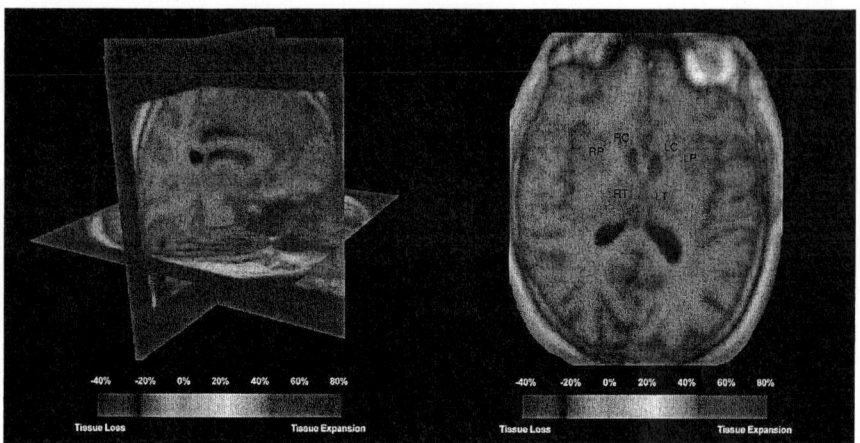

Fig. 2. 3D Jacobian map of the semantic dementia patient shows the active right temporal lobe atrophy (left panel), and deep nuclei involvement (right panel; see text)

Table 1. Statistics of inverse consistency error. * denotes the displacement/deformation obtained by switching the order of the source/target. The numbers are reported with respect to the 64x64x64 resolution of the FFT parameterization of the displacement

	Forward mapping (inverse consistent)			
	$|u_x - u_x^*|$	$|u_y - u_y^*|$	$|u_z - u_z^*|$	$|h - h^*|$
Maximum	0.3893	0.8290	0.4345	0.8616
Mean	0.0047	0.0071	0.0049	0.0115
	Backward mapping (inverse consistent)			
	$|u_x^{-1} - u_x^{-1*}|$	$|u_y^{-1} - u_y^{-1*}|$	$|u_z^{-1} - u_z^{-1*}|$	$|h^{-1} - h^{-1*}|$
Maximum	0.2751	0.8009	0.4145	0.8107
Mean	0.0048	0.0071	0.0047	0.0115
	Forward mapping (inverse inconsistent)			
	$|u_x - u_x^*|$	$|u_y - u_y^*|$	$|u_z - u_z^*|$	$|h - h^*|$
Maximum	0.8343	0.8894	0.9616	0.9617
Mean	0.0323	0.0297	0.0360	0.0685
	Backward mapping (inverse inconsistent)			
	$|u_x^{-1} - u_x^{-1*}|$	$|u_y^{-1} - u_y^{-1*}|$	$|u_z^{-1} - u_z^{-1*}|$	$|h^{-1} - h^{-1*}|$
Maximum	0.8499	0.9009	0.9884	0.9579
Mean	0.0322	0.0288	0.0362	0.0674

the log(J) distribution is symmetric around mean zero. To this end, a permutation test was performed where 10,000 samples were generated by randomly flipping the sign of each element in the observed distribution (under the null hypothesis that the observed is symmetric around zero). The test statistic was the mean value of the re-sampled distribution. No re-sampled test statistic (maximum 7.67e-5; minimum – 8.23e-5) was as extreme as the observed statistic, and thus the null hypothesis was rejected with statistical significance. We then relaxed the null hypothesis and tested the symmetry of log(J) distribution using another permutation test (random flipping around the observed mean −0.0011) with skewness as the test statistic. The left panel in the second row of Fig. 4 shows the histogram of the re-sampled statistics. The one-sided p-value is 0.067, and thus the null hypothesis (symmetric around its negative mean) cannot be rejected at the 5% significance level. By contrast, a similar skewness permutation test performed on the log(J) values under the inconsistent mapping yielded a p<0.0001. Thus, a statistically significant skewness was detected in the case of inconsistent mapping compared to its inverse consistent counterpart.

Finally, we examined the differences in the log(J) distributions obtained from inverse consistent versus inconsistent mappings. As discussed in previous sections, one would argue that, by equally penalizing positive and negative log(J) values, an inverse

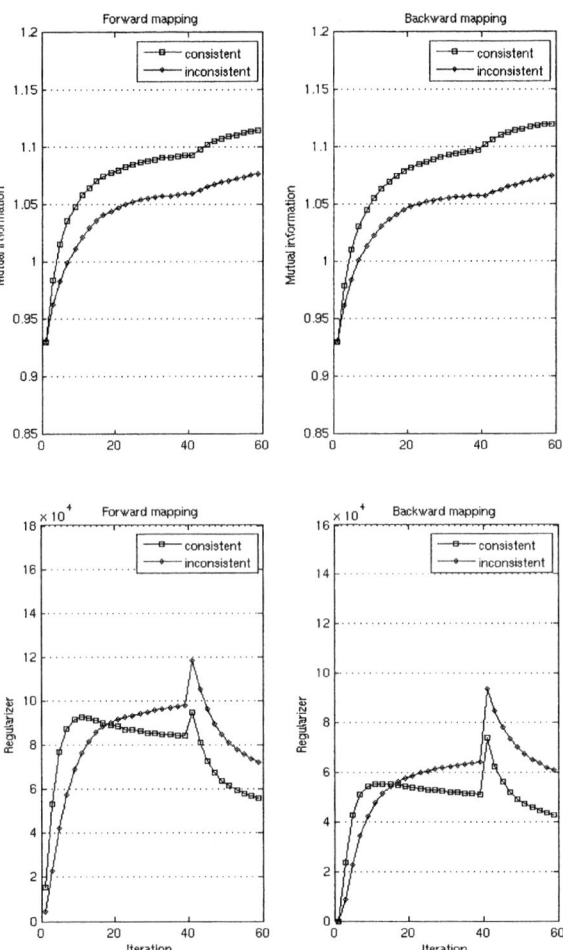

Fig. 3. The Mutual Information (the first row) and the regularizer (the second row) are plotted against the iteration number (x axis) in both the forward (left panel) and backward (right panel) direction. The transient increase of the values around iteration 40 is due to the upsampling of the displacement FFT parameterization

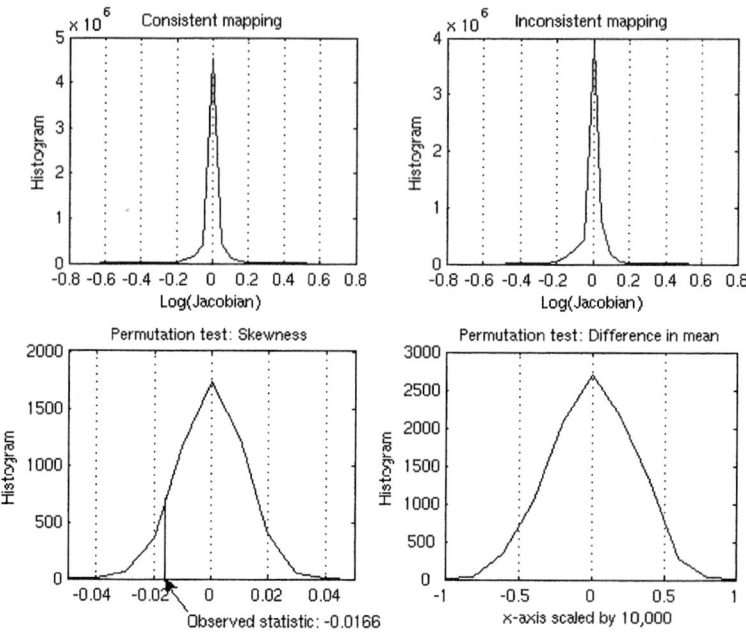

Fig. 4. Skewness of Logged Jacobian distributions. The first row shows the histogram of the log(J) values of the inverse consistent mapping constructed using the proposed algorithm (left panel), and the corresponding histogram using the inconsistent matching (right panel). Second Row: A permutation test is performed to determine if the consistent matching yields log(J) values symmetric around its mean (left panel shows the histogram of the re-sampled skewness statistic) with a one-sided p-value of 0.067. Another permutation test is performed to determine if the two distributions in the first row are statistically different. The right panel shows the histogram of the re-sampled test statistic (the values scaled by 10^4) where no re-sampled statistic is as extreme as the observed (i.e., p<0.0001)

consistent mapping would shift the mean log(J) value rightward (less negative). We formally tested the statistical significance of this shift using a third permutation test (right panel in the second row of Fig. 4). The test statistic in this case was the difference of the mean log(J) values between consistent and inconsistent mappings with the observed statistic 6.066e-4. 10,000 samples of this test statistic were calculated by generating two re-sampled distributions using random shuffling of each element in the two observed distributions (under the null hypothesis that the two distributions are identical and share the same mean). Again, not a single re-sampled test statistic (max 9.44e-5, min −8.73e-5) was as extreme as the observed, and thus a statistically significant difference was detected between the two observed distributions.

4 Conclusion

In this paper, we developed an inverse consistent image registration approach by applying variation calculus principles to the forward mapping only. We characterized the statistical properties of the Jacobian maps, both empirically and by applying the Kullback-Liebler distance to the set of material density functions in both target and source coordinates. We showed that the mean value of any log Jacobian map is always negative except for the trivial case where the Jacobian map is identically one on the whole image domain (incompressible flow). By contrast, any non-trivial log Jacobian map pulled back to the source coordinate must have a positive mean value. Thus, contrary to common belief, the values of any non-trivial Jacobian map do not follow a log normal distribution with zero mean. We also showed that compared to inconsistent matching, consistent matching reduces the skewness and increases the mean value of the log(J) distribution (making it more symmetric and thus allowing more unbiased detection of expanding and shrinking regions). Moreover, the statistical theory of these distributions has strong ties with formulations in information theory. Our conclusion has important consequences when performing statistical tests on maps of tissue change in both longitudinal and inter subject/group studies.

We also proposed a new algorithm that implements consistent matching in an intuitive manner without introducing extra penalty functions/parameters. Furthermore, the proposed algorithm provides a general recipe for inverting body forces back and forth between the forward and backward directions, and thus is applicable to any image registration schemes that compute displacement fields using incremental updating. We tested the proposed algorithm using longitudinal MRI images in a case of semantic dementia and demonstrated promising results for tracking atrophic processes in the brain.

Acknowledgements. This work was funded in part by NIH Grants R21 EB001561, R21 RR019771, and P41 RR13642. The authors would like to thank Dr. David Shattuck and Dr. Soo-Jin Lee for their valuable comments and suggestions.

References

1. P. M. Thompson and A. W. Toga, "A framework for computational anatomy," *Computing and Visualization in Science*, vol. 5, pp. 13-34, 2002.
2. U. Grenander and M. I. Miller, "Computational anatomy: An emerging discipline," *Quarterly of Applied Mathematics*, vol. 56, pp. 617-694, 1998.
3. R. P. Woods, J. C. Mazziotta, and S. R. Cherry, "MRI-PET registration with automated algorithm," *J. Comput. Assist. Tomogr.*, vol. 17, no. 4, pp. 536–546, 1993.
4. P. Cachier and D. Rey. *Symmetrization of the Non-Rigid Registration Problem using Inversion-Invariant Energies: Application to Multiple Sclerosis.* In MICCAI'00, Lecture Notes in Computer Science, vol. 1935, pp 472-481, Pittsburgh, Pennsylvania, USA, October 200.
5. D. Rey, G. Subsol, H. Delingette, and N. Ayache. Automatic Detection and Segmentation of Evolving Processes in 3D Medical Images: Application to Multiple Sclerosis. In IPMI'99, Lecture Notes in Computer Science, vol. 1613, pp 154-167, Visegrád, Hungary, June 1999.
6. G. E. Christensen and H. J. Johnson, "Consistent image registration," *IEEE Transactions on Image Processing*, vol. 20, pp. 568-582, 2001.
7. J. Ashburner, J. Anderson, and K. Friston, "High-dimensional image registration using symmetric priors," NeuroImage, vol. 9, pp. 619-628, 1999.
8. W.M. Wells, P. Viola, H. Atsumi, S. Nakajima, and R. Kikinis, " Multi-modal volume registration by maximization of mutual information" Med. Image Anal. vol. 1(1), pp. 35-51, 1996.

Robust Nonrigid Multimodal Image Registration Using Local Frequency Maps*

Bing Jian[1], Baba C. Vemuri[1], and José L. Marroquin[2]

[1] Department of Computer and Information Science and Engineering,
University of Florida, Gainesville, FL, 32611 USA
{bjian, vemuri}@cise.ufl.edu
[2] Centro de Investigacion en Matematicas, A.C.Apostado Postal 402,
Guanajuato, Mexico 36020
jlm@cimat.mx

Abstract. Automatic multi-modal image registration is central to numerous tasks in medical imaging today and has a vast range of applications e.g., image guidance, atlas construction, etc. In this paper, we present a novel multi-modal 3D non-rigid registration algorithm where in 3D images to be registered are represented by their corresponding local frequency maps efficiently computed using the Riesz transform as opposed to the popularly used Gabor filters. The non-rigid registration between these local frequency maps is formulated in a statistically robust framework involving the minimization of the integral squared error a.k.a. L_2E (L_2 error). This error is expressed as the squared difference between the true density of the residual (which is the squared difference between the non-rigidly transformed reference and the target local frequency representations) and a Gaussian or mixture of Gaussians density approximation of the same. The non-rigid transformation is expressed in a B-spline basis to achieve the desired smoothness in the transformation as well as computational efficiency.

The key contributions of this work are (i) the use of Riesz transform to achieve better efficiency in computing the local frequency representation in comparison to Gabor filter-based approaches, (ii) new mathematical model for local-frequency based non-rigid registration, (iii) analytic computation of the gradient of the robust non-rigid registration cost function to achieve efficient and accurate registration. The proposed non-rigid L_2E-based registration is a significant extension of research reported in literature to date. We present experimental results for registering several real data sets with synthetic and real non-rigid misalignments.

1 Introduction

Image registration is a central algorithm to many image processing tasks and has a vast range of applications including, but not limited to, medical image analysis, remote sensing, optical imaging, etc. In this section, we will briefly review existing algorithms reported in literature for achieving multi-modal registration. We will point out their limitations and hence motivate the need for a new and efficient computational algorithm for achieving our goal.

---

* This research was in part supported by RO1-NS 42075.

1.1 Previous Work

Image registration methods in literature to date may be classified into feature-based and "direct" methods. Most feature-based methods are limited to determining the registration at the feature locations and require an interpolation at other locations. If however, the transformation/registration between the images is a global transformation e.g., rigid, affine etc. then, there is no need for an interpolation step. However, in the case of a nonrigid transformation, it is necessary to interpolate. Also, the accuracy of the registration is dependent on the accuracy of the feature detector.

Several feature-based methods involve detecting surfaces landmarks [1], edges, ridges etc. (see [2] for references). Most of these assume a known correspondence with the exception of the work in Chui et.al., [1]. Work reported in Irani et.al., [3] uses the energy (squared magnitude) in the directional derivative image as a representation scheme for matching achieved using the SSD cost function. Recently, Liu et.al., [4] reported the use of local frequency in a robust statistical framework using the integral squared error a.k.a., L_2E. The primary advantage of L_2E over other robust estimators in literature is that there are no tuning parameters in it. The idea of using local phase was also exploited by Mellor et. al., [5], who used mutual information (MI) to match local-phase representation of images and estimated the non-rigid registration between them. However, robustness to significant non-overlap in the field of view (FOV) of the scanners was not addressed. For more on feature-based methods, we refer the reader to the survey by Maintz et.al., [2].

In the context of "direct" methods, the primary matching techniques for intra-modality registration involve the use of normalized cross-correlation, modified SSD, and (normalized) mutual information (MI). Recently, Roche et.al., [6] developed a correlation ratio based algorithm for registering MR scans with ultra-sound images. The results presented were quite impressive however, the issue of robustness to variations in the FOVs of the scanners was not adequately addressed. Direct methods such as, variants of optical flow-based registration that accommodate for varying illumination maybe used for inter-modality registration and we refer the reader to [7, 8] for such methods. Guimond et. al., [9] reported a multi-modal brain warping technique that uses Thirion's Demons algorithm [10] with an adaptive intensity correction. The technique however was not tested for robustness with respect to significant non-overlap in the FOVs.

A popular "direct" approach is based on the concept of maximizing mutual information (MI) pioneered by Viola and Wells [11] and Collignon et al., [12] and modified in Studholme et al., [13]. Reported registration experiments in these works are quite impressive for the case of rigid motion. In [14], Studholme et.al., presented a normalized MI scheme for matching multi-modal image pairs misaligned by a rigid motion. Normalized MI was shown to cope with image pairs not having exactly the same FOV, an important and practical problem. The problem of being able to handle non-rigid deformations in the MI framework is a very active area of research and some recent papers reporting results on this problem are [5, 15, 16, 17, 18, 19]. Computational efficiency and accuracy (in the event of significant non-overlaps) are issues of concern in all the MI-based non-rigid registration methods.

1.2 Overview of Proposed Registration Method

In this paper, we develop a multi-modal registration technique which is based on a *local frequency* representation of the image data. A *local frequency* image representation can be obtained by filtering the image with Gabor filters and then computing the gradient of the phase of the filtered images. As an alternative to the Gabor filter, we use the Riesz transform (see section (2), which is computationally more efficient. Once, we compute this local frequency representation for each of the two (source and target) images to be registered, we are ready to find the registration transformation which will best match these representations. Several matching criteria may be defined and we developed a statistically robust measure called the $L_2 E$ defined as the squared difference between the true density of the residual – defined as the squared difference between the transformed source and the target local frequency representations – and a Gaussian density approximation of the same. This matching criteria is minimized over a class of smooth transformations expressed in a B-spline basis. *The algorithm we have developed is well suited for situations where the source and target images have FOVs with large non-overlapping regions (which is quite common in practise)*. This formulation leads to a nonlinear cost function whose optimization yields the desired non-rigid registration. Several experiments with synthetic and real 3D data sets are presented to depict the performance of our algorithm.

Rest of the paper is organized as follows: in section 2.1, we present the local frequency computation using the Riesz transform and section 2.2 contains the details of our model for matching the local frequency representations. In section 2.3, we present the numerical algorithm and section 3 contains the experimental results on 2D/3D medical image data sets. Finally, we conclude in section 4.

2 Proposed Registration Method

2.1 Computing Local Frequency Using Riesz Transform

For multi-modal image registration, the relation between the brightness of the corresponding pixels is usually complicated: multiple intensity values in one modality image may map into single intensity in another modality; image feature existing in one image may not have correspondence in the other image, etc. However, multi-modal image data, acquired either with different sensors, or with the same sensor, mainly differ in the low frequency components. High frequency components, on the other hand, normally correspond to the physical structure of the object being imaged, and thus are good at expressing the commonality existing within the multi-sensor image pair. In the local frequency representation on which our algorithm is based, edges and ridges will have high values (since they are associated with high frequency components) and will be the dominant features for the matching stage.

In 1-D case, the local (instantaneous) frequency is well defined as the rate of change in phase of analytical signal obtained by Hilbert transform. However, the estimation of local frequency for higher dimensional images is still an important and open problem in the field of signal processing and computer vision. Quadrature filters are widely used as an approach to computing local phase and frequency in an image.

In this work, we present a novel formulation for computing the local-frequency using the Riesz transform which can be regarded as a generalization of the Hilbert transform in higher dimension. The key feature of this formulation is the fact that unlike the Gabor filter based technique, we do not need a bank of filters for computing the local frequency representation. A 3-D generalization of the Hilbert transform may be obtained by the vector sum of 3 Riesz transforms:

$$H_3(I) = \mathcal{F}^{-1}\left[\left(\sum_{k=1}^{3} \frac{-iu_k}{|u|} e_k\right) \mathcal{F}[I]\right] \quad (1)$$

where $I(x,y,z)$ is the given 3D image and $u = (u_1, u_2, u_3)^T$ is the spatial frequency vector, e_k is the unit vector in the direction of the kth coordinate axis, and $\mathcal{F}$ is the Fourier transform operator. This may be rewritten as:

$$H_3(I) = \mathcal{F}^{-1}\left[\frac{\mathcal{F}[\nabla I]}{|u|}\right] \quad (2)$$

After some detailed analysis [20], it is possible to show that the righthand side of equation (2) can be approximated as:

$$\frac{\nabla I}{\sqrt{\omega_1^2(x,y,z) + \omega_2^2(x,y,z) + \omega_3^2(x,y,z)}} = \frac{\nabla I(x,y,z)}{|\omega(x,y,z)|} \quad (3)$$

where $\omega_k(x,y,z)$ is the kth component of the local frequency. The frequency magnitude may therefore be estimated as:

$$|\omega(x,y,z)| \approx \frac{|\nabla I(x,y,z)|}{|H_3(I)(x,y,z)|} \quad (4)$$

where H_3 is computed using (1). In order to make this approximation less sensitive to noise, we use a smoothing operator on both the computation of the ∇I and H_3. It should be remarked that a precise computation of ∇I is crucial for the correct approximation of $|\omega|$; the best results are obtained when this computation is performed in the frequency domain.

In this way, the estimation of $|\omega|$ requires one forward 3-D Fourier transform and 6 inverse 3-D Fourier transforms, plus 2 separable 3-D convolutions. This can be done in $O(N\log N)$ time, where N is the number of voxels in the image. In comparison, the Gabor filter bank requires $O(4Nm^3k)$ time – where, $m3$ is the convolution kernel size and k is the number of filters. In our implementation $m3 >> logN$. Additional advantages of our approach accrue in the form of storage savings since, there is a large storage requirement in the Gabor filter-based approach described in Liu et al., [4] to keep the responses of a large filter bank at each lattice point for computing the max. local freq. response. No such filterbanks are used in our approach for computing the local frequency response.

Our current implementation uses FFTW[1] package which is a very efficient implementation. Even for 3D volumes ($210 \times 210 \times 120$), the computation can be done in

---

[1] www.fftw.org

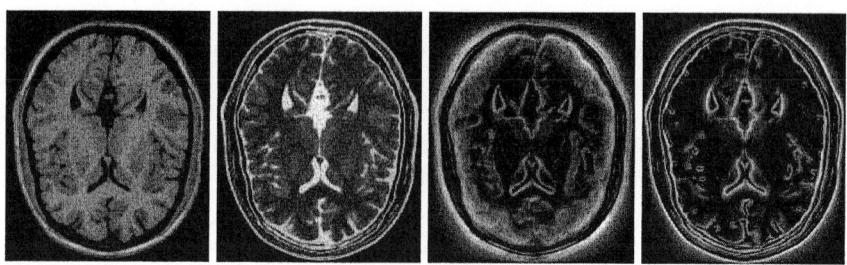

Fig. 1. Left: a pair of T1 and T2 images; Right: their corresponding local frequency maps

1 minute, under a Linux system running on a PC equipped with a 2.6GHZ Pentium4. Figure (1) illustrates two examples of computed local frequency in 2D for two T1 and T2 slices obtained from BrainWeb [21]. Note the richness of the structure in the representation.

2.2 Matching Local Frequency Representations

Let I_1 and I_2 be two images to be registered, and assume the deformation field from I_1 to I_2 is $\mathbf{u} = \mathbf{u}(\mathbf{x})$, i.e. the point $\mathbf{x}$ in I_1 corresponds to the $\mathbf{x} + \mathbf{u}(\mathbf{x})$ in I_2. Denote by $\mathbf{F_1}$ and $\mathbf{F_2}$ the local frequency representations corresponding to I_1 and I_2 respectively. The corresponding local frequency constraint is given by

$$(\mathbf{I} + \mathbf{J}(\mathbf{u})^\mathbf{T})\mathbf{F_1}(\mathbf{x} + \mathbf{u}(\mathbf{x})) = \mathbf{F_2}(\mathbf{x}) + \epsilon(\mathbf{x}) \tag{5}$$

where $\mathbf{J}(\mathbf{u})$ is the Jacobian matrix of deformation field.

Note the above equation holds for the vector-valued frequency representation. However, experiments show that the vector-valued representation is much more sensitive to the noise than the magnitude of frequency and the Jacobian matrix term makes the numerical optimization computationally expensive. Applying Mirsky's theorem from matrix perturbation theory [22] which states $\sqrt{\sum_i (\tilde{\sigma}_i - \sigma_i)^2} \leq \|\mathbf{J}(\mathbf{u})^\mathbf{T}\|_F$ where $\tilde{\sigma}_i - \sigma_i$ is the difference in the singular values between the perturbed matrix $(\mathbf{I} + \mathbf{J}(\mathbf{u})^\mathbf{T})$ and $\mathbf{I}$, and imposing the regularization condition that $\mathbf{J}(\mathbf{u})$ is small, we can approximate the $\|(\mathbf{I} + \mathbf{J}(\mathbf{u})^\mathbf{T})\mathbf{F}(\mathbf{x})\|$ by $\|\mathbf{F}(\mathbf{x})\|$ to get the following simplified form:

$$\|\mathbf{F_1}(\mathbf{x} + \mathbf{u}(\mathbf{x}))\| = \|\mathbf{F_2}(\mathbf{x})\| + \epsilon(\mathbf{x}) \tag{6}$$

where $\|\cdot\|$ gives the magnitude of local frequency.

Instead of the popular SSD approach, we develop a statistical robust matching criterion based on the minimization of the integral squared error(ISE) or simply L_2E between a Gaussian model and the true density function of the residual. Traditionally, the L_2E criterion originates in the derivation of the nonparametric least squares Cross-validation algorithm for choosing the bandwidth h for the kernel estimate of a density and has been employed as the goodness-of-fit criterion in nonparametric density estimation. Recently, Scott [23] exploited the applicability of L_2E to parametric problems and demonstrated its robustness behavior and nice properties of practical importance.

In the parametric case, given the r.v. ϵ from (6) with unknown density $g(\epsilon)$, for which we introduce the Gaussian model $f(\epsilon|\theta)$, we may write the L_2E estimator as

$$\hat{\theta}_{L_2E} = \arg\min_\theta \int [f(\epsilon|\theta) - g(\epsilon)]^2 dx \tag{7}$$

Simply expand above equation and notice the fact that $\int g(\epsilon)^2 dx$ does not depend on θ and $\int f(\epsilon|\theta)g(\epsilon)dx = E_g[f(\epsilon|\theta)]$ is the so called expected height of the density which can be approximated by the estimator $\frac{1}{n}\sum_{i=1}^n f(\epsilon_i|\theta)$, hence the proposed estimator minimizing the L_2 distance will be

$$\hat{\theta}_{L_2E} = \arg\min_\theta [\int f(\epsilon|\theta)^2 dx - \frac{2}{n}\sum_{i=1}^n f(\epsilon_i|\theta)]. \tag{8}$$

For Gaussian distributions, we have closed form for the integral in the bracketed quantity in (8) and hence can avoid numerical integration which is a practical limitation not only in computation time but also in accuracy. Thus, we get the following criterion $L_2E(\mathbf{u}, \sigma)$ from (8) for our case,

$$\frac{1}{2\sqrt{\pi}\sigma} - \frac{2}{N}\sum_{i=1}^N exp\left\{-\frac{(\|\mathbf{F}_1(\mathbf{x} + \mathbf{u}(\mathbf{x}))\| - \|\mathbf{F}_2(\mathbf{x})\|)^2}{2\sigma^2}\right\} \tag{9}$$

Equation (9) differs from the standard SSD approach in that the quadratic error terms are replaced by robust potentials (in this case, inverted Gaussians), so that the large errors are not unduly overweighed, but rather are treated as outliers and given small weight.

Generally, a regularization term is needed for nonrigid registration problem to impose the local consistency or smoothness on the deformation field $\mathbf{u}$. In case $\mathbf{u}$ is assumed to be differentiable, this regularization term could be defined as a certain norm of its Jacobian $\mathbf{J}(\mathbf{u})$. For simplicity, the Frobenius norm of Jacobian of deformation field $\|\mathbf{J}(\mathbf{u})\|_\mathbf{F}^2$ is used here. Altogether, the proposed non-rigid image registration method is expressed by the following optimization problem:

$$\hat{\theta} = \arg\min_{\theta=[\mathbf{u},\sigma]} L_2E(\mathbf{u}, \sigma) + \lambda\|\mathbf{J}(\mathbf{u})\|_\mathbf{F}^2 \tag{10}$$

where λ is the Lagrange multiplier and σ is the parameter controlling the shape of the residual distribution modelled by a zero mean Gaussian $\phi(x|0, \sigma)$. Unlike other robust estimators, this shape parameter σ need not be set by the user, but rather it is automatically adjusted during the numerical optimization. Deformation field $\mathbf{u}$, in this work, is expressed for computational efficiency, by a B-Spline model controlled by a small number of displacement estimates which lie on a coarser control grid.

2.3 Numerical Implementation

The numerical implementation is achieved using nonlinear optimization techniques to solve equation (10). In our current implementation, we handle the minimization over σ

and u separately. At each step, the σ is the minimizer of the L_2 distance between the true density and model density of residual distribution given fixed u. A zero vector is used as the initial guess for u. In each iteration, we evaluate the gradient of $E(\mathbf{u}) = L_2 E(\mathbf{u}, \sigma) + \lambda \|\mathbf{J}(\mathbf{u})\|_{\mathbf{F}}^2$ with respect to each of the parameters in u using *analytical formulae* which can be computed in laboratory frame:

$$\nabla_{\mathbf{u}} L_2 E = \frac{2}{N * \sigma^2} \sum_{i=1}^{N} \left\{ exp\left\{ -\frac{\mathbf{D}_i^2}{2\sigma^2} \right\} \mathbf{D}_i \mathbf{G}_i \right\} \qquad (11)$$

$$\nabla_{\sigma} L_2 E = -\frac{1}{2\sqrt{\pi \sigma^2}} - \frac{2}{N} \sum_{i=1}^{N} \left\{ exp\left\{ -\frac{\mathbf{D}_i^2}{2\sigma^2} \right\} \frac{\mathbf{D}_i^2}{\sigma^3} \right\} \qquad (12)$$

where

$$\mathbf{D}_i = \|\mathbf{F_1}(\mathbf{x_i} + \mathbf{u}(\mathbf{x_i}))\| - \|\mathbf{F_2}(\mathbf{x_i})\|$$

is the frequency magnitude error at pixel i,

$$\mathbf{G}_i = (\nabla \|\mathbf{F_1}\|)(\mathbf{x_i} + \mathbf{u}(\mathbf{x_i}))$$

is the spatial gradient of $(\|\mathbf{F_1}\|)$. Then, a block diagonal matrix is computed as approximation of Hessian matrix by leaving out the second-derivative terms and observing that the overall Hessian matrix is sparse multi-banded block-diagonal. Finally, a preconditioned gradient descent technique is used to update the parameter estimates. In this step, an accurate line search derived by Taylor approximation is performed.

The numerical optimization approach is outlined as follows:

- Set $i = 0$ and give an initial guess for deformation field $\mathbf{u_0}$;
- Gaussian fitting: $\sigma_i = \arg\min L_2 E(\mathbf{u_i}, \sigma)$, this step involves a quasi-Newton nonlinear optimization;
- Update deformation estimates: $\mathbf{u}_{i+1} = \mathbf{u}_i + \Delta \mathbf{u}$, this step involves a preconditioned gradient descent method close to that used by [7];
- Iterate: $i = i + 1$
- Stopping criteria: $\|\Delta \mathbf{u}\| \approx 0$

3 Experimental Results

In this section we present three sets of experiments. The first set constitutes of a 2-D example to depict the robustness of $L_2 E$. The second set contains experiments with 2-D MR T1- and T2- weighted data obtained from the Montreal Neurological Institute database [21]. The data sets were artificially misaligned by known non-rigid transformations and our algorithm was used to estimate the transformation. The third set of experiments was conducted with 3-D real data for which no ground truth was available.

3.1 Robustness Property of the $L_2 E$ Measure

In this section, we demonstrate the robustness property of $L_2 E$ and, hence, justify the use of the $L_2 E$ measure in the registration context.

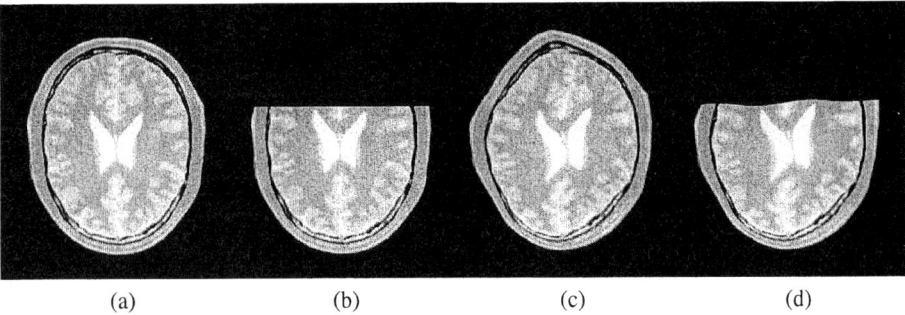

Fig. 2. Depiction of the robustness property of the L_2E measure. From left to right: (a): a 2-D MR slice of size 257×221; (b): the source image obtained from (a) by cutting the top third of image; (c): transformed (a) serving as the target; (d) warped source image with the estimated deformation

In order to depict the robustness property of L_2E, we designed a series of experiments as follows: with a 2-D MR slice as the source image, the target image is obtained by applying a known nonrigid transformation to the source image. Instead of matching the original source image and transformed image, we cut more than 1/3 of the source image (to simulate the affect of significant non-overlap in the FOVs), and use it and the transformed image as the input to the registration algorithms. Figure 2 depicts an example of this experiment. In spite of missing more than 33% of one of the two images being registered, our algorithm yields a low average error of 1.32 and a standard deviation of 0.97 in the estimated deformation field over the uncut region. *The error here is defined by the magnitude of the vector difference between ground truth and estimated deformation fields.* For comparison purposes, we also tested the MI and the SSD method on the same data set in this experimental setup. The nonrigid mutual information registration algorithm was implemented following the approach presented in [24]. And in both the MI and SSD method, the nonrigid deformations are modeled by B-Splines with the same configuration as in our method. However, both the MI and the SSD method fail to give acceptable results due to the significant non-overlap between the data sets.

3.2 Inter-modality Registration

For problem of inter-modality registration, we tested our algorithm on two MR-T1 and -T2 2D image slices from the BrainWeb site [21] of size 181×217. These 2 images are originally aligned with each other and are shown in Figure (1) as well as their corresponding local frequency maps computed via the application of the Riesz transform described earlier. In this experiment, a set of synthetic nonrigid deformation fields were generated using four kinds of kernerl-based spline representations: cubic B-spline, elastic body spline, thin plate spline and volume spline. In each case, we produced 15 randomized deformations where the possible values of each direction in deformation vary from -15 to 15 in pixels. The left half of Table 1 shows the statistics of the difference between the ground truth and estimated deformation fields. For purpose of compari-

Table 1. Statistics of the errors between ground truth displacement fields and estimated deformation fields obtained using our method and the MI method on pairs of T1-T2 MR images

Statistics (in pixels)	Our Method			MI Method		
	mean	std. dev.	median	mean	std. dev.	median
Thin Plate Spline	2.03	1.83	1.33	2.02	1.81	1.31
Elastic Body Spline	1.98	1.87	1.28	1.99	1.87	1.27
Volume Spline	2.13	2.03	1.53	2.12	2.04	1.52
Cubic B-Spline	1.29	1.18	0.79	1.27	1.17	0.79

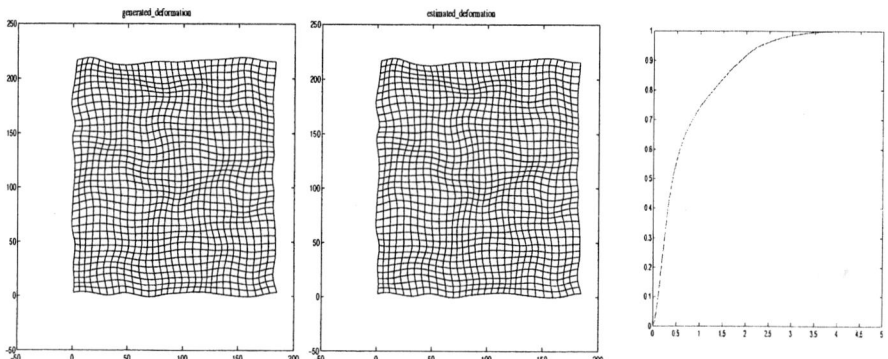

Fig. 3. From left to right: the ground truth deformation field; the estimated deformation field; the cumulative distribution of the estimated error in pixels

son, in this setup we also tested the nonrigid mutual information registration algorithm which was used in the previous experiment. As shown in the right half of Table 1, MI-based nonrigid registration produces almost same accuracy in the results as our method for this fully overlapped data sets. However, the strength of our technique does not lie in registering image pairs that are full overlapped. Instead, it lies in registering data pairs with significant non-overlap, as shown in Figure 2. Figure 3 shows plots of the estimated B-Spline deformation along with the ground truth as well as the cumulative distribution of the estimated error. Note that the error distribution is mostly concentrated in the small error range indicating the accuracy of our method.

3.3 3D Data Example

To conclude our experimental section, we show results on a 3D example for which no ground truth deformations are available. The data we used in our experiments is a pair of MR images of brains from different rats. The source image is $(46.875 \times 46.875 \times 46.875)$ micron resolution with the field of view $(2.4 \times 1.2 \times 1.2 cm)$, while the target is 3D diffusion-weighted image with $(52.734 \times 52.734 \times 52.734)$ micron resolution with the field of view $(2.7 \times 1.35 \times 1.35 cm)$. Both the images have the same acquisition matrix $(256 \times 512 \times 256)$.

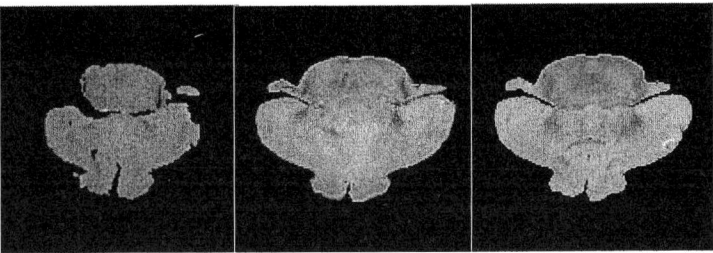

Fig. 4. Nonrigid registration of an MR-T1 & MR-DWI mouse brain scan. Left to Right: an arbitrary slice from the source image, a slice of the transformed source overlayed with the corresponding slice of the edge map of the target image and the target image slice

Figure 4 shows the registration results for the dataset. As is visually evident, the misalignment has been fully compensated for after the application of the estimated deformation. The registration was performed on reduced volumes ($128 \times 128 \times 180$) which took around 10 minutes to obtain the results illustrated in figure 4 with the control knots placed every $16 \times 16 \times 16$ voxels by running our C++ program on a 2.6GHZ Pentium PC. Validation of non-rigid registration on real data with the aid of segmentations and landmarks obtained manually from a group of trained anatomists are the goals of our ongoing work.

4 Conclusions

In this paper, we presented a novel algorithm for non-rigid 3D multi-modal registration. The algorithm used the local frequency representation of the input data and applied a robust matching criteria to estimate the non-rigid deformation between the data. The key contributions of this paper lie in, (i) efficient computation of the local frequency representations using the Riesz transform, (ii) a new mathematical model for local-frequency based non-rigid registration, and (iii) the efficient estimation of 3D non-rigid registration between multi-modal data sets possibly in the presence of significant non-overlapping between the data. To the best of our knowledge, these features are unique to our method. Also the robust framework used here namely, the L_2E measure, has the advantage of providing an automatic dynamic adjustment of the control parameter of the estimator's influence function. This makes the L_2E estimator robust with respect to initializations. Finally, we presented several real data (with synthetic and real non-rigid misalignments) experiments depicting the performance of our algorithm.

Acknowledgments

This work benefited from the use of the ITK[2], an open source software developed as an initiative of the U.S. National Library of Medicine. Authors would like to thank

---

[2] www.itk.org

Dr. S.J. Blackband, Dr. S. C. Grant both of the Neuroscience Dept, UFL and Dr. H. Benveniste of SUNY, BNL for providing us with the mouse DWI data set. This research was supported in part by the NIH grant RO1 NS42075.

References

1. Chui, H., Win, L., Schultz, R., Duncan, J., Rangarajan, A.: A unified non-rigid feature registration method for brain mapping. Medical Image Analysis **7** (2003) 112–130
2. Maintz, J.B.A., Viergever, M.A.: A survey of medical image registration. Medical Image Analysis **2** (1998) 1–36
3. Irani, M., Anandan, P.: Robust Multi-sensor Image Alignment. In: International Conference on Computer Vision, Bombay, India (1998) 959–965
4. Liu, J., Vemuri, B.C., Marroquin, J.L.: Local frequency representations for robust multimodal image registration. IEEE Transactions on Medical Imaging **21** (2002) 462–469
5. Mellor, M., Brady, M.: Non-rigid multimodal image registration using local phase. In: Medical Image Computing and Computer-Assisted Intervention - MICCAI 2004, Saint-Malo, France (2004) 789–796
6. Roche, A., Pennec, X., Malandain, G., Ayache, N.: Rigid registration of 3-d ultrasound with mr images: A new approach combining intensity and gradient information. IEEE Transactions on Medical Imaging **20** (2001) 1038–1049
7. Szeliski, R., Coughlan, J.: Spline-based image registration. Int. J. Comput. Vision **22** (1997) 199–218
8. Lai, S.H., Fang, M.: Robust and efficient image alignment with spatially-varying illumination models. In: IEEE Conference on Computer Vision and Pattern Recognition. (1999) II: 167–172
9. Guimond, A., Roche, A., Ayache, N., Menuier, J.: Three-Dimensional Multimodal Brain Warping Using the Demons Algorithm and Adaptive Intensity Corrections. IEEE Trans. on Medical Imaging **20** (2001) 58–69
10. Thirion, J.P.: Image matching as a diffusion process: an analogy with maxwell's demons. Medical Image Analysis **2** (1998) 243–260
11. Viola, P.A., Wells, W.M.: Alignment by maximization of mutual information. In: Fifth Intl. Conference on Computer Vision, MIT, Cambridge (1995)
12. Collignon, A., Maes, F., Delaere, D., Vandermeulen, D., Suetens, P., Marchal, G.: Automated multimodality image registration based on information theory. Information Processing in Medical Imaging (Y. Bizais, C. Barillot and R. Di Paola, eds.) (1995)
13. Studholme, C., Hill, D., Hawkes, D.J.: Automated 3D registration of MR and CT images in the head. Medical Image Analysis **1** (1996) 163–175
14. Studholme, C., Hill, D.L.G., Hawkes, D.J.: An overlap invariant entropy measure of 3D medical image alignment. Pattern Recognition **32** (1999) 71–86
15. Rueckert, D., Frangi, A.F., Schnabel, J.A.: Automatic construction of 3d statistical deformation models of the brain using non-rigid registration. IEEE Trans. Med. Imaging **22** (2003) 1014–1025
16. Hermosillo, G., Chefd'hotel, C., Faugeras, O.: Variational methods for multimodal image matching. Int. J. Comput. Vision **50** (2002) 329–343
17. Rueckert, D., Sonoda, L.I., Hayes, C., Hill, D.L.G., Leach, M.O., Hawkes, D.J.: Nonrigid registration using free-form deformations: Application to breast mr images. IEEE Trans. on Medical Imaging **18** (1999) 712–721
18. Leventon, M.E., Grimson, W.E.L.: Multimodal volume registration using joint intensity distributions. In: Proc. Conference on Medical Image Computing and Compter–Assisted Intervention (MICCAI), Cambridge, MA (1998) 1057–1066

19. Gaens, T., Maes, F., Vandermeulen, D., Suetens, P.: Non-rigid multimodal image registration using mutual information. In: Proc. Conference on Medical Image Computing and Compter-Assisted Intervention (MICCAI). (1998) 1099–1106
20. Servin, M., Quiroga, J.A., Marroquin, J.L.: General n-dimensional quadrature transform and its application to interferogram demodulation. Journal of the Optical Society of America A **20** (2003) 925–934
21. CA, C., Kwan, K., Evans, R.: Brainweb: online interface to a 3-d mri simulated brain database (1997)
22. Stewart, G., Sun, J.: Matrix Perturbation Theory. Academic Press (1990)
23. Scott, D.: Parametric statistical modeling by minimum integrated square Error. Technometrics **43** (2001) 274–285
24. Mattes, D., Haynor, D.R., Vesselle, H., Lewellen, T.K., Eubank, W.: Non-rigid multimodality image registration. In: Proc. SPIE, Medical Imaging 2001: Image Processing. Volume 4322., Bellingham, WA (2001) 1609–1620

Imaging Tumor Microenvironment with Ultrasound

Mallika Sridhar[1] and Michael F. Insana[1,2]

[1]University of California, Davis CA 95616, USA
msridhar@ucdavis.edu
[2]University of Illinois at Urbana-Champaign, Urbana IL 61801,USA
mfi@uiuc.edu

Abstract. Recent advances in molecular biology are providing new opportunities for breast cancer imaging. Our approach uses ultrasound to image viscoelastic features of tumors. These features describe microenvironmental factors that stimulate signaling pathways in tumors that ultimately affect metastatic potential and response to traditional therapeutics. This paper explains the motivation for the approach, describes measurements in phantoms and patients, and defines measurement sensitivity using hydrogels with tissue-like features.

1   Viscoelastic Imaging of the Tumor Microenvironment

Cancer cells communicate locally with other cells and the extracellular matrix (ECM) using molecular signals. Communication is essential if a cancerous tumor is to grow and metastasize [Ele01]. Molecular signaling controls many facets of tumor progression related to outcome including growth rate, degree of invasiveness, and metastatic potential. Signals are generated in response to the tissue *microenvironment*, which is determined by cell phenotype, spatial organization, and biochemical and metabolic activities. Current trends in cancer imaging aim to visualize the signaling pathways and the tumor microenvironment to better understand disease progression and design targeted imaging and therapeutic agents. The goal of cancer imaging is to exploit disease-specific object contrast mechanisms that provide specific information for tumor detection and disease management decisions.

Molecular imaging techniques are well suited for this task. Successful techniques enhance object contrast for molecular-scale events by targeting circulating *imaging probes* for attachment to specific sites of disease. Standard modalities then image the energy emitted or reflected from the attached probes. One approach to molecular imaging employs integrin-based imaging probes to identify regions of enhanced angiogenic (new blood vessel) activity [Day04].

A less direct approach is to image the causes or effects of molecular signaling. Metabolic and structural features of the tumor microenvironment are naturally targeted for imaging because of their key roles in the signaling process. For example, ^{18}F-PET probes are applied to quantify changes in tumor cell metabolism that are highly correlated with histological markers [Abb04]. Also, with confocal and multi-photon microscopy, it is possible to visualize the effects of ECM-cell signaling on stromal microstructure, in vivo [Voy01]. The optical methods use autofluorescence to generate the contrast necessary to study ECM structure, whereas the other methods depend on the development of targeted probes.

Our ultrasonic approach provides images of viscoelastic features that describe the tumor microenviroment without contrast enhancement. Tissues are mechanically stressed while we image time-varying strains at near-B-mode spatial resolution from sequential frames of echo data. Strain images are analyzed to separately map the elastic and viscous properties of tissues, as described below.

Elastic properties, we hypothesize, indicate disease-specific changes in collagen density and structural organization. Stromal-epithelial cell signaling modifies fibroblast cell activity to increase production of ECM component proteins [Ele01]. These changes begin a cascade of events that include formation of a stiff desmoplastic reaction surrounding the tumor mass. Desmoplasia is the effect sensed during manual palpation, a common screening procedure for breast cancer. To sense the elastic changes, ultrasound is used to track local displacements in 1-100 μm range [Nig02, Ber03].

Viscous features indicate pH-induced changes from highly metabolic and poorly perfused regions of the tumor. For example, acidic conditions lead to protonation of the side-chains on collagen molecules that affect cross linking [Ush00] and vicinal water structure [Pol01]. Viewing soft tissues as a water-based polymer, reduced pH softens the medium (lower shear modulus) and causes it to creep (viscous flow) faster when held under a load. Viscous properties could reveal regional variations in cell metabolism and oxygenation since these properties are highly correlated with pH. Fast growing tumors often generate acidic regions that enhance genetic instability leading to metastatic progression and reduced therapeutic responsiveness [Gil02]. This paper describes the image science of viscoelastic imaging for assessing functional features of breast cancer development. Our goal is to understand what material property information is available with viscoelasticity imaging. Feature sensitivity is assessed using collagen hydrogels with known material properties that are similar to those of breast tissues.

1.1 Physical Models: Gelatin

There is a fibrous collagen matrix within breast tissues and other organs that provides mechanical integrity as well as signaling sources and receptors. Without the matrix, tissues would be viscous fluids. The 3-D organization of the collagen molecules determine the structural stability of the matrix. The structure depends on the density of surface charges during assembly, which strongly depends on the microenvironment. Consequently, the viscoelastic response of breast tissue to a mechanical deformation can describe the concentration of collagen, extracellular pH, and any other effect that changes the balance of surface charge.

To develop imaging methods we use gelatin as a test material [Hal97, Mad03]. The homogeneity and structural simplicity of the type I collagen in this hydrogel allow for interpretation of viscoelastic properties in terms of molecular-scale structure and forces while preserving essential features of the polymer structure. Much is already known about the physical chemistry of hydrogels [Roe02, Cha96, Ell04]. Like proteins in tissue stroma, the collagen molecules in gelatin have charged hydrophilic surfaces that adsorb water. The collagen molecules cross link by bonding at charged sites along the amino acid backbone. The dimensional stability of the gel depends on the interplay of covalent bond, hydrogen bond, electrostatic, and van der Waals forces [Ush00].

On a macroscopic scale, hydrogels, like tissues, are incompressible viscoelastic solids. Bulk material properties are determined by the shear modulus G since deformations produce changes in shape but not volume. The elastic properties of hydrogels depend on the degree of cross linking between collagen molecules. Covalently-bonded cross links are very stable; they do not change with elastic deformations. However, the weaker bonds generate an initial elastic response that creeps over time. As shown in the results section, the viscous creep is biexponential with the shorter relaxation time T_1 between 0.1 and 10 s and the longer relaxation time T_2 in the range of 100 s. It has been postulated that T_1 indicates properties of vicinal water flow and T_2 described the relaxation of weakly bonded cross links [Sri04].

During gelation, collagen self assembles into structures at many spatial scales. Native structures emerge only within a narrow range of environmental conditions. Confocal microscopy has shown that greater collagen concentration increases fibril density without affecting fibril length or diameter [Roe02]. However, a shift in pH away from the isoelectric point (pI) [1] induces a transition to a more amorphous structure. The congealed polymer has shorter and thicker fibrils under acidic conditions and longer and thinner fibrils under basic conditions. When pH $\neq$ pI, the added charges compete for the weakly bound sites of molecular cross linking, thus weakening the matrix. Elastic measurements alone do not define pH, but when combined with viscous creep time constants, a unique description emerges. Viscoelastic imaging can describe average properties of environmentally induced effects occurring at the molecular scale.

2 Methods

2.1 Gelatin Samples

Tissue-like gelatin samples were prepared for either mechanical testing or viscoelastic imaging as described previously [Hal97]. 26 ml of propyl alcohol and 14 g of type A, 275 bloom, animal-hide gelatin were added to 200 ml distilled water. The solution was heated at 60°C until visually clear before adding 0.3 ml of formaldehyde to increase collagen cross linking. pH values were adjusted between 3 and 8 (isoelectric point pI = 5) by adding an acid (HCl) or a base

---

[1] pI is defined as the pH of a protein at which there are equal numbers of positive and negative charges at the molecular surfaces.

(NaOH). The solution was poured into a testing container and cooled to initiate gelation. These samples were used for materials testing 24 hours after congealing.

For imaging experiments, 9.1 g of graphite powder is added to the molten gel and thoroughly mixed to provide tissue-like ultrasonic absorption and backscatter. Most of the collagen molecules assemble into a triple helix fibril structure. The fibrils are cross linked into a random network trapping graphite particles and water. Graphite scatters ultrasound but does not affect structures that determine mechanical properties. Conversely the structural matrix only weakly interacts with ultrasound. Imaging samples were aged 5 days before measurements to increase stiffness. From an earlier analysis of gelatin elasticity [Hal97], we adjusted image-based measurements to match mechanical-testing measurements for differences in sample age.

2.2 Viscoelastic Modeling

A continuum description of material properties is appropriate at our resolution scale. The constitutive equation relating material properties to time-dependent stress $\sigma(t)$ and strain $\epsilon(t)$ as measured along one axis of a cubic volume is a differential equation [Tsc89],

$$\sum_{n=0}^{N} a_n \frac{d^n \sigma}{dt^n} = \sum_{m=0}^{M} b_m \frac{d^m \epsilon}{dt^m} . \qquad (1)$$

For linear time-invariant behavior of the material, the coefficients a_n and b_m are constant. They are model parameters related to the material properties we seek to measure.

Assuming the system is initially at rest, $\sigma = \epsilon = 0$ for $t < 0$, we apply the one-sided Laplace transform to (1) to find

$$\tilde{a}(s)\tilde{\sigma}(s) = \tilde{b}(s)\tilde{\epsilon}(s) , \qquad (2)$$

where $\tilde{\sigma}(s) \triangleq \mathcal{L}\sigma(t) = \int_0^\infty dt\, \exp(-st)\sigma(t)$ and $\tilde{a}$ and $\tilde{b}$ are polynomials in s: $\tilde{a}(s) = \sum_n a_n s^n$, $\tilde{b}(s) = \sum_m b_m s^m$. From (2)

$$\tilde{\epsilon}(s) = \tilde{R}(s)\,\tilde{\sigma}(s) \text{ and } \tilde{\sigma}(s) = \tilde{Q}(s)\,\tilde{\epsilon}(s) , \text{ where } \tilde{R}(s) = \frac{\tilde{a}(s)}{\tilde{b}(s)} = \tilde{Q}^{-1}(s) . \quad (3)$$

Eq (3) is Hooke's law for linear, time-varying viscoelastic solids as described in the complex s-plane. Here, R is the shear retardance; its inverse is Q, the shear relaxance.

Two experiments are described by (3). In one, we stimulate the medium with a known, time-varying stress, measure the resulting strain, and the material properties are computed. This is the *viscous creep experiment* and $R(t) = \mathcal{L}^{-1}\{\tilde{R}(s)\}$ is the impulse response of the system. In the other, we stimulate the medium with a known strain and the stress is measured. This is a *stress relaxation experiment* and $Q(t)$ is the impulse response. Materials testing equipment, such as a cone viscometer, can measure R or Q to validate imaging experiments where only R can be measured.

At this point, we return to our physical model of hydrogel mechanical behavior and add some 19th century physics. A standard creep experiment applies a uniaxial step stress to a sample, $\sigma(t) = \sigma_0\, u(t)$. The initial effect is to elastically deform the matrix. Over time, water flows and the stretched cross links relax, thus generating a bi-exponential, time-varying strain called viscous creep (Fig. 1a). Water flow through the compressed polymer gives one viscoelastic response, like a shock absorber. This is represented mathematically by a Voigt retardance unit, $\tilde{R}_w(s) = R_1/(1+T_1 s)$, where $T_1 = \eta_1 R_1$ is the relaxation time for the first viscous component and η_1 is its coefficient of viscosity ([Tsc89], Ch 3). The weaker hydrogen and electrostatic bonds contribute a second viscoelastic response, $\tilde{R}_{ch}(s) = R_2/(1+T_2 s)$. Finally, covalently-bonded cross links are very stable; they do not creep under a load and thus contribute a purely elastic response over the measurement time: $\tilde{R}_{cc}(s) = R_0$. Note that R_i, T_i, η_i for $i = 0, 1, 2$ are all constants. The three component retardances assemble in series and in combination with (3) for a step stress stimulus gives strain in the time domain as

$$\epsilon(t) = R_0 \sigma_0 + R_1 \sigma_0 (1 - \exp(-t/T_1)) + R_2 \sigma_0 (1 - \exp(-t/T_2))\,. \tag{4}$$

Out of five possible parameters we display three, $R_0\sigma_0$, T_1, and T_2. $R_0\sigma_0$ is the instantaneous strain that describes elastic response of the medium. T_1 and T_2 are viscous relaxation time constants for water flow and cross linking mechanisms as described above. We postulate that these three parameters can describe the local biochemical environment of cancerous tissues.

2.3 Viscoelastic Measurements

Three types of measurements were performed on gelatin samples. A cone viscometer (standard materials testing device) was used to apply and sense the average stress and strain (Fig. 1a). Strain is measured for 120 s at a sampling rate of 3 Hz after stimulating the sample with a ramp stress. Samples were allowed to relax for 300 s before the measurement was repeated. Average measurements $\hat{\epsilon}(t)$ were fit to (4) is estimate parameters $R_0\sigma_0$, T_1 and T_2 as a function of pH. Results from the viscometer studies were used to understand and validate contrast mechanisms for imaging.

They also indicated the temporal resolution and acquisition times required for effective viscoelastic imaging. Its near-ideal geometry and high sensitivity provided an upper bound on sensitivity to pH-induced changes.

To gain further confidence in our estimates, we applied standard indentation techniques (Fig. 1b) to estimate elastic moduli [Kar01]. Cylindrical gelatin samples, 60 mm in diameter and 6 mm in height, were placed on a digital force plate. A flatended, cylindrical indentor 1.5 mm in radius was pressed into the top surface of samples under computer control at a constant speed of 0.02 mm/s. After cycling 10 times, the indenter position and the resultant force were recorded (Fig. 1b). The force-displacement data were applied to an equation developed for the specific measurement geometry to estimate the elastic modulus Q_0 [Hay72, Kar01].

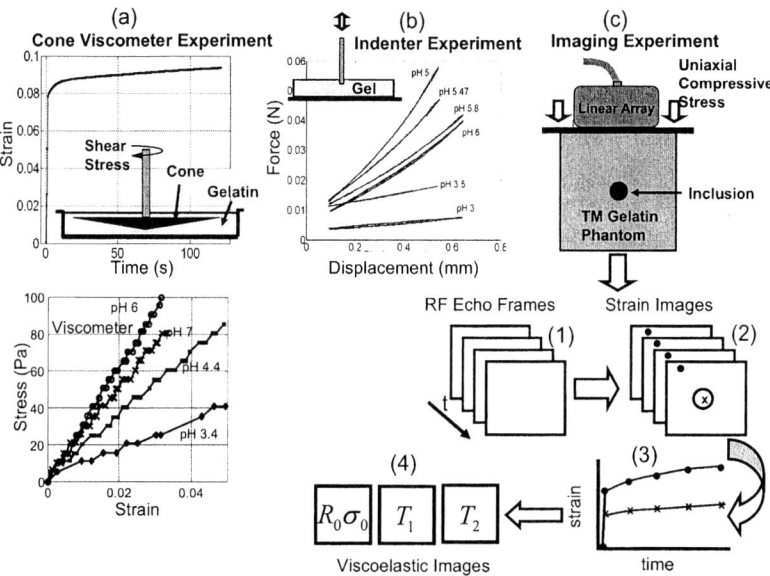

Fig. 1. Three experiments: (a) and (b) are used to validate imaging experiment (c). (a) A cone viscometer applies a shear force to measure creep (top) and stress-strain curves (bottom) for samples at different pH. (b) Indenter applies compressive force to measure force-displacement that are related to stress-strain curves. (c) Ultrasonic viscoelastic imaging (steps 1-4). Imaging array applies a compressive force while acquiring RF echo frames. RF frames are processed to form strain image sequence. Pixels in the target (x) and background (o) are fit to bi-exponential curves to generate viscoelastic images

We image viscoelastic parameters by applying a stress field to the surface of tissues and phantoms with an ultrasound transducer while recording frames of radiofrequency (RF) echo signals (Fig. 1c). A linear array transducer is flush mounted to a compression plate and positioned with a computer controlled motion system. Echo frames were recorded at 13 fps synchronous to the transducer motion from a Siemens Antares ultrasound system with an Ultrasound Research Interface (URI). Strain was computed between sequential RF frames using either a correlation-based algorithm [Cha98] or a regularized optical flow algorithm [Bar04]. The spatial resolution for strain is normally determined by the correlation window length, but ultimately is limited by the pulse bandwidth. For each pixel in the strain image sequence, values are plotted as a function of time. Those curves are fit to (4) using techniques described in [Sri04] to estimate three images displaying the parameters $R_0\sigma_0$, T_1, and T_2.

2.4 Free-Hand Clinical Viscoelastic Imaging

To estimate material properties, we use simple sample geometries and precise movements to mechanically stimulate samples. However, the same precision is impractical in clinical applications. Studies have shown it is possible to apply a stress to a phantom using a hand-held transducer that varies less than 5% up over the 20 s imaging time [Sri04a]. Some drift is acceptable provided pathology-specific contrast can be maintained.

3 Results

Figures 2 (a-c) display measurements of elastic modulus Q_0 and relaxation time constants T_1, T_2 from Eqs. (3) and (4) versus pH as measured by the three techniques described in Fig. 1: viscometer, indenter, and ultrasonic viscoelastic imaging. The collagen matrix structure of each sample was adjusted by varying the pH *before* the gel congealed, so the properties are spatially homogeneous. Principal strains give the relationship between the shear modulus obtained in the viscometer studies G and the elastic modulus from indenter and imaging measurements Q_0 for these incompressible gels: $Q_0 = 3G$ [Tsc89].

Elastic modulus estimates are similar for all three techniques below the iso-electric point; however, viscometer values exceed the indenter and imaging results at pH > 5. Gel stiffness is greatest at the isoelectric point where the shape of the collagen fibrils and their surface charge distributions provide dense cross links via fragile hydrogen and electrostatic bonds. Gelatin softens at lower and higher pH values because cross-link sites compete for binding locations with the excess charges.

Relaxation time constant estimates increase linearly over the same pH range. The correlation coefficients listed suggest a linear dependence on pH, however for the relaxation time constant T_1, a step function at the iso-electric point could also describe its pH response. The viscometer yielded a slope $\Delta T_1/\Delta pH = 2.34$ that is smaller than $\Delta T_2/\Delta pH = 41.42$, showing that T_2 is more sensitive to pH changes. The slopes for the imaging experiments are lower than those for the viscometer most likely because the total measurement time is shortened from 200 s (viscometer) to 20 s (imaging), or perhaps because of differences in signal-to-noise ratios and experimental uncertainties. The acquisition time for imaging is limited by the memory of the on-board processor, although it can be extended if the acquisition depth and frame rate are reduced.

Similar trends in the three parameters were observed for stress rates between 20 – 1000 Pa/s (curves not shown), however, the time constants progressively decreased with stress rate. The relaxation parameters did not change as the peak applied stress was varied between 20 – 100 Pa, confirming that we are in the linear, viscoelastic measurement region for these materials. The strain response is nonlinear for greater applied stress; e.g., see Fig. 1 (b).

To generate the data of Fig. 2 (a-c), we adjusted pH before the gels congealed to alter the 3D structure of the matrix as it formed [Ush00]. We found no literature to predict what happens if we inject acids or bases into congealed gelatin *after* the matrix structure has been set. Our intention was to generate a focal region with varying pH for imaging experiments, although it was unclear if or how pH affects a formed matrix. This question was partially addressed in Fig. 2 (d-g) and (h-m), where small volumes of either a strong acid or strong

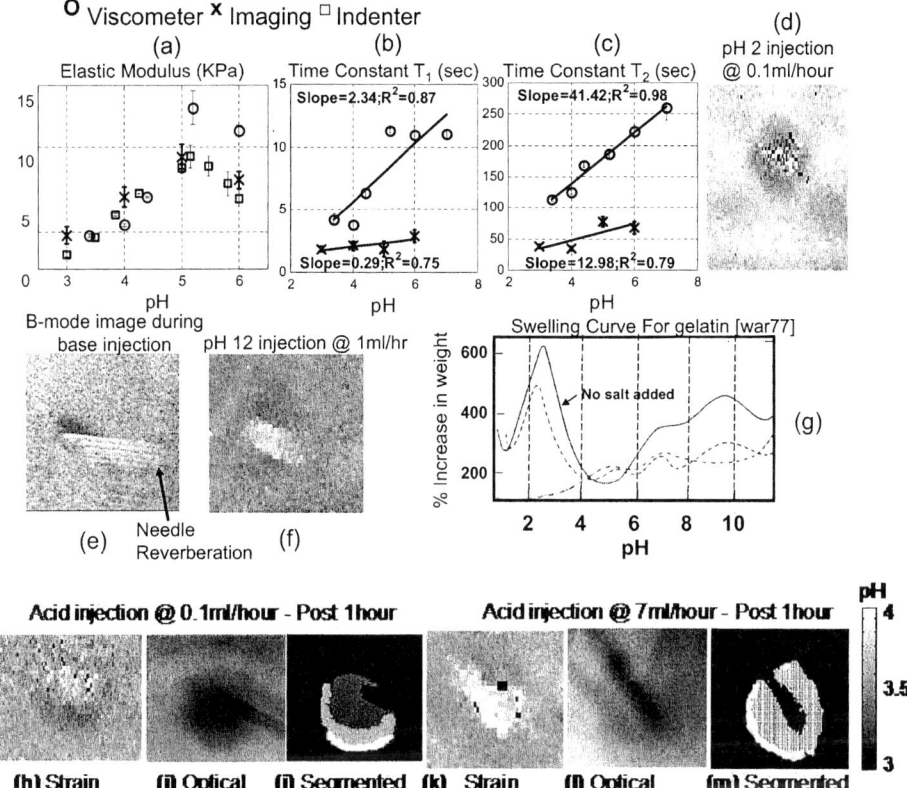

Fig. 2. (a-c) Estimates of elastic modulus, T_1 and T_2 for homogeneous gelatin samples whose pH was adjusted during manufacturing. Viscometer, indenter and imaging experiments are compared. Slopes and R^2 values result from linear regression. The B-scan in (e) shows the needle and the 2 mm fluid bolus (dark region). (d,f,h,k) Strain images of acid and base injections into pI = 5 gelatin. Curve in (g) shows the variation in swelling with pH [War77]. Gray-scale optical and color segmented images are shown in (i,l) and (j,m) respectively. The colorbar represents the pH scale only for segmented images

base were slowly infused into isoelectric gelatin. In the B-scan of Fig. 2 (e), you can see the fluid volume surrounding the needle. We withdrew the needle and waited one hour for the fluid to diffuse, then we imaged strain: Fig. 2 (d,f,h,k). A needle-type pH probe was used to estimate local gel pH after imaging. Near the infusion site, the gel seemed to soften (bright regions in strain images) for extreme pH values (pH 1 and pH 12) due to local breakdown of collagen structure as was expected from Fig. 2(a). Neutral-pH fluid injections produced no detectable strain contrast, thereby confirming that the softening is pH related and not just from the presence of the added fluid. Close comparison of Figs. 2 (h) and (k) shows that contrast depends on infusion rate. At high flow rates, the injected solution produces significant softening whereas at lower flow rates acids have time to diffuse away from the injection site in addition to being buffered (pH $\simeq$ 2) by gelatin. The buffering reduces the change in pH, which lowers strain contrast (compare Figs. 2 (h) and (k)), but it also changes the balance of free charge such that the region around the infusion site draws water from its surrounding and swells and stiffens according to Figs. 2 (g). This creates the dark ring around the infusion site as seen in the strain image of Fig. 2 (h). Thus the softening effects of pH on the collagen matrix compete with the stiffening induced by the osmotic gradients of added charge.

To test the above theories, we first infused a pH 2 fluid into another gel sample, where we found a dark lesion consistent with swelling (Fig. 2 (d)). Buffering and diffusion were monitored when pH 3 acids dissolved in a universal indicator pH dye (Auspex Scientific) were injected into transparent gels. Color changes correlated with pH were captured over time using a digital camera. Examples of such optical images for different flow rates at 1 hour are shown in Figs. 2 (i), (l). Acids infused at high flow rates homogeneously buffered by approximately 1 pH unit whereas at low flow rates only acids that had diffused away underwent buffering. Figs. 2 (j), (m) show these regions and were estimated by applying color-segmentation algorithms to Figs 2 (i), (l). Although all processing was done in color, all images were converted into gray-scale.

Furthermore, although the relaxation times were sensitive to pH-induced matrix changes from adding an acid or base prior to congealing (Figs. 2 (b,c)), we found little or no change in T_1 or T_2 images for acid injections into congealed gelatin.

In the body, the most dangerous tumors have highly metabolic regions with inadequate perfusion and poorly formed lymphatics. These edematous and acidic regions provide an unstable environment for cell growth. Extracellular pH in tissue can fall from the normal isoelectric value of pH 7.4 to 6.4 locally in heterogeneous tumors [Gil02]. If tissues are similar to these gels, then we can expect a variation in relaxation times equal to the slope values. There are no breast tissues measurements equivalent to those of gels in Fig. 2 (a-c). Our plan to obtain this information is to use gelatin to validate the viscoelastic imaging technique and then image lesions in vivo to estimate the viscous relaxation times of tissues.

Clearly we are just beginning to understand how pH effects the structure of collagen matrices. Nevertheless, to see what effects we can expect in vivo, we scanned a few patients undergoing sonographically-guided breast biopsy. One patient presented a single nonpalpable mass that was detected mammographically. That lesion appeared sonographically as a hypoechoic regions that was later determined to be benign (Fig. 3 (a)). The strain image of that lesion (Fig. 3 (b)) showed what appeared to be two moderately stiff lesions. We fit the time varying strain sequence to a mono-exponential function and displayed that relaxation-time image in Fig. 3 (c). The bright regions corresponding to lesion areas in the strain image show longer relaxation times, consistent with the dense collagen matrix of a fibrotic lesion. The chi-squared (χ^2) image provided an indication of how well the time-varying strain data fit a mono-exponential – bright areas of χ^2

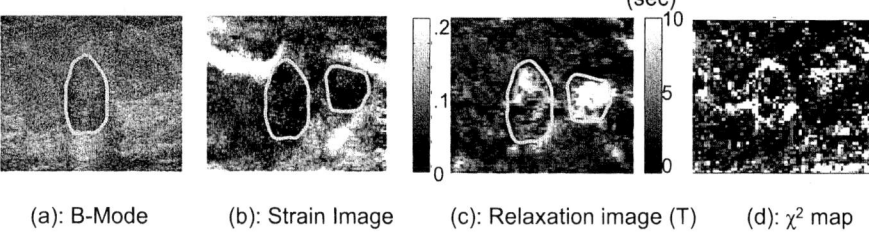

(a): B-Mode   (b): Strain Image   (c): Relaxation image (T)   (d): χ^2 map

Fig. 3. (a) B-mode breast image with a fibroadenoma. The corresponding (b) strain, (c) relaxation time, (d) and χ^2 images. Lesion margins are outlined

near the lesion margins indicate a poor fit as you might expect near a boundary between two tissue types.

We were surprised to see two lesions in the viscoelastic images, since only one appeared in the sonogram and mammogram. Although only the large lesion was biopsied, our clinical collaborators felt that a second lesion was possible. The image set of Fig. 3 shows that the fibroadenoma is slightly hypoechoic, somewhat stiffer than surrounding tissues, and less viscous than the surround regions that relaxed more quickly. In our experience, tissues usually creep much more than does gelatin for the same applied stress. Consequently, tissue are more viscous and therefore could provide higher contrast for relaxation time than that observed in gelatin phantoms.

4 Summary

Ultrasound is highly sensitive to the collagenous tissue matrix (stroma) that determines the mechanical properties of breast tissue and plays an important signaling role in the development of malignant disease. By mechanically stressing this matrix, we observe time-varying deformation patterns that describe the local biochemical environment. For example, it is possible to image metabolically driven pH variations that are known to trigger the molecular signals that promote genetic instability. There is accumulating evidence to show that elasticity imaging can reveal the fibrotic and desmoplastic reactions of the body specific to malignant growth [Ple00, Sin00, Nig02]. This report expands on that method to include viscoelastic properties that image functional features of tumor growth such as pH.

To explore the capabilities of viscoelastic imaging, we used gelatin, a collagen hydrogel, to mimic some acoustic and mechanical features of breast tissue. The characteristics of water movement and relaxing cross links that determine stability of the matrix under a load, provided a physical model for viscoelastic mechanisms. This physical model is consistent with the bi-exponential, time-varying strain curve observed experimentally in response to a uniaxial step stress.

The dependence of elastic modulus on pH showed a peak near pH = 5, the isoelectric pH, whereas the relaxation time constants increased linearly with pH. The long time constant T_2 varied much more with pH than T_1. When the molecular surface charges are unbalanced, as they are for pH values away from pI, charge repulsion does not allow the collagen molecules to form their normal tightly-folded structure. Additionally, the excess surface charge preferentially interacts with polar water molecules rather than other cross link sites on the protein [Ush00]. These occur on either side of the isoelectric point and result in a peak modulus value at pI and decreased values on either side. Furthermore, the changes in the binding structure that alters cross-linking mechanisms primarily affects T_2. In particular interactions with water occur in acidic regions and could result in shorter time constants as seen with the viscometer results.

It seems that detection sensitivity to pH is reduced for relaxation constant images compared with viscometer measurements. The loss of sensitivity could result from a number of factors such as reduced acquisition time, more complex imaging geometry, signal averaging during curve fitting, different experimental errors and uncertainty in force compensation. We suspect that shortening of the total acquisition time is the major effect. The situation is analogous to MRI where TR and TE can affect contrast in T1- and T2-weighted MR images. There needs to be a balance between the artifacts generated by long measurement times (analogous to TR in MRI) and the bias in relaxation times generated by short measurement times. However, the high sensitivity and near-ideal geometry of the viscometer measurements allow them to serve as an upper limit for imaging sensitivity.

While creating focal regions of varying pH in congealed isoelectric gels for imaging, we observed a breakdown of the collagen matrix, resulting in soft regions. However upsetting the charge balance by shifting the pH caused local swelling from osmotic gradients that stiffen tissues. Thus, pH induces changes in simple gelatin can be complex. Note that for this type I collagen gel, the pI was intentionally reduced from pI =7.4 in its natural in vivo state to pH $\sim$ 5 during manufacturing of gelatin powder as a preservative mechanism gainst bacterial growth. Nevertheless, measurements encompassing pH = pI, regardless of the value of pI, should be equivalent from the point of view of matrix stability.

The clinical example showed there are measurable effects in benign breast tumors but it is too early to know what the effects reveal about the tissues. We plan to continue our use of gelatin to develop viscoelastic imaging to probe for the first time the viscoelastic properties of breast tissue and interpret the results in terms of the local biochemical environment.

References

[Abb04] Abbey CK, Borowsky AD, McGoldrick ET, Gregg JP, Maglione JE, Cardiff RD, Cherry SR: In vivo positron-emission tomography imaging of progression and transformation in a mouse model of mammary neoplasia. Proc. Natl. Acad. Sci. USA **101** (2004) 11438–11443

[Bar04] Pellot-Barakat C, Frouin F, Insana MF, Herment Alan: Ultrasound Elastography Based on Multiscale Estimations of Regularized Displacement Fields. IEEE Trans Medical Imaging. **23** (2004) 153-163

[bar82] Barsky S, Grotendorst GR and Liotta LA: Increased content of type V collagen desmoplasia of human breast carcinoma. Am. J. Pathology **108** (1982) 276-283

[Ber03] Bercoff J, Chaffai S, Tanter M, Sandrin L, Catheline S, Fink M, Gennisson JL, Meunier M: In vivo breast tumor detection using transient elastography. Ultrasound Med. Biol. **29** (2003) 1387-1396

[Cha96] Chachra D, Gratzer PF, Pereira CA, Lee JM: Effect of applied uniaxial stress on rate and mechanical effects of cross-linking is tissue derived biomaterials. Biomaterials **17** (1996) 1865-1875

[Cha98] Chaturvedi P, Insana MF, Hall TJ: Testing the limitations of 2-D local companding in strain imaging using phantoms. IEEE Trans. Ultrason., Ferro., Freq., Control **45** (1998) 1022-1031

[Day04] Dayton P, Pearson D, Clark J, Simon S, Schumann P, Zutshi R, Matsunaga T, Ferrara K: Ultrasonic detection of alphaVbeta3 expressing-cells with targeted contrast agents. Mol. Imaging **3** (2004) 125-134

[Ele01] Elenbaas B, Weinberg RA: Heterotypic signaling between epithelial tumor cells and fibroblasts in carcinoma formation. Exp. Cell Res. **264** (2001) 169-184

[Ell04] Elliott JE, Macdonald M, Nie J, Bowman CN: Structure and swelling of poly(acrylic acid) hydrogels: effect of pH, ionic strength, and dilution on the crosslinked polymer structure. Polymer **45** (2004) 1503-1510

[Gil02] Gilles RJ, Raghunand N, Karczmar GS, Bhujwalla ZM: MRI of the tumor microeviroment. J. Mag. Res. Imag. **16** (2002) 430-450

[Hal97] Hall TJ, Bilgen M, Insana MF, Krouskop TA: Phantom materials for elastography. IEEE Trans. Ultrason., Ferro., Freq. Control **44** (1997) 1355-1365

[Hay72] Hayes WC, Keer LM, Herrmann G, Mockros LF: A mathematical analysis for indentation tests of articular cartilage. J. Biomech., **5** (1972) 541 - 551.

[Kar01] Kargel C, Trummer B, Plevnik G, Pellot-Barakat C, Mai JJ, Insana MF: Is ultrasonic imaging a sensitive indicator of spatially varying elastic anisotropy? Proc. IEEE Ultrason. Symp. **01CH37263C** (2001) 1659-1662

[Mad03] Madsen EL, Frank GR, Krouskop TA, Varghese T, Kallel F, Ophir J: Tissue-mimicking oil-in-gelatin dispersions for use in heterogeneous elastography phantoms. Ultrason. Imaging **25** (2000) 17-38

[Nig02] Nightingale K, Soo MS, Nightingale R, Trahey G: Acoustic radiation force impulse imaging. Ultrasound Med. Biol. **28** (2002) 227-235

[Ple00] Plewes DB, Bishop J, Samani A, Sciarretta J: Visualization and quantification of breast cancer biomechanical properties with magnetic resonance elastography. Phys. Med. Biol. **45** (2000) 1591-1610

[Pol01] Pollack GH: Cells, Gells, and the Engines of Life. Ebner and Sons, Seattle WA

[Roe02] Roeder BA, Kokini K, Sturgis JE, Robinson JP, Voytik-Harbin SL: Tesile mechanical properties of 3-D type I collagen extracellular matrices with varied microstructure. Trans. ASME **124** (2002) 214-222

[Sin00] Sinkus R, Lorenzen J, Schrader D, Lorenzen M, Dargatz M, Holz D: High-resolution tensor MR elastography for breast tumour detection. Phys. Med. Biol. **45** (2000) 1649-1664

[Sri04]   Sridhar M, Du H, Pellot-Barakat C, Simon SI, Insana MF: Ultrasonic mechanical relaxation imaging of pH in biopolymers. Proc. SPIE **5373** (2004) 929–932
[Sri04a] Sridhar M, Du H, Pellot-Barakat C, Tsou J, Insana MF: Ultrasonic Imaging of Biochemical Changes in Tissues. Proc. IEEE Ultrasonics Symposium *In Press*
[Tsc89]   Tschoegl NW, Phenomenological Theory of Linear Viscoelastic Behavior. An Iintroduction, Springer, New York (1989)
[Ush00]   Usha R, Ramasami T: Effect of pH on dimensional stability of rat tail tendon collagen fiber. J. Appl. Polym. Sci. **75** (2000) 1577–1584
[Voy01]   Voytik-Harbin SL, Rajwa B, Robinson JP: Three-dimensional imaging of extracellular matrix and extracellular matrix-cell interactions. Methods Cell Biol. **63** (2001) 583–597
[War77]   Ward AG, Courts A: The Science and Technology of Gelatin; Academic Press, New York, **1977**.

PDE-Based Three Dimensional Path Planning for Virtual Endoscopy

M. Sabry Hassouna and A.A. Farag

Computer Vision & Image Processing Laboratory (CVIP),
University of Louisville, Louisville, Kentucky
{msabry, farag}@cvip.uofl.edu

Abstract. Three dimensional medial paths or curve skeletons ($\mathcal{CS}$) are an essential component of any virtual endoscopy (VE) system, because they serve as flight paths for a virtual camera to navigate the human organ and to examine its internal structures. In this paper, we propose a novel framework for computing flight paths of tubular structures for VE using partial differential equation (PDE). The method works in two passes. In the first pass, the overall topology of the organ is analyzed and its important topological nodes are identified, while in the second pass, the actual flight paths are computed by tracking them starting from each identified node. The proposed framework is robust, fully automatic, computationally efficient, and computes $\mathcal{CS}$ that are centered, connected, thin, and less sensitive to boundary noise. We have extensively validated the robustness of the proposed method both quantitatively and qualitatively against several synthetic phantoms and clinical datasets.

1 Introduction

Virtual endoscopy (VE) is an integration of medical imaging and virtual reality. VE gives a computer-based alternative to standard radiological image viewing and to traditional fiber optic endoscopy for examining the interior structures of human organs. Unlike traditional fiber optic endoscopy, which is confined to the interior of a hollow organ, VE enables navigation between the inner and outer mucosal layers. VE has many advantages, such as being less invasive, cost-effective, free of risks and side effects. Therefore, VE is ideal for screening purposes and surgical planning. The computation of flight paths from volumetric objects is still a challenging process due to the complex nature of the anatomical structures.

Compared with 2D skeletonization methods, few methods have been proposed for extracting $\mathcal{CS}$, which can be classified as: (1) Ridge based and scale space methods for intensity data, (2) Topological thinning and distance transform methods for segmented data, and (3) Hybrid methods for both types of data. We will review only recent representative methods of each class.

Aylward and Bullitt [1] proposed a $\mathcal{CS}$ tracking approach for intensity images. The Eigen vectors of the Hessian matrix are used to estimate the local orientation of the vessels, and a normal plane is iteratively updated to follow the vessel's cross-section. The method generates $\mathcal{CS}$ that are thin and connected. However, it requires user interaction and a set of heuristics to handle branching and end points.

Deschamps and Cohen [2] relate the problem of finding $\mathcal{CS}$ to that of finding paths of minimal action in 3D intensity images, which can be found by first solving the Eikonal equation using the fast marching method and then following the gradient descent between two points selected by a user on the branch of interest. The method is fast and generates good quality $\mathcal{CS}$ but is limited to one branch at a time. For tree structures, it generates trajectories rather than $\mathcal{CS}$ [3].

Bitter et al. [4] proposed a penalized-distance algorithm to extract $\mathcal{CS}$ from volumetric data. A graph is first built from a coarse approximation of the 3D skeleton. Each edge of the graph is assigned a weight which is a function of both the Euclidean distance from a user defined source point and from the object's boundary. The $\mathcal{CS}$ are then extracted using Dijkstra's shortest path algorithm [5]. The parameters of the weight factor are specified heuristically for each object preventing the algorithm from automation.

Siddiqi et al. [6] extracted $\mathcal{CS}$ by thinning the object's medial surface, which has been computed by thresholding the negative average outward flux of the gradient field of the distance map. They have presented nice $\mathcal{CS}$ for vascular trees. However, the accuracy of computing $\mathcal{CS}$ becomes a function of the accurate computation of the object's medial surface. In addition, the user has to choose a suitable threshold value to guarantee connected skeleton.

Zhou and Toga [7] proposed a voxel coding technique, in which each voxel is assigned two codes. One is the distance from the object's boundary, while the other is the distance from a user defined point. The object is divided into a set of clusters, where each cluster is assumed to be the object cross section, whose center is the voxel of maximum distance from the boundary. $\mathcal{CS}$ are initially extracted as trajectories and then centered using some criteria. The algorithm guarantees connected paths. However, as the complexity of the object increases, the clusters are no longer normal to the $\mathcal{CS}$, and hence centeredness is not guaranteed.

In this paper, we present a PDE-based framework for computing flight paths of tubular structures for VE. The proposed framework is an enhanced version of our recent work [8]. The key idea is to propagate from a medial voxel that belongs to the $\mathcal{CS}$ of the organ, wave fronts of different speeds. The first front propagates with a moderate speed to capture the organ's topology, while the second one propagates much faster at medial voxels such that $\mathcal{CS}$ intersect the propagating fronts at those voxels of maximum positive curvatures, which are identified by solving an ordinary differential equation. Unlike previous methods, the new technique automatically and consistently handles complex anatomical structures with arbitrary number of loops.

2   Higher-Accuracy Fast Marching Method (HAFMM)

Consider a closed curve Γ propagating normal to itself with a speed $F(\mathbf{x})$ in one direction only. The front motion is governed by a nonlinear partial differential equation, known as the Eikonal equation Eq. (1).

$$||\nabla T(\mathbf{x})||F(\mathbf{x}) = 1.0 \qquad (1)$$

$T(\mathbf{x})$ is the time at which the front crosses the voxel $\mathbf{x}$. The *Fast marching method* (FMM) [9] is a computational technique that approximates the solution of Eq. (1). The idea of the algorithm is to introduce an order in the selection of the grid points based on the fact that the arrival time $T(\mathbf{x})$ at any grid point depends on the neighbors with smaller values. In this paper, we employ the HAFMM [10], which is an accurate version of the original FMM. It uses second-order approximation of the gradient whenever points are available, but reverts to a first-order approximation in the other cases.

3 The Proposed High Speed Propagation Model

One of the essential applications of the fast marching methods is the computation of distance fields with sub-pixel accuracy, which can be classified as distance from boundary (DFB) field, which computes at each voxel its minimum distance from the object's boundary, and distance from source point (DFS) field, which computes at each voxel its minimum distance from a known source point.

In this paper, we propose a new speed function Eq. (2) for the propagating fronts such that $\mathcal{CS}$ intersect them at those voxels of maximum positive curvatures. $\lambda(\mathbf{x})$ is a *medial descriptor function* that assigns each medial voxel a higher weight than a non-medial one, $D(\mathbf{x})$ is the minimum distance from the object's boundary, and α controls the front convexity at medial voxels.

$$F(\mathbf{x}) = e^{\alpha \, \lambda(\mathbf{x})} \quad (2)$$

$$\lambda(\mathbf{x}) = D(\mathbf{x}) + \frac{1.0}{1.0 + \|\nabla D(\mathbf{x})\|}$$

Assume that we want to compute the curve skeleton between the two medial voxels A and B of the single branch structure of Figure 1(a). Let A be a point source P_S that transmits a wave front W_α that evolves over time in the normal direction inside the object. Since the medial voxels A, z, and B have higher distances from the object's boundary than those of the non-medial voxels x, y, u, and v, let $\lambda(A) = \lambda(z) = R$ and $\lambda(u) = \lambda(v) = \lambda(x) = \lambda(y) = R - \Delta$, where $0 < \Delta < R$ and Δ is the minimum distance between two neighboring voxels. In order to study the role of α, we solve Eq.(1) around P_S numerically [10] with $T(A) = 0$. The solution is given by Eq.(3).

$$\begin{aligned} T(x) = T(y) &= e^{-\alpha R} + e^{-\alpha(R-\Delta)} \\ T(u) = T(v) &= e^{-\alpha(R-\Delta)} \\ T(z) &= e^{-\alpha R} \end{aligned} \quad (3)$$

Consider the following cases with $\Delta = 1.0$:

1. $\alpha = 0$: $T(u) = T(v) = T(z)$ and the voxels u, v, and z form the front W_0, whose positive curvature is κ_0 at the front tip z.
2. $\alpha = 1$: $T(u) = T(v) \simeq 2.7 T(z)$. Since $T(z) < T(u)$ and the voxels of the front have equal travel times from the source point P_S, then the front W_1 that passes by z must have a shorter base than that of W_0 which passes by u as shown in Figure 1(a). As a consequence, W_1 has more positive curvature $\kappa_1 > \kappa_0$ at z.
3. $\alpha = \infty$: As α increases indefinitely we get,

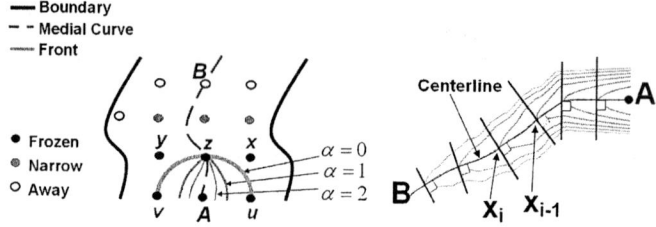

Fig. 1. (a) Single branch structure (b) A curve skeleton intersects the propagating fronts at those voxels of maximum positive curvatures

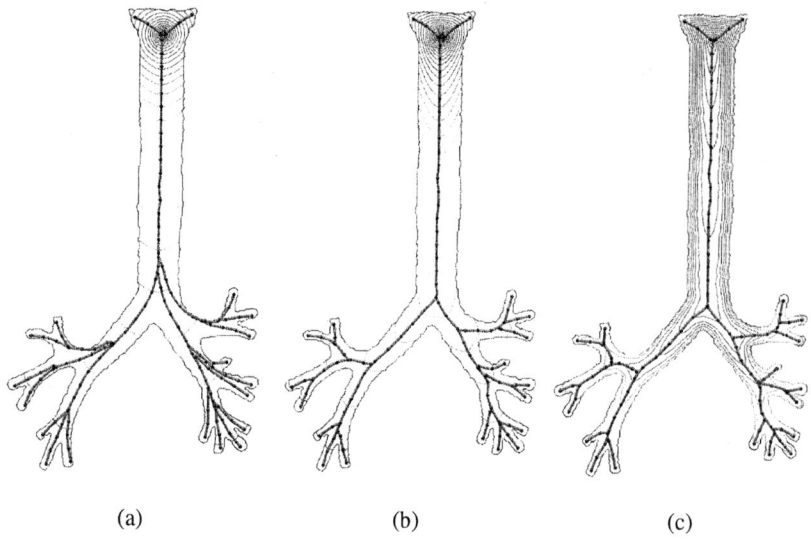

Fig. 2. Trajectories converge to $\mathcal{CS}$ with increasing α (a) $\alpha = 0.1$ (b) $\alpha = 0.3$ (c) $\alpha = 0.8$

$$\lim_{\alpha \to \infty} \frac{F(z)}{F(u)} = \lim_{\alpha \to \infty} \frac{e^{\alpha R}}{e^{\alpha(R-1.0)}} = \lim_{\alpha \to \infty} e^{\alpha} = \infty \qquad (4)$$

$$\lim_{\alpha \to \infty} \frac{T(z)}{T(u)} = \lim_{\alpha \to \infty} \frac{e^{-\alpha R}}{e^{-\alpha(R-1.0)}} = \lim_{\alpha \to \infty} e^{-\alpha} = 0 \qquad (5)$$

Under fast propagation, the interpretation of Eq.(4) is that, each medial voxel is moving much faster than a non-medial one. Hence, it is one of the tips of the moving front. On the other hand, the interpretation of Eq.(5) is that, the front has very short base as well as very high curvature at medial voxels.

The propagating front is monotonically increasing in time; there is only one global minimum over the cumulative cost field T, that is P_S, which has zero travel time. Then, the path between B and A can be found by backtracking from B along the gradient of T until A is reached. Let $\mathbf{x}_i$ and $\mathbf{x}_{i-1}$ be two medial voxels as shown in Figure 1(b). Since medial voxels have equal distances from the object's boundary, then the propagating front at $\mathbf{x}_i$ is symmetric around the line segment $\overrightarrow{\mathbf{x}_{i-1}\mathbf{x}_i}$ and perpendicular to it. Also, since the propagating fronts are level sets, then the direction of the gradient at each medial voxel is normal to its front. Therefore, by backtracking from $\mathbf{x}_i$ along the gradient of T, we reach $\mathbf{x}_{i-1}$. As a consequence, the path between A and B is the medial curve or $\mathcal{CS}$ that connects them.

The idea of the proposed speed model is to distinguish medial voxels from others by making them the front tips of maximum positive curvatures. In fact, this distinction already exists even at low speed propagation as long as we are dealing with a single tube-like structure [3]. Unfortunately, at low speed propagation, this distinction disappears near a branching or a merging node, where the propagating fronts at joint $\mathcal{CS}$ superimpose, resulting in a new wave front whose tip is not necessarily a medial voxel. This fact is illustrated in Figure 2, where trajectories converge to $\mathcal{CS}$ with increasing α.

4 Medial Descriptor Function $\lambda(\mathbf{x})$

A medial descriptor function $\lambda(\mathbf{x})$ is a scalar function that distinguishes medial voxels from others, while satisfying two conditions. Let $\mathbf{x}$ be a medial voxel, while $\mathbf{y}$ is non-medial one.

Condition 1: $\lambda(\mathbf{x}) \geq \lambda(\mathbf{y})$
Condition 2: If $D(\mathbf{y}_i) \geq D(\mathbf{y}_j)$, then $\lambda(\mathbf{y}_i) \geq \lambda(\mathbf{y}_j)$.

The first condition guarantees that a medial voxel is moving faster than its non-medial neighbors and hence it is the tip of the moving front. The second condition guarantees that the moving front is smooth and a non-medial voxel can not be the front tip with positive curvature. In this paper, we propose two different medial descriptor functions: the smoothing $\lambda_1(\mathbf{x})$ and the salient $\lambda_2(\mathbf{x})$.

4.1 The Smoothing Medial Descriptor Function $\lambda_1(\mathbf{x})$

This function assigns each voxel in the object its minimum distance $D(\mathbf{x})$ from the object's boundary as given by Eq. (6).

$$\lambda_1(\mathbf{x}) = D(\mathbf{x}) \qquad (6)$$

The function has been called smoothing because the distance is monotonically increasing gradually from the boundary of the object to its center. It is obvious that both conditions are satisfied without a proof.

4.2 The Salient Medial Descriptor Function $\lambda_2(\mathbf{x})$

For a moving front with a unit speed, the solution of Eq. (1) is proportional to $D(\mathbf{x})$ [9]. Therefore $\|\nabla D(\mathbf{x})\| = 1.0$ except at local maximum voxels ($\mathcal{CS}$), where the gradient is theoretically zero. According to Eq. (7), $\lambda_2(\mathbf{x})$ assigns medial voxels higher weights than any other voxel, therefore, the first condition is satisfied. All non-medial voxels have equal gradient magnitude $\|\nabla D(\mathbf{x})\| = 1.0$, therefore, the second condition is also satisfied. The distance field is continuous at the medial voxels but is not differentiable

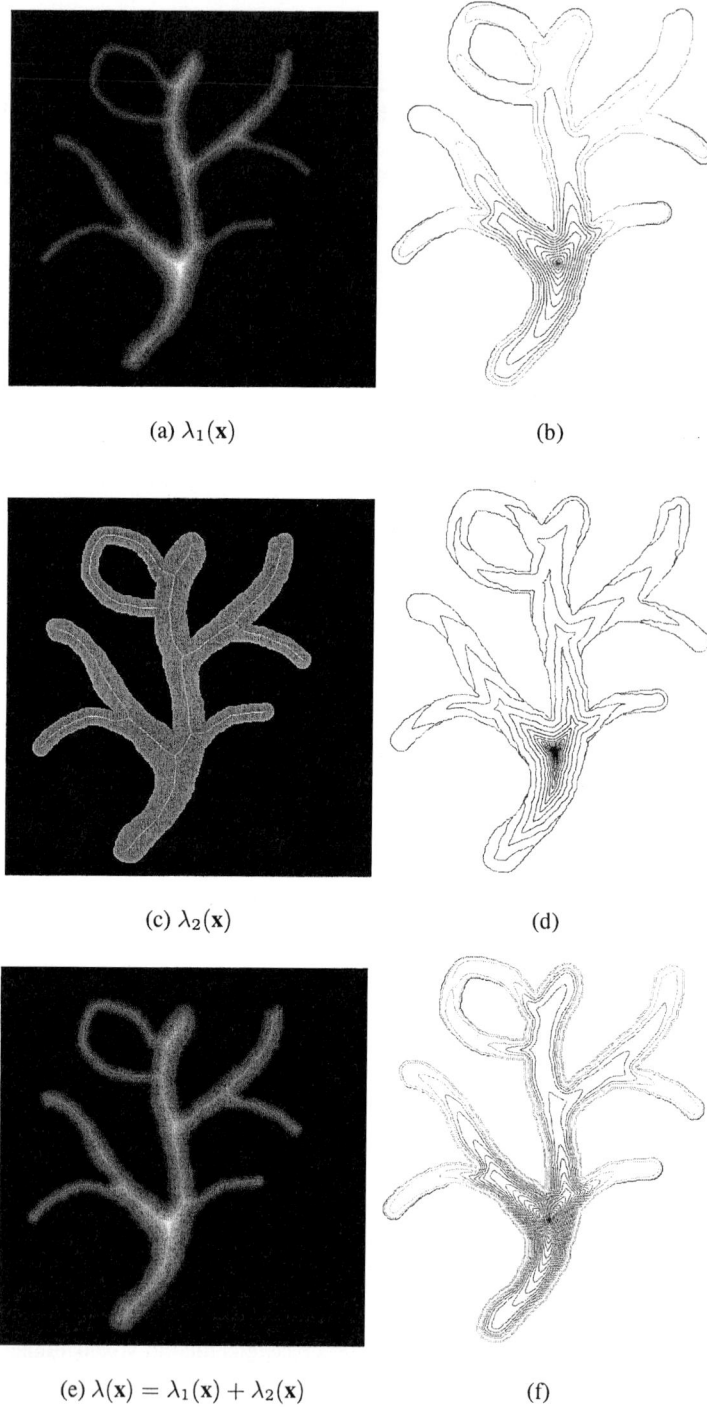

(a) $\lambda_1(\mathbf{x})$ (b)

(c) $\lambda_2(\mathbf{x})$ (d)

(e) $\lambda(\mathbf{x}) = \lambda_1(\mathbf{x}) + \lambda_2(\mathbf{x})$ (f)

Fig. 3. (a,c,e) Illustration of the proposed $\lambda(\mathbf{x})$'s of a 2D shape. (b,d,f) Propagation with the corresponding $\lambda(\mathbf{x})$'s

and hence it is slightly blurred. Salient features are those which have a low probability of being mis-classified with any other feature. This descriptor has been called salient because it identifies only salient medial voxels with sufficiently small gradient values.

$$\lambda_2(\mathbf{x}) = \frac{1.0}{1.0 + \|\nabla D(\mathbf{x})\|} \qquad (7)$$

Although $\lambda_1(\mathbf{x})$ does not provide much distinction between medial and non-medial voxels, it provides a smooth transition between them. On the other hand, $\lambda_2(\mathbf{x})$ identifies salient medial voxels of sufficiently small gradient values as shown in Figure 3(c). If we propagate a front from a source point using only $\lambda_2(\mathbf{x})$ as shown in Figure 3(d), the resulting fronts will be very sharp at medial voxels because all non-medial voxels are moving with nearly constant speed but less than that of the medial ones. Unfortunately, the gradient at sharp locations of the front is not defined leading to instable numerical analysis. To solve the problem, we augment $\lambda_1(\mathbf{x})$ as a smoothing term since it adds a monotonic increasing distance to each non-medial voxel, and hence they do not move any more with a constant speed. In Figure 3(e), we show that by augmenting the proposed medial descriptors, we get a new distance field whose medial voxels are more distinguished than those of Figure 3(a). The right hand side of Figure 3 shows the different shapes that the front may take experiencing different medial descriptors. Notice that by augmenting the proposed descriptors, we get fronts with large curvature at medial voxels but are still differentiable as shown in Figure 3(f).

5 Identification of Topological Nodes

In order to extract the entire $\mathcal{CS}$ of an object, we have to identify first its important topological nodes such as merging and extreme nodes. In this paper, we propose a method for identifying those nodes automatically. Initially, we compute the minimum distance field $D(\mathbf{x})$ with sub-pixel accuracy using the HAFMM by propagating a unit speed front from the object's boundary towards its center. Then, we select automatically one of its $\mathcal{CS}$ voxels and consider it a point source P_S that transmits a moderate speed wave front Eq.(8). P_S is selected as the voxel of global maximum $D(\mathbf{x})$.

$$F(\mathbf{x}) = D^\beta(\mathbf{x}) \quad 0 < \beta \leq 1.0 \qquad (8)$$

The solution of Eq.(1) under the moderate speed wave will result in a new real-valued distance field $D_1(\mathbf{x})$. We discretize $D_1(\mathbf{x})$ by computing its integer values. Therefore, the object's basic element is converted from a voxel to a cluster. Each cluster consists of connected voxels with the same discretized distance value. Two clusters are adjacent if they share a common voxel. Now, we can construct the cluster graph whose root is the cluster containing P_S with zero cluster value. The cluster graph contains two main types of clusters; Extreme cluster ($Xcluster$), which exists at the tail of the cluster graph and Merging cluster ($Mcluster$), which has at least two adjacent clusters (Successors) with the same distance value but less one than the distance value of $Mcluster$. The medial voxel of a cluster is computed by searching the cluster for the voxel with maximum $D(\mathbf{x})$. Extreme and merging nodes are the medial voxels of the associated

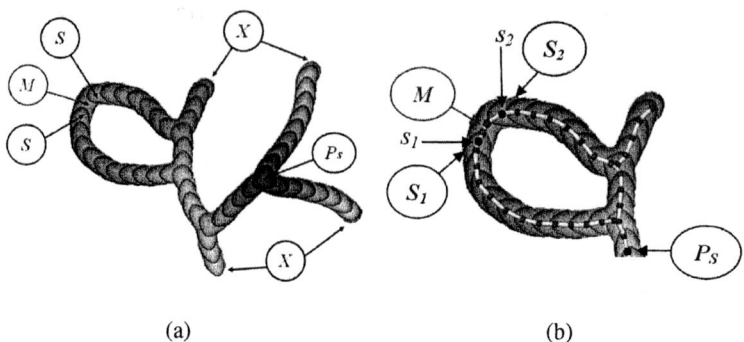

Fig. 4. (a) Cluster Graph (b) Curve skeletons around a loop

clusters. Figure 4(a) shows a cross section of the cluster graph of a 3D tree structure with one loop, where X, M, and S represent extreme, merging, and successor clusters, respectively.

6 Extraction of Curve Skeletons

In order to extract the $\mathcal{CS}$ between two medial voxels A and B, we initialize A to zero travel time and then propagate a high speed wave inside the object until B is reached. Finally, we backtrack from B along the gradient of $T(\mathbf{x})$ until A is found. The extraction process is the solution of the ordinary differential equation Eq.(9). $C(t)$ traces out the $\mathcal{CS}$, which is found by solving Eq.(9) using Runge-Kutta of order 2. The error of the method is $O(h^3)$, where h is the integration step. To ensure connected $\mathcal{CS}$, h is set to a small value; $h = 0.1$.

$$\frac{dC}{dt} = -\frac{\nabla T(\mathbf{x})}{|\nabla T(\mathbf{x})|}, \quad C(0) = B \qquad (9)$$

For $C_i = [x_i, y_i, z_i]^T$,

$$f(C_i) = -\frac{\nabla T(C_i)}{\|\nabla T(C_i)\|}, \quad k_1 = hf(C_i), \quad C_{i+1} = C_i + hf\left(C_i + \frac{k_1}{2}\right) \qquad (10)$$

If the object contains loops, we first extract their $\mathcal{CS}$ followed by those that originate from extreme nodes. Each loop in the object is associated with one merging cluster M of the cluster graph. For illustration, let M have only two successors S_1 and S_2 as shown in Figure 4(b). In order to extract the $\mathcal{CS}$ of this loop, three steps are required. In the first step, we compute the medial voxel s_1 of S_1 and consider the entire voxels of both M and S_2 as part of the object's background (construct holes) such that there is a unique $\mathcal{CS}$ from s_1 to P_S. Finally, we propagate a fast wave from P_S until s_1 is reached and then extract the $\mathcal{CS}$ between them. In the second step, we extract the $\mathcal{CS}$ between s_2 and P_S in a similar fashion to the first step except that we consider the entire voxels of both M and S_1 as part of the object's background and those of S_2 as part of the object's foreground. In the third step, we propagate a fast wave from s_1 until s_2 is reached and then extract the $\mathcal{CS}$ between them. The same concept can be generalized for a merging cluster with several successors.

The proposed framework can be summarized as follows: (1) Construct the minimum distance field $D(\mathbf{x})$, (2) Find the point source P_S, (3) Propagate a moderate speed wave from P_S, discretize the resultant distance field $D_1(\mathbf{x})$, and construct the cluster graph, (4) Identify extreme and merging nodes, (5) Construct a new distance field $D_2(\mathbf{x})$ from P_S by propagating a fast speed wave, (6) If the object contains loops, extract their $\mathcal{CS}$, and finally, (7) Extract those $\mathcal{CS}$ that originate from extreme nodes and ends with P_S or on a previously extracted path.

7 Validation

We have quantitatively validated the proposed method against ground truth $\mathcal{CS}$ that are generated analytically to model different 3D synthetic phantoms. Each phantom is created by centering a sphere of a fixed or varying radius at each ground truth voxel. The voxels of the ground truth and those extracted by the proposed method are represented by white and black spheres, respectively, while overlapped voxels are represented by light grey color. The phantoms are designed to measure the performance of the method when the anatomical structures have the following geometrical or topological properties: (1) high curvature and torsion (e.g., blood vessels), (2) sudden change in the organ's cross section (e.g., colon or aneurysm in vessels), and (3) several branching nodes (e.g., blood vessels and tracheobronchial trees). To study the sensitivity of the proposed method to noise, 50% of phantom's boundary were corrupted with additive noise to simulate acquisition or segmentation error as shown in the first row of Figure 5. A quantitative analysis was carried out by computing the amount of overlap, average, and maximum distance between the ground truth and computed $\mathcal{CS}$ for both noise-free and noisy phantoms. The quantitative results are presented in Table 1. Although the amount of overlap was less than 90 %, the average and maximum distance never exceed 0.35 and 1.41 mm (e.g., one voxel), respectively. In the presence of noise, the amount of overlap has been decreased by only 5 %, while the average and maximum distance has been increased slightly. For both noise-free and noisy cases, the computed $\mathcal{CS}$ were always adjacent to the ground truth ones, which is quite acceptable for flight paths, therefore, the proposed method has low sensitivity to boundary noise.

We have also validated the proposed method qualitatively against several clinical datasets as shown in Figure 5(d-j). Notice the complexity of the datasets and the accuracy of the computed $\mathcal{CS}$ especially around loops and near branching nodes.

Table 1. Quantitative validation of noise-free and noisy phantoms

Phantom	Vessels		Spiral		Colon	
State	Noise-Free	Noisy	Noise-Free	Noisy	Noise-Free	Noisy
Percentage of Overlap	75 %	70 %	90 %	86 %	70 %	65 %
Average Distance (mm)	0.35	0.45	0.08	0.17	0.24	0.52
Maximum Distance (mm)	1.41	2.0	1.0	1.41	1.0	2.0

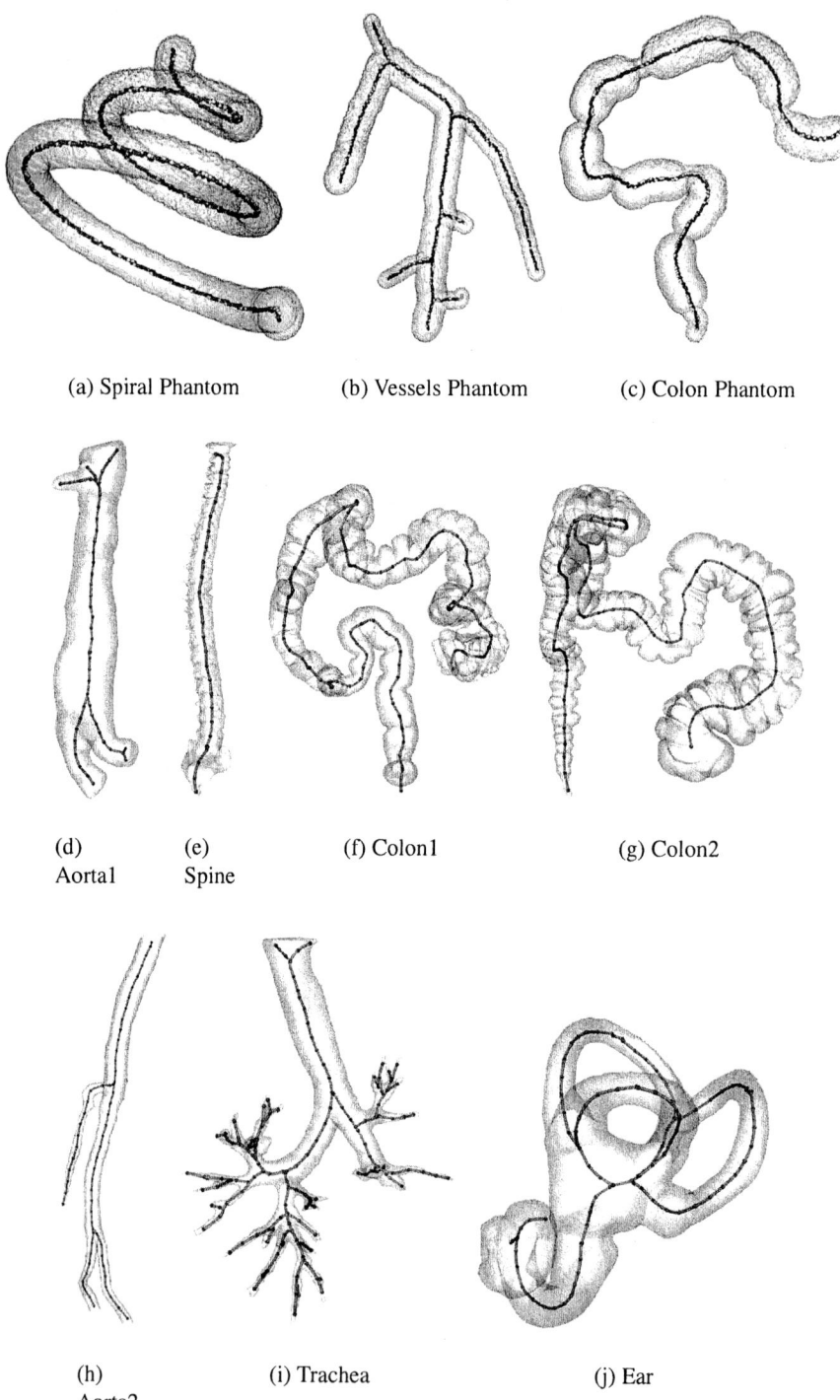

Fig. 5. Computed CS of (a-c) Synthetic phantoms (d-j) Clinical datasets

8 Discussion

Our experiments have been carried out on a single 400Mhz SGI infinite reality supercomputer. The volume sizes and running times in seconds of the tested datasets are presented in Table 2. We have implemented a general virtual endoscopy application to test the quality of the computed flight paths as shown in Figure 6. The surface of the organ has been color-coded by its mean curvature to facilitate the screening exam.

The proposed model is controlled by two main parameters α in Eq.(2) and β in Eq.(8). Theoretically α should be very high such that trajectories converge to $\mathcal{CS}$. Practically, a small value of α can still achieve the goal because $\lambda(\mathbf{x})$ highly distinguishes medial voxels from others. The experimental results showed that for $\alpha \geq 0.5$, trajectories converge to $\mathcal{CS}$. We can safely automate the algorithm by setting $\alpha = 1.0$.

β controls the thickness and orientation of the individual clusters in the cluster graph. As β increases, clusters become perpendicular to the desired $\mathcal{CS}$ (because the wave is fast at medial voxels) as well as their thickness increases. It is recommended to keep the thickness as small as possible to capture the small details of the object. Ex-

Table 2. Sizes and running times of different clinical datasets using the proposed method

Anatomical Organ	Actual Volume	Processed Voxels	Time in Sec.
Colon 1	$157 \times 248 \times 180$	517462	127
Colon 2	$184 \times 253 \times 231$	742563	216
Trachea	$145 \times 248 \times 198$	185491	70
Aorta 1	$84 \times 145 \times 365$	128086	40
Aorta 2	$130 \times 259 \times 97$	297954	55
Spine	$253 \times 49 \times 55$	53771	13
Ear	$162 \times 241 \times 125$	588823	114

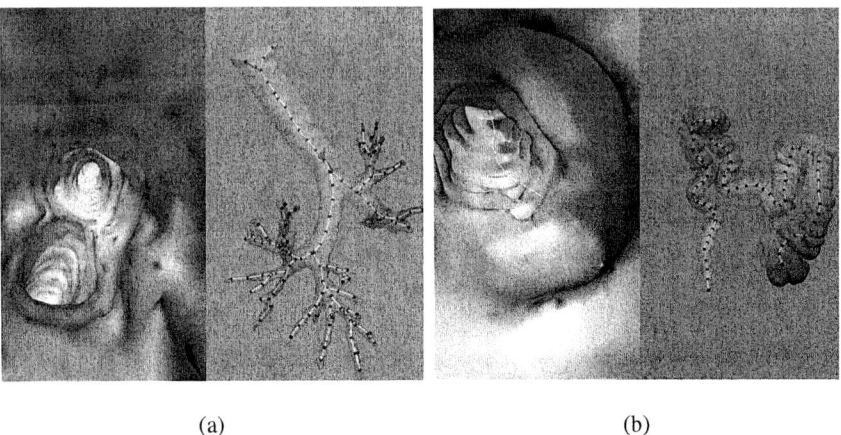

(a) (b)

Fig. 6. Internal views by the virtual camera for (a) Trachea (b) Colon

perimental results showed that $\beta = 0.5$ provides a balance between reasonable cluster thickness and perpendicular clusters that capture the large curvature parts of the organ.

The core of our method is the HAFMM, which is used in computing all distance fields. Fortunately, the complexity of the HAFMM for n voxels is $O(nlogn)$. Therefore, our method is computationally efficient.

9 Conclusion

In this paper, we have presented a robust, fully automatic, and fast method for computing flight paths of tubular structures for VE applications. The computed flight paths enjoy several features such as being centered, connected, thin, and less sensitive to noise. Unlike previous methods, our technique can handle complex anatomical structures with arbitrary number of loops. The robustness of the proposed method is demonstrated by correctly extracting all the CS of the tested clinical datasets as well as the successful validation against synthetic phantoms of different complexity.

References

1. Aylward, S.R., Bullitt, E.: Initialization, noise, singularities, and scale in height ridge traversal for tubular object centerline extraction. IEEE Trans. Medical Imaging **21** (2002) 61–75
2. Deschamps, T., Cohen, L.: Fast extraction of minimal paths in 3d images and applications to virtual endoscopy. Medical Image Analysis **5** (2001)
3. Deschamps, T.: Curve and Shape Extraction with Minimal Path and Level-Sets techniques - Applications to 3D Medical Imaging. PhD thesis, Université Paris-IX Dauphine (2001)
4. Bitter, I., Kaufman, A.E., Sato, M.: Penalized-distance volumetric skeleton algorithm. IEEE Transactions on Visualization and Computer Graphics **7** (2001) 195–206
5. Dijkstra, E.W.: A note on two problems in connexion with graphs. Numerische Mathematik **1** (1959) 269–271
6. Bouix, S., Siddiqi, K., Tannenbaum, A.: Flux driven fly throughs. In: Computer Vision and Pattern Recognition. (2003) 449–454
7. Zhou, Y., Toga, A.W.: Efficient skeletonization of volumetric objects. IEEE Transactions on Visualization and Computer Graphics **5** (1999) 196–209
8. Hassouna, M.S., Farag, A.: Robust centerline extraction framework using level sets. In: Proc. of IEEE Conference on Computer Vision and Pattern Recognition, San Diego, CA (2005)
9. Adalsteinsson, D., Sethian, J.: A fast level set method for propagating interfaces. Journal of Computational Physics **118** (1995) 269–277
10. Sethian, J.: Level Sets Methods and Fast Marching Methods. 2nd edn. Cambridge University Press (1999)

Elastic Shape Models for Interpolations of Curves in Image Sequences*

Shantanu H. Joshi[1], Anuj Srivastava[2], and Washington Mio[3]

[1] Department of Electrical Engineering, Florida State University,
Tallahassee, FL 32310, USA
[2] Department of Statistics, Florida State University, Tallahassee, FL 32306, USA
[3] Department of Mathematics, Florida State University, Tallahassee, FL 32306, USA

Abstract. Many applications in image analysis are concerned with the temporal evolution of shapes in video sequences. In situations involving low-contrast, low-quality images, human aid is often needed to extract shapes from images. An interesting approach is to use expert help to extract shapes in certain well-separated frames, and to use automated methods to extract shapes from intermediate frames. We present a technique to interpolate between expert generated shapes. This technique preserves salient features in the interpolated shapes, and allows analysts to model a continuous evolution of shapes, instead of a coarse sampling generated by the expert. The basic idea is to establish a correspondence between points on the two end shapes, and to construct a geodesic flow on a shape space maintaining that correspondence. This technique is demonstrated using echocardiographic images and infrared human gait sequences.

1 Introduction

Image-based shape analysis plays an ever increasing role in medical diagnosis using non-invasive imaging. Shapes and shape variations of anatomical parts are often important factors in detecting normality/abnormality of imaged patients. More generally, an important goal in image analysis is to classify and recognize objects of interest present in observed images. Imaged objects can be characterized in many ways: according to their colors, textures, shapes, movements, and locations. The past decade has seen large efforts in modeling and analysis of pixel values or textures in images to attain these goals albeit with limited success. An emerging opinion in the scientific community is that global features such as shapes be used to discriminate between images of objects. Characterization of complex objects using their global shapes is fast becoming a major tool in computer vision and medical image analysis. In case the interest lies in analyzing shapes of silhouettes in images, it is often neccessary to extract curves depicting these silhouettes before or during the analysis.

---

* Research supported in part by (FRG) DMS-0101429 and ARO W911 NF-04-01-0268.

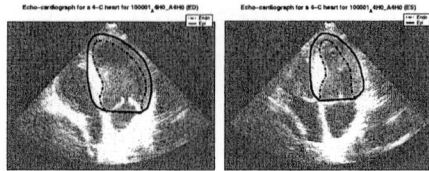

Fig. 1. Expert traced curves, denoting epi (solid lines) and endo(broken lines) -cardial borders, over ED (left) and ES (right) frames of an echocardiographic image sequence

In case of video sequences containing dynamic objects, an interesting problem is to analyze a sequence of evolution of shapes. The problem modifies to extraction, tracking, and analysis of shapes of **dynamic curves**. A statistical framework for analysis of such dynamic shapes requires modeling and estimating stochastic processes on shape spaces. In general this problem requires extraction of curves from each individual image frame. However, an efficient alternative is to manually extract shapes from images that are separated by a fixed interval, say T, using expert assistance and then interpolate between those extracted shapes to fill in the remaining frames. In this paper we present a technique that not only interpolates between observed shapes but also retains important local features, such as corners and bends while preserving the global shape structures.

In order to motivate shape-based image analysis, two interesting applications are presented below.

1. **Echo-cardiographic Image Sequences**[1]: Consider the two images displayed in Figure 1, acquired as the end diastolic (ED) and end systolic (ES) frames from a sequence of echocardiographic images during systole, taken from the apical four chamber view. Note that systole is the squeezing portion of the cardiac cycle and that the typical acquisition rate in echocardiography is 30 image frames/second. Among other things, a cardiologist is interested in temporal evolution of cardiac boundaries: epicardial and endocardial, to analyze a patient's health. Superimposed on both images are expert tracings of the epicardial (solid lines) and endocardial borders (broken lines) of the left ventricle of the heart. From these four borders, indices of cardiac health, including chamber area, fractional area change, and wall thickness, can be easily computed. Since a manual tracing of these borders is too time consuming to be practical in a clinical setting, these borders are currently generated for research purposes only. The current clinical practice is to estimate these indices subjectively or (at best) make a few one-dimensional measurements of wall thickness and chamber diameter. A major goal in echocardiographic image analysis has been to develop and implement automated methods for computing these two sets of borders as well as the sets of borders for the 10-15 image frames that are typically acquired between ED and ES. Different

---

[1] Special thanks to Dr. David Wilson, Department of Mathematics, University of Florida Gainesville for the use of the echo-cardiographic images.

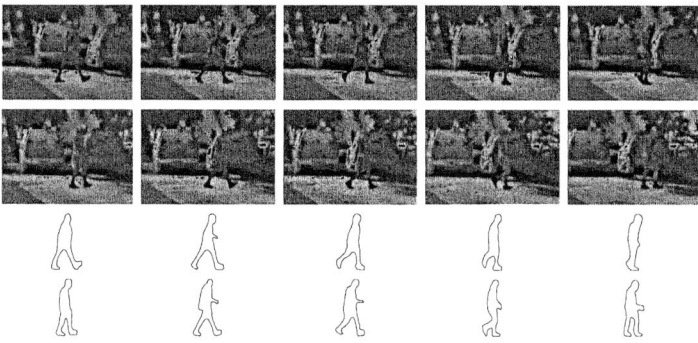

Fig. 2. Top two rows: an infrared image sequence showing human gait for a test subject. Bottom two rows show the corresponding evolution of silhouettes in these images

aspects of past efforts [6, 1] include both the construction of geometric figures to model the shape of the heart as well as validation. While it is difficult for cardiologists to generate borders for all the frames, it is possible for them to provide borders for the first and the last frames in a cardiac cycle. Since it is not uncommon for the heart walls to exhibit diskinetic (i.e. irregular) motion patterns, the boundary variations in the intermediate frames can be important in a diagnosis. Our goal is to estimate epicardial and endocardial boundaries in the intermediate frames given the boundaries at the ED and ES frames.

2. **Gait Analysis for Human Recognition**: Another application requiring characterization of shape evolution is recognition of humans using gait sequences. Image sequences that capture walking patterns of humans, are used to analyze gaits under the hypothesis that gait can be used to recognize people up to a reasonable accuracy. The use of night-vision cameras, such as an infrared camera, is popular in such surveillance applications. In view of the low-contrast and low-quality of infrared images, one often needs human assistance for shape extraction. Shown in Figure 2 is an example of an infrared image sequence of human gait. As earlier, a human can extract shapes form well-separated time frames, and we seek an automated technique to interpolate between those frames. A need for interpolation may also arise when the capture rate is slow, and the shape changes a lot from frame to frame. When this happens, in order to register shapes across two shape sequences, interpolation between observed shapes helps to provide a continuum of shapes for matching.

1.1 Past Work

Shape interpolation has seldom been studied explicitly as a topic of research, although many methods provide techniques for interpolating between shapes. A large part of the past efforts has been restricted to finite dimensional or "landmark-based" analysis of shapes. Here shapes are represented by a discrete

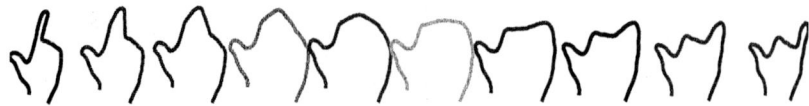

Fig. 3. Geodesic path between hand gestures under the bending metric

sampling of the object contour [2, 5] and key points or landmarks are defined on the curve. This process however requires an expert intervention, as automatic detection of landmarks is not straightforward. Since the analysis depends heavily on the landmarks chosen, this approach is limited in its scope. Also, shape interpolation with geodesics in this framework lacks a physical interpretation, and does not provide interesting intermediate shapes.

More recently, a geometric approach by Klassen et al. [3] represents shapes as constrained functions, and analyzes shapes in resulting nonlinear spaces. In particular, they represent a closed curve by its angle function θ and impose constraints ($\int \exp(j\theta(s))ds = 0$, $\theta(s)ds = \pi$, etc) to form a pre-shape space. It is important to note that all curves in this approach have arc-length, or unit speed, parametrization. A further equivalence of all curves, that differ in the placement of origin, results in the complete shape space. To analyze shapes, this method uses computation of geodesic paths between arbitrary closed curves in this space, and statistics, such as mean and tangent covariance, can be computed accordingly. In view of arc-length parametrization, these geodesic paths exhibit **bending** of one shape into another; no stretching or compression is allowed. Although appropriate in many situations, this approach may not produce interesting results in cases involving elastic curves, where the curves more naturally can stretch and compress to form a better match, than by simply bending. Paths generated by bending are liable to lose important features, such as corners, in going from one shape into another. This is illustrated by Figure 3 that shows a typical geodesic path between two hand gestures. The intermediate shapes shown in Figure 3 do not preserve local features like tip of the fingers etc. Elastic formulation of shapes which relaxed the unit-speed curve restriction was proposed by Mio and Srivastava [4]. Since the main goal of this paper is to interpolate between biological shapes, we explore this new approach that utilizes elastic curves to analyze such shapes.

2 Geometric Representation of Elastic Shapes

In this paper we allow for curves to have variable-speed parameterizations [4], resulting in local stretching and compression of curves when they are being compared. The framework is similar to that used by Klassen et al. [3], except that the shape representation now includes a speed function ϕ, in addition to the angle function θ. Additionally, the Riemannian metric is modified to account for this change in representation.

2.1 Shape Representations

Let $\alpha\colon [0, 2\pi] \to \mathbb{R}^2$ a smooth, non-singular parametric curve in the sense that $\alpha'(t) \neq 0$, $\forall t \in [0, 2\pi]$. In addition we also assume that the rotation index of this curve is 1. We can write its velocity vector as $\alpha'(t) = e^{\phi(t)} e^{j\theta(t)}$, where $\phi\colon [0, 2\pi] \to \mathbb{R}$ and $\theta\colon [0, 2\pi] \to \mathbb{R}$ are smooth, and $j = \sqrt{-1}$. The function ϕ is the *speed* of α expressed in logarithmic scale, and θ is the angle function as earlier. $\phi(t)$ is a measurement of the rate at which the interval $[0, 2\pi]$ was stretched or compressed at t to form the curve α; $\phi(t) > 0$ indicates local stretching near t, and $\phi(t) < 0$ local compression. The arc-length element of α is $ds = e^{\phi(t)} dt$. Curves parameterized by arc length, i.e., traversed with unit speed, are those with $\phi \equiv 0$. We will represent α via the pair (ϕ, θ) and denote by $\mathcal{H}$ the collection of all such pairs.

Parametric curves that differ by rigid motions or uniform scalings of the plane, or by orientation-preserving re-parameterizations are to be viewed as representing the same shape. Since the functions ϕ and θ encode properties of the velocity field of the curve α, the pair (ϕ, θ) is clearly invariant to translations of the curve. The effect of a rotation is to add a constant to θ keeping ϕ unchanged, and scaling the curve by a factor $k > 0$ changes ϕ to $\phi + \log k$ leaving θ unaltered. To obtain invariance under uniform scalings, we restrict pairs (ϕ, θ) to those representing curves of length 2π. To get rotational invariance, we fix the average value of angle functions with respect to the arc-length element to be, say, π. In other words, we restrict shape representatives to pairs (ϕ, θ) satisfying the conditions

$$\mathcal{C} = \{(\phi, \theta) \in \mathcal{H} : \int_0^{2\pi} e^{\phi(t)} dt = 2\pi, \ \frac{1}{2\pi}\int_0^{2\pi} \theta(t) e^{\phi(t)} dt = \pi, \ \int_0^{2\pi} e^{\phi(t)} e^{j\theta(t)} dt = 0\}, \tag{1}$$

$\mathcal{C}$ is called the *pre-shape space* of planar elastic strings.

There are two possible ways of re-parameterizing a closed curve, without changing its shape.

1. **Shift of Origin**: One way is to change the placement of origin $t = 0$ on the curve. This change can be represented as the action of a unit circle $\mathbb{S}^1$ on a shape (ϕ, θ), according to:

$$r \cdot (\phi(t), \theta(t)) = (\phi(t - r), \theta(t - r) + r), \text{ for } r \in \mathbb{R} \tag{2}$$

2. **Non-uniform Speed Parametrizations of Curves**: Re-parameterizations of α that preserve orientation and the property that α is non-singular are those obtained by composing α with an orientation-preserving diffeomorphism $\gamma\colon [0, 2\pi] \to [0, 2\pi]$ such that $\gamma_t(t) > 0, \forall t \in [0, 2\pi]$; the action of γ on α is to produce the curve β which is represented by $(\phi \circ \gamma + \log \gamma_t, \theta \circ \gamma)$, where $\circ$ denotes composition of maps. Hence, reparameterizations define an action (a right action, to be more precise) of the group $\mathcal{D}_I$ of orientation-preserving diffeomorphisms of the interval $[0, 2\pi]$ on $\mathcal{H}$ by

$$(\phi, \theta) \circ \gamma = (\phi \circ \gamma + \log \gamma_t, \theta \circ \gamma). \tag{3}$$

The space of all (shape preserving) re-parameterizations of a shape in $\mathcal{C}$ is thus given by $\mathbb{S}^1 \times \mathcal{D}_I$.

2.2 Riemannian Metric

In order to compare curves quantitatively, we assume that they are made of an elastic material and adopt a metric that measures how difficult it is to reshape a curve into another taking into account the elasticity of the string. Infinitesimally, this can be done using a *Riemmanian structure* on $\mathcal{H}$. Since $\mathcal{H}$ is a linear space, its tangent space at any point is the space $\mathcal{H}$ itself. Thus, for each (ϕ, θ), we wish to define an inner product $\langle \, , \, \rangle_{(\phi,\theta)}$ on $\mathcal{H}$. We adopt the simplest Riemannian structure that will make diffeomorphisms $\gamma \in \mathcal{D}_I$ act by 'rigid motions' (or, isometries) on $\mathcal{H}$, much like the way translations and rotations act on standard Euclidean spaces. Given $(\phi, \theta) \in \mathcal{H}$, let h_i and f_i, $i = 1, 2$, represent infinitesimal deformations of ϕ and θ, respectively so that (h_1, f_1) and (h_2, f_2) are tangent vectors to $\mathcal{H}$ at (ϕ, θ). For $a, b > 0$, define

$$\langle (h_1, f_1), (h_2, f_2) \rangle_{(\phi,\theta)} = a \int_0^1 h_1(t) h_2(t) \, e^{\phi(t)} \, dt + b \int_0^1 f_1(t) f_2(t) \, e^{\phi(t)} \, dt. \quad (4)$$

It can be shown that re-parameterizations preserve the inner product, i.e., $\mathbb{S}^1 \times \mathcal{D}_I$ acts on $\mathcal{H}$ by isometries, as desired. This inner product leads to the norm

$$\|(h, f))\|_{(\phi,\theta)} = \sqrt{\langle (h, f), (h, f) \rangle_{(\phi,\theta)}}$$

The elastic properties of the curves are built-in to the model via the parameters a and b, which can be interpreted as *tension* and *rigidity coefficients*, respectively. Large values of the ratio $\chi = a/b$ indicate that strings offer higher resistance to stretching and compression than to bending; the opposite holds for smaller χ.

3 Geodesic Paths Between Elastic Shapes

The task of computing geodesic paths between any two shapes, say (ϕ_1, θ_1) and (ϕ_2, θ_2), is accomplished in two steps. The first step seeks an optimal alignment, or registration, between the two shapes, and the second step finds a geodesic path in $\mathcal{C}$ maintaining that optimal alignment.

3.1 Optimal Alignment Between Shapes

As a first step, we seek an optimal alignment between the pairs by solving the problem:

$$(\hat{\gamma}, \hat{r}) = \underset{\mathbb{S}^1 \times \mathcal{D}_I}{\operatorname{argmin}} \left(\|(\phi_1, \theta_1) - (r \cdot ((\phi_2, \theta_2) \circ \gamma))\|_{(\phi_1, \theta_1)} \right) \quad (5)$$

This is a joint optimization problem over $\mathbb{S}^1 \times \mathcal{D}_I$. The following steps show the computation of an optimal diffeomorphism ($\hat{\gamma}$) for any two closed pair of

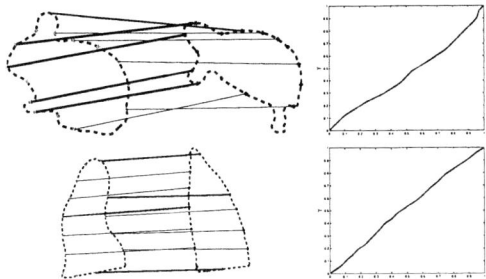

Fig. 4. Examples of alignment between two shapes alongwith the corresponding γ

shapes. The shapes are assumed to be discretized to N samples for the purpose of computer representation.

Let s_1, s_2 be two shapes. $s_1 \equiv (\phi_1, \theta_1)$, $s_2 \equiv (\phi_2, \theta_2)$. $s_1, s_2 \in \mathbb{R}^N \times \mathbb{R}^N$.

1. Compute

$$\gamma^r = \operatorname*{argmin}_{\gamma} \|s_1 - r \cdot s_2 \circ \gamma\|_{s_1}, \text{ for each } r \in (1, ...N-1) \quad (6)$$

2. The optimal $(\hat{\gamma}, \hat{r})$ is given as,

$$(\hat{\gamma}, \hat{r}) = \operatorname*{argmin}_{r \in (1,...N-1)} \|s_1 - r \cdot s_2 \circ \gamma^r\|_{s_1} \quad (7)$$

The γ in Step 1 above, is solved for using Dynamic Programming in the search space of $\mathcal{D}_I$. Figure 4 shows examples of the alignment between pairs of shapes obtained using the above procedure. The optimal $\hat{\gamma}$ used to form the alignment is shown in the right panel. It is noted that similar key features across different shapes are matched successfully. For example, the tip of the nose as well as one foot is aligned between the shapes of the rabbit and the turtle. The bottom row of Figure 4 shows the correspondence between two endo-cardial curves during the End-Diastole cycle. In this case, the apex of each curve as well as the the centers of the mitral valve are matched together. The non-identity nature of γ exhibits local stretching and compression.

3.2 Geodesic Paths Between Shapes in $\mathcal{C}$

Now that optimal registration between the shape pairs is established, we derive an approach for computing geodesic paths between them in $\mathcal{C}$. Similar to ideas presented in [3], we use a shooting method to construct geodesic paths in $\mathcal{C}$. Given two shapes s_1 and s_2 as above, let $\Psi_t(\phi_1, \theta_1, h, f)$ denote the geodesic flow starting from s_1 in the direction (h, f). The shooting method solves for (h, f) such that $\Psi_1(\phi_1, \theta_1, h, f) = (\tilde{\phi}_2, \tilde{\theta}_2)$, where $(\tilde{\phi}_2, \tilde{\theta}_2) = \hat{r} \cdot (\phi_2, \theta_2) \cup \hat{\gamma}$. After choosing an initial direction, we iteratively refine this direction in such a way that a miss function, denoting the distance (in $\mathcal{H}$) between the shape reached and (ϕ_2, θ_2), is minimized to zero.

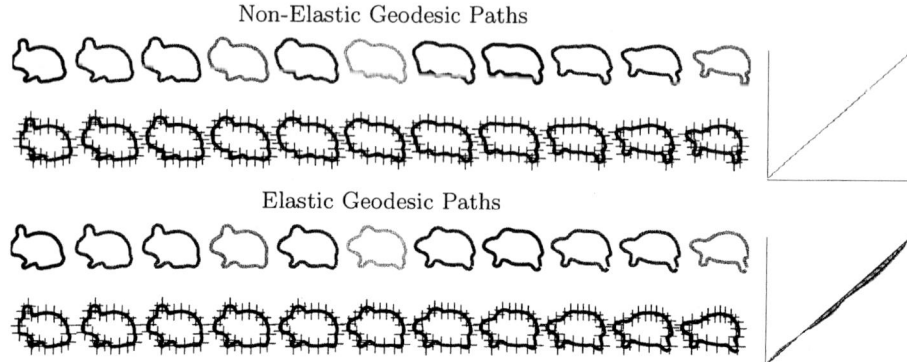

Fig. 5. Top two rows (left to right), show the geodesic evolution when stretching is penalized. Bottom two rows show the evolution when bending is penalized. The right panel shows the corresponding γ

Figure 5 shows two examples of geodesic paths traversed from left to right for different values of χ in this framework. As a first example, we set χ to be large and a resulting geodesic is shown in the top two rows of Figure 5. The evolution from left to right is via bending, with virtually no stretching. This observation is supported by a plot of $\hat{\gamma}$ which resembles the identity function. The tick marks show the sampling along the path of the curve. In contrast, we set χ to a low value for the second example, with the resulting geodesic shown in the bottom two rows. In this case the graph of the diffeomorphism clearly shows non-uniform speed along the length of the curve. This is also evident from regions of dense and sparse sampling along the curve. This path correctly aligns important features in the two shapes, and preserves them in the evolution from one to another. For example, the tip of the nose remains aligned and common key features such as feet are preserved throughout the intermediate shapes in the geodesic. This demonstrates the strength of this method to match features in shapes via local deformations.

4 Shape Interpolations in Image Sequences

A closed contour α has two sets of descriptors associated with it: a shape descriptor denoted by $(\phi, \theta) \in \mathcal{C}$ and a vector $z \in \mathcal{Z}$ of nuisance variables. In our approach, interpolation between two closed curves is performed via interpolations between their shapes and nuisance components, respectively. The interpolation of shape is obtained using geodesic paths, while that of the nuisance components is obtained using linear methods. Let $\alpha_1 = (\phi_1, \theta_1, z_1)$ and $\alpha_2 = (\phi_2, \theta_2, z_2)$ be the two closed curves, and our goal is to find a path $\Phi : [0,1] \mapsto \mathcal{C} \times \mathcal{Z}$ such that $\Phi_0 = (\phi_1, \theta_1, z_1)$ and $\Phi_1 = (\phi_2, \theta_2, z_2)$. For example, in Figure 1, the endocardial boundary (broken curves) of the ED and ES frames can form α_1 and α_2, respectively. Alternatively, one can treat the epicardial boundaries (solid curves) of ED and ES frames as α_1 and α_2 as well. The different components are interpolated as follows:

1. **Shape Component**: Given the two shapes (ϕ_1, θ_1) and (ϕ_2, θ_2) in $\mathcal{C}$, we use the shooting method to find the geodesic that starts from the first and reaches the other in unit time. This results in the flow $\Psi_t(\phi_1, \theta_1, h, f)$ such that $\Psi_0(\phi_1, \theta_1, h, f) = (\phi_1, \theta_1)$ and $\Psi_1(\phi_1, \theta_1, h, f) = (\phi_2, \theta_2)$. This also results in a re-parametrization of (ϕ_2, θ_2) such that the origins (points where $s = 0$) on the two curves are now registered. With a slight abuse of notation we will also call the new curve (ϕ_2, θ_2). Let a shape along this path be given by $(\phi_t, \theta_t) = \Psi_t(\phi_1, \theta_1, h, f)$. Since this shape lies in $\mathcal{C}$, the average value of θ_t for all t is π.
2. **Translation**: If p_1, p_2 represent the locations of the origins on the two curves, i.e. $p_i = \alpha_i(0)$, $i = 1, 2$, then the linear interpolation between them is given by $p(t) = (1-t)p_1 + tp_2$.
3. **Orientation**: For a closed curve α_i, the average orientation is defined by $\beta_i = \frac{1}{2\pi}\int_0^{2\pi} \frac{1}{j}\log(\dot{\alpha}_i(s))ds$, $i = 1, 2$, $j = \sqrt{-1}$. Given β_1 and β_2, a linear interpolation between them is $\beta(t) = (1-t)\beta_2 + t\tilde{\beta}_2$, where $\tilde{\beta}_2 = \text{argmin}_{\beta \in \{\beta_2 - 2\pi, \beta_2, \beta_2 + 2\pi\}} |\beta - \beta_1|$.
4. **Scale**: If ρ_1 and ρ_2 are the lengths of the curves α_1 and α_2, then a linear interpolation on the lengths is simply $\rho(t) = (1-t)\rho_1 + t\rho_2$.

Using these different components, the resulting geodesic on the space of closed curves is given by $\{\Phi_t : t \in [0, 1]\}$ where:

$$\Phi_t(s) = p(t) + \rho(t)\int_0^s e^{j(\theta_t(\tau) - \pi + \beta(t))} e^{\phi_t} d\tau .$$

Shown in Figure 6 is a sequence of 12 image frames for the same patient as displayed in Figure 1. Again, each image frame has a set of epicardial and endocardial borders overlaid on the image. In Figure 6, borders in the first and last frames have been traced by an expert, while the borders on the intermediate frames have been generated using the path Φ_t, one each for epicardial and endocardial boundaries. Note that the endocardial border is more distorted than

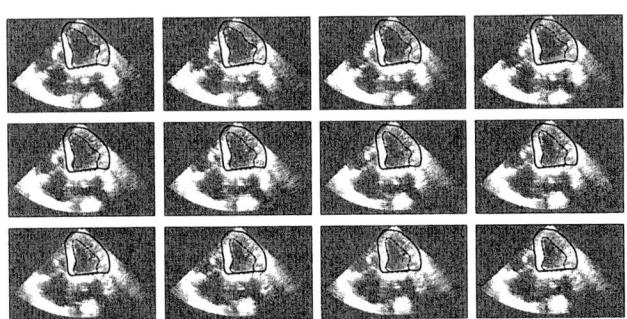

Fig. 6. Interpolation of echo-cardial curves between ED and ES using geodesics

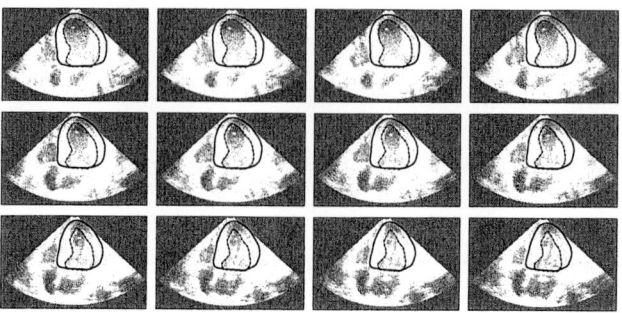

Fig. 7. Interpolation of echo-cardial curves between ED and ES using geodesics

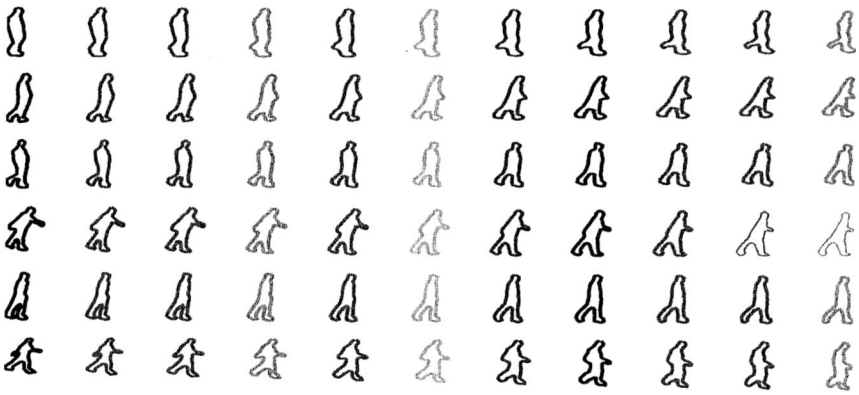

Fig. 8. Geodesic interpolation of human motion

the epicardial border in the transition. In view of the geodesic paths in $\mathcal{C}$ that incorporate elastic stretching as well as bending, it is observed, that the apex of both curves as well as any sharp corners or edges are continuously aligned along the path. Similarly, Figure 7 shows another example of such an interpolation.

As another application of this approach, it was used to interpolate shapes of human motion. Each row of Figure 8 shows a geodesic path for a single subject, where the first shape is the start of a gait sequence that culminates in the last shape at the end of the cycle. Here the first and the last shapes in each row are extracted manually from IR images. Interestingly enough, this technique performs well even in the case where the feet are joined together at the start and spread wide apart at the end of the sequence.

5 Statistics of Elastic Shapes

There are various techniques to compute the mean of a collection of shapes. One way is to compute an extrinsic mean, that involves embedding the non-linear

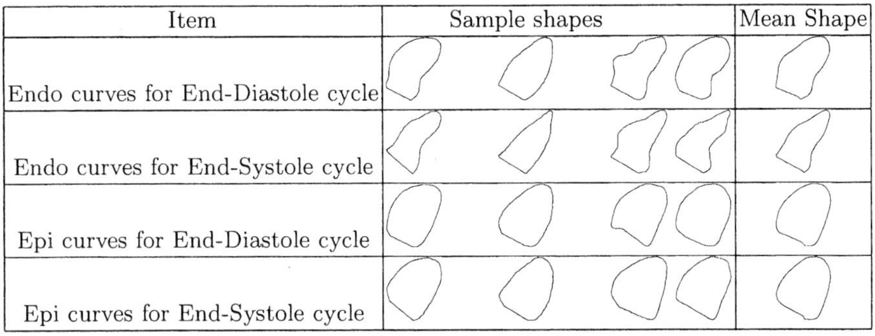

Item	Sample shapes				Mean Shape
Endo curves for End-Diastole cycle					
Endo curves for End-Systole cycle					
Epi curves for End-Diastole cycle					
Epi curves for End-Systole cycle					

Fig. 9. Mean shapes of echo-cardial curves at different cycles

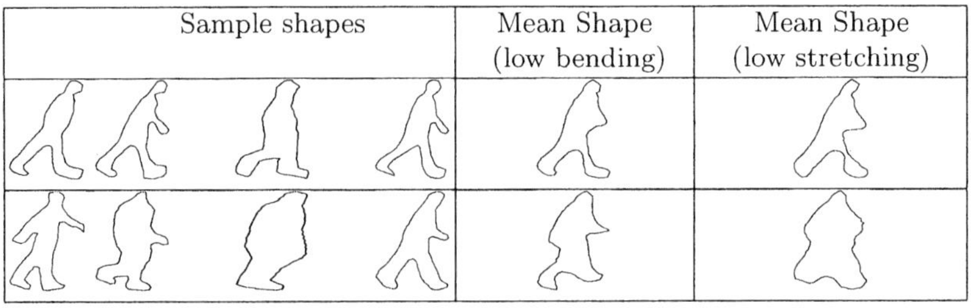

Sample shapes				Mean Shape (low bending)	Mean Shape (low stretching)

Fig. 10. For each row, the center panel shows the mean shape after low stretching, whereas the last panel shows the average shape after high bending

manifold in a larger vector space e.g.($\mathbb{L}^2 \times \mathbb{L}^2$), computing the Euclidean mean in that space, and then projecting it down to the manifold. However, we use an intrinsic notion of mean (Karcher mean) that does not require an Euclidean embedding. For a collection $(\phi, \theta)_i, i = 1, ..., n$ in $\mathcal{C}$, let $d((\phi, \theta)_i, (\phi, \theta)_j)$ be the geodesic distance between shapes i and j. The Karcher mean is defined as the element $\mu \in \mathcal{S}$ that minimizes the quantity $\sum_{i=1}^{n} d((\phi, \theta), (\phi, \theta)_i)^2$. The notion of a well-defined average shape is pertinent to carry out any statistical analysis on the space of shapes. In particular, the mean shape can be used in clustering and classification of for endo- and epi-cardial curves. It also serves as a useful tool in forming inferences based on normal and abnormal cardiac curves. Figure 9 shows a few sample means of cardiac curves computed at different cycles. It is observed, that the mean of shapes that have certain common features such as corners and bends, tends to retain those features.

Another interesting example is that of the mean of sample human shapes. In Figure 10, the center panel for each row shows the mean shape due to higher stretching than bending, whereas the last panel, shows the average shape due to higher bending as compared to stretching. For the diverse poses of human shapes in the second row of Figure 10, the mean shape in the center panel retains local features such as arms, and feet, whereas higher bending in the last panel, grossly smoothes the average and bears no resemeblance to either of the sample shapes.

6 Conclusion

Based on an elastic model for closed shapes, geodesic flows were constructed to interpolate between a given pair of shapes. This interpolation was successfully applied between echo-cardial curves for the ED and the ES cycles. From the results of human gait interpolation, it is evident that the geodesic paths maintain the correspondence between key features present in both the shapes. Further a framework for statistical analysis of shapes was examined. The mean shape of endo- as well as epi-cardial curves preserves corners as well as edges present in the original shapes. In case of averages of human shapes, it was seen that greater bending resulted in smoothing of the overall shape, whereas higher stretching helped the mean shape to serve as a better representative of a given mix of shapes.

References

1. Y. Chen, H. Tagare, Thiruvenkadam S., D. Huang, D. Wilson, K. Gopinath, R. Briggs, and M. Geiser. Using prior shapes in geometric active contours in a variational framework. *International Journal of Computer Vision*, 50:315–328, 2002.
2. I. L Dryden and K.V. Mardia. *Statistical Shape Analysis*. John Wiley & Son, 1998.
3. E. Klassen, A. Srivastava, W. Mio, and S. H. Joshi. Analysis of planar shapes using geodesic paths on shape spaces. *IEEE Pattern Analysis and Machiner Intelligence*, 26:372–383, 2004.
4. W. Mio and A. Srivastava. Elastic-string models for representation and analysis of planar shapes. In *Proc. IEEE Computer Vision and Pattern Recognition*, 2004.
5. C. G. Small. *The Statistical Theory of Shape*. Springer, 1996.
6. D.C. Wilson, M. Geiser, and Larocca J. Automated analysis of echocardiographic apical 4-chamber images. In *International Society for Optical Engineering in Mathematical Modeling, Estimation, and Imaging*, pages 128–139, 2000.

Segmenting and Tracking the Left Ventricle by Learning the Dynamics in Cardiac Images*

W. Sun[1], M. Çetin[1], R. Chan[2], V. Reddy[2], G. Holmvang[2], V. Chandar[1], and A. Willsky[1]

[1] Laboratory for Information and Decision Systems,
Massachusetts Institute of Technology, Cambridge, MA USA
[2] Cardiovascular MR-CT Program, Massachusetts General Hospital,
Harvard Medical School, Boston, MA USA
waltsun@mit.edu

Abstract. Having accurate left ventricle (LV) segmentations across a cardiac cycle provides useful quantitative (e.g. ejection fraction) and qualitative information for diagnosis of certain heart conditions. Existing LV segmentation techniques are founded mostly upon algorithms for segmenting static images. In order to exploit the dynamic structure of the heart in a principled manner, we approach the problem of LV segmentation as a recursive estimation problem. In our framework, LV boundaries constitute the dynamic system state to be estimated, and a sequence of observed cardiac images constitute the data. By formulating the problem as one of state estimation, the segmentation at each particular time is based not only on the data observed at that instant, but also on predictions based on past segmentations. This requires a dynamical system model of the LV, which we propose to learn from training data through an information-theoretic approach. To incorporate the learned dynamic model into our segmentation framework and obtain predictions, we use ideas from particle filtering. Our framework uses a curve evolution method to combine such predictions with the observed images to estimate the LV boundaries at each time. We demonstrate the effectiveness of the proposed approach on a large set of cardiac images. We observe that our approach provides more accurate segmentations than those from static image segmentation techniques, especially when the observed data are of limited quality.

1 Introduction

Of the cardiac chambers in the heart, the left ventricle (LV) is quite frequently analyzed because its proper function, pumping oxygenated blood to the entire body, is vital for normal activity. One quantitative measure of the health of the LV is ejection fraction (EF). This statistic measures the percentage volume of blood transmitted out of the LV in a given cardiac cycle. To compute EF, we need

---
* This work supported by NSF ITR grant 0121182 & AFOSR grant FA9550-04-1-0351.

to have segmentations of the LV at multiple points in a cardiac cycle; namely, at end diastole (ED) and end systole (ES). In addition, observing how the LV evolves throughout an entire cardiac cycle allows physicians to determine the health of the myocardial muscles. Segmented LV boundaries can also be useful for further quantitative analysis. For example, past work [7, 18] on extracting the flow fields of the myocardial wall assumes the availability of LV segmentations throughout the cardiac cycle.

Automatic segmentation of the left ventricle (LV) in bright blood breath-hold cardiac magnetic resonance (MR) images is non-trivial because the image intensities of the cardiac chambers vary due to differences in blood velocity [24]. In particular, blood that flows into the ventricles produces higher intensities in the acquired image than blood which remains in the ventricles [9]. Locating the LV endocardium is further complicated by the fact that the right ventricle and aorta often appear jointly with the LV in many images of the heart. Similarly, automatic segmentation of low signal-to-noise ratio (SNR) cardiac images (e.g. body coil MR or ultrasound) is difficult because intensity variations can often obscure the LV boundary.

Several approaches exist for LV segmentation. Goshtasby and Turner [9], as well as Weng et al. [27] and Geiger et al. [8], apply intensity thresholding and then a local maximum gradient search to determine the final segmentation. Such gradient-based methods rely primarily on local information. When the image statistics inside an object's boundary are distinctly different from those outside, the use of region statistics may be more appropriate, especially if the discontinuity at the boundary is weak or non-uniform. Tsai et al. [26] consider region-based segmentations of the LV. Chakraborty et al. [3] consider combining both gradient and region techniques in the segmentation of cardiac structures. Similarly, Paragios [20] uses gradient and region techniques to segment two cardiac contours, the LV endocardium and epicardium. In all three papers, active contours (or curve evolution) [2, 4, 13, 15, 16, 19], a technique which involves evolving a curve to minimize (or maximize) a related objective functional, are used to determine the segmentation. In our work, we also take advantage of region-based information and curve evolution.

Static segmentation methods are limited by the data available in an individual frame. During a single cardiac cycle, which lasts approximately 1 second, the heart contracts from end diastole (ED) to end systole (ES) and expands back to ED. Over this time, MR systems can acquire approximately 20 images of the heart. Because adjacent frames are imaged over a short time period (approximately 50 ms), the LV boundaries exhibit strong temporal correlation. Thus, previous LV boundaries may provide information regarding the location of the current LV boundary. Using such information is particularly useful for low SNR images, where the observation from a single frame alone may not provide enough information for a good segmentation. There exists some past work which simply uses the previous frame's LV boundary as the prediction for the boundary in the current frame [8, 12]. Meanwhile, Zhou et al. [28] consider LV shape tracking by combining predictions, obtained through linear system dynamics assumed known, with observations. Their technique uses landmark points to represent the LV boundaries, which introduces the issue of correspondence. All uncertainties are assumed to be Gaussian. Senegas et al. [21] use a Bayesian framework for tracking using a sample-based approach to estimate the densities. They use spherical harmonics for the shape model, and a simple linear model to approximate the cardiac dynamics.[1] In our work, we use non-linear dynamics in the recursive estimation of the LV boundary. We represent the LV by level sets to avoid issues inherent with marker points [23] and apply principal components analysis on the level sets to determine a basis to represent the shapes. Furthermore, we propose a method for learning a non-trivial dynamic model of the LV boundaries and apply this model to obtain predictions. Finally, we compute the maximum *a posteriori* (MAP) estimate using curve evolution.

In particular, we propose a principled Bayesian approach for recursively estimating the LV boundaries across a cardiac cycle. In our framework, LV boundaries constitute the dynamic system state we estimate, and a cardiac cycle of mid-ventricular images constitutes the data. From a training set of data, we learn the dynamics using an information-theoretic criterion [11]. More specifically, this involves finding a non-parametric density estimate of the current boundary conditioned on previous boundaries. The densities are approximately represented by using sample-based (i.e. particle filtering [1]) methods.

For the test data, we apply a particle filter to recursively estimate the LV boundary. Starting with the segmentations at the initial frames, we use the non-linear dynamic model learned from the training data to predict the boundary at the next frame. We then incorporate the image observation of this frame to produce a posterior density estimate of the LV boundary at each frame, which involves computing the MAP estimate at each frame using curve evolution. This procedure is then repeated for each subsequent frame. We apply the proposed

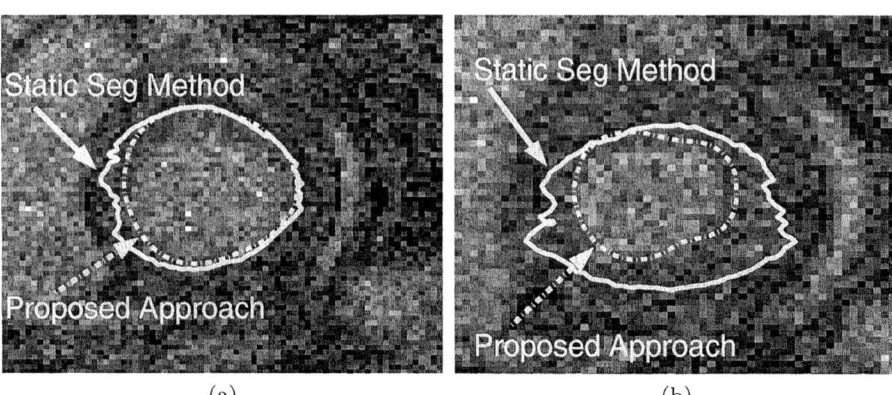

(a)   (b)
Fig. 1. (a) Segmentation of the fourth frame in the cardiac cycle. (b) Segmentation of the eighth frame (near end systole) in the cardiac cycle

---

[1] We thank the reviewer who brought Senegas et al.'s related work to our attention.

algorithm to high and low SNR cardiac data to illustrate that our technique works in both regimes. We also demonstrate the improvements provided by the proposed method over results obtained from static LV segmentation methods, as shown in Figure 1.

2 Framework and Methodology

We formulate the LV segmentation and tracking problem as an estimation of the posterior distribution at each time t_0 based on data from $t = 1$ to $t = t_0$. First, let y_t be the image data which are measurements of the blood and tissue intensity field f_t. Then, define X_t as the dynamic system state which contains information about the LV boundary at t. The segmentation problem involves finding the (f_t, X_t) pair which maximizes $p(f_t, X_t|Y_t)$, where $Y_t = [y_1, y_2, \ldots, y_t]$. We then recursively compute X_t to track the LV boundary across the entire cardiac cycle.

Mathematically, we apply Bayes' Theorem to the posterior $p(f_t, X_t|Y_t)$. Assuming that X_t is a Markov process and observing that $p(Y_{t-1})$ and $p(Y_t)$ do not depend on X_t, we have

$$p(f_t, X_t|Y_t) \propto p(y_t|f_t, X_t)p(f_t|X_t)p(X_t|Y_{t-1}) \qquad (1)$$

$$= p(y_t|f_t, X_t)p(f_t|X_t)\int_{X_{t-1}} p(X_t|X_{t-1})\int_{f_{t-1}} p(f_{t-1}, X_{t-1}|Y_{t-1})df_{t-1}dX_{t-1},$$

where $p(y_t|f_t, X_t)$ is the likelihood term, $p(f_t|X_t)$ is the field prior, and $p(X_t|Y_{t-1})$ is the prediction density. From Eqn. (1), we observe the recursive nature of the problem (i.e. $p(f_t, X_t|Y_t)$ is written as a function of $p(f_{t-1}, X_{t-1}|Y_{t-1})$).

Given this framework, applying it to the LV tracking problem is not straightforward. One of the challenges involves the presence of arbitrary, non-Gaussian probability densities. In Section 3, we discuss the use of a sample-based approach

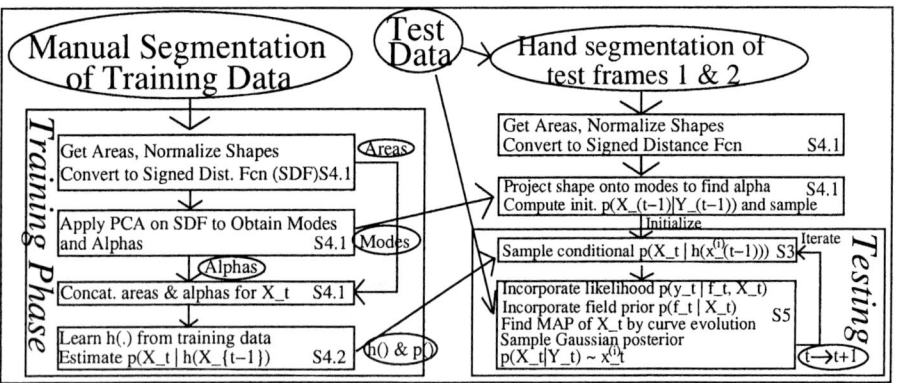

Fig. 2. Block diagram of our technique illustrating both the training and testing phases. Section data inside each block indicate where we describe the specific actions in text

to non-parametrically represent the densities in Eqn. (1). In addition, the dynamic model of the LV boundaries, hence the forward density $p(X_t|X_{t-1})$, needs to be learned using statistics from the training data. We discuss the procedure for learning in Section 4. Finally, we explain in Section 5 how we practically compute the MAP estimate of X_t and use this information to produce a segmentation as well as an estimate of the posterior $p(f_t, X_t|Y_t)$. Experimental results are shown in Section 6, and we summarize the work in Section 7. Figure 2 shows a block diagram representation of the algorithmic framework we propose.

3 Sample-Based Methods

Because many of the densities in Eqn. (1) have no simple closed-form, we use sample-based methods, such as particle filters [1, 5, 6, 14], to approximate these densities. Such methods represent a probability density using a set of weighted samples drawn from that density. Suppose we have an equally-weighted set of N samples $x_{t-1}^{(i)}$ that represent $p(X_{t-1}|Y_{t-1})$, a term which appears as part of $p(X_t|Y_{t-1})$ in the formulation according to

$$p(X_t|Y_{t-1}) = \int_{X_{t-1}} p(X_t|X_{t-1}) p(X_{t-1}|Y_{t-1}) dX_{t-1}. \tag{2}$$

From the conditional distribution $p(X_t|X_{t-1})$ (assume known for now), we next obtain M samples $x_{t|t-1}^{(i,j)}$ from $p(X_t|X_{t-1} = x_{t-1}^{(i)})$ for each i. Since the sample points for $p(X_{t-1}|Y_{t-1})$ are equally-weighted, $p(X_t|Y_{t-1})$ can similarly be approximated by the $N \times M$ equally-weighted samples $x_{t|t-1}^{(i,j)}$.

To complete the recursion as shown in Eqn. (1), we make an approximation for the marginalization of f_{t-1}. In particular, we choose the f_{t-1} which maximizes the posterior rather than marginalizing over f_{t-1}. Thus, we have

$$p(X_{t-1}|Y_{t-1}) = \int_{f_{t-1}} p(f_{t-1}, X_{t-1}|Y_{t-1}) df_{t-1} \approx \max_{f_{t-1}} p(f_{t-1}, X_{t-1}|Y_{t-1}). \tag{3}$$

In the above discussion, we have described how, given $p(f_{t-1}, X_{t-1}|Y_{t-1})$, we can obtain $p(X_t|Y_{t-1})$ assuming $p(X_t|X_{t-1})$ is known. In the next section, we explain how we estimate $p(X_t|X_{t-1})$ through learning the system dynamics.

4 Learning the Dynamics

A number of approaches can be taken to learn the dynamics of an evolving system. We can consider purely physics-based models to constrain and explain the dynamics of a given problem [17, 22]. The drawback is that systems that accurately model physics may require high dimensional states and/or a complex set of differential equations that model the interaction between adjacent masses in the system. Alternatively, we may assume a statistical model that can either be parametric or non-parametric. For the former, the challenge is

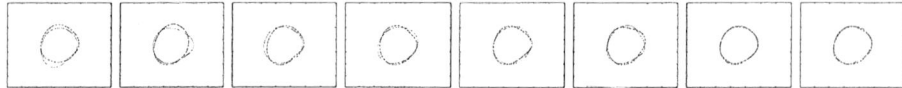

Fig. 3. Illustration of LV shape variability. $\pm 1\sigma$ for the first eight primary modes of variability (left to right). Solid curve represents $+1\sigma$ while dashed represents -1σ

to find a parametric model that is well-matched to the problem structure and captures the statistical variability inherent in the problem. For richer modeling capacity, one can turn to non-parametric models, which can be computationally difficult. In Section 4.2, we explain our non-parametric, yet computationally tractable approach to learning the dynamics of LV boundaries. Before discussing this method, we first provide a description of the system state X_t.

4.1 Implicit Parametric Shape Model and State Representation

The set of LV boundaries have different internal areas and different shapes across a cardiac cycle and between patients. We want to represent these boundaries in a simple, low-dimensional, yet accurate, manner. To accomplish this, we use principal components analysis (PCA) on the shape variability to obtain a basis for the shapes [16]. We then represent each shape by a linear combination of the basis elements. The tracking problem reduces to learning the time evolution of the coefficients of the basis elements.

Starting with a training set of manually-segmented and registered data, we determine the area of each LV. Normalizing with respect to area, we create signed distance functions whose zero level sets are the shapes [23]. Leveraging on Leventon's PCA on shapes [16], we obtain a mean shape $\bar{\psi}$ and the primary modes of variability ψ_i (for i=1,2, ..., K, where K is the number of shapes in the dataset) across the entire training set. In effect, we use a single basis to represent the shapes across the entire cardiac cycle. Figure 3 shows the eight primary modes of variability from the training set used in the experimental results presented in Section 6. For a given signed distance function ψ in the training set, $\psi = \bar{\psi} + \sum_{i=1}^{K} \alpha_i \psi_i$, where α_i's are a set of constants. It is known that for shapes which do not vary greatly, the primary few modes of variability can explain the majority of the variability of the data. In our training set, the first eight modes explain 97% of the variability in our specific training set of data. Thus, we approximately represent each ψ by the eight element vector $\boldsymbol{\alpha} = [\alpha_1; \alpha_2; \ldots; \alpha_8]^T$. By using PCA, a given curve (LV segmentation) can be approximately represented by a vector containing its area A and $\boldsymbol{\alpha}$.

Given this representation, we define the state X_t with the notion that the dynamics are a second-order system. This choice is made because higher-order systems require a larger state, while first-order systems do not adequately capture whether we are in the diastolic or systolic phase. Thus, we represent our state X_t as an eighteen-dimensional vector containing the area of the LV and the shape variabilities at frames t and $t-1$, namely $X_t = [A_t; \boldsymbol{\alpha}_t^T; A_{t-1}; \boldsymbol{\alpha}_{t-1}^T]^T$.

4.2 A Maximally-Informative Statistic

We propose learning the dynamics from a training set of data based on a technique [11] which produces a non-parametric density estimate of $p(X_t|X_{t-1})$. This estimate is obtained by using an information-theoretic criterion to maximize the predictive power of the observations.

Since the dimensionality of the conditional density may be large, we consider only the portion of the state X_{t-1} that is statistically pertinent to the prediction of X_t. Thus, we introduce a function $h(X_{t-1})$ which seeks to reduce dimensionality yet capture all information in X_{t-1} that relates to X_t (achieved exactly only when $I(X_t; X_{t-1}) = I(X_t; h(X_{t-1}))$, where $I(X_t, X_{t-1})$ is the mutual information between X_t and X_{t-1}). We can then create an estimate of $p(X_t|h(X_{t-1}))$ as an equally-informative yet simpler representation of $p(X_t|X_{t-1})$.

In practice, we constrain h to be linear, which likely precludes it from being a sufficient statistic. However, we choose the parameters of h such that $I(X_t; h(X_{t-1}))$ is maximized, thus making h maximally-informative within this class. Details regarding h and the maximization are in [25]. Once the parameters of h are determined, we obtain a kernel density estimate of $p(X_t|h(X_{t-1}))$, where for kernel size we use the plug-in method of Hall et al. [10].

5 Finding the MAP Estimate by Curve Evolution

Now, we incorporate the data at time t to obtain the posterior $p(f_t, X_t|Y_t)$. Given equally-weighted samples $x_{t|t-1}^{(i,j)}$ for $p(X_t|Y_{t-1})$ as described in Section 3, one could in principle weight the particles by the likelihood and field priors to obtain a representation of $p(f_t, X_t|Y_t)$. Such an approach may work if the training data are rich. However, when we have a limited amount of training data, we make the assumption that the posterior distribution of X_t is Gaussian and determine this distribution by first computing its MAP estimate to determine the mean parameter (since we do not have a method in place to compute the posterior covariance, we approximate it to be a diagonal matrix with individual variances determined empirically from the shape variability in the training data). Maximizing $p(f_t, X_t|Y_t)$ to obtain the MAP estimate is equivalent to minimizing

$$E(f_t, X_t) = -\log p(y_t|f_t, X_t) - \log p(f_t|X_t) - \log p(X_t|Y_{t-1}), \quad (4)$$

which involves a likelihood term $p(y_t|f_t, X_t)$, the prior on the field $p(f_t|X_t)$, and a prediction term $p(X_t|Y_{t-1})$. We discuss each term in Eqn. (4) individually.

5.1 Likelihood Term

Because we are interested in locating the boundary, we apply a simple observation model which assumes that the intensities are piecewise constant, with a bright intensity representing blood and a darker one representing the myocardium. Intensity variations in the observation, such as those due to differences in blood velocity [9], are modeled through a multiplicative random field (other choices of noise models can be handled in our framework, with the result being a different observation model). Mathematically, the observation model is

$$y_t(z) = \begin{cases} f_t^{R_{in}(X_t)} \cdot n(z), & z \in R_{in}(X_t) \\ f_t^{R_{out}(X_t)} \cdot n(z), & z \in R_{out}(X_t), \end{cases} \quad (5)$$

where $f_t^{R_{in}(X_t)}$ and $f_t^{R_{out}(X_t)}$ are the constant, but unknown, field intensities for the blood pool region inside, R_{in}, and the myocardial region immediately outside (within five pixels), R_{out}, of the LV boundary, respectively, and $n(z)$ is spatially independent, identically distributed lognormal random field with $\log n(z)$ a Gaussian random variable having zero mean and variance σ_n^2. Note that we explicitly indicate the dependence of the regions on X_t. Given the field intensity $f_t^{R(X_t)}$ and the observation model of Eqn. (5), $\log y_t(z)$ is normally distributed with mean $\log f_t^{R(X_t)}$ and variance σ_n^2. Thus,

$$p(y_t|f_t, X_t) \propto \quad (6)$$

$$exp(-\int_{z \in R^{in}(X_t)} \frac{(\log y_t(z) - \log f_t^{R_{in}(X_t)})^2}{2\sigma_n^2} dz - \int_{z \in R^{out}(X_t)} \frac{(\log y_t(z) - \log f_t^{R_{out}(X_t)})^2}{2\sigma_n^2} dz).$$

Since we have a second order model, X_t contains LV boundary information at both t and $t-1$. For the likelihood term, the regions R_{in} and R_{out} are determined by the boundary information from time t.

5.2 Field Priors

In applications where it is possible to extract prior field information, we incorporate a field prior into the problem. The mean log intensity inside is approximately stationary across a cardiac cycle. We compute the mean and variance of the log intensity inside (u and σ_u^2, resp.) and that immediately outside the curve (v and σ_v^2, resp.) from the training data and use this as a field prior to obtain

$$p(f_t|X_t) \propto exp(-\frac{(\log f_t^{R_{in}} - u)^2}{2\sigma_u^2}) exp(-\frac{(\log f_t^{R_{out}} - v)^2}{2\sigma_v^2}). \quad (7)$$

5.3 Prediction Term

Next, we want to provide a model for the prediction term. In Section 3, we described having equally-weighted samples $x_{t|t-1}^{(i,j)}$ to approximately represent our prediction term $p(X_t|Y_{t-1})$. We model this prediction density with a Parzen density estimate using these sample points. Mathematically,

$$p(X_t|Y_{t-1}) = \frac{1}{MN} \sum_{(i,j)} k(X_t; x_{t|t-1}^{(i,j)}, \sigma^2) = \frac{1}{MN} \sum_{(i,j)} \frac{1}{\sqrt{2\pi}\sigma} exp(\frac{-d^2(X_t, x_{t|t-1}^{(i,j)})}{2\sigma^2}),$$
$$(8)$$

where $k(X; \mu, \sigma^2)$ represents a Gaussian kernel with mean μ and variance σ^2 as determined from the bandwidth [10], MN is the number of samples, and $d(X_t, x)$ is a *distance* measure [25] between X_t and sample x.

5.4 Curve Evolution

Having the likelihood, prediction, and prior as above, and defining $F_t^i(X_t) = \log f_t^{R_{in}(X_t)}$ and $F_t^o(X_t) = \log f_t^{R_{out}(X_t)}$, Eqn. (4) becomes

$$E(f_t, X_t) = \alpha \left(\int_{z \in R_{in}(X_t)} \frac{(\log y_t(z) - F_t^i(X_t))^2}{2\sigma_n^2} dz + \int_{z \in R_{out}(X_t)} \frac{(\log y_t(z) - F_t^o(X_t))^2}{2\sigma_n^2} dz \right)$$

$$+ \beta \left(\frac{(F_t^i(X_t) - u)^2}{2\sigma_u^2} + \frac{(F_t^o(X_t) - v)^2}{2\sigma_v^2} \right) + \gamma \log \left(\frac{1}{MN} \sum_{(i,j)} \frac{1}{\sqrt{2\pi}\sigma} exp \left(\frac{-d^2(X_t, x_{t|t-1}^{(i,j)})}{2\sigma^2} \right) \right), \tag{9}$$

where α, β, γ are weighting parameters specified based on the quality of data. For instance, in low SNR images, α is less heavily-weighted relative to β and γ. Details of the minimization process, which involves coordinate descent and curve evolution, may be found in [25].

6 Experimental Results

We apply the proposed technique on 2-D mid-ventricular slices of data, although it is also applicable to 3-D with a corresponding increase in computational complexity. The dataset we use contains twenty frame time sequences of breath-hold cardiac MR images, each representing a single cardiac cycle. We do not consider arrhythmia because only patients having sustained and hemodynamically-stable arrhythmia can be practically imaged and analyzed. Such a condition is very rare. Anonymized data sets of were obtained from the Cardiovascular MR-CT Program at Massachusetts General Hospital.

6.1 Training

As discussed in Section 4.1, we represent each manually segmented LV from the training set (a total of 840 frames) by a shape variability vector $\boldsymbol{\alpha}$ and an area A. We obtain the state X_t for each frame t in the cardiac cycle. Then, we learn the dynamics of our system by maximizing $I(X_t; h(X_{t-1}))$, where we approximate h by a linear function, and use gradient ascent on the parameters of h to find the maximum. We obtain a density estimate of $p(X_t|h(X_{t-1}))$ for use in test data.

6.2 Testing

We take sequences of twenty frames (ones not included in the training set), each a single cardiac cycle, as input for testing. For initialization, we assume that a user provides a segmentation of the first two frames in the sequence. The segmentations can be approximate segmentations using some automated method, an expert hand-segmentation, or predicted using a segmentation from a neighboring 2-D slice of the same patient at the same time. From these segmentations, we obtain the initial posterior $p(f_2, X_2|Y_2)$. Using particle filters and curve evolution as described, we recursively estimate the posterior for each frame.

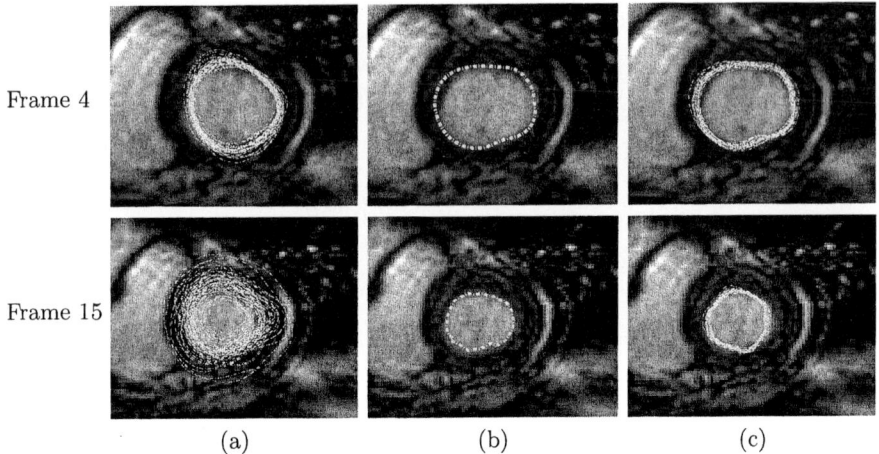

Fig. 4. (a) Curves representing predictions of the LV segmentation (observed MR image in background). (b) Segmentation of an MR image by obtaining the MAP estimate of X_t. (c) Curves representing samples of the posterior density $p(f_t, X_t | Y_t)$

6.3 Results

In Figure 4, we show the segmentation and tracking of the LV based on a test image sequence. Figure 4(a) shows LV boundaries extracted from samples of $p(X_t | h(X_{t-1}))$. Due to space constraints, we show two representative frames from the cardiac cycle. Note that these predictions are obtained based on segmentations from previous frames and on the learned dynamic model, but before incorporating the data shown in Figure 4(a). Figure 4(b) shows the MAP estimate of X_t, which involves incorporating the observed data. This estimate is obtained by minimizing Eqn. (9) and provides what qualitatively appears to be a reasonable segmentation of the LV boundary. Quantitatively, we measure accuracy by computing the symmetric difference between the segmentation and the manually-segmented truth normalized by the area of the truth. Here, the average value across the cardiac cycle of test data is 0.04. Finally, Figure 4(c) shows equally-weighted samples of the posterior density $p(X_t | Y_t)$. This example shows good results, but since the quality of the images are very good, static segmentation methods yield results similar to those shown in Figure 4(b).

We now consider low SNR images where static segmentation may not produce reasonable results. To simulate low SNR conditions, we add independent, lognormal multiplicative noise to MR images to produce a noisy dataset. Using dynamics trained from the MR image training set and initializing again using hand-segmentations on the first two frames, we estimate the LV boundaries. Figure 5 shows segmentations for a full cardiac cycle by taking the MAP estimate of X_t overlaid on the corresponding noisy MR data. The segmentations appear to provide accurate localizations of the LV boundaries despite low quality data.

Figure 1 provides a visual comparison between our approach and one using static segmentation. Only two frames are shown due to space limitations, but

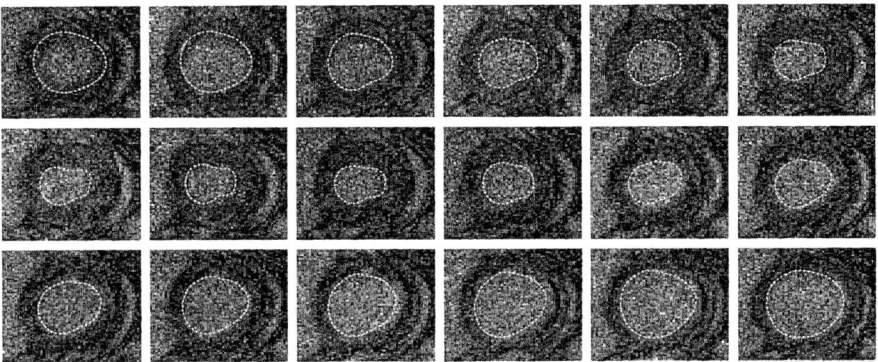

Fig. 5. MAP estimate of segmentations from frame 3 to 20 of a full cardiac cycle

they are representative of the results obtained throughout the cardiac cycle. Quantitatively across the entire cardiac cycle, the normalized symmetric difference from our approach is 0.08, while that for static segmentation is 0.17. The static segmentation method is obtained by replacing the $p(X_t|Y_{t-1})$ term in our formulation with a curve length prior and is similar to the region-based segmentations described in the introduction [3, 20, 26]. In both illustrations, incorporating dynamics into the segmentation process using the approach we propose results in better estimates than those using a static segmentation method.

7 Conclusion

We have proposed a principled method to recursively estimate the LV boundary across a cardiac cycle. In the training phase, we learn the dynamics of the LV by obtaining a non-parametric density estimate for the system dynamics. From this, we produce predictions which, used in conjunction with the observations from a new frame, estimate the LV boundary in this frame. The process is repeated through a cardiac cycle. This approach uses information from temporal neighbors to produce better segmentations than using observations at the current frame alone. We have illustrated this method on high and low SNR images. Our formulation produces reasonable estimates using either set of measurements.

A number of extensions to this work may be considered. For instance, our ongoing work considers the generalization to general non-parametric densities for the posterior when a rich enough training set is available. Also, in the learning phase, one might be interested in explicitly incorporating physical constraints to the dynamic system. Adding such constraints may help to eliminate boundary estimates which are known to be physically impossible. In addition, other forms of the function h may be considered. More general non-linear functions may yield a more informative statistic at the cost of greater computational complexity, while a time-varying one may be more informative if sufficient training data is available. In this work, we have posed the problem as a forward recursive filter.

Our current work considers improving the estimates by the use of smoothing. Finally, we note that although we track only 2-D slices of the LV in this paper, a natural experimental extension involves applying the technique to 3-D LV data.

References

1. S. Arulampalam, S. Maskell, N. Gordon, and T. Clapp, "A tutorial on particle filters for on-line non-linear/non-Gaussian Bayesian tracking," *IEEE Transactions on Signal Processing*, 50:2 (2002) 174:188.
2. V. Caselles, F. Catte, T. Coll, and F. Dibos, "A geometric model for active contours in image processing," *Numerische Mathematik*, 66 (1993) 1-31.
3. A. Chakraborty, L. Staib, and J. Duncan, "Deformable boundary finding in medical images by integrating gradient and region information," *IEEE Transactions on Medical Imaging*, 15 (1996) 859-870.
4. Y. Chen, H. D. Tagare, S. Thiruvenkadam, F. Huang, D. Wilson, K. S. Gopinath, and R. W. Briggs, "Using prior shapes in geometric active contours in a variational framework," *Int'l Journal of Computer Vision*, 50:3 (2002) 315-328.
5. A. Doucet, S. J. Godsill, and C. Andrieu, "On sequential Monte Carlo sampling methods for Bayesian filtering," *Statistics and Computing*, 10:3 (2000) 197-208.
6. P. M. Djuric, J. H. Kotecha, J. Zhang, Y. Huang, T. Ghirmi, M. F. Bugallo, and J. Miguez, "Particle filtering," *IEEE Signal Processing Magazine*, 20:5 (2003) 19-38.
7. J. S. Duncan, A. Smeulders, F. Lee, and B. Zaret, "Measurement of end diastolic shape deformity using bending energy," *Computers in Cardiology*, (1988) 277-280.
8. D. Geiger, A. Gupta, L. A. Costa, and J. Vlontzos, "Dynamic programming for detecting, tracking and matching deformable contours," *IEEE Transactions on Pattern Analysis and Machine Intelligence*, 17:3 (1995) 294-302.
9. A. Goshtasby and D. A. Turner, "Segmentation of cardiac cine MR images for extraction of right and left ventricular chambers," *IEEE Transactions on Medical Imaging*, 14:1 (1995) 56-64.
10. P. Hall, S. J. Sheather, M. C. Jones, and J. S. Marron, "On optimal data-based bandwidth selection in kernel density estimation," *Biometrika*, 78:2 (1991) 263-269.
11. A. Ihler, "Maximally Informative Subspaces," MS Thesis, MIT (2000).
12. M. Jolly, N. Duta, and G. Funka-Lea, "Segmentation of the left ventricle in cardiac MR images," *Proc of the IEEE Int'l Conf on Computer Vision*, 1 (2001) 501-508.
13. M. Kass, A. Witkin, and D. Terzopoulos, "Snakes: Active contour models," *Int'l Journal of Computer Vision*, (1987) 321-331.
14. J. H. Kotecha and P. M. Djuric, "Gaussian particle filtering," *IEEE Transactions on Signal Processing*, 51:10 (2003) 2592-2601.
15. G. Kuhne, J. Weickert, O. Schuster, and S. Richter, "A tensor-driven active contour model for moving object segmentation," *Proceedings of the 2001 IEEE Int'l Conference on Image Processing*, 2 (2001) 73-76.
16. M. Leventon, E. Grimson, and O. Faugeras, "Statistical shape influence in geodesic active contours," *Proc IEEE Conf on Comp Vision & Patt Rec*, 1 (2000) 316-323.
17. A. McCulloch, J. B. Bassingthwaighte, P. J. Hunter, D. Noble, T. L. Blundell, and T. Pawson, "Computational biology of the heart: From structure to function," *Progress in Biophysics and Molecular Biology*, 69:2-3 (1998) 153-155.
18. J. C. McEachen II and J. S. Duncan, "Shape-based tracking of left ventricular wall motion," *IEEE Transactions on Medical Imaging*, 16:3 (1997) 270-283.

19. N. Paragios and R. Deriche, "Geodesic Active Contours and Level Sets for the Detection and Tracking of Moving Objects," *IEEE Transactions on Pattern Analysis and Machine Intelligence,* 22 (2000) 266-280.
20. N. Paragios, "A variational approach for the segmentation of the left ventricle in cardiac image analysis," *Int'l Journal of Computer Vision,* 50:3 (2002) 345-362.
21. J. Senegas, T. Netsch, C. A. Cocosco, G. Lund, and A. Stork, "Segmentation of Medical Images with a Shape and Motion Model: A Bayesian Perspective," *Computer Vision Approaches to Medical Image Analysis (CVAMIA) and Mathematical Methods in Biomedical Image Analysis (MMBIA) Workshop,* (2004) pp. 157-168.
22. M. Sermesant, C. Forest, X. Pennec, H. Delingette, and N. Ayache, "Deformable biomechanical models: Applications to 4D cardiac image analysis," *Medical Image Analysis,* 7:4 (2003) 475-488.
23. J. A. Sethian, "Level Set Methods: Evolving Interfaces in Geometry, Fluid Mechanics, Computer Vision, and Material Science," *Cambridge Univ. Press,* 1996.
24. G. K. von Schutthess, "The effects of motion and flow on magnetic resonance imaging," In *Morphology and Function in MRI,* Ch. 3 (1989) 43-62.
25. W. Sun, M. Cetin, R. Chan, V. Reddy, G. Holmvang, V. Chandar, A. Willsky, "Segmenting and Tracking the Left Ventricle by Learning the Dynamics in Cardiac Images," *MIT LIDS Technical Report 2642,* (Feb 2005).
26. A. Tsai, A. Yezzi, W. Wells, C. Tempany, D. Tucker, A. Fan, W. E. Grimson, and A. Willsky, "A shape-based approach to the segmentation of medical imagery using level sets," *IEEE Transactions on Medical Imaging,* 22:2 (2003) 137-154.
27. J. Weng, A. Singh, and M. Y. Chiu, "Learning-based ventricle detection from cardiac MR & CT images," *IEEE Trans on Medical Imaging,* 16:4 (1997) 378-391.
28. X. S. Zhou, D. Comaniciu, and A. Gupta, "An information fusion framework for robust shape tracking," *IEEE Transactions on Pattern Analysis and Machine Intelligence,* 27:1 (2005) 115-129.

3D Active Shape Models Using Gradient Descent Optimization of Description Length

Tobias Heimann[1], Ivo Wolf[1], Tomos Williams[2], and Hans-Peter Meinzer[1]

[1] Div. Medical and Biological Informatics,
German Cancer Research Center, 69120 Heidelberg, Germany
t.heimann@dkfz.de
[2] Div. of Imaging Science, Stopford Building, Oxford Road,
University of Manchester, M13 9PT, UK

Abstract. Active Shape Models are a popular method for segmenting three-dimensional medical images. To obtain the required landmark correspondences, various automatic approaches have been proposed. In this work, we present an improved version of minimizing the description length (MDL) of the model. To initialize the algorithm, we describe a method to distribute landmarks on the training shapes using a conformal parameterization function. Next, we introduce a novel procedure to modify landmark positions locally without disturbing established correspondences. We employ a gradient descent optimization to minimize the MDL cost function, speeding up automatic model building by several orders of magnitude when compared to the original MDL approach. The necessary gradient information is estimated from a singular value decomposition, a more accurate technique to calculate the PCA than the commonly used eigendecomposition of the covariance matrix. Finally, we present results for several synthetic and real-world datasets demonstrating that our procedure generates models of significantly better quality in a fraction of the time needed by previous approaches.

1 Introduction

Since their introduction by Cootes et al. [1], Active Shape Models (ASMs) have become popular tools for automatic segmentation of medical images. The main challenge of the approach is the point correspondence problem in the model construction phase: On every training sample for the ASM, landmarks have to be placed in a consistent manner. While manual labeling is a time-consuming but feasible solution for 2D models with a limited number of landmarks, it is highly impractical in the 3D domain: Not only is the required number of landmarks higher than in the 2D case, but it also becomes increasingly difficult to identify and pinpoint corresponding points, even for experts.

Several automated methods to find the correspondences in 3D have been proposed. Brett and Taylor [2] use a pairwise corresponder based on a symmetric version of the ICP algorithm. All training shapes are decimated to generate sparse polyhedral approximations and then merged in a binary tree, which is used to propagate landmark positions. Shelton [3] measures correspondence between surfaces in arbitrary dimensions by a cost function which is composed of three parts representing Euclidean distance, surface deformation and prior information. The function is minimized using a multi-resolution approach that matches highly decimated versions of the meshes first and iteratively refines the results. Paulsen and Hilger [4] match a decimated template mesh to all training shapes using thin plate spline warping controlled by a small set of manually placed anatomic landmarks. The resulting meshes are relaxed to fit the training shapes by a Markov random field regularization. Another approach based on matching templates is presented by Zhao and Teoh [5]: They employ an adaptive-focus deformable model to match each training shape to all others without the need for manually placed landmarks. The shape yielding the best overall results in this process is subsequently used to determine point correspondences, enhanced by a "bridge-over" procedure for outliers.

A common characteristic of these methods is that they base their notion of correspondence on general geometric properties, e.g. minimum Euclidean distance and low distortion of surfaces. A different approach is presented by Davies et al. [6] who propose to minimize a cost function based on the minimum description length of the resulting statistical shape model. In a recent comparison [7], this approach has shown to be superior to other correspondence methods. However, the optimization of the MDL criterion for 3D shapes is complex to implement and computationally expensive. In this paper, we present an optimized procedure for minimizing the description length which is easier to implement and more efficient than the current method.

2 Fundamentals

2.1 Active Shape Models

The most popular kind of ASMs uses point distribution models (PDMs), which represent each d-dimensional training sample as a set of n landmarks. For every sample, landmark positions are defined by a single vector $\mathbf{x}$, storing the coordinates for landmark i at (x_i, x_{i+n}, x_{i+2n}). The vectors of all training samples form the columns of the landmark configuration matrix $\mathbf{L}$. Applying principal component analysis (PCA) to this matrix delivers the principal modes of variation $\mathbf{p}_m$ in the training data. Restricting the model to the first c modes, all valid shapes can be approximated by the mean shape $\bar{\mathbf{x}}$ and a linear combination of displacement vectors:

$$\mathbf{x} = \bar{\mathbf{x}} + \sum_{m=1}^{c} y_m \mathbf{p}_m \qquad (1)$$

Cootes used an eigenvector decomposition of the covariance matrix of $\mathbf{L}$ to calculate the PCA [1], a method commonly employed for this purpose. However, the same results can also be achieved by a singular value decomposition (SVD), which is numerically more stable and thus more accurate when the covariance matrix is ill-conditioned [8].

Theorem 1. *Any $m \times n$ real matrix $\mathbf{A}$ with $m \geq n$ can be written as the product*

$$\mathbf{A} = \mathbf{U}\mathbf{D}\mathbf{V}^{\mathbf{T}} \quad (2)$$

where $\mathbf{U}$ and $\mathbf{V}$ are column orthogonal matrices of size $m \times n$ and $n \times n$, respectively, and $\mathbf{D}$ is a $n \times n$ diagonal matrix. Then $\mathbf{U}$ holds the eigenvectors of the matrix $\mathbf{A}\mathbf{A}^{\mathbf{T}}$ and $\mathbf{D}^2$ the corresponding eigenvalues.

Without calculating the covariance matrix, the PCA can thus be obtained by the SVD of the matrix $\mathbf{A} = \frac{1}{\sqrt{s-1}}(\mathbf{L} - \bar{\mathbf{L}})$, where s is the number of samples and $\bar{\mathbf{L}}$ a matrix with all columns set to $\bar{\mathbf{x}}$. In addition to the increased accuracy, the matrices $\mathbf{U}$ and $\mathbf{V}$ allow calculating gradient information for the eigenvalues which we will use during the optimization stage of the model-building process.

2.2 Correspondence by Minimizing Description Length

A prerequisite for statistical shape models is a set of landmark points located at corresponding positions on all training shapes. To quantify this correspondence, the MDL approach introduced by Davies et al. [9] defines a cost function F which is based on the minimum description length of the generated model. In this work, we use a simplified version of the MDL as proposed by Thodberg [10], where F is defined as:

$$F = \sum_m \mathcal{L}_m \quad \text{with} \quad \mathcal{L}_m = \begin{cases} 1 + \log(\lambda_m/\lambda_{\text{cut}}) & \text{for } \lambda_m \geq \lambda_{\text{cut}} \\ \lambda_m/\lambda_{\text{cut}} & \text{for } \lambda_m < \lambda_{\text{cut}} \end{cases} \quad (3)$$

This formulation features one free parameter λ_{cut} which represents the expected noise in the training data. Since all shapes are rescaled to produce a mean shape with RMS radius $r = 1/\sqrt{n}$ for the PCA, the optimal value for λ_{cut} depends on the original average radius of the training shapes $\bar{r}$:

$$\lambda_{\text{cut}} = \left(\frac{\sigma}{\bar{r}}\right)^2, \quad (4)$$

where σ is the standard deviation of noise in the training data. In coherence with the voxel quantization error, Thodberg choses $\sigma = 0.3$ and uses $\bar{r} = 100$ in all his experiments. While we adopt the same σ-value, we modify $\bar{r}$ depending on the resolution of the images from which the training shapes are extracted.

3 Mesh Parameterization

To define an initial set of correspondences and a means of manipulating them efficiently, we need a convenient parameter domain for our training shapes. For closed 2D objects, the natural choice for this parameter domain is the arc-length position on the contour: Choosing an arbitrary starting point and normalizing the total arc-length to 1, all positions on the contour (i.e. all potential landmark positions) can be described by a single parameter $p \in [0..1]$.

In order to minimize complexity for the parameterization of 3D shapes, we will restrict the discussion to closed two-manifolds of genus 0 (i.e. surfaces without holes and self-intersections). Objects of this class are topologically equivalent to a sphere and comprise most shapes encountered in medical imaging (e.g. liver, kidneys and lungs). The task is to find a one-to-one mapping which assigns every point on the surface of the mesh a unique position on the unit sphere, described by two parameters longitude $\theta \in [0..2\pi]$ and latitude $\phi \in [0..\pi]$.

The mapping of an arbitrary shape to a sphere inevitably introduces some distortion. There are a number of different approaches which attempt to minimize this distortion, typically preserving either local angles or facet areas while trying to minimize distortions in the other. An overview of recent work on this topic can be found in [11].

For an initial parameterization, Davies uses diffusion mapping, a simplified version of the method described by Brechbühler [12] which is neither angle- nor area-preserving. Due to our optimization strategy (Sect. 4), our focus lies on preserving angles: Moving neighboring points on the parameterization sphere in a specific direction, we expect the corresponding landmarks on the training shape to move in a coherent direction as well. This behavior is guaranteed by conformal mapping functions, transformations that preserve local angles.

3.1 Creating a Conformal Mapping

Definition 1. *Each training sample for the ASM is represented as a triangulated mesh $K = (V, E)$ with vertices $u, v \in V$ and edges $[u, v] \in E$. The vertex positions are specified by $\mathbf{f} : V \to R^3$, an embedding function defined on the vertices of K. A second function $\mathbf{\Omega} : V \to R^3$ specifies the coordinates as mapped on the unit sphere, $\forall v \in V : |\mathbf{\Omega}(v)| = 1$.*

Gu et al. present a variational method to create a conformal parameterization in [13]. From an initial Gauss map, where $\mathbf{\Omega}(v)$ represents the normal vector of v, they use a gradient descent optimization to minimize the string energy of the mesh, defined as:

$$\mathcal{E}(K, \mathbf{\Omega}) = \sum_{[u,v] \in E} k_{u,v} \|\mathbf{\Omega}(u) - \mathbf{\Omega}(v)\|^2 \tag{5}$$

Minimizing the string energy with all edge weights $k_{u,v}$ set to 1 yields the barycentric mapping, where each vertex is positioned at the center of its neighbors. Subsequently, a conformal mapping can be obtained using edge weights depending on the opposing angles α, β of the faces adjacent to $[u, v]$ as in:

$$k_{u,v} = \frac{1}{2} \left(\cot \alpha + \cot \beta \right) \tag{6}$$

During the optimization process, all vertices must constantly be projected back onto the sphere by $\mathbf{\Omega}(u) = \mathbf{\Omega}'(u)/|\mathbf{\Omega}'(u)|$. The formal correctness of this approach was later proved in [14].

3.2 Mapping Landmarks

Following the preceding sections, the parameterization is defined by a spherical mesh with the same topology as the training sample. In order to obtain the 3D position for an arbitrary landmark at the spherical coordinates (θ, ϕ), which is generally not a vertex, we have to find the intersection between a ray from the origin to (θ, ϕ) and the parameterization mesh. Since mapping landmarks is the most computationally expensive part of the model-building process, an intelligent search strategy of ordering the triangles according to the likelihood of ray intersection speeds up the algorithm considerably. Intersected triangle indices for each landmark are cached and, in the case of a cache miss, neighboring triangles are given priority when searching for the ray intersection. To test a triangle for intersection, we use the method described in [15], which conveniently produces the barycentric coordinates of the intersection point. The same coordinates used on the respective triangle of the training mesh yield the final landmark position.

4 Optimizing Landmark Correspondences

With an initial conformal parameterization Ω_i for each training sample i, we can acquire the necessary landmarks by mapping a set of spherical coordinates to each shape. To optimize the point correspondences with the MDL criterion, two possibilities are available: We can either change the individual Ω_i and maintain a fixed set of global landmarks or modify individual landmark sets Ψ_i.

In this work, we opted for the first alternative, which has the advantage that the correspondence is valid for any set of points placed on the unit sphere. Therefore, it is possible to alter number and placement of landmarks on the unit sphere at any stage of the optimization, e.g. to better adapt the triangulation to the training shapes. Moreover, we do not need to worry about the correct ordering of landmarks: Since the valid set on the unit sphere is fixed, ensuring a one-to-one mapping to the training shapes is sufficient.

4.1 Re-parameterization

To modify the individual parameterizations in an iterative optimization process, we need a transformation function of the type $\Omega' = \Phi(\Omega)$. In [6], Davies et al. use symmetric theta transformations for that purpose: Employing a wrapped Cauchy kernel with a certain width and amplitude, landmarks near the kernel position are spread over the sphere, while landmarks in other regions of the surface are compressed. By accumulating the effects of thousands of kernels at different positions, arbitrary parameterizations can be created.

While this re-parameterization method produces the required effect, it is an inefficient means of modifying surface parameterizations. The main disadvantage is that it is a global modification, i.e. adding one new kernel modifies all landmark positions on the object. Intuitively, it would be desirable to keep established landmark correspondences stable. Therefore, we suggest a new method for modifying parameterization functions based on kernels with strictly local effects.

We will assume that we know a principal direction $(\Delta\theta, \Delta\phi)$ in which the vertices of a local neighborhood on the parameterization mesh should move to improve landmark correspondences. Then we define a Gaussian envelope function to change each spherical coordinate by $c(x,\sigma) \cdot (\Delta\theta, \Delta\phi)$ with

$$c(x,\sigma) = \begin{cases} e^{\frac{-x^2}{2\sigma^2}} - e^{\frac{-(3\sigma)^2}{2\sigma^2}} & \text{for } x < 3\sigma \\ 0 & \text{for } x \geq 3\sigma \end{cases} \quad (7)$$

The variable x denotes the Euclidean distance between the center of the kernel and the specific vertex of the parameterization mesh, while σ specifies the size of the kernel. The movements are cut off at 3σ to limit the range and keep the modification local. During the course of the optimization, σ is decreased to optimize larger regions at the beginning and details at the end. Three examples for possible kernel configurations with different σ-values are shown in Fig. 1.

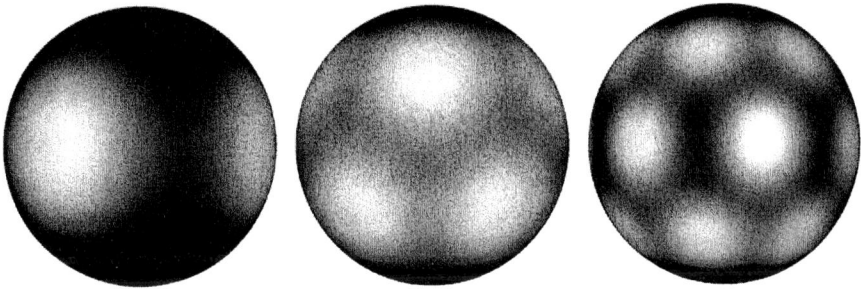

Fig. 1. Kernel configurations for σ values of 0.4, 0.3 and 0.2. Bright intensities mark regions with large vertex movements, dark ones those with no modification

The proposed method of modification does not work if a kernel includes one of the poles of the spherical parameterization mesh ($\phi = 0$ or $\phi = \pi$) because vertices would all move either toward or away from this point, depending on $\Delta\phi$. Nevertheless, the positions of the different kernels have to change in the course of the optimization in order to guarantee an equal treatment for all vertices of the parameterization mesh. This limitation is overcome by defining specific kernel configurations as shown in Fig. 1, which do not cover the pole sections of the sphere. By keeping these configurations fixed and instead rotating all parameterizations and the global landmark collection by a random rotation matrix, the relative kernel positions are changed without touching a pole. The random rotation matrices for these operations are acquired using the method described in [16].

4.2 Calculating MDL Gradients

Given a kernel at a certain position, we need the direction $(\Delta\theta, \Delta\phi)$ for the movement which minimizes the cost function. Since all modifications of the parameterization change landmark positions on the training sample, the first step is to quantify the effect landmark movements have on the MDL value. As shown in [17], the work of Papadopoulo and Lourakis on estimating the Jacobian of the SVD [18] can be used for that purpose, calculating the gradients of the MDL objective function with respect to individual landmarks.

The calculation of the singular value derivatives does not add a significant computational overhead. Given the centered and un-biased landmark configuration matrix $\mathbf{A}$ from Sect. 2.1, the derivative for the m-th singular value d_m is calculated by:

$$\frac{\partial d_m}{\partial a_{ij}} = u_{im} \cdot v_{jm} \tag{8}$$

The scalars u_{im} and v_{jm} are elements of the matrices $\mathbf{U}$ and $\mathbf{V}$ from (2). Since our MDL cost function uses $\lambda_m = d_m^2$, we can derive the MDL gradients as

$$\frac{\partial F}{\partial a_{ij}} = \sum_m \frac{\partial \mathcal{L}_m}{\partial a_{ij}} \quad \text{with} \quad \frac{\partial \mathcal{L}_m}{\partial a_{ij}} = \begin{cases} 2u_{im}v_{jm}/d_m & \text{for } \lambda_m \geq \lambda_{\text{cut}} \\ 2d_m u_{im} v_{jm}/\lambda_{\text{cut}} & \text{for } \lambda_m < \lambda_{\text{cut}} \end{cases} \tag{9}$$

This derivation yields a 3D gradient for every landmark, revealing the influence of its movements on the cost function. Two examples of the resulting gradient fields are visualized in Fig. 2.

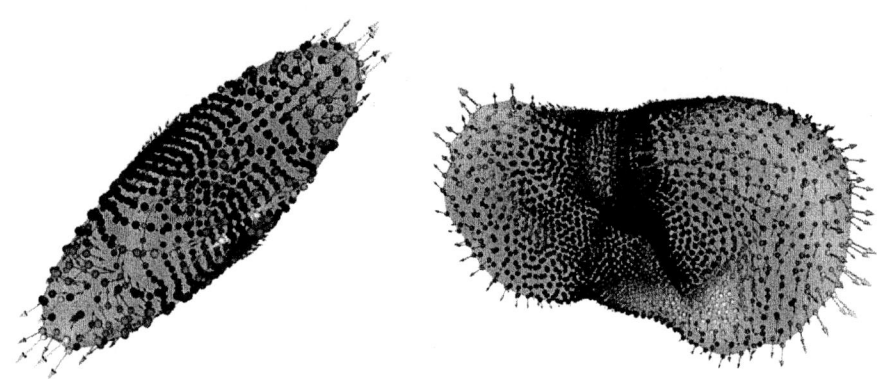

Fig. 2. Gradients of the MDL cost function visualized for two sample shapes. The value of the directional derivative is color-coded ranging from black for weak gradients to white for the strongest gradients

4.3 Putting It All Together

The final step is to transform the calculated gradient fields into optimal kernel movements $\mathbf{k} = (\Delta\theta, \Delta\phi)$ on the parameterization mesh. Using the chain rule, we get:

$$\frac{\partial F}{\partial \mathbf{k}} = \frac{\partial F}{\partial a_{ij}} \frac{\partial a_{ij}}{\partial \mathbf{k}} \tag{10}$$

We use finite differences to estimate the surface gradients $\partial a_{ij}/\partial \mathbf{k}$.

Both Davies [19] and Thodberg [10] describe cases in which the MDL optimization can lead to landmarks piling up in certain regions or collapsing to a point. Davies keeps one shape as a master example with fixed landmarks to prevent this effect while Thodberg suggests adding a stabilizing term to the cost function. Since we have never observed the problematic behavior with our new re-parameterization, we do not employ any of these methods.

In addition to modifying the mapping functions Ω_i by re-parameterization, other variables which influence landmark positions can be included in the optimization. The rotation of each mapping Ω_i determines the position of the first landmark on the training shape and the relative orientation of all others. By calculating gradients for rotating the parameterization mesh around the three Euclidean axes and using those instead of the surface gradients $\partial a_{ij}/\partial \mathbf{k}$ in (10), we have an efficient method to optimize this variable.

Other possibilities for optimization include scale and rotation of the individual training shapes, which are normally determined by a generalized procrustes matching. While we do optimize scale in our procedure, we did not notice significant improvements in the resulting MDL values due to this step.

5 Results

5.1 Datasets

We tested the presented method on several synthetic and real-life datasets. Synthetic data has the advantage that the global minimum of the MDL function is known, since it can be calculated from the correspondences inherent for generated data. A tabular description of all employed datasets is given in Tab. 1.

Table 1. The collection of datasets used for the evaluation

	Cuboids	Ellipsoids	Lungs	Livers
Origin	synthetic	synthetic	clinical	clinical
Mean size (radius in voxels)	100	100	25	70
Number of samples	20	20	18	21
Perceived sample variance	low	medium	medium	high
Sample complexity (# vertices)	486	962	3250–5000	1500–2000
Model complexity (# landmarks)	642	642	2562	2562

5.2 Performance Measures

In [19], Davies describes three measures to quantify the quality of the created shape model: Generalization ability, specificity and compactness. The same measures are also used in the comparison of different correspondence methods by Styner et al. [7].

Generalization ability quantifies the capability of the model to represent new shapes. It can be estimated by performing a series of leave-one-out tests on the training set, measuring the distance of the omitted training shape to the closest match of the reduced model. Specificity describes the validity of the shapes the model produces. The value is estimated by generating random parameter values from a normal distribution with zero mean and the respective standard deviation from the PCA. The distance of the generated shape to the closest match of the training set is averaged over a number of 10,000 runs. Compactness simply measures the accumulative variance of the model. All measures are defined as functions of the number of modes or parameters used by the model and displayed as piecewise linear graphs. Smaller values indicate better models.

While generalization ability and specificity are well-established qualities inherent to a good model, compactness is an implementation specific measure: The MDL approach assumes that low variances result in a good ASM, but this is no imminent truth. We therefore restrict our evaluation to the first two measures.

5.3 Comparison with Current Standard

For all datasets described in Sect. 5.1, Active Shape Models have been generated using the gradient descent technique (GD) proposed in this paper and using the current standard approach (STD) by Davies [19]. Our GD-algorithm was implemented in C++ and run on a 3.0GHz Intel Pentium 4 with Windows XP and 512MB of memory. The code makes use of the Hyper-Threading architecture to optimize several samples concurrently. The STD-experiments were performed using the original Matlab code on a 2.8GHz Intel Xenon with Linux and 2GB of memory. After optimization, the global landmark sets of the GD-optimized models were adjusted to match the landmark distributions of the STD-models. For the evaluation, all models were rescaled to the same dimensions as the average training sample. The results of the experiments are summarized in Tab. 2. For our GD-optimization, we list additional intermediate values for the point at which the MDL values surpasses the results of the STD-method.

The GD-optimization reaches the same MDL values as the converged STD-method up to 5,000 times faster and produces distinctly better final results. Generalization ability and specificity values for all datasets are displayed in Fig. 3. In accordance with the MDL values, models optimized with our GD-method exhibit significantly better generalization ability and specificity values.

Table 2. Resulting MDL values at different stages of optimization using the gradient descent (GD) and standard (STD) method for all datasets. Times are given in hours and minutes

Optimization	Cuboids		Ellipsoids		Lungs		Livers	
	Time	MDL	Time	MDL	Time	MDL	Time	MDL
Initial values	0:00	1305	0:00	1288	0:00	1216	0:00	2323
STD (converged)	63:24	1297	63:24	1284	432:00	1203	432:00	2275
GD (intermediate)	0:01	1246	0:01	1254	0:05	1180	0:07	2263
GD (converged)	0:36	1243	2:43	1247	17:03	1160	14:45	2140

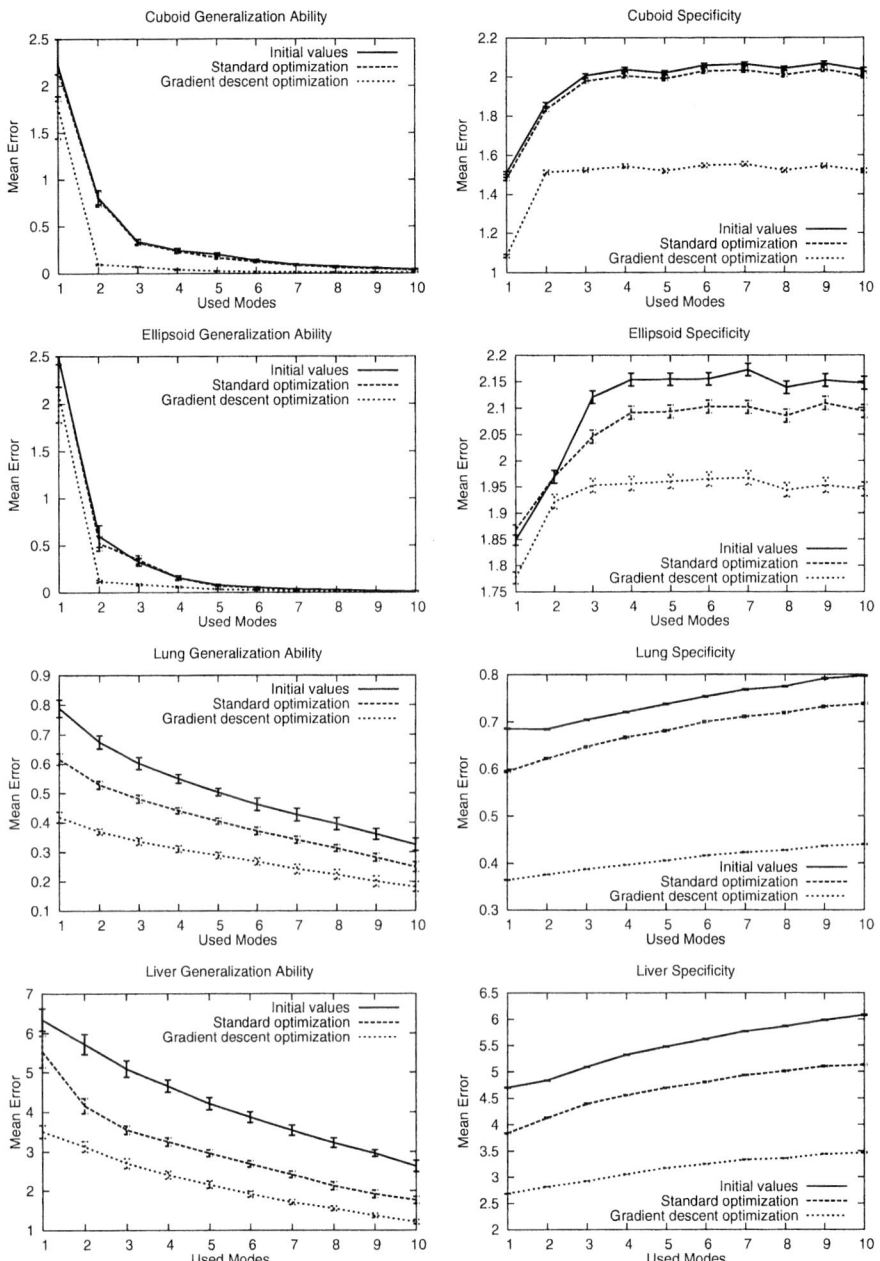

Fig. 3. Graphs of generalization ability and specificity for different numbers of modes for all datasets. In addition to the results after standard optimization and our gradient descent method, the initial values before optimization are displayed as orientation

6 Conclusions

As demonstrated in the preceding section, our gradient descent optimization produces significantly better models than the current standard approach while at the same time being several orders of magnitude faster. Highly detailed models containing over 2,500 landmarks can be successfully optimized in less than 20 hours on a normal desktop PC. This significant performance gain opens up new possibilities for building larger and more detailed 3D ASMs. Excluding the platform difference, a major part of the improvements can be attributed to our novel method of local parameter modification controlled by the estimated gradients of the MDL cost function. As the lower MDL values after optimization indicate, our method is less sensitive to convergence to local minima than the original approach. It offers an efficient, robust and versatile approach to automatic model building that should further propagate the use of 3D ASMs in clinical practice. To represent more complex shapes (e.g. brain ventricles), the mesh surface could be cut and parameterized over multiple domains instead of a single sphere.

Future research will investigate in how far the established correspondences can be used to reorganize landmarks after the optimization in order to represent the geometry of the model optimally with a minimum number of points. Additionally, the stability of our re-parameterization method against landmark collapse has to be verified using a larger number of test datasets.

Acknowledgements

The work reported here was partially funded by the German Research Foundation through SFB 414: Information Technology in Medicine. Special thanks to Rhodri H. Davies for many inspiring discussions about MDL optimization. The original MR lung data was kindly provided by Christian Plathow, the 3D meshes were created by Max Schöbinger. The CT liver data and segmentations were supplied by Matthias Thorn and Jan-Oliver Neumann.

References

1. Cootes, T.F., Taylor, C.J., Cooper, D.H., Graham, J.: Active shape models – their training and application. Computer Vision and Image Understanding **61** (1995) 38–59
2. Brett, A.D., Taylor, C.J.: A method of automated landmark generation for automated 3D PDM construction. Image and Vision Computing **18** (2000) 739–748
3. Shelton, C.R.: Morphable surface models. Int. Journal of Computer Vision **38** (2000) 75–91
4. Paulsen, R.R., Hilger, K.B.: Shape modelling using markov random field restoration of point correspondences. In: Proc. IPMI. (2003) 1–12
5. Zhao, Z., Teoh, E.K.: A novel framework for automated 3D PDM construction using deformable models. In: Proc. SPIE Medical Imaging. Volume 5747. (2005)

6. Davies, R.H., Twining, C.J., Cootes, T.F., Waterton, J.C., Taylor, C.J.: 3D statistical shape models using direct optimisation of description length. In: Proc. European Conference on Computer Vision, Part III, Springer (2002) 3–20
7. Styner, M., Rajamani, K.T., Nolte, L.P., Zsemlye, G., Székely, G., Taylor, C.J., Davies, R.H.: Evaluation of 3D correspondence methods for model building. In: Proc. IPMI. (2003) 63–75
8. Kalman, D.: A singularly valuable decomposition: The SVD of a matrix. College Math Journal **27** (1996) 2–23
9. Davies, R.H., Twining, C.J., Cootes, T.F., Waterton, J.C., Taylor, C.J.: A minimum description length approach to statistical shape modelling. IEEE trans. Medical Imaging **21** (2002) 525–537
10. Thodberg, H.H.: Minimum description length shape and appearance models. In: Proc. IPMI. (2003) 51–62
11. Floater, M.S., Hormann, K.: Surface parameterization: a tutorial and survey. In Dodgson, N.A., Floater, M.S., Sabin, M.A., eds.: Advances in Multiresolution for Geometric Modelling. Mathematics and Visualization. Springer, Berlin, Heidelberg (2005) 157–186
12. Brechbühler, C., Gerig, G., Kübler, O.: Parametrization of closed surfaces for 3-D shape description. Computer Vision and Image Understanding **61** (1995) 154–170
13. Gu, X., Wang, Y., Chan, T.F., Thompson, P.M., Yau, S.T.: Genus zero surface conformal mapping and its application to brain surface mapping. In: Proc. IPMI. (2003) 172–184
14. Gotsman, C., Gu, X., Sheffer, A.: Fundamentals of spherical parameterization for 3D meshes. ACM Trans. Graph. **22** (2003) 358–363
15. Möller, T., Trumbore, B.: Fast, minimum storage ray-triangle intersection. Journal of Graphics Tools **2** (1997) 21–28
16. Arvo, J.: Fast random rotation matrices. In Kirk, D., ed.: Graphics Gems III. Academic Press (1992) 117–120
17. Ericsson, A., Åström, K.: Minimizing the description length using steepest descent. In: Proc. British Machine Vision Conference. (2003) 93–102
18. Papadopoulo, T., Lourakis, M.I.A.: Estimating the Jacobian of the singular value decomposition: Theory and applications. In: Proc. European Conference on Computer Vision, Springer (2000) 554–570
19. Davies, R.H.: Learning Shape: Optimal Models for Analysing Shape Variability. PhD thesis, University of Manchester, Manchester, UK (2002)

Capturing Anatomical Shape Variability Using B-Spline Registration

Thomas H. Wenckebach, Hans Lamecker, and Hans-Christian Hege

Zuse Institute Berlin (ZIB), Takustr. 7, 14195 Berlin, Germany
{wenckebach, lamecker, hege}@zib.de
www.zib.de/visual

Abstract. Registration based on B-spline transformations has attracted much attention in medical image processing recently. Non-rigid registration provides the basis for many important techniques, such as statistical shape modeling. Validating the results, however, remains difficult - especially in intersubject registration. This work explores the ability of B-spline registration methods to capture intersubject shape deformations. We study the effect of different established and new shape representations, similarity measures and optimization strategies on the matching quality. To this end we conduct experiments on synthetic shapes representing deformations which typically may arise in intersubject registration, as well as on real patient data of the liver and pelvic bone. The experiments clearly reveal the influence of each component on the registration performance. The results may serve as a guideline for assessing intensity based registration.

1 Introduction

Motivation. Detailed analysis of anatomical shape variability frequently depends on identification of corresponding points on different shapes. Morphological studies, like neuroanatomical studies of the brain, generation of anatomical atlases, and many other applications demand such information. In recent times statistical shape modeling has been proven a successful method in medical image processing. The performance of statistical shape models crucially depends on the way anatomical regions of different shapes are mapped to each other. Anatomical correspondence across different subjects is not well understood, and hence much harder to validate than in intrasubject matching.

Volumetric registration of medical data using B-spline transformations has been widely applied in medical image processing [1, 2, 3, 4, 5]. In many cases registration is performed directly on (tomographic) image data which implicitly contains the shape of the object. In this work we will explore the capability of B-spline based registration methods to capture shape variability. Therefore we focus on registration of surfaces, where the deformation model itself can be studied more accurately without interference originating from image-related mismatches. Particularly in intersubject registration large deformations may

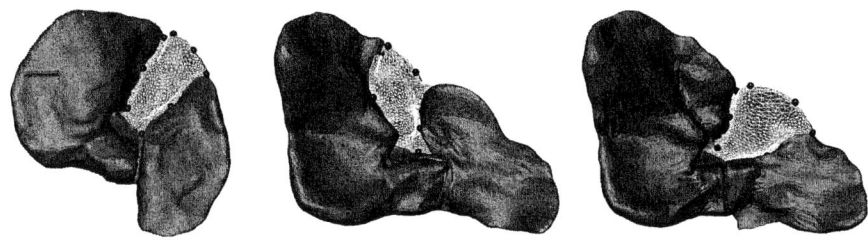

Fig. 1. Comparison of different liver registrations with equal surface distance: *Left:* Template. *Mid:* Triangulation registration with boundary constraints (similar result for distance field registration), *Right:* Triangulation registration without boundary constraints (similar result for label field) leads to incorrect anatomical matching

occur. Anatomically corresponding structures may differ geometrically or may be separated widely, see for instance Fig. 1.

Contributions. The aim of this work is to study the influence of different shape representations, similarity measures as well as optimization strategies on the performance of the B-spline based registration framework. To this end we define a set of pairs of synthetic shapes that represent deformations which typically may arise in intersubject registration. Moreover, we consider two anatomical shapes of different variability: liver consists of soft tissue, and its shape is subject to respiratory state, patient pose, and configuration of neighbouring organs, while pelvic bone is basically a rigid structure. Here, additional anatomical expert knowledge is available for validation. We evaluate the performance measured in terms of surface distance after registration, regularity of the deformation map, robustness and landmark placement. These experiments clearly reveal strengths and weaknesses of the different components under investigation.

Previous Work. Fleute et al. [6] first used intersubject non-rigid registration for building a statistical shape model of the knee. They employed the algorithm by Szeliski and Lavallée [1] using asymmetric surface distance as similarity measure. Frangi et al. applied Rückert's registration [2] based on label fields for CT bone, MRI brain data [7], and cardiac images [8]. They compare their method to the work of Brett et al. [9], who use a symmetric variant of the rigid iterative closest-points algorithm (ICP) [10] for brain data. Non-rigid extensions to ICP have been reported recently [11,12]. Rohlfing et al. [3] employed the algorithm by Rückert for construction of an anatomical atlas of the honey bee.

The capability of the deformation model has not been analyzed thoroughly up to now. It was assumed that correspondences based on B-spline registration are fold-over free [7] as opposed to those obtained by the ICP approach of Brett et al. We show this to be generally not the case. Usually, validation is performed indirectly by assessing the performance of the derived shape models or in terms of the implemented similarity measures. Rohlfing et al. evaluate the quality (sharpness, entropy) of the averaged intensity image obtained by their registration. Frangi et al. [8] consider landmark correspondence.

Instead of surfaces, lower dimensional structures such as landmarks [13] or feature curves [14] are in use. Unfortunately, for many organs like the liver such descriptions are difficult to derive due to a lack of characteristic shape features. Incorporation of geometric features into ICP can be found in [15, 16]. Wang et al. [17] base their semi-automatic matching on curvature classifiers.

A fundamentally different approach to non-rigid matching is based on mappings of two-dimensional manifolds [18, 19, 20], as opposed to volumetric mappings.

2 Algorithmic Overview

The task of volumetric registration is to find a spatial mapping $\mathbf{T} : \mathbb{R}^3 \to \mathbb{R}^3$ between a *template* shape X and a *target* shape Y, such that X and Y resemble each other as much as possible. The similarity of X and Y is defined by some cost function $E(\mathbf{T}, X, Y)$. We will study the following shape representations:

Label fields (LF). $A{:}\Omega_A \to \mathcal{L}_A$ with $\mathcal{L}_A \subset \mathbb{Z}$ implicitly contain the boundary along voxels belonging to different segments $\mathcal{L}_A$ ($= \{0, 1\}$ for binary images). Label fields with smooth boundaries are generated by scan-conversion of triangulated surfaces.

Signed distance fields (SDF). $A{:}\Omega_A \to \mathcal{D}_A$ with $\mathcal{D}_A \subset \mathbb{R}$ encoding for each voxel the spatial distance to the closest point of a surface. It's level sets implicitly represent a family of shapes. A is computed via euclidean distance mapping [21].

Triangulated surfaces (TS).5 $\mathcal{S}_A \subset \mathbb{R}^3$ are the only parametric shape representations considered in this work. Triangulated surfaces are typically generated by segmentations of tomographic data using the marching cubes algorithm.

In the framework of parametric registration, the transformation $\mathbf{T}$ is composed of an affine transformation $\mathbf{T}_{\text{affine}}$ as well as a B-spline deformation $\mathbf{T}_{\text{B-spline}}$. The latter is defined on a 3D discrete uniform control point grid (CPG) with cubic B-spline interpolation between adjacent control points, see [2, 4] for details. The B-spline deformation model appears suitable for intersubject registration, because it provides smooth deformations when a physical model is not known.

The optimal transformation $\mathbf{T}$ for a given cost function E is determined by a nonlinear multilevel optimization scheme. The CPG is refined iteratively, providing a parameter pyramid, while at the same time there is a data pyramid consisting of several sampled versions of the shapes. The main intention of this approach is to prevent optimization from being trapped in a local minimum of the similarity criterion. By means of B-spline CPG refinement global deformations are corrected at the beginning, while local deformations are iteratively resolved later on. The minimum $\mathbf{T}^*$ of the cost function E is found by employing a gradient descent-like search strategy. Instead of numerically approximating the gradient, a *search-direction* is computed by scanning the whole parameter space within some capture range depending on the level within the data pyramid [22].

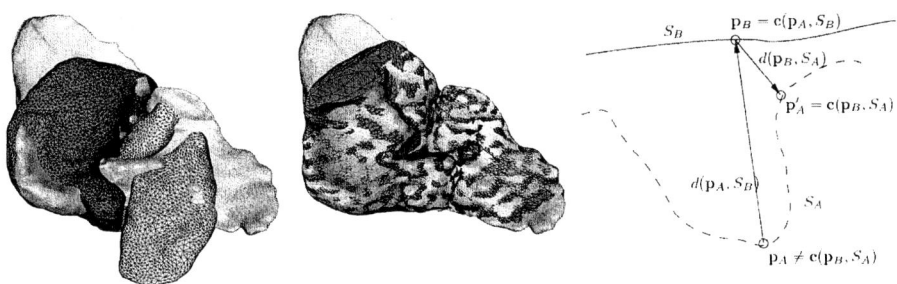

Fig. 2. Problem of asymmetric distance measures. *Left:* Initial template and target. *Mid:* Result with one-sided surface distance. *Right:* Schematic view

The general cost function of the registration consists of a term measuring shape similarity D, a regularization term R smoothing the transformation, plus additional boundary constraints:

$$E(\mathbf{T}, X, Y) = D(\mathbf{T}(X), Y) + \lambda R(\mathbf{T}) + \text{boundary constraints} ,\qquad(1)$$

where the shape similarity D consists of a weighted sum of different measures:

Similarity Measure 1 (Label Consistency). Given label fields A, B, with labels $\mathcal{L} = \{1, \ldots, L\}$ and image domain Ω, let $p_{AB}(l, m)$ denote the probability of cooccurence of labels $l, m \in \mathcal{L}$ in the overlap domain $\Omega_{A,B}$. Label consistency [8] is measured by

$$D_{\mathcal{L}}(A, B) = \sum_{l=1}^{L} p_{AB}(l, l) .\qquad(2)$$

Similarity Measure 2 (Grey-Value Difference). For distance fields A and B, grey-value difference is defined as

$$D_{\mathcal{D}}(A, B) = \frac{1}{|\Omega_{A,B}|} \sum_{\mathbf{x} \in \Omega_{A,B}} [A(\mathbf{x}) - B(\mathbf{x})]^2 .\qquad(3)$$

For triangulations $\mathcal{S}_A$ and $\mathcal{S}_B$ let $d_s(\mathbf{p}, \mathcal{S}_B) = \min_{\mathbf{q} \in B} \|\mathbf{p} - \mathbf{q}\|_2$ denote the distance of a point $\mathbf{p}$ on $\mathcal{S}_A$ to the surface $\mathcal{S}_B$. Based on d_s, we define the closest point $\mathbf{c}$ on $\mathcal{S}_B$ to $\mathbf{p}$ on $\mathcal{S}_A$ by $\mathbf{c}(\mathbf{p}, \mathcal{S}_B) = \arg\min_{\mathbf{q} \in \mathcal{S}_B} \|\mathbf{p} - \mathbf{q}\|_2$. Obviously, this correspondence is asymmetric (cf. Fig. 2, right). We propose to use a symmetric surface distance as the fundamental similarity measure for shapes:

Similarity Measure 3 (Surface Distance) is defined by

$$D_s(\mathcal{S}_A, \mathcal{S}_B) = \frac{1}{|\mathcal{S}_A| + |\mathcal{S}_B|} \left(\sqrt{\sum_{\mathbf{p} \in \mathcal{S}_A} d_s(\mathbf{p}, \mathcal{S}_B)^2} + \sqrt{\sum_{\mathbf{q} \in \mathcal{S}_B} d_s(\mathbf{q}, \mathcal{S}_A)^2} \right) .\qquad(4)$$

Note that measures employed on triangulations should be symmetric in order to match convex or concave regions as illustrated in Fig. 2, left. This implies a considerable algorithmic complexity in contrast to the conventional asymmetric

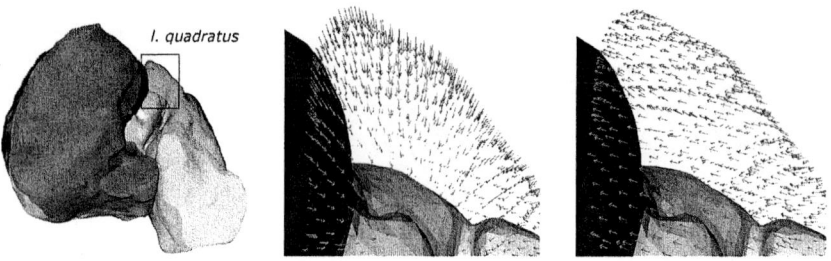

Fig. 3. Ambiguity induced by a spatial attractor. The anatomically corresponding region in the middle (l. quadr.) is hardly pronounced on the target. *Left:* Overview. *Mid:* Close-up: displacements for correct solution. *Right:* Displacements for bad solution

scheme: the latter can be implemented efficiently using a distance map of the target surface, while the former requires at any partial derivative calculation a search for closest points.

Local geometric characterizations of surfaces are often included in the cost function to improve the matching. Particularly in intersubject registration, situations are common where anatomical structures are pronounced to a highly different degree, yet spatially aligned closely (cf. Fig. 3). Such problems may be avoided by incorporating the normal vector fields $\mathbf{n}_A$ and $\mathbf{n}_B$ of the surfaces:

Similarity Measure 4 (Normal Deviation) is defined by

$$D_n(\mathcal{S}_A, \mathcal{S}_B) = \frac{1}{|\mathcal{S}_A| + |\mathcal{S}_B|} \left(\sum_{\mathbf{p} \in \mathcal{S}_A} d_n(\mathbf{p}, \mathcal{S}_B)^2 + \sum_{\mathbf{q} \in \mathcal{S}_B} d_n(\mathbf{q}, \mathcal{S}_A)^2 \right), \quad (5)$$

with $d_n(\mathbf{p}, \mathcal{S}_B) = 1 - \mathbf{n}_A(\mathbf{p}) \cdot \mathbf{n}_B(\mathbf{c}(\mathbf{p}, \mathcal{S}_B))$.

Other commonly used local geometric characterizations are based on the principal curvatures κ_1 and κ_2 of a surface. Koenderink and van Doorn [23] introduced two suitable classifiers: the so-called shape index $S = \frac{2}{\pi} \arctan \frac{\kappa_1 + \kappa_2}{\kappa_2 - \kappa_1}$ with $\kappa_2 \neq \kappa_1$ separates a surface into convex, hyperbolic and concave areas, and transitions between these; the range is continuous within $[-1, 1]$. Note that S is invariant under global scaling of the surface. The curvedness $C = \sqrt{\frac{\kappa_1^2 + \kappa_2^2}{2}}$ is a suitable classifier when scale is of interest. It also has some advantages over the mean curvature: the mean curvature vanishes at points where $\kappa_1 = -\kappa_2$ and its magnitude is not intuitive, since it does not grow proportionally with the radius of a sphere. Both defects are cured by the curvedness C. Misregistrations as shown in Fig. 4 can be avoided by using such information.

Similarity Measure 5 (Curvature Similarity). Let curv denote either the shape index S or the curvedness C. Curvature similarity is defined as

$$D_{\mathrm{curv}}(\mathcal{S}_A, \mathcal{S}_B) = \frac{1}{|\mathcal{S}_A| + |\mathcal{S}_B|} \left(\sum_{\mathbf{p} \in \mathcal{S}_A} d_c(\mathbf{p}, \mathcal{S}_B)^2 + \sum_{\mathbf{q} \in \mathcal{S}_B} d_c(\mathbf{q}, \mathcal{S}_A)^2 \right), \quad (6)$$

with $d_c(\mathbf{p}, \mathcal{S}_B) = \mathrm{curv}(\mathbf{p}) - \mathrm{curv}(\mathbf{c}(\mathbf{p}, \mathcal{S}_B))$.

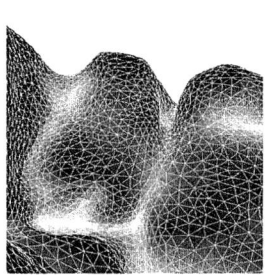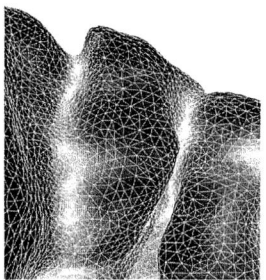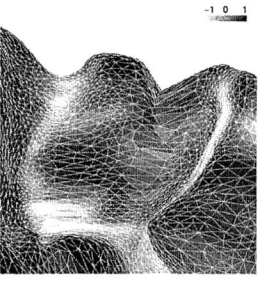

Fig. 4. Plain LF registration. *Left:* Target. *Mid:* Template. *Right:* Misregistration (shape index colouring of original template is transferred to deformed template)

Regularization (Grid Energy). Large deformations in intersubject registration, as well as over-refinement of the CPG may lead to irregular B-spline deformations. Therefore, in some applications we use a regularization term R in the cost function, which models the bending energy of a thin metal plate (biharmonic model, see [1, 2]).

Boundary Constraint (Landmarks). We encountered situations in intersubject registration where all of the above similarity measures with or without regularization fail to achieve a reasonable registration. In this case, boundary constraints expressed by the sum of squared differences of manually specified corresponding landmarks on the template and the target shape may guide the optimization towards a better solution. In practice, reliable placement of landmarks on organs like the liver is possible in rare cases, only.

3 Results

Implementation. All components of the algorithm are implemented in one software framework in optimized C++ code. Increased performance is achieved by exploiting separability of B-spline interpolation and incremental evaluation of similarity measures. Adaptive CPG refinement is accomplished by switching off control points away from the template surface (for TS and LF registration only).

As a benchmark for evaluating the matching capability of the B-spline registration framework we identify three classes of deformations typically arising in intersubject registration:

Large deformations occur when corresponding structures lie spatially far apart, even after affine registration. As an example, consider Fig. 4: the concave structure ("valley") should be coloured in blue after successful matching. Instead, it is mapped to the convex region to the right. The "cigar"/"banana" pair in Fig. 5 exemplifies this problem.

Spatial attractors may cause ambiguities in the registration. In Fig. 3 the lobus quadratus of the template shape might be deformed towards the left (lobus dex-

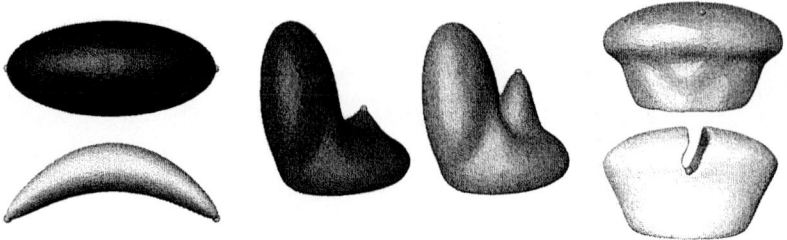

Fig. 5. Synthetic test shapes with target points (available for download at www.zib.de/wenckebach/ipmi05). *Left:* Problem 1: cigar/banana. *Mid:* Problem 2: two hills. *Right:* Problem 3: muffins

ter), or down towards the anatomically correct region, which is hard to detect on the target. This situation is represented by "two hills" shapes in Fig. 5.

Absent features on one shape, which exist on the other, inevitably introduce some degree of arbitrariness. In the liver, neighbouring organs or vessels often cause deformations to a very different degree (cf. Fig. 9). Such cases are accentuated in an extreme fashion by the "muffin" shapes in Fig. 5.

We consider the following criteria in our evaluation of registration performance: a necessary requirement for a correct matching is a value for surface distance D_s close to zero. Moreover, the transformation **T** should be regular, i.e. the determinant of the Jacobian $|J_T|$ must be positive for each CPG cell. Additionally, for synthetic shapes we examine the euclidean distance of manually defined target points (*target point deviation* d_t in percentage of the shape diameter).

3.1 Experiments: Synthetic Shapes

The optimization starts on a coarse CPG ($5 \times 5 \times 5$), which is successively refined to $19 \times 19 \times 19$. The results of all experiments are sensitive to the initial CPG resolution. As a general rule, we found that matching quality improves when the resolution of the CPG is adapted to the frequency content of the shape.

The step width for the search direction is iteratively decreased from 10 % of shape diameter on the initial to 0.05 % on the final level. A higher initial CPG resolution was necessary for LF and SDF registration of the muffins. In all cases the surface distance vanishes after registration except for the muffin shapes using SDF or LF registration. Regularity is violated whenever using TS registration. Moreover, all experiments show that registration is *not* robust with respect to the weighting of the geometric similarity measures.

Banana. For TS registration, the best result is shown in Fig. 6, left ($d_t = 3.3\,\%$). Carefully adjusting the weight of curvedness in the cost function improves matching the cusps. Yet, distortions are spread unevenly over the surface and there is little regularity. Amplifying the grid energy reduces surface distortion at the cost of larger target point deviation ($d_t = 8.3\,\%$). SDF registration combined

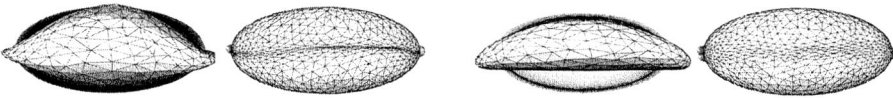

Fig. 6. Results banana. *Left:* TS registration with curvedness (1st level, result). *Right:* Combination of SDF and TS registration with curvedness (1st level, result)

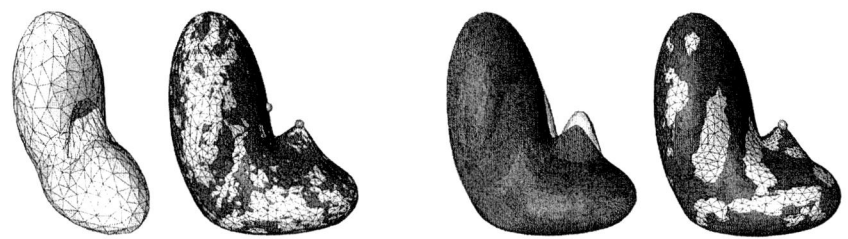

Fig. 7. Results two hills. *Left:* TS registration (1st level, result). *Right:* TS with normal deviation (1st level, result)

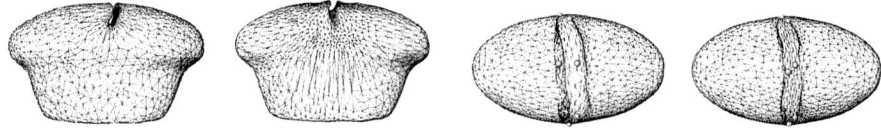

Fig. 8. Results muffin. *From left to right:* LF, SDF (surface distortion), TS registration (severe surface foldings), TS with normal deviation (improved matching)

with curvedness yields better results ($d_t = 2.8\%$), cf. Fig. 6 right. Neither shape index ($d_t = 47.8\%$) nor normal deviation ($d_t = 11.7\%$) lead to improvements.

Two Hills. Shape representation plays a crucial role in this example: SDF registration yields nearly perfect target point deviation of $d_t = 0.7\%$, whereas LF works satisfactorily only with a much larger initial search width ($d_t = 9.3\%$). TS registration leads to large mismatches with $d_t = 13.3\%$, which is improved by using normal deviation ($d_t = 1\%$) or shape index ($d_t = 1.3\%$), cf. Fig. 7. Curvedness performs better ($d_t = 0.7\%$) at the cost of enormous surface distortions; grid energy alleviates this. Both shape index and curvedness produce irregular deformations.

Muffin. Implicit representations require higher CPG resolution to accomplish a satisfactory target point deviation (LF: $d_t = 6.3\%$, SDF: $d_t = 7.9\%$). TS registration has larger target point deviation of $d_t = 8.4\%$, which is improved by considering normal deviation ($d_t = 5.8\%$); curvature measures yield no improvements. TS registration produces severe surface foldings, while SDF registration shows massive surface distortions (cf. Fig. 8). SDF registration will often fail in such cases, since deformations along the surface are ill-defined. Grid energy fails to alleviate this problem due to unacceptable matching quality.

The performance in terms of CPU time is – in all cases – best using LF or TS registration with one-sided surface distance. SDF representation is worse by a factor of 5, while symmetric TS registration increases the runtime by a factor of 20, due to the complexity of evaluating the two-sided surface distance.

3.2 Experiments: Anatomical Shapes

The optimization starts on a CPG of about 100 mm grid spacing, which is successively refined to 5 mm. For the LF representation an increased search width is employed. No geometric similarity measures are incorporated into the cost function, as this would require an extensive parameter study for the relative weights within the cost function.

Liver. The sample consists of 24 individuals. All shapes are registered to one target shape. Registration based on distance fields is always performed in combination with regularization to avoid distortions as present in the muffin example (cf. Fig. 8). The grid energy is applied adaptively on the last two levels of the optimization ($\lambda = 0.002/0.01$).

Anatomical mismatch is measured by the overlap d_o of corresponding anatomical regions (patches) of the liver. The surface distance is computed among corresponding patches only, and afterwards divided by D_s: the smaller d_o, the better the anatomical match. Although these regions cannot in general be specified uniquely, this measure is less sensitive to errors than individual landmark placement. The following regions were defined by medical experts (cf. Fig. 9): (1) lower left lobe, (2) lower right lobe plus caudate lobe, (3) lower quadratic lobe and (4) whole upper part of the liver. Cases of large anatomical mismatches (cf. Fig. 1) could be resolved by using landmark based boundary constraints. A typical result is shown in Fig. 9. Quantitative results are given in Tab. 1.

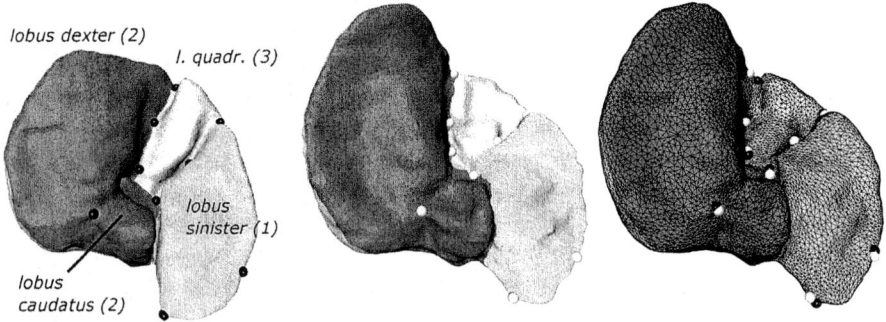

Fig. 9. SDF registration for the liver. Anatomically corresponding regions can be identified by their colour; target point locations indicate matching errors. *Left:* Template after affine registration. *Mid:* Target. *Right:* Resulting deformed template. The "valleys" of the template are not matched perfectly, yet the transformation remains regular; surface distortion is moderate, anatomical matching is satisfactory

Table 1. Results for registration of real patient data (GE grid energy). Maximum and median of surface distance over the whole set, as well as the mean percentage of surface distance above a threshold of 2 mm is given. Average CPU times refer to a SGI system with 500 MHz MIPS R14k processor. For liver data, a histogram of anatomical mismatch (log. scale) is provided

shape class	method	D_s [mm] max	D_s [mm] med	> 2[%] mean	CPUtime [hh:mm:ss]
liver	LF	0.71	0.49	4.73	00:42:45
	SDF GE	1.27	0.44	3.84	25:11:33
	TS	0.44	0.32	0.71	11:40:49
pelvic bone	LF	0.74	0.61	4.75	01:22:04
	SDF	0.83	0.45	1.98	03:10:09
	TS	0.38	0.34	0.33	31:35:24

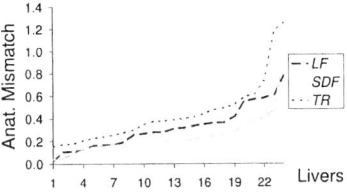

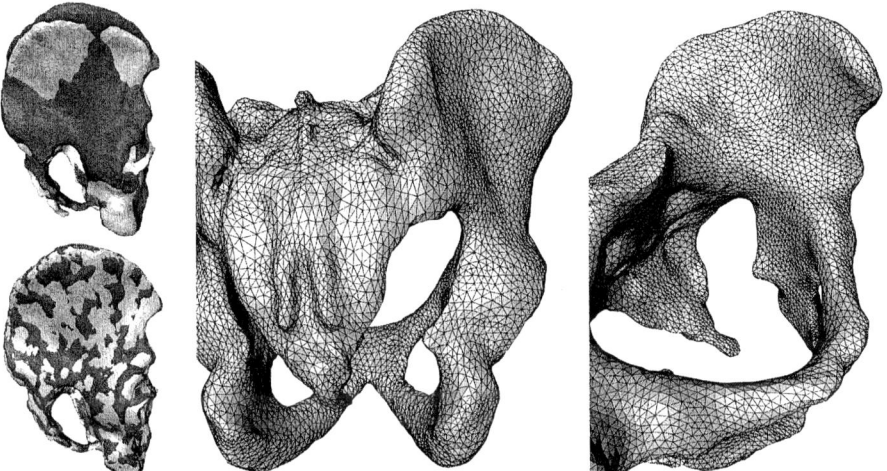

Fig. 10. SDF registration for pelvic bone. *Left:* Initial setting, result. *Mid, right:* Deformed template (with little surface distortion)

Pelvic Bone. The sample comprises 17 male individuals. The target shape is reconstructed from the male visible human data set. One exemplary result is shown in Fig. 10. Quantitative results over the whole sample are given in Tab. 1. The deformation map is fold-over free for all shape representations. Visual inspection shows virtually no anatomical mismatch in all cases apart from the LF registrations, where the variability of the bending of the sacrum is not captured correctly (only 6 correct results).

4 Discussion and Conclusion

We studied the ability of a registration framework based on B-spline transformations to capture intersubject shape variability. To this end we identified three different classes of typical deformations, which we represented by three different synthetic shapes. Moreover, two anatomical objects of different degrees of variability were examined. For our experiments we varied the essential components of the framework: shape representation, similarity measure and optimization strategy. The performance was measured in terms of surface distance between the deformed template and the target shape, regularity of the transformation $\mathbf{T}$, robustness and correspondence of landmark points or regions.

Optimization Strategies. The resolution of the CPG plays a crucial role. Although B-spline transformations are indeed capable of capturing large shape deviations, the control point spacing should be adapted to the frequency content of the shapes. This was shown by the banana/cigar example, where most of the deformation takes place around the cusps. Harmonic analysis of the shapes may be a suitable pre-processing step for building adaptive control grids.

Similarity Measures. Using the symmetric surface distance is very costly, yet may be needed in cases where deformations are large. Weighting the terms in the cost function is a difficult task, especially between surface distance and geometric features. Although it seems fairly clear for the synthetic shapes, which geometric similarity is feasable to use, one cannot deduce from this the correct cost function for the anatomical examples. Completely different cost functions may certainly be more suitable for other applications. We found that the grid energy as a regularizer often is too restrictive to recover large deformations. To prevent large surface distortions, yet obtain good matchings, regularizers constraining deformation in the tangential directions of the shapes rather than in the normal direction should be employed.

Shape Representations. Of all shape representations used the SDF approach performed best. Triangulation based registration often lead to irregular transformations, while label field registration yielded deficient matchings, both in terms of target point deviation for the synthetic shapes and of anatomical correspondence for the medical examples. This can be explained by the fact that distance fields contain more information than triangulated surfaces or label fields: the latter encode a single 2-dimensional manifold while distance fields contain a continuous set of manifolds by extending the surface into $\mathbb{R}^3$, which is beneficial in the optimization process.

Since the shape of anatomical structures is contained only implicitly in medical image data (e.g. MRI or CT), it is a-priori uncertain whether B-spline transformations represent the appropriate deformation model. The results of our experiments may serve as a guideline for assessing such intensity based registration tasks.

Future work will be directed towards combining SDF representations with different regularizers. Moreover, cost functions with different structures than the one used here should be explored. As a general rule, any a-priori anatomical knowledge available should be included to support intersubject registration.

Acknowledgements. We thank the developers of Amira [24], a software framework for advanced visual data analysis, that has been used for this work. Funding for T.H. Wenckebach and H. Lamecker has been provided by Deutsche Forschungsgemeinschaft (DFG) through the research center MATHEON.

References

1. Szeliski, R., Lavallée, S.: Matching 3-d anatomical surfaces with non-rigid deformations using octree-splines. IJCV **18(2)** (1996) 171–186
2. Rückert, D., Sonoda, L.I., Hayes, C., Hill, D.L.G., Leach, M.O., Hawkes, D.J.: Non-rigid registration using free-form deformations: Application to breast MR images. IEEE Trans Med Imaging **18(8)** (1999) 712-721
3. Rohlfing, T., Brandt, R., Maurer, C.R., Menzel, R.: Bee brains, B-splines and computational democracy: Generating an average shape atlas. Proc. IEEE Workshop on Mathematical Methods in Biomedical Image Analys (2001) 187–194
4. Kybic, J., Unser, M.: Fast parametric elastic image registration. IEEE Trans Med Imaging **12(11)** (2003) 1427-1441
5. Kabus, S., Netsch, T., Fischer, B., Modersitzki, J: B-spline registration of 3D images with Levenberg-Marquardt optimization. Proc. SPIE MI **5370** (2004) 304–313
6. Fleute, M., Lavallée, S., Julliard, R.: Incorporating a statistically based shape model into a system for computed-assisted anterior cruciate ligament surgery. MIA **3(3)** (1999) 209–222
7. Frangi, A.F., Rückert, D., Schnabel, J.A., Niessen, W.J.: Automatic 3D ASM construction via atlas-based landmarking and volumetric elastic registration. Proc. IPMI (2001) 78–79
8. Frangi, A.F., Rückert, D., Schnabel, J.A., Niessen, W.J.: Multiple-object three-dimensional shape models: Application to cardiac modeling. IEEE Trans Med Imaging **21(9)** (2002) 1151–1166
9. Brett, A.D., Taylor, C.J.: A method of automated landmark generation for automated 3D PDM construction. Imag Vis Comp **18(9)** (2000) 739-48
10. Besl, P.J., McKay, N.D.: A method for registration of 3-D shapes. IEEE Trans PAMI **14(2)** (1992) 239-256
11. Chui, H., Rangarajan, A.: A new point matching algorithm for non-rigid registration. CVIU **89(2–3)** (2003) 114–141
12. Xie, Z., Farin, G.: Image registration using hierarchical B-splines. IEEE Trans. on Visualization and Computer Graphics **10(1)** (2004) 85–94
13. Paulsen, R.R., Hilger, K.: Shape modelling using Markov random field restoration of point correspondences. Proc. IPMI (2003) 1–12
14. Subsol, G., Thirion, J.-P., Ayache, N.: A scheme for automatically building three-dimensional morphometric anatomical atlases: Application to skull atlas. MIA **2(1)** (1998) 37–60
15. Rusinkiewicz, S., Levoy, M.: Efficient variants of the ICP algorithm. Proc. of Third International Conference on 3D Digital Imaging and Modelling (2001) 145–152
16. Sharp, G.C., Lee, S.W., Wehe, D.K.: ICP registration using invariant features. IEEE Trans PAMI **24(1)** (2002) 90–102
17. Wang, Y., Peterson, B.S., Staib, L.H.: Shape-based 3D surface correspondence using geodesics and local geometry. Proc. CVPR (2000) 644–651
18. Kelemen, A., Székely, G., Gerig, G.: Three-dimensional model-based segmentation of brain MRI. IEEE Trans Med Imaging **18(10)** (1999) 828–839

19. Davies, R.H., Twining, C.J., Cootes, T.F., Waterton, J.C., Taylor, C.J.: 3D statistical shape models using direct optimisation of description length. Proc. 7th ECCV **3** (2002) 3–20
20. Lamecker, H., Lange, T., Seebaß, M.: A statistical shape model for the liver. Proc. MICCAI (2002) 422–427
21. Borgefors, G.: Distance transformations in digital images. Computer Vision, Graphics, and Image Processing **34** (1986) 344-371
22. Rohlfing, T.: Multimodale Datenfusion für die bildgesteuerte Neurochirurgie und Strahlentherapie. PhD thesis, Technische Universität Berlin (2000)
23. Koenderink, J.J., van Doorn, A.J.: Surface shape and curvature scales. IVC **10(8)** (1992) 557–565
24. Stalling, D., Westerhoff, M., Hege, H.-C.: Amira: A highly interactive system for visual data analysis. In: Hansen, C.D., Johnson C.R. (eds.): The Visualization Handbook (2005) 749–767

A Riemannian Approach to Diffusion Tensor Images Segmentation

Christophe Lenglet[1], Mikaël Rousson[2], Rachid Deriche[1], Olivier Faugeras[1],
Stéphane Lehericy[3], and Kamil Ugurbil[3]

[1] I.N.R.I.A, 2004 route des lucioles, 06902 Sophia-Antipolis, France
{clenglet, der, faugeras}@sophia.inria.fr
[2] Siemens Corporate Research, 755 College Road East, Princeton, NJ 08540, USA
rousson@scr.siemens.com
[3] CMRR, University of Minnesota, 2021 6th Street SE, Minneapolis, MN 55455, USA
{lehericy, kamil}@cmrr.umn.edu

Abstract. We address the problem of the segmentation of cerebral white matter structures from diffusion tensor images. Our approach is grounded on the theoretically well-founded differential geometrical properties of the space of multivariate normal distributions. We introduce a variational formulation, in the level set framework, to estimate the optimal segmentation according to the following hypothesis: Diffusion tensors exhibit a Gaussian distribution in the different partitions. Moreover, we must respect the geometric constraints imposed by the interfaces existing among the cerebral structures and detected by the gradient of the diffusion tensor image. We validate our algorithm on synthetic data and report interesting results on real datasets. We focus on two structures of the white matter with different properties and respectively known as the corpus callosum and the corticospinal tract.

1 Introduction

Diffusion magnetic resonance imaging is a relatively new modality [1] able to quantify the anisotropic diffusion of water molecules in highly structured biological tissues. As of today, it is the only non-invasive method that allows us to distinguish the anatomical structures of the cerebral white matter. Diffusion tensor imaging [2] models the probability density function of the three-dimensional molecular motion, at each voxel of a diffusion MR image, by a normal distribution of 0-mean and whose covariance matrix is given by the diffusion tensor. Numerous algorithms have been proposed to perform a robust estimation of this tensor field (see [3] and references therein). Among other applications, DTI is extremely useful in order to identify the neural connectivity patterns of the human brain [4], [5], [6]. Most of the existing techniques addressing this last issue work on a fiber-wise basis. In other words, they do not take into account the global coherence that exists among fibers of a given tract. Recent work by Corouge et al. [7] has proposed to cluster and align fibers by local shape parameterization so that a statistical analysis of the tract geometrical and physiological properties can be carried out. This work relies on the extraction of a set of streamlines by the method proposed in [4] which is known to be sensible to noise and unreliable in areas of fiber crossings. For these reasons, we propose to directly perform the segmentation of diffusion tensor images in order to extract neural fiber bundles. To our knowledge, the only approaches addressing the issue of white matter internal structures segmentation are [8], [9], [10], [11], [12], [13], [14] and [15]

We hereafter draw a quick state of the art of these techniques. Zhukov et al. [8] define an invariant anisotropy measure in order to drive the evolution of a level set and isolate strongly anisotropic regions of the brain. Alternatively, Wiegell et al. [9], Feddern et al. [10], Rousson et al. [11], Wang et al. [12] and [13], Lenglet et al. [14], and Jonasson et al. [15] use or propose different measures of dissimilarity between full diffusion tensors. In [9], [12] and [11], the authors use the Frobenius norm of the difference of tensors. A spatial coherence or a regularity term was used in the first two methods, respectively in a k-means algorithm or an active contour model to perform the segmentation of different cerebral structures such as the thalamus nuclei or the corpus callosum. The third method used a region-based surface propagation. In [12], a generalization of the region-based active contours to matrix-valued images is proposed. It is consequently restricted to the 2D case. In [10], partial differential equations based on mean curvature motion, self-snakes and geodesic active contour models are extended to two-dimensional and three-dimensional tensor-valued images. This method still relies on the Euclidean metric between tensors. The authors apply this framework to the regularization and segmentation of diffusion tensor images. In [15], the authors introduce a geometric measure of dissimilarity by computing the normalized tensor scalar product of two tensors, which can be interpreted as a measure of overlap. Finally, the methods exposed in [13] and [14] rely on the symmetrized Kullback-Leibler divergence to derive an affine invariant dissimilarity measure between diffusion tensors.

Contribution: Our main contributions are threefold: First, the major difference with all the existing approaches is the rigorous differential geometrical framework, strongly rooted in the information geometry and used to express a Gaussian law between diffusion tensors. We overcome the classical hypothesis considering covariance matrices as a linear space. Hence, we define relevant statistics to model the distribution of diffusion tensors. We also use a consistent gradient of the tensor field to detect the boundaries of various structures in the white matter. We then propose a variational formulation of the segmentation problem, in the level set framework, to evolve a surface toward the optimal partition of the data. We finally validate our approach on synthetic and real datasets.

Organization of the Paper: Section 2 first reviews necessary material related to the Riemannian geometry of the multivariate normal model. It then introduces the numerical schemes used to approximate a Gaussian law for diffusion tensors. We finally describe how to compute the gradient of a tensor field. Section 3 sets up the Bayesian formulation of the segmentation problem that we use throughout this paper. Section 4 presents and discusses experimental results on synthetic and real DTI datasets.

2 Statistics and Geometry of Diffusion Tensors Fields

As in [16], we can consider the family of three-dimensional normal distributions with 0-mean as the 6-dimensional parameter space of variances-covariances $\mathcal{M} = \{\theta : \theta = (\theta_1, ..., \theta_6) \in \mathbb{R}^6\}$. This simply translates the fact that, for diffusion MRI, the average displacement of spins in a voxel is zero. We identify $\mathcal{M}$ with $S^+(3, \mathbb{R})$, the set of 3×3 real symmetric positive-definite matrices, e.g. covariance matrices whose independent components are denoted by θ_i.

Following the work by Rao [17] and Burbea-Rao [18], where a Riemannian metric was introduced in term of the Fisher information matrix, it is possible to define notions such as the geodesic distance, the curvature, the mean, and the covariance matrix. The basis of the tangent space $T_\Sigma S^+(3, \mathbb{R}) = S_\Sigma(3, \mathbb{R})$ at $\Sigma \in S^+(3, \mathbb{R})$ is taken to be as in [19] and denoted by E_i, $i = 1, ..., 6$.

We now detail the geometry of $S^+(3, \mathbb{R})$ and propose an original formulation for a generalized Gaussian law on this manifold. Relying on the explicit, and very simple, expression of the squared geodesic distance gradient, we show how to compute the spatial gradient of a diffusion tensor image.

2.1 Differential Geometry of Multivariate Normal Distributions

The fundamental mathematical tools needed to derive our numerical schemes were detailed in [19], [20], [21], [22], [23] and [24]. Without employing the information geometry associated to the Fisher information matrix but instead, identifying $S^+(3, \mathbb{R})$ with the quotient space $GL^+(3, \mathbb{R})/SO(3, \mathbb{R})$, other works such as [25] and [26] recently used similar ideas to derive statistical or filtering tools on tensors fields.

Metric Tensor, Geodesics and Geodesic Distance: The metric tensor for $S^+(3, \mathbb{R})$, derived from the Fisher information matrix is given by the following theorem:

Theorem 1. *The Riemannian metric for the space $S^+(3, \mathbb{R})$ of multivariate normal distributions with zero mean is given, $\forall \Sigma \in S^+(3, \mathbb{R})$ by:*

$$g_{ij} = g(E_i, E_j) = \langle E_i, E_j \rangle_\Sigma = \frac{1}{2}\mathrm{tr}(\Sigma^{-1} E_i \Sigma^{-1} E_j) \quad i,j = 1, ..., 6 \quad (1)$$

In practice, this means that for any tangent vectors A, B, their inner product relative to Σ is $\langle A, B \rangle_\Sigma = \frac{1}{2}\mathrm{tr}(\Sigma^{-1} A \Sigma^{-1} B)$.

We recall that, if $\Sigma : t \mapsto \Sigma(t) \in S^+(3, \mathbb{R})$, $\forall t \in [t_1, t_2] \subset \mathbb{R}$ denotes a curve segment in $S^+(3, \mathbb{R})$ between two normal distributions parameterized by Σ_1 and Σ_2, its length is expressed as: $\mathcal{L}_\Sigma(\Sigma_1, \Sigma_2) = \int_{t_1}^{t_2} \left(\sum_{i,j=1}^{6} g_{ij}(\Sigma(t)) \frac{d\theta_i(t)}{dt} \frac{d\theta_j(t)}{dt} \right)^{1/2} dt$
As stated for example in [24], the geodesic starting from $\Sigma(t_1) \in S^+(3, \mathbb{R})$ in the

direction $V = \dot{\Sigma}(t_1) \in S(3,\mathbb{R})$ is given by:

$$\Sigma(t) = \Sigma(t_1)^{1/2} \exp\left(t\Sigma(t_1)^{-1/2} V \Sigma(t_1)^{-1/2}\right) \Sigma(t_1)^{1/2} \; \forall t \in [t_1, t_2] \quad (2)$$

We recall that the geodesic distance $\mathcal{D}$ between any two element Σ_1 and Σ_2 is the length of the minimizing geodesic between Σ_1 and Σ_2:

$$\mathcal{D}(\Sigma_1, \Sigma_2) = \inf_{\Sigma} \{\mathcal{L}_\Sigma(\Sigma_1, \Sigma_2) : \Sigma_1 = \Sigma(t_1), \Sigma_2 = \Sigma(t_2)\}$$

It is given by the following theorem, whose original proof is available in an appendix of [27] but different versions can also be found in [19] and [23].

Theorem 2. *(S.T. Jensen, 1976)*
Consider the family of multivariate normal distributions with common mean vector but different covariance matrices. The geodesic distance between two members of the family with covariance matrices Σ_1 and Σ_2 is given by

$$\mathcal{D}(\Sigma_1, \Sigma_2) = \sqrt{\frac{1}{2}\mathrm{tr}(\log^2(\Sigma_1^{-1/2}\Sigma_2\Sigma_1^{-1/2}))} = \sqrt{\frac{1}{2}\sum_{i=1}^{m}\log^2(\eta_i)}$$

where η_i denote the m eigenvalues of the matrix $\Sigma_1^{-1/2}\Sigma_2\Sigma_1^{-1/2}$.

2.2 A Gaussian Distribution for Diffusion Tensors

We now show how to compute the empirical mean [28], [29] and the empirical covariance matrix on $S^+(3,\mathbb{R})$ to define a Gaussian law on that manifold.

Intrinsic Mean:

Definition 1. *The normal distribution parameterized by $\overline{\Sigma} \in S^+(3,\mathbb{R})$ and defined as the empirical mean of N distributions Σ_k, $k = 1,...,N$, achieves the minimum of the sum of squared distances $\mu : S^+(3,\mathbb{R}) \to \mathbb{R}^+$ defined by*

$$\mu(\Sigma, \Sigma_1, ..., \Sigma_N) = \frac{1}{N}\sum_{k=1}^{N}\mathcal{D}^2(\Sigma_k, \Sigma)$$

Karcher proved in [28] that such a mean, known as the Riemannian barycenter, exists and is unique for manifolds of non-positive sectional curvature. This was shown to be the case for $S^+(3,\mathbb{R})$ in [19]. A closed-form expression of the mean cannot be obtained [24] but a gradient descent algorithm was proposed in [16]. A flow is derived from an initial guess $\overline{\Sigma}_0$ toward the mean of a subset of $S^+(3,\mathbb{R})$:

$$\overline{\Sigma}_{t+1} = \overline{\Sigma}_t^{1/2} \exp\left(-\frac{dt}{N}\overline{\Sigma}_t^{1/2}\left(\sum_{k=1}^{N}\log(\Sigma_k^{-1}\overline{\Sigma}_t)\right)\overline{\Sigma}_t^{-1/2}\right)\overline{\Sigma}_t^{1/2} \quad (3)$$

Intrinsic Covariance Matrix: Based on the explicit solution of the geodesic distance, we can compute $\Lambda \in S^+(6,\mathbb{R})$, the empirical covariance matrix relative to the mean $\overline{\Sigma}$ of N elements of $S^+(3,\mathbb{R})$. As in [30], we associate to Σ_k the unique tangent vector $\beta_k \in S(3,\mathbb{R})$, seen as an element of $\mathbb{R}^6$ and identified with the gradient of the squared geodesic distance function $\beta_k = \nabla \mathcal{D}^2(\Sigma_k, \overline{\Sigma}) = \overline{\Sigma} \log\left(\Sigma_k^{-1}\overline{\Sigma}\right)$ [24]. It follows:

Definition 2. *Given N elements of $S^+(3,\mathbb{R})$ and their mean value $\overline{\Sigma}$, the empirical covariance matrix relative to $\overline{\Sigma}$ is defined as:* $\Lambda = \frac{1}{N-1}\sum_{k=1}^{N}\beta_k\beta_k^T$

Generalized Gaussian Distribution on $S^+(3,\mathbb{R})$: The notion of Gaussian law was generalized to random samples of primitives belonging to a Riemannian manifold in [29]. Following theorem 4 therein:

Theorem 3. *The generalized Gaussian distribution in $S^+(3,\mathbb{R})$ for a covariance matrix Λ of small variance $\sigma^2 = \text{tr}(\Lambda)$ is of the form:*

$$p(\Sigma|\overline{\Sigma},\Lambda) = \frac{1+O(\sigma^3)+\epsilon(\frac{\sigma}{\xi})}{\sqrt{(2\pi)^6|\Lambda|}} \exp\frac{-\beta^T\gamma\beta}{2} \quad \forall \Sigma \in S^+(3,\mathbb{R})$$

β *is defined as* $\nabla\mathcal{D}^2(\Sigma,\overline{\Sigma})$ *and expressed in vector form. The concentration matrix is* $\gamma = \Lambda^{-1} - \mathcal{R}/3 + O(\sigma) + \epsilon(\frac{\sigma}{\xi})$, *with $\mathcal{R}$ the Ricci tensor at the mean $\overline{\Sigma}$. ξ is the injectivity radius at $\overline{\Sigma}$ and ϵ is such that $\lim_{0+} r^{-\omega}\epsilon(r) = 0 \,\forall \omega \in \mathbb{R}^+$.*

In section 3, we will use our estimates of $\overline{\Sigma}$ and Λ together with the above theorem to evaluate the probability of a diffusion tensor to belong to a given subset of the diffusion tensor image. The computation of $\mathcal{R}$ is performed on the basis of closed-form expressions for the metric and the Riemann tensor [19],[16].

2.3 Gradient of a Diffusion Tensor Image

We end this section with the definition of the gradient of a tensor field. From now on $\Sigma : \Omega \subset \mathbb{R}^3 \mapsto S^+(3,\mathbb{R})$ denotes the diffusion tensor image such that $\Sigma(x)$ is a diffusion tensor for all $x \in \Omega$. The spatial gradient of Σ can be estimated from the intrinsic gradient of the squared geodesic distance:

$$\nabla^{\pm}_{k=1,2,3}\Sigma(x) \simeq \frac{1}{|e_k|}\nabla\mathcal{D}^2\left(\Sigma(x \pm e_k), \Sigma(x)\right) = \frac{1}{|e_k|}\Sigma(x)\log\left(\Sigma(x \pm e_k)^{-1}\Sigma(x)\right)$$

where the e_k are the elements of the canonical basis of $\mathbb{R}^3$ and are used to access the neighbors of $\Sigma(x)$ on the discrete grid. The $+$ and $-$ respectively denote the forward and backward finite differences. We make use of central finite differences so that the gradient in the direction e_k (we recall that it is a symmetric matrix) is given by: $\nabla_k\Sigma(x) \simeq \frac{1}{2}\left(\nabla_k^+\Sigma(x) - \nabla_k^-\Sigma(x)\right)$. It is then straightforward to obtain the norm of the gradient as:

$$|\nabla\Sigma(x)|^2 = \sum_{k=1}^{3}|\nabla_k\Sigma(x)|^2_{\Sigma(x)} = \frac{1}{2}\sum_{k=1}^{3}\text{tr}\left(\left(\Sigma(x)^{-1}\nabla_k\Sigma(x)\right)^2\right)$$

We will use this information in section 3 to localize the boundaries between structures of the brain white matter.

3 Segmentation by Surface Evolution

Our goal is to compute the optimal 3D surface separating an anatomical structure of interest from the rest of a diffusion MRI dataset. The statistical surface evolution, as developed in [31], is a well-suited framework for our segmentation problem. We hereafter summarize the basic notions of this technique.

3.1 Bayesian Formulation for Image Partitioning

Following general works on image segmentation [32],[33], [34], we seek the optimal partition of the image domain Ω by maximizing the *a posteriori* frame partition probability $p(\mathcal{P}(\Omega) \,|\, \Sigma)$ for the observed diffusion tensor image Σ. The Bayes rule allows to express this probability as:

$$p(\mathcal{P}(\Omega) \,|\, \Sigma) \propto p(\Sigma \,|\, \mathcal{P}(\Omega)) p(\mathcal{P}(\Omega)). \tag{4}$$

This formulation yields a separation of the image-based cues from the geometric properties of the boundary given by $\mathcal{P}(\Omega)$. While being valid for any number of regions, we restrict this formulation to binary partitions: the structure of interest and the background. The image partition can be represented as the zero-crossing of a level set function ϕ [35],[36]. Noting $\mathcal{B}$ the interface between the two regions Ω_{in} and Ω_{out}, ϕ is constructed as the signed distance function to $\mathcal{B}$:

$$\begin{cases} \phi(x) = 0, & \text{if } x \in \mathcal{B} \\ \phi(x) = \mathcal{D}_{Eucl}(x, \mathcal{B}), & \text{if } x \in \Omega_{in} \\ \phi(x) = -\mathcal{D}_{Eucl}(x, \mathcal{B}), & \text{if } x \in \Omega_{out}, \end{cases}$$

where $\mathcal{D}_{Eucl}(x, \mathcal{B})$ stands for the Euclidean distance between x and $\mathcal{B}$. Hence, the optimal partition is obtained by maximizing: $p(\phi|\Sigma) \propto p(\Sigma|\phi) p(\phi)$. At this stage, these two terms still need to be defined. For this purpose, several assumptions on the structure of interest need to be introduced. In the following, a smoothness constraint is imposed with the term $p(\phi)$ while $p(\Sigma|\phi)$ expresses the likelihood of the diffusion tensors to be inside, outside or on the boundary of the structure. This yields an optimization criterion similar to the *Geodesic Active Regions* presented in [34].

3.2 Smoothness Constraint

The second term of (4) expresses the probability of the interface to represent the structure of interest and can be used to introduce prior shape knowledge. For the segmentation of diffusion tensor images, we have no high level prior information but we can use this term to impose shape regularity. Such a constraint can be obtained by favoring structures with a smaller surface $|\mathcal{B}|$ with $p(\phi) \propto \exp(-\nu|\mathcal{B}|)$. This can be expressed with ϕ by introducing the Dirac function [37]:

$$p(\phi) \propto \exp\left(-\nu \int_\Omega \delta(\phi) |\nabla \phi(x)| \, dx\right). \tag{5}$$

3.3 Data Term

To further specify the image term $p(\Sigma|\phi)$, we introduce several hypothesis. First, for a given level set ϕ, we can classify the voxels into three classes: inside, outside or on the boundary. Then, we can define the probability density functions of a diffusion tensor for each class: p_{in}, p_{out} and p_b. Assuming the diffusion tensors to be independent and identically distributed realizations of the corresponding random process, the data term is given by:

$$p(\Sigma|\phi) = \prod_{x\in\Omega_{in}} p_{in}(\Sigma(x)) \cdot \prod_{x\in\Omega_{out}} p_{out}(\Sigma(x)) \cdot \prod_{x\in\mathcal{B}} p_b(\Sigma(x)) \quad (6)$$

This gives two types of probability distributions: region-based with $p_{in/out}$ and boundary-based with p_b. p_{in} and p_{out} are given by the generalized Gaussian distribution of Theorem 3. The parameters of these laws may be known a priori but in the absence of such information, they are introduced as unknown parameters. Regarding p_b, the probability should be close to one for high gradients of the diffusion tensors field and around zero for small variations. This leads to:

$$p_b(\Sigma(x)) \propto \exp\left(-g_\alpha\left(|\nabla\Sigma(x)|\right)\right),$$

with $g_\alpha(u) = 1/(\epsilon+u^\alpha)$. This boundary term is the basis of several works referred to as active contours [38] and, often, $\alpha = 1$ or 2 is chosen while ϵ is set to a small constant. For the sake of readability, we will use the notation $g_\alpha(\Sigma(x))$.

3.4 Energy Formulation

Maximizing the *a posteriori* segmentation probability is equivalent to minimizing its negative logarithm. Integrating the regularity constraint (5) and the image term (6), we end up with the following energy:

$$E(\phi, \overline{\Sigma}_{in/out}, \Lambda_{in/out}) = \nu \int_\Omega \delta(\phi)|\nabla\phi|\, dx + \int_\Omega \delta(\phi)|\nabla\phi|g_\alpha(\Sigma(x))\, dx$$
$$- \int_{\Omega_{in}} \log p(\Sigma(x)|\overline{\Sigma}_{in}, \Lambda_{in})dx - \int_{\Omega_{out}} \log p(\Sigma(x)|\overline{\Sigma}_{out}, \Lambda_{out})dx.$$

The boundary term of this energy corresponds to the Geodesic Active Contours [38] and naturally includes a regularization[1] on the interface. Following [39], [40], an alternate minimization is employed to perform the optimization for the two types of unknown parameters. For given statistical parameters, the Euler-Lagrange equations are computed to derive the implicit front evolution:

$$\frac{\partial\phi}{\partial t} = \delta(\phi)\left((\nu + g_\alpha(\Sigma))\operatorname{div}\left(\frac{\nabla\phi}{|\nabla\phi|}\right) + \frac{\nabla\phi}{|\nabla\phi|}\cdot\nabla g_\alpha(\Sigma) + \log\frac{p(\Sigma|\overline{\Sigma}_{in},\Lambda_{in})}{p(\Sigma|\overline{\Sigma}_{out},\Lambda_{out})}\right), \quad (7)$$

while the statistics can be updated after each evolution of ϕ from their empirical estimates, as described in section 2. More details on this optimization can be found in [36], [40].

---

[1] The regularity term (5) could be included in p_b by replacing g_α by $g_{\alpha,\nu} = \nu + g_\alpha$.

4 Results and Validation

4.1 Experimental Setup

In practice, there is a few important points that must be carefully taken care of when implementing and running our segmentation algorithm: When dealing with real DTI data, we use a mask of the brain so that the tensors statistics of Ω_{out} are not corrupted by the signal from the outside of the brain. With regard to the initialization of the algorithm, we always take one to three small spheres of radius 2 voxels placed inside the structure that we seek to segment.

Next, there are two parameters that have to be chosen: The first one is the value of ν in equation 5. It constrains the smoothness of the surface and is usually set in the range 5 to 10. The second parameter arises from the hypothesis of theorem 3 regarding the trace of the covariance matrix Λ. This quantity must be small for the generalized Gaussian law to hold. In other words, this means that we restrict ourselves to concentrated distributions. Hence, we set a threshold for the variance which, whenever reached, induces the end of the update for the statistical parameters. We let the surface evolve while using a fixed mean and covariance matrix to model the distribution of the tensors in $\Omega_{in/out}$.

Finally, we were able to improve the computational efficiency of the method by noticing and verifying that, within the limits of theorem 3, the term involving the Ricci tensor $\mathcal{R}/3$ can be neglected. We found a difference of at least 2 orders of magnitude between Λ^{-1} and $\mathcal{R}/3$.

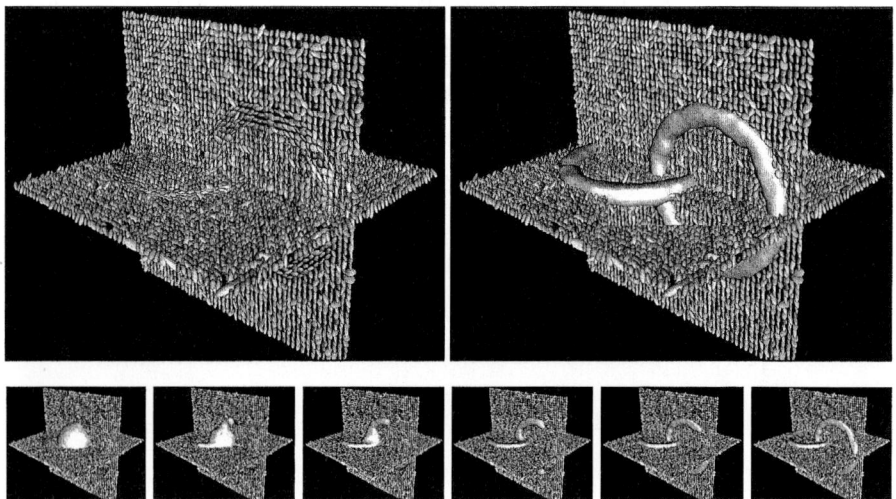

Fig. 1. Segmentation of 2 tori in a noisy synthetic tensor field: [TOP LEFT] Initial data [TOP RIGHT] Final segmentation [BOTTOM] Surface evolution

A Riemannian Approach to Diffusion Tensor Images Segmentation

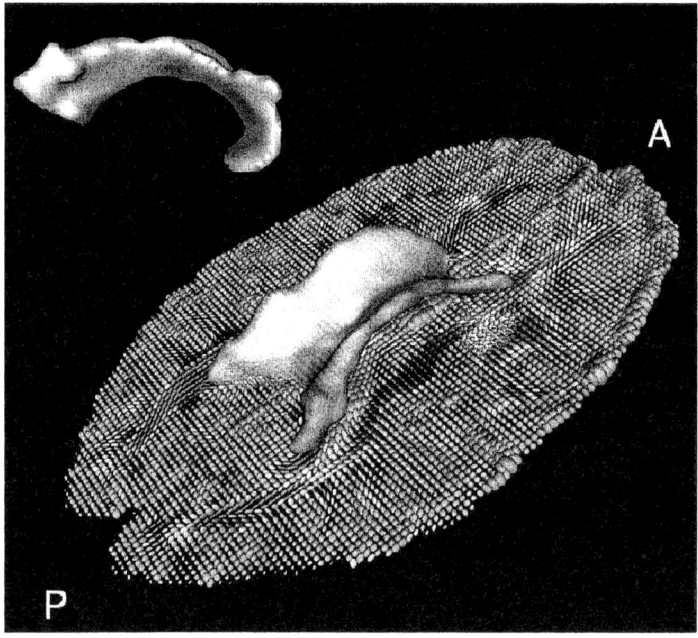

Fig. 2. Segmentation of the corpus callosum (A: anterior, P: posterior)

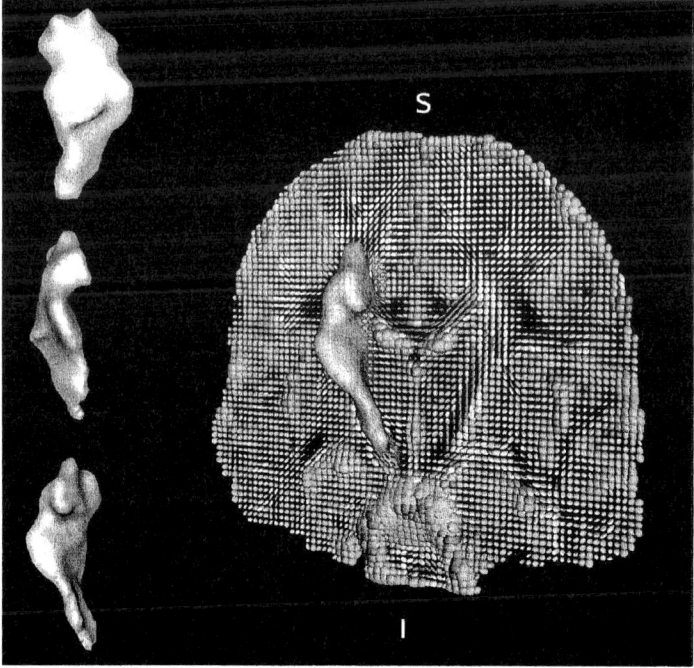

Fig. 3. Segmentation of the left corticospinal tract (I: inferior, S: superior)

4.2 Synthetic Data

In order to validate the algorithm on data for which ground truth is available, we have generated a $50 \times 50 \times 50$ synthetic tensor field composed of a background with a privileged orientation and 2 tori whose internal tensors are oriented according to the tangential direction of the principal circle of the tori. Eigenvectors and eigenvalues of the tensors are independently corrupted by Gaussian noise (figure 1). Despite the large orientational variation and the fairly high level of noise, our method is able to correctly extract the structures for different initializations.

4.3 Real Data

Diffusion weighted images were acquired on a 3 Tesla Siemens Magnetom Trio whole-body scanner. We used 12 gradients directions with a b-factor of $1000s/mm^2$, $TR = 9.2s$ and $TE = 92ms$. Voxel size is $2 \times 2 \times 2mm$.

The corpus callosum is a very important part of the brain that connects areas of each hemisphere together. By initializing our segmentation with only 2 small spheres within this structure, we managed to extract the volume presented on figure 2. Finally, we focused on a different part of the white matter, known as the internal capsule. Mainly oriented in the inferior-superior direction, the posterior part of this fiber bundle includes the corticospinal tract for which we present, on figure 3, the result of the segmentation obtained with our method. We also tested, on this particular example, the overall influence of the boundary term p_b. It turns out that, as expected, if we do not use this term in the energy, the resulting segmentation incorporates undesired regions of the brain such as the anterior and posterior parts of the corona radiata. This shows that the interface detection part of our method does play an important role to discriminate relevant structures. Visual inspection of the results obtained on several datasets and comparison with neuroanatomical knowledge validated the proposed segmentations.

5 Conclusion

We have presented a novel statistical and geometric approach to the segmentation of diffusion tensor images seen as fields of multivariate normal distributions. We focused on the differential geometrical properties of the space of normal distributions to derive a generalized Gaussian law on that manifold. This allowed us to model the distribution of a subset of diffusion tensors. Together with a constraint on the variations of the tensor field, we have embedded this information in a statistical surface evolution framework to perform the segmentation of inner structures of the cerebral white matter. This method achieved very good results on synthetic data and was able to capture fine details in real DTI datasets.

Acknowledgments. This work was supported by grants NSF-0404617 US-France (INRIA) Cooperative Research, NIH-R21-RR019771, NIH-RR08079, the MIND Institute and the Keck foundation.

References

1. Le Bihan, D., Breton, E., Lallemand, D., Grenier, P., Cabanis, E., Laval-Jeantet, M.: MR imaging of intravoxel incoherent motions: Application to diffusion and perfusion in neurologic disorders. Radiology (1986) 401–407
2. Basser, P., Mattiello, J., Le Bihan, D.: MR diffusion tensor spectroscopy and imaging. Biophysica (1994) 259–267
3. Tschumperlé D., Deriche, R.: Variational frameworks for DT-MRI estimation, regularization and visualization. In: Proc. ICCV (2003) 116–122
4. Mori, S., Crain, B., Chacko, V., Zijl, P.V.: Three-dimensional tracking of axonal projections in the brain by magnetic resonance imaging. Annals of Neurology 45 (1999) 265–269
5. Behrens, T., Johansen-Berg, H., Woolrich, M., Smith, S., Wheeler-Kingshott, C., Boulby, P., Barker, G., Sillery, E., Sheehan, K., Ciccarelli, O., Thompson, A., Brady, J., Matthews, P.: Non-invasive mapping of connections between human thalamus and cortex using diffusion imaging. Nat. Neuroscience 6 (2003) 750–757
6. Lenglet, C., Deriche, R., Faugeras, O.: Inferring white matter geometry from diffusion tensor MRI: Application to connectivity mapping. In: Proc. ECCV (2004) 127–140
7. Corouge, I., Gouttard, S., Gerig, G.: A statistical shape model of individual fiber tracts extracted from diffusion tensor MRI. In: Proc. MICCAI (2004) 671–679
8. Zhukov, L., Museth, K., Breen, D., Whitaker, R., Barr, A.: Level set segmentation and modeling of DT-MRI human brain data. Journal of Electronic Imaging 12:1 (2003) 125–133
9. Wiegell, M., Tuch, D., Larson, H., Wedeen, V.: Automatic segmentation of thalamic nuclei from diffusion tensor magnetic resonance imaging. NeuroImage 19 (2003) 391–402
10. Feddern, C., Weickert, J., Burgeth, B., Welk, M.: Curvature-driven PDE methods for matrix-valued images. Technical Report 104, Department of Mathematics, Saarland University, Saarbrücken, Germany (2004)
11. Rousson, M., Lenglet, C., Deriche, R.: Level set and region based surface propagation for diffusion tensor MRI segmentation. In: Proc. Computer Vision Approaches to Medical Image Analysis, ECCV Workshop (2004) 123–134
12. Wang, Z., Vemuri, B.: Tensor field segmentation using region based active contour model. In: Proc. ECCV (2004) 304–315
13. Wang, Z., Vemuri, B.: An affine invariant tensor dissimilarity measure and its application to tensor-valued image segmentation. In: Proc. CVPR (2004) 228–233
14. Lenglet, C., Rousson, M., Deriche, R.: Segmentation of 3D probability density fields by surface evolution: Application to diffusion MRI. In: Proc. MICCAI (2004) 18–25
15. Jonasson, L., Bresson, X., Hagmann, P., Cuisenaire, O., Meuli, R., Thiran, J.: White matter fiber tract segmentation in DT-MRI using geometric flows. Medical Image Analysis (2004) In press.
16. Lenglet, C., Rousson, M., Deriche, R., Faugeras, O.: Statistics on multivariate normal distributions: A geometric approach and its application to diffusion tensor MRI. Research Report 5242, INRIA (2004)
17. Rao, C.: Information and accuracy attainable in the estimation of statistical parameters. Bull. Calcutta Math. Soc. 37 (1945) 81–91
18. Burbea, J., Rao, C.: Entropy differential metric, distance and divergence measures in probability spaces: A unified approach. Journal of Multivariate Analysis 12 (1982) 575–596

19. Skovgaard, L.: A Riemannian geometry of the multivariate normal model. Technical Report 81/3, Statistical Research Unit, Danish Medical Research Council, Danish Social Science Research Council (1981)
20. Burbea, J.: Informative geometry of probability spaces. Expositiones Mathematica **4** (1986) 347–378
21. Eriksen, P.: Geodesics connected with the fisher metric on the multivariate manifold. Technical Report 86-13, Inst. of Elec. Systems, Aalborg University (1986)
22. Calvo, M., Oller, J.: An explicit solution of information geodesic equations for the multivariate normal model. Statistics and Decisions **9** (1991) 119–138
23. Förstner, W., Moonen, B.: A metric for covariance matrices. Technical report, Stuttgart University, Dept. of Geodesy and Geoinformatics (1999)
24. Moakher, M.: A differential geometric approach to the geometric mean of symmetric positive-definite matrices. SIAM J. Matrix Anal. Appl. **26:3** (2005) 735–747
25. Fletcher, P., Joshi, S.: Principal geodesic analysis on symmetric spaces: Statistics of diffusion tensors. In: Proc. Computer Vision Approaches to Medical Image Analysis, ECCV Workshop (2004) 87–98
26. Pennec, X., Fillard, P., Ayache, N.: A Riemannian framework for tensor computing. Research Report 5255, INRIA (2004)
27. Atkinson, C., Mitchell, A.: Rao's distance measure. Sankhya: The Indian Journal of Stats. **43** (1981) 345–365
28. Karcher, H.: Riemannian centre of mass and mollifier smoothing. Comm. Pure Appl. Math **30** (1977) 509–541
29. Pennec, X.: Probabilities and statistics on Riemannian manifolds: A geometric approach. Research Report 5093, INRIA (2004)
30. Charpiat, G., Faugeras, O., Keriven, R.: Approximations of shape metrics and application to shape warping and shape statistics. Research Report 4820, INRIA (2003)
31. Rousson, M.: Cues integrations and front evolutions in image segmentation. PhD thesis, Université de Nice-Sophia Antipolis (2004)
32. Leclerc, Y.: Constructing simple stable description for image partitioning. International Journal of Computer Vision **3** (1989) 73–102
33. Zhu, S., Yuille, A.: Region competition: Unifying snakes, region growing, and Bayes/MDL for multiband image segmentation. IEEE Transactions on Pattern Analysis and Machine Intelligence **18** (1996) 884–900
34. Paragios, N., Deriche, R.: Geodesic active regions: a new paradigm to deal with frame partition problems in computer vision. Journal of Visual Communication and Image Representation **13** (2002) 249–268
35. Osher, S., Sethian, J.: Fronts propagating with curvature dependent speed: Algorithms based on the Hamilton-Jacobi formulation. Journal of Computational Physics **79** (1988) 12–49
36. Chan, T., Vese, L.: Active contours without edges. IEEE Transactions on Image Processing **10** (2001) 266–277
37. Zhao, H., Chan, T., Merriman, B., Osher, S.: A variational level set approach to multiphase motion. Journal of Computational Physics **127** (1996) 179–195
38. Caselles, V., Kimmel, R., Sapiro, G.: Geodesic active contours. The International Journal of Computer Vision **22** (1997) 61–79
39. Kass, M., Witkin, A., Terzopoulos, D.: Snakes: Active contour models. In: Proc. ICCV (1987) 259–268
40. Rousson, M., Deriche, R.: A variational framework for active and adaptative segmentation of vector valued images. In: Proc. IEEE Workshop on Motion and Video Computing (2002) 56–62

Coil Sensitivity Estimation for Optimal SNR Reconstruction and Intensity Inhomogeneity Correction in Phased Array MR Imaging

Prashanthi Vemuri[1], Eugene G. Kholmovski[1], Dennis L. Parker[1], and Brian E. Chapman[2]

[1] UCAIR, Department of Radiology, University of Utah, SLC, USA
{pvemuri, ekhoumov, parker}@ucair.med.utah.edu
[2] Department of Radiology, University of Pittsburgh, PA, USA
chapmanbe@upmc.edu

Abstract. Magnetic resonance (MR) images can be acquired by multiple receiver coil systems to improve signal-to-noise ratio (SNR) and to decrease acquisition time. The optimal SNR images can be reconstructed from the coil data when the coil sensitivities are known. In typical MR imaging studies, the information about coil sensitivity profiles is not available. In such cases the sum-of-squares (SoS) reconstruction algorithm is usually applied. The intensity of the SoS reconstructed image is modulated by a spatially variable function due to the non-uniformity of coil sensitivities. Additionally, the SoS images also have sub-optimal SNR and bias in image intensity. All these effects might introduce errors when quantitative analysis and/or tissue segmentation are performed on the SoS reconstructed images. In this paper, we present an iterative algorithm for coil sensitivity estimation and demonstrate its applicability for optimal SNR reconstruction and intensity inhomogeneity correction in phased array MR imaging.

1 Introduction

Phased array coils (multiple receiver coil systems) have been extensively used for acquisition of MR images owing to their benefit of increased SNR, extended field-of-view (FOV), and reduced acquisition time. The optimal way to merge individual coil information into the composite image in terms of the maximum SNR has been proposed by Roemer et al. [1], where each voxel value is obtained by the combination of voxel by voxel coil data with each coil's contribution weighted by the corresponding coil sensitivity. This algorithm can only be applied when the coil sensitivities are known. To find coil sensitivity profiles additional reference scans are required. Increase in imaging time and possible discrepancies between estimated and the true coil sensitivity profiles due to patient motion between reference and imaging scans make this approach difficult to use in clinical practice. Thus, the SoS algorithm [1] is typically used for image reconstruction from multi-coil data where the resulting (composite) image is obtained by the square root of the sum of the squares of the individual coil images. In comparison with the images reconstructed by the SNR optimal approach [1], the SoS reconstructed images are modulated by a spatially variable function due to the non-uniformity of coil sensitivities and have systematic error (bias) in signal intensity which necessitate intensity inhomogeneity correction and bias compensation before using the images for quantitative analysis.

A multitude of post processing algorithms [2-6] have been proposed to correct the intensity inhomogeneity in the SoS images. In all these techniques, it is assumed that the intensity inhomogeneity can be represented by a slowly varying function of position. The intensity inhomogeneity in the SoS image is estimated by fitting a low degree polynomial to the SoS image or from the low resolution image obtained by filtering out the higher frequency contributions in the frequency domain representation of the SoS image. Finally, the intensity inhomogeneity is corrected by dividing the SoS image by the estimate. Reliability of the given approach directly depends on the validity of the approximation of the intensity inhomogeneity in the SoS reconstructed images by a slowly varying function.

The sensitivity of the individual coil element (which is typically a circular loop) can be described by a unimodal, smoothly varying function of position [7]. Such a function can be accurately represented by a low degree polynomial. However, the intensity inhomogeneity in the SoS images must be characterized by the square root of the sum of squares of the individual coil sensitivities. Thus, the sensitivity modulation in the SoS images is multimodal and has a large number of higher order terms. Therefore, it cannot be reliably approximated by a low order polynomial. In this paper, we have proposed to estimate the intensity inhomogeneity in the individual coil images instead of the intensity inhomogeneity in the corresponding SoS image. Using this approach, consistent estimates of coil sensitivities can be found by fitting low order polynomial function to the image regions occupied by a dominant tissue type. Furthermore, the resulting estimates can be used not only for inhomogeneity correction in the SoS image but also for optimal SNR reconstruction.

2 Theory

The complex image acquired by the i-th coil can be described as a product of the true image $I(r)$ and the complex coil sensitivity $S_i(r)$ with additive Gaussian noise:

$$R_i(r) = I(r)S_i(r) + N_i(r), \quad i = 1, 2, .., L \tag{1}$$

where r denotes the position in the image space, L is the number of coils in the coil array and $N_i(r)$ is the complex Gaussian noise. When the coil sensitivities are known, the optimal SNR image $I_{OPT}(r)$ is given by [1]:

$$I_{OPT}(r) = \frac{\mathbf{R}(r)\psi^{-1}\mathbf{S}^H(r)}{\mathbf{S}(r)\psi^{-1}\mathbf{S}^H(r)} \tag{2}$$

where $\mathbf{R}(r)$ is the row vector of coil images: $\mathbf{R}(r) = [R_1(r), R_2(r),..., R_L(r)]$; $\mathbf{S}(r)$ is the row vector of coil sensitivities: $\mathbf{S}(r) = [S_1(r), S_2(r),..., S_L(r)]$; ψ is a Hermitian L by L matrix which describes the coupling and noise correlations between the coil elements and H denotes a Hermitian transpose. In the cases where the coil sensitivities are unknown, the SoS algorithm is applied:

$$I_{SoS}(r) = \sqrt{\mathbf{R}(r)\mathbf{\psi}^{-1}\mathbf{R}^H(r)} \qquad (3)$$

Even though SoS images are within 10% of the maximum SNR limits of the optimal SNR reconstruction [1], the intensity of the SoS reconstructed image is modulated by a spatially variable function due to the non-uniformity of coil sensitivities, which limits the usage of the images for quantitative analysis and segmentation. To resolve this problem, the algorithm proposed in this paper estimates the sensitivity profiles of the individual coil elements by iteratively identifying the image region occupied by a dominant tissue type and fitting low order polynomial function to image intensity in the region. Finally, Eq. [2] is used to combine the individual coil images to obtain the optimal SNR image without any intensity inhomogeneity.

2.1 Preliminary Steps: Un-Biasing, Estimation of Individual Coil Phase Maps and Noise Correlation Matrix

The developed iterative algorithm has achieved more reliable results when the preliminary steps described in detail below have been applied before the algorithm initialization.

The acquired coil images are corrupted by sensitivity inhomogeneity as well as complex Gaussian noise. Hence, it is important to remove the noise related bias in the magnitude coil images before they are used to estimate the corresponding sensitivity maps. The noise bias in each coil image is calculated by evaluating the standard deviation of noise from the histogram of the image. Then, the bias is removed by using the technique proposed in [8]. The resulting unbiased coil images $R_i^c(r)$ are used instead of the original coil images $R_i(r)$ for the sensitivity estimation.

For SNR optimal reconstruction it is essential to know both magnitude and phase of coil sensitivities. The phase variation in the coil images is mainly linear in nature [9] and can be accurately estimated from the low resolution complex coil images. It is to be noted that an apodization function (e.g. Hamming window) needs to be used to reduce the effect of Gibbs artifact when the phase map of each individual coil $\hat{\theta}_i(r)$ is estimated.

The noise correlation matrix $\mathbf{\psi}$ can be found using either a pre-scan noise calibration [1] or from a set of noise samples in the image field-of-view (FOV) [10]. In the case when sufficient numbers of noise samples are not present in the FOV, the noise correlation matrix can be assumed to be an identity matrix.

2.2 Iterative Technique for Coil Sensitivity Estimation

The developed technique has three main steps: First, dominant tissue spatial distribution (the region of support) is identified; second, for each coil element, the sensitivity maps $S_i(r)$ is estimated by fitting low degree polynomial function to the image intensity in the region of support and finally, the sensitivity maps are used in Eq. [2] to reconstruct the new image estimate. Since the estimation of the coil sensitivity profiles crucially depends on the identification of the region of support, an iterative algorithm has been developed where the first iteration of the algorithm is initialized by the SoS image: $I_{OPT}^{(0)}(r) = I_{SoS}(r)$. On subsequent iterations the current image estimate with substantially suppressed intensity inhomogeneity is used to refine the region of support.

The flowchart for the algorithm is shown in Fig. 1 and the main steps of this algorithm are explained in detail below.

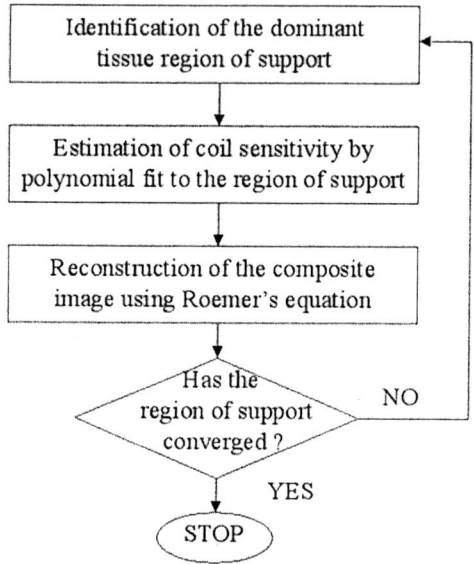

Fig. 1. Flow chart of the algorithm

2.2.1 Identification of the Region of Support
In high SNR MR images, the intensity distribution can be described as a linear combination of Gaussian distributions. The given assumption has been widely used in a number of statistics-based techniques for segmentation of brain tissues in the MR images [11-13]. A similar approach is utilized in our method to identify a spatial distribution of the dominant tissue type. The detailed description is illustrated in the context of brain MRI.

The histogram h of the brain MRI image can be modeled by a linear combination of Gaussian distributions:

$$h = \sum_{k=1}^{4} \alpha_k G(\mu_k, \sigma_k) \qquad (4)$$

where $G(\mu_k, \sigma_k)$ is the Gaussian distribution of the k-th tissue type ($k=1$ corresponds to air/bone, $k=2$ to CSF, $k=3$ to gray matter and $k=4$ to white matter) with mean μ_k and variance σ_k. α_k is the number of voxels corresponding to each tissue type within the image. It can be assumed that the intensity value corresponding to the global maximum of the image histogram (excluding the histogram peak related to tissue free image areas) corresponds to the mean of the dominant tissue type. Assuming for simplicity that the dominant tissue is white matter ($k=4$). Then, the region of support in the n-th iteration, $M^{(n)}(r)$, is identified using the image estimate $I_{OPT}^{(n-1)}(r)$ obtained at the $(n-1)$-th iteration as follows:

$$M^{(n)}(r) = \begin{cases} 1 & \mu_4 - 2\sigma_4 < I_{OPT}^{(n-1)}(r) < \mu_4 + 2\sigma_4 \\ 0 & \text{otherwise} \end{cases} \quad (5)$$

where μ_4 is equal to the image intensity value corresponding to the peak of the image intensity distribution (histogram) of $I_{OPT}^{(n-1)}(r)$. Identification of the dominant tissue region support is preferable rather than identifying other tissue spatial distributions as dominant tissue region would present a larger number of voxels spread throughout the image. This way more precise estimates of coil sensitivities can be found.

2.2.2 Estimation of Coil Sensitivities

Each coil image is modulated by complex coil sensitivity. The estimation of the phase maps $\hat{\theta}_i(r)$ is done as a preliminary step of the algorithm (Sec 2.1) and the magnitude of the coil sensitivity is estimated in the current step of the algorithm.

In the absence of noise and image intensity modulation due to non-uniform coil sensitivities, the image intensity distribution should consist of a few peaks corresponding to different tissue types. Hence, when the image region defined by $M^{(n)}(r)$ is considered, the image intensity in the region should be equal to μ_4. But in the images acquired by phased array coils the intensity distribution is mainly spread due to coil sensitivity non-uniformity. To restore the original intensity distribution, the coil sensitivities should be identified and their influence on the composite image intensity should be compensated.

For each individual coil image, an estimate of the image intensity modulation due to the coil sensitivity magnitude $|\hat{S}_i^n(r)|$ is found by fitting a polynomial function to image intensity values in the region of support $M^{(n)}(r)$. A least-squares algorithm is used for polynomial fit because it is optimal for Gaussian noise found in MR images [14]. The estimate of the complex coil sensitivity is given by:

$$\hat{S}_i^{(n)}(r) = |\hat{S}_i^{(n)}(r)| e^{j\hat{\theta}_i(r)} \quad (6)$$

2.2.3 Reconstruction of Composite Image

Once the sensitivity maps are found, new image estimate is calculated using the following equation:

$$I_{OPT}^{(n)}(r) = \frac{R(r)\psi^{-1}(\hat{S}^{(n)}(r))^H}{\hat{S}^{(n)}(r)\psi^{-1}(\hat{S}^{(n)}(r))^H} \quad (7)$$

where $\hat{S}^{(n)}(r) = [\hat{S}_1^{(n)}(r), \hat{S}_2^{(n)}(r), ..., \hat{S}_L^{(n)}(r)]$. The images obtained in this step of the algorithm have substantially suppressed intensity inhomogeneity in comparison with the original SoS images.

2.2.4 Termination of the Algorithm

In each iteration, coil sensitivity maps and image estimate are updated based on the current region of support. Then the image estimate is used to re-identify the region of support for the next iteration. This process is repeated till the region of support does not change anymore; i.e. there are no more points added or removed from the identified dominant tissue region of support. This would cause the estimated sensitivity map to remain constant yielding the same image estimate. At this point when the region of support converges, the algorithm is terminated.

2.3 Application to Multi-contrast MR Images

The proposed technique can also be applied for inhomogeneity correction and reconstruction of multi-contrast images when they are acquired using the same coils over the same imaging volume. The only difference in the algorithm would be the identification of the dominant tissue spatial distribution.

Since all of the multi-contrast images are modulated by the same coil sensitivities, the ratios between them are practically free from coil sensitivity intensity modulation and can be used to identify the dominant tissue spatial distribution. Given $C1_i(r)$, $C2_i(r)$,...,$CK_i(r)$, $i=1,...L$ are individual coil images from a multi-contrast study with K different contrasts and $C1_{OPT}^{(n-1)}(r), C2_{OPT}^{(n-1)}(r),..., CK_{OPT}^{(n-1)}(r)$ are the corresponding composite images obtained by the $(n-1)$-th algorithm iteration and arranged in the order of decreasing SNR. The region of support of the dominant tissue in the n-th iteration, $M^{(n)}(r)$, is identified using the ratio of the highest SNR images as follows:

$$M^{(n)}(r) = \begin{cases} 1 & \gamma - 0.05 < \dfrac{C2_{OPT}^{(n-1)}(r)}{C1_{OPT}^{(n-1)}(r) + \varepsilon} < \gamma + 0.05 \\ 0 & \text{otherwise} \end{cases} \quad (8)$$

where γ is the value of the ratio corresponding to the dominant tissue distribution and ε is a small value used as a regularization parameter.

Polynomial fit to the regions of the highest SNR images $C1_i^{(n-1)}(r)$ defined by the region of support $M^{(n)}(r)$ is used for obtaining the sensitivity map estimates $\hat{S}_i^{(n)}(r)$ as explained in Sec 2.2.2. These maps are used to reconstruct each of the different contrast images using Eq. [7] and this process is repeated till the region of support converges.

3 Results

The proposed technique was tested on computer generated as well as real MR images acquired on a 1.5 Tesla GE SIGNA Lx 8.4 MR scanner (GE Medical Systems, Waukesha, WI) with NV/CVi gradients and on a 3 Tesla Siemens Trio MR scanner (Siemens Medical Solutions, Erlangen, Germany) with Sonata gradients using standard clinical imaging pulse sequences. Both phantom and patient data were acquired. Informed consent was obtained from all human subjects in accordance with our institution's human subject policies. All computations were carried out on a Ultra-

80 computer with 450 MHz processor (Sun-Microsystems Inc.) using MATLAB (The Mathworks, Natick, MA).

In all the studies, third degree polynomials were used in the proposed algorithm to model coil sensitivities. The results obtained by the application of the proposed method were compared with the images reconstructed using the conventional SoS algorithm. In each of the cases presented, the original SoS and intensity inhomogeneity corrected images have been scaled to have the same mean in the region of support identified at the final algorithm iteration. The standard deviation (STD) of image intensity in the region of support was used as a figure of merit for a quantitative description of the algorithm performance.

3.1 Computer Simulation

For quantitative comparison of our algorithm operating on individual coil images with the standard intensity inhomogeneity correction techniques operating on the SoS image, computer simulations were performed. The simulations were done assuming that a uniform circular object was imaged using a four-coil receiver system. Identical circular loop coils were generated using the model presented in [7]. The degree of intensity inhomogeneity was varied by adjusting the coil radius. The STD in the image area occupied by the object was evaluated for the SoS image and in the intensity inhomogeneity corrected images. The results presented in Fig. 2 demonstrate that our algorithm gives better intensity inhomogeneity correction than the standard approach.

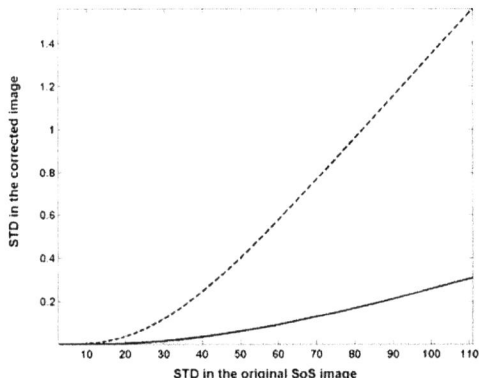

Fig. 2. STD of the corrected images vs. the STD in the original SoS image. Solid line corresponds to our algorithm, dashed line corresponds to the standard technique

3.2 Phantom Data

An eight-channel head coil (MRI Devices, Waukesha, WI) was used for phantom imaging on the Siemens 3 Tesla MR scanner. To test the efficacy of our algorithm, a uniform phantom filled with mineral oil was imaged using a 2D turbo spin-echo pulse sequence. The images were reconstructed using SoS (Fig. 3a) and the proposed technique (Fig. 3b). Our algorithm converged after three iterations when the complete image area occupied by the phantom was identified as the region of support. The image histograms shown in Fig. 3c and the intensity profiles shown in Fig. 3d demonstrate close to perfect phantom intensity uniformity after application of our algorithm. STD of image intensity in the region of support for the SoS and the proposed algorithm was 196.1 and 60.1, respectively.

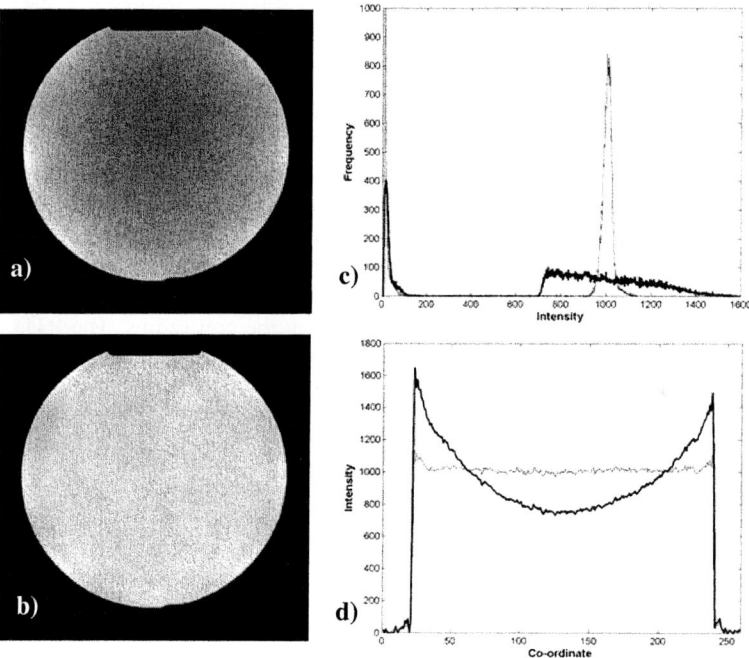

Fig. 3. The phantom images reconstructed using **a:** SoS and **b:** the proposed technique. **c:** Histograms of the images shown in **a** (solid line) and **b** (dashed line). **d:** Intensity profiles through the center of the images shown in **a** (solid line) and **b** (dashed line)

3.3 Human Data

Brain Imaging. Patient images were acquired using the same pulse sequence as well as the hardware as the phantom images (Sec 3.2). Images were reconstructed by the SoS algorithm and the proposed iterative technique. The image region occupied by the dominant tissue, white matter, was used as the region of support. The algorithm converged after four iterations. For better white matter visualization, both images were scaled to a user defined intensity window. The intensity inhomogeneity modulation in the SoS image is easily observed in Fig. 4a. The proposed algorithm improved image intensity uniformity (Fig. 4b) and substantially reduced STD from 183.3 to 58.8. Naive intensity based segmentation was performed on both the images. The results shown in Fig 4c and 4d demonstrate that the images reconstructed by the new algorithm give substantially more trustworthy segmentation than the SoS images.

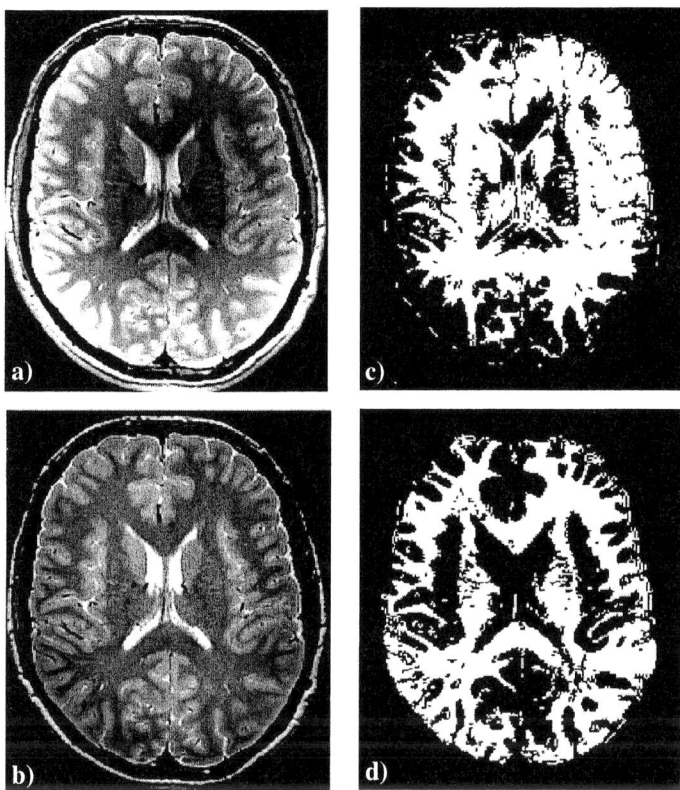

Fig. 4. The brain image reconstructed using **a:** SoS and **b:** the proposed technique. White matter segmentation results **c:** SoS and **d:** the proposed technique

Multi-Contrast Carotid Imaging. A specially designed bilateral four-channel phased array coil was used for imaging the carotid arteries on GE 1.5 Tesla MR scanner. Images were obtained using a triple contrast pulse sequence [15] that allows acquisition of spatially co-registered proton density (PD), T1-, and T2-weighted images in one scan. These images were used to test the algorithm performance for correction of intensity inhomogeneity in multi-contrast datasets. The decreasing order of SNR in these images was PD, T1, and T2. Due to incomplete fat signal saturation in T1 images, the ratio of T2 to PD images was used to identify the dominant tissue (in this case, muscle) region of support for the estimation of the coil sensitivities. The algorithm convergence was achieved in three iterations. As can be seen in Fig. 5, the vessel wall and surrounding tissues visualization drastically improves by the application of the proposed algorithm allowing robust tissue segmentation. STD of image intensity in the region of support for SoS reconstructed PD, T1-, and T2-weighted images was 70.0, 67.2, and 86.3 respectively. The images reconstructed by our algorithm have considerably decreased intensity inhomogeneity in comparison with the SoS images resulting in STD equal to 29.0, 30.0 and 60.3 for PD, T1-, T2-weighted images, respectively. Higher STD value for T2 image in comparison with STD in PD and T1 images is caused by substantially lower SNR of the T2 image.

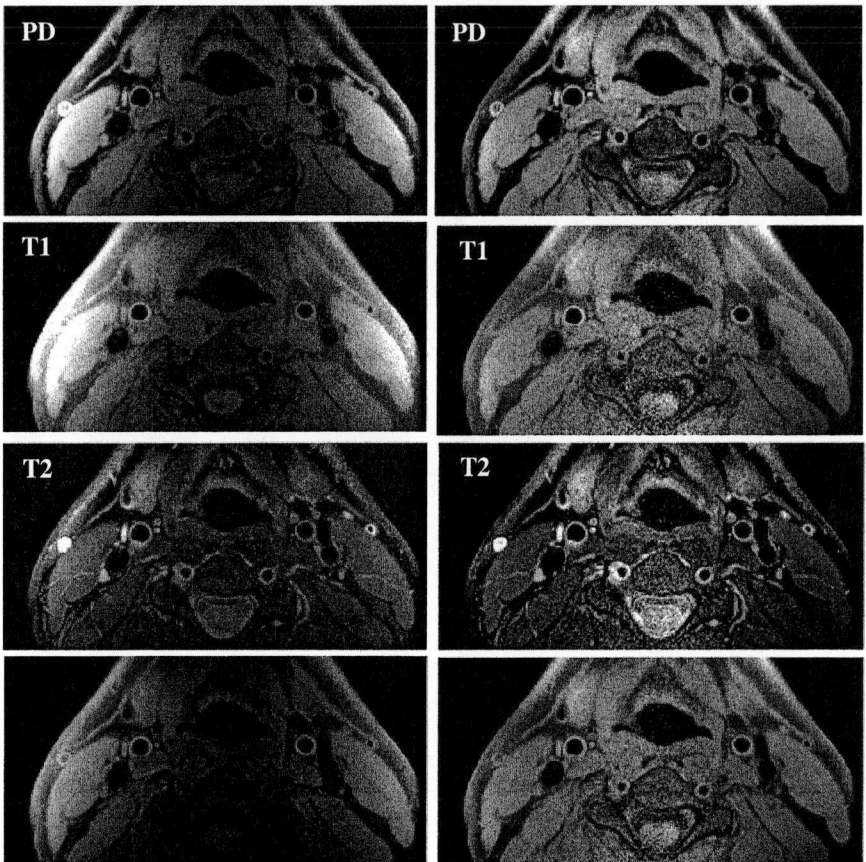

Fig. 5. PD, T1, T2 and color composite images from triple contrast scan of the carotid arteries. The images reconstructed using: SoS (left row); new algorithm (right row). Color coding used for composite images: PD=red, T1=green, T2=blue

4 Conclusions and Discussion

Intensity inhomogeneity compensation is an important preliminary step before performing quantitative analysis and/or segmentation on MR images acquired by a multi-coil receiver system. In this paper, an iterative algorithm for coil sensitivity estimation for optimal SNR reconstruction and intensity inhomogeneity correction in phased array MR imaging has been presented. The algorithm iteratively identifies the image region occupied by the dominant tissue type, fits a polynomial function to this region in each coil image to estimate the coil sensitivity, and then combines coil images and the corresponding coil sensitivity estimates to achieve the SNR optimal reconstruction. The estimate of the coil sensitivity is refined in each iteration based on the knowledge of the composite image reconstructed in the previous step. The major advantage of the algorithm is that it does not require additional reference scans to perform SNR optimal reconstruction but estimates the sensitivity maps based on the individual coil data generated by an MR scanner. Hence, it can be used in a typical clinical scan scenario without any time penalty for additional reference scans. The application of the proposed algorithm to real MR phantom as well as human datasets has demonstrated considerable suppression of intensity inhomogeneity in all processed images in comparison with the original SoS images.

The proposed technique is computationally efficient as well as completely automated. It does not involve any operator intervention at any stage of the algorithm. The algorithm typically requires from three to five iterations to converge. To speedup processing high resolution three-dimensional datasets, the data should be sub-sampled to make it computationally efficient for estimating the coefficients of the three-dimensional fit. Processing a 512x512x100 image volume from high resolution MR angiography study took less than 50 seconds of computational time after sub-sampling by a factor of four in all dimensions.

The performance of the proposed method crucially depends on the identification of the image regions occupied by the dominant tissue type. It is essential that the tissue is represented not only by the significant number of imaging voxels but also the voxels are distributed across the entire image to guarantee reliable results of polynomial fitting. The assumption that the image contains dominant tissue is valid in many typical MR imaging applications such as brain, breast, spine, and neck studies. However, it is quite problematic to identify dominant tissue distributed throughout the entire image in heart or liver studies where cross-sectional images of the entire torso are usually acquired. In such cases, an additional preliminary step is required to choose the image region containing the anatomical structure of interest (e.g. heart for cardiac MR imaging). Then, the algorithm can be applied to the user chosen image region without any further modifications. This approach can be extended to the entire image by subdividing it into smaller sub-regions with substantial representation of some tissue type in each of them. This way, fitting to multiple tissue types can be realized.

The selection of the region of interest should also be utilized if the image to process is corrupted by aliasing (wrap-around) artifacts due to insufficient data sampling in phase encoding direction. In such cases, intensity inhomogeneity in the coil images cannot be described by slowly varying functions of position resulting in suboptimal performance of the proposed algorithm. After the image region without aliasing is selected our method can be successfully applied.

Acknowledgements

This work is supported in part by NIH grants R01 HL48223 and HL57990 and Seimens Medical Solutions.

References

1. Roemer, P.B., Edelstein, W.A., Hayes, C.E., Souza, S.P., Mueller, O.M.: The NMR Phased-Array. *Magnetic Resonance in Medicine,* 16:192–225, 1990.
2. Murakami, J.W., Hayes, C.E., Weinberger, Ed.: Intensity Correction of Phased-Array Surface Coil Images. *Magnetic Resonance in Medicine*, 35:585-590, 1996.

3. Meyer, C.R., Bland, P.H., Pipe, J.: Retrospective Correction of Intensity Inhomogeneities in MRI. *IEEE Transactions on Medical Imaging*, 14:36-41, 1995.
4. Sled, J.G., Zijdenbos, A.P., Evans, A.C.: A Nonparametric Method for Automatic Correction of Intensity Non-uniformity in MRI data. *IEEE Transactions on Medical Imaging*, 17:87-97, 1998.
5. Han, C., Hatsukami, T.S., Yuan, C.: A Multi-scale Method for Automatic Correction of Intensity Non-Uniformity in MR Images. *Journal of Magnetic Resonance Imaging*, 13:428-436, 2001.
6. Vokurka, E.A., Thacker, N.A., Jackson, A.: A Fast Model Independent Method for Automatic Correction of Intensity Non-uniformity in MRI Data. *Journal of Magnetic Resonance Imaging*, 10:550-562, 1999.
7. Smythe, W.R.: Static and Dynamic Electricity. McGraw Hill, New York, 1968.
8. Gudbjartsson, H., Patz, P.: The Rician Distribution of Noisy MRI Data. *Magnetic Resonance in Medicine*, 34:910-914, 1995.
9. Ahn, C.B., Cho, Z.H.: A New Phase Correction Method in NMR Imaging Based on Autocorrelation and Histogram Analysis. *IEEE Transactions on Medical Imaging*, 6:32-36, 1987.
10. Pruessmann, K.P., Weiger, M., Scheidegger, M.B., Boesiger, P.: SENSE: Sensitivity Encoding for Fast MRI. *Magnetic Resonance in Medicine*, 42:952-962, 1999.
11. Liang, Z., MacFall, J.R., Harrington, D.P.: Parameter Estimation and Tissue Segmentation from Multispectral MR images. *IEEE Transactions on Medical Imaging*, 13:441-449, 1994.
12. Wells, W.M., Grimson, W.E.L., Kikinis, R., Jolesz, F.A.: Adaptive Segmentation of MRI Data. *IEEE Transactions on Medical Imaging*, 15:429-442, 1996.
13. Wilson, D.L., Noble, J.A.: An Adaptive Segmentation Algorithm of Time-of-flight MRA Data. *IEEE Transactions on Medical Imaging*, 18:938-945, 1999.
14. Press, W.H., Flannery, B.P., Teukolsky, S.A., Vetterling, W.T.: Numerical Recipes in C : The Art of Scientific Computing. Cambridge University Press, New York, 1996.
15. Kim, S.E., Kholmovski, E.G., Jeong, E.K., Buswell, H.R., Tsuruda, J.S., Parker, D.L.: Triple Contrast Technique for Black Blood Imaging with Double Inversion Preparation. *Magnetic Resonance in Medicine*, 52:1379-1387, 2004.

Many Heads Are Better Than One: Jointly Removing Bias from Multiple MRIs Using Nonparametric Maximum Likelihood

Erik G. Learned-Miller and Vidit Jain

Department of Computer Science,
University of Massachusetts, Amherst, MA 01003, USA
elm@cs.umass.edu
http://www.cs.umass.edu/~elm

Abstract. The correction of multiplicative bias in magnetic resonance images is an important problem in medical image processing, especially as a preprocessing step for quantitative measurements and other numerical procedures. Most previous approaches have used a maximum likelihood method to increase the probability of the pixels in a single image by adaptively estimating a correction to the unknown image bias field. The pixel probabilities are defined either in terms of a pre-existing tissue model, or nonparametrically in terms of the image's own pixel values. In both cases, the specific location of a pixel in the image does not influence the probability calculation. Our approach, similar to methods of joint registration, simultaneously eliminates the bias from a set of images of the same anatomy, but from different patients. We use the statistics from the same location across different patients' images, rather than within an image, to eliminate bias fields from all of the images simultaneously. Evaluating the likelihood of a particular voxel in one patient's scan with respect to voxels in the same location in a set of other patients' scans disambiguates effects that might be due to either bias fields or anatomy. We present a variety of "two-dimensional" experimental results (working with one image from each patient) showing how our method overcomes serious problems experienced by other methods. We also present preliminary results on full three-dimensional volume correction across patients.

1 Introduction

The problem of bias fields in magnetic resonance (MR) images is an important problem in medical imaging. We illustrate the problem in Figure 1 using a synthetic image from BrainWeb [10] and an artificial bias field. When a patient is imaged in the MR scanner, the goal is to obtain an image which is a function solely of the underlying tissue (left of Figure 1). However, typically the desired anatomical image is corrupted by a multiplicative bias field (second image) that is caused by engineering issues such as imperfections in the radio frequency coils used to record the MR signal. The result is a corrupted image (third image). (See [1] for background information on bias fields.) The goal of bias correction is to estimate the uncorrupted image from the corrupted image.

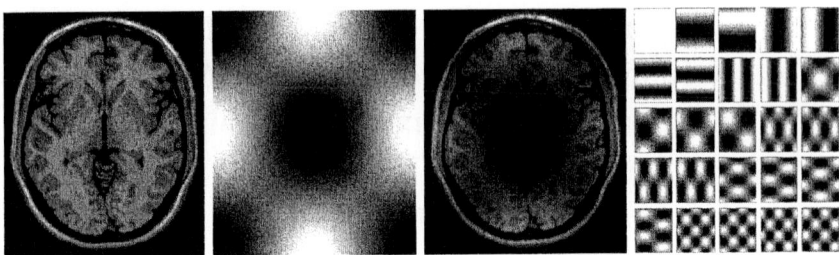

Fig. 1. On the left is an idealized mid-axial MR image of the human brain with little or no bias field. The second image is a simulated low-frequency bias field. It has been exaggerated for ease of viewing. The third image is the result of pixelwise multiplication of the image by the bias field. On the right is the set of basis images used to parameterize smooth bias fields for the slice-based algorithm

Radiologists appear to be remarkably immune to the effects of bias fields under many circumstances.[1] This is probably because radiologists seem to make mostly *relative intensity* judgments based upon local image information. They use so-called window-level adjustments to optimize local contrast for discriminating various properties of the tissues in a specific region. Bias fields, however, are a major problem for automated computer applications like registration, segmentation or pre-screening which depend upon similar tissues having consistent values across a scan. In these applications, the actual numeric brightness value assigned to a tissue is critical and directly affects whether such algorithms will work.

A variety of statistical methods have been proposed to address this problem. Wells et al. [9] developed a statistical model using a fixed number of tissues, with the brightness distribution for each tissue type (in a bias-free image) represented by a one-dimensional Gaussian distribution or by a nonparametric distribution. An expectation-maximization (EM) procedure was then used to simultaneously estimate the bias field, the tissue type, and the residual noise. While this method works well in many cases, it has several drawbacks: (1) Models must be developed *a priori* for each type of acquisition (for each different setting of the MR scanner), for each new area of the body, and for different patient populations (like infants and adults). (2) Models must be developed from "bias-free" images, which may be difficult or impossible to obtain in many cases. (3) The model assumes a fixed number of tissues, which may be inaccurate. For example, during development of the human brain, there is continuous variability between gray matter and white matter. In addition, a discrete tissue model does not handle so-called partial volume effects in which a pixel represents a combination of several tissue types. This occurs frequently since many pixels occur at tissue boundaries.

Tissue-free modeling approaches have also been suggested, as for example by Viola [11]. In that work, a nonparametric model of brightness values was developed from a single image. Using the observation that the entropy of the pixel brightness distribution

---

[1] Anecdotally, moderate bias fields do not seem to significantly effect radiologists' ability to make diagnoses.

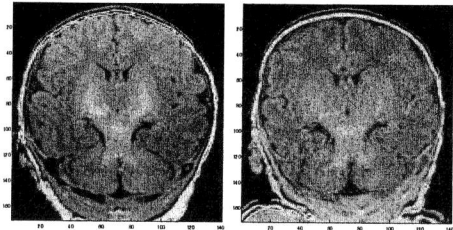

Fig. 2. The infant brain image on the left shows a coronal MR image with a strong bias field. The image is too bright at the top and too dark at the bottom. This is easy to see and can be corrected successfully by a variety of bias correction techniques. The right image, however, is a more difficult case. In particular, the subtle increase in intensity in the middle of the image is, from an algorithmic point of view, difficult to categorize. Is it a subtle increase in intensity due to a low frequency bias field, or is it a slight increase in intensity due to say, partial myelination of white matter in a developing infant? Due to the location of the increased intensity, a radiologist would usually guess that this is developing white matter in an infant brain, but algorithms that do not take into account spatial location and the appearance of other similar scans cannot make such an assessment. It is exactly this sort of information which is leveraged by our algorithm

for a *single image* is likely to increase when a bias field is added, Viola's method postulates a bias-correction field by minimizing the entropy of the resulting pixel brightness distribution. This approach addresses several of the problems of fixed-tissue models, but has its own drawbacks: (1) The statistical model may be weak, since it is based on data from only a single image. (2) There is no mechanism for distinguishing between certain low-frequency image components and a bias field. That is, the method may mistake signal for noise in certain cases when removal of the true signal reduces the entropy of the brightness distriibution. We illustrate this problem in Figure 2.

The present method, first presented in [5] overcomes or improves upon problems associated with both of these methods and their many variations (see, e.g., [1] for recent techniques). It models tissue brightness nonparametrically, but uses data from multiple images to provide improved distribution estimates and alleviate the need for bias-free images for making a model. Most importantly, it conditions the distributions on spatial location, taking advantage of a rich information source ignored in other methods. Experimental results demonstrate the effectiveness of our method.

2 The Image Model and Problem Formulation

We assume we are given a set **I** of observed images I_i with $1 \leq i \leq N$, as shown on the left side of Figure 3. Each of these images is assumed to be the product of some bias-free image L_i and a smooth bias field $B_i \subset \mathcal{B}$. We shall refer to the bias-free images as *latent images* (also called *intrinsic images* by some authors). The set of all latent images shall be denoted **L** and the set of unknown bias fields **B**. Then each observed image can be written as the product $I_i(x,y) = L_i(x,y) * B_i(x,y)$, where (x,y) gives the pixel coordinates of each point, with P pixels per image.

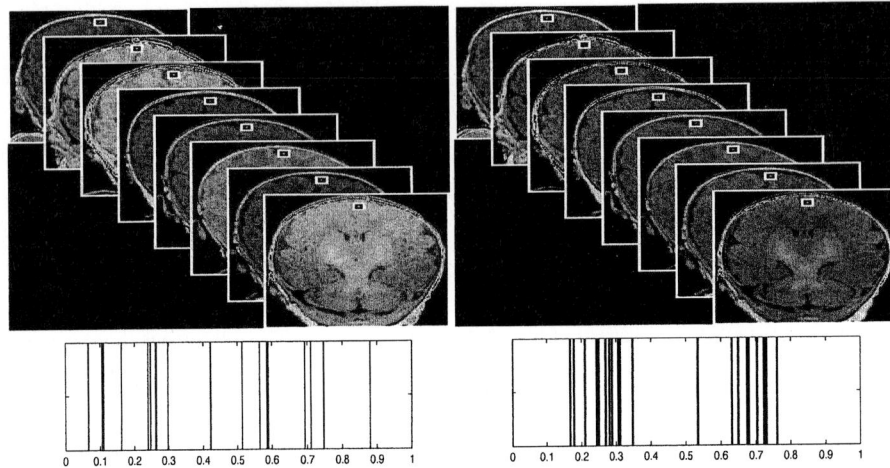

Fig. 3. Top left. A set of mid-coronal brain images from eight different infants, showing clear signs of bias fields. A *pixel-stack*, a collection of pixels at the same point in each image, is represented by the small square near the top of each image. The plot beneath the images shows the values of the pixels in the pixel stack (plus points from an additional 13 images). Note the wide distribution (high entropy) of brightness values in the stack. The estimated entropy of this distribution was -0.4980. **Top right.** The same mid-coronal images after bias correction. Note the uniformity of the images and the higher concentration (lower entropy) of brightness values from the pixel stack. The estimated entropy for these samples was -0.8389

Consider again Figure 3. A *pixel-stack* through each image set is shown as the set of pixels corresponding to a particular location in each image (not necessarily the same tissue type). Our method relies on the principle that the pixel-stack values are likely, on average, to have lower empirical entropy when the bias fields have been removed. We now explain what exactly this means and why it should be true.

2.1 Entropy, Nonparametric Distributions, and Maximum Likelihood

Consider some infinite set of images taken from a fixed population, such as mid-coronal images of infants between zero and two years of age. Now pick a particular location in each image, such as the middle pixel. The distribution over *tissue values* at this location, across the images, is a random variable (call it T). We might expect white matter, cerebrospinal fluid, vasculature, or a handful of other tissue at this location, each with some relative frequency. The *entropy* (defined formally below) of this random variable gives us a measure of the variability of tissues at this location.

In MR images with no bias fields, each tissue is mapped to a fairly consistent brightness value, another random variable (call it L, for latent image brightness). Thus, the entropy of the tissue types at a particular spatial location is closely related to the entropy of brightness values in bias-free MRs at that location. An empirical sample of true brightness values from such a set of images is in the lower right of Figure 3.

Now consider what happens when random bias fields are *introduced* into each image (going from right to left in Figure 3). If we consider the random variable B to be the contribution of a random bias field to each image, then we will be perturbing the original distribution of brightness values L to values $L \times B$. This tends to spread out the brightness values in the pixel stack, increasing their empirical entropy, as shown by the set of samples on the lower left of Figure 3. In fact, in dealing with an infinite sample, it can be proven [3] that the entropy of a random variable (brightness) will always increase (or remain the same) when an independent random variable is added to it.[2]

The idea that entropy increases when random variables are added together has another interpretation in terms of probability theory. In particular, the average log probability density (which is just the negative entropy) of points in a distribution of one random variable is guaranteed to be *higher* than the average log probability density of another random variable which is the original random variable plus an independent source of randomness. In other words, the probability density of our data under a bias-free distribution should be higher than the probability of our data under distribution that include bias. This is only guaranteed when we have an infinite amount of data, but is usually true even for the case of finite data. This is true irrespective of the form of the distributions. That is, these ideas make no assumptions about the *parametric form* of the distributions, and are thus completely nonparametric. It is these ideas upon which our method is based. We now describe the specifics of our model and method.

2.2 The Model

The latent image generation model assumes that each pixel is drawn from a fixed distribution $p_{x,y}(\cdot)$ which gives the probability of each gray value at the the location (x, y) in the image. Furthermore, we assume that all pixels in the latent image are independent, given the distributions from which they are drawn. It is also assumed that the bias fields for each image are chosen independently from some fixed distribution over bias fields. Unlike most models for this problem which rely on statistical regularities within an image, we take a completely orthogonal approach by assuming that pixel values are independent given their image locations, but that pixel-stacks in general have low entropy when bias fields are removed.

We formulate the problem as a maximum a posteriori (MAP) problem, searching for the most probable bias fields given the set of observed images. Letting $\mathcal{B}$ represent the 25-dimensional product space of smooth bias fields (corresponding to the 25 basis images of Figure 1), we wish to find

$$\arg\max_{\mathbf{B} \in \mathcal{B}} P(\mathbf{B}|\mathbf{I}) \stackrel{(a)}{=} \arg\max_{\mathbf{B} \in \mathcal{B}} P(\mathbf{I}|\mathbf{B}) P(\mathbf{B}) \qquad (1)$$

$$\stackrel{(b)}{=} \arg\max_{\mathbf{B} \in \mathcal{B}} P(\mathbf{I}|\mathbf{B}) \qquad (2)$$

$$\stackrel{(c)}{=} \arg\max_{\mathbf{B} \in \mathcal{B}} P(\mathbf{L}(\mathbf{I}, \mathbf{B})) \qquad (3)$$

---

[2] Here we are *multiplying* random variables rather than adding them, so this result does not strictly apply. However, when one of the random variables is near 1 (as is the bias random variable) and we force its mean to be 1, this result will usually hold even for multiplication.

$$= \arg\max_{B \in \mathcal{B}} \prod_{x,y} \prod_{i=1}^{N} p_{x,y}(L_i(x,y)) \qquad (4)$$

$$= \arg\max_{B \in \mathcal{B}} \sum_{x,y} \sum_{i=1}^{N} \log p_{x,y}(L_i(x,y)) \qquad (5)$$

$$\stackrel{(d)}{\approx} \arg\min_{B \in \mathcal{B}} \sum_{x,y} H(p_{x,y}) \qquad (6)$$

$$\stackrel{(e)}{\approx} \arg\min_{B \in \mathcal{B}} \sum_{x,y} \hat{H}_{\text{Vasicek}}(L_1(x,y), ..., L_N(x,y)) \qquad (7)$$

$$= \arg\min_{B \in \mathcal{B}} \sum_{x,y} \hat{H}_{\text{Vasicek}}\left(\frac{I_1(x,y)}{B_1(x,y)}, ..., \frac{I_N(x,y)}{B_N(x,y)}\right). \qquad (8)$$

Here H is the Shannon entropy $(-E(\log P(x)))$ and $\hat{H}_{\text{Vasicek}}$ is a sample-based entropy estimator discussed below. (a) is just an application of Bayes rule. (b) assumes a uniform prior over the allowed bias fields. The method can easily be altered to incorporate a non-uniform prior. (c) expresses the fact that the probability of the observed image given a particular bias field is the same as the probability of the latent image associated with that observed image and bias field. The approximation (d) replaces the empirical mean of the log probability at each pixel with the negative entropy of the underlying distribution at that pixel. This entropy is in turn estimated (e) using the entropy estimator of Vasicek [8] directly from the samples in the pixel-stack, without ever estimating the distributions $p_{x,y}$ explicitly.

The inequality (d) becomes an equality as N grows large by the law of large numbers, while the consistency of Vasicek's entropy estimator [2] implies that (e) also goes to equality with large N. (See [2] for a review of entropy estimators.)

2.3 The Entropy Estimatior

The entropy estimator used is similar to Vasicek's estimator [8], given (up to minor details) by

$$\hat{H}_{\text{Vasicek}}(Z^1, ..., Z^N) = \frac{1}{N-m} \sum_{i=1}^{N-m} \log\left(\frac{N}{m}(Z^{(i+m)} - Z^{(i)})\right), \qquad (9)$$

where Z^i's represent the values in a pixel-stack, $Z^{(i)}$'s represent those same values in rank order, N is the number of values in the pixel-stack and m is a function of N (like $N^{0.5}$) such that m/N goes to 0 as m and N go to infinity. These entropy estimators are discussed at length elsewhere [4].

To understand the intuition behind this estimator, consider the case when $m = 1$. In this case $Z^{(i+m)} - Z^{(i)}$ just represents the distance between two adjacent samples. The result of Vasicek's estimator is just proportional to the sum of the log of these distances. Thus, if many points are clustered in one area, many of these values will be small resulting in a low entropy. If points are spread out, then many of these values will be large, resulting in a large entropy.

3 The Algorithm

Using these ideas, it is straightforward to construct algorithms for joint bias field removal. As mentioned above, we chose to optimize Equation (8) over the set of band-limited bias fields. To do this, we parameterize the set of bias fields using the sine/cosine basis images shown on the right of Figure 1:

$$B_i = \sum_{j=1}^{25} \alpha_j \phi_j(x,y).$$

We optimize Equation (8) by *simultaneously* updating the bias field estimates (taking a step along the numerical gradient) for each image to reduce the overall entropy. That is, at time step t, the coefficients α_j for each bias field are updated using the latent image estimates and entropy estimates from time step $t-1$. After all α's have been updated, a new set of latent images and pixel-stack entropies are calculated, and another gradient step is taken. Though it is possible to do a full gradient descent to convergence by optimizing one image at a time, the optimization landscape tends to have more local minima for the last few images in the process. The appeal of our joint gradient descent method, on the other hand, is that the ensemble of images provides a natural smoothing of the optimization landscape in the joint process. It is in this sense that our method is "multi-resolution", proceeding from a smooth optimization in the beginning to a sharper one near the end of the process.

We now summarize the algorithm:

1. Initialize the bias field coefficients for each image to 0, with the exception of the coefficient for the DC-offset (the constant bias field component), which is initialized to 1. Initialize the gradient descent step size δ to some value.
2. Compute the summed pixelwise entropies for the set of images with initial "neutral" bias field corrections. (See below for method of computation.)
3. Iterate the following loop until no further changes occur in the images.
   (a) For each image:
      i. Calculate the numerical gradient $\nabla_\alpha H_{\text{Vasicek}}$ of (8) with respect to the bias field coefficients (α_j's) for the current image.
      ii. Set $\alpha = \alpha + \delta \nabla_\alpha \hat{H}_{\text{Vasicek}}$.
   (b) Update δ (reduce its value according to some schedule).

Upon convergence, it is assumed that the entropy has been reduced as much as possible by changing the bias fields, unless one or more of the gradient descents is stuck in a local minimum. Empirically, the likelihood of sticking in local minima is reduced by increasing the number of images (N) in the optimization. In our experiments described below with only 21 real infant brains, the algorithm appears to have found a global minimum of all bias fields to the extent that this can be discerned visually.

Note that for a set of *identical* images, the pixel-stack entropies are not increased by multiplying each image by the same bias field (since all images will still be the same). More generally, when images are approximately equivalent, their pixel-stack entropies are not signficantly affected by a "common" bias field, i.e. one that occurs in all of the images.[3] This means that the algorithm cannot, in general, eliminate all bias fields from a set of images, but can only *set all of the bias fields to be equivalent*. We refer to any constant bias field remaining in all images after convergence as the *residual bias field*.

Fortunately, there is an effect that tends to minimize the impact of the residual bias field in many test cases. The residual bias field tends to consist of components for each α_j that approximate the mean of that component across images. For example, if half of the observed images have a positive value for a particular component's coefficient, and half have a negative coefficient for that component, the residual bias field will tend to have a coefficient near zero for that component. Hence, the algorithm naturally eliminates bias field effects that are non-systematic, i.e. that are not shared across images.

If the same type of bias field component occurs in a majority of the images, then the algorithm will not remove it, as the component is indistinguishable, under our model, from the underlying anatomy. In such a case, one could resort to within-image methods to further reduce the entropy. However, there is a risk that such methods will remove components that actually represent smooth gradations in the anatomy. This can be seen in the bottom third of Figure 5, and will be discussed in more detail below.

4 Slice-Based Experiments

To test our algorithm, we ran two sets of experiments, the first on images with simulated bias fields, and the second on real brain images. In the first experiment, we started with a single brain image and created a set of "different" brain images by first adding different

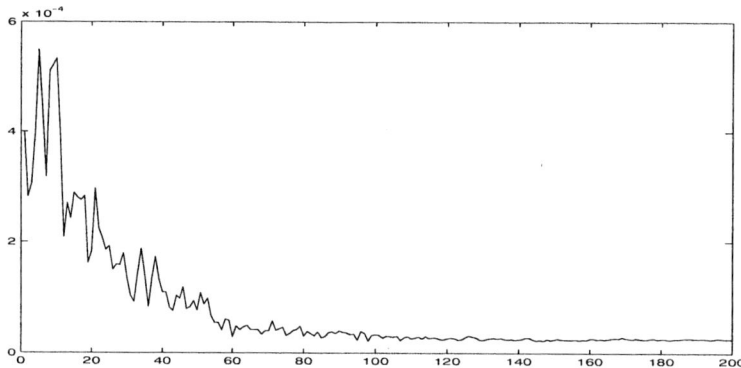

Fig. 4. Typical convergence of the variance of the difference between bias field coefficient estimates and their true values, across images. This convergence implies that the true bias field is recovered up to some "shared" component

---

[3] Actually, multiplying each image by a bias field of small magnitude can artificially reduce the entropy of a pixel-stack, but this is only the result of the brightness values shrinking towards zero. Such artificial reductions in entropy can be avoided by normalizing a distribution to unit variance between iterations of computing its entropy, as is done in this work.

known bias fields to each image and then randomly translating the images from zero to five pixels in a random direction. The random translation creates an image set in which the pixel stacks have variability similar to a true set of images, but for which the latent images are still known.

If our algorithm works as claimed, then the final recovered images should not necessarily be equal to the original images (since shared bias components cannot be detected) but should recover bias fields that, up to some shared bias field, are equivalent to the originally introduced bias fields. Another way to say this is that the difference $\hat{\alpha} - \alpha$ between the estimated biasfield coefficients $\hat{\alpha}$ and the original bias field coefficients α for each image should be constant across images. If this is true, than the variance of these differences across images should go to zero as the algorithm runs. Figure 4 demonstrates that this is exactly what happens in our experiments. The plot shows that as the algorithm runs, the difference between the estimated bias field coefficients and the true bias field coefficients becomes equal (its variance goes to zero).

More interesting are the results on real images, in which the latent images come from different patients. We obtained 21 pre-registered[4] infant brain images (top of Figure 5) from Brigham and Women's Hospital in Boston. Large bias fields can be seen in many of the images. Probably the most striking is a "ramp-like" bias field in the sixth image of the second row. (The top of the brain is too bright, while the bottom is too dark.) Because the brain's white matter is not fully developed in these infant scans, it is difficult to categorize tissues into a fixed number of classes as is typically done for adult brain images; hence, these images are not amenable to methods based on specific tissue models developed for adults (e.g. [9]).

The middle third of Figure 5 shows the results of our algorithm on the infant brain images. (These results must be viewed in color on a good monitor to fully appreciate the results.) While a trained technician can see small imperfections in these images, the results are remarkably good. All major bias artifacts have been removed.

It is interesting to compare these results to a method that reduces the entropy of each image individually, without using constraints between images. Using the results of our algorithm as a starting point, we continued to reduce the entropy of the pixels *within* each image (using a method akin to Viola's [11]), rather than across images. These results are shown in the bottom third of Figure 5. Carefully comparing the central brain regions in the middle section of the figure and the bottom section of the figure, one can see that the butterfly shaped region in the middle of the brain, which represents developing white matter, has been suppressed in the lower images. This is most likely because the entropy of the pixels *within a particular image* can be reduced by increasing the bias field "correction" in the central part of the image. In other words, the algorithm strives to make the image more uniform by removing the bright part in the middle of the image. However, our algorithm, which compares pixels across images, does not

---

[4] It is interesting to note that registration is not strictly necessary for this algorithm to work. The proposed MAP method works under very broad conditions, the main condition being that the bias fields do not span the same space as parts of the actual medical images. It is true, however, that as the latent images become less registered or differ in other ways, that a much larger number of images is needed to get good estimates of the pixel-stack distributions.

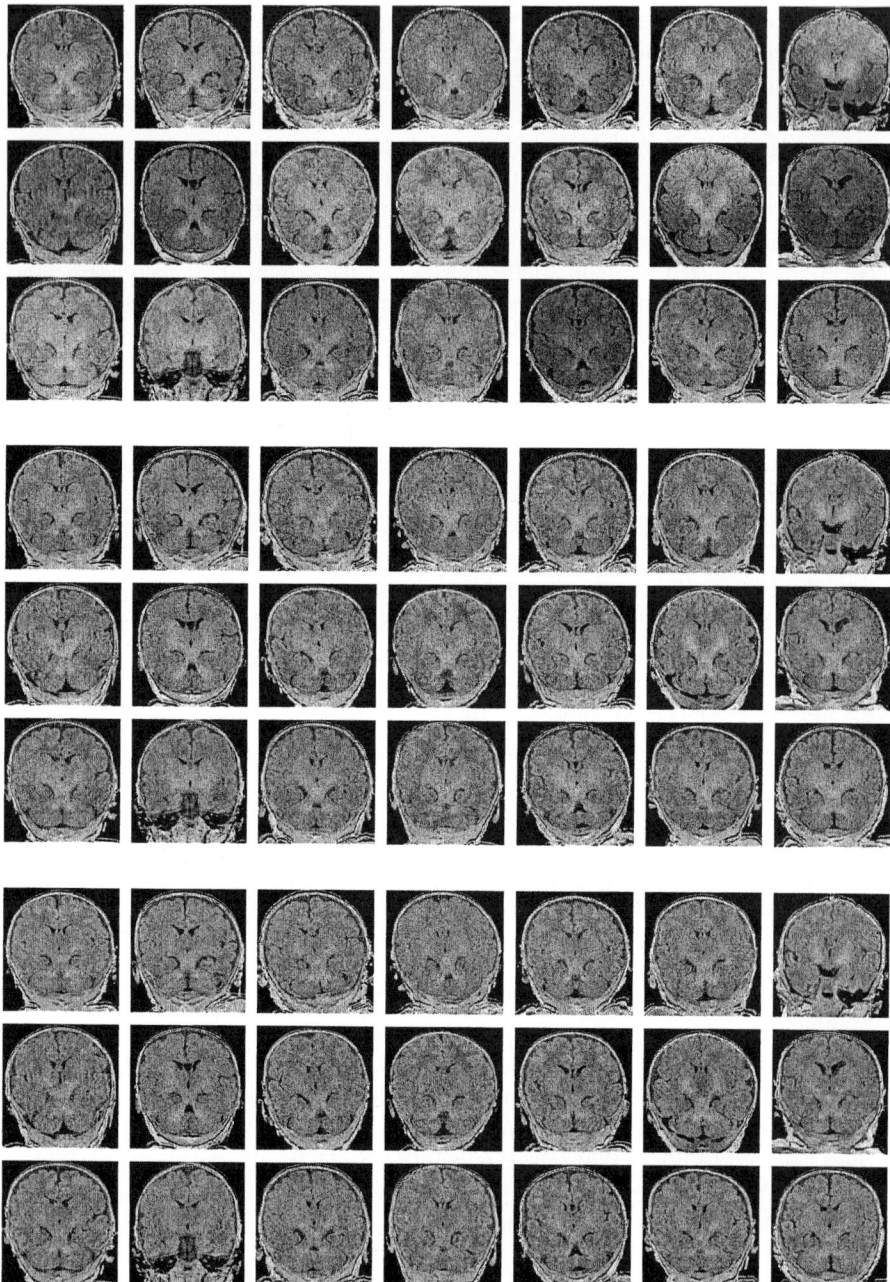

Fig. 5. NOTE: This image must be viewed in color (preferably on a bright display) for full effect. **Top.** Original infant brain images. **Middle.** The same images after bias removal with our algorithm. Note that developing white matter (butterfly-like structures in middle brain) is well-preserved. **Bottom.** Bias removal using a single image based algorithm. Notice that white matter structures are repressed

suppress these real structures, since they occur across images. Hence coupling across images can produce superior results.

5 Volumetric Bias Removal

Extending this basic method to work with a full series of images from each patient, rather than a single image from each patient, is straightforward and requires only minor modifications to the source code. First, we must parameterize the set of smooth three-dimensional bias fields, which means we need a three-dimensional Fourier basis of volumes. In this work, we used 3-D bases consisting of either 27 or 125 basis volumes, representing bias fields limited, respectively, to either one Hertz or two Hertz in spatial frequency. The 125-volume basis is analogous to the basis shown in Figure 1.

To understand the advantage of correcting bias across volumes rather than across sets of slices one at a time, consider what happens when a set of patient scans are corrected one slice at a time (still grouped across patients of course). In this case, the estimates of bias fields may change sharply from one image to the next within the same patient, ignoring the fact that bias fields tend to be smooth in all three dimensions. This can be avoided by forcing the volumetric bias fields to be parameterized by a smooth three-dimensional basis that enforces smoothness of the bias fields in all directions, and gives us another constraint with which to separate the patients' true anatomical data from smooth bias fields.

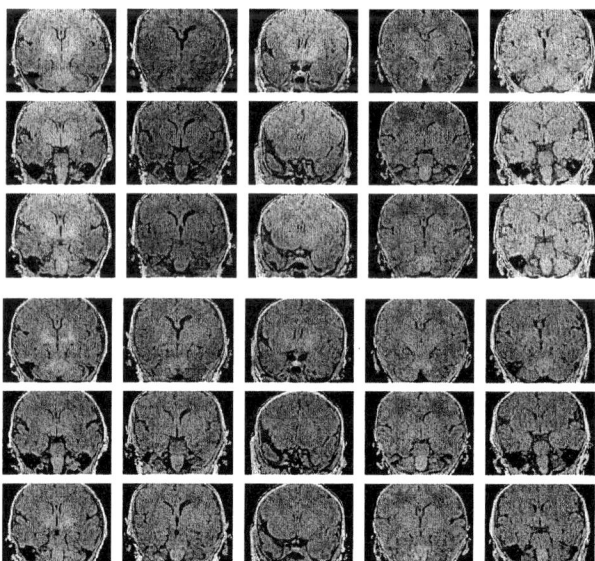

Fig. 6. This figure shows the results of our volumetric joint bias removal algorithm. 15 patient volumes were used, and the bias in each volume was reduced using the 27-component basis volumes for smooth three-dimensional bias fields. The top half of the figure shows 3 images in each column from 5 different patients (rows). The bottom shows the corrected images

In Figure 6, we show the results of our volumetric bias removal algorithm. The bias removal algorithm was done using the 27-volume basis on 15 patients simultaneously. Results are shown for 3 slices from each of five patients. In future work, we plan to make specific comparisons of volumetric joint bias removal techniques with sequential slice-based joint bias removal to see if the former offers any significant advantage.

The idea of minimizing pixelwise entropies to remove nuisance variables from a set of images is not new. In particular, Miller et al. [6, 7] presented an approach they call *congealing* in which the sum of pixelwise entropies is minimized by *separate affine transforms* applied to each image. Our method can thus be considered an extension of the congealing process to non-spatial transformations. We are currently combining such approaches to do registration and bias removal simultaneously.

This work uses information unused in other methods, i.e. information across images. This suggests an iterative scheme in which both types of information, both within and across images, are used. Local models could be based on weighted neighborhoods of pixels, *pixel cylinders*, rather than single pixel-stacks, in sparse data scenarios. For "easy" bias correction problems, such an approach may be overkill, but for difficult problems in bias correction, where the bias field is difficult to separate from the underlying tissue, as discussed in [1], such an approach could produce critical extra leverage.

We thank Dr. Terrie Inder and Dr. Simon Warfield for graciously providing the infant brain images for this work. The images were obtained under NIH grant P41 RR13218. Also, we thank Neil Weisenfeld and Sandy Wells for helpful discussions. This work was partially supported by Army Research Office grant DAAD 19-02-1-0383.

References

1. Fan, A., Wells, W., Fisher, J., Cetin, M., Haker, S., Mulkern, C., Tempany, C., Willsky, A.: A unified variational approach to denoising and bias correction in MR. IPMI, 2003.
2. Beirlant, J., Dudewicz, E., Gyorfi, L. and van der Meulen, E.: Nonparametric entropy estimation: An overview. *Int. J. of Math. and Stat. Sci., 6.* pp.17-39. 1997.
3. Cover, T. and Thomas J. *Elements of Information Theory.* Wiley, 1991.
4. Learned-Miller, E. G. and Fisher, J.: ICA using spacings estimates of entropy. *Journal of Machine Learning Research*, Volume 4, pp. 1271-1295, 2003.
5. Learned-Miller, E. G. and Ahammad, P.: Joint MRI Bias Removal Using Entropy Minimization Across Images. *Neural Information Processing Systems 17*, pp. 761-768, 2005.
6. Miller, E. G., Matsakis, N., Viola, P. A.: Learning from one example through shared densities on transforms. *IEEE Conference on Computer Vision and Pattern Recognition.* 2000.
7. Miller, E. G.: Learning from one example in machine vision by sharing probability densities. Ph.D. thesis. Massachusetts Institute of Technology. 2002.
8. Vasicek, O.: A test for normality based on sample entropy. *Journal of the Royal Statistical Society Series B, 31.* pp. 632-636, 1976.
9. Wells, W. M., Grimson, W. E. L., Kikinis, R., Jolesz, F.: Adaptive segmentation of MRI data. *IEEE Transactions on Medical Imaging, 15.* pp. 429-442, 1996.
10. Collins, D.L., Zijdenbos, A.P., Kollokian, J.G., Sled, N.J., Kabani, C.J., Holmes, C.J., Evans, A.C.: Design and Construction of a realistic digital brain phantom. IEEE Transactions on Medical Imaging, 17. pp. 463-468, 1998.
11. Viola, P.A. : Alignment by maximization of mutual information. Ph.D. Thesis. Massachusetts Institute of Technology. 1995.

Unified Statistical Approach to Cortical Thickness Analysis

Moo K. Chung[1], Steve Robbins[2], and Alan C. Evans[2]

[1]Department of Statistics, University of Wisconsin-Madison
[2]Montreal Neurological Institute, McGill University, Canada
mchung@stat.wisc.edu, {stever, alan}@bic.mni.mcgill.ca

Abstract. This paper presents a unified image processing and analysis framework for cortical thickness in characterizing a clinical population. The emphasis is placed on the development of data smoothing and analysis framework. The human brain cortex is a highly convoluted surface. Due to the convoluted non-Euclidean surface geometry, data smoothing and analysis on the cortex are inherently difficult. When measurements lie on a curved surface, it is natural to assign kernel smoothing weights based on the geodesic distance along the surface rather than the Euclidean distance. We present a new data smoothing framework that address this problem implicitly without actually computing the geodesic distance and present its statistical properties. Afterwards, the statistical inference is based on the random field theory based multiple comparison correction. As an illustration, we have applied the method in detecting the regions of abnormal cortical thickness in 16 high functioning autistic children.

1 Introduction

The human cerebral cortex has the topology of a 2D highly convoluted grey matter shell of average thickness of 3mm. The thickness of the grey matter shell is usually referred as the *cortical thickness* and can be obtained from magnetic resonance images (MRI). The cortical thickness can be used as an anatomical index for quantifying cortical shape variations. The thickness measures are obtained after a sequence of image processing steps which are described briefly here. The first step is to classify each voxel into three different tissue types: cerebrospinal fluid (CSF), grey matter, and white matter. The CSF/grey matter interface is called the *outer cortical surface* while the grey/white matter interface is called the *inner cortical surface*. These two surfaces bound the gray matter. The mainstream approach in representing the cortical surface has been to use a fine triangular mesh that is constructed from deformable surface algorithms [10] [14]. Cortical thickness is estimated by computing the distance between the two triangular meshes [11] [14]. In our study, we have used the method presented in [14]. In order to compare cortical thickness measures across subjects, it is necessary to align the cortical surfaces via surface registration algorithms [16] [20].

For cross-comparison between subjects, surfaces are registered into the *template surface* which serves as reference coordinates.

The image segmentation, thickness computation and surface registration procedures are expected to introduce noise in the thickness measure. In order to increase the signal-to-noise ratio (SNR) and smoothness of data for the random field theory, some type of data smoothing is necessary. For 3D whole brain MRIs, Gaussian kernel smoothing is widely used to smooth data, in part, due to its simplicity in numerical implementation. The Gaussian kernel weights an observation according to its Euclidean distance. However, data residing on the convoluted brain surface fails to be isotropic in the Euclidean sense. On the curved surface, a straight line between two points is not the shortest distance so one may incorrectly assign less weights to closer observations. So when the observations lie on the cortical surface, it is more natural to assign the weights based on the geodesic distance along the surface. Previously *diffusion smoothing* has been developed for smoothing data along the cortex before the random field based multiple comparison correction [1] [6] [7]. By solving a diffusion equation on a manifold, Gaussian kernel smoothing can be indirectly generalized. Although diffusion smoothing has been used widely in image analysis starting with [15], most of previous work is about surface fairing [19]. There is a very few publications that smooth out observations defined on surface for data analysis [1] [3] [6] [7]. The drawback of the previous diffusion smoothing approach is the need for setting of up a finite element method (FEM) to solve the diffusion equation numerically and making the algorithm converges [6]. To address this problem, we have developed a simpler and more efficient method based on the heat kernel convolution on a manifold.

As an illustration, the method was applied to groups of autistic and normal subjects, and we were able to detect the regions of statistically significant cortical thickness difference between the groups.

2 Heat Kernel Smoothing

The cortical surface $\partial\Omega$ can be assumed to be a C^2 Riemannian manifold [12]. Let $p = X(u^1, u^2) \in \partial\Omega$ be the parametric representation of $\partial\Omega$. We assume the following model on thickness measure Y:

$$Y(p) = \theta(p) + \epsilon(p),$$

where $\theta(p)$ is a mean thickness function and $\epsilon(p)$ is a zero-mean random field, possibly a Gaussian white noise process, with covariance function $R_\epsilon(p, q)$. The Laplace-Beltrami operator Δ corresponding to the surface parameterization $p = X(u^1, u^2) \in \partial\Omega$ is given by

$$\Delta = \frac{1}{\det g^{1/2}} \sum_{i,j=1}^{2} \frac{\partial}{\partial u^i}\left(\det g^{1/2} g^{ij} \frac{\partial}{\partial u^j}\right),$$

where $g = (g_{ij})$ is the Riemannian metric tensor. Solving equation $\Delta\psi = \lambda\psi$, we order eigenvalues $0 = \lambda_0 \leq \lambda_1 \leq \lambda_2 \leq \cdots$ and corresponding eigenfunc-

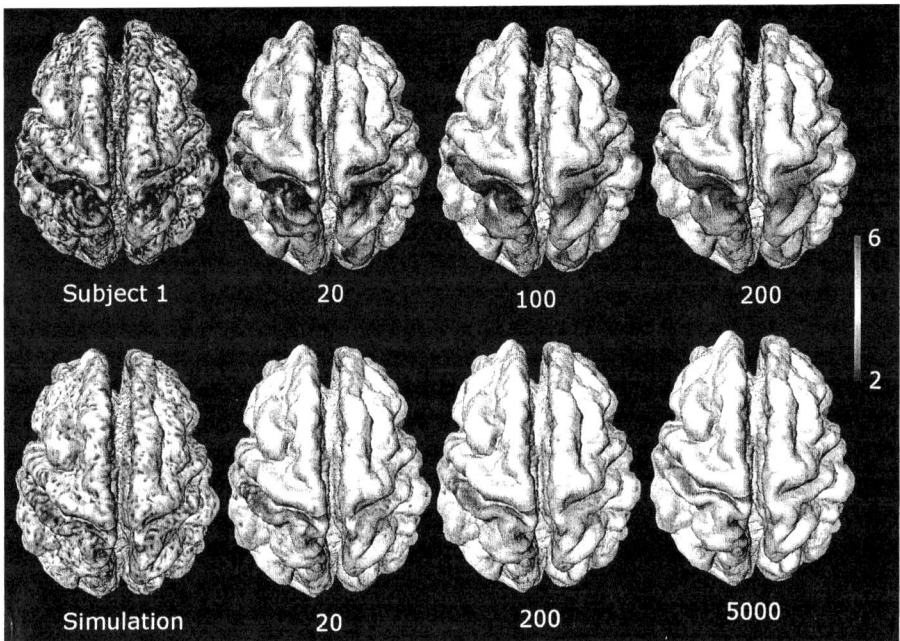

Fig. 1. Top: Heat kernel smoothing of cortical thickness with $\sigma = 1$ and $k = 20, 100, 200$ iterations. Bottom: Heat kernel smoothing on simulated data with $\sigma = 1$ and $k = 20, 200, 5000$ iterations. The mean thickness and the variance are estimated from 12 normal subject data and Gaussian white noise is added to the mean function

tions $\psi_0, \psi_1, \cdots$. The eigenfunctions ψ_j form orthonormal basis of $L^2(\partial\Omega)$, the L^2 space of functions defined on $\partial\Omega$. On the unit sphere, the eigenvalues are $m(m+n-1)$ and the corresponding eigenfunctions are spherical harmonics Y_{lm} ($|m| \leq l, 0 \leq l$) [21]. On an arbitrary surface, the explicit representation of eigenvalues and eigenfunction are only obtained through numerical methods. Based on orthonormal basis, the *heat kernel* $K_\sigma(p, q)$ is analytically given as

$$K_\sigma(p,q) = \sum_{j=0}^{\infty} e^{-\lambda_j \sigma} \psi_j(p)\psi_j(q), \tag{1}$$

where σ is the bandwidth of the kernel [2] [17] . When $g_{ij} = \delta_{ij}$, the heat kernel becomes the Gaussian kernel, which is the probability density of $N(0, \sigma^2)$. natural extension of the Gaussian kernel. This can be interpreted as the transition probability density for an isotropic diffusion process with respect to the surface area element [22]. The kernel is symmetric, i.e. $K_\sigma(p,q) = K_\sigma(q,p)$ and isotropic with respect to the geodesic distance $d(p,q)$.

Definition 1. *Heat kernel smoothing of cortical thickness Y is the convolution:*

$$K_\sigma * Y(p) = \int_{\partial\Omega} K_\sigma(p,q) Y(q) \, dq. \tag{2}$$

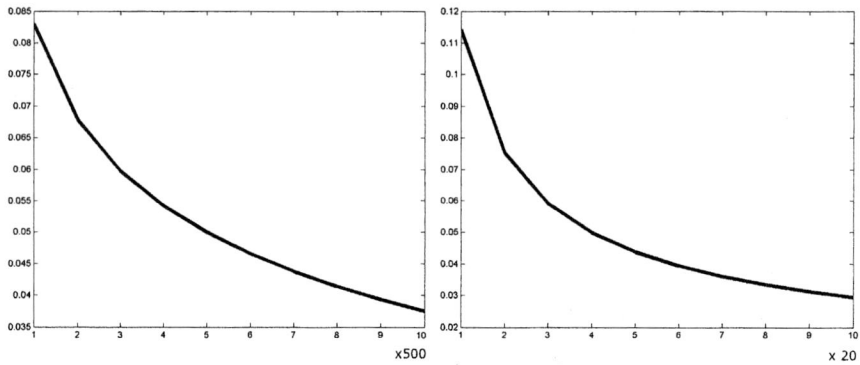

Fig. 2. Left: Within-subject variance plotted over the number of iterations of heat kernel smoothing with $\sigma = 1$. Decreasing variance implies the convergence of the heat kernel smoothing to the mean thickness (Theorem 4). Right: Between-subject variance plotted over the number of iterations illustrating Theorem 5

It can be written in terms of basis function expansion:

$$K_\sigma * Y(p) = \sum_{j=0}^{\infty} \alpha_j \phi_j(p),$$

where $\alpha_j = e^{-\lambda_j \sigma} \int_{\partial \Omega} \phi_j(q) Y(q) \, dq$. We also define the *heat kernel estimator* of unknown signal $\theta(p)$ to be $\hat{\theta}_\sigma(p) = K_\sigma * Y(p)$. As $\sigma \to 0$, $K_\sigma(p, q)$ becomes the Dirac delta function $\delta(p, q)$ so the heat kernel estimator becomes unbiased as $\sigma \to 0$, i.e. $\lim_{\sigma \to 0} \mathbb{E}\hat{\theta}_\sigma(p) = \theta(p)$. As σ gets larger, the bias increases. However the total bias over all cortex is always zero, i.e. $\int_{\partial \Omega} [\theta(p) - \mathbb{E}\hat{\theta}_\sigma(p)] \, dp = 0$. Let us list important nontrivial properties of heat kernel smoothing.

Theorem 1. *$K_\sigma * Y$ is the unique solution of the following isotropic diffusion equation at time $t = \sigma^2/2$:*

$$\frac{\partial f}{\partial t} = \Delta f, \; f(p, 0) = Y(p), p \in \partial \Omega \qquad (3)$$

This is a well known result [17]. This theorem implies that the heat kernel smoothing isotropically assigns weights on $\partial \Omega$.

Theorem 2.

$$K_\sigma * Y(p) = \arg \min_{\theta(p) \in L^2(\partial \Omega)} \int_{\partial \Omega} K_\sigma(p, q) [Y(q) - \theta(p)]^2 \, dq.$$

The proof can be found in [5]. This shows that the heat kernel smoothing can be formulated as a regression on a manifold.

Theorem 3.
$$\underbrace{K_\sigma * \cdots * K_\sigma}_{k \text{ times}} *Y = K_{\sqrt{k}\sigma} * Y.$$

This can be seen as a scale space property of diffusion. From Theorem 1, $K_\sigma * (K_\sigma * Y)$ can be taken as the diffusion of signal $K_\sigma * Y$ after time $\sigma^2/2$ so that $K_\sigma * (K_\sigma * Y)$ is the diffusion of signal Y after time σ^2. Hence

$$K_\sigma * K_\sigma * Y = K_{\sqrt{2}\sigma} * Y.$$

Arguing inductively we see that the general statement holds. We will denote the k-fold iterated kernel as $K_\sigma^{(k)} = \underbrace{K_\sigma * \cdots * K_\sigma}_{k \text{ times}}$. This is the basis of our iterated heat kernel smoothing. Heat kernel with a large bandwidth will be performed by iteratively applying heat kernel smoothing with a smaller bandwidth. For instance iterated heat kernel smoothing with $\sigma = 1$ and $k = 200$ will generate heat kernel smoothing with the effective bandwidth of $\sqrt{200} = 14.14$mm. Figure 1 shows the process of iterated heat kernel smoothing.

Theorem 4.
$$\lim_{\sigma \to \infty} K_\sigma * Y = \frac{\int_{\partial\Omega} Y(q)\, dq}{\mu(\partial\Omega)}.$$

Here $\mu(\partial\Omega)$ is the total surface area of $\partial\Omega$. This theorem shows that when we choose large bandwidth, heat kernel smoothing converges to the sample mean of data on $\partial\Omega$. Figure 1 (bottom) shows the convergence of heat kernel smoothing to the within-subject mean cortex 4mm as the bandwidth increases. Figure 2 (left) shows the convergence of the within-subject variance indirectly implying $K_\sigma * Y$ converges to a constant, which is the average thickness over the cortex.

It is natural to assume the measurements $Y(p)$ and $Y(q)$ to have less correlation when p and q are away so we assume the covariance function to be $R_\epsilon(p,q) = \rho(d(p,q))$ for some nondecreasing function ρ. Then we can show the variance reduction property of heat kernel smoothing.

Theorem 5. $\mathbf{Var}[K_\sigma * Y(p)] \leq \mathbf{Var}Y(p)$ for each $p \in \partial\Omega$.

Figure 2 (right) shows the between-subject variance decreases as σ increases.

The problem with the heat kernel smoothing on an arbitrary surface is that the explicit analytic form of the heat kernel is unknown. To address this problem we use the *parametrix expansion* of the heat kernel [17] [22]:

$$K_\sigma(p,q) = \frac{1}{(2\pi\sigma)^{1/2}} \exp\Big[-\frac{d^2(p,q)}{2\sigma^2}\Big][1 + O(\sigma^2)] \tag{4}$$

for small $d(p,q)$. This expansion spells out the exact form of the kernel for small bandwidth. When the metric is flat, the heat kernel becomes a Gaussian kernel, reconfirming that heat convolution is a generalization of Gaussian kernel. The expansion is the basis of our heat kernel smoothing formulation. Heat kernel smoothing with a large bandwidth will be decomposed into iterated kernel

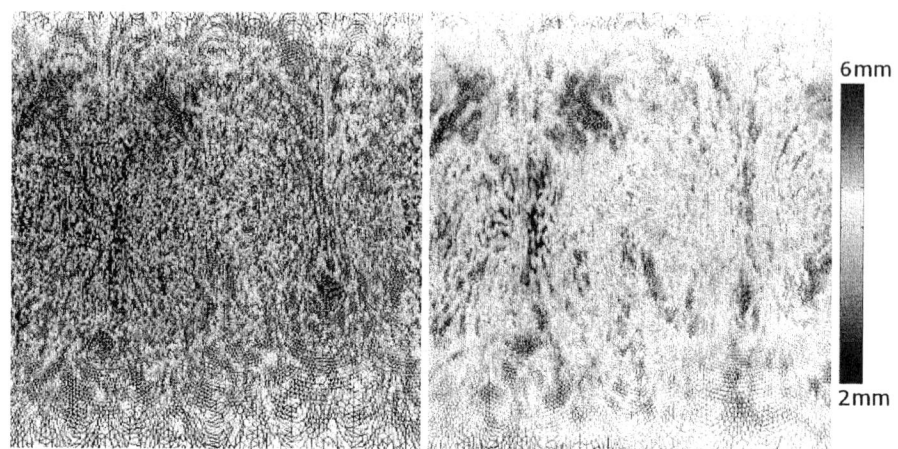

Fig. 3. Thickness maps are projected onto a unit square. Left: original noisy thickness map. Right: Heat kernel smoothing with $\sigma = 1$ and $k = 200$ iterations

smoothing. We will truncate and normalize the heat kernel using the first order term. For each $p \in \partial \Omega$, we define

$$\widetilde{K}_\sigma(p,q) = \frac{\exp\left[-\frac{d^2(p,q)}{2\sigma^2}\right] \mathbf{1}_{B_p}(q)}{\int_{B_p} \exp\left[-\frac{d^2(p,q)}{2\sigma^2}\right] dq}, \qquad (5)$$

where $\mathbf{1}_{B_p}$ is an indicator function defined on a small compact domain containing B such that $\mathbf{1}_{B_p}(q) = 1$ if $q \in B_p$ and $\mathbf{1}_{B_p}(q) = 0$ otherwise. Note that for each fixed p, $\widetilde{K}_\sigma(p,q)$ defines a probability distribution in B_p and it converges to $K_\sigma(p,q)$ as $\sigma \to 0$ in B_p. This implies

$$\widetilde{K}_\sigma^{(k)} * Y(p) \to K_\sigma^{(k)} * Y(p) \text{ as } \sigma \to 0.$$

For a discrete triangular mesh, we can take B_p to be a set of points containing p and its neighboring nodes $q_1, \cdots, q_m$, and take a discrete measure on B_p, which still make (5) a probability distribution. This can be viewed as a *Gaussian kernel Nadaraya-Watson* type smoothing extended to manifolds [4]. Figure 3 shows a flattened thickness map illustrating how heat kernel smoothing can enhance the thickness pattern by increasing the signal-to-noise ratio.

3 Random Field Theory on Cortical Manifold

Here we will describe how to perform multiple comparisons on $\partial \Omega$ using the random field theory. The random field theory based approach is widely used for correcting multiple comparisons in 3D whole brain volume but rarely used on 2D cortical manifolds [1] [7] [8] [24]. First we combine both the autistic and the

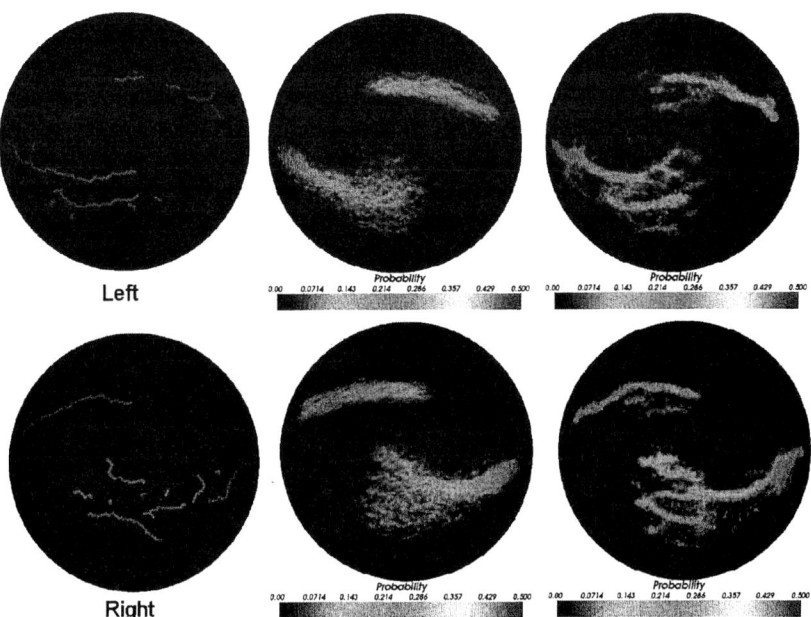

Fig. 4. Automatically generated traces of the central and superior temporal sulcal fundi [3]. The first column shows the traces generated for the template surface. The second column shows the probability of sulcal matching based on 149 normal subjects before any surface normalization. The third column shows the probabilities after surface normalization. The first row is the left hemisphere and the second row is the right hemisphere. Note that the distribution is much more spatially concentrated and the matching probabilities are much greater after normalization

control subjects in a single indexing j and set up a general linear model (GLM) on cortical thickness Y_j for subject j:

$$K_\sigma * Y_j(p) = \lambda_1(p) + \lambda_2(p) \cdot \text{age}_j + \lambda_3(p) \cdot \text{volume}_j + \beta(p) \cdot \text{group}_j + \epsilon_j \quad (6)$$

is used. Here dummy variable group is 1 for the autistic subjects and 0 for the normal subjects. volume is the total gray matter volume for subject j. The total gray matter volume is estimated by computing the volume bounded by the both outer and inner surfaces [8]. The error is modeled as a smooth Gaussian random field which is viewed as the heat kernel convolution with Gaussian white noise, i.e. $\epsilon_j = K_\sigma * W$. Then we test the group difference by performing a hypothesis testing:

$$H_0 : \beta(p) = 0 \text{ for all } p \in \partial\Omega$$

v.s.

$$H_1 : \beta(p) \neq 0 \text{ for some } p \in \partial\Omega.$$

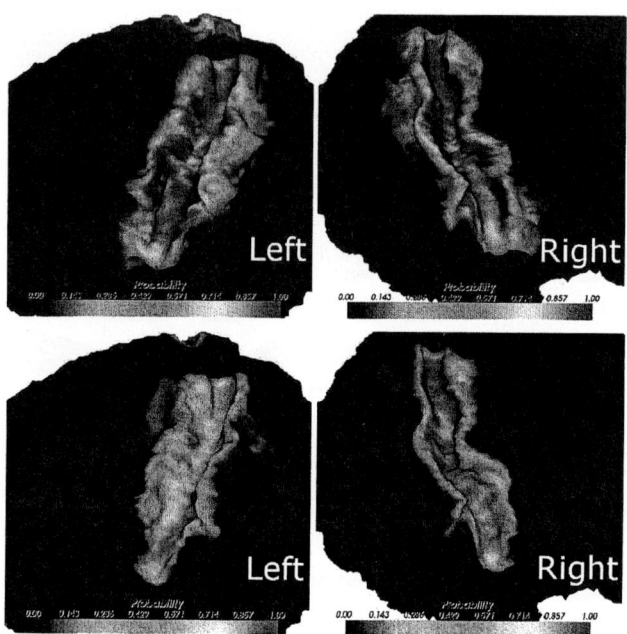

Fig. 5. Probability of sulcal matching, after normalization, for 39 manually identified central sulci defined as the surface region surrounded by gyri, not just the fundus. The views are illustrated on a slightly-opened version of the template cortical surface in order to better view inside the sulcus. The warping in 2D localizes the central sulcus nearly completely inside the template central sulcus. Left (right) figure is the left (right) central sulci

The test statistic is the ratio of the sum of the squared residual errors under the null and alternate models. Under H_0, the test statistic is a F random random field with 1 and $n = n_1 + n_2 - 4$ degrees of freedom [23]. The null hypothesis is the intersection of collection of hypothesis $H_0 = \bigcap_{p \in \partial \Omega} H_0(p)$, where $H_0(p) : \beta(p) = 0$ for each fixed p. The type I error for the multiple comparisons is then given by

$$\alpha = P\Big(\bigcup_{p \in \partial \Omega} \{F(p) > h\} \Big) = 1 - P\Big(\bigcap_{p \in \partial \Omega} F(p) \leq h\} \Big)$$
$$= 1 - P(\sup_{p \in \partial \Omega} F(p) \leq h) = P(\sup_{p \in \partial \Omega} F(p) > h)$$

for some h. The resulting p-value is usually called the *corrected p-value*. The distribution of $\sup_{p \in \partial \Omega} F(p)$ is asymptotically given as

$$P(\sup_{p \in \partial \Omega} F(p) > h) \approx \sum_{d=0}^{2} \phi_d(\partial \Omega) \rho_d(h) \qquad (7)$$

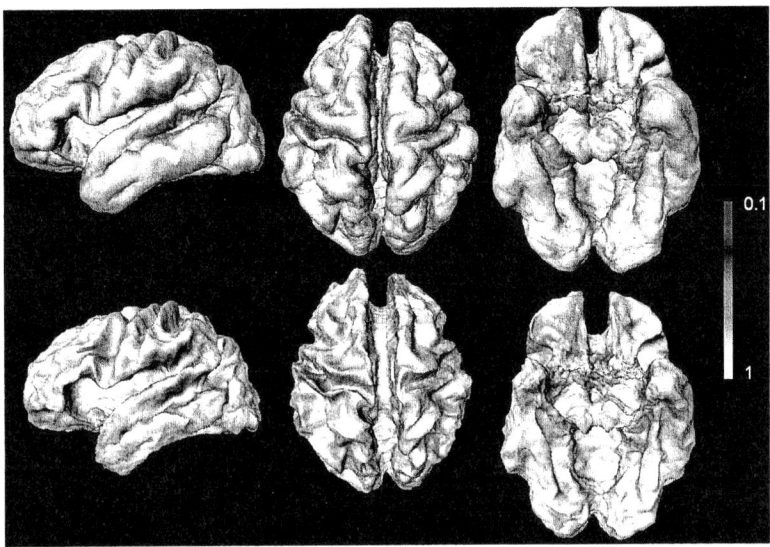

Fig. 6. Corrected p value maps of F-test removing the effect of age and relative gray matter volume difference projected onto the average outer (top) and inner surfaces (bottom). It shows relatively asymmetric thickness difference between two groups

where ϕ_d are the d-dimensional Minkowski functionals of $\partial\Omega$ and ρ_d are the d-dimensional Euler characteristic (EC) density of F-field with $\alpha = 1$ and $\beta = n$ degrees of freedom [23]. The Minkowski functionals are $\phi_0 = 2, \phi_1 = 0, \phi_2 =$ area$(\partial\Omega)/2 = 49,616$mm^2, the half area of the template cortex $\partial\Omega$. The EC density is given by

$$\rho_0(h) = \int_h^\infty \frac{\Gamma(\frac{\alpha+\beta}{2})}{\Gamma(\frac{\alpha}{2})\Gamma(\frac{\beta}{2})} \frac{\alpha}{\beta} \left(\frac{\alpha x}{\beta}\right)^{\frac{(\alpha-2)}{2}} \left(1 + \frac{\alpha x}{\beta}\right)^{-\frac{(\alpha+\beta)}{2}} dx,$$

$$\rho_2(h) = \frac{\lambda}{2\pi} \frac{\Gamma(\frac{\alpha+\beta-2}{2})}{\Gamma(\frac{\alpha}{2})\Gamma(\frac{\beta}{2})} \left(\frac{\alpha h}{\beta}\right)^{\frac{(\alpha-2)}{2}} \left(1 + \frac{\alpha h}{\beta}\right)^{-\frac{(\alpha+\beta-2)}{2}}$$

$$\times \left[(\beta-1)\frac{\alpha h}{\beta} - (\alpha-1)\right]$$

where λ measures the smoothness of fields ϵ and given as $\lambda = 1/(2\sigma^2)$. The resulting corrected p-values maps for F field is shown in Figure 6. The main use of the corrected p-value maps are the localization and visualization of thickness difference.

4 Application

T_1-weighted MR scans were acquired for 16 autistic and 12 control subjects on a 3-Tesla GE SIGNA scanner. They are all right-handed males. 16 autistic subjects were diagnosed with high functioning autism (HFA). The average age is 17.1 ± 2.8 is for the control subjects and 16.1 ± 4.5 for the autistic subjects. The complete description of the data set, image acquisition parameters, the subsequent image processing routines, and the interpretation of the resulting statistical parametric maps is provided in [5]. Each image underwent several image preprocessing steps. Image intensity nonuniformity was corrected using nonparametric nonuniform intensity normalization method [18]. Then using the automatic image processing pipeline, the image was spatially normalized into the Montreal neurological institute (MNI) stereotaxic space using a global affine transformation. Subsequently, an automatic tissue-segmentation algorithm based on a supervised artificial neural network classifier was used to classify each voxel as cerebrospinal fluid (CSF), gray matter, or white matter [13]. Brain substructures such as the brain stem and the cerebellum were removed automatically. Triangular meshes for inner and outer cortical surfaces were obtained by a deformable surface algorithm [14]. Such a *deformable surface* approach has the advantage that the surface topology can be fixed to be spherical and the deformation process can maintain a non-intersecting surface at all times, obviating the need for topology correction [9]. The mesh starts as an ellipsoid located outside the brain and is shrunk to obtain the inner cortical surface. Then the inner surface is expanded, with constraints, to obtain the outer cortical surface. The triangular meshes are not constrained to lie on voxel boundaries. Instead, the triangular meshes can cut through a voxel, which serves to reduce discretization error and partial volume effect. Thickness is measured using the natural anatomical homology between vertices on the inner and outer cortical surface meshes, since the outer surface is obtained by deforming the inner surface.

Afterwards, thickness measures are smoothed with heat kernel smoothing with parameters $\sigma = 1$ and $k = 200$ giving the effective smoothness of $\sqrt{200} = 14.14$ mm. A surface-to-surface registration to a template surface was performed to facilitate vertex-by-vertex inter-subject thickness comparison. We have formulated it as a registration problem of two functional data on a unit sphere [20]. First a mapping from a cortical surface onto the sphere is established while recording the mapping. Then cortical curvatures are mapped onto the sphere. The two curvature functions on the sphere are aligned by solving a regularization problem that tries to minimize the discrepancy between two functions while maximizing the smoothness of the alignment in such a way that the pattern of gyral ridges are matched smoothly. This alignment is projected back to the original surface using the recorded mapping. This regularization mechanism produces a smooth deformation field, with very little folding. The deformation field is parameterized using a triangulated mesh and the algorithm proceeds in a coarse-to-fine manner, with four levels of mesh resolution. Figure 4 and Figure 5 illustrate the effectiveness of this surface registration algorithm by computing the probability of matching superior temporal sulcal fundi and central sulci.

After smoothing out thickness measurements, statistical analysis is performed following the procedures described in the previous section. The resulting corrected p-value map (< 0.1) for the F statistic is projected onto the template surface for visualization. Figure 6 shows statistically significant regions of cortical thickness between two groups. After removing the effect of age and total grey matter volume difference, the statistically significant regions of thickness decreases are highly localized at the right inferior orbital prefrontal cortex, the left superior temporal sulcus and the left occipito-temporal gyrus in autistic subjects.

5 Conclusions

This paper has introduced heat kernel smoothing and its statistical properties for data analysis on the cortical manifolds. The technique can be used in smooth out data that is necessary in the random field theory based multiple comparison correction. We have applied the methodology in detecting the regions of abnormal cortical thickness in a group of autistic subjects; however, the approach is not limited to a particular clinical population. The algorithm is implemented in MATLAB and freely available to download on the web http://www.stat.wisc.edu/~mchung/softwares/hk. A sample cortical mesh for a subject and its thickness measures can be also downloaded from the same website for other researchers.

Acknowledgement

Authors wish to thank Kim Dalton and Richard J. Davidson of the Waisman Laboratory for Brain Imaging and Behavior, University of Wisconsin-Madison for providing the data illustrated in this study.

References

1. A. Andrade, Kherif, J. F., Mangin, K.J. Worsley, A. Paradis, O. Simon, S. Dehaene, D. Le Bihan, and J-B. Poline. Detection of fmri activation using cortical surface mapping. *Human Brain Mapping*, 12:79–93, 2001.
2. N. Berline, E. Getzler, and Vergne M. *Heat kernels and dirac operators*. Springer-Verlag, 1991.
3. A. Cachia, J.-F. Mangin, Riviére D., D. Papadopoulos-Orfanos, F. Kherif, I. Bloch, and J. Régis. A generic framework for parcellation of the cortical surface into gyri using geodesic voronoï diagrams. *Image Analysis*, 7:403–416, 2003.
4. P. Chaudhuri and J. S. Marron. Scale space view of curve estimation. *The Annals of Statistics*, 28:408–428, 2000.
5. M.K. Chung, S. Robbins, Davidson R.J. Alexander A.L. Dalton, K.M., and A.C. Evans. Cortical thickness analysis in autism with heat kernel smoothing. *NeuroImage*, 2005 in press.
6. M.K. Chung and J. Taylor. Diffusion smoothing on brain surface via finite element method. In *Proceedings of IEEE International Symposium on Biomedical Imaging (ISBI)*, 2004.

7. M.K. Chung, K.J. Worsley, S. Robbins, and A.C. Evans. Tensor-based brain surface modeling and analysis. In *IEEE Conference on Computer Vision and Pattern Recognition (CVPR)*, volume I, pages 467–473, 2003.
8. M.K. Chung, K.J. Worsley, S. Robbins, T. Paus, Taylor, J.N. J., Giedd, J.L. Rapoport, and A.C. Evans. Deformation-based surface morphometry applied to gray matter deformation. *NeuroImage*, 18:198–213, 2003.
9. A.M. Dale and B. Fischl. Cortical surface-based analysis i. segmentation and surface reconstruction. *NeuroImage*, 9:179–194, 1999.
10. C. Davatzikos and R.N. Bryan. Using a deformable surface model to obtain a shape representation of the cortex. *Proceedings of the IEEE International Conference on Computer Vision*, 1995.
11. S.E. Jones, B.R. Buchbinder, and I. Aharon. Three-dimensional mapping of cortical thickness using laplace's equation. *Human Brain Mapping*, 11:12–32, 2000.
12. S.C. Joshi, J. Wang, M.I. Miller, D.C. Van Essen, and U. Grenander. On the differential geometry of the cortical surface. *Vision Geometry IV*, pages 304–311, 1995.
13. K. Kollakian. Performance analysis of automatic techniques for tissue classification in magnetic resonance images of the human brain. Technical Report Master's thesis, Concordia University, Montreal, Quebec, Canada, 1996.
14. J.D. MacDonald, N. Kabani, D. Avis, and A.C. Evans. Automated 3-d extraction of inner and outer surfaces of cerebral cortex from mri. *NeuroImage*, 12:340–356, 2000.
15. P. Perona and J. Malik. Scale-space and edge detection using anisotropic diffusion. *IEEE Trans. Pattern Analysis and Machine Intelligence*, 12:629–639, 1990.
16. S.M. Robbins. Anatomical standardization of the human brain in euclidean 3-space and on the cortical 2-manifold. Technical Report PhD thesis, School of Computer Science, McGill University, Montreal, Quebec, Canada, 2003.
17. S. Rosenberg. *The Laplacian on a Riemannian Manifold*. Cambridge University Press, 1997.
18. J.G. Sled, A.P. Zijdenbos, and A.C. Evans. A nonparametric method for automatic correction of intensity nonuniformity in mri data. *IEEE Transactions on Medical Imaging*, 17:87–97, 1988.
19. N. Sochen, R. Kimmel, and R. Malladi. A general framework for low level vision. *IEEE Transactions on Image Processing*, 7:310–318, 1998.
20. P.M. Thompson and A.W. Toga. A surface-based technique for warping 3-dimensional images of the brain. *IEEE Transactions on Medical Imaging*, 15:1–16, 1996.
21. G. Wahba. *Spline models for observational data*. SIAM, 1990.
22. F.-Y. Wang. Sharp explict lower bounds of heat kernels. *Annals of Probability*, 24:1995–2006, 1997.
23. K.J. Worsley. Local maxima and the expected euler characteristic of excursion sets of χ^2, f and t fields. *Advances in Applied Probability.*, 26:13–42, 1994.
24. K.J. Worsley, J.E. Taylor, F. Tomaiuolo, and J. Lerch. Unified univariate and multivariate random field theory. *NeuroImage*, 2005.

zHARP: Three-Dimensional Motion Tracking from a Single Image Plane

Khaled Z. Abd-Elmoniem[1], Matthias Stuber[12], Nael F. Osman[12], and Jerry L. Prince[12]

[1] Department of Electrical and Computer Engineering,
Johns Hopkins University, Baltimore, MD 21218, USA
[2] Department of Radiology and Radiological Sciences,
Johns Hopkins School of Medicine, Baltimore, MD 21287, USA
{khaled, mstuber1, nael, prince}@jhu.edu

Abstract. Three-dimensional imaging and quantification of myocardial function are essential steps in the evaluation of cardiac disease. We propose a tagged magnetic resonance imaging methodology called zHARP that encodes and automatically tracks myocardial displacement in three dimensions. Unlike other motion encoding techniques, zHARP encodes both in-plane and through-plane motion in a single image plane without affecting the acquisition speed. Postprocessing unravels this encoding in order to directly track the 3-D displacement of every point within the image plane throughout an entire image sequence. Experimental results include a phantom validation experiment, which compares zHARP to phase contrast imaging, and an *in vivo* study of a normal human volunteer. Results demonstrate that the simultaneous extraction of in-plane and through-plane displacements from tagged images is feasible.

1 Introduction

The use of magnetic resonance imaging (MRI) for the quantification of regional function of the heart based on the measurement of motion has great potential for clinical adoption. Primary limiting factors to date are the lengthy image acquisition protocols and tedious postprocessing procedures required to yield regional motion measures. This paper addresses both of these limitations in a novel combined imaging and postprocessing method based on tagged magnetic resonance imaging and harmonic phase (HARP) processing [1, 2].

Three main MR imaging protocols that have been used for the quantification of myocardial motion: myocardial tagging, displacement encoding with stimulated echoes (DENSE) [3, 4], and phase contrast (PC) velocity encoding techniques [5, 6]. In tagging, myocardial spins are modulated at end-diastole in a prespecified pattern. Later in the cardiac cycle, the displaced tag lines are imaged and tracked using postprocessing algorithms in order to compute displacement and strain images. This technique permits rapid imaging and visualization as well as fast, automatic computation of in-plane (i.e., two-dimensional) motion measures using HARP. To date, however, there has been no extension to three-dimensions in an equally efficient and automatic way.

Phase contrast imaging adds to every myocardial spin a phase value proportional to the velocity in the encoding direction. PC imaging times are generally long and phase distortion leads to significant measurement errors. Also, since velocity rather than displacement is the measured quantity, computation of displacement and strain (as opposed to strain rate) at later times in a sequence is typically corrupted by numerical integration errors. PC is readily extended to three-dimensions though imaging time becomes prohibitively long.

DENSE encodes position in a manner similar to MR tagging through the use of stimulated echoes. Automatic processing analogous to HARP can then be used to compute displacement and strain. The acquisition protocol of DENSE supports higher spatial resolution than that of conventional HARP techniques, but the computation of in-plane motion is sensitive to through-plane motion in DENSE, unlike conventional tagging techniques.

To date, extension of these three basic approaches to three dimensions has required extensive additional data collection over that of 2-D imaging; and, except for PC, the result yields only sparse motion information. In all three cases, long imaging times may be prohibitive due to patient breath-holding constraints or may produce sub-optimal results due to gross misregistration of images collected over a long period of time.

In this paper, we present a novel MRI methodology called zHARP, which images and automatically tracks the 3-D myocardial displacement of all points in an image plane. A pulse sequence for acquiring an image that encodes both in-plane and through-plane motion without affecting the acquisition speed of the underlying pulse sequence is presented. An automatic algorithm, based on the harmonic phase (HARP) concept, that tracks the 3-D displacements of every point in the image plane through the entire image sequence, is also presented. The zHARP methodology is validated in both phantom and human studies.

2 Methods

2.1 Pulse Sequence

ZHARP uses a slice-following 3-D tagging imaging sequence. The pulse sequence is similar to the standard slice-following CSPAMM (SF-CSPAMM) sequence [7] except that a small z-encoding gradient is applied immediately before the readout and again with the opposite polarity to the second orthogonal CSPAMM acquisition, as shown in Fig. 1. This gradient adds a z-position dependent phase φ_z to every material point in the acquired slice. This additional phase is linearly related to the distance of the point from the isocenter of the scanner. Susceptibility and general field inhomogeneities lead to an additional (artifactual) phase accumulation φ_e. This erroneous phase is identical in both the horizontally and vertically tagged images, however, and it will be shown to (mathematically) vanish in the computation of both in-plane and through-plane displacements.

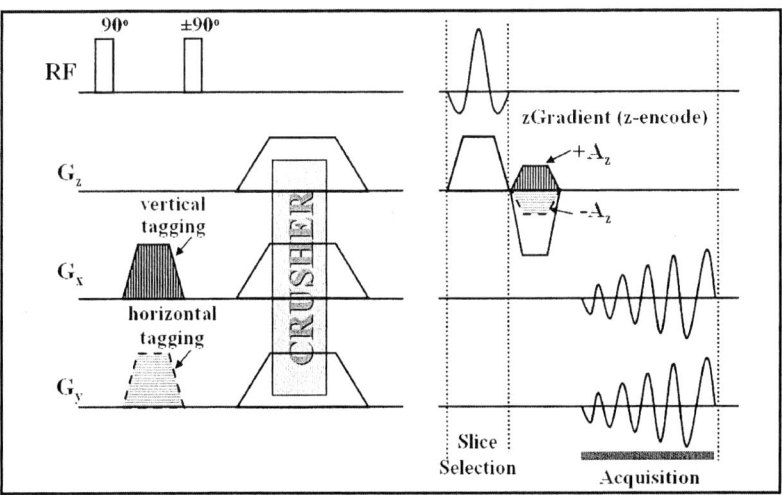

Fig. 1. ZHARP pulse sequence: A typical CSPAMM tagging spiral acquisition sequence with and added z-encode gradient with magnitude $|A_z|$ in the slice-select direction. A $+A_z$ and a $-A_z$ gradients are added to the vertical and horizontal tagging sequences, respectively

2.2 ZHARP Formulation

The zHARP z-encode gradient has the same strength for both A and B CSPAMM acquisitions. Upon (complex signal acquisition and) subtraction, the signal from the untagged tissue is removed, just as in standard CSPAMM. However, the tagged tissue now has a z-phase, acquired at the imaging moment. Accordingly, the z-encoded CSPAMM image $I(\mathbf{r}, t)$ at $\mathbf{r}(x, y)$ and time t can be represented as

$$I(\mathbf{r},t) = 2 \int_{\bar{z}(\mathbf{r})-\triangle/2}^{\bar{z}(\mathbf{r})+\triangle/2} \rho(\mathbf{r},t) e^{j\varphi_e(\mathbf{r})} \cos(\boldsymbol{\omega}^\mathrm{T} \mathbf{p}(\mathbf{r},t)) e^{j\kappa_z(\mathbf{r})z(\mathbf{r})} dz, \quad (1)$$

where $\bar{z}$ is the (tag) slice position, $\triangle$ is the (tag) slice thickness, $\rho(\mathbf{r},t)$ is the effective spin density, $\boldsymbol{\omega}$ is the tag frequency, $\mathbf{p}(\mathbf{r},t)$ is the reference map (the position of the 3-D spatial point $\mathbf{r}$ at the reference time), and κ_z is the z-encode frequency.

If the frequency κ_z is small enough and the slice thin enough, then we have the approximation

$$I(\mathbf{r},t) \approx 2\rho(\mathbf{r},t) e^{j\varphi_e(\mathbf{r})} \cos(\boldsymbol{\omega}^\mathrm{T} \mathbf{p}(\mathbf{r},t)) e^{j\kappa_z(\mathbf{r})\bar{z}(\mathbf{r})}. \quad (2)$$

Letting $\varphi_z(\mathbf{r}) = \kappa_z(\mathbf{r})\bar{z}(\mathbf{r})$, (2) becomes

$$I(\mathbf{r},t) \approx 2\rho(\mathbf{r},t) e^{j\varphi_e(\mathbf{r})} e^{j\varphi_z(\mathbf{r})} \cos(\boldsymbol{\omega}^\mathrm{T} \mathbf{p}(\mathbf{r},t)). \quad (3)$$

This is the usual CSPAMM image multiplied by $e^{j\varphi_e(\mathbf{r})} e^{j\varphi_z(\mathbf{r})}$, which means that the $\bar{z}$ position of every myocardial material point in the slice is now encoded in the phase of the complex image I without affecting the usual CSPAMM magnitude content. For simplicity of notation in the following, we omit the argument of $\varphi_e(\mathbf{r})$ and $\varphi_z(\mathbf{r})$.

2.3 ZHARP Images

An image plane is scanned twice in order to compute the in-plane motion, first with vertical tagging, $\boldsymbol{\omega} = \omega_x(1,0,0)$, and then with horizontal tagging, $\boldsymbol{\omega} = \omega_y(0,1,0)$. A positive z-encode gradient is applied to the first scan and a negative one is applied to the second scan. Using the relation

$$\mathbf{p}(\mathbf{r},t) = \mathbf{r} - \mathbf{u}(\mathbf{r},t), \qquad (4)$$

where $\mathbf{u}$ is the displacement, (3) becomes

$$I_x(\mathbf{r},t) \propto \rho(\mathbf{r},t) e^{j\varphi_e} e^{j\varphi_z} \cos(\omega_x x - \varphi_x), \qquad (5)$$
$$I_y(\mathbf{r},t) \propto \rho(\mathbf{r},t) e^{j\varphi_e} e^{-j\varphi_z} \cos(\omega_y y - \varphi_y), \qquad (6)$$

for the first and second scans, where $\varphi_x = \omega_x u_x$ and $\varphi_y = \omega_y u_y$. In these equations, the phases φ_x and φ_y are called either the displacement-encoding phases or the harmonic phase (HARP) maps in the x and y directions, respectively [2].

2.4 ZHARP Algorithm

ZHARP uses two steps to extract the 3-D displacement of each material point.

Step 1. Extraction of Displacement-Encoding Phase Maps. At first glance, it appears to be impossible to sort out the in-plane and through-plane motion components from the image data in (5) and (6). It can be done, however, by applying the 2-D HARP concept [2,1] to both the negative and positive harmonic peaks of I_x and I_y. This idea is illustrated in the block diagram of Fig. 2. Whereas in conventional HARP, there would be only two harmonic phases that are computed, one for the horizontally tagged image and one for the vertically tagged image, in zHARP there are four computed harmonic phases, ϕ_A, ϕ_B, ϕ_C, and ϕ_D. Furthermore, these computed phases include not only the harmonic phases, φ_x and φ_y arising from object in-plane motion, but also the phases arising from our explicit z-encoding, φ_z, and from erroneous phase sources, φ_e.

Referring to Fig. 2, we see that the computed harmonic phases form a system of linear equations,

$$\phi_A = \varphi_e + \varphi_z - \varphi_x, \qquad (7)$$
$$\phi_B = \varphi_e + \varphi_z + \varphi_x, \qquad (8)$$
$$\phi_C = \varphi_e - \varphi_z - \varphi_y, \qquad (9)$$
$$\phi_D = \varphi_e - \varphi_z + \varphi_y. \qquad (10)$$

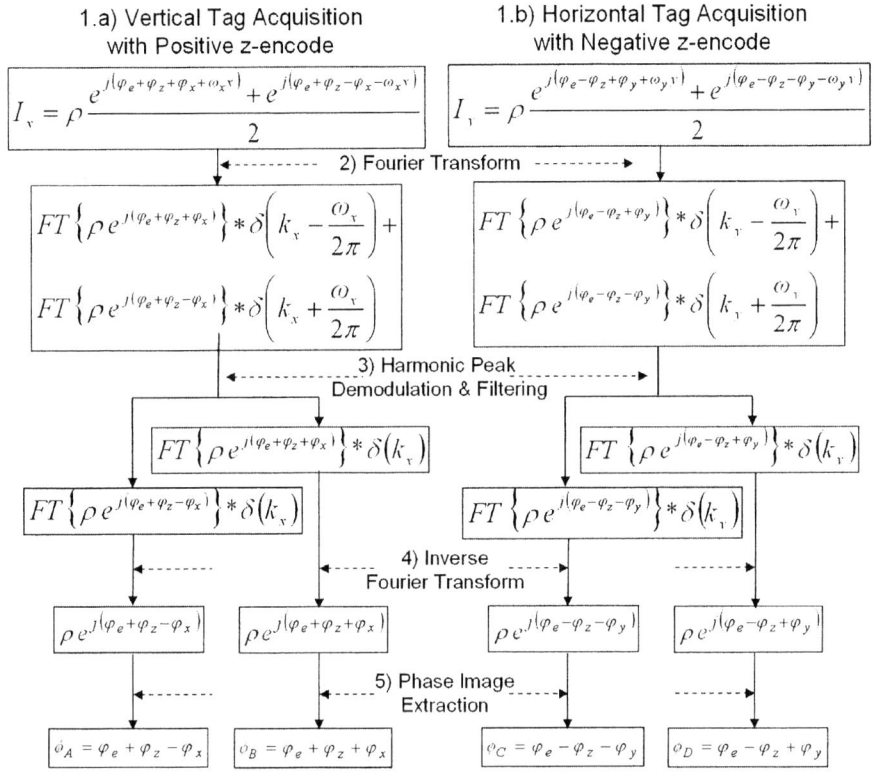

Fig. 2. Extraction of displacement-encoding phase maps. Left flowchart: Extraction of ϕ_A and ϕ_B of from vertically tagged images I_x. Right flowchart: Extraction of ϕ_C and ϕ_D of from horizontally tagged images, I_y. The $*$ and δ symbols represent linear convolution and the impulse function, respectively

This system is readily solved for the desired phases that are related to motion, yielding

$$\varphi_x = (\phi_B - \phi_A)/2, \tag{11}$$

$$\varphi_y = (\phi_D - \phi_C)/2, \tag{12}$$

$$\varphi_z = ((\phi_A + \phi_B) - (\phi_C + \phi_D))/4. \tag{13}$$

Step 2. 3-D Motion Tracking. Consider a material point located at $\mathbf{r}_m$ at time t_m. The principle of 2-D HARP tracking [1] is based on the fact that HARP phase is a material property, and therefore that the apparent in-plane position of this point at time t_{m+1}, given by $\mathbf{r}_{m+1}$, can be determined by the following relations

$$\varphi_x(\mathbf{r}_{m+1}, t_{m+1}) = \varphi_x(\mathbf{r}_m, t_m), \tag{14}$$

$$\varphi_y(\mathbf{r}_{m+1}, t_{m+1}) = \varphi_y(\mathbf{r}_m, t_m). \tag{15}$$

Now consider a point on the image plane $\mathbf{r}_0$ at the time t_0 of tag application. Since the phases φ_x and φ_y are found using (11) and (12), 2-D HARP tracking can be used to track the apparent in-plane position of $\mathbf{r}_0$ throughout the image sequence [1]. This yields a sequence of points in the image plane given by $\{\mathbf{r}_0, \ldots, \mathbf{r}_m, \mathbf{r}_{m+1}, \ldots\}$. This is a standard HARP result, a tracking of the apparent 2-D position of an arbitrary point in the plane [1]. Importantly, it is shown here that it is possible to obtain this result despite the presence of an explicit z-encode and the presence of phase anomalies.

Because slice following is used, it is now possible to recover the z position of $\mathbf{r}_0$ throughout the sequence. We note that at the time of tag (and z-encode) application, we have

$$\varphi_z(\mathbf{r}_0, t_0) \approx \kappa_z z_0. \tag{16}$$

At a later time, if the z phase does not wrap, then we have the relation

$$\varphi_z(\mathbf{r}_{m+1}, t_{m+1}) - \varphi_z(\mathbf{r}_m, t_m) \approx \kappa_z(z_{m+1} - z_m). \tag{17}$$

Rearranging, and using the wrapping operator $\mathcal{W}$ defined in [1] (which recovers the correct net phase difference), yields

$$z_{m+1} = z_m + \frac{1}{\kappa_z}\mathcal{W}\{\varphi_z(\mathbf{r}_{m+1}, t_{m+1}) - \varphi_z(\mathbf{r}_m, t_m)\}, \tag{18}$$

which can be used in an iterative fashion to track the z position of $\mathbf{r}_0$ throughout the sequence.

Together, these two steps describe the algorithmic component of zHARP. It is evident that a single point or an arbitary collection of points in an image slice can be tracked in three dimensions using this imaging and processing methodology.

3 Experiments and Results

The pulse sequence was implemented on a Philips 1.5 T Intera MRI scanner. Image processing was performed off-line on a personal computer. Three experiments were conducted: two phantom experiments and a normal human volunteer.

3.1 1-D z Displacement of Phantom

The pulse sequence and the algorithm were first tested on a water-filled-bottle phantom moving sinusoidally (1″ peak-to-peak) in parallel to the main magnetic field (z direction) at a rate of 52 cpm. The orientations of the acquired slice, so-called short axis (SA) slice, and also the long axis (LA) slice are shown in Fig. 3. Fourteen axial-plane cardiac phases were acquired during the first 466 ms of each cycle. Fig. 4 shows the zHARP algorithm steps applied to the 14th frame and how the through-plane and in-plane displacements were extracted. In this experiment, only though-plane displacement occurred and was measured.

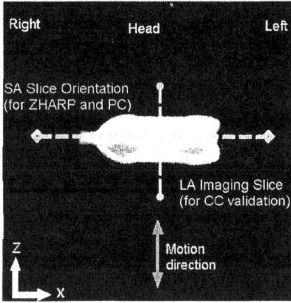

Fig. 3. Short axis (SA) and long axis (LA) slice orientations for the experiment in Sec. 3.1. Motion is along the B_o filed of the magnet. SA slice is along the bottle axis of symmetry and perpendicular to the direction of motion. LA slice is perpendicular to axis of symmetry

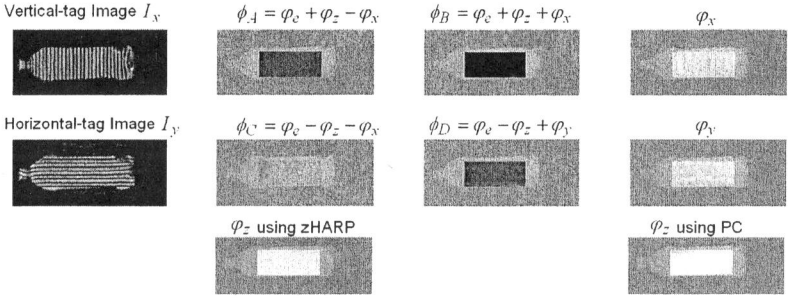

Fig. 4. Displacement phase maps extraction for the experiment in Sec. 3.1. Phase maps are shown at a rectangular region of interest (ROI) in the middle of the bottle. The magnitude image of the bottle is shown in the background of the ROI

For comparison, the phantom was also imaged using a conventional PC method and a z displacement map was obtained thereafter by integration (see Fig. 5).

Through-plane motion in the SA slice is shown as in-plane horizontal shift in the LA slice as shown in Fig. 5. As a reference standard, z displacement was also computed using a cross correlation method (CC) applied to the LA tagged dataset. Fig. 6 compares the mean displacement value and the standard deviation obtained from PC, zHARP, and CC. Relative RMS error between PC and CC was 10.7% and between zHARP and CC was only 4.0%.

3.2 2-D Combined x and z Displacement

In the second experiment, the phantom and the imaged slice were tilted by 43° about the anterior-posterior axis while the phantom was moving along the B_o field direction. In addition, a stationary water phantom was inserted

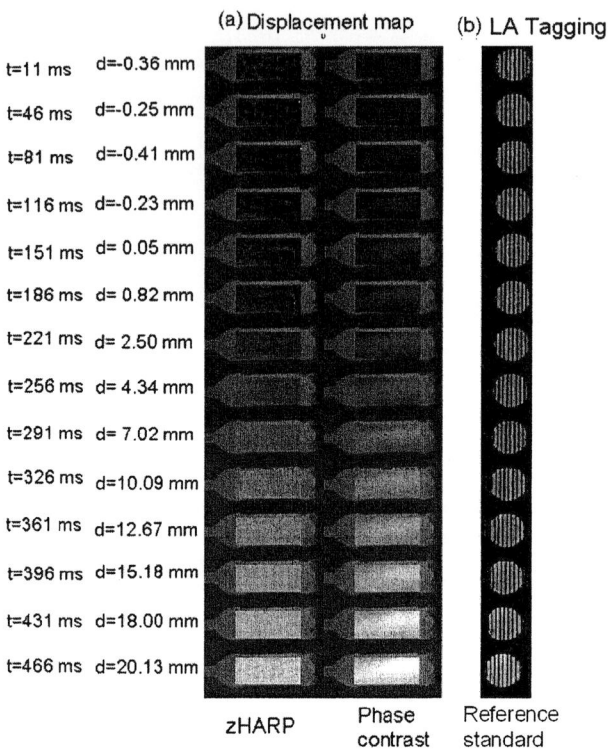

Fig. 5. Z-displacement (φ_z) maps extraction for the experiment in Sec. 3.1. through the 14 CINE images. t: time, d:displacement. (a) φ_z left: using zHARP and right: using phase contrast. (b) Reference standard dataset; tagged long axis slices that used for displacement calculations using cross correlation method

above the imaging coil for comparison. In this tilted placement, both in-plane x displacement and through-plane z motion components were generated (see Fig. 7). Fig. 8 shows the displacement profile through a motion cycle. Both x and z displacement maps are shown and, as expected, both displacements follow a sinusoidal pattern. Because of the tilting-setup, $|\text{mean}(x \text{ displacement})| = \tan(43°) \times |\text{mean}(z \text{ displacement})|$ at any time. The total displacement profile $\sqrt{|z - \text{displacement}|^2 + |x - \text{displacement}|^2}$ is shown with 1″ peak-to-peak total displacement as expected.

A rectangular mesh of points was constructed over the stationary and moving phantoms and tracked throughout the cycle. Tracking results of sample timeframes are shown in Fig. 9 with the acquisition time shown to the left. The frames show both a SA slice in the moving phantom (in the center of the image) and a part of the stationary phantom (at the bottom of the image). In-plane motion in the x direction is shown as a shift from one time frame to another. Through-plane motion is displayed as the color of the tracked point with the color palette shown to the right. Notice the yellow color of the stationary phantom

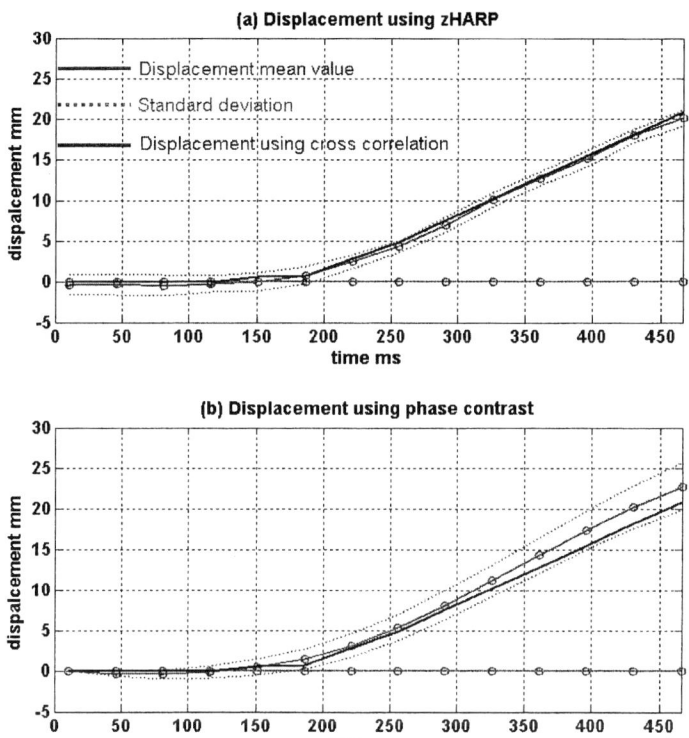

Fig. 6. Z-displacement (φ_z) profile in the first 460ms of the phantom motion cycle. (a) Using zHARP. (b) Using phase contrast (PC). Notice the increasing standard deviation and the drift of the PC values from the cross correlation values

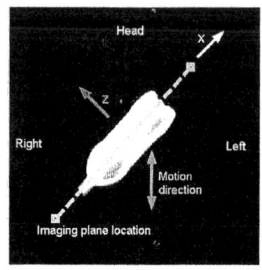

Fig. 7. Short axis (SA) and long axis (LA) slice orientations for the experiment in Sec. 3.2

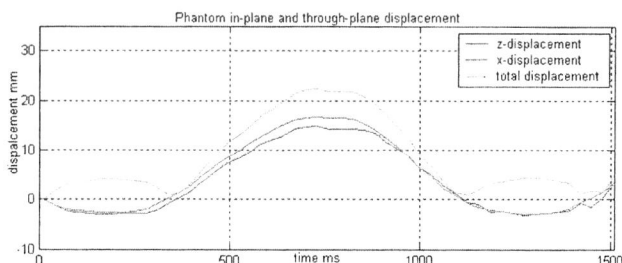

Fig. 8. Average in-plane and through-plane displacement profiles with time and the total $1''$ peak-to-peak displacement

and the change of the moving phantom from yellow ($z = 0$) to green ($z = -ve$) then to red ($z = +ve$) then to green ($z = -ve$) (compare with the profile in Fig. 8).

3.3 Normal volunteer

The data presented in this section was obtained from a 26-year-old healthy adult male subject with a heart rate of approximately 80 bpm. The scanning was done after a written consent and IRB approval. Four ECG leads were placed on the chest for triggering of the pulse sequence by the R-wave. The patient position was head first and supine. An oblique, equatorial short-axis, 6mm-thick slice of the left ventricle was scouted. The location and orientation of the slice is shown in Fig. 10(a). Twelve systolic images of size 256×256 were acquired starting from end-diastole to end-systole with a square FOV of 35cm and temporal resolution of 30ms. The first and last time-frames were scanned 11ms and 341ms, respectively,

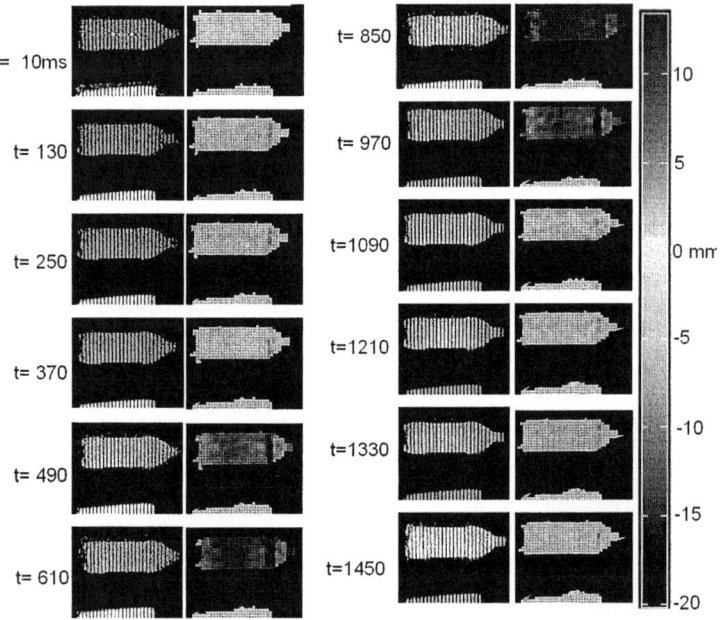

Fig. 9. SA CINE time-frames and tracking. Left: Sample tagged images at different time instants of the motion cycle (notice the horizontal motion of the phantom). Middle: The corresponding zHARP mesh tracking. In-plane tracking (shown as a shift in the phantom position from frame to frame) and through-plane tracking is shown as a change in coloring. Right: The color palette using for representing through-plane motion tracking

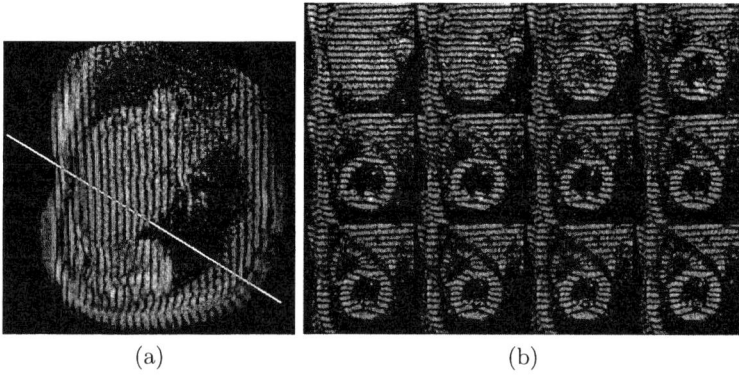

Fig. 10. Data used in the experiment of Sec. 3.3. (a) A four-chambers slice (4C). The line shown is the intersection between the shown 4C and the acquired SA slice. (b)From right to left: The twelve zHARP SA time-frames used in the experiment

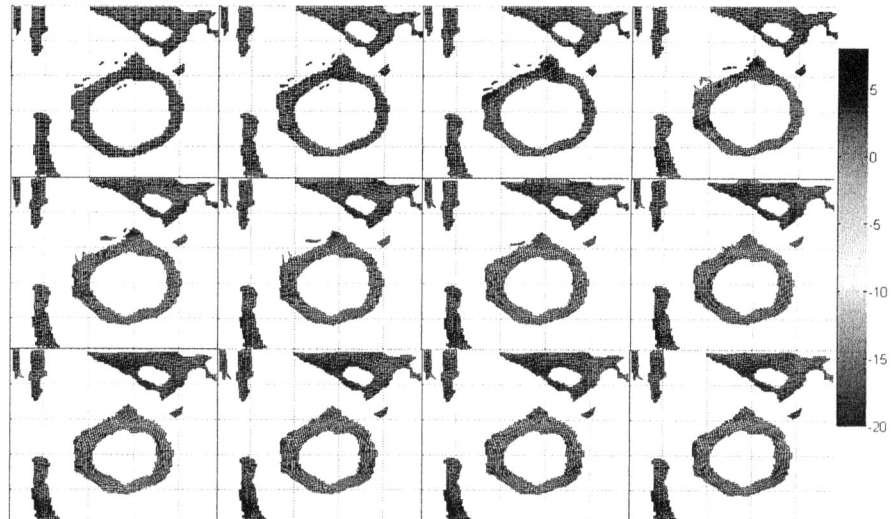

Fig. 11. Mesh tracking result. In-plane displacements are shown as twisting and binding of the mesh grid lines. Through-plane displacement is shown as the colors of the points

after the R-wave trigger. Figure 10(b) shows the 97 × 97 LV region-of-interest (ROI) dataset as they look in the acquired horizontal tag zHARP.

A 97 × 97 mesh of points was tracked on the ROI data. Results in Fig. 11 show in-plane twisting of the mesh and color-encoded z-displacement. Figure 12 shows the though-plane displacement profile of selected tracked points around the LV myocardium.

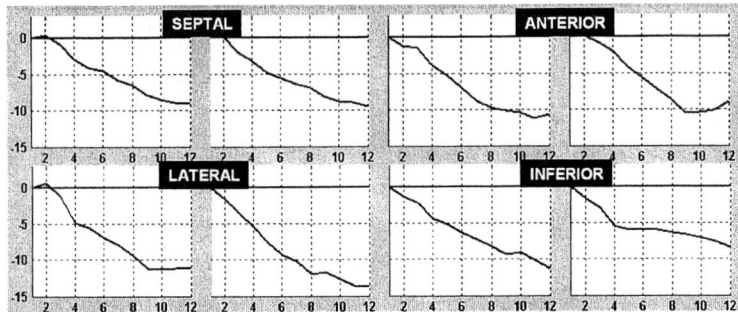

Fig. 12. CW: z Displacement tracking results for points around the myocardium for the experiment in Sec. 3.3. Vertical axes are in mm and horizontal axes are the time-frame index

4 Conclusion

In this work, we modified the slice following CSPAMM MRI acquisition process by adding a z phase encode. Using HARP processing on four spectral peaks, both the in-plane and through-plane motions can be recovered. Key advantages of this approach include the ability to compute dense 3-D motion from only a single acquired image orientation and no increase in imaging time over that of slice following CSPAMM. In contrast to the PC method, where tracking errors accumulate over time, zHARP shows a consistent tracking performance throughout the time of tag persistence.

Combining this technique with a multi-slice acquisition will provide a layer-cake of 3D tracked points which can be used to track the heart and compute a variety of strains. It may therefore be possible to significantly reduce the number of planes that are acquired, and still obtain an accurate assessment of the state of the LV and RV myocardium.

Acknowledgments

This research was funded by the National Heart, Lung, and Blood Institute under Grant R01 HL47405.

Notice — Jerry L. Prince and Nael F. Osman are founders of and own stock in Diagnosoft, Inc., a company that seeks to license the HARP technology. The terms of this arrangement are being managed by the Johns Hopkins University in accordance with its conflict of interest policies.

References

1. Osman, N.F., Kerwin, W.S., McVeigh, E.R.,Prince, J.L.: Cardiac Motion Tracking Using CINE Harmonic Phase (HARP) Magnetic Resonance Imaging. Magn. Reson. Med. **42**(6) (1999) 1048–1060

2. Osman, N.F., McVeigh, E.R.,Prince, J.L.: Imaging heart motion using harmonic phase MRI. IEEE Trans. Med. Imag., **19**(3) (2000) 186–202
3. Aletras, A.H., Wen, H.: DENSE: Displacement Encoding with Stimulated Echoes in Cardiac Functional MRI. J. Magn. Reson. **173** (1999) 247-252
4. Aletras, A.H., Wen, H.: Mixed echo train acquisition displacement encoding with stimulated echoes: an optimized DENSE method for in vivo functional imaging of the human heart. Magn. Reson. Med. **46** (2001) 523–534
5. Pelc, N.J., Herfkens, R.J., Shimakawa, A., Enzmann, D.R.: Phase contrast cine magnetic resonance imaging. Magn. Reson. Q. **7** (1991) 229-254
6. Pelc, N.J., Sommer F.G., Li, K.C., Brosnan, T.J., Herfkens, R.J., Enzmann, D.R.: Quantitative magnetic resonance flow imaging. Magn. Reson. Q. **10** (1994) 125-147
7. Fischer, S.E., McKinnon, G.C., Scheidegger, M.B.: True Myocardial Motion Tracking. Magn. Reson. Med. **31** (1994) 401

Analysis of Event-Related fMRI Data Using Diffusion Maps

Xilin Shen and François G. Meyer

University of Colorado at Boulder, Boulder CO 80309, USA

Abstract. The blood oxygen level-dependent (BOLD) signal in response to brief periods of stimulus can be detected using event-related functional magnetic resonance imaging (ER-fMRI). In this paper, we propose a new approach for the analysis of ER-fMRI data. We regard the time series as vectors in a high dimensional space (the dimension is the number of time samples). We believe that all activated times series share a common structure and all belong to a low dimensional manifold. On the other hand, we expect the background time series (after detrending) to form a cloud around the origin. We construct an embedding that reveals the organization of the data into an activated manifold and a cluster of non-activated time series. We use a graph partitioning technique–the normalized cut to find the separation between the activated manifold and the background time series. We have conducted several experiments with synthetic and in-vivo data that demonstrate the performance of our approach.

1 Introduction

The goal of functional neuroimaging is to map the activity of the brain in space and time. Functional magnetic resonance imaging (fMRI) has become one of the main tools for noninvasive assessment of human brain functions since its invention in the early 1990s. Event-related fMRI makes it possible to study the transient changes triggered by cognitive and sensory stimulation. Unlike block paradigm, event-related fMRI allows mixing of different task conditions on a trial-by-trial basis and provides a means of examining the dynamics and time-course of neural activity under various conditions.

However, the increase in the signal during an event-related fMRI experiment only lasts for a short period of time. The analysis is further complicated by the variation in the shape and amplitude of the hemodynamic response across different cortical regions [1]. Therefore, methods of analysis that rely on a specific model of the hemodynamic response will not be optimal. Several methods [2], [3] address this problem by considering a family of hemodynamic responses constructed from a set of basis functions. Others [4], [5] sought solutions via nonparametric data-driven methods.

Here, we regard the fMRI data as a very large set of time series $x_i(t)$ in $\mathbb{R}^T$, indexed by their position i. After removing the low frequency components from the time series in the preprocessing, we assume any significant changes in the fMRI signal are related to the experimental paradigm. Although the experiment could recruit several cortical regions with different temporal responses, we restrict our attention to scenarios with no more than one type of temporal response. We now consider the set of all activated time series taken from the same cortical region. We assume that this set constitutes a manifold in $\mathbb{R}^T$. Clearly, if we were to use a parametric model for the hemodynamic response, the set of all hemodynamic responses generated from all the possible values of the parameters would form a manifold. The fact that the activated time series belong to a manifold in $\mathbb{R}^T$ has two implications. First, the activated time series reside only in a very small part of $\mathbb{R}^T$. Second, the activated time series are similar to each other, and one can go smoothly from one to the other one. In practice, the activated times series are corrupted by noise, and the associated manifold may exhibit some roughness.

A meaningful geometric description of the data in $\mathbb{R}^T$ would exhibit the presence of the activated manifold, and thus would have the power to discriminate between the activated and the non-activated time series. The diffusion maps method [6] is known to be capable of generating efficient representations of complex geometric structures. In particular, it can be applied to describe the geometry of a low dimensional manifold in high dimensions. In this work, we apply this technique to event-related fMRI data. The diffusion maps provide us with an embedding of the dataset. We then use a graph partitioning technique called the normalized cut [7] to separate the activated time series from the background time series. Because the normalized cut is closely related to the diffusion maps, it provides a natural method to perform the clustering of the time series. The paper is organized as follows. In the next section, we give a brief review to diffusion maps and the way we modify the graph construction. In section 3, we describe the normalized cut criterion and its relation to the diffusion maps. Results of experiments conducted on synthetic and in-vivo ER-fMRI data are presented in section 4.

2 Diffusion Maps and Graph Construction

The problem of finding meaningful structures and geometric descriptions of a data set has been the central interest in many areas like information retrieval, artificial intelligence and statistical data analysis. Different techniques have been developed to construct a representation for data lying on a low-dimensional manifold embedded in a high-dimensional space, among which are the classical linear methods including Principle Component Analysis (PCA) and Multidimensional Scaling (MDS), and the kernel methods like Local Linear Embedding (LLE) [8], Laplacian eigenmaps [9], and Hessian eigenmaps [10]. Most recently, Coifman and Lafon [6] have shown that all kernel methods are special cases of a general framework based on a diffusion process. By defining a random walk on the data set, they associate a Markov matrix to this data set. The spectral analysis of the Markov matrix provides a family of mappings which they termed "diffusion maps".

2.1 Diffusion Maps, Diffusion Distances

To construct the diffusion maps, we consider two time series $x(t)$ and $y(t)$ as being the nodes of a graph G. For two distinct nodes of the graph G we define a weight function $K(x,y)$ that measures the similarity between the time series according to

$$K(x,y) = \exp(-\frac{\|x-y\|^2}{\sigma}),$$

where $\|x-y\|^2 = \sum_t (x(t) - y(t))^2$. K is a symmetric, positive semi-definite matrix. We define the diffusion matrix: $A = D^{-1}K$ where D is a diagonal matrix with $d_{xx} = \sum_y k(x,y)$. By definition, this matrix is row-stochastic and can be viewed as the transition matrix of a random walk on the data set. Moreover, we can show that this random walk is reversible, which is the same to say that A is conjugate to a symmetric matrix:

$$\tilde{A} = D^{\frac{1}{2}} A D^{-\frac{1}{2}} \qquad (1)$$

Then we define the diffusion distance between x and y at time m by:

$$D_m^2(x,y) = \tilde{a}^m(x,x) + \tilde{a}^m(y,y) - 2\tilde{a}^m(x,y) \qquad (2)$$
$$= \sum_{j \geq 0} \lambda_j^{2m} (\phi_j(x) - \phi_j(y))^2 \qquad (3)$$

where $\{\lambda_j\}$ and $\{\phi_j\}$ are the eigenvalues and eigenvectors of $\tilde{A}$, and $1 = \lambda_0 \geq \lambda_1 \geq \lambda_2 \geq ... \geq 0$. The quantity $\tilde{a}^m(x,y)$ denotes the entry of $\tilde{A}$ for row x and column y and it represents the probability of transition from x to y in m steps. The diffusion distance $D_m^2(x,y)$ is then a sum over all paths of length less than or equal to m between x and y. The value of $D_m^2(x,y)$ decreases when the number of paths between x and y gets larger. So it is a measure of connectivity of the points in the graph and it is robust to noise.

Last we introduce the family of diffusion maps $\{\Phi_m\}$ by

$$\Phi_m(x) = \begin{pmatrix} \lambda_0^m \phi_0(x) \\ \lambda_1^m \phi_1(x) \\ \cdot \\ \cdot \\ \cdot \end{pmatrix} \qquad (4)$$

The diffusion maps convert diffusion distances into Euclidean distances:

$$\|\Phi_m(x) - \Phi_m(y)\|^2 = \sum_{j \geq 0} \lambda_j^{2m}(\phi_j(x) - \phi_j(y))^2 = D_m^2(x,y) \qquad (5)$$

This embedding is related to the way a random walk propagates over the data set. In particular, it is sensitive to all sorts of bottleneck effects, therefore it is able to discover different clusters in the data set.

2.2 Modified Way of Constructing the Graph

Before applying the diffusion maps described in the previous section to fMRI data, we need to construct the adjacency graph. We consider each time series to be a node in the graph, and we put an edge between a pair of time series x and y if they are similar. Similarity can be defined by the Euclidean distance between the two time series, $\|x - y\|^2 = \sum_t (x(t) - y(t))^2$. We connect the two nodes x and y of the graph if x is among the n nearest neighbors of y, or y is among the n nearest neighbors of x. This approach is chosen for its simplicity and is guaranteed to give well connected graphs.

However, this definition of connectivity is not adapted to data set with low SNR, which is the case of fMRI data. Indeed, if the data are noisy, this approach will create many unfaithful connections between activated time series and non-activated time series, thereby severely obscuring the geometric structure of the data set. The idea can be better illustrated by the following computation. Suppose we have activated voxels i, j and non-activated voxel k. The time series from these voxels are given by:

$$x_i(t) = s_i(t) + n_i(t)$$
$$x_j(t) = s_j(t) + n_j(t)$$
$$x_k(t) = n_k(t)$$
$$t = 1, 2, ..., T$$

where $s(t)$ is the signal time course generated by the hemodynamic response of an activated voxel, and $n(t)$ is the noise. The T dimensional distance between the time series are:

$$d_{ij} = x_i(t) - x_j(t) = (s_i(t) - s_j(t)) + (n_i(t) - n_j(t))$$
$$d_{ik} = x_i(t) - x_k(t) = s_i(t) + (n_i(t) - n_k(t))$$

If the variability of the signal across different activated voxels is small, then $(s_i(t) - s_j(t))$ is close to a zero. So d_{ij} can be viewed as a noise vector, while d_{ik} contains an additional term: the signal information $s_i(t)$. But the Euclidean norm maps the T dimensional vector to a single number. Under cases of high SNR, we have $\|d_{ij}\|^2 < \|d_{ik}\|^2$ with high probability. However as the SNR decreases, this inequality becomes much weaker, making it more difficult to differentiate between two activated time series and an activated time series and a background time series. Graphs constructed via the n nearest neighbors (with the Euclidean norm) are flawed in the sense that the connection between nodes does not always reflect the intrinsic organization of the original data.

We keep the Euclidean norm to compare time series, but we enforce the existing the spacial correlation present in the fMRI data during the construction of the graph. Indeed, truly activated voxels tend to be spatially clustered. Therefore, we add additional edges to the adjacency graph obtained by the nearest neighbor search. If two voxels are neighbors spacially, then the corresponding time series will be connected in the graph, irrespective of the Euclidean between these time series. In summary, the criteria for putting an edge between a pair of nodes in the graph is summarized as follows:

Put an edge between the nodes x and y if

- $\|x-y\|^2$ *is among the n smallest values of* $\|x-z\|^2$, *for all* $z \in G$ *or,*
- $\|x-y\|^2$ *is among the n smallest values of* $\|y-z\|^2$, *for all* $z \in G$ *or,*
- *if* $\|p(x) - p(y)\|^2 \leq r$, *where* $p(x)$ *is the spatial position of the voxel from which the time series x originates.*

By imposing this spacial neighborhood criterion, we strengthen the connections within the activated nodes as well as the connections within the non-activated nodes in the graph. This feature is very important for the diffusion process performed over the graph afterward: a random walk starting from an activated node will have much higher probability landing on another activated node rather than a non-activated node in a given number of steps. Fig. 2 shows the improvement in revealing the structure of the data set by the modified approach of the graph construction.

3 Normalized Cut

3.1 Segmentation by the Normalized Cut

Now that we have a description of the geometry of the dataset provided by the diffusion maps, separating the activated voxels from the non-activated voxels becomes a clustering problem. A closely related algorithm for clustering under a general graph-theoretic framework has been recently proposed [7]. Given a weighted graph $G = (V, E)$, we seek to partition the vertices into two disjoint subsets $A, B, A \cap B = \emptyset, A \cup B = V$, so that the similarity within each subset A and B is high and across A and B is low. Shi et al defined the following disassociation measure called the normalized cut ($Ncut$),

$$Ncut(A, B) = cut(A, B)\left(\frac{1}{vol(A)} + \frac{1}{vol(B)}\right)$$

$$cut(A, B) = \sum_{u \in A, v \in B} w(u, v)$$

$$vol(A) = \sum_{u \in A, v \in V} w(u, v)$$

The optimal partitioning of the graph can be obtained by minimizing $Ncut$ over all possible subsets A and B. The combinatorial problem turns out to be NP-complete. However, we can relax the optimization problem by allowing the indicator function to take real values. The problem reduces then to minimizing the Laplacian of the graph, which can be computed efficiently. It is shown in [7] that

$$minNcut(A, B) = min_\mathbf{f} \frac{\mathbf{f}^T \mathbf{L} \mathbf{f}}{\mathbf{f}^T \mathbf{D} \mathbf{f}} \qquad (6)$$

with the condition $\mathbf{f}^T \mathbf{D} \mathbf{1} = \mathbf{0}$, where $\mathbf{L}$ is the Laplacian of the graph. We can minimize (6) by solving the following generalized eigensystem,

$$\mathbf{Lf} = \lambda \mathbf{Df}. \tag{7}$$

The second smallest eigenvector $\mathbf{f}_2$ of the above eigensystem is the real valued solution to the normalized cut problem. However, since the eigenvectors take on continuous values, they are no longer indicator functions. We can still split the graph into two components by clustering the nodes according to the sign of $\mathbf{f}_2(i)$.

3.2 Relationship to Diffusion Maps

The normalized cut approach is one of the clustering techniques developed in the field of spectral graph theory [11]. Interestingly, the solution obtained in the previous section has very close ties to diffusion maps. Let $\mathbf{g} = \mathbf{D}^{\frac{1}{2}} \mathbf{f}$, assuming $\mathbf{D}$ is invertible,

$$\frac{\mathbf{f}^T \mathbf{L} \mathbf{f}}{\mathbf{f}^T \mathbf{D} \mathbf{f}} = \frac{\mathbf{g}^T \mathbf{D}^{-\frac{1}{2}} \mathbf{L} \mathbf{D}^{-\frac{1}{2}} \mathbf{g}}{\mathbf{g}^T \mathbf{g}} = \frac{\mathbf{g}^T \tilde{\mathbf{L}} \mathbf{g}}{\mathbf{g}^T \mathbf{g}} \tag{8}$$

Recall that in section 2, we have defined a symmetric version of the diffusion matrix $\tilde{A}$ in (1). It is easy to verify that $\tilde{\mathbf{L}} = \mathbf{I} - \tilde{\mathbf{A}}$. So the eigenvectors for $\tilde{\mathbf{L}}$ are the exactly the same ones for $\tilde{\mathbf{A}}$. Partitioning the graph subject to the normalized cut criterion using the embedding given by the diffusion maps is in a certain sense equivalent to itinerating the diffusion process over the graph, but with updated weight function dependent on the diffusion distances between pairs of points.

4 Experiment and Results

4.1 Details About the Implementation of the Algorithm

Given an fMRI dataset, we set up a weighted graph $G = (V, E)$ by taking each time series as a node and connecting pairs of nodes according to the criterion defined in 2.2. In the experiment we connect each node to 6 of its nearest neighbors in terms of the Euclidean distance and 4 of its spacial neighbors taking $r = 1$. The similarity kernel $k(x,y) = exp(-\frac{\|x-y\|^2}{\sigma})$ is chosen for its relative simplicity and isotropic property. The value of σ is typically set to 10 to 20 percent of the total range of the Euclidean distance between pairs of time series. Then the diffusion maps are constructed by computing the eigenvectors of the diffusion matrix $\tilde{A}$ in (1). We eliminate the first eigenvector, and keep the following four eigenvectors to characterize the structure of the data. The selection is justified by the fact that we expect to find only one activated manifold in the dataset. Furthermore, four degrees of freedom should provide enough richness to characterize this manifold. Now we use the new coordinates to rebuild the weighted graph. By splitting the second smallest eigenvectors of the Laplacian matrix, we obtain the partition of the graph. In the final step, we label the activated voxels and examine the corresponding time series. Notice the fact that usually the cluster of the activated voxels has much smaller size than the cluster of the non-activated voxels. We can use this cue to quickly tell the two clusters apart. Further examination of the time series from the activated voxels is necessary to ensure that the activation detected is indeed related to the experiment paradigm.

4.2 Artificial Event-Related Data

We first apply our approach to an artificial data set of event-related fMRI. The fMRI signal time series are generated by convolving a stimulus time course with the hemodynamic filter $h(t)$ of SPM [12].

$$h(t) = (\frac{t}{d})^a exp(-\frac{t-d}{b}) - c(\frac{t}{d'})^{a'} exp(-\frac{t-d'}{b'}) \qquad (9)$$

where $d = ab$ is the time to peak, $d' = a'b'$ is the time to undershoot, with $a = 6, a' = 12$ and $b = b' = 0.9s; c = 0.35$. This model has become the most frequent one since it models both activation, undershoot and that both modes are not symmetrical. The signal time series $s(t)$ is shown in the upper plot of Fig. 1(c). It remains deterministic for all activated voxels.

The synthetic data set contains $N = 30 \times 30 = 900$ brain voxels with one small activated focus of 13 voxels, see Fig. 1(a) for the spacial localization of the activation region. We add white Gaussian noise to the signal $s(t)$ to create the activated time series, and use white Gaussian noise for non-activated time series. Four data sets with SNR= $0.6, 0.7, 0.8, 1$ were generated. We apply the diffusion maps followed by the normalized cut to each data set.

Fig. 2 compares the result of diffusion process on graphs constructed with and without spacial information. At SNR= 0.8, the diffusion process on a graph constructed without the spacial information fails to reveal any interesting structure of the data set. As one can observe in the upper row in Fig. 2, the red stars that represent the activated time series are buried by the black circles which

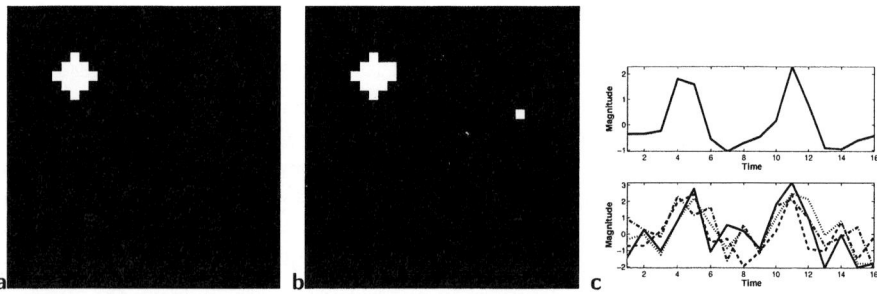

Fig. 1. Left: the true activation map with activated voxels in white and non-activated voxels in black; Middle: activation map for a data set with SNR= 0.8, obtained using our method; Right: (upper) the event-related signal time course $s(t)$, (lower) some of the activated time courses detected

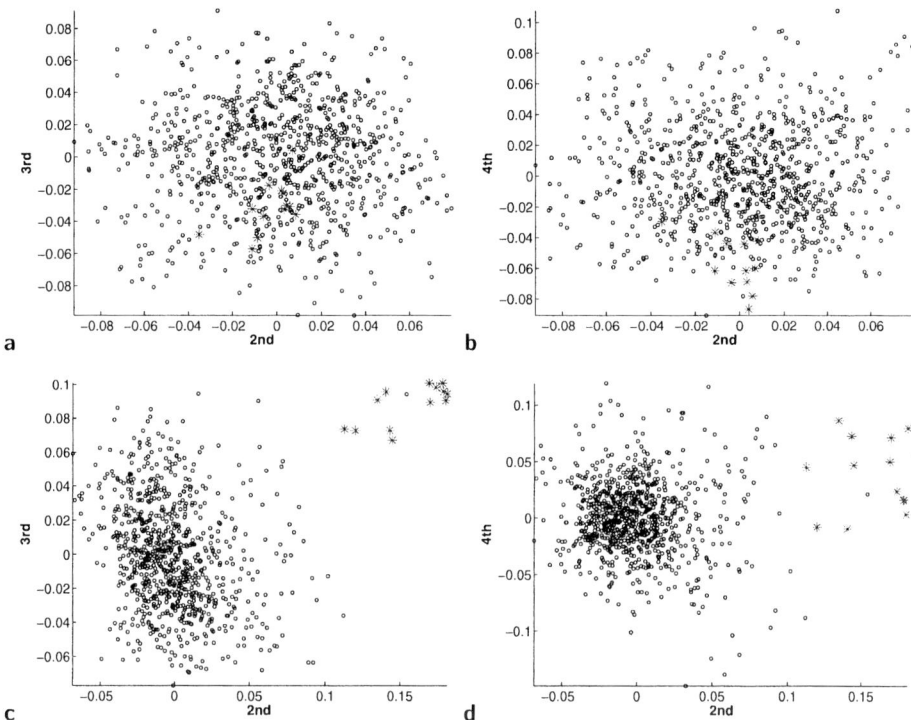

Fig. 2. Upper: diffusion on graph constructed without spacial information; Lower: diffusion on graph constructed with spacial information. The majority are non activated nodes represented by black circles. The activated nodes are represented by red stars

represent the non-activated time series. While for exactly the same data set, by imposing the connections between spacial neighbors, there is a considerable improvement in separating the activated nodes from the non-activated nodes, see the lower row in Fig. 2. Fig. 1(b) shows the activation map obtained for this data set, and the lower plot in Fig. 1(c) displays some of the activated time series detected.

We now compare the performance of our approach with the method of regression. The comparison is based on the number of true and false positives for each value of SNR. The true activation rate is the ratio between the number of true positives detected by the algorithm and the total number of true positives. The false activation rate is the ratio between the number of false positives detected by the algorithm and the total number of true negatives. For each SNR, we generate 10 independent data sets and the averaged statistics are shown in Fig. 3.

The Regression Method. Since we have the absolute knowledge of the signal time series $s(t)$ of the synthetic data set, we can regress each time series onto the signal time series, and apply a Student t-test to the regression coefficient to test

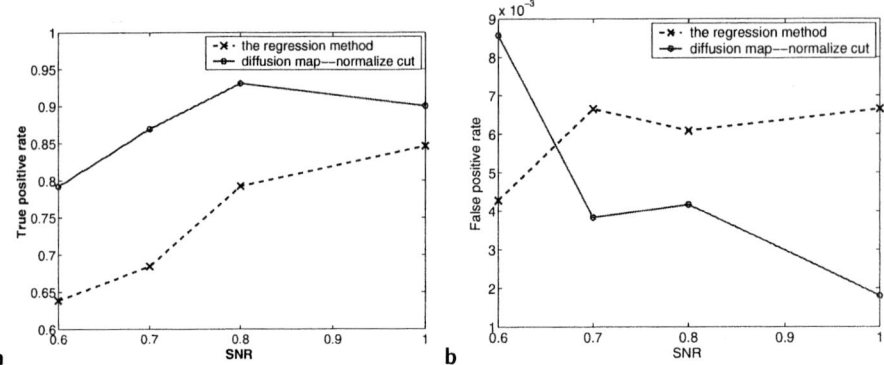

Fig. 3. True activation rate (a) and false activation rate (b) obtained with our diffusion-normalized cut method and the regression method

its significance. The null hypothesis is that the regression coefficient is not significant, which means the time series is not from an activated voxel. The activation map based on the regression method is obtained by thresholding the p value at $p = 0.005$. Knowing exactly the signal time series is a very strong condition which could never be realized in real fMRI experiment. We should expect the method of regression to give the best performance one can expect statistically. Fig. 3(a) shows that our method does very well in terms of detecting the activation. But it suffers from a high false positive rate when the SNR drops below 0.7. One thing worth mentioning here is that once the SNR is greater than 0.7, the false positives detected by our method are always spatially isolated, as is shown in Fig 1(b). This makes it possible to further reduce the number of false positives.

4.3 In-Vivo ER-fMRI Data

We present here the results of an experiment conducted with event-related fMRI data, provided by Dr. Gregory McCarthy (Brain Imaging and Analysis Center, Duke University), demonstrate prefrontal cortex activation in the presence of infrequent events. Visual stimuli were presented to the subjects: most of the images were squares. Infrequent events (targets) consisted in the appearance of circles at random times. Occasionally, images of everyday objects (novels) were also presented. A picture was displayed every 1.5 seconds. The subject was asked to mentally count the number of occurrences of the circles and report that number at the end of each run for total of 10 runs. The experiment was designed to study whether the processes that elicit P300, an event-related potential caused by infrequent target events whose amplitude is dependent on the preceding sequence of stimuli, could also be measured by fMRI. The data was acquired with a gradient echoplanar EPI sequence (TR=1500ms, TE=45ms, NEX=1, FOV=40×20cm, slice thickness =7mm, and imaging matrix 128×64). More details about the experiment are available in [13].

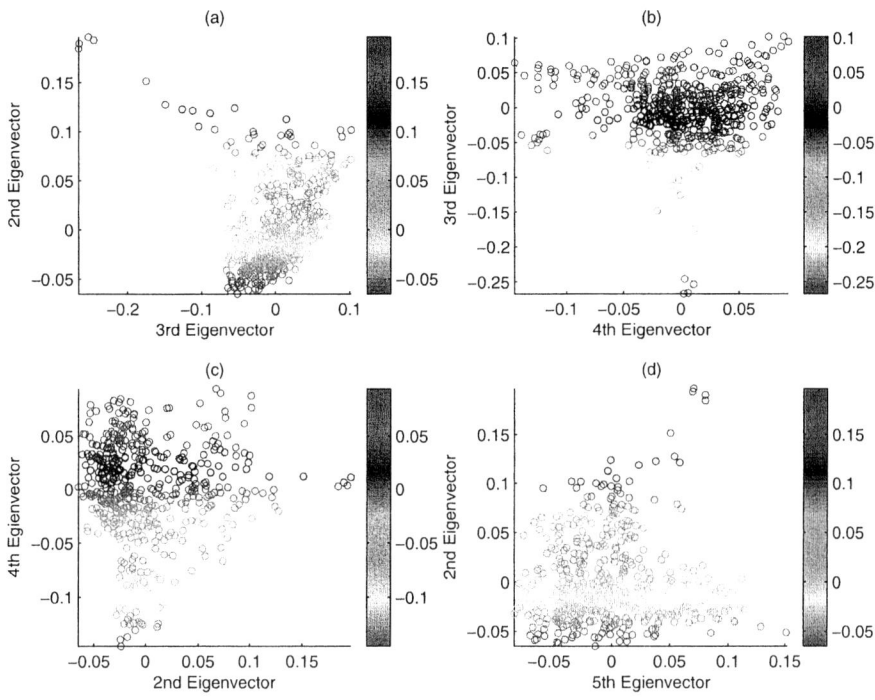

Fig. 4. The first few coordinates given by the diffusion maps

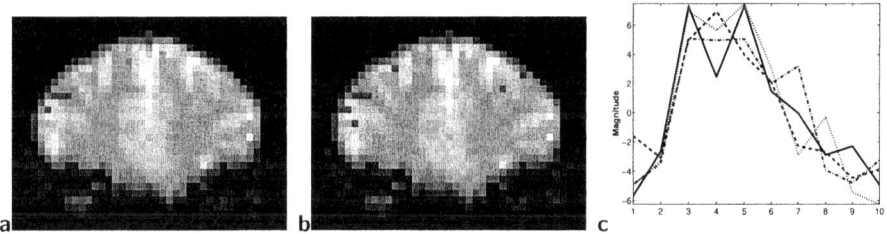

Fig. 5. Left: activation map generated using our method; Middle: activation map generated using the correlation analysis. Right:Time series from the activated voxels

In order to demonstrate the application of our approach to the study of activations by infrequent events, we extract 10-image segments consisting of the 10 consecutive images starting at the target onset. We have in each run about 5 to 6 targets for a total of 49 targets (the data for the 10th run were lost). These segments of images were averaged in order to increase the SNR. The mean value of the time series was removed voxel-wise before we applied our approach. Fig. 4 shows the data structure represented by the first few coordinates provided by the diffusion maps.

A small cluster of four voxels well detached from the mass of the point cloud can be seen in Fig. 4 especially in sub-plot(a). It indicates the presence of activated time series. The activation map generated using our approach is shown in Fig. 5(a). It is compared with the activation map generated by a correlation analysis, shown in Fig. 5(b). We compute the correlation between the time series and the hemodynamic response model defined in (9). The correlation threshold is 0.6. Meanwhile the time series from the four activated voxels are shown in Fig. 5(c).

5 Conclusion

We have presented in this paper a new approach that detects activation in an fMRI dataset. We view all the time series as vectors in a high dimensional space (the dimension is the number of time samples). We assume that all activated times series share a common structure and all belong to a low dimensional manifold. We constructed an embedding that reveals the organization of the data into an activated manifold and a cluster of non-activated time series. We use a graph partitioning technique–the normalized cut to find the separation between the activated manifold and the background time series.

Unlike most fMRI data analysis methods our approach does not require any model of the hemodynamic response or any *a priori* information. It could also be applied to block designed fMRI experiment. In fact, because the signal in block designed experiment has a stronger statistical power, we should expect our method to perform well. In our current implementation, we assume that there is only one type of activation. This assumption makes the presentation of the method simpler, and leads to easier implementation. The approach extends naturally to multiple activations associated with different hemodynamic responses. Although we focused our attention on event-related fMRI, our approach could be applied to the analysis of other biomedical datasets.

Acknowledgments. The authors are extremely grateful to Dr. Mauro Maggioni and Dr. Stéphane Lafon for discussions of the theory and the implementation of diffusion maps. This work was supported by the program on Multiscale Geometry and Analysis in High Dimensions at the Institute of Pure and Applied Mathematics (IPAM) at UCLA.

References

1. Aguirre, G.K., Zarahn, E., D'esposito, M., "The variability of human BOLD hemodynamic responses" Neuroimage **8** (1998) 360–369
2. Josephs O, Turner R, Friston K, "Event-related fMRI" Human Brain Mapping **5** (1997) 243–248
3. Friston, K.J., Fletcher, P., Josephs, O., Holmes, A., Rugg, M.D., Turner, R., "Event-related fMRI: characterizing differential responses" Neuroimage **7** (1998) 30–40

4. Clare, S., Humberstone, M., Hykin, J., Blumhardt, L., Bowtell, R., Morris, P., "Detecting activations in event-related fMRI using analysis of variance" Magne. Reson. Med. **42** (1999) 1117–1122
5. Meyer, F.G., Chinrungrueng, J., "Analysis of Event-related fMRI data using best clustering bases" Medical Imaging **22** (2003) 933–939
6. Coifman, R.R., Lafon, S., "Diffusion Maps" submitted to Applied and Computational Harmonic Analysis (2004)
7. Shi, J., Malik, J., "Normalized Cuts and Image Segmentation" Pattern Analysis and Machine Intelligence **22** no.8 (2000) 888–905
8. Roweis, S.T., Saul, L.K., "Nonlinear dimensionality reduction by local linear embedding" Science **290** (2000) 2323-2326
9. Belkin, M., Niyogi, P., "Laplacian eigenmaps for dimensionality reduction and data representation" Neural computation **13** (2003) 1373–1396
10. Donoho, D.L., Grimes, C., "Hessian eigenmaps: new locally linear embedding techniques for high-dimensional data" Proceedings of the National Academy of Science **100** (2003) 5591-5596
11. Chung, F.R.K., Spectral Graph Theory Am. Math. Soc. (1997)
12. Friston, K.J., Ashburner, J., SPM 97 course notes (1997)
13. McCarthy, G., Luby, M., Gore, J., Goldman-Rakic, P., "Infrequent events transiently activate human prefrontal and parietal cortex as measured by functional MRI." Journal of Neurophysiology **77** (1997) 1630–1634

Automated Detection of Small-Size Pulmonary Nodules Based on Helical CT Images

Xiangwei Zhang[1], Geoffrey McLennan[2], Eric A. Hoffman[3], and Milan Sonka[1]

[1] Dept. of Electrical Engineering, University of Iowa, Iowa City, IA, 52242, USA
[2] Department of Internal Medicine, University of Iowa, Iowa City, IA, 52242, USA
[3] Department of Radiology, University of Iowa, Iowa City, IA, 52242, USA

Abstract. A computer-aided diagnosis (CAD) system to detect small-size (from $2\,mm$ to around $10\,mm$) pulmonary nodules in helical CT scans is developed. This system uses different schemes to locate juxtapleural nodules and non-pleural nodules. For juxtapleural nodules, morphological closing, thresholding and labeling are performed to obtain volumetric nodule candidates; gray level and geometric features are extracted and analyzed using a linear discriminant analysis (LDA) classifier. To locate non-pleural nodules, a discrete-time cellular neural network (DTCNN) uses local shape features which successfully capture the differences between nodules and non-nodules, especially vessels. The DTCNN was trained using genetic algorithm (GA). Testing on 17 cases with 3979 slice images showed the effectiveness of the proposed system, yielding sensitivity of 85.6% with 9.5 FPs/case (0.04 FPs/image). Moreover, the CAD system detected many nodules missed by human visual reading. This showed that the proposed CAD system acted effectively as an assistant for human experts to detect small nodules and provided a "second opinion" to human observers.

1 Introduction

Lung cancer is one of the most lethal kinds of cancer worldwide. Its cure depends critically on disease detection in the early stages. Computed tomography (CT) technology is an important tool for detection and diagnosis of pulmonary nodules. Due to the large amount of image data created by thoracic CT examination, interpreting lung CT images to detect nodules is a very challenging task for the radiologists. Computer-aided diagnosis (CAD) is considered as a promising tool to aid the radiologists in lung nodule CT interpretation.

Many techniques of nodule detection have been developed based on chest radiographs or CT images. Giger [1] obtained nodules using multiple gray-level thresholding and a rule-based approach. Armato [2] introduced some 3D features, and performed feature analysis by a linear discriminant analysis (LDA) classifier. Kanazawa [3] used fuzzy clustering and a rule-based method. Penedo [4] set up 2 Neural networks (NNs), with the first one detecting the suspected areas, and the second one acting as a classifier. Template-based methods were used to detect nodules by Lee [5]. A prior model [6] was developed by Brown to find nodules on the baseline scan and located nodules in the follow up scans.

According to locations, nodules can be divided into two groups: juxtapleural nodules (nodules attached to pleura) and non-pleural nodules. Usually, a juxtapleural nodule distorts the transversal (axial) lung contour and yields an indented part, a human observer is able to find this abnormality by a tracking procedure along the contour. This method does not work for non-pleural nodules. A small-sized nodule tends to be ignored by a human observer, when located near vessels or airways, especially when attached to them.

Based on previous observations, we propose to deal with juxtapleural nodules and non-pleural nodules respectively. In order to find nodules in initial stages and compensate for readings of radiologists, detection of small-sized nodules (from $2\,mm$ to around $10\,mm$) is of our main interest.

2 Overall Scheme

The overall scheme of nodule detection is outlined in Fig. 1. There are three fundamental steps: preprocessing, juxtapleural nodule detection, and non-pleural nodule detection. The preprocessing consists of isotropic resampling (implemented by trilinear interpolation) and lung segmentation. The isotropic data are more suitable for 3D processing, and also simplify the structure of the DTCNN. The cubic voxel size of $0.7\,mm$ is always produced. And the lung area is extracted from the thoracic CT data [7], so that the successive processing is restricted to the pulmonary zone. In the detection of juxtapleural nodules, morphological closing is applied to the original segmented lung mask to include juxtapleural nodules; then thresholding and labeling are performed to yield 3D volumetric nodule candidates; finally, gray level features and 3D global geometric features are extracted and fed into a LDA classifier to confirm or refute a nodule. In the detecting non-pleural nodules, first optimal thresholding is applied to the whole lung to obtain the non-air part, which consists of nodules, vessels, airway walls and other high attenuation structures. For each voxel belonging to the non-air part, local shape index feature is computed. A DTCNN trained using genetic

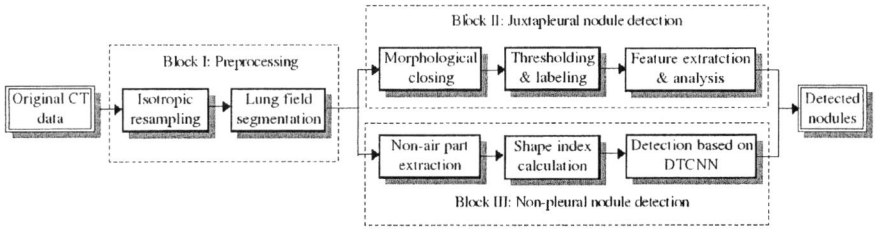

Fig. 1. Overall scheme of the whole pulmonary nodule CAD system

algorithm (GA) is applied to the local geometric feature to extract nodule areas. 3D labeling is operated to give the positions of detected nodules.

3 Juxtapleural Nodule Detection

3.1 Juxtapleural nodule candidate generation

In the preprocessing, the lung field extracted from the thoracic CT data [7] includes two 3D connected components, indicating left and right lung, shown in Fig. 2 (b). Note that in this step, a juxtapleural nodule is usually treated as being outside the lung field, shown in Fig. 2 (b).

Morphological closing can be used to include the indented area of a juxtapleural nodule, shown in Fig. 2 (c). Note that the closing operation should be applied to left and right lungs individually so that no regions between the two lung parts are included. Considering the isometric property of the resampled CT data, the structural element can be easily chosen as a sphere (3D) or a circle (2D). Due to heart motion effect, many undesired areas near the heart will be included if 3D morphological closing is used. Experiments showed that a simple

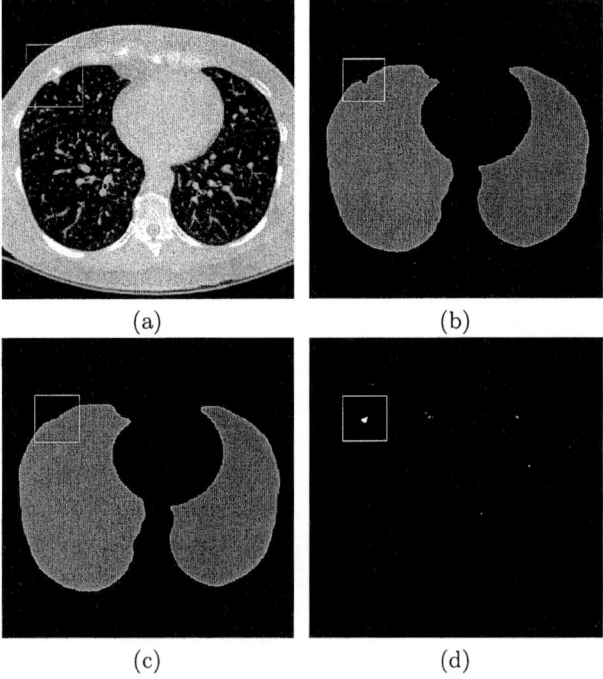

Fig. 2. Juxta-pleural nodule candidate generation. (a) An original CT section image with a juxtapleural nodule; (b) Segmented lung mask image; (c) Lung mask after 2D closing; (d) Juxta-pleural nodule candidates created by thresholding

2D closing in the transversal section image is able to include true nodule areas without introducing too many false nodule areas caused by heart motion effect. Considering the voxel size of 0.7 mm and the nodule size of our interest (from 2 mm to around 10 mm), a circular structural element with radius of 15 voxels is large enough to include the major part of a juxta-pleural nodule.

Optimal thresholding [8] is used to automatically determine a threshold for segmentation between the background (air part) and objects (high intensity part, including nodules). The threshold is detected iteratively. Let T^t be the threshold at iteration step t, and μ_b^t and μ_o^t be the mean gray-level of background and objects. μ_b^t and μ_o^t are obtained by applying T^t to the image. Then for the next step $t+1$, the threshold is updated by $T^{t+1} = (\mu_b^t + \mu_o^t)/2$. This updating procedure is iterated until the threshold does not change, i.e., $T^{t+1} = T^t$. The initial threshold value T^0 is chosen as the mean value of the whole image. 3D component analysis is followed to organize the connected high intensity image voxels into 3D objects, but only the objects attached to the lung wall are of interest. The size property is used to remove the candidates that have very large volume or very small volume, for example, the main part of the vessel tree is usually the largest object in the lung. The results of the previous processing are the nodule candidate objects, shown in Fig. 2 (d).

3.2 Feature Extraction

Given the 3D volume of the nodule candidates, gray level features including highest value, lowest value, average value, standard deviation can be obtained directly. Seven geometric features are also extracted: volume size, surface area, AspectRatio, Sphericity, m_1, m_2, $mRatio$.

$$AspectRatio = \frac{Maximum\ Diameter}{Minimum\ Diameter}, \quad sphericity = \frac{(\frac{3Size}{4\pi})^{1/3}}{(\frac{SurfaceArea}{4\pi})^{1/2}}. \quad (1)$$

The rth contour sequence moments and central moments m_r, μ_r are defined as

$$m_r = \frac{1}{N}\sum_{i=1}^{N}(z(i))^r, \quad \mu_r = \frac{1}{N}\sum_{i=1}^{N}(z(i) - m_1)^r \quad (2)$$

where $z(i)$ is the distance between the center and boundary surface point i. N is the number of points on the boundary surface. $mRatio$ is simply defined as m_2/m_1.

3.3 Feature Analysis

Leave one case out method is used for training and testing. In this scheme, the classifier was trained based on nodule candidates in all but one case, and the nodule candidates in the remaining case was employed to test the trained classifier. The procedure of training and processing was repeated until each case has been already utilized as the testing case. The idea of choosing this scheme instead of common leave one (candidate) out is that each clinical case is independent of other cases, but a nodule candidate is possibly dependent on other candidates in the same case. In this work, LDA, neural network (NN), and support vector machine (SVM) are tried to do the classification.

4 Non-pleural Nodule Detection

4.1 Local Shape Features

Basic observations show that most non-pleural nodules usually take a sphere-like shape, while vessels and airways are tubular structures. See, for example, Fig. 3. This shape difference usually was used as a feature of a segmented object, i.e., a global feature of a suspected nodule area (SNA), as in the detection of juxtapleural nodules. In order to avoid treating a non-isolated nodule as part of other structures, a local shape feature associated with each voxel is used. By assuming the surface of interest to be a level surface locally, local shape features can be computed for each voxel.

A local shape can be completely described by its two principal curvatures, i.e., the maximal and minimal curvatures k_1, k_2. Equivalently, the Gaussian curvature K and the mean curvature H can describe a local shape, like in the HK

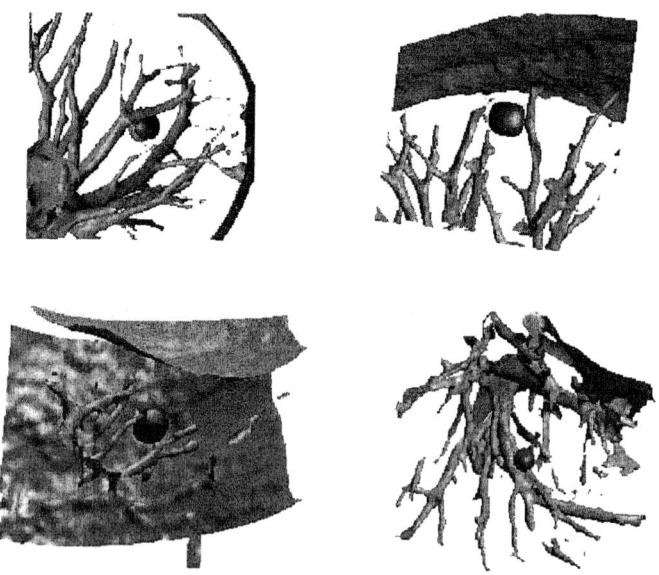

Fig. 3. Iso-surface rendering of anatomical structures in the pulmonary zone. The spherical like objects located close to the center of each image are nodules; the tubular structures are vessels; the planar shapes are pleural surface. Note that the nodules are illustrated in a darker gray level

segmentation introduced by Besl [9]. Neither the k_1, k_2 nor the HK curvature pair capture the intuitive notion of "local shape" very well, as two parameters are needed to "tell" the local shape. Koenderink [10,11] proposed two measures of local surface, "shape index" S and "curvedness" C. The shape index is scale-invariant and captures the intuitive notion of "local shape", whereas the curvedness specifies the amount of curvature. The S and C are defined as:

$$S = \frac{2}{\pi} \cdot arctan \frac{k_1 + k_2}{k_1 - k_2}, \quad C = \sqrt{\frac{k_1^2 + k_2^2}{2}}, \quad \text{for } k_1 \geq k_2 \tag{3}$$

SC scheme decouples the shape and the magnitude of the curvatures. This is done by transforming a k_1, k_2 Cartesian coordinate description of a local shape into a polar coordinate description. Every distinct shape, except for the plane, corresponds to a unique value of S. Specifically, $S = 1$ indicates a cap (like spherical nodules); $S = 0.5$ (ridge) corresponds to cylindrical shapes (like vessels). The SC scheme has been successfully been used to detect colonic polyps in virtual colonoscopy[12].

Many derivations of curvature computation for level surface have been developed [13,14,15]. The resulting formula is essentially identical and a concise derivation is given in [15]. The Gaussian curvature K and the mean curvature H have the following formulas:

$$K = \frac{1}{(f_x^2 + f_y^2 + f_z^2)^2} \{ f_x^2(f_{yy}f_{zz} - f_{yz}^2) + 2f_yf_z(f_{xy}f_{xz} - f_{xx}f_{yz})$$
$$+ f_y^2(f_{xx}f_{zz} - f_{xz}^2) + 2f_xf_z(f_{xy}f_{yz} - f_{xz}f_{yy})$$
$$+ f_z^2(f_{xx}f_{yy} - f_{xy}^2) + 2f_xf_y(f_{xz}f_{yz} - f_{xy}f_{zz}) \} \tag{4}$$

$$H = \frac{-1}{2(f_x^2 + f_y^2 + f_z^2)^{3/2}} \{ (f_y^2 + f_z^2)f_{xx} + (f_x^2 + f_z^2)f_{yy} + (f_x^2 + f_y^2)f_{zz}$$
$$- 2f_xf_yf_{xy} - 2f_xf_zf_{xz} - 2f_yf_zf_{yz} \} \tag{5}$$

The principal curvatures can be computed from K and H as follows:

$$k_{1,2} = H \pm \sqrt{H^2 - K} \tag{6}$$

The estimation of partial derivatives is implemented by directly convolving the intensity image with the corresponding derivatives of the Gaussian filter.

Because most small-sized nodules show a sphere-like structure, the shape index of each voxel belonging to nodules should be around the value of 1. Similarly, vessels have tube-like structures, represented by the shape index value of 0.5. Due to the existence of structural noise, the difference of the shape index value between a nodule and vessels only makes sense for a population of voxels, rather than a single voxel. What is needed is an information processing system that synthesizes the information in a neighborhood of a voxel to give a decision on the voxel's class, either nodule or non-nodule. In this work, discrete-time cellular neural networks (DTCNN) act as this classification system.

Considering the high intensity property of nodules, the local shape based detection can be applied only to the bright parts inside the lung, i.e., a region of interest (ROI) can be obtained to reduce the processing. Optimal thresholding [8] described before is used to determine the threshold.

4.2 Discrete-Time Cellular Neural Networks

The discrete-time cellular neural network (DTCNN) [16, 17] was introduced as a discrete-time version of the CNN [18, 19]. This first-order, discrete-time dynamical system consists of multiple identical cells on regular spaced positions. The dynamics of a cell is described by the following discrete-time state equation:

$$X(n+1) = AY(n) + BU + I \qquad (7)$$

where X indicates the inner state of the cell, Y the output, and U the input of the cell. n is a nonnegative integer indicating the time step. A is the feedback template; B is the control (input) template. I is a constant bias parameter. The output is described by the following piecewise-linear function:

$$Y(n) = \frac{1}{2}(|X(n)+1| - |X(n)-1|) \qquad (8)$$

The two templates A, B and bias I completely determine the behavior of a DTCNN with given inputs and initial conditions.

The DTCNN can be interpreted as an iterative filter. For the one-step filter in Equation (7), a new voxel value, $X(n+1)$ are determined directly by the old voxel values in the corresponding neighborhood. The r-neighborhood of the cell $C(i,j,k)$ is a cubic region of dimensions $(2r+1) \times (2r+1) \times (2r+1)$ around the center position (i,j,k). This neighborhood is usually chosen to be as small as possible, typically, $r = 1$. Therefore, a one-step filter can only extract the very local properties. The propagation property of iterative filter asserts that the output image value after n iterations can be indirectly influenced by a neighborhood n times larger than the original neighborhood.

In our nodule detection application, a 3D DTCNN is built with the same structure and size as the segmented lung, with each cell representing a voxel at a corresponding position. The neighborhood of the DTCNN is chosen as $3 \times 3 \times 3$, $r = 1$. With the aim of quickly detecting nodules in their initial stages (diameters around or under $10\,mm$), the iteration time $N = 9$ of the DTCNN is chosen. This results in an affected neighborhood with size $19 \times 19 \times 19$, which is sufficient to cover the various sizes of nodules of our interest. In this work, the output reached when the iteration stops is defined as the settled output, denoted as $Y(N)$.

Because CNN's default input and initial condition values are in the interval $[-1, 1]$, a normalization is needed to make the data suitable for usage in CNN. The shape index value range $[0.5, 1]$ is linearly transformed to $[-1, 1]$, and all the values from the interval $[-1, 0.5]$ are mapped to the value of -1. Considering that the output value of 1 corresponds to the nodule class, this normalization method actually gives the voxels with the shape index values near 1 a larger initial probability of being a nodule. Based on this idea, the DTCNN can be viewed as a system with the initial state of each cell being the shape index value of the corresponding voxel. With the iterations increasing, the information in larger neighborhoods is utilized to make the decision, until either the state reaches a stable equilibrium point or the iterations stop.

4.3　DTCNN Learning Based on Genetic Algorithm

Due to the piecewise-linear nonlinearity of DTCNN, derivative based methods, such as the gradient descent procedure cannot be used for training of DTCNN. Kozek [20] proposed genetic algorithm (GA) for CNN learning. By minimizing the differences between the settled output and the desired output, this input-output approach guarantees that the settled output finally approaches the desired output from the initial state.

For each nodule used for training, the image data in a neighborhood are extracted. The choice of the neighborhood size is a tradeoff between the learning load and the capability of decreasing the potential FPs. One extreme choice is the whole lung, but this is not practical due to the heavy load. In our scheme, $31 \times 31 \times 31$ (edge about $20\,mm$) neighborhood is chosen. Accurate segmentation of nodules requires a lot of domain knowledge, so a simple method of creating the desired output image (DOI) is used instead. An ellipsoid having value 1 inside and value -1 outside is generated for each nodule, with the center and the size are adapted to overlap the nodule as much as possible.

Genetic algorithm [21] are stochastic optimization techniques that simulate the mechanisms of natural selection and genetics. GA uses binary strings (chromosomes) to encode points in parameter space. Chromosomes are evaluated by a predefined fitness function to quantify the performance of each possible solution. A higher fitness corresponds to a better solution. Searching from a population of chromosomes, GA tries to combine information in good chromosomes to get the optimal solution.

Instead of using the most commonly used cost function of the Euclidean distance type [20], a more complex metric [22] is used. This method measures sensitivity and specificity of a classification scheme by a pair of parameters, ρ^1 and ρ^2. For simplicity, we denote the desired nodule area, i.e., the area with value 1, as D_j for the jth training image; similarly, the recognized nodule area is indicated by R_j; and the intersection between D_j and R_j is represented as $D_j \cap R_j$. Then $\rho_j^1 = (D_j \cap R_j)/D_j$, and $\rho_j^2 = (D_j \cap R_j)/R_j$. Another consideration is the convergence speed of the DTCNN. We propose a scheme to penalize an oscillated solution. For the jth training image, an oscillation index is defined as

$$O_j = \frac{1}{2k} \sum_{i=1}^{k} |y_i(N-1) - y_i(N)| \qquad (9)$$

It measures the difference between the settled output and the output at previous step. The value of O_j falls in the interval $[0,1]$. The fitness functions of a chromosome are defined for a single training image j and for all the training images:

$$f_j = \rho_j^1 \rho_j^2 (1 - O_j), \quad f(p) = \frac{1}{m} \sum_{j=1}^{m} f_j \tag{10}$$

Here m is the number of the training images. The ultimate fitness function is the average of the fitness values for all the training images.

5 Experimental Results

The database consisted of 19 CT scans in lung cancer screening trial. These cases were selected according to radiology reports showing the existence of lung nodules. The slice size is 512×512 (x, y) pixels, the in-plane resolution, same for x and y directions, ranges from $0.54\,mm$ to $0.93\,mm$. The axial (z) reconstruction interval varied from $0.70\,mm$ to $1.30\,mm$. The 19 cases were divided into two groups: one group with 2 scans was used for training of DTCNN; the remaining 17 cases were used for evaluation. The 17 scans were visually read by a pulmonologist, who was asked to find all nodules and give their locations.

The detection of juxtapleural nodules consisted of candidate creation and classification. In the candidate creation step, 29 from 31 juxtapleural nodules in the 17 scans were included, a sensitivity of 93.6% with 145 FPs/case. For the classification step, LDA, feedforward neural networks, linear support vector machine with recursive feature elimination (SVM-RFE) were tried. And LDA gave the best results. The reason for this is probablly due to the curse of dimensionality, as the number of samples is small comparing to the number of features. ROC of the LDA using *leave one case out* scheme is shown in Fig. 4 (a). The area under the ROC is 0.9735. An operating point with sensitivity of 89.7% (26 from 29) and specificity of 95.4% on this ROC curve resulted in an overall sensitivity of 83.9% (26 from 31) with an average of 6.7 FPs per case, Fig. 4 (b).

In the detection of non-pleural nodules, 5 nodules from the two CT scans formed the training data according to the procedure in Section 4.3. Totally 111

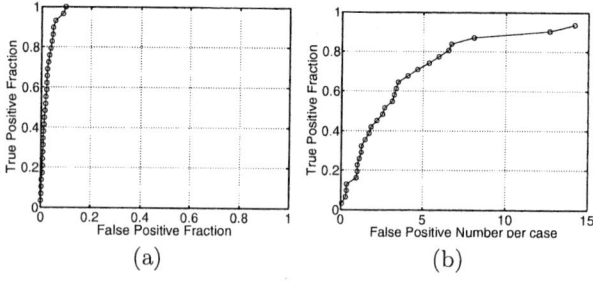

Fig. 4. ROC curves of juxtapleural nodule detection. (a) ROC curve of the LDA; (b) ROC curve of the juxtapleural nodule detection system (including both the candidate creation and classification)

possible nodule positions were given in the 17 testing cases by the CAD. This 111 positions included 20 from the 30 nodules found by the pulmonologist, a sensitivity of 66.7%.

One important thing is the presence of nodules missed by the human reader but identified by the CAD. The pulmonologist annotating nodules in the initial session visually reviewed the CAD results to confirm nodules that were identified by the CAD system. Pleural based focal opacities were confirmed by the human reader as nodule or nodule-like focal opacities if identified by a CAD system as actionable, and therefore in need of a subsequent visual reading. Linear pleural opacities that were part of fissures were not included as significantly identifiable in the visual scanning. Apical opacities were not identified as significantly findable/actionable lesions. 11 juxtapleural nodules, which were undetected in the first visual reading were identified as true nodules in the second review. 13 areas were indicated as nodule-like focal opacity pleural lesions. For the non-pleural nodules, 32 nodules undetected in the first reading were identified as true nodules in the second review after they were identified by the CAD system, and 8 additional positions were identified as very suspicious areas. The detection results of the human reader and the CAD are shown in Table 1. The CAD system detected many nodules originally missed by the human visual reading. This demonstartes that the proposed CAD system performed effectively as a radiologist's assistant to detect small nodules in the pulmonary CT images.

This facts motivated an alternative evaluation method. The union of the nodules detected in the first visual reading and the nodules confirmed in the second visual review was considered as the truth. Accordingly, for juxtapleural nodule detection (previously chosen operating point), 37 from 42 true nodules were detected by the CAD, a sensitivity of 88.1% with an average of 6.1 FPs/case; furthermore, if the nodule like focal opacities are considered as TPs, the sensitivity of our CAD increased to 90.9% (50 from 55) with 5.3 FPs/case. For non-pleural nodule detection, the total number of true nodules in these 17 cases were 62. The human reader detected 30 of these 62 nodules, a sensitivity of 48.4%, whereas our CAD system located 52, a sensitivity of 83.9%. The number of total FPs by CAD in these 17 cases was 59, corresponding to 3.5FPs/case. If the 8 very suspicious areas were considered as TPs, the sensitivity of our CAD increased to 85.7%, and the total number of FPs dropped to 51, equivalent to 3FPs/case.

Considering juxtapleural and non-pleural nodules together, a overall sensitivity of 85.6% (89 from 104) with 9.5 FPs/case was attained. If the possible lesions are treated as TPs rather than FPs, the sensitivity increased to 88% (110 from 125) with 8.3 FPs/case.

Table 2 shows the performance comparison of our scheme with several other methods of detecting pulmonary nodules in CT images. Although no strict conclusion on the superiority can be given due to the differences of the test images, the comparison is of interest. The statistical results show that our method attained a much higher sensitivity and much lower FP rate than multiple thresholding method [2] and template matching scheme [5]. A prior model method [6] gave a similar sensitivity and FP rate, but the results were obtained on a much

Table 1. The number of correctly detected lesions in terms of locations and detection method (Nodule (Nodule like))

Location/reader	Human	CAD	Human−CAD	CAD−Human	CAD+Human
Juxtapleural	31	37(50)	5	11(24)	42(55)
Non-pleural	30	52(60)	10	32(40)	62(70)

Table 2. Performance comparisons between several nodule detection CAD systems

Methods	Nodule size/number	Sensitivity	FP
Multiple thresholding [2]	$3-28mm/187$	70%	$3/slice$
Template matching [5]	$5-30mm/98$	72%	$30/case$
Prior model [6]	$5-30mm/36$	86%	$11/case$
This work	$2-15mm/104$	85.6%	$9.5/case$

smaller dataset. In addition, the goal of our work presented here is to detect nodules as early as possible, so the CT scans used were collected in a lung cancer screening trial for asymptomatic subjects. The nodules in these cases are all small-size nodules (most of them are from $2\,mm$ to $10\,mm$). Detecting small-size nodules is more difficult and often leads to a lower sensitivity and higher FP rate.

6 Conclusion

A new CAD system was proposed to locate small nodules in high resolution helical CT scans. Morphological closing, thresholding and 3D component analysis were used to obtain juxtapleural nodule candidates, gray level and geometric features were analyzed using a LDA classifier. Leave one case out method was utilized to evaluate the LDA. This juxtapleural nodule detection method was able to obtain a sensitivity 88.1% with an average of 6.1 FPs/case. To locate non-pleural nodules, a DTCNN based scheme was developed. This method employed the local shape feature to perform voxel classification. The DTCNN was trained using genetic algorithm (GA). The non-pleural nodule finding scheme attained sensitivity of 83.9% with an average 3.5 FPs/case. By evaluating the two subsystems together, an overall performance of 85.6% sensitivity with 9.5 FPs/case (0.04 FPs/image) will be attained. Furthermore, the CAD system located many nodules missed by the human reading. This showed that the proposed CAD system was an effective assistant for human experts to detect small nodules and provide a valuable "second opinion" to the human observer.

References

1. Giger, M.L., Bae, K.T., MacMahon, H.: Computerized detection of pulmonary nodules in computed tomography images. Investigate. Radiol. **29** (1994) 459–465
2. Armato, S.G., Giger, M.L., Moran, C.J., Blackburn, J.T., Doi, K., MacMahon, H.: Computerized detection of pulmonary nodules on CT scans. Radiographics **19** (1999) 1303–1311
3. Kanazawa, K., Kawata, Y., Niki, N., Satoh, H., Ohmatsu, H., Kakinuma, R., Kaneko, M., Moriyama, N., Eguchi, K.: Computer-aided diagnostic system for pulmonary nodules based on helical CT images. In Doi, K., MacMahon, H., Giger, M.L., Hoffmann, K., eds.: Computer-Aided Diagnosis Medical Imaging. Elsevier, Amesterdam, The Netherlands (1999) 131–136
4. Penedo, M.G., Carreira, M.J., Mosquera, A., Cabello, D.: Computer-aided diagnosis: a neural-network-based approach to lung nodule detection. IEEE Transactions on Medical Imaging **17** (1998) 872–880
5. Lee, Y., Hara, T., Fujita, H., Itoh, S., Ishigaki, T.: Automated detection of pulmonary nodules in helical CT images based on an improved template-matching technique. IEEE Transactions on Medical Imaging **20** (2001) 595–604
6. Brown, M.S., McNitt-Gray, M.F., Goldin, J.G., Suh, R.D., Sayre, J.W., Aberle, D.R.: Patient-specific models for lung nodule detection and surveillance in CT images. IEEE Transactions on Medical Imaging **20** (2001) 1242–1250
7. Hu, S., Hoffman, E.A., Reinhardt, J.M.: Automatic lung segmentation for accurate quantitation of volumetric X-ray CT images. IEEE Transactions on Medical Imaging **20** (2001) 490–498
8. Ridler, T.W., Calvard, S.: Picture thresholding using an iterative selection method. IEEE Transactions on Systems, Man and Cybernetics **8** (1978) 630–632
9. Besl, P.J., Jain, R.C.: Segmentation through variable-order surface fitting. IEEE Trans. Patt. Anal. Machine Intell. **10** (1988) 167–192
10. Koenderink, J.J.: Solid Shape. The MIT Press, London (1990)
11. Koenderink, J.J., van Doorn, A.J.: Surface shape and curvature scales. Image and Vision Computing **10** (1992) 557–565
12. Yoshida, H., Nappi, J.: Three-dimensional computer-aided diagnosis scheme for detection of colonic polyps. IEEE Transactions on Medical Imaging **20** (2001) 1261–1274
13. Monga, O., Benayoun, S.: Using partial derivatives of 3D images to extract typical surface features. Computer Vision and Image Understanding **61** (1995) 171–189
14. Thirion, J.P., Gourdon, A.: Computing the differential characteristics of isointensity surfaces. Computer Vision and Image Understanding **61** (1995) 190–202
15. Turkiyyah, G., Stori, D., Ganter, M., Chen, H., Vimawala, M.: An acceleration triangulation method for computing the skeletons of free from solid models. Computer-Aided Design **29** (1997) 5–19
16. Harrer, H., Nossek, J.A., Stelzl, R.: An analog implementation of discrete time cellular neural networks. IEEE Transactions on Neural Networks **3** (1992) 466–476
17. Harrer, H., Nossek, J.A.: Discrete time cellular neural networks. Int. J. Circuit Theory and Applicat. **20** (1992) 453–467
18. Chua, L.O., Yang, L.: Cellular neural networks: theory. IEEE Transactions on Circuits and Systems **35** (1988) 1257–1272
19. Chua, L.O., Yang, L.: Cellular neural networks: applications. IEEE Transactions on Circuits and Systems **35** (1988) 1273–1290

20. Kozek, T., Roska, T., Chua, L.O.: Genetic algorithm for CNN template learning. IEEE Transactions on Circuits and Systems **40** (1988) 392–402
21. Goldberg, D.E.: Genetic Algorithms in Search, Optimization, and Machine learning. Addison-Wesley, Reading, MA (1989)
22. Potocnik, B., Zazula, D.: Automated analysis of a sequence of ovarian ultrasound images. Part I, segmentation of single 2D images. Image and Vision Computing **20** (2002) 217–225

Nonparametric Neighborhood Statistics for MRI Denoising

Suyash P. Awate and Ross T. Whitaker

School of Computing, University of Utah, Salt Lake City, UT 84112, USA
{suyash, whitaker}@cs.utah.edu

Abstract. This paper presents a novel method for denoising MR images that relies on an optimal estimation, combining a likelihood model with an adaptive image prior. The method models images as random fields and exploits the properties of independent Rician noise to learn the higher-order statistics of image neighborhoods from corrupted input data. It uses these statistics as priors within a Bayesian denoising framework. This paper presents an information-theoretic method for characterizing neighborhood structure using nonparametric density estimation. The formulation generalizes easily to simultaneous denoising of multimodal MRI, exploiting the relationships between modalities to further enhance performance. The method, relying on the information content of input data for noise estimation and setting important parameters, does not require significant parameter tuning. Qualitative and quantitative results on real, simulated, and multimodal data, including comparisons with other approaches, demonstrate the effectiveness of the method.

1 Introduction

Over the last several decades, magnetic resonance (MR) imaging technology has benefited from a variety of technological developments resulting in increased resolution, signal to noise ratio (SNR), and acquisition speed. However, fundamental trade-offs between resolution, speed, and SNR combined with scientific, clinical, and financial pressures to obtain more data more quickly, result in images that still exhibit significant levels of noise. In particular, the need for shorter acquisition times, such as in dynamic imaging, often undermines the ability to obtain images having both high resolution and high SNR. Furthermore, the efficacy of higher-level, post processing of MR images, including tissue classification and organ segmentation, that assume specific models of tissue intensity (e.g. homogeneous), are sometimes impaired by even moderate noise levels. Hence, denoising MR images remains an important problem. From a multitude of statistical and variational denoising formulations proposed, no particular one appears as a clear winner in all relevant aspects, including the reduction of randomness and intensity bias, structure and edge preservation, generality, reliability, automation, and computational cost. The paper proposes a method for denoising MR magnitude data modeling images as random fields, but unlike statistical methods in literature, *it does not rely on a specific, ad-hoc image prior*. Instead, it estimates the higher-order signal statistics from the neighborhood statistics of the noisy input data by deconvolving the latter with the noise statistics. It then uses these statistics as priors within an optimal Bayesian denoising framework.

2 Related Work

A multitude of variational/nonlinear PDE-based methods have been developed for a wide variety of images and applications [15, 14], with some of these having applications to magnetic resonance imaging (MRI) [8, 11, 7]. However, such methods impose certain kinds of *models* on local image structure, and these models are often too simple to capture the complexity of anatomical MR images. Also they do not take into account the bias introduced by Rician noise. Furthermore, they usually involve manual tuning of *critical* free parameters that control the conditions under which the models prefer one sort of structure over another; this has been an impediment to the widespread adoption of these techniques.

The wavelet literature addresses image denoising extensively [16]. Healy *et al.* [9] were among the first to apply soft-thresholding based wavelet techniques for denoising MR images. Hilton *et al.* [10] applied a threshold-based scheme for functional MRI data. Nowak [13], operating on the square magnitude MR image, includes a Rician noise model in the threshold-based wavelet denoising scheme and thereby corrects for the bias introduced by the noise.

Several statistically based image processing algorithms rely on information theory such as the *mean-shift* algorithm [3]. It is a *mode seeking* process that operates only on image intensities (scalar/vector valued) and does not account for the neighborhood structure. As such it has been used for image segmentation, but not for reconstruction. Some MR nonuniformity correction methods are based on the quantification of information content in MR images [19, 12]. They follow from the observation that nonuniformities increase the entropy of the 1D *gray scale* probability density functions (PDFs). However, entropy measures on first-order image statistics are insufficient for denoising; thus this paper extends the information theoretic strategy to higher-order PDFs.

Another class of statistical methods are based on Markov random fields [24, 22]. The proposed method also exploits the Markov property of the images, but rather than imposing an ad-hoc image model, it *estimates* the relevant conditional PDFs from the input data. We show that incorporating spatial information, via neighborhood statistics, is effective for MRI denoising *and* that the process can be bootstrapped from the image data, making a very general algorithm with less tuning of critical free parameters.

Previous work in estimation theory has addressed the use of optimal image estimation using neighborhood probabilities [21]. That work focuses on *discrete* functions and relies on inverting the channel transition matrix (noise model) to give a closed form estimate for source statistics. The proposed method addresses continuous-valued signals, which is essential for medical imaging applications, and thus entails deconvolving nonparametric approximations to PDFs via entropy reduction. It also addresses the effect of noise in the neighborhoods that are used to condition the estimate, hence making it more effective for reducing additive/multiplicative noise, which is important in medical image processing.

The method in this paper builds on our previous work in [1]. That work lays down the foundations for unsupervised learning of higher-order image statistics and proposes entropy reduction as a denoising heuristic for independent additive zero-mean Gaussian noise for single gray scale images. This paper uses entropy reduction coupled with the Rician noise model as a means to recover higher-order image statistics from noisy input data. It exploits such statistics for optimal Bayesian denoising of MR images, with a method for computing the expectation of the posterior. It also addresses the question of how to utilize multimodal data within this optimal framework.

3 Neighborhood Statistics for MRI Denoising

This section begins with an overview of the random-field image model and then describes the formulation that uses *a priori* information of higher-order (neighborhood) statistics within an optimal Bayesian estimation framework. The next section (Section 4) describes a way of bootstrapping this process by generating such priors from the noisy data itself.

3.1 Random Field Image Model

A random field/process [5] is a family of random variables $X(\Omega; T)$, for some index set T, where, for each fixed $T = t$, the random variable $X(\Omega; t)$ is defined on the sample space Ω. If we let T be a set of points defined on a discrete Cartesian grid and fix $\Omega = \omega$, we have a realization of the random field called the *digital image*, $X(\omega, T)$. In this case $\{t\}_{t \in T}$ is the set of pixels in the image. For 2-dimensional images t is a two-vector. We use a shorthand to denote random variables $X(\Omega; t)$ by $X(t)$. We denote a specific realization $X(\omega; t)$ (the digital image), as a deterministic function $x(t)$.

If we associate with T a family of pixel neighborhoods $N = \{N_t\}_{t \in T}$ such that $N_t \subset T$, $t \notin N_t$, and $u \in N_t$ if and only if $t \in N_u$, then N is called a neighborhood system for the set T and points in N_t are called neighbors of t. We define a random vector $Y(t) = \{X(t)\}_{t \in N_t}$, denoting its realization by $y(t)$, corresponding to the set of intensities at the neighbors of pixel t. We denote the noiseless image by $X(\omega, T)$ and its associated set of neighborhood intensities by $Y(\omega, T)$. Correspondingly, for the observed noisy image, we use $\tilde{X}(\omega, T)$ and $\tilde{Y}(\omega, T)$. For the formulation in this paper, we assume the noiseless image to be generated from a stationary ergodic process (in practice this assumption can be relaxed, somewhat). For notational simplicity, we use the short hand for random variables $X(t)$ as X and their realizations $x(t)$ as x, dropping the index t.

3.2 Bayesian Estimation with Higher-Order Statistical Priors

The proposed strategy relies on several pieces of technology that interact to provide accurate, practical models of image statistics. For clarity the discussion

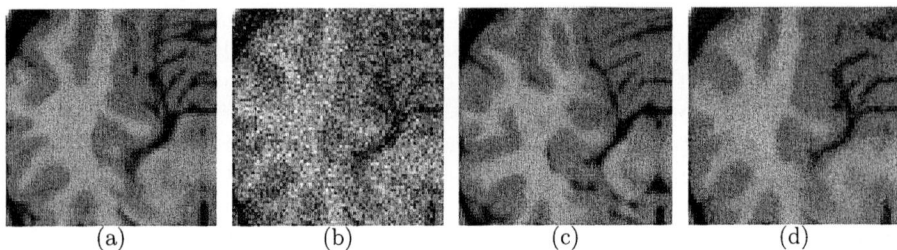

Fig. 1. Insets of (a) the noiseless image, (b) the noisy image (SNR 12db), (c) one of the two images forming the higher-order *prior*, and (d) the denoised image (SNR 23db)

begins at a high level allowing for certain available models and estimates; successive sections discuss how each of these pieces is developed from the input data. Our goal is to estimate the true intensity x from the observed noisy intensity $\tilde{x}$ by exploiting the neighborhood intensities. We begin with the simplest case where we know the *uncorrupted* neighborhood intensities y. We consider Bayesian estimation with the prior $P(X|Y = y)$ and the likelihood $P(\tilde{X} = \tilde{x}|X)$. Assuming again, for simplicity, that we know the prior, Bayes rule gives the posterior as

$$P(X|\tilde{X} = \tilde{x}, Y = y) = \frac{1}{\eta} P(\tilde{X} = \tilde{x}|X) P(X|Y = y) \qquad (1)$$

where $\eta = P(\tilde{X} = \tilde{x}|Y = y)$ is a normalization factor. For a squared error loss function the optimal estimate is the posterior mean $\hat{x} = E[X|\tilde{X} = \tilde{x}, Y = y]$.

In practice, two problems undermine this strategy. The first concerns obtaining the conditional PDFs that give the priors for an image. We propose to model these nonparametrically using Parzen windowing with samples of image neighborhoods, as described in subsequent sections. These samples can come from either a suitable database of high SNR images (e.g. different images of the same modality and anatomy) or from the noisy input image itself, using a bootstrapping process described in Section 4. The second problem is that, even if we know the priors, we know only $\tilde{y}$ for the input data (not y). To address this issue, we start with $\tilde{y}$ as an approximation for y and iterate on the posterior estimates to a fixed point where the posterior estimate for each pixel is consistent with the prior given by the estimates of its neighbors. Thus, as the iterations proceed, the noise in the pixel intensities reduces and the neighborhoods give progressively better estimates of the prior. The proposed algorithm is therefore:

1. The input image I comprises a set of intensities $\{\tilde{x}\}_{t \in T}$ and neighborhoods $\{\tilde{y}\}_{t \in T}$. These values form the initial values ($I^0 = I$) of a sequence of images $I^0, I^1, I^2, \ldots$, with corresponding intensities $\hat{x}^0, \hat{x}^1, \hat{x}^2, \ldots$ and neighborhoods $\hat{y}^0, \hat{y}^1, \hat{y}^2, \ldots$.
2. Compute the likelihood PDF $P(\tilde{X} = \tilde{x}|X)$, as described in Section 3.4.
3. For each pixel in the current image I^m, estimate the higher-order prior $P(X|Y = \hat{y}^m)$, as described in Section 3.3.
4. Construct a new image I^{m+1} with intensities $\hat{x}^{m+1}$ as the posterior mean $\hat{x}^{m+1} = E[X|\tilde{X} = \tilde{x}, Y = \hat{y}^m]$.

5. If $\| I^{m+1} - I^m \| > \delta$ (small threshold), go to Step 3, otherwise I^{m+1} is the output.

Figure 1 shows a demonstration of this concept on simulated MRI data from the BrainWeb [2] project. We corrupt a T1 image with Rician noise and use two other similar, but not identical, images as priors. We use 9×9 neighborhoods. Figure 1(c) is one of the two images representing the nonparametric prior model (Parzen windows, 500 local random samples for each t), and Figure 1(d) is the output image. This example shows the power of the prior—the denoised image exhibits structures that are barely visible in the noisy version. The coming sections describe the underlying technology in this estimation process, and give an algorithm for generating data-driven prior models *without an example*.

3.3 Modeling the Prior: Nonparametric Density Estimation

Bayesian estimation using higher-order statistics entails the estimation of higher-order conditional PDFs. Despite theoretical arguments suggesting that density estimation beyond a few dimensions is impractical, the empirical evidence from the statistics literature is more optimistic [17, 1]. The results in this paper confirm that observation. Moreover, stationarity implies that the random vector (X, Y) exhibits identical marginal PDFs, leading to more accurate density estimates [17]. In addition, the neighborhoods in natural images have a lower-dimensional topology in the high-dimensional feature space [4] that aids in density estimation.

We use the Parzen-window nonparametric density estimation technique [6] with an n-dimensional Gaussian kernel $G_n(z, \Psi_n)$, where n is the neighborhood size. Having no a priori information on the structure of the PDFs, we choose an isotropic Gaussian, i.e. $\Psi_n = \sigma_P I_n$, where I_n is the $n \times n$ identity matrix. Using optimal values of the Parzen-window parameters is critical for success, and that can be difficult in such high-dimensional spaces; we have developed a method for automatically choosing this parameter, as described Section 4.3.

For a stationary ergodic process, the estimated prior is

$$P(X|\tilde{Y} = \tilde{y}_i) = \frac{\sum_{t_j \in A_i} G_n(\tilde{y}_i - y_j, \Psi_n) G_1(x_j, \Psi_1)}{\sum_{t_j \in A_i} G_n(\tilde{y}_i - y_j, \Psi_n)} \quad (2)$$

where the set A_i is a small subset of T, chosen at random for each t_i, and x_j and y_j are shorthand for $x(t_j)$ and $y(t_j)$ respectively. This results in a stochastic approximation for the conditional PDFs and the corresponding posteriors.

3.4 Approximating the Rician Likelihood

The Rician PDF of the MRI intensities does not lend itself to analytical, closed-form representations of quantities, such as the likelihood and the posterior expectation, which we need for each iteration of this algorithm. In practice we have found that the shape of the PDF is less important than having good estimates of variance and bias. Therefore, we develop a method of approximating Rician noise (via the likelihood) by additive Gaussian noise with a signal-dependent

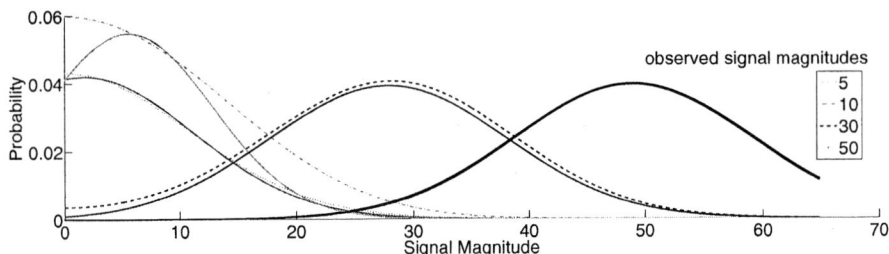

Fig. 2. Gaussians (solid lines) approximating likelihood functions (non-solid lines) for different observed signal magnitudes (underlying noise $\equiv N(0, 100)$).

mean and variance. For the underlying independent noise $N(0, \sigma^2)$, and σ estimated using the method described by Nowak [13], the likelihood is

$$P\left(\tilde{X} = \tilde{x} | X = x\right) = \frac{\tilde{x}}{\sigma^2} \exp(-\frac{\tilde{x}^2 + x^2}{2\sigma^2}) I_0(\frac{\tilde{x}x}{\sigma^2}) \qquad (3)$$

where $I_0(\cdot)$ is the zero-order modified Bessel function of the first kind. For a discrete set of observed signal magnitudes $\tilde{x}$, we fit a Gaussian to the likelihoods via a Levenberg-Marquardt optimization scheme. In this way, we create (in a preprocessing step) a lookup table mapping $\tilde{x}$ to the parameters of the Gaussian approximation, and interpolate the parameters between sample points as needed in subsequent likelihood calculations. At high SNR the means are close to $\tilde{x}$ while at low SNR the means are substantially lower. Figure 2 shows the likelihood PDFs and the approximated Gaussians for various observed signal magnitudes.

3.5 Computing the Posterior Mean

Equations 1 and 2, and the Gaussian approximated likelihood, give the posterior

$$P(X|\tilde{X} = \tilde{x}, \tilde{Y} = \tilde{y}_i) = \frac{1}{\eta} \frac{\sum_{t_j \in A_i} G_n(\tilde{y}_i - y_j, \Psi_n) G_1(x_j, \tilde{\sigma}_P^2)}{\sum_{t_j \in A_i} G_n(\tilde{y}_i - y_j, \Psi_n)} G_1(\tilde{x}_L, \tilde{\sigma}_L^2), \qquad (4)$$

where $\tilde{\sigma}_P^2$ is the Parzen-window kernel variance, and $\tilde{x}_L$ and $\tilde{\sigma}_L^2$ are the mean and variance of the Gaussian approximation to the likelihood (from the lookup table). The posterior mean is given by a sum of expectations of Gaussian products:

$$E[X|\tilde{X} = \tilde{x}, \tilde{Y} = \tilde{y}_i] = \frac{\sum_{t_j \in A_i} G_n(\tilde{y}_i - y_j, \Psi_n) K_{ij} M_{ij}}{\sum_{t_j \in A_i} G_n(\tilde{y}_i - y_j, \Psi_n) K_{ij}}; \qquad (5)$$

$$K_{ij} = \frac{\exp(-A_{ij}(C_{ij} - B_{ij}^2/4))}{\sqrt{2\pi(\tilde{\sigma}_P^2 + \tilde{\sigma}_L^2)}}; M_{ij} = \frac{B_{ij}}{2};$$

$$A_{ij} = \frac{\tilde{\sigma}_P^2 + \tilde{\sigma}_L^2}{2\tilde{\sigma}_P^2 \tilde{\sigma}_L^2}; B_{ij} = 2\frac{x_j \tilde{\sigma}_P^2 + \tilde{x}_L \tilde{\sigma}_L^2}{\tilde{\sigma}_P^2 + \tilde{\sigma}_L^2}; C_{ij} = \frac{x_j^2 \tilde{\sigma}_P^2 + \tilde{x}_L^2 \tilde{\sigma}_L^2}{\tilde{\sigma}_P^2 + \tilde{\sigma}_L^2};$$

where we exploit the property that the Gaussian is its own *conjugate*.

4 Bootstrapping Neighborhood Statistics from Noisy Input Data

So far we discussed denoising with higher-order statistical priors. In the absence of noiseless/high-SNR example images, we must estimate these from the noisy input image. If we wish to construct an approximation to the prior (neighborhood statistics) from the input data, we must address the affects of noise on this PDF. We approximate Rician noise as (nonstationary) additive Gaussian. Hence the proposed method derives from the effects of additive Gaussian noise on PDFs. Additive noise in the signal corresponds to a *convolution* of the PDFs of the signal and noise. Therefore, for probability densities, noise reduction corresponds to deconvolving the PDF of the input data by the PDF of the noise.

4.1 Estimating Neighborhood Statistics

Rician noise affects the conditional PDFs in two ways: (a) it introduces a bias (shift), and (b) it increases its entropy $h(\tilde{X}|\tilde{Y} = \tilde{y})$ [18]. Hence, we propose entropy reduction coupled with bias correction in an attempt to recover the PDFs. Of course, entropy reduction might also partly eliminate the normal variability in the image. However, we are motivated by the observation that noiseless images tend to have very low entropies relative to their noisy versions. Thus, entropy reduction first affects the noise substantially more than the image statistics. We propose bias correction by shifting intensities $\tilde{x}$ towards their likelihood mean $E[\tilde{X} = \tilde{x}|X]$. For the case of zero noise these two values coincide, thereby eliminating the need for any correction. Otherwise, we move $\tilde{x}$ towards its likelihood mean with a force proportional to the difference. Thus, to restore the conditional PDFs of the input, we minimize the functional

$$\sum_{t \in T} \left[\lambda_1 \left(h(\tilde{X}|\tilde{Y} = \tilde{y}) \right) + \lambda_2 \left(\tilde{x} - E[\tilde{X} = \tilde{x}|X] \right)^2 / 2 \right]. \qquad (6)$$

The first term in the functional sharpens the conditional PDFs, and the second term aids in bias correction. We use an iterative gradient-descent optimization scheme with finite forward differences. The PDF restoration proceeds as follows:

1. The input image I comprises a set of intensities $\{\tilde{x}\}_{t \in T}$. These values form the initial values of a sequence of images $I^0, I^1, I^2, \ldots$.
2. Using the current image I^m, construct a new image I^{m+1} with intensities $\tilde{x}^{m+1} = \tilde{x}^m - \lambda_1 \partial h / \partial \tilde{x}^m - \lambda_2 \left(\tilde{x}^m - E[\tilde{X} = \tilde{x}^m|X] \right)$.
3. If the estimated noise level (as per the method in [13]) in I^{m+1} is zero, then stop. Otherwise, go to Step 2.

We call the final image generated by this process as the *PDF-restored* image. This image forms the *example* image, from which samples are taken to model the prior conditional probabilities in Equation 2. In practice, the results are somewhat insensitive to the values of λ_1 and λ_2, and we choose λ_1, as described in Section 5, related to a mean-shift update.

4.2 Entropy Minimization via Gradient Descent

Entropy is the expectation of negative log-probability, and therefore we can approximate it with the sample mean [20]. For a stationary ergodic process, we approximate the entropy of the conditional PDF as

$$h(\tilde{X}|\tilde{Y} = \tilde{y}_i) \approx -\frac{1}{|T|} \sum_{t_i \in T} \log \left[\frac{\sum_{t_j \in A_i} G_{n+1}(\tilde{w}_i - \tilde{w}_j, \Psi_{n+1})}{|A_i| P(\tilde{Y} = \tilde{y}_i)} \right] \quad (7)$$

where $\tilde{w}_i = (\tilde{x}_i, \tilde{y}_i)$, A_i is a small subset of T, chosen at random; as done in Section 3.3 for computing the prior. A variety of practical issues associated with this strategy, are discussed in Section 4.3. The gradient descent for w_i is

$$\frac{\partial \tilde{x}_i}{\partial t} = -\frac{1}{|T|} \frac{\partial \tilde{w}_i}{\partial \tilde{x}_i} \sum_{t_j \in A_i} \frac{G_{n+1}(\tilde{w}_i - \tilde{w}_j, \Psi_{n+1})}{\sum_{t_k \in A_i} G_{n+1}(\tilde{w}_i - \tilde{w}_k, \Psi_{n+1})} \Psi_{n+1}^{-1}(\tilde{w}_i - \tilde{w}_j) \quad (8)$$

where $\partial \tilde{w}_i / \partial \tilde{x}_i$ projects the $n+1$ dimensional vector $\tilde{w}_i$ onto the dimension associated with the element $\tilde{x}_i$. In previous work [1] we have shown that, a timestep of $|T|\sigma_P^2$ corresponds to a mean-shift procedure on the conditional PDFs; that is, each data value moves to the weighted average of the sample data.

4.3 Implementation Issues

This section discusses several practical issues that are crucial for the effectiveness of the entropy reduction and prior estimation on image neighborhoods. A more detailed discussion on these issues is given in [1].

Parzen-Window Kernel Width: Parzen-window density estimates, using finitely many samples, are greatly sensitive to the value of the Gaussian kernel σ_P [6]. The particular choice of σ_P is related to the sample size $|A_i|$ in the stochastic approximation. We automatically compute an *optimal* σ_P, that minimizes the average entropy of all conditional PDFs in the image, via a Newton-Raphson optimization scheme. Our experiments show that for sufficiently large $|A_i|$ additional samples do not significantly affect the estimates of entropy and σ_P, and thus $|A_i|$ can also be generated automatically from the input data.

Stationarity and Local Sampling Strategies: In practice, image statistics are not homogeneous, and statistics for most images are more accurately modeled as piecewise stationary ergodic. Thus the set A_i of samples used to evaluate entropy and process pixel t_i should consist of pixels that are spatially near t_i. To achieve this, we choose a unique set of samples for each pixel t_i at random from a Gaussian distribution on the image coordinates, centered at t_i with standard deviation 30. Thus, the set A_i comprises pixels biased to be more near t_i. This strategy gives consistently better results than uniform sampling, and we have found that the it performs well for virtually any choice of the standard deviation that encompasses more than several hundred pixels. For this sampling strategy, $|A_i|$ is automatically computed to be 500 for all examples in the paper.

Neighborhood Shape and Size: Larger neighborhoods generally yield better results but take longer to compute. Typically 9×9 neighborhoods suffice, and we use them for the results in this paper. To obtain rotational invariance we use a metric in the feature space (neighborhood mask) that controls the influence of each neighborhood pixel by making distances in this space less sensitive to neighborhood rotations. Likewise image boundaries are handled through anisotropic metrics that do not distort the neighborhood statistics of the image.

Computation: The computational complexity of the proposed method is significant: $O(|T||A_i|E^D)$ where D is the image dimension and E is the extent of the neighborhood along a dimension. This is exponential in E, and our current results are limited to 2D images. The literature suggests some potential improvements (e.g. [23]). However, the purpose of this paper is to introduce the theory and methodology—algorithmic improvements are the subject of future work.

5 Experiments and Results

We show results using (a) real T1 noisy data, as well as (b) simulated MR data (181×217 pixels) obtained via BrainWeb [2] for unimodal and multimodal denoising. We simulate Rician noise by adding zero-mean Gaussian noise to the real and imaginary parts of the simulated MR data and taking the magnitude. For entropy minimization in the functional 6, the time step $\lambda_1 = |T|\sigma^2$ ($\equiv$ mean-

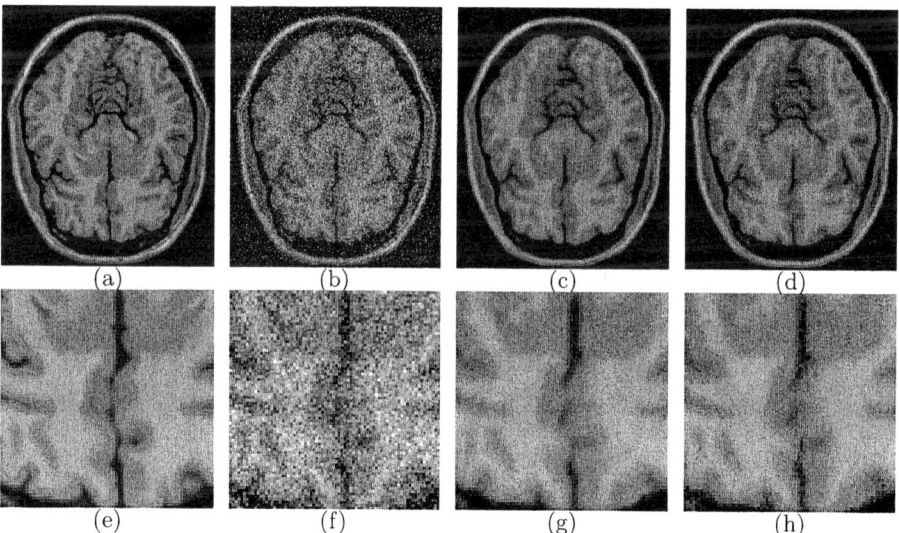

Fig. 3. (a) Noiseless T1 image. (b) Noisy image (gray matter SNR 12db, normalized squared error 1.0). (c) PDF-restored image (13 iterations) (as described in Section 4.1). (d) Denoised image (5 iterations, gray matter SNR 23db, normalized squared error 0.16). (e)-(h) show zoomed insets of images (a)-(d)

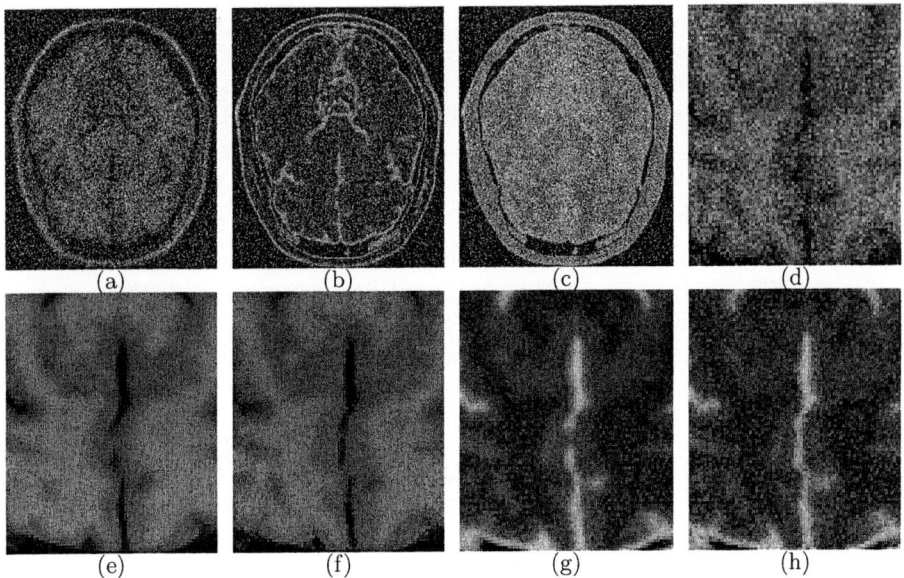

Fig. 4. Multimodal denoising. (a)-(c) Noisy T1, T2, PD images (signal intensity range 0:100, underlying noise $N(0, 400)$) (d) Zoomed inset of noisy T1 image. (e),(f) Zoomed insets of PDF-restored (as described in Section 4.1) and denoised T1 images. (g),(h) Zoomed insets of PDF-restored and denoised T2 images

shift update) can lead to oscillations, because of interactions of neighborhoods from one iteration to the next. We have found that a time step of $\lambda_1 = 0.2|T|\sigma^2$ alleviates this effect. We fix $\lambda_2 = 0.2$. We compute SNR as $20\log(x/\sigma)$ where x is the signal magnitude and the (estimated) underlying noise PDF is $N(0, \sigma^2)$. Each iteration on these data sets takes about 2 minutes on a Pentium-IV machine.

Multimodal denoising entails a simultaneous denoising of T1, T2, and PD images in a coupled manner, treating the combination of images as an image of vectors with the PDFs in the *combined* probability space. Although this paper shows results with multimodal images that are well aligned, we have evidence that the denoising is fairly robust to minor misregistration errors. The results show that incorporating more information in the denoising framework, via images of multiple modalities, produces consistently better results.

Figure 3 shows a denoising example using T1 data (SNR 12db) for the gray matter. With a normalized sum of squared pixel errors for the noisy image as 1.0, the denoised image has a squared error of 0.16. In general, the PDF-restored image (as described in Section 4.1) appears more smooth than the denoised image and may have less error. However the restoration of the neighborhood PDFs can produce some loss of structure, and the subsequent Bayesian estimation, which retains a fidelity to the input data, helps retain some of those details. We can see this behavior in the regions corresponding to the cerebro spinal fluid. This is even more clear in the next denoising example in Figure 4. With the same underlying noise PDF the normalized squared errors for the T2 and PD

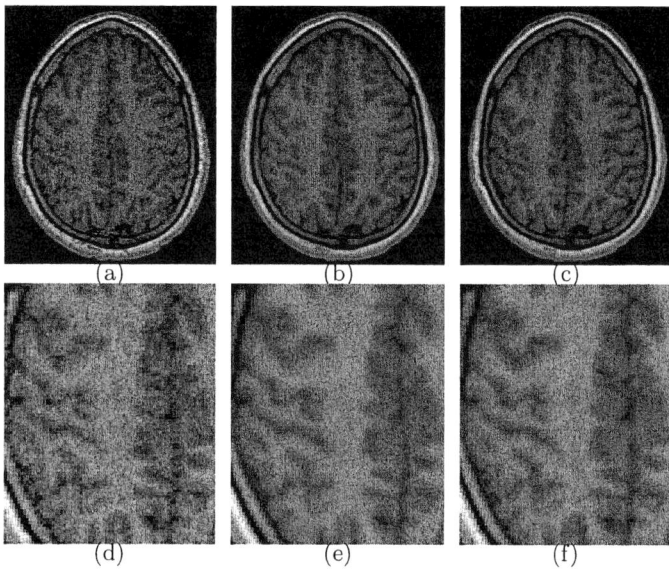

Fig. 5. (a) Real noisy image. (b) PDF-restored image (as described in Section 4.1). (c) Denoised image. (d)-(f) are zoomed insets of (a)-(c)

modalities are 0.3 and 0.19, respectively. Performing multimodal denoising with T1, T2, and PD data gives improved normalized squared errors of 0.10, 0.29, and 0.16, respectively.

Figure 4 shows T1, T2 and PD images (signal intensity range 0:100) with the underlying noise PDF as $N(0, 400)$. The SNR is 6db for the gray matter. Here, with a normalized squared error for the noisy image as 1.0, the squared error for the T1, T2, and PD denoised images are 0.08, 0.32, and 0.09 respectively. The squared error for T1 is significantly better than results in [13] for an equivalent gray matter SNR. Multimodal denoising, using T1, T2 and PD all together, gives normalized squared errors as 0.06, 0.17 and 0.07, respectively. Figure 5 shows results using real T1 noisy MRI data.

Acknowledgments

This work was supported by the NSF grant EIA0313268 and the NSF CAREER grant CCR0092065.

References

1. S. Awate and R. Whitaker. Higher-order image statistics for unsupervised, information-theoretic, adaptive, image filtering. *To appear in Proc. IEEE Int. Conf. Computer Vision Pattern Recog. 2005.*

2. D. Collins, A. Zijdenbos, V. Kollokian, J. Sled, N. Kabani, C. Holmes, and A. Evans. Design and construction of a realistic digital brain phantom. *IEEE Trans. Med. Imag.*, 17(3):463–468, 1998.
3. D. Comaniciu and P. Meer. Mean shift: A robust approach toward feature space analysis. *IEEE Trans. Pattern Anal. Mach. Intell.*, 24(5):603–619, 2002.
4. V. de Silva and G. Carlsson. Topological estimation using witness complexes. *Symposium on Point-Based Graphics*, 2004.
5. E. Dougherty. *Random Processes for Image and Signal Processing*. Wiley, 1998.
6. R. Duda, P. Hart, and D. Stork. *Pattern Classification*. Wiley, 2001.
7. A. Fan, W. Wells, J. Fisher, M. Çetin, S. Haker, R. Mulkern, C. Tempany, and A. Willsky. A unified variational approach to denoising and bias correction in mr. In *Info. Proc. Med. Imag.*, pages 148–159, 2003.
8. G. Gerig, R. Kikinis, O. Kubler, and F. Jolesz. Nonlinear anisotropic filtering of mri data. *IEEE Trans. Med. Imag.*, 11(2):221–232, 1992.
9. D. Healy and J. Weaver. Two applications of wavelet transforms in magnetic resonance imaging. *IEEE Trans. Info. Theory*, 38(2):840–860, 1992.
10. M. Hilton, T. Ogden, D. Hattery, G. Jawerth, and B. Eden. Wavelet denoising of functional MRI data. pages 93–114. 1996.
11. M. Lysaker, A. Lundervold, and X. Tai. Noise removal using fourth-order partial differential equation with applications to medical magnetic resonance images in space and time. *IEEE Trans. Imag. Proc.*, 2003.
12. J. Mangin. Entropy minimization for automatic correction of intensity nonuniformity. In *IEEE Work. Math. Models Biomed. Imag. Anal.*, pages 162–169, 2000.
13. R. Nowak. Wavelet-based rician noise removal for magnetic resonance imaging. *IEEE Trans. Imag. Proc.*, 8:1408–1419, '99.
14. S. Osher and R. Fedkiw. *Level Set Methods and Dynamic Implicit Surfaces*. Springer, 2003.
15. P. Perona and J. Malik. Scale-space and edge detection using anisotropic diffusion. *IEEE Trans. Pattern Anal. Mach. Intell.*, 12(7):629–639, July 1990.
16. J. Portilla, V. Strela, M. Wainwright, and E. Simoncelli. Image denoising using scale mixtures of gaussians in the wavelet domain. *IEEE Trans. Imag. Proc.*, 12(11):1338–1351, 2003.
17. D. Scott. *Multivariate Density Estimation*. Wiley, 1992.
18. C. Shannon. A mathematical theory of communication. *Bell System Tech. Journal*, 27:379–423, July 1948.
19. J. Sled, A. Zijdenbos, and A. Evans. A nonparametric method for automatic correction of intensity nonuniformity in mri data. *IEEE Trans. Med. Imag.*, 17:87–97, 1998.
20. P. Viola and W. Wells. Alignment by maximization of mutual information. In *Proc. Int. Conf. Comp. Vision*, pages 16–23, 1995.
21. T. Weissman, E. Ordentlich, G. Seroussi, S. Verdu, and M. Weinberger. Universal discrete denoising: Known channel. *HP Labs Tech. Report HPL-2003-29*, 2003.
22. W. Wells, E. Grimson, R. Kikinis, and F. Jolesz. Adaptive segmentation of mri data. In *Proc. Int. Conf. on Comp. Vision*, pages 59–69, 1995.
23. C. Yang, R. Duraiswami, N. Gumerov, and L. Davis. Improved fast gauss transform and efficient kernel density estimation. In *Proc. Int. Conf. Comp. Vision*, pages 464–471, 2003.
24. Y. Zhang, M. Brady, and S. Smith. Segmentation of brain mr images through a hidden markov random field model and the expectation-maximization algorithm. *IEEE Trans. Med. Imag.*, 20(1), 2001.

Construction and Validation of Mean Shape Atlas Templates for Atlas-Based Brain Image Segmentation

Qian Wang[1], Dieter Seghers[1], Emiliano D'Agostino[1], Frederik Maes[1], Dirk Vandermeulen[1], Paul Suetens[1], and Alexander Hammers[2]

[1] Katholieke Universiteit Leuven, Faculties of Medicine and Engineering, Medical Image Computing - ESAT/PSI, University Hospital Gasthuisberg, Herestraat 49, B-3000 Leuven, Belgium
Qian.Wang@uz.kuleuven.ac.be

[2] Division of Neuroscience and Mental Health, MRC Clinical Sciences Centre, London, United Kingdom

Abstract. In this paper, we evaluate different schemes for constructing a mean shape anatomical atlas for atlas-based segmentation of MR brain images. Each atlas is constructed and validated using a database of 20 images for which detailed manual delineations of 49 different subcortical structures are available. Atlas construction and atlas based segmentation are performed by non-rigid intensity-based registration using a viscous fluid deformation model with parameters that were optimally tuned for this particular task. The segmentation performance of each atlas scheme is evaluated on the same database using a leave-one-out approach and measured by the volume overlap of corresponding regions in the ground-truth manual segmentation and the warped atlas label image.

1 Introduction

Segmentation of brain structures in three-dimensional (3D) magnetic resonance (MR) images is important for image-based brain morphometry. Manual delineation by trained experts is time consuming and susceptible to intra- and inter-rater subjectivity. On the other hand, automated segmentation approaches relying only on image intensity information cannot cope with the complexity of the image data and the variability of the structures under study. Robust automated approaches require model-based strategies that incorporate prior knowledge about the intensity and shape characteristics of the objects to be segmented. In atlas-based segmentation this knowledge is represented as an annotated image or atlas, which is warped to the image under study by an appropriate spatial transformation, such that volumes of interest (VOI) defined in the atlas are correctly projected onto the anatomically corresponding structures in the study image. In its simplest form, the atlas consists of an actual image (template) acquired from a single individual and its associated VOI label image. However, such an atlas is intrinsically biased towards the anatomy of a single subject.

To account for the significant biological variability that exists across subjects, a statistical or probabilistic atlas has to be constructed from a database of examples that is representative for the population under study. While different voxel-wise attributes can be considered for statistical modelling, such as image intensity, anatomical region label or local shape variability, an intensity-based template is needed to enable the use of automated voxel similarity based registration approaches for template-to-study image warping. Based on the fact that the spatial normalization procedures are limited by regularization constraints in the amount of deformation, the "best" template should minimize (some measure of) the deformation from the template to all subjects in the population. The template can therefore be constructed as the "geometrical average" of the group of images [1].

A popular intensity-based brain template, that is widely used for functional and morphometrical studies, is the MNI template distributed with SPM [2], which was constructed by linear registration of a large set of normal brain MR images. Other approaches [3,1] construct a mean shape template iteratively starting from an affine average, whereby in each iteration all images in the set are aligned with the average image obtained in the previous iteration. Linear registration, however, can not compensate for local inter-subject shape variability and the resulting intensity-averaged template is necessarily blurred in regions where this variability is large, such as the cortex. Guimond et al. [4] proposed a method for constructing a mean shape template based on averaging of the deformation fields obtained by non-rigid image registration between one reference image and all other images in the database. They evaluated the impact of the choice of the reference image on the final atlas template and found this to be not significant. However, only 5 images were used for template construction and the global indices used to measure the difference of atlas templates constructed from different reference images can not assess local shape differences, which are crucial for atlas-based segmentation. Kochunov et al. [5] construct a mean shape template by defining a "minimal deformation target" (MDT) that is constructed by deforming a single reference image in the set such that the deformed image minimizes the average deformation to all images in the set. The reference image is selected such that its MDT is optimal in some sense among all the MDT images that can be constructed from the set. Nevertheless, optimal MDT is still biased towards the anatomy of the reference image from which it was constructed. Rohlfing et al. [6] compared different strategies for intensity-based template selection in the context of atlas-based segmentation of 3D confocal microscopy images of bee brains, namely by registration of the study images to an individual intensity image, to a shape-averaged intensity-based template, to the most similar intensity image from the database, and to all intensity images from the database followed by multi-classifier decision fusion (MUL). The MUL strategy was found to score the best, but is computationally much more expensive than when a single template is used.

In this paper, we evaluate different strategies for template and label atlas construction for atlas-based segmentation of human MR brain images, using a database of 20 images with detailed manual delineations of 49 different subcortical structures [7]. For each template constructed from the intensity images in the database, an associated region label atlas is constructed from the corresponding manual segmentations. Inter-subject image registration for template construction and template-to-image registration for atlas-based segmentation are performed using the same state-of-the-art non-rigid image registration (NRR) algorithm based on maximization of mutual information (MI) constrained by a viscous fluid deformation model [8] with parameters that were optimally tuned for this particular task. The segmentation performance of each atlas scheme is evaluated on the same database using a leave-one-out approach and measured by the volume overlap of corresponding regions in each of the manual segmentations and the warped atlas label image.

2 Material and Methods

2.1 Image Database

The set of 20 high-resolution normal brain MR images (10 females, 10 males, median age 31 years) used in this study was acquired at the National Society for Epilepsy, Chalfont St Peter, Buckinghamshire, UK [7]. All images have voxel sizes around 0.937 mm^3 and image dimensions of $[165-195] \times [198-199] \times [155-175]$. Each brain was manually segmented into 49 sub-structures as illustrated in figure 3. These include major brain structures such as the ventricles, cerebellum or corpus callosum, as well as the major lobes and gyri and the deep gray matter structures such as hippocampus, putamen, caudate nucleus and thalamus. The volume of the structures varies between about 183 cm^3 (left frontal lobe) to about 0.3 cm^3 (nucleus accumbens).

The images are first globally aligned by affine registration of each image to the SPM T1-weighted MR template using maximization of MI [9]. Probabilistic white matter (WM), gray matter (GM) and cerebrospinal fluid (CSF) segmentation maps are obtained for each image by automated intensity-based tissue classification using the method described in [10]. These maps are summed to construct a brain mask that is used to eliminate non-brain voxels from further analysis.

2.2 Non-rigid Image Registration

Inter-subject image registration for atlas construction and atlas-to-image registration for atlas-based segmentation are performed using the NRR algorithm of D'Agostino et al. [8]. The method is based on maximization of MI of corresponding voxel intensities and is constrained by a viscous fluid deformation model. The Navier Stokes equation of the viscous fluid model is solved approximately by spatial convolution of the MI force field with a Gaussian kernel ψ_σ of width σ. To preserve the topology of the deforming image, regridding is applied whenever the Jacobian of the deformation field becomes negative. The width of the spatial smoothing kernel ψ_σ controls the smoothness of the deformation: for too small a value, the deformation is not sufficiently constrained and the algorithm converges prematurely; for too large a value, the force field is over-smoothed, and small features will be lost. An optimal value of $\sigma = 7$ voxels was determined by evaluating the performance of the NRR algorithm for inter-subject registration of the MR brain images in the database as a function of σ, using volume overlap between the warped manual segmentations as evaluation criterion [11]. This value for σ was adopted for all registrations in this study.

2.3 Atlas Construction

Let I_1 to I_N denote the $N = 20$ pre-processed images in the database. With each image I_i is associated a set of $K = 49$ binary label images L_{ik} obtained by manual segmentation of region k in image i. Let T_{ij} denote the deformation field that results from non-rigid registration of source image I_i to target image I_j. The deformed source image I_i after warping to the space of I_j is represented as $\tilde{I}_{ij} = T_{ij}(I_i)$. Several schemes for construction of a mean shape average template are evaluated in this paper:

AT0: Individual Brain Image. Each of the individual brain images I_i and its label images L_{ik} are used as template and label atlas respectively for atlas-based segmentation of all other images in the database.

AT1: Minimal Deformation Target. The MDT template derived from image I_i is defined as $MDT_i = \bar{T}_i(I_i)$ with $\bar{T}_i = \frac{1}{N}\sum_{j=1}^{N} T_{ij}$ the average deformation of I_i when warped to all images in the database. The MDT template requires the least amount of deformation to all images in the database [5]. Ideally, an identical MDT brain should be obtained regardless of the initial image from which it was constructed. However, because the registration algorithm is topology preserving, each MDT_i will inevitably be biased towards the topology of the corresponding I_i.

AT2: Intensity-Averaged MDT. Instead of transforming an individual brain I_i by the mean deformation $\bar{T}_i$ to obtain MDT_i, $AT2_i = \bar{T}_i(\bar{I}_i)$ is obtained by transforming the intensity-averaged template $\bar{I}_i = \frac{1}{N}\sum_{j=1}^{N} \tilde{I}_{ji}$ to its MDT shape. $\bar{I}_i$ is constructed by voxel-wise averaging of all images I_j in the database after warping to I_i. Hence, some bias of $AT2_i$ towards I_i from which it was constructed can not be excluded.

AT3: Population-Averaged MDT. If all the individuals are representative of the same (normal) population under study and if the image quality of all images is similar, all MDT_i templates are very close to each other, except for some unresolved residual topological variations. These are removed by voxel-wise averaging over all subjects: $AT3 = \frac{1}{N}\sum_{i=1}^{N} MDT_i$. To compensate for global intensity differences between different MDTs, inter-subject intensity normalization is performed prior to averaging [12].

The construction of the corresponding label atlases requires some consideration. If atlases for AT1 and AT2 are constructed by direct application of the mean shape MDT transform to the manually segmented label image, the manual segmentation errors in the original label image would be propagated, and possibly amplified, into the atlas, which negatively affects segmentation performance. Instead, all images in the database are registered to the AT1, AT2 or AT3 template and the individual binary label images are warped accordingly by trilinear interpolation and subsequent binarization by thresholding at a value of 50%. A statistical probabilistic anatomical map (SPAM) R_k is constructed for each region k individually by averaging the warped label images of all subjects within the space of the atlas.

We compare these mean shape atlas schemes with an atlas-based segmentation strategy based on multi-classifier decision fusion (MUL) [6]. With MUL, each individual image in the database of N segmented images is used in turn as template to segment the study image. The final labelling for each voxel in the study image is decided by majority voting over all N segmentations. This is an alternative solution to atlas-based image segmentation that does not require an intensity-averaged template. We evaluated two different MUL strategies, one using the original images I_i and labels L_{ik} as templates and atlases (MUL0) and one using the corresponding MDT_i templates and MDT labels instead (MUL1). For MUL1, corresponding label images are obtained by directly warping L_{ik} to the MDT space, as we anticipate that the MUL decision fusion will introduce some smoothing anyway.

2.4 Validation

The atlas schemes AT0, AT1, AT2 and AT3 are evaluated for atlas-based segmentation. The intensity-based template is non-rigidly registered to each of the study MR images I_i, yielding deformation fields T_i. These are used to warp the atlas SPAMs R_k for each region k into the subject space using trilinear interpolation of probability values. Binary segmentation maps S_{ik} are derived from the warped SPAMs by setting $S_{ik} = 1$ in each voxel were region k has the highest probability over all SPAMs. The volume overlap between the manual ground truth segmentation L_{ik} and the atlas-based segmentation S_{ik} is evaluated for each region k by the region similarity index (RSI):

$$RSI_{ik} = \frac{V(L_{ik} \& S_{ik})}{V(L_{ik} \| S_{ik})} \quad (1)$$

The mean $\bar{RSI}_k$ obtained by averaging RSI_{ik} over all images i indicates the performance of a particular atlas scheme for segmentation of region k. We use the global similarity index (GSI) obtained by averaging across all $K = 49$ regions as a global performance indicator for the algorithm:

$$GSI = \frac{1}{K} \sum_{k=1}^{K} \bar{RSI}_k \quad (2)$$

3 Results

Figure 1 shows two different individual brains (AT0) and their corresponding AT1 (i.e. MDT) and AT2 templates, as well as the population-averaged AT3 template. AT1 and AT2 are in the same mean shape space, transformed by the same average deformation, but AT2 is a bit blurred due to inter-subject intensity averaging. The mean shape transformation compensates for shape differences between individual brains. As a result, the AT1 and AT2 templates derived from different individual brain images are largely similar in shape (as is apparent for the ventricles for instance). Nevertheless, the topology of the initial brain image is preserved in the corresponding templates in both cases and local topological differences are still present in different AT1 and AT2 templates as indicated in figure 1. The intensity averaging applied to construct AT2 can not fully remove this bias. AT3 is designed to further reduce this bias by averaging over the topologies of all individuals.

To examine the impact of topological differences in the initial images on the mean shape templates derived from them, 20 different AT2 templates were constructed using different individual brains as reference. This set of AT2s was then voxel-wise averaged after intensity normalization, and voxel-wise intensity variance was calculated subsequently as shown in figure 2. The voxel-wise averaged AT2 looks quite similar to AT3 and both are conceptually identical. From figure 2, we can see that the ventricle structures have almost identical shape in all

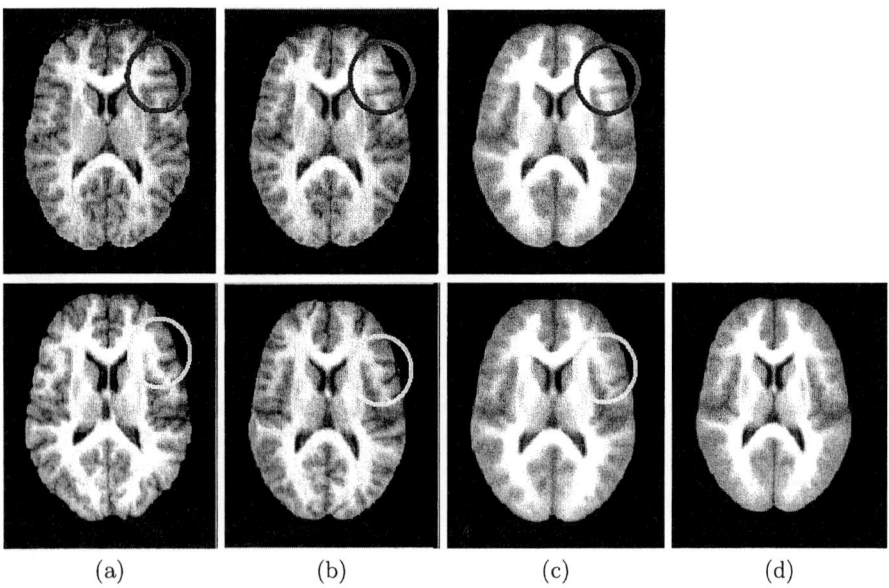

(a) (b) (c) (d)

Fig. 1. (a) Brain images for two individuals (top and bottom); (b) MDT and (c) AT2 brain templates derived from (a); (d) population-averaged AT3 brain. The unique topologies of each brain are maintained in their MDT and AT2 templates

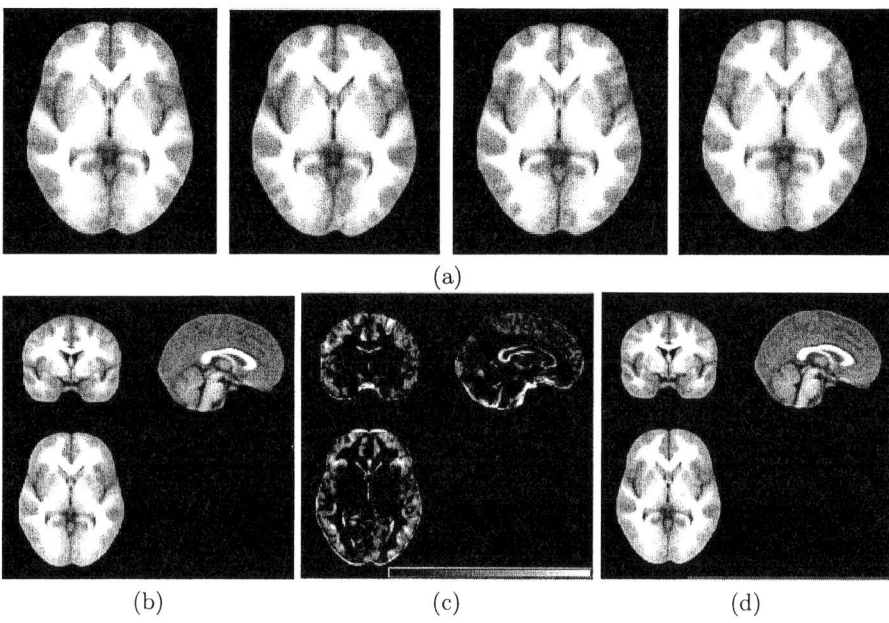

Fig. 2. (a) Four AT2 templates constructed using 4 different initial individual brain images; (b) Voxel-wise averaging of 20 intensity-normalized AT2 templates and (c) the voxel-wise intensity variance map; (d) AT3 template, shown here for comparison with (b). The intensity variance between different AT2 templates is near zero in the ventricular region, while significant variability exists in the cortical areas

AT2 templates, as indicated by near zero variance in that area. However, the neo-cortical area shows large variability in the variance map, which is caused by unresolved topology-specific bias remaining in each AT2.

Figure 3(a) illustrates the quality of the manual segmentations for two images in the database. Slice by slice delineation introduces local irregularities in the segmentation maps that are difficult to avoid. The label image constructed for AT3 by maximum probability fusion of 49 region SPAMs is shown in figure 3(b). The AT3 label image is much smoother than the manual delineation of individual brains and removes most of the irregularities in the manual segmentaion.

Figure 4 summarizes the performance of the atlas schemes AT0, AT1, and AT2, all constructed from I_1, together with AT3, for segmentation of the 19 other images in the dataset. The figure shows that, using an average RSI threshold of 70%, AT0, AT1, AT2 and AT3 are able to segment 16, 22, 28 and 30 regions (out of total 49) respectively. The GSI values are 64.8%, 67.0%, 67.5% and 70.0% respectively.

Figure 5 summarizes the performance of AT0 (I1), AT1 (MDT1), AT2 and AT3 for segmentation of the deep gray matter structures. AT3 performs systematically better than the other schemes for each structure. The average RSI values vary between 50% for the smallest structures (nucleus accumbens) to 77% for the largest ones (thalamus).

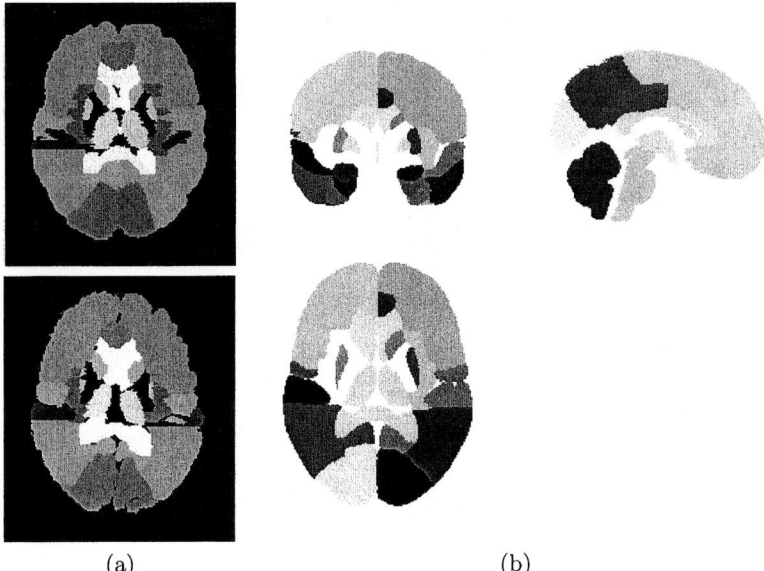

Fig. 3. (a) Manual segmentation for two images in the database; (b) Maximum probability label image of the AT3 atlas constructed from SPAMs of 49 regions computed from the 20 segmentations in the database

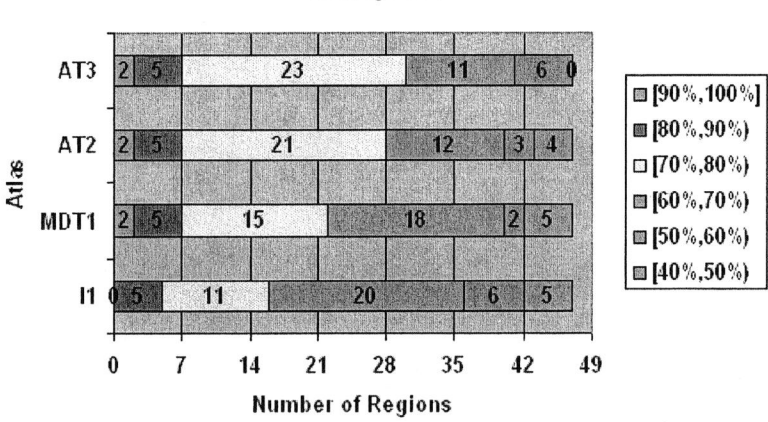

Fig. 4. Performance of different template construction schemes for atlas-based segmentation. Each color bar in this figure represents the number of regions that, using a particular atlas, were segmented with an average RSI value in the ranges indicated by the color of the bar. Figure shows only the statistics for average RSI larger than 40%. The graph compares the AT0, AT1 and AT2 templates, constructed from the first image in the database, with the population-averaged AT3 template

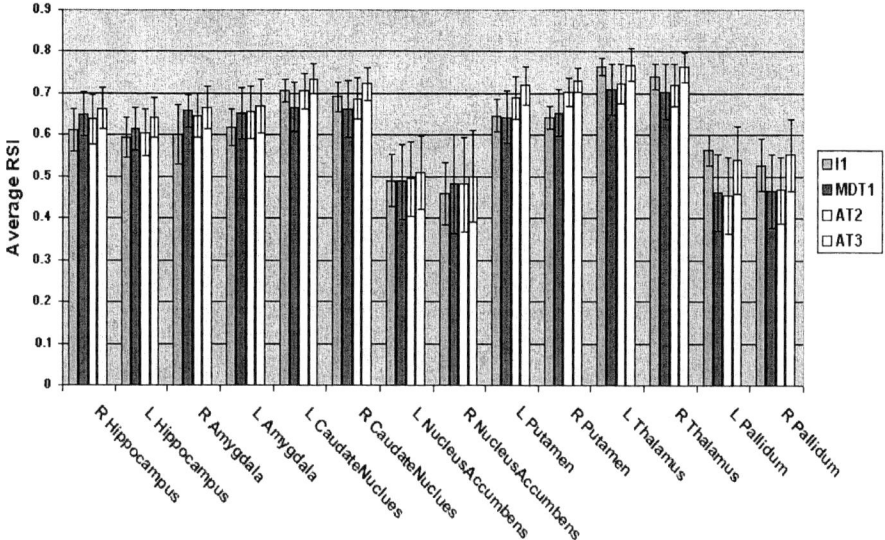

Fig. 5. Performance of AT0 (I1), AT1 (MDT1), AT2 and AT3 for segmentation of the deep gray matter structures

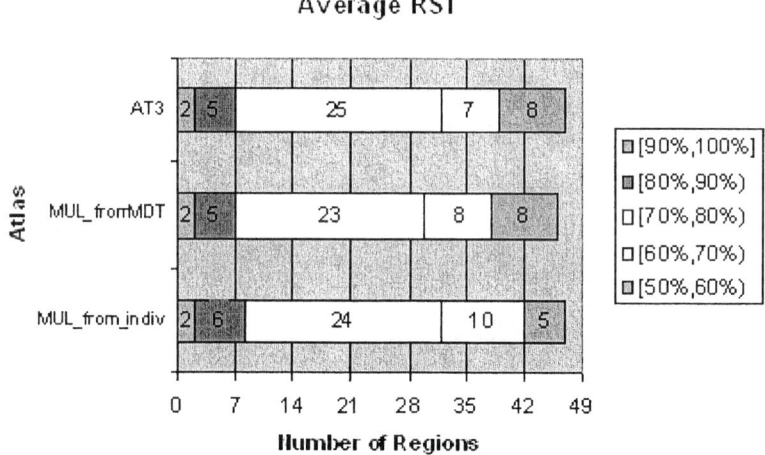

Fig. 6. As figure 4, but comparing AT3 to multi-decision fusion segmentation using the original images (MUL0) or their MDTs (MUL1) as templates, evaluated for 5 images in the database. Figure shows only the regions with an average RSI larger than 50%

The impact of the choice of the initial image used for atlas construction on the atlas-based segmentation performance was evaluated by using each of the 20 images in the database in turn as template AT0 for segmentation of the 19 other images in the dataset. The GSI values varied between 58% and 65%, compared to 70.0% for AT3.

Figure 6 compares the segmentation performance of the mean shape AT3 atlas with the MUL0 and MUL1 segmentation strategies for 5 images in the dataset. For these 5, both AT3 and MUL0 succeed at segmenting 32 regions with an average RSI larger than 70%, while only 30 for MUL1. The overall GSI obtained with each method over all atlas regions is 70% for AT3, 72% for MUL0 and 69% for MUL1. MUL0 scored somewhat better than AT3, but the difference is small compared to the much higher computational complexity of MUL versus AT3. For AT3, only one template-to-study image registration has to be computed, while for MUL each of the templates (19 in our experiment) needs to be warped to the study image. Somewhat surprisingly, MUL1, which uses the MDT images, scores worse than MUL0 which uses the original images. A possible explanation may be that the label images associated with the MDT templates in MUL1 were not derived from SPAMs, but by warping of the original segmentations into MDT space. If the same approach is applied for the AT1 label image, the GSI of AT1 atlas-based segmentation drops from 67.0% to 63.9%.

4 Discussion and Conclusion

In this paper, several schemes for brain atlas construction were evaluated by the ability of the constructed intensity template and label atlas to accurately segment 49 brain regions by atlas-based segmentation using intensity-based NRR. Our results indicate that a carefully designed intensity-averaged template (AT3), which explicitly attempts to remove residual topological differences after nonlinear alignment and intensity rectification, has better segmentation performance compared to individual templates (AT0) and average templates whose shape is derived from only a single individual image (AT1 and AT2). The NRR algorithm used in the atlas construction is able to resolve local shape variability. The constructed average shape template therefore retains local features in more detail and is less blurred compared to templates constructed by affine alignment only (e.g. SPM). The performance of AT3 for atlas-based segmentation of human brain images was shown to be comparable to that of a MUL strategy, but at a much lower computational cost.

The validation study can be extended in several aspects. Firstly, other atlas construction schemes could have been included. In [6] for instance, a mean shape template was constructed for the bee brain by first performing an affine registration of all images to a common reference image, followed by non-rigid warping of the same set of images to the intensity averaged image obtained after affine registration. This process was iterated until convergence using the average brain from a previous iteration as template. However, for human brain images that show substantial inter-subject variability, the averaging of affinely coregistered images introduces significant blurring that is likely to affect the accuracy of subsequent NRR steps. Hence, this scheme was not considered here. In [4], the AT2 atlas, constructed in MDT space starting from a single individual reference image, is iteratively refined by warping all images again to the AT2 template, while in [5] the reference image is selected such that the MDT template is optimal with respect to all images in the set. Both approaches aim at reducing the influence of the initial reference image used for template construction. The effect of iterating the template construction procedure and the selection of an optimal MDT should be further investigated and validated.

Secondly, the simplistic similarity index used here to measure volume overlap assumes a one-to-one correspondence between objects, and does not account for the nature of errors in case of imperfect label overlap. Various spatial correspondence indices using information theory have been proposed in [13] that can evaluate global, local and individual correspondences between observed and reference objects. Lastly, there should also be some formal distance analysis of different atlases.

The intensity-based NRR method applied here has been shown to perform well for inter-subject MR brain image registration [8]. Nevertheless, the algorithm can be improved in several aspects and the impact thereof on atlas construction and atlas-based segmentation performance should be investigated. For instance, instead of intensity-based alignment by maximization of MI, alternative similarity measures can be used that incorporate voxel label information in the registration process, aiming at aligning corresponding voxel labels rather than voxel intensities [14], so that the registration will not be affected by poor image quality. An average transformation derived from the label images can subsequently be applied to the corresponding intensity images to create an intensity-averaged brain template [15]. Moreover, the development of reliable registration algorithms that can match label images directly to intensity images [16] may completely eliminate the need to construct an average intensity image for atlas-based segmentation, such that one can focus on building a probabilistic label atlas from the available manual segmentations by label-based registration.

Also, the viscous fluid regularization model imposes identical regularization behaviour everywhere in the image domain. Instead, a spatially varying regularization scheme could be adopted, for instance based on a statistical deformation model, which would allow the deformation of anatomical structures to be constrained differently in different parts of the brain. Such a model can be constructed by statistical analysis of the deformation fields obtained by inter-subject registration [17]. Future work will therefore focus on augmenting the AT3 atlas with local shape variability information.

Acknowledgments. This work is supported by the Flemish Institute for the Promotion of Innovation by Science and Technology in Flanders (IWT, project IWT/GBOU/020195), by the K.U.Leuven (projects /OF/GOA/1999/05 and /OF/GOA/2004/05) and by the Fund for Scientific Research - Flanders (FWO-Vlaanderen, project FWO/G.0258.02).

References

1. P.M. Thompson and A.W. Toga. A framework for computational anatomy. *Computing and Visualization in Science*, 5:13–34, 2002.
2. Statistical parameter mapping. http://www.fil.ion.ucl.ac.uk/spm/spm99.html.
3. John Ashburner. *Computational Neuroanatomy*. PhD thesis, University College London, 2000.
4. A. Guimond, J. Meunier, and J.-P. Thirion. Automatic computation of average brain models. In *MICCAI'98*, pages 631–640, 1998.
5. P. Kochunov, J.L. Lancaster, P. Thompson, R. Woods, J. Mazziotta, J. Hardies, and P. Fox. Regional spatial normalization: toward an optimal target. *Journal of Computer Assisted Tomography*, 25(5):805–816, 2001.
6. T. Rohlfing, R. Brandt, R. Menzel, and C.R. Maurer Jr. Evaluation of atlas selection strategies for atlas-based image segmentation with application to confocal microscopy images of bee brains. *NeuroImage*, 21:1428–1442, 2004.
7. A. Hammers, R. Allom, M.J. Koep, S.L. Free, R. Myers, L. Lemieux, T.N. Mitchell, D.J. Brooks, and J. Duncan. Three-dimensional maximum probability atlas of the human brain, with particular reference to the temporal lobe. *Human Brain Mapping*, 19(4):224–247, 2003.
8. E. D'Agostino, F. Maes, D. Vandermeulen, and P. Suetens. A viscous fluid model for non-rigid image registration using mutual information. *Medical Image Analysis*, 7:565–575, 2003.
9. F. Maes, A. Collignon, D. Vandermeulen, G. Marchal, and P. Suetens. Multimodality image registration by maximization of mutual information. *IEEE Transactions on Medical Imaging*, 16(2):187–198, 1997.
10. K. Van Leemput, F. Maes, D. Vandermeulen, and P. Suetens. Automated model-based tissue classification of MR images of the brain. *IEEE Trans. Med. Img.*, 18(10):897–908, 1999.
11. Q. Wang, E. DAgostino, D. Seghers, F. Maes, D. Vandermeulen, and P. Suetens. Large-scale validation of non-rigid registration algorithms in a brain image segmentation framework. Technical Report KUL/ESAT/PSI/0502, KU Leuven, Dept. of Electrical Engineering, 2005.
12. D. Seghers, E. D'Agostino, F. Maes, D. Vandermeulen, and P. Suetens. Construction of a brain template from MR images using state-of-art registration and segmentation techniques. In *MICCAI'04*, pages 696–703, 2004.
13. F. Bello and A.C.F. Colchester. Measuring global and local spatial correspondence using information theory. In *MICCAI'98*, pages 964–973, 1998.
14. E. D'Agostino, F. Maes, D. Vandermeulen, and P. Suetens. An information theoretic approach for non-rigid image registration using voxel class probabilities. In *MICCAI'03*, pages 812–820, 2003.
15. T. Rohlfing, R. Brandt, C.R. Maurer Jr., and R. Menzel. Bee brains, b-splines and computational democracy: generating an average shape atlas. In *IEEE Workshop on Mathematical Methods in Biomedical Image Analysis*, pages 187–194, 2001.
16. E. D'Agostino, F. Maes, D. Vandermeulen, and P. Suetens. Non-rigid atlas-to-image registration by minimization of class-conditional image entropy. In *MICCAI'04*, volume 3216 of *Lecture Notes in Computer Science*, pages 745–753, 2004.
17. D. Rueckert, A.F. Frangi, and J.A. Schnabel. Automatic construction of 3-D statistical deformation models of the brain using nonrigid registration. *IEEE Trans.Med. Img.*, 22(8), 2003.

Multi-figure Anatomical Objects for Shape Statistics

Qiong Han, Stephen M. Pizer, Derek Merck, Sarang Joshi, and Ja-Yeon Jeong

Medical Image Display and Analysis Group,
University of North Carolina at Chapel Hill, NC 27599, USA
han@cs.unc.edu

Abstract. Multi-figure m-reps allow us to represent and analyze a complex anatomical object by its parts, by relations among its parts, and by the object itself as a whole entity. This representation also enables us to gather either global or hierarchical statistics from a population of such objects. We propose a framework to train the statistics of multi-figure anatomical objects from real patient data. This training requires fitting multi-figure m-reps to binary characteristic images of training objects. To evaluate the fitting approach, we propose a Monte Carlo method sampling the trained statistics. It shows that our methods generate geometrically proper models that are close to the set of Monte Carlo generated target models and thus can be expected to yield similar statistics to that used for the Monte Carlo generation.

1 Introduction

The shape statistics of simple objects with one part have been widely studied. Methods using various representations have been proposed and shown to be effective [1, 2]. However, many anatomical objects have multiple named parts, e.g., the prostate (fig. 1-a) has two seminal vesicles attached to it and the liver (fig. 1-b) has left and right lobes. Due to the inherent complexity of objects made from multiple parts, previous statistical descriptions of such objects concentrated on their global structure [1, 3] or on the extremely local behavior of geometric primitives, such as points, without reference to the parts' inter-relations [4, 5].

M-reps [6] have been successfully used to represent anatomical objects and complexes of objects [7, 8, 9]. An m-rep consists of one or more medial sheets, with the part corresponding to each sheet called a *figure*. Previous work on m-reps has been restricted to single figure objects. Computing statistics of such m-reps via *principal geodesic analysis* (PGA) [2, 14] has proved useful.

Medial description is also well suited to represent an object with parts [7, 10], e.g., an object with a protrusion subfigure, i.e., additive figure to the host (fig. 1-c), or an indentation subfigure, i.e., subtractive figure from the host (fig. 1-d). We use multi-figure m-reps to represent objects with multiple parts.

In the m-rep of a multi-figure object, each object part is geometrically represented by a single figure m-rep, and the figures of the object are connected by

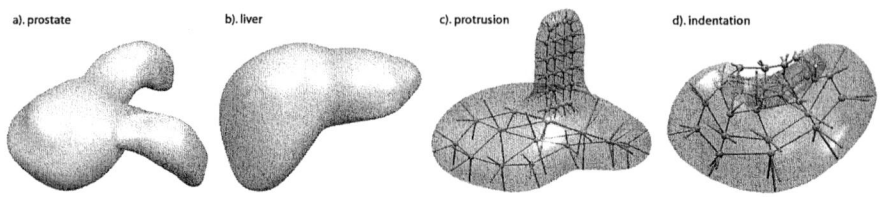

Fig. 1. a) A prostate with two seminal vesicle protrusions. b) A liver represented by the union of the left and right lobes. c) An object with protrusion. d) A kidney with the renal pelvis as an indentation subfigure. Object *a* has three single-figure parts while objects *b-d* have two such parts

the hinge geometry briefly reviewed in section 2.2. As with the single figure case, the multi-figure m-rep describes an object at successively smaller scales following a coarse-to-fine hierarchy, for which the two top levels are 1) the object and 2) each individual figure and relations among the figures. In the top level the object is simply the union of its parts, enabling efficient analysis of the complex object as a whole. In addition, we can talk about individual part properties, such as shapes and volumes. Statistically, variation of the object within a population can be also measured in a multi-scale fashion. For example, we can investigate the variation of livers as well as of left liver lobes only.

In the process of training object statistics, we assume that each training object is given by a single binary characteristic image. We need to extract the m-rep for each object and then do PGA on the set of resulting m-reps. An efficient and reliable m-rep extraction method based on deformable model fitting is described in section 3.

The multi-figure m-rep captures the natural hierarchy within a complex object. This form of representation also allows statistical analysis following the same hierarchy. While this approach can begin with global statistics on the union of the object parts, we describe a statistical description of the parts and their inter-relations via a hierarchical approach based on the *residue*. In section 4 we first sketch the global approach and then the residue approach. Both approaches are applied to the extracted multi-figure m-reps and the results are shown in section 5.1.

To evaluate the method of fitting m-reps to binary images, we propose a Monte Carlo technique and a means of data analysis based on geodesic differences between sample m-reps and the m-reps extracted from corresponding binary images. This data analysis method and its results are described in section 5.3.

We discuss incorporating the statistics into the training process to improve the quality of the extracted m-reps and conclude the paper in section 6.

2 Representing Multi-figure Objects

In the multi-figure representation, each part of the object is represented by a single figure m-rep, which is briefly reviewed in the next subsection.

2.1 Single Figure M-Rep

An m-rep is an extension of the Blum medial locus [11]; in the extension the medial locus forms the primitive description. The simplest geometric object is represented by a single continuous medial sheet with boundary. A discrete m-rep is formed by sampling the medial sheet over a spatially regular lattice to form a mesh of medial *atoms* (fig. 2-left), where each atom consists of a position on the medial sheet, and two equal length spokes. An internal medial atom is defined as a 4-tuple $\{\underline{x}, r, \underline{s}_0, \underline{s}_1\}$, consisting of the hub position $\underline{x} \in \mathbb{R}^3$, the spoke length $r \in \mathbb{R}^+$, and the two spoke directions as two unit vectors $\underline{s}_0, \underline{s}_1 \in S^2$ (fig. 2-middle). The medial atoms on the edge of the medial sheet correspond to crests of the object boundary. Such an end atom adds a bisector spoke of length ηr with a corresponding crest sharpness parameter $\eta \in \mathbb{R}^+$ (fig. 2-right). In section 3.1 we briefly review the mathematical background behind our representation.

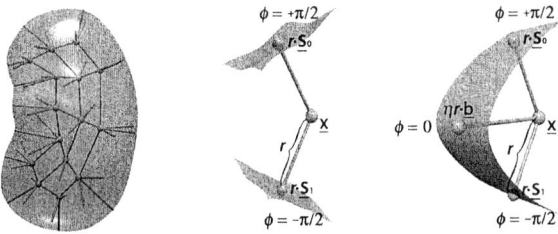

Fig. 2. Left: a single figure m-rep for a kidney and the object boundary implied by it. Middle: an internal medial atom. Right: an end atom. The local implied boundary is incident to and orthogonal to the spoke ends

Given an m-rep figure, a smooth object surface is generated to interpolate the boundary positions and normals implied by the atom spokes; presently a subdivision method [12] is used to generate the object boundary. If u, v parametrizes the medial sheet, the implied boundary is parametrized by (u, v, ϕ), where ϕ designates the side of the figure from the top ($\phi = +\frac{\pi}{2}$) to the bottom ($\phi = -\frac{\pi}{2}$) and changes continuously across crests ($\phi \in [-\frac{\pi}{2}, +\frac{\pi}{2}]$) (fig. 2-right).

The single figure m-rep scheme has been extended to handle the complex of non-overlapping, single figure objects. Next we briefly review extending the representation to multi-figure m-rep objects.

2.2 The Multi-figure M-Rep Object with Hinge Geometry

As detailed in [10], a multi-figure object is represented by a *directed acyclic graph* (DAG) of figures, each represented by a single figure m-rep. Subfigures can be recursively attached to their hosts to form any desired object DAG. This allows representation of arbitrarily complex objects, although most anatomical objects are adequately represented by a tree of two or three levels. The host and subfigure are determined according to anatomic naming and the tightness of posterior

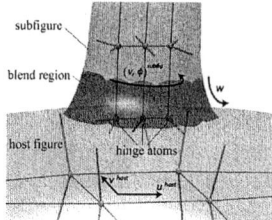 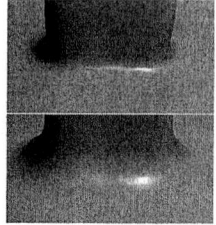

Fig. 3. Left: the host figure/subfigure arrangement, with the subfigure (six medial atoms appearing) on top, the host figure (four medial atoms showing) below, and the blend region shown darker. **Right:** different shapes of the blend region

probabilities of the figures. In this paper we restrict our examples to objects with a single host figure and a single subfigure, e.g., the liver with the right lobe as the host and the left lobe as the subfigure. In the rest of this subsection we review how two figures are connected by the hinge geometry. Via the hinge the deformation of a host figure is propagated to its subfigure. A subfigure also has its own deformation which does not affect its host. A smooth surface boundary is then generated for the entire object by a method called *blending*.

Hinge Geometry. The subfigure is attached to its host by a $1D$ curve of hinge atoms, which, when sampled, form an end row or column of the subfigure atom mesh. Each hinge atom rides on the medially implied boundary of the host, with known figural coordinates of the host figure. The hinge geometry is an extension of the Blum medial locus that avoids the instability against boundary noise of the low-volume portion of branches. The host/subfigure arrangement is demonstrated in (fig. 3-left). The single hinge geometry allows both additive and subtractive subfigures (fig. 1-a-d).

With the two types of subfigure transformations below, we are able to represent and describe multi-figure objects with variable inter-figure relations.

Host Figure Implied Subfigure Transformation. As the host figure deforms, the hinge atoms at the fixed (u, v, ϕ) in the host figure's coordinates change their locations and orientations. Since each subfigure atom can be represented as transformations of its neighboring atoms, the deformation of the host figure is propagated to the subfigure starting from the hinge atoms.

Hinge-Relative Subfigure Transformations. The subfigure can also translate, rotate, hinge, scale, and elongate on the host figure boundary while the host stays put. These basic hinge-relative transformations all take place in the host's figural coordinates and are at the subfigure scale levels. They form a key component of the coarse-to-fine hierarchy.

2.3 Blending

Blending, a well-studied field within computer graphics, is necessary if a smooth surface is to be generated from a host figure and its intersecting subfigure. To blend a subfigure with its host, an interpolating subdivision method is used to generate the implied boundary of each single figure. Each host figure and its attached subfigure meet and merge into each other. Designated sections from both figures are removed and replaced by a smooth region called the blend (fig. 3-left). The blend between the two figures is parameterized by (w, v, ϕ), where v and ϕ are the same as those in the subfigure coordinates and w ranges from $+1$, at the subfigure, to -1, at the host. Two parameters delimiting the top and the bottom of the blend control the shape of the blend region (fig. 3-right).

3 Fitting Multi-figure M-Reps to Binary Images

The extraction of an m-rep from a binary characteristic image for statistical training is done by fitting a deformable m-rep template M_0 into the binary image. A large-scale-to-small optimization process over transformations associated with each respective stage is applied to the m-rep template. We define the objective function and then detail the transformations associated with each fitting stage in the following subsections. Firstly we review some mathematical background of the m-rep geometry; more details can be found in [2].

3.1 Background Theory Review

As the primitive in an m-rep, each internal(end) medial atom can be understood as a point on the manifold $\mathcal{M}_{int}(1)$ ($\mathcal{M}_{end}(1)) = \mathbb{R}^3 \times \mathbb{R}^+ \times S^2 \times S^2(\times \mathbb{R}^+)$. Let $\mathcal{M}(1)$ denote the manifold for a medial atom without specifying whether it is an internal or end atom. Thus an m-rep of n medial atoms can be seen as a point on the manifold $\mathcal{M}(n) = [\mathcal{M}(1)]^n$.

The space $\mathcal{M}(n)$ is a particular type of manifold known as a Riemannian symmetric space, which simplifies the calculation of geodesics and distances. Let $dis(y, z) : \mathcal{M}(n) \times \mathcal{M}(n) \to \mathbb{R}^+ \cup \{0\}$ denote the geodesic distance, i.e., the locally shortest distance on the manifold $\mathcal{M}(n)$, between two points $y, z \in \mathcal{M}(n)$. There are a pair of maps Exp_y and Log_y that map between $\mathcal{M}(n)$ and the tangent space $T_y\mathcal{M}(n)$ at y, and are inverse of each other. $T_y\mathcal{M}(n)$ can be identified with $\mathbb{R}^{8n+n_{ext}}$ with n_{ext} as the number of end atoms in y and z.

- $\text{Log}_y(z)$ maps the point z to the tangent space $T_y\mathcal{M}(n)$ at y. The geodesic distance between y and z is preserved and calculated via the Log map.

$$dis(y, z) = \|\text{Log}_y(z)\| \tag{1}$$

- $\text{Exp}_y(\underline{v})$ maps the tangent vector $\underline{v} \in T_y\mathcal{M}(n)$ to the point on $\mathcal{M}(n)$ along the geodesic curve $\gamma_{\underline{v}}(t)$. The distance is preserved as $dis(y, \text{Exp}_y(\underline{v})) = \|\underline{v}\|$.

Given dis, we can calculate the Fréchet mean $\overline{M}$ of N points (m-reps) $\{M_i | M_i \in \mathcal{M}(n), i = 1, 2, ..., N\}$ by minimizing the average squared geodesic distance:

$$\overline{M} = \text{Mean}(M_i) = \arg\min_{M \in \mathcal{M}(n)} \frac{1}{N} \sum_{i=1}^{N} \|\text{Log}_M(M_i)\|^2 \tag{2}$$

In the residue approach described in section 4.2, we need to calculate the difference between m-reps via the difference between their corresponding atoms. Let $\underline{a}_1, \underline{a}_2 \in \mathcal{M}(1)$ be two corresponding atoms. Then their difference is

$$\underline{a}_1 \ominus \underline{a}_2 = g_{\underline{a}_2}^{-1} \circ \underline{a}_1 \in \mathcal{M}(1), \tag{3}$$

where $g_{\underline{a}_2}^{-1} \in G(1)$ is the composition of hub translation, spoke magnification(s), and spoke rotations determining an atom transformation and, $G(1)$ denotes the Lie-group of such transformations.

Assume an m-rep template $\in \mathcal{M}(n)$ has n medial atoms $\{\underline{a}_i\}$. $G(n) = [G(1)]^n$ acts smoothly on $\mathcal{M}(n)$ as the transformation between m-reps. The difference between two m-reps $M_1, M_2 \in \mathcal{M}(n)$ from the same template is defined as

$$M_1 \ominus M_2 = \prod_{j=1}^{n} (\underline{a}_{1j} \ominus \underline{a}_{2j}) \in \mathcal{M}(n) \tag{4}$$

3.2 Objective Function

The objective function measuring the mismatch between the m-rep and binary image [15] is a sum of three terms: an m-rep-to-binary boundary distance, a term penalizing irregularity of the m-rep atoms, and a term for achieving correspondence across the m-reps in a training population.

Binary Image Match. A distance map image $D(\underline{x}) : \mathbb{R}^3 \to \mathbb{R}^+ \cup \{0\}$ is calculated for each given binary image I_b by an extension of the Danielsson distance mapping [13] to 3D. The binary image match term is then calculated by the integral of the distance map on the m-rep implied object surface $\mathcal{B}$, except that at the boundary locations where the surface normal differs from the distance gradient by more than a certain threshold, $D(\underline{x})$ is replaced by the distance along the surface normal to the nearest binary object boundary location. $L(M, D)$ measures how well M fits into the distance map image D.

$$L(M, D) = \alpha \cdot \frac{1}{\text{area}(\mathcal{B}(M))} \int_{\mathcal{B}(M)} D^2(\underline{x}) d^2 A \tag{5}$$

Regularity Penalty. This term penalizes non-uniform spacing and changes in spoke length and orientation of the medial atom. It leads to proper object geometry and correspondence across the training cases.

$$\text{Reg}(M) = \beta \cdot \sum_{i=1}^{n} \|\text{Log}_{\underline{a}_i}(\text{Mean}(\text{N}(\underline{a}_i)))\|^2 \tag{6}$$

For each medial atom $\underline{a}_i$, the regularity is calculated as the squared geodesic distance between $\underline{a}_i$ and the Fréchet mean (eqn. 2) of its neighboring atoms $\text{N}(\underline{a}_i)$. The penalties are then accumulated for all the medial atoms of the object.

Correspondence to a Reference M-Rep The reference penalty depends on the geodesic distance between the current M and the reference m-rep M_0, which the fitting starts with in our present implementation. This term explicitly penalizes weak correspondence across m-reps.

$$\text{Ref}(M) = (1 - \alpha - \beta) \cdot \|\text{Log}_{M_0}(M)\|^2 \tag{7}$$

In equations (5)-(7), $\alpha, \beta \geqslant 0$, and $\alpha + \beta \in [0, 1]$. The complete objective function is the combination of the three terms:

$$\text{Obj}(M, D) = \text{L}(M, D) + \text{Reg}(M) + \text{Ref}(M) \tag{8}$$

A two-figure m-rep is used as the example in the following subsections. Assume a two-figure m-rep template M_0 has host figure F_1 and subfigure F_2, and each figure $F_i \subset M_0$ has atoms $\{\underline{a}_j^i | i = 1, 2, j = 1, 2, ..., n_i\}$.

3.3 Extraction Framework

The objective function is then optimized over the following sequence of transformations, successively finer in scale, applied to the m-rep template.

- Initial alignment of M_0 by $T_1 \in \mathbb{R}^3 \times \mathbb{R}^+ \times SO(3)$, calculated by the template M_0 and the distance map image D;
- **object stage:** $T_{obj} \in \mathbb{R}^3 \times \mathbb{R}^+ \times SO(3)$, on the entire object;
- **host figure:** the host F_1 is the target and the subfigure is deformed by an implied transformation $T_{host\_implied} \in \mathbb{R}^3 \times \mathbb{R}^+ \times SO(3)$;
  - figural stage: $T_{host\_fig} \in \mathbb{R}^3 \times \mathbb{R}^+ \times SO(3)$, on the host figure;
  - atom stage: $T_{host\_atom} \in G(n_1)$, on the host figure atoms $\underline{a}_{1,2,...,n_1}^1$;
- **subfigure stage:** the subfigure F_2 is the target in this stage;
  - figural stage: $T_{sub\_fig} \in \mathbb{R}^3 \times \mathbb{R}^+ \times SO(3)$, on the subfigure. At the end of this stage, the hinge atoms are projected onto the host figure surface;
  - atom stage: $T_{sub\_atom} \in G(n_2)$, on the subfigure atoms $\underline{a}_{1,2,...,n_2}^2$.

input:
a two-figure m-rep template M_0 with host figure F_1 and subfigure F_2;
a distance map images D_i: calculated from the given binary images. I_{bi}.
output:
extracted two-figure m-reps M_i from the images D_i.
framework:
for each D_i {
1. Calculate T_1 by the 1st and 2nd moments of M_0 and D_i, $M_1 = T_1 \circ M_0$;
2. $T_2 = \arg\min_{T_{obj}}(\text{Obj}(T_{obj} \circ M_1, D_i))$, $M_2 = T_2 \circ M_1$;
3. $T_3 = \arg\min_{T_{host\_fig}}(\text{Obj}(T_{host\_fig} \circ F_1 \subset M_2, D_i))$, $M_3 = T_3 \circ M_2$;
4. $T_4 = \arg\min_{T_{host\_atom}}(\text{Obj}(T_{host\_atom} \circ F_1 \subset M_3, D_i))$, $M_4 = T_4 \circ M_3$;
5. $T_4' = T_{host\_implied}$, $M_4' = T_4' \circ F_2 \in M_4$;
6. $T_5 = \arg\min_{T_{sub\_fig}}(\text{Obj}(T_{sub\_fig} \circ F_2 \subset M_4', D_i))$, $M_5 = T_5 \circ M_4'$;
7. M_5' = hinge atoms in $F_2 \subset M_5$ are projected to the surface of $F_1 \subset M_5$;
8. $T_6 = \arg\min_{T_{sub\_atom}}(\text{Obj}(T_{sub\_atom} \circ F2 \subset M_5', D_i))$, $M_i = T_6 \circ M_5'$;
}

This framework can be extended to arbitrary levels of hierarchy. However in this paper, our data and experiments focus on objects with two-figures. Next we describe the statistical analysis on the extracted multi-figure m-reps.

4 Statistics of Multi-figure Objects

As reviewed in section 3.1, an m-rep consisting of n atoms is a point on the manifold $\mathcal{M}(n)$. The principal geodesic analysis has been proposed to do statistical analysis for single figure object in such a space [2]. Briefly, given N m-reps $\{M_i | M_i \in \mathcal{M}(n)\}$, the Fréchet mean $\overline{M}$ is first calculated using (2). Let $u_i = \mathrm{Log}_{\overline{M}}(M_i)$, then the covariance matrix is given by $\Sigma = \frac{1}{N} \sum_{i=1}^{N} u_i u_i^T$. The PGA is computed as $\{\underline{p}_k, \lambda_k \mid \underline{p}_k \in T_{\overline{M}} \mathcal{M}(n)$ are the principal geodesic directions, $\lambda_k \in \mathbb{R}$ are the variances$\} = \{$eigenvectors/eigenvalues of $\Sigma\}$.

4.1 Global Statistics

Assume that a multi-figure object O has N figures as $\{F_i, i = 1, 2, ..., N\}$ and each figure F_i has n_i medial atoms. Treat O as the union of all its figures and let n_O be the total number of atoms in O. The global statistics of such objects are computed by the mean object $\overline{O}$ and the PGA in $\mathcal{M}(n_O)$.

4.2 Hierarchical Statistics Based on Residue

For multi-figure m-rep statistics we follow the hierarchical statistical framework for multi-objects detailed in [14]. In the case of two-figure object O consisting of figures F_1 and F_2 with n_1, n_2 atoms, respectively, the host and subfigure are like the single figure objects in the complexes of multi-objects, and the hinge atoms act as the augmenting atoms that relate the host figure's changes to the sympathetic subfigure changes. Let $n_O = n_1 + n_2$. Three definitions are needed to sketch how two-figure object statistics are represented and computed.

- Residue: difference between two m-reps by the operation $\ominus$ (eqn. 3,4);
- Augmentation: $U_1 = F_1 \cup A_1$ denotes the union of host figure atoms and the hinge atoms A_1 in the subfigure F_2;
- Projection: an m-rep M can be projected into the PGA subspace by $\pi_H(M) \approx \mathrm{Exp}_{\overline{M}} \sum_{i=1}^{k} \langle \underline{p}_i, \mathrm{Log}_{\overline{M}}(M) \rangle \underline{p}_i$.

There are three parts PGA_g, PGA_h, and PGA_s in the hierarchical statistics for a two-figure object.

1. PGA_g: statistics on the n_O atoms making up the entire object. This captures the global shape variation of the object. This variation is removed from both the host figure atoms and the subfigure atoms before steps 2 and 3;
2. PGA_h: statistics on the residue of the union U_1 of the host figure atoms and the hinge atoms in the subfigure. This describes the remaining variation of U_1 after the projection to the global variation PGA_g has been removed;
3. PGA_s: statistics on the residue of subfigure F_2 after the residual changes in the host figure are propagated to the subfigure and have then been removed. The variation in the host figure is computed by projection to PGA_h, and the propagation is computed via the hinge atoms.

We applied both the global and the hierarchical statistical analysis to the extracted m-reps of livers. The results are shown in the next section.

5 Results and Evaluation

5.1 The Data and Results

We use 15 expert segmented binary images of livers. A two-figure m-rep template is fit into the images by the framework described in section 3. There are 3×7 and 3×4 sampled atoms in the host figure and subfigure, respectively. Three atoms in the subfigure are used as the hinge atoms. The total of 33 liver atoms lie in a manifold of 290-dimensions. The extracted m-reps $M_{1,2,...,15}$ are used for the shape statistics. Fig. 4-left shows the cumulative variances in the principal modes of the global statistics; 4-right shows the variations of the livers in the host and subfigure residue statistics as parts of the hierarchical statistics.

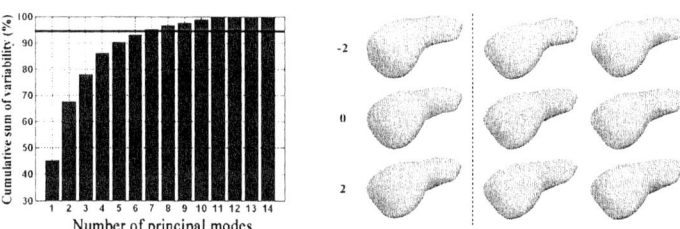

Fig. 4. Left: accumulated sum of the variances from the global stats PGA_g: the first 7 modes capture over **95%** of the total variability. **Right:** the residue shape variation after the global variation is removed: each column shows the liver -2 standard deviations from the residue mean along the respective eigenmode, the residue mean, and the liver $+2$ standard deviations from the mean. The left column shows the first principal mode of the host residue stats PGA_h; the other two columns show the first two modes of the subfigure residue stats: PGA_s describes the remaining shape variation of the subfigure after the global and host-implied variation have been removed

5.2 Generate New M-Reps Using the Monte Carlo Method

In order to evaluate the extraction method, we need binary images for which we know the true m-reps. A sampling scheme based on a Monte Carlo method, described next, is used to generate sample m-reps from the trained statistics. Sample binary images used as target images are then created as the interior of the sampled m-reps.

Assume the PGA statistics on the extracted training m-reps (with n atoms) are the mean m-rep $\overline{M}$, the first N_{PGA} principal variances $\{\lambda_{1,2,...,N_{PGA}}\}$, and the corresponding first N_{PGA} normalized principal geodesic directions $\{\underline{p}_{1,2,...,N_{PGA}}\}$, which is a subset of all the principal directions and sufficient to describe the variability of the m-rep shape space. New m-reps are generated by using the PGA as the population distribution $p(M)$ and sampling from it via the Monte Carlo method.

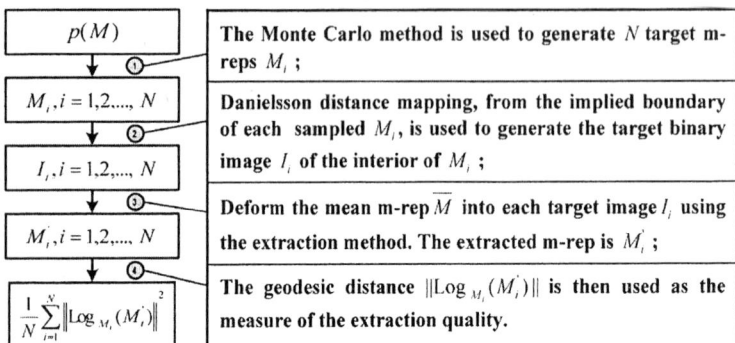

Fig. 5. Diagram flow to evaluate the extraction process given an initial population distribution $p(M)$

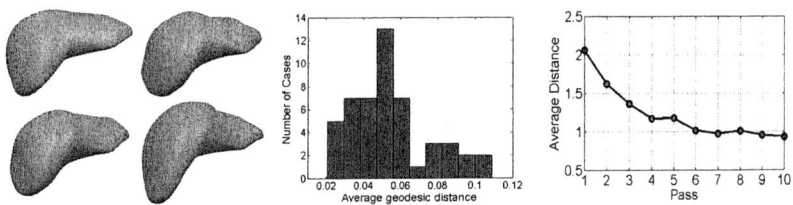

Fig. 6. Left: 4 of the 50 sampled m-reps used in the evaluation. **Middle**: evaluation results of the extraction framework shown as a histogram of geodesic distances between the extracted m-reps M'_i and the m-reps M_i as the truth. **Right**: in the first ten passes of the multi-pass extraction using the shape statistics, the fitting quality improves while the average distance from the m-rep implied surface points to the closest contour points in the binary image decreases. The distance is in the unit of image voxel

1. Generate a Gaussian vector $\underline{\alpha} = (\alpha_{1,2,...,N_{PGA}})$, with each α_i sampled from the standard normal distribution $\mathcal{N}(0,1)$;
2. Apply $\underline{\alpha}$ as the components on the principal directions for a tangent vector $\underline{v} = \sum_{i=1}^{N_{PGA}} \alpha_i \sqrt{\lambda_i} \cdot \underline{p}_i$ in the tangent space $T_{\overline{M}}(\mathcal{M}(n))$ at the mean $\overline{M}$;
3. The exponential map is used to map $\underline{v}$ to the m-rep manifold as a sampled m-rep $M = \text{Exp}_{\overline{M}}(\underline{v})$.

5.3 Evaluation

The diagram in fig. 5 details this evaluation using the Monte Carlo sample generation described in the previous section 5.2.

50 liver m-reps (fig. 6-left) were generated using the Monte Carlo sampling method. The evaluation results are shown in fig. 6-middle as a histogram of the mismatch (geodesic distance) between the extracted m-reps and their corresponding m-reps as the truth, which the target images are created from. The

average geodesic distance across all the livers is 0.054, in the units of the average boundary displacement implied by all the atoms together. And the averaged m-rep-to-binary distance is 0.674 image voxel for all the 50 m-reps.

6 Discussion and Conclusion

Our examples suggest that extracted m-reps are good enough to be useful in applications requiring statistical analysis, such as segmentation by the posterior optimization of m-reps or the characterization of the geometric differences between object populations.

We have observed that by the incorporation of the PGA statistics into a multi-pass training, the fitting quality can be improved. The first pass uses the same method described in section 3.3 to extract the m-reps. A following new pass uses the shape statistics trained on the extracted m-reps from the previous pass as the shape prior. Assume the PGA from a previous pass is given by $\{\overline{M}, \lambda_j, \underline{p}_j\}$. In a new pass, m-reps are extracted from the same images by the optimization over the coefficients of the principal directions in the following objective function, combining the object-to-image mismatch and the squared Mahalanobis distance as the present log shape prior.

$$\underset{(\alpha_1, \alpha_2, \ldots, \alpha_{N_{pgc}})}{\arg\min} \; L(M_i = \mathrm{Exp}_{\overline{M}}(\sum_{j=1}^{N_{PGA}} \alpha_j \sqrt{\lambda_j} \cdot \underline{p}_j), D_i) + \sum_{j=1}^{N_{PGA}} \frac{\alpha_j^2}{\lambda_j} \quad (9)$$

Results (fig. 6-right) indicate that the first several passes of the fitting with statistics improve the quality of the extracted m-reps. Y axis in fig. 6-right is the average image match distance (defined in section 3.2) over all the 15 images. The decreasing distance in the first 10 passes indicates the improvement of the extraction. However, the convergence of this process is still under research.

We have shown a framework to extract the medial descriptions represented by multi-figure m-reps from binary characteristic images of multi-figure objects, especially the objects with two-figures as demonstrated in the result section 5.1. A Monte Carlo method has been designed to evaluate the extraction process. We have also shown how to do either global or hierarchical statistical analysis on multi-figure objects. We are evaluating our method when applied to the objects represented by a tree of more than one subfigures (fig. 1-a), as well as the objects also with indentation subfigure(s) (fig. 1-d). The bias and reliability of the statistical framework and the convergence of the multi-pass fitting are also subjects of research.

Acknowledgement

We thank Keith Muller for advice on Monte Carlo generation of m-reps and analysis of their results, P. Thomas Fletcher, Conglin Lu, and Rohit Saboo for m-reps statistics and Monte Carlo methodology, Stephen Aylward and the CADDLab in Radiology Department of UNC for the liver binary characteristic images, Delphi Bull for the help on organizing the reference list. The work reported here was done under the partial support of NIH grant P01 EB02779.

References

1. Cootes, T.F., Taylor, C.J., Cooper, D.H., and Graham, J.: Active shape models - their training and application. Computer Vision and Image Understanding. 61(1): 38-59, 1995.
2. Fletcher, P.T., Lu, C., Pizer, S.M., and Joshi, S.: Principal geodesic analysis for the nonlinear study of shape. IEEE Transactions on Medical Imaging (TMI), 23(8): 995-1005, Aug 2004.
3. Gerig, G., Styner, M., Weinberger, D., Jones, D., and Lieberman, D. : Shape analysis of brain ventricles using SPHARM. IEEE Workshop on Mathematical Methods in Biomedical Image Analysis (MMBIA), 171-178, 2001.
4. Csernansky, J.C., Joshi, S., Wang, L., Gado, M., PhilipMiller, J., Grenander, U., and Miller, M.I.: Hippocampal morphometry in schizophrenia by high dimensional brain mapping. National Academy of Science, 95: 11406-11411, Sept 1998.
5. Styner, M., Gerig, G., Lieberman, J., Jones, D., and Weinberger, D.: Statistical shape analysis of neuroanatomical structures based on medial models. Medical Image Analysis (MEDIA), 7(3): 207-220, 2003.
6. Pizer, S.M., Fletcher, T., Fridman, Y., Fritsch, D.S., Gash, A.G., Glotzer, J.M., Joshi, S., Thall, A., Tracton, G., Yushkevich, P., and Chaney, E.L.: Deformable m-reps for 3D medical image segmentation. Int. J. Comp. Vis. - Special UNC-MIDAG issue (IJCV), 55(2): 85-106, Nov-Dec 2003.
7. Pizer, S.M., Fletcher, P.T., Joshi, S., Gash, A.G., Stough, J., Thall, A., Tracton, G., and Chaney E.L.: A method and software for segmentation of anatomic object ensembles by deformable m-reps. To appear, Medical Physics, 2005.
8. Rao, M., Stough, J., Chi, Y-Y., Muller, K., Tracton, G.S., Pizer, S.M., and Chaney E.L.: Comparison of human and automatic segmentations of kidneys from CT images. Int. J. Rad. Onc., Biol., Physics, 61(3): 954-960, 2005.
9. Chaney, E.L., Pizer, S.M., Joshi, S., Broadhurst, R., Fletcher, R., Gash, G., Han, Q., Jeong, JY., Lu, C., Merck, D., Stough, J., Tracton, G., MD Bechtel, J., Rosenman, J., Chi, YY., and Muller, K.: Automatic male pelvis segmentation from CT images via statistically trained multi-object deformable m-rep models. Abstract and presentation at Annual Meeting of American Society for Therapeutic Radiology and Oncology (ASTRO), 2004.
10. Han, Q., Lu, C., Liu, S., Pizer, S.M., Joshi, S., and Thall, A.: Representing multi-figure anatomical objects. IEEE International Symposium on Biomedical Imaging (ISBI), 1251-1254, 2004.
11. Blum, H. and Nagel, R.: Shape description using weighted symmetric axis features. Pattern Recognition, 10: 167-180, 1978.
12. Thall, A.: Fast C^2 interpolating subdivision surfaces using iterative inversion of stationary subdivision rules. http://midag.cs.unc.edu/pub/papers/Thall TR02-001.pdf, 2002.
13. Danielsson, P.E.: Euclidean distance mapping. Computer Graphics and Image Processing, 14: 227-248, 1980.
14. Pizer, S.M., Jeong, J., Lu, C., Muller, K. and Joshi, S.: Estimating the statistics of multi-object anatomic geometry using inter-object relationships. Proc. Workshop on Deep Structure, Singularities and Computer Vision, Springer LNCS, 2005.
15. Merck, D., Gash, G., Joshi S., and Pizer, S.M: On single figure statistical m-rep model construction. Submitted for publication, http://midag.cs.unc.edu/GeomModFS.html, 2005.

The Role of Non- overlap in Image Registration

Jonas August and Takeo Kanade

Healthcare Robotics Center,
The Robotics Institute Carnegie Mellon University,
Pittsburgh, Pennsylvania

Abstract. Here we model the effect of non-overlapping voxels on image registration, and show that a major defect of overlap-only models—their limited capture range—can be alleviated. Theoretically, we introduce a maximum likelihood model that combines histograms of overlapping and non-overlapping voxels into a common joint distribution. The convex problem for the joint distribution is solved via iterative application of replicator equations that converge monotonically. We then focus on rigidly aligning images with unknown translation, where we present a fast FFT-based method for computing joint histograms for all relative translations of an image pair. We then apply this method to standard overlap-only information theoretic registration criteria such as mutual information as well as to our variants that exploit non-overlap. Our experimental results show that global optima correspond to the correct registration generally only when non-overlapping image regions are included.

1 Introduction

This paper addresses a long-standing complaint with intensity-based image registration methods: they generally converge correctly only if given an initial guess within a limited "capture range" of the correct alignment. We are led to ask: even if processing were free but *no* initial guess were given, do current registration criteria select the correct alignment? Unfortunately not, since the global optima of information theoretic registration criteria such as entropy may be far away from the correct result [5–p. R27]. Here we suggest a fix.

Spurious global optima can arise when there is too little overlap of the image pair for reliable estimation of the joint distribution of corresponding voxels. We thus revisit the concept of overlap beginning in §2, where we review a common probabilistic registration model that assumes full overlap and which explains why the joint histogram of the image pair can be used as an estimate of the joint distribution of intensities of corresponding voxels. In §3, we generalize this model to allow for merely partial overlap, and it is here we see terms in the likelihood that depend on the *non-overlapping* voxels. The revised model gives rise to a joint distribution that trades off the joint histogram on the overlapping voxels with univariate histograms from the non-overlapping voxels, unlike [7, 9]. In §4, we solve for this joint distribution using a monotonically-convergent iterative scheme, i.e., where no step size is required.

To solve for the alignment itself, we focus on the case of unknown translation. In §5, we compute the *globally optimal* alignment to within one voxel using a fast FFT-based method for computing joint and non-overlap histograms over all translations. This also makes it practical to visualize various registration criteria over the entire set of transformations, not only those within a local neighborhood of a potential solution. These complex registration landscapes (§6) highlight the difficulties that registration search strategies must confront, and put into question the feasibility of local search for fully automatic (full capture range) image registration. We suggest that global methods not based on local search will be necessary in the absence of a good initial guess. In hindsight, the standard practice of ignoring the non-overlap seems strange since it uses different image data to evaluate competing alignments that differ in overlap. This violates the principle that all hypotheses be compared using the same information.

2 Idealized Registration Configuration: Full Overlap

To introduce our argument and notation, we start with the simpler situation where the effects of overlap are ignored. Let $u : X \to \{1, \ldots, M\}$ and $v : Y \to \{1, \ldots, N\}$ be the two images to be aligned, where region X (resp. Y) is the finite cardinality set of possible voxels (locations) and M (resp. N) is the number of possible intensities for image u (resp. v). Typically, X and Y are the vertices of a finite lattice in 2- or 3-dimensions. Thus $u_x = u(x)$ is the intensity (in the range $\{1, \ldots, M\}$) at voxel $x \in X$ and $v_y = v(y)$ is the intensity (in the range $\{1, \ldots, N\}$) at voxel $y \in Y$.

The goal of intensity-based image registration is to optimally choose that spatial transformation $y = T(x)$ that maps between the two image regions so that u_x and $v_{T(x)}$, the intensities at corresponding voxels x and $T(x)$, are in some sense correlated, suggesting that their joint distribution will be important. We assume that the intensities for pairs of corresponding voxels are independent and identically distributed (IID), i.e., if $x' \neq x$, then $(u_x, v_{T(x)})$ and $(u_{x'}, v_{T(x')})$ are IID, each pair having joint distribution (probability mass function) $p(m,n) = p_{m,n}, m \in \{1, \ldots, M\}, n \in \{1, \ldots, N\}$. Further assuming full overlap, i.e., that the mapping $T : X \to Y$ is one-to-one and onto, the likelihood (joint probability) of the two images is therefore

$$\text{Prob}\{u, v | \text{full overlap}\} = \prod_{x \in X} p(u_x, v_{T(x)}),$$

and the log likelihood is

$$L_{\text{full}} := \sum_{x \in X} \log p(u_x, v_{T(x)}). \qquad (1)$$

Recall the identity $\sum_n \delta(k, n) = 1$, where the Kronecker delta function $\delta(k, n)$ is equal to 1 if $k = n$ and is 0 otherwise. We apply this identity twice to obtain

$$L_{\text{full}} = \sum_{x \in X} \left[\sum_m \delta(u_x, m) \right] \left[\sum_n \delta(v_{T(x)}, n) \right] \log p(u_x, v_{T(x)}). \qquad (2)$$

By changing the order of summation (permissible because all sums are finite), we can write

$$L_{\text{full}} = \sum_{m,n} a^T_{m,n} \log p_{m,n}, \quad \text{where } a^T_{m,n} := a_{m,n} := \sum_{x \in X} \delta(u_x, m) \delta(v_{T(x)}, n) \quad (3)$$

is the joint histogram (raw, unnormalized counts) of intensity pairs at corresponding voxels for transformation T. Observe that $\sum_{m,n} a_{m,n} = |X|$, the number of voxels in X. To determine the unknown joint distribution p, we solve an optimization problem: maximizing the (log) likelihood. We first show L_{full} is well behaved, and then show the solution is the normalized histogram.

Proposition 1. L_{full} *is a concave function of* p.

Proof. Observe in (3) that L_{full} is a nonnegatively-weighted sum of the concave function log [4]. □

Let S be the **simplex of distributions**[1]

$$S := \{ p \in \mathbb{R}^{MN} :$$
$$p_{m,n} \geq 0, \forall m, n; \quad \text{[Nonnegativity constraint]} \quad (4)$$
$$\sum_{m,n} p_{m,n} = 1 \}. \quad \text{[Normalization constraint]} \quad (5)$$

Observe that set S is convex.

Proposition 2. *Fix transformation T and suppose $a^T_{m,n} > 0$, for all m, n. Then normalized histogram $p^* = a^T/|X|$ is the global optimum of the convex problem*

$$\max_p L_{\text{full}}(T, p) \text{ subject to } p \in S.$$

Proof. We first ignore the nonnegativity constraint but later check that it is satisfied. Applying the method of Lagrange multipliers to the constrained optimization problem (now with only the normalization equality constraint having the Lagrange multiplier γ), we seek the maximum of $\phi(p, \gamma) = L_{\text{full}} + \gamma(\sum_{m,n} p_{m,n} - 1)$. Recall that the first-order necessary conditions for optimality are obtained by setting to zero the partial derivatives of ϕ with respect to the unknowns. Differentiating w.r.t. $p_{m,n}$, we get $a^T_{m,n}/p^*_{m,n} + \gamma^* = 0$, and therefore $p^*_{m,n} = -a^T_{m,n}/\gamma^*$. Differentiating w.r.t. γ we get the normalization constraint (5), and thus $p^*_{m,n} = a^T_{m,n}/\sum_{k,l} a^T_{k,l} = a^T_{m,n}/|X|$. Since $a^T_{m,n}$ is strictly positive, so is $p^*_{m,n}$, and therefore the nonnegativity constraint is not active at p^* and can be ignored. Since L_{full} is concave in p, the unique stationary point p^* is the global maximizer. □

---

[1] Here all distributions are normalized and histograms are unnormalized, unless otherwise stated.

The following consequence of Prop. 2 may be viewed as a justification, first shown in [7], for the use of minimum entropy for (fully overlapping) image registration: the transformation T that minimizes the empirical entropy of distribution $a^T/|X|$ maximizes the likelihood.

Corollary 1. $L^*_{\text{full}}(T) := \max_p L_{\text{full}}(T,p) = -|X|\,\text{entropy}\,(a^T/|X|)$.

3 Realistic Registration Configuration: Partial Overlap

Now we include the effect of partial overlap of the two images. There are three regions to consider: (a) the voxels that overlap, as before; (b) the voxels in image u that do not map to voxels in image v; and (c) the voxels in image v that do not get mapped to from image u. Even if the only dependencies are between corresponding voxel intensities, as before, what distributions should be used for the non-overlapping regions (b) and (c)? We suggest that no new information about the non-overlapping voxels should be assumed; a non-overlapping voxel is to be treated just the same as an overlapping voxel pair, but where one voxel of the pair was not observed. In other words, the reason why there are no corresponding v-voxels for the non-overlapping u-voxels is that we have limited our region of interest (ROI) for image v, and vice versa. Thus we obtain the probability for intensity u_x at non-overlapping voxel x by marginalizing the joint distribution: sum the joint probability of u_x and v_y over all possible values of the unknown v_y. Specifically, if $p(m,n) = p_{m,n}$ is the joint distribution for intensities $u_x = m$ and $v_y = n$ at corresponding voxels x and y, then the intensity $u_x = m$ at non-overlapping voxel x is distributed according to the marginal distribution $\sum_n p(m,n)$. Similarly, the intensity $v_y = n$ at non-overlapping voxel y is distributed according to the marginal distribution $\sum_m p(m,n)$.

When we explicitly consider partial overlap, both the domain of definition and the mapping rule can vary (Fig. 1); thus the alignment transformation is $T: A_T \to Y$, where domain $A_T \subset X$ is the set of voxels in image u that map to voxels in image v. Note that $T(A_T) \subset Y$ is the set of voxels in image v that

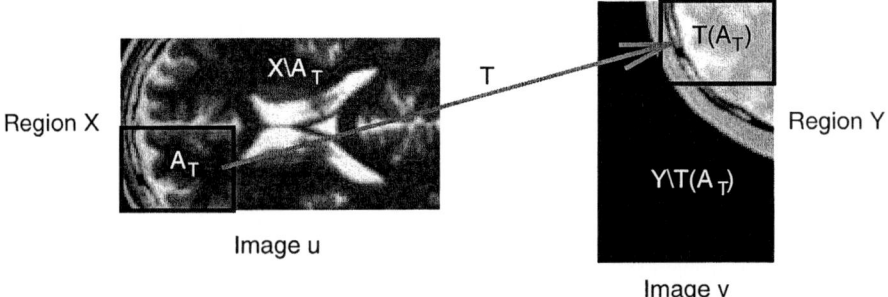

Fig. 1. Partially overlapping images u and v represent different regions of interest in the patient. See text for notation

get mapped to. Thus the non-overlapping portion of image u is $X \setminus A_T$, i.e., everything in X but A_T; similarly, the non-overlapping part of image $v(y)$ is $Y \setminus T(A_T)$. Again assuming IID distributions, the probability of the image pair u, v at transformation T is

Prob$\{u, v|$partial overlap$\}$

$$= \left[\prod_{x \in A_T} p(u_x, v_{T(x)})\right] \times \left[\prod_{x \in X \setminus A_T} \sum_n p(u_x, n)\right] \times \left[\prod_{y \in Y \setminus T(A_T)} \sum_m p(m, v_y)\right].$$

Again using the Kronecker identity and changing order of summation as in the fully-overlapping case, the log likelihood is

$$L_{\text{partial}} = \sum_{x \in A_T} \log p(u_x, v_{T(x)})$$
$$+ \sum_{x \in X \setminus A_T} \log \sum_n p(u_x, n) + \sum_{y \in Y \setminus T(A_T)} \log \sum_m p(m, v_y) \quad (6)$$
$$= \sum_{m,n} a_{m,n}^T \log p_{m,n}$$
$$+ \sum_m b_m^T \log \sum_n p_{m,n} + \sum_n c_n^T \log \sum_m p_{m,n}, \quad (7)$$

where we define

$$a_{m,n}^T := a_{m,n} := \sum_{x \in A_T} \delta(u_x, m) \delta(v_{T(x)}, n) \quad (8)$$
$$b_m^T := b_m := \sum_{x \in X \setminus A_T} \delta(u_x, m) \quad (9)$$
$$c_n^T := c_n := \sum_{y \in Y \setminus T(A_T)} \delta(v_{T(x)}, n), \quad (10)$$

the (T-dependent) joint histogram for the overlapping region, and the histograms for the non-overlapping regions of image u and v, respectively. Again we can maximize this likelihood L_{partial} to determine the unknown joint distribution p. But unlike §2, clearly some sort of numerical optimization will be needed to compute this $p \in S$: we have to trade off the effects of the overlapping versus the non-overlapping histograms. Fortunately, objective function L_{partial} is well-behaved, leading to a convex problem for p.

Proposition 3. L_{partial} *is a concave function of* p.

Proof. Since log is concave and $\sum_n p_{m,n}$ is affine in p, their composition $\log \sum_n p_{m,n}$ is concave in p; similarly for $\log \sum_m p_{m,n}$ [4]. Thus, L_{partial}, a nonnegatively-weighted sum of concave functions, is concave. □

Before introducing our optimization strategy in §4, we suggest how this optimal p be used.

Proposal 1 (Non-Overlap Imperative) *Given partially overlapping images u and v, to evaluate information-theoretic image comparison measures such as joint entropy and mutual information, use the distribution p that maximizes L_{partial} instead of the overlap-only-based normalized joint histogram.*

4 Replicator Equations for Combining Histograms

Now we present an iterative method for estimating the distribution p that maximizes the log likelihood L_{partial} for partial overlap. We suppress T for now as it will be optimized for after we have optimized for p at each fixed T. Since our problem is to maximize concave L_{partial} over convex set S, we could attempt to exploit the arsenal of convex programming. Instead, we suggest an iterative technique with a simple implementation, where the iteration cost is low (unlike other second-order methods that might apply) and which requires no tuning of parameters at all. Specifically, the **replicator equations** for updated distribution p' are similar to a gradient ascent on the log likelihood, except the gradient multiplicatively—not additively—updates the previous distribution p, and the result is normalized to sum to one to remain in the simplex of distributions:

$$p'_{m,n} := \frac{p_{m,n} L_{m,n}}{\sum_{i,j} p_{i,j} L_{i,j}}, \text{ where } L_{m,n} := \frac{\partial L_{\text{partial}}}{\partial p_{m,n}} = \frac{a_{m,n}}{p_{m,n}} + \frac{b_m}{\sum_j p_{m,j}} + \frac{c_n}{\sum_i p_{i,n}}. \quad (11)$$

Observe that this simplex-preserving multiplicative update method converges in one step to the the result in Prop. 2 if b and c are both zero. More importantly, in contrast to the undesirable instability of (additive) gradient ascent when too large a step size is chosen, each multiplicative update increases the log likelihood *without choosing a step size*.

Definition 1. *Continuous mapping $f : D \to D$ is* **growth transformation** *for objective function $\phi : D \to \mathbb{R}$ if $\phi(f(p)) \geq \phi(p)$, for all $p \in D$.*

The concept of growth transformation was used in papers by Baum and coworkers [2,3] and Pelillo [6] to characterize the dynamics of replicator equations, which are a particular class of relaxation labeling processes [8], for certain polynomial objective functions ϕ that arise in evolutionary game theory, computer vision and parameter estimation for Markov chains. Although our objective function L_{partial} is non-polynomial, we have obtained the same result.

Proposition 4. *Update (11) is a growth transformation for $L_{\text{partial}} : S \to \mathbb{R}$.*

Explicitly, this states that $L_{\text{partial}}(p') \geq L_{\text{partial}}(p)$, for any distribution $p \in S$ and its update p' from (11): we can depend on the update to monotonically improve the log likelihood. We have proved Prop. 4 using the log-sum and arithmetic-geometric means inequalities [1].

Because the replicator equations describe a growth transformation for L_{partial}, the choice of initial distribution p^0 that starts the iterations is unimportant, but to avoid degeneracies we suggest that all components be non-zero. We use the normalized version of overlap histogram a as the initial condition in our experiments. To maximize L_{partial}, we iteratively apply the replicator equations until a termination condition is satisfied. In our experiments, we simply stopped after completing only two iterations.

5 FFTs for Global Optimization of Translation

Designers of information theoretic objective functions for image registration have not insisted that global optima approximate the true solution, and have instead focused on local optima. Perhaps this bias stems from the seeming intractability of computing the global optimum. To illustrate, even when T is restricted to a translation and $n = |X| \approx 10^5$ to 10^9 is the number of voxels, $O(n)$ operations are required to compute the joint histogram at each of $O(n)$ possible translations, for an apparent total of $O(n^2)$ operations to find the global optimum! These two onerous $O(n)$ are usually [10] reduced to $O(1)$ by (i) using statistical sampling to approximate the joint distribution and (ii) abandoning global optimization entirely for local, greedy search.

Here we introduce a method to allow exact global optimization of translation for information theoretic objectives in only $O(k\, n \log n)$ operations, where $k = MN$ is the number of bins in the joint histogram. This technique applies to both the full overlap and partial overlap likelihoods, as well as to any registration method that that requires computation of the joint distribution, such as entropy, mutual information [10], and normalized mutual information [9]. The trade-off is histogram resolution for image resolution, which is often acceptable because the joint histogram requires crude quantization just to maintain sufficient bin counts for reliability.

The main idea is that the (m,n)-th bin of the joint histogram is the cross-correlation $a_{m,n}^T = \sum_x f(x)g(x+t) =: \text{corr}_{f,g}(t)$ between two binary vectors $f(x) := \delta(u_x, m)$ and $g(y) := \delta(v_y, n)$, where $y = T(x) := x + t$ for translation t. The translation is a 2- or 3-dimensional vector depending on the dimensionality of images u and v. Zero-padding f and g to an appropriate size l^2 or l^3 for 2- or 3-d, resp., we can avoid wrap-around artifacts in assuming their periodicity, and thus apply Fourier methods. Specifically, if the discrete Fourier transform of f at spatial frequency vector ω is $\hat{f}(\omega) := \sum_x f(x) e^{-2\pi i \omega \cdot x / l}$, and z^* is the complex conjugate of $z \in \mathbb{C}$, we know that $\widehat{\text{corr}_{f,g}}(\omega) = \hat{f}^*(\omega) \hat{g}(\omega)$. Thus for the (m,n)-th bin, computing $a_{m,n}^T$ over all translations takes $O(n \log n)$ work using the FFT. By performing this over all k bins we can calculate the joint histogram over all translations in $O(k\, n \log n)$ time.

The non-overlap histograms b^T and c^T require a similar approach, because they depend on the non-constant region of overlap A_T. (We cannot simply compute the histograms for each image; we need a histogram for each possible overlap.) For b^T, our computation is based on a cross-correlation between f and a mask (of ones) the size of image v. For c^T, the cross-correlation is between a u-sized mask and g. Each also requires $O(k\, n \log n)$ computations.

Given the overlap and non-overlap histograms, for each translation we can solve the optimization problem for p in §4 with $O(k)$ work, and all translations with $O(k\,n)$ work. Evaluating any of the optimization criteria L_{full}, L_{partial}, entropy, mutual information or normalized mutual information is only $O(k\,n)$ more work and the selection of its global optimum takes $O(n)$ time for a grand total of $O(k\,n \log n)$ operations.

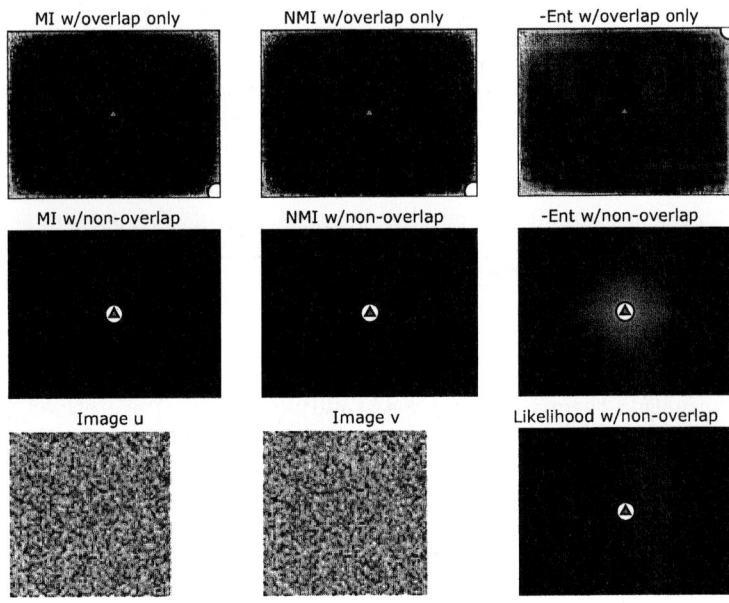

Fig. 2. A correlated pair of uniform noise images (bottom left). Registration landscapes (other images) indicate confidence (via color: blue=low, red=high) in a translation represented by (horizontal,vertical) position of the colored pixel. Top row shows registration landscapes for criteria computed using joint distribution of overlapping voxels only (left to right: mutual information (MI), normalized mutual information (NMI), and L_{full}=weighted negative entropy (-Ent)). The same criteria are shown in middle row, except non-overlapping pixels were also included to compute joint distribution p via minimization of L_{partial} (see §4). Bottom right shows evaluation of optimized $L^*_{\text{partial}}(T)$ at translation T. The white circle and green triangle indicate the computed global optimum of landscape and ground truth translation, respectively. Observe that criteria computed using only the overlap (top) incorrectly have global optima in the corners due to spurious responses from small sample effects, i.e., the image pair overlaps by only a few pixels near the corners of these landscapes. The non-overlapping pixels help make criteria calculations more reliable (middle row and bottom right), so that the global optima are correct. *For all landscapes in this paper, the green triangle hides a spike with a local optimum, but only for the non-overlap-based landscapes is this also a global optimum*

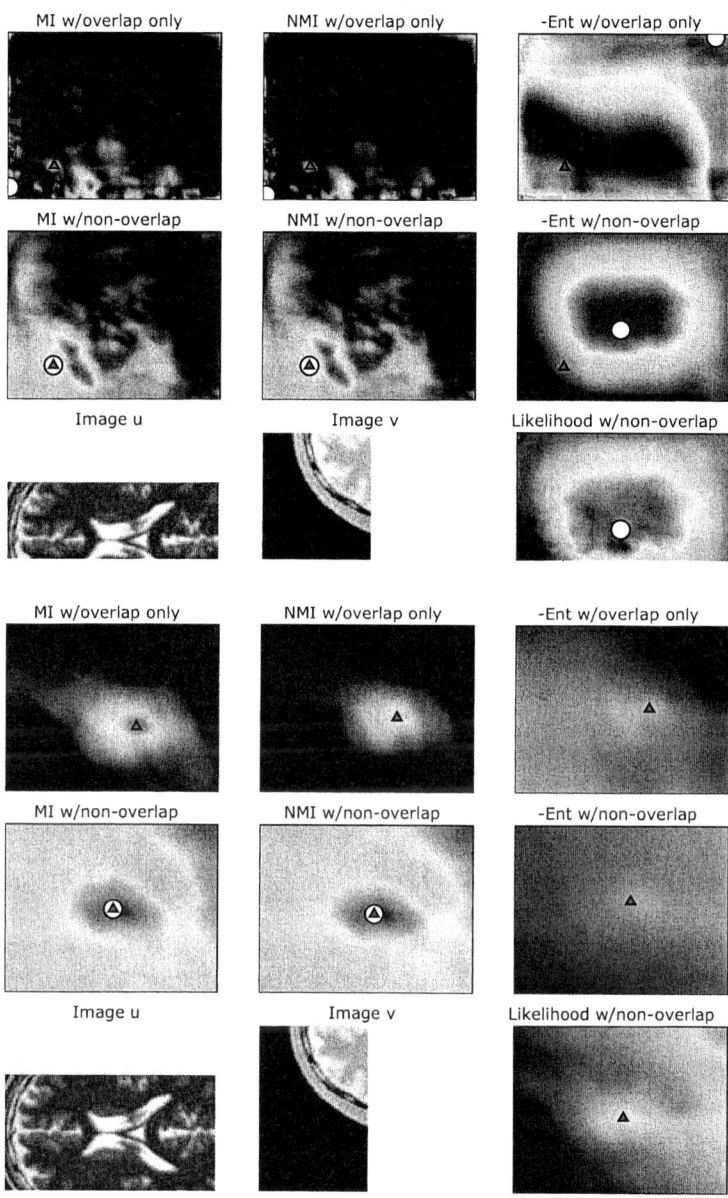

Fig. 3. T2- and PD-weighted MRIs images of human head with restricted ROIs. Top 3x3 image grid shows entire registration landscapes (see Fig. 2 for explanation), while bottom 3x3 grid shows zoom of vicinity of ground truth showing nearby local peak. Most current registration methods use a local search strategy for finding this peak. However, the many spurious peaks, especially in overlap-only landscapes, confound local search unless a close initial guess is provided. The large background in image v is a major violation of the homogeneity/IID assumption. Fig. 5 reduces these artifacts by automatically masking out the background

6 Experimental Results

To test the effect of including non-overlapping image portions, we evaluated several registration criteria over all 2-d translations, thus computing a "registration landscape". For joint distribution estimates using overlapping image portions only, the criteria included mutual information, normalized mutual information, and L_{full}. For the non-overlap-based joint distribution computed by optimizing L_{partial} w.r.t. p, these criteria, as well as L_{partial}, were also used to form landscapes. For joint distribution $q = (q_{m,n})$, the formula for mutual information is $\text{MI}(q) = \text{entropy}(\sum_m q_{m,n}) + \text{entropy}(\sum_n q_{m,n}) - \text{entropy}(q)$, and for normalized mutual information it is $\text{NMI}(q) = [\text{entropy}(\sum_m q_{m,n}) + \text{entropy}(\sum_n q_{m,n})]/\text{entropy}(q)$. All joint histograms had 16 uniformly-spaced bins to which we added 0.1 to avoid degeneracy. Computations (in Numerical Python under GNU/Linux) used up to 0.5GB and took tens of seconds on a 2.4GHz Intel Xeon. We began with a synthetic example where each image started as a common uniform(0,1) noise field, to which independent uniform(0,1) noise was added (Fig. 2). Figs. 3, 4, and 5 show registration results for T1-, T2-, and PD-weighted MRIs of the same brain (images from http://www.bic.mni.mcgill.ca/brainweb). To combat the spatially nonhomoge-

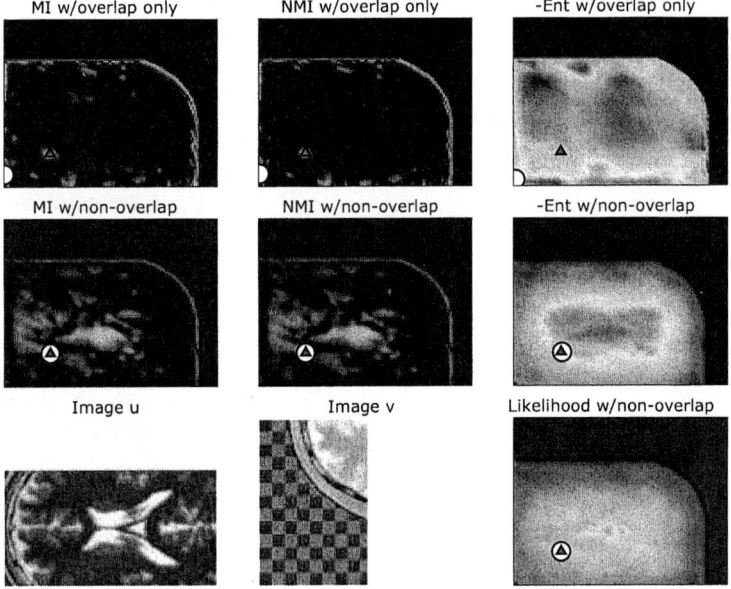

Fig. 4. T2- and PD-weighted MRIs images of human head with restricted ROIs, *with background elimination* via thresholding. Checkerboard indicates background, which was masked out of histogram computations to ensure greater statistical spatial homogeneity. Registration landscapes using non-overlap pixels (middle row and bottom right) have correct global optima; overlap-only landscapes still have only correct local optima

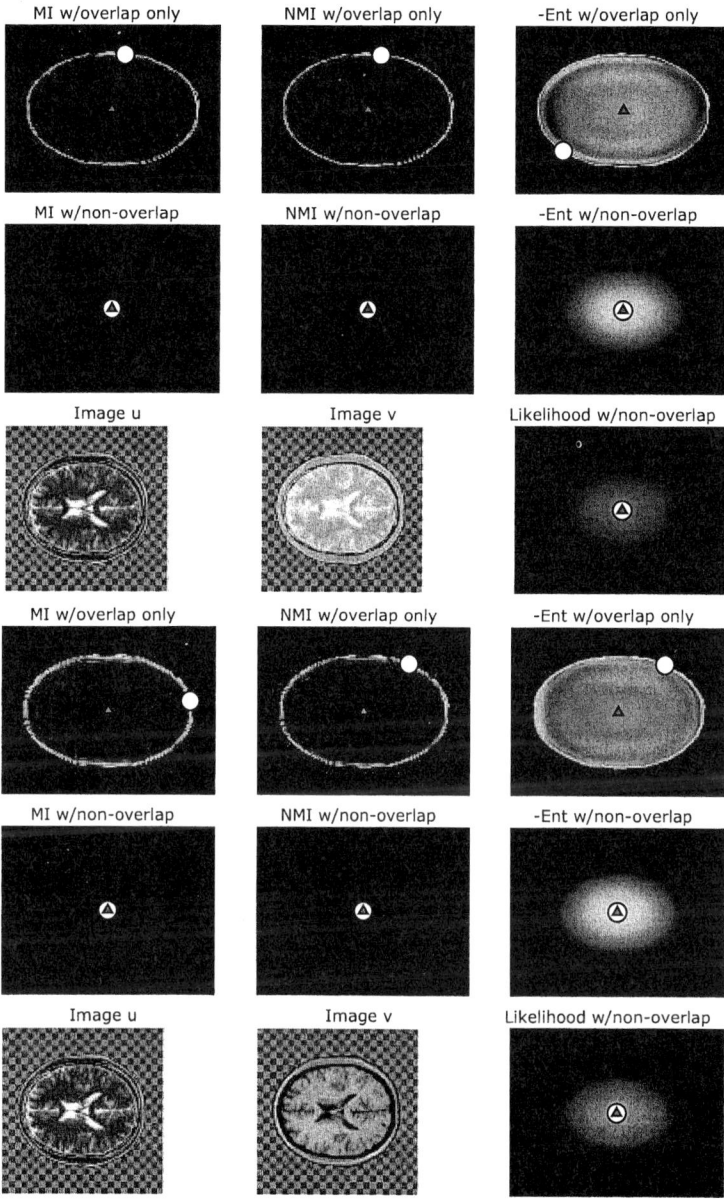

Fig. 5. T2- and PD-weighted MRIs (top 3x3 grid) and T2- and T1-weighted MRIs (bottom 3x3 grid), with full ROI and background-elimination. The spurious global optima for overlap-only landscapes occur on the outer rim of the Minkowski sum of the masks of the two brain regions and are due to small sample effects, similar to the noisy corner/border responses in Fig. 2. Registration landscapes using non-overlap pixels here also have correct global optima, as well as much smoother response in the periphery

neous statistics induced by the black background, the images in Fig. 4 and 5 were thresholded at 2 out 256 gray levels, and the supra-threshold mask was regularized by morphologically closing and then opening by a 3-pixel disk, with the background of the resulting masked image indicated by a checkerboard. Histograms were then computed using only non-background pixels. In contrast to the concave dependency of L_{partial} and L_{full} on distribution p, observe that the landscapes are highly non-concave functions of translation T. Thus it will be difficult to significantly increase the capture range of standard methods that locally search for T. Unsurprisingly, local search usually finds only local optima.

References

1. J. August and T. Kanade. The theory of non-overlap in image registration. Technical report, The Robotics Institute, Carnegie Mellon University, 2005.
2. L. E. Baum and J. A. Eagon. An inequality with applications to statistical estimation for probabilistic functions of markov processes and to a model for ecology. *Bull. Amer. Math. Soc.*, 73:360–363, May 1967.
3. L. E. Baum and G. R. Sell. Growth transformations for functions on manifolds. *Pacific J. Math.*, 27:211–227, 1968.
4. S. Boyd and L. Vandenberghe. *Convex Optimization*. Cambridge UP, 2004.
5. D. L. Hill, P. G. Batchelor, M. Holden, and D. J. Hawkes. Medical image registration. *Physics in Medicine and Biology*, 46:R1–R45, 2001.
6. M. Pelillo. The dynamics of nonlinear relaxation labeling processes. *J. Math. Imaging and Vision*, 7:309–323, 1997.
7. A. Roche, G. Malandain, and N. Ayache. Unifying maximum likelihood approaches in medical image registration. *Intl. J. Imaging Syst. Technol.*, 11:71–80, 2000.
8. A. Rosenfeld, R. A. Hummel, and S. W. Zucker. Scene labeling by relaxation operations. *IEEE Transactions on Systems, Man, and Cybernetics*, 6(6):420–433, 1976.
9. C. Studholme, D. L. G. Hill, and D. J. Hawkes. An overlap invariant entropy measure of 3d medical image alignment. *Pattern Recognition*, 32:71–86, 1999.
10. P. Viola and W. M. Wells III. Alignment by maximization of mutual information. *International Journal of Computer Vision*, 24(2):137–154, 1997.

Multimodality Image Registration Using an Extensible Information Metric and High Dimensional Histogramming

Jie Zhang and Anand Rangarajan

Dept. of Computer & Information Science & Engineering,
University of Florida, Gainesville, FL 32611-6120
{jiezhang, anand}@cise.ufl.edu

Abstract. We extend an information metric from intermodality (2-image) registration to multimodality (multiple-image) registration so that we can simultaneously register multiple images of different modalities. And we also provide the normalized version of the extensible information metric, which has better performance in high noise situations. Compared to mutual information which can even become negative in the multiple image case, our metric can be easily and naturally extended to multiple images. After using a new technique to efficiently compute high dimensional histograms, the extensible information metric can be efficiently computed even for multiple images. To showcase the new measure, we compare the results of direct multimodality registration using high-dimensional histogramming with repeated intermodality registration. We find that registering 3 images simultaneously with the new metric is more accurate than pair-wise registration on 2D images obtained from synthetic magnetic resonance (MR) proton density (PD), MR T1 3D volumes from Brain Web. We perform the unbiased registration of 5 multimodality images of anatomy, CT, MR PD, T1 and T2 from Visible Human Male Data with the normalized metric and high-dimensional histogramming. Our results demonstrate the efficacy of the metrics and high-dimensional histogramming in affine, multimodality image registration.

1 Introduction

An information *metric* was proposed and used for multimodality image registration in our previous work [1]. Compared to mutual information [2, 3, 4], the information metric can be easily and naturally extended to multiple random variables and hence can be used to register multiple images simultaneously. (There is no easy and natural corresponding extension for mutual information.) Mutual information of multiple random variables [5] is not necessarily nonnegative, which renders it inadequate as an image similarity measure. Others [6, 7, 8] have proposed different nonnegative definitions, but they are not natural extensions of the mutual information of two random variables and do not embody the true (in our eyes) spirit of mutual information: shared information between multiple images. Hence, using mutual information to simultaneously register multiple images is not appropriate despite the fact that mutual information is a very good measure (though not a metric) for registering two images. Our goals in the paper are: first, we wish to perform an unbiased registration of multimodality images and second, we hope to demonstrate that multimodality (multiple images) registration can achieve better accuracy than repeated intermodality (two images) registration.

In order to compute the information metric, we need to estimate the high dimensional probability mass function (PMF) so as to compute the Shannon entropy of multiple random variables. Due to the curse of dimensionality, and especially when derivatives of the PMF are required, it is difficult to accurately estimate a high dimensional probability distribution. The simplest PMF estimation approach is histogramming and has been used in database research such as multiple-attribute-data query [9]. In multimodality image registration, despite the fact that we only need to estimate the entropy (of the form $p \log p$) from the PMF, high dimensional histogramming is not prevalent and due to this, there is almost no previous work on simultaneous, multimodality image registration. In this paper, we use an efficient technique to compute high dimensional histograms so as to efficiently compute the Shannon entropy of multiple images. The technique can compute high dimensional histograms in $O(N)$ time where N is the number of samples (simultaneously drawn from all images). We also show a relationship between the maximum number of bins allowed along each axis of the high dimensional histogram such that the histogram will converge to the true PMF in the high dimensional space as $N \to \infty$.

In the following sections, we describe the information metric and the high dimensional histogramming technique.

2 Multimodality Registration Using the Extensible Metric

Before we move to multimodality registration, we briefly introduce some concepts and the basic registration framework using a metric (technically a pseudometric) in intermodality (2-image) registration. More details about the new metric for intermodality registration can be found in our previous work [1].

2.1 Intermodality Registration Using a Metric

The image similarity metric ρ in the intermodality (2-image) case is the sum of two conditional entropies. For two random variables X and Y,

$$\rho(X,Y) = H(X|Y) + H(Y|X) = 2H(X,Y) - H(X) - H(Y) \qquad (1)$$

where $H(\cdot)$ is the entropy of a random variable $[H(X) = -E\{\log(p(X)\}]$, where $p(X)$ is the PMF of X, and $E\{\cdot\}$ denotes the expectation of a random variable. We also proposed two normalized versions of the metric: The first is

$$\tau(X,Y) = \frac{\rho(X,Y)}{H(X,Y)}. \qquad (2)$$

$\tau(X,Y)$ is also a pseudometric [10]. And $0 \leq \tau(X,Y) \leq 1$, $\tau(X,Y)=0$ if $X=Y$; $\tau(X,Y)=1$ if X and Y are independent. The second normalized version of the metric $\rho(X,Y)$ is

$$\eta(X,Y) = \frac{\rho(X,Y)}{H(X)+H(Y)}. \quad (3)$$

And $0 \leq \eta(X,Y) \leq 1$, $\eta(X,Y) = 0$ if $X = Y$; $\eta(X,Y) = 1$ if X and Y are independent. But $\eta(X,Y)$ does not satisfy the triangle inequality and hence it is not a metric (or pseudometric).

From the definition in (1), we see that ρ is very similar to mutual information (MI) (4) in the 2-image case except that the metric has one more joint entropy term, which means the metric gives joint entropy more weight than the marginal entropy in comparison to mutual information

$$MI(X,Y) = H(X) + H(Y) - H(X,Y) = \frac{H(X)+H(Y)-\rho(X,Y)}{2}. \quad (4)$$

And we have found that minimizing the normalized metric τ or η is *equivalent* to maximizing the normalized mutual information (NMI) [11] (5) in the 2-image case

$$NMI(X,Y) = \frac{H(X)+H(Y)}{H(X,Y)} = 2 - \tau(X,Y). \quad (5)$$

Consequently, from our perspective, NMI is not *ad hoc* since it is inversely proportional to a pseudometric.

Now we move to our main topic—multimodality image registration.

2.2 Extension to the Multimodality Case

From the definition of the information metric for two random variables (1), we can *easily* extend the metric to multiple random variables in two different ways. The first extension, for n random variables $X_1, X_2, \ldots X_n$,

$$\rho(X_1, X_2, \ldots, X_n) = \sum_{i=1}^{n} H(X_i | X_1, \ldots, X_{i-1}, X_{i+1}, \ldots, X_n) \quad (6)$$

and the second is,

$$\mu(X_1, X_2, \ldots, X_n) = \sum_{i=1}^{n} H(X_1, \ldots, X_{i-1}, X_{i+1}, \ldots, X_n | X_i). \quad (7)$$

And after dividing by either the joint entropy $H(X_1, X_2, \ldots, X_n)$ or by the sum of the marginals $\sum_{i=1}^{n} H(X_i)$, we get their normalized counterparts.

If we want to simultaneously register three images $I^{(1)}$, $I^{(2)}$ and $I^{(3)}$, we obviously need to find more transformations. We define the biased case as one where $I^{(1)}$ is the reference image and fixed in the registration and we seek two optimal affine transformations—T_2^* for image $I^{(2)}$ and T_3^* for image $I^{(3)}$ by minimizing the metric (8).

$$\{T_2^*, T_3^*\} = \arg \min_{\{T_2, T_3\}} \rho(I^{(1)}, I^{(2)}(T_2), I^{(3)}(T_3)). \tag{8}$$

We define the unbiased case as one where there is no reference image and we seek three optimal affine transformations—T_1^* for image $I^{(1)}$, T_2^* for image $I^{(2)}$ and T_3^* for image $I^{(3)}$ by minimizing the metric (9).

$$\{T_1^*, T_2^*, T_3^*\} = \arg \min_{\{T_1, T_2, T_3\}} \rho(I^{(1)}(T_1), I^{(2)}(T_2), I^{(3)}(T_3)) \tag{9}$$

where $I^{(1)}(T_1)$ is the transformed image of image $I^{(1)}$ using affine transformation T_1, $I^{(2)}(T_2)$ is the transformed image of image $I^{(2)}$ using affine transformation T_2 and $I^{(3)}(T_3)$ is the transformed image of image $I^{(3)}$ using affine transformation T_3. Equivalent minimizations can be carried out for the normalized counterparts of ρ and μ.

3 Computing the Entropy of Multiple Random Variables

The multimodality image registration measures ρ, μ and their normalized versions are all entropy-based measures. Consequently, all these measures require the computation of the joint entropy of many random variables—henceforth termed "multi-dimensional entropy."

The approach in [12] used minimum spanning trees (MST) to estimate the α-entropy in image registration. The MST-based approach directly estimates entropy without estimating the high dimensional PMF. But computing an MST for a graph with many edges is very expensive $[O(E \log E)]$ where E is the number of voxels and furthermore, the method cannot compute the normalized versions of the information measure. (Also the method computes the Renyi entropy instead of the Shannon entropy.) Indirect methods compute entropy by first estimating the high dimensional PMF. While histogramming is a popular approach for estimating the PMF, it has not been used for computing the high dimensional entropy in image registration, mainly because *naive implementations are exponential in complexity in the dimensionality of random variables.* Our technique for computing high dimensional histograms (to be explained below) overcomes the aforementioned dimensionality problem. Its computational complexity is $O(N)$ where N is the number of samples drawn from (corresponding) pixel locations over a set of images. The $O(N)$ computational complexity is much smaller than some popular high dimensional PMF estimation methods such as Parzen windows $O(N^2)$, Gaussian mixture models $O(NK)$ where K is the number of clusters, etc. An approximation to the Parzen window entropy can be computed in $O(NM)$, $M < N$ using fast Gauss transforms [13], but you have to first cluster the samples. To our knowledge, this approach has not been explored in medical image registration. Its advantage over the high dimensional histogramming technique is that it is analytically differentiable.

We now describe the high dimensional histogramming approach. Assume we have M images $I^{(m)}$, $m \in \{1, \ldots, M\}$ and the number of histogram bins for the

m^{th} image $I^{(m)}$ is $K^{(m)}$, $m \in \{1,\ldots,M\}$. The total number of bins in the multi-dimensional histogram of M images is $\prod_{m=1}^{M} K^{(m)}$, which will be very large if M or $K^{(m)}$ is large. But in the space of the joint histogram of M images, most of the bins of the joint histogram are empty. Empty bins do not contribute anything when we compute the high dimensional Shannon entropy (since $p \log p \to 0$ as $p \to 0$.) Hence, using $\prod_{m=1}^{M} K^{(m)}$ bins in the space of the joint histogram of M images is impractical and furthermore is unnecessary since we only need know the non-empty bins.

Assume a bounded range $[I_{min}^{(m)}, I_{max}^{(m)}]$ for image $I^{(m)}$. Let $B_i^{(m)}$ be the binned intensity value of image $I^{(m)}$ at location i, $i \in \{1,\ldots,N\}$:

$$B_i^{(m)} = \left\lfloor (K^{(m)} - 1) \times \frac{I_i^{(m)} - \min_{1 \leq j \leq N}\{I_j^{(m)}\}}{\max_{1 \leq j \leq N}\{I_j^{(m)}\} - \min_{1 \leq j \leq N}\{I_j^{(m)}\}} + 1 \right\rfloor, \forall m. \quad (10)$$

From (10), we see that the binned intensity values of image $I^{(m)}$ are integers in $\{1,\ldots,K^{(m)}\}$. Let $L^{(m)}$ be the minimum length of digital bits which can represent $K^{(m)}$, $m \in \{1,\ldots,M\}$. Then we get a new code $C_i = B_i^{(1)} B_i^{(2)} \cdots B_i^{(M)}$ with length $\sum_{m=1}^{M} L^{(m)}$, which is a concatenation of the binned intensity values of *all* images at location i, $i \in \{1,\ldots,N\}$. The number of different elements of the set $\{C_i, i \in \{1,\ldots,N\}\}$ is the number of non-empty bins of the joint histogram of M images. Hence we can use $\{C_i, i \in \{1,\ldots,N\}\}$ to generate the joint histogram of M images by counting the number of identical C_is in the code set. That this is valid is guaranteed by the following theorem.

Theorem 1: $C_i = C_j$ if and only if $B_i^{(m)} = B_j^{(m)}$ $\forall m \in \{1,\ldots,M\}$, $\forall i, j \in \{1,\ldots,N\}$. [Proof omitted due to lack of space.]

The number of bins $K^{(m)}$ is the only free parameter in our method but it is also very important. Below, following [14], we propose a criterion for limiting the maximum number of bins in the histogram.

Theorem 2: Let $U_1, U_2, \ldots, U_N$ be i.i.d. random variables in $\Re^M$ with PMF f. Let $\mathcal{P}$ be a partition of $\Re^M$ into cubes of size h, and define the histogram PMF estimator by

$$f_N(u) = \frac{1}{Nh^M} \sum_{i=1}^{N} I_{\{U_i \in A(u)\}} \quad (11)$$

where $A(u)$ is the set in $\mathcal{P}$ that contains u and I is the indicator function of a set. Then the estimate is *universally consistent* in L_1 if $h \to 0$ and $Nh^M \to \infty$ as $N \to \infty$, that is, for any f the L_1 error of the estimate $\int |f_N(u) - f(u)|\, du$ converges to zero in probability, or equivalently, for any $\epsilon > 0$,

$$\lim_{N \to \infty} \Pr\left(\int |f_N(u) - f(u)|\, du \geq \epsilon\right) = 0. \quad (12)$$

For our case, the domain of PMF is a bounded subset of $\Re^M$, namely $[0,1]^M$. If we use the same number $K^{(m)} = K$ bins for each image in the set, then

$h = \frac{1}{K}$. Thus $h \to 0$ is equivalent to $K \to \infty$ and $Nh^M \to \infty$ is equivalent to $\frac{N}{K^M} \to \infty$, for which $K < N^{\frac{1}{M}}$ is necessary. Let $K = N^{\frac{1}{M+\alpha}}$, then as $K \to \infty$, $\frac{N}{K^M} = N^{\frac{\alpha}{M+\alpha}} \to \infty$ for any $\alpha > 0$ as $N \to \infty$, which satisfies the condition of the theorem. Hence we use $K = N^{\frac{1}{M+\alpha}}$ for some $\alpha > 0$ as a criterion in our high dimensional histogram. In plain English, Theorem 2 essentially says that if you have more samples, then use more bins for the histogram but the rate of increase of the number of bins should be slower than the rate of increase of the number of samples. (The simplification of $K^{(m)} = K$ has been used for the sake of exposition. An extension to different $K^{(m)}$ is straightforward.)

From Theorem 1, we know that to compute the high dimensional histogram, we only need to count the number of identical C_i in the set $\{C_i, i \in \{1, \ldots, N\}\}$. From Theorem 2, we know that for any $C_i, i \in \{1, \ldots, N\}, C_i \in [1, N]$. We can count the number of identical C_i in the set $\{C_i, i \in \{1, \ldots, N\}\}$ by traversing N samples once. Thus the time complexity of computing high dimensional histograms is $O(N)$.

4 Experimental Results

4.1 Multimodality vs. Intermodality: Simultaneous Registration of 3 Images and Pair-Wise Registration on Synthetic PD, T2 and T1 MR Images

In the registration experiments of this section, we use the powerful Brainweb simulated MRI volumes for a normal brain [15]. The main advantage of using simulated MR data is that the ground truth is known. The size of each image is 256mm×256mm.

We decompose an affine transformation matrix into a product of shear, scale and rotations. Let $T = \begin{bmatrix} a & b & 0 \\ c & d & 0 \\ e & f & 1 \end{bmatrix}$ be an affine transformation. $\begin{bmatrix} a & b \\ c & d \end{bmatrix} = \begin{bmatrix} 2^s & 0 \\ 0 & 2^s \end{bmatrix}$ $R(\theta) \begin{bmatrix} 2^t & 0 \\ 0 & 2^{-t} \end{bmatrix} R(\phi)$, where s and t are scale and shear parameters, and $R(\theta) = \begin{bmatrix} \cos(\theta) & -\sin(\theta) \\ \sin(\theta) & \cos(\theta) \end{bmatrix}$, $R(\phi) = \begin{bmatrix} \cos(\phi) & -\sin(\phi) \\ \sin(\phi) & \cos(\phi) \end{bmatrix}$ are two rotation matrices. In our experiments, the range of shear and scale parameters is [-1 1], the range of rotation parameters are [-45 45] degrees and the range of translations is [-10 10] mm. In this decomposition of an affine transformation, reflections are not allowed.

In the experiments, we use the following ten measures to register 3 triplets of 2D slices of 3D PD, T2 and T1 MR brain volume images.

1. $\rho(X, Y, Z) = H(X|Y, Z) + H(Y|X, Z) + H(Z|X, Y)$
2. $\mu(X, Y, Z) = H(X, Y|Z) + H(Y, Z|X) + H(Z, X|Y)$
3. $\tau(X, Y, Z) = \frac{\rho(X,Y,Z)}{H(X,Y,Z)}$
4. $\eta(X, Y, Z) = \frac{\rho(X,Y,Z)}{H(X)+H(Y)+H(Z)}$

5. $\kappa(X,Y,Z) = \frac{\mu(X,Y,Z)}{H(X,Y,Z)}$
6. $\sigma(X,Y,Z) = \frac{\mu(X,Y,Z)}{H(X)+H(Y)+H(Z)}$
7. modified mutual information: $mMI(X,Y,Z) = H(X) + H(Y) + H(Y) - H(X,Y,Z)$
8. sum of pair-wise mutual information: $pMI(X,Y,Z) = MI(X,Y)+MI(Y,Z)+MI(Z,X)$
9. modified normalized information: $mNMI(X,Y,Z) = \frac{H(X)+H(Y)+H(Y)}{H(X,Y,Z)}$
10. sum of pair-wise normalized mutual information: $pNMI(X,Y,Z) = NMI(X,Y)+NMI(Y,Z)+NMI(Z,X)$

The slices are chosen in the axial direction. We then transform the MR T2 image with an affine transformation $\hat{T}_1 = \begin{bmatrix} 1.2496 & -0.39666 & 0 \\ 0.39666 & 0.93006 & 0 \\ 4 & 4 & 1 \end{bmatrix}$, with $s_1 = 0.2$, $t_1 = 0.2$, $\theta_1 = 10$, $\phi_1 = 10$, $e_1 = 4$ and $f_1 = 4$. We also transform the MR T1 image with an affine transformation $\hat{T}_2 = \begin{bmatrix} 1.4205 & -0.88097 & 0 \\ 0.88097 & 0.67935 & 0 \\ 8 & 8 & 1 \end{bmatrix}$, with $s_2 = 0.4$, $t_2 = 0.4$, $\theta_2 = 20$, $\phi_2 = 20$, $e_2 = 8$ and $f_2 = 8$. We have done two experiments with these data. Each experiment is repeated 30 times with different Gaussian noise. We add Gaussian noise with zero mean and standard deviation 0.1 in the first experiment and zero mean and standard deviation 0.2 in the second experiment. (The intensity range of all images is normalized to the [0,1] interval.) We use a coarse-to-fine brute force search strategy to find the optimal T_1^* and T_2^*. The finest search resolution of scale and shear is 0.05. The finest search resolution of rotation is 0.5 degrees in the first experiment and 1 degree in the second experiment. The finest search resolution of translation is 1 mm. The registration measures are computed only in the overlap area of the three images with bilinear interpolation used for transforming the image intensities.

To compare each measure and validate the registration results, we compute the mean error of each parameter of two affine transformations recovered by ten measures and the sum of $\left\|\hat{T}_1 - T_1^*\right\| + \left\|\hat{T}_2 - T_2^*\right\|$ of 30 experiments.

Figure 1 depicts the sum of $\left\|\hat{T}_1 - T_1^*\right\| + \left\|\hat{T}_2 - T_2^*\right\|$ of 30 noise trials in the first set of experiments. From the results, we see that multimodality registration is more accurate than repeated pair-wise (intermodality) registration. And the normalized metric η has best performance. Table 1 shows the mean error of each parameter of two affine transformations recovered with the ten measures of 30 noise trials in the second experiment. Figure 2 shows the sum of $\left\|\hat{T}_1 - T_1^*\right\| + \left\|\hat{T}_2 - T_2^*\right\|$ of 30 noise trials in the second experiment. From the results, we see that the two non-normalized metrics ρ and μ failed in recovering scale because of high noise. But the normalized metric η (which is based on ρ) still has best performance. And multimodality registration is more accurate than repeated pair-wise registration.

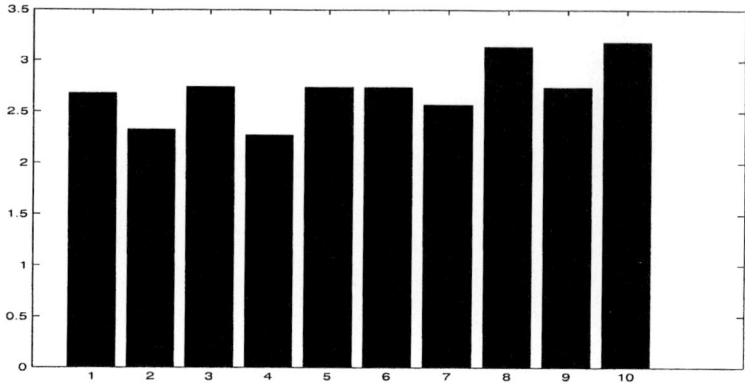

Fig. 1. Plots of sum of $\left\|\hat{T}_1 - T_1^*\right\| + \left\|\hat{T}_2 - T_2^*\right\|$ of 30 trials recovered by ten measures in the first experiment with noise std. 0.1. Numbers 1 to 10 represent ρ, μ, τ, η, κ, σ, mMI, pMI, mNMI and pNMI—the ten registration measures

Table 1. Mean errors of different affine parameters in the second experiment with Gaussian noise with mean 0 and std. 0.2

measures	error of transformation on MR T2						error of transformation on MR T1					
	s	t	θ	ϕ	e	f	s	t	θ	ϕ	e	f
ρ	0.24	0.01	2.53	1.53	2.53	0.7	0.11	0.02	3.77	2.4	1.73	1.2
μ	0.64	0.06	10.57	3.03	5.93	1.57	0.42	0.08	4.87	3.53	2.97	2.03
τ	0	0	1.1	1.33	1.93	0.43	0.0033	0.0083	3.83	1.67	1.833	0.97
η	0	0	0.97	1.33	1.93	0.33	0.0017	0.0083	2.8	1.23	1.77	0.93
κ	0	0	1.03	1.2	2.07	0.37	0.005	0.0117	3.53	1.43	2.13	0.7
σ	0	0	1.03	1.2	2.07	0.37	0.005	0.0117	3.53	1.43	2.13	0.7
mMI	0	0	1.1	1.2	2.03	0.37	0.005	0.0117	3.93	1.4	2	0.9
pMI	0	0	1.2	1.37	2.17	0.3	0.005	0.013	7.43	1.8	2	0.67
mNMI	0	0	1.03	1.2	2.07	0.37	0.005	0.0117	3.53	1.43	2.13	0.7
pNMI	0	0	1.16	1.37	2.17	0.3	0.005	0.0133	7.4	1.8	2.23	0.77

With these experiments on synthetic PD, T2 and T1 MR 2D images, we see that these ten measures have similar performance in low noise experiments. Generally, they can correctly recover scale and shear parameters but have error in recovering rotation and translation. And we see that multimodality registration is more accurate than repeated pair-wise registration. In the high noise case, the two non-normalized metrics failed to recover scale because they prefer small overlaps of images. The normalized metric η still has best performance. And these experimental results also show that minimizing the normalized metric κ or σ is equivalent to maximizing the modified normalized mutual information.

In our following experiments, we will only use the normalized measure η.

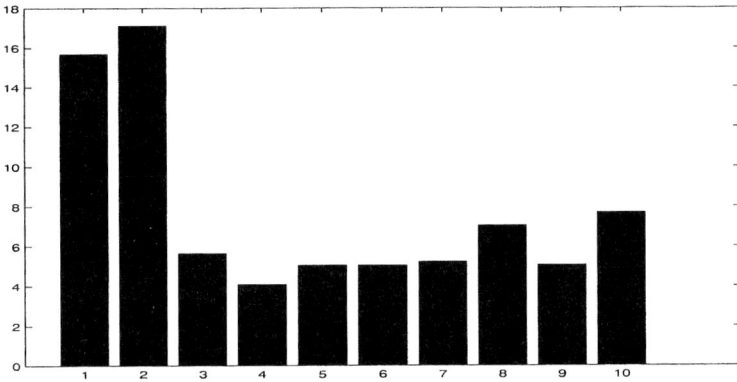

Fig. 2. Plots of sum of $\left\|\hat{T}_1 - T_1^*\right\| + \left\|\hat{T}_2 - T_2^*\right\|$ of 30 trials recovered by ten measures in the second experiment with noise 0.2. Numbers 1 to 10 represent ρ, μ, τ, η, κ, σ, mMI, pMI, mNMI and pNMI—the ten registration measures

4.2 Unbiased Multiple Image Registration of Visible Human Data

---
Algorithm 1 Iterated sequential search
---
1. sequentially search ten translations which minimize η corresponding to 5 images;
2. sequentially search ten scaling and shear parameters which minimize η for 5 images;
3. sequentially search ten rotations which minimize η for 5 images;
4. if η decreases in this iteration then go to 1; else end.

In this section, we register pentads of images of head slice from Visible Human Male Data. For the pentad, the first image is the photograph of anatomical slice, the second is the CT image, the third is an MR PD image, the fourth is an MR T1 image and the fifth is an MR T2 image. The slice number of the pentads in the Visible Human Male Data is 1165. Because ground truth is unknown, we register 5 images simultaneously without bias. That means that each image gets an affine transformation and we minimize the normalized metric η on five affine transformations:

$$\{T_1^*, T_2^*, T_3^*, T_4^*, T_5^*\} = \arg\min_T \eta(I^{(1)}(T_1), I^{(2)}(T_2), I^{(3)}(T_3), I^{(4)}(T_4), I^{(5)}(T_5)) \tag{13}$$

where $T = \{T_1, T_2, T_3, T_4, T_5\}$ and T_1, T_2, T_3, T_4 and T_5 are five affine transformations. $I^{(m)}(T_m)$ is the transformed image of image $I^{(m)}$ using affine transformation T_m, $m \in \{1, ..., 5\}$. Since the time complexity of searching for 30 parameters of 5 affine transformations is high, we used iterated sequential search using algorithm 1 for each parameter until the normalized measure η achieves the minimum. The color images of the anatomical slice are converted to grayscale and the intensity of images is normalized to the interval $[0, 1]$ prior to registration.

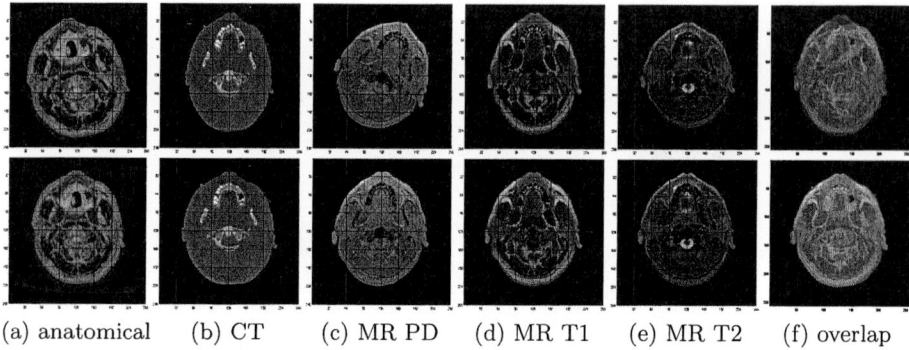

(a) anatomical (b) CT (c) MR PD (d) MR T1 (e) MR T2 (f) overlap

Fig. 3. The first row is the set of images before registration; the second row is the set after registration. [Dataset index: VHD #1165.]

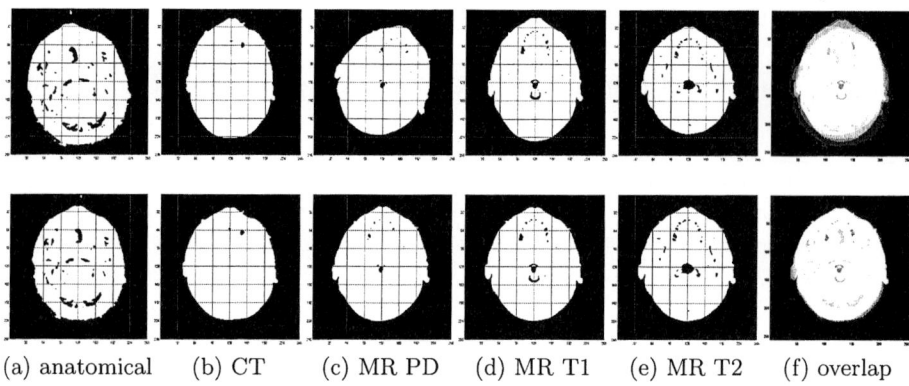

(a) anatomical (b) CT (c) MR PD (d) MR T1 (e) MR T2 (f) overlap

Fig. 4. Segmented images before (1st row) and after (2nd row) registration. [Dataset index: VHD #1165.]

The normalized measure η is computed only in the overlap area of the three images with bilinear interpolation used for transforming the image intensities. The image size is 256 by 256. (The pixel size is 0.32mm square for a photograph of anatomical slice and 1mm for MR and CT images.) The histogram of each image used 8 bins. High dimensional histograms are computed using the technique in section 3.

In Figure 3, we show the images before and after registration. In order for human perception to gauge the results of registration, we add a grid to the images. A careful examination of the images before and after registration reveals that the images are indeed better aligned. For a quantitative evaluation of the registration, we coarsely segment these images by basically segmenting the object from the background in the images. Then we represent these segmented images as binary images as shown in Figure 4. (Object is with intensity value 1

Table 2. Results of unbiased registration of anatomical slice, CT, MR PD, T1 and T2 images.[Dataset index: VHD #1165.]

	Anatomy	CT	MR PD	MR T1	MR T2
s	-0.1	0.01	0.02	-0.03	0.07
t	-0.01	0.09	-0.01	0.08	-0.02
θ	-7	3	20	0	0
ϕ	-1	-2	0	0	0
e	4	2	-1	0	0
f	-9	1	0	0	0

Table 3. Number of pixels in nonoverlap region of segmented images before and after registration. upper triangle is before registration and lower triangle is after registration. [Dataset index: VHD #1165.]

nonoverlap	Anatomic	CT	MR PD	MR T1	MR T2
Anatomic	0	8250	8721	7719	9449
CT	2372	0	4173	1915	3853
MR PD	2984	1530	0	4446	3632
MR T1	2980	1234	1118	0	4292
MR T2	3390	1700	1434	800	0

and background is with intensity value 0.) We evaluate the quality of the registration by comparing the number of pixels in the nonoverlap region of pairwise segmented images before and after registration. From these results in Table 3, we see that the number of pixels in the nonoverlap region of segmented pairwise images after registration is much less prior to registration. Provided that the segmentation errors are not significant and these can also be gauged by human perception, we see the images are better aligned after registration. Also, from the segmented images in Figure 4, we see that these images are better aligned after registration.

From the affine transformations achieved in the registration as shown in Table 2, we see that the affine transformations of all three images include a certain amount of shear. This serves as a very preliminary justification for using an affine mapping.

From these anecdotal evaluation results, we see that minimizing the normalized measure η and computing high dimensional histograms works well for the simultaneous (and unbiased) registration of multimodality images.

5 Conclusions

We have presented an information metric for intermodality image registration, which can be easily extended to the multimodality case as opposed to mutual information which is not so easily extended. The information metric is a linear combination of conditional entropies and has the properties of symmetry, non-negativity and triangle inequality. Normalized versions of this extensible information metric are also proposed and used for multimodality image registration. We derive and use a new efficient technique for computing high dimensional histograms so as to efficiently compute the joint entropy of multiple images. We then demonstrate how the high dimensional histogramming technique can be used to simultaneously register many images without being biased to a reference image. The high dimensional histogramming technique can also be used for feature-based multimodality image registration (where a vector of features is available at each voxel) and for non-rigid multimodality image registration. These represent attractive topics for further research.

Acknowledgements

This work was partially supported by NSF IIS 0307712. We thank Tim Cootes and Derek Hill for helpful conversations.

References

1. Zhang, J., Rangarajan, A.: Affine image registration using a new information metric. In: IEEE Computer Vision and Pattern Recognition (CVPR). Volume 1. (2004) 848–855
2. Viola, P., Wells III, W.M.: Alignment by maximization of mutual information. In: Fifth Intl. Conf. Computer Vision (ICCV), IEEE Press (1995) 16–23
3. Collignon, A., Vandermeulen, D., Suetens, P., Marchal, G.: 3D multi–modality medical image registration using feature space clustering. In Ayache, N., ed.: Computer Vision, Virtual Reality and Robotics in Medicine. Volume 905 of Lecture Notes in Computer Science., Springer–Verlag (1995)
4. Pluim, J.P.W., Maintz, J.B.A., Viergever, M.A.: Mutual-information-based registration of medical images: A survey. IEEE Trans. on Medical Imaging 22 (2003) 986–1004
5. Cover, T., Thomas, J.: Elements of Information Theory. John Wiley and Sons, New York, NY (1991)
6. Studholme, C., Hill, D.L.G., Hawkes, D.J.: Incorporating connected region labelling into automated image registration using mutual information. In Amini, A.A., Bookstein, F.L., Wilson, D.C., eds.: Mathematical methods in biomedical image analysis (MMBIA). IEEE Computer Soc. Press (1996) 23–31
7. Boes, J.L., Meyer, C.R.: Multi-variate mutual information for registration. In Taylor, C., Colchester, A., eds.: Medical image computing and computer-assisted intervention (MICCAI). Volume 1679 of Lecture notes in Computer Science. Springer-Verlag (1999) 606–612
8. Lynch, J.A., Peterfy, C.G., White, D.L., Hawkins, R.A., Genant, H.K.: MRI-SPECT image registration using multiple MR pulse sequences to examine osteoarthritis of the knee. In Hanson, K.M., ed.: Medical Imaging: Image Processing. Volume 3661 of Proc. SPIE. SPIE (1999) 68–77
9. Poosala, V., Ioannidis, Y.: Selectivity estimation without the attribute value independence assumption. In: 23rd VLDB conference. (1997) 486–495

10. Rajski, C.: A metric space of discrete probability distributions. Information and Control **4** (1961) 371–377
11. Studholme, C., Hill, D.L.G., Hawkes, D.J.: An overlap invariant entropy measure of 3D medical image alignment. Pattern Recognition **32** (1999) 71–86
12. Neemuchwala, H., Hero, A., Carson, P., Meyer, C.: Local feature matching using entropic graphs. In: IEEE International Symposium on Biomedical Imaging. (2004)
13. Yang, C., Duraiswami, R., Gumerov, N., Davis, L.: Improved fast Gauss transform and efficient kernel density estimation. In: Ninth IEEE International Conference on Computer Vision (ICCV). Volume 1. (2003) 464–471
14. Devroye, L., Gyorfi, L., Lugosi, G.: A Probabilistic Theory of Pattern Recognition. Springer (1997)
15. Collins, D.L., Zijdenbos, A.P., Kollokian, V., Sled, J.G., Kabani, N.J., Holmes, C.J., Evans, A.C.: Design and construction of a realistic digital brain phantom. IEEE Trans. Med. Imag. **17** (1998) 463–468

Spherical Navigator Registration Using Harmonic Analysis for Prospective Motion Correction

C. L. Wyatt[1], N. Ari[2], and R.A. Kraft[3]

[1] Virginia Tech
clwyatt@vt.edu
[2] GE Medical Systems
[3] Wake Forest University School of Medicine

Abstract. Spherical navigators are an attractive approach to motion compensation in Magnetic Resonance Imaging. Because they can be acquired quickly, spherical navigators have the potential to measure and correct for rigid motion during image acquisition (prospectively as opposed to retrospectively). A limiting factor to prospective use of navigators is the time required to estimate the motion parameters. This estimation problem can be separated into a rotational and translational component. Recovery of the rotational motion can be cast as a registration of functions defined on a sphere. Previous methods for solving this registration problem are based on optimization strategies that are iterative and require k-space interpolation. Such approaches have undesirable convergence behavior for prospective use since the estimation complexity depends on both the number of samples and the amount of rotation. We propose and demonstrate an efficient algorithm for recovery of rotational motion using spherical navigators. We decompose the navigator magnitude using the spherical harmonic transform. In this framework, rigid rotations can be recovered from an over-constrained system of equations, leading to a computationally efficient algorithm for prospective motion compensation. The resulting algorithm is compared to existing approaches in simulated and actual navigator data. These results show that the spherical harmonic based estimation algorithm is significantly faster than existing methods and so is suited for prospective motion correction.

1 Introduction

Subject motion is a significant problem in many applications of Magnetic Resonance Imaging (MRI), in particular those that use combinations of long TR acquisitions and large gradients. Several techniques are available for motion correction or reduction including physiological gating [9], fast imaging [4], navigator echoes [11], and registration [16], and are often used in combination. Because navigator echoes can be acquired quickly, they are an attractive approach to

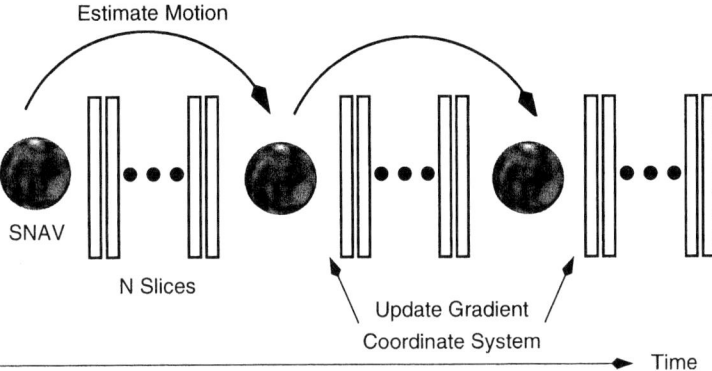

Fig. 1. Generic 2D multi-slice MRI sequence using SNAVs for prospective motion correction

prospective motion correction, that is correction for motion during the imaging sequence. Prospective motion correction does not suffer from interpolation artifacts and is important where spin history artifacts are of concern, as post-processing methods cannot correct them [2].

Navigator echoes are a sparse samplings of k-space that take advantage of the Fourier properties of rigid coordinate transformations. They are interspersed between portions of the acquisition, such as between volumes (Fig. 1). When used prospectively, motion parameters, estimated from successive navigators, are used to update the gradient coordinate system before the next series of slices is acquired.

Navigators are distinguished by the k-space sampling trajectory employed. Orbital (2D) navigators [7] sample k-space in circular trajectories, generally in orthogonal planes. However, orbital navigators are sensitive to out-of-plane motion and cannot recover arbitrary rotations [12]. Spherical (3D) navigators (SNAVs) [15], which sample a spherical shell of k-space, can accurately recover arbitrary rotations and are the focus of this paper.

Recovery of rotational motion from successive navigator acquisitions, either prospectively or retrospectively, requires registration. Previous work has focused on iterative matching algorithms for aligning magnitude navigator data to estimate the rotational motion[15, 1]. These iterative techniques, while providing accurate results over a range of angles, are difficult to implement for prospective motion correction due to their computational requirements and convergence behavior. These issues limit the clinical application of SNAVs for prospective motion correction.

This paper presents an approach to SNAV registration based on spherical harmonic analysis that was motivated by a recent solution to motion estimation from catadioptric image sequences in computer vision [13]. The resulting algorithm has several advantages over existing methods of navigator registration: no need for k-space interpolation, simple computational structure suitable for real-time implementation, and the ability to recover a wide range of arbitrary rotation angles. The paper is organized as follows. First we describe the spherical navigator model and existing motion recovery algorithms. We then develop a motion estimation algorithm using the discrete spherical harmonic transform. This algorithm is then tested in both synthetic and real navigator data. We conclude with a discussion of the results and additional potential applications.

2 Spherical Navigator Echoes

A spherical navigator signal can be modeled as a sampling of the Fourier transform, $F(k_x, k_y, k_z) \in \mathbb{C}$, of the object space on the sphere of radius ρ. Without loss of generality we consider the unit sphere, S^2, and the locus of frequencies on its surface:

$$F(\boldsymbol{k}) \quad \text{where} \quad \boldsymbol{k} = [k_x(t)\ k_y(t)\ k_z(t)]^T \in S^2 . \tag{1}$$

Given two navigator signals, we refer to the source, F_S as the signal before a rigid transformation in the object space, and the target, F_T, as the signal after. The Fourier property of rigid transformations allows recovery of rigid motion between these successive navigator acquisitions. Consider a rigid coordinate transformation in the object domain,

$$\begin{bmatrix} x' \\ y' \\ z' \end{bmatrix} = \mathbf{M} \begin{bmatrix} x \\ y \\ z \end{bmatrix} + \begin{bmatrix} \Delta x \\ \Delta y \\ \Delta z \end{bmatrix},$$

where $\mathbf{M}$ is a matrix representing a rotation from the orthogonal group, $SO(3)$, and $[\Delta x\ \Delta y\ \Delta z]^T$ is a translation. Rigid transformations in object space lead to an equivalent rotation of the k-space coordinates, $\boldsymbol{k}$, and a linear phase shift:

$$F(k_x'(t), k_y'(t), k_z'(t)) = F(k_x(t), k_y(t), k_z(t)) \exp^{-i2\pi(\Delta x k_x + \Delta y k_y + \Delta z k_z)}, \tag{2}$$

where $\boldsymbol{k}' = \mathbf{M}\boldsymbol{k}$.

The effect of translational motion can be separated from rotational motion by treating the magnitude and the phase of F independently. Taking the logarithm of the phase component leads to an overdetermined system of linear equations, the solution of which is the translation component [15].

In this paper we are primarily concerned with recovering the rotational component of the motion using the magnitude of F_S and F_T. This component of the rigid motion estimation is more complex than estimating the translation. The SNAV rotation estimation problem may may be viewed as a registration of two functions defined on S^2. Previous work on navigators has focused on iterative algorithms that minimizes an objective function comparing a rotated source navigator to the target navigator. For example, Welch et al. [15] use downhill simplex minimization of the squared difference between the source and target navigator magnitudes. In [1] several different objective functions are considered with the downhill simplex minimization algorithm and hierarchical schemes. A drawback of this type of motion recovery is the need to interpolate the navigator at each iteration, with increasing computation time as the number of SNAV samples increases. Also, the number of iterations required to locate the minimum increases as the rotation angle increases, making it difficult to predict the total computation time. In the following section, we develop a similar approach to rotational motion recovery that uses the spherical harmonic transform of the SNAV, rather the magnitude component directly.

3 Harmonic Analysis on the Unit Sphere

We treat the magnitude spherical navigator as being in the set of square integrable functions defined on the unit sphere, $f(\theta, \phi) \in L^2(S^2)$, where $\theta \in [0, \pi)$ is the colatitude coordinate and $\phi \in [0, 2\pi)$ is the longitude coordinate. Surface spherical harmonics are a Fourier expansion of the functions in $L^2(S^2)$ and have been studied extensively in the context of quantum mechanics and geophysics. The description of spherical harmonics that follows is based on [5, 8, 13] and the text [3].

3.1 Spherical Harmonic Transform

The $2L+1$ spherical harmonics, $Y_l^m : S^2 \mapsto \mathbb{C}$, for each $L \geq 0$, form an orthonormal basis for any $f \in L^2(S^2)$.

$$Y_l^m(\theta, \phi) = (-1)^m \sqrt{\frac{(2l+1)(l-m)!}{4\pi(l+m)!}} P_l^m(cos(\theta)) \exp^{im\phi}, \qquad (3)$$

where l is the degree of the harmonic, $|m| \leq l$, and P_l^m are the associated Legendre Polynomials. Thus, any $f(\theta, \phi)$ can be expanded in this basis, with coefficients $f(l, m)$, as:

$$f(\theta, \phi) = \sum_{l \in \mathbb{N}} \sum_{m \leq l} f(l, m) Y_l^m(\theta, \phi) \qquad (4)$$

$$f(l, m) = \int_\theta \int_\phi f(\theta, \phi) \bar{Y}_l^m(\theta, \phi) d\theta d\phi. \qquad (5)$$

If $f(\theta, \phi)$ is bandlimited with bandlimit, B, then a sampled version, $\hat{f}$, with at least $2B$ samples in θ and ϕ, is sufficient to recover the original f. This is equivalent to the Nyquist theorem in Fourier analysis and leads to a discrete spherical harmonic transform, first developed in Driscoll and Healy [5],

$$\hat{f}(l, m) = \frac{\sqrt{2\pi}}{2B} \sum_{j=0}^{2B-1} w_j P_l^m(\cos \theta_j) \sum_{k=0}^{1B-1} \exp^{-im\phi_k} f(\theta_j, \phi_k), \qquad (6)$$

where $|m| \leq l$, $\theta_j = \pi(2j+1)/4B$, and $\phi_k = 2\pi k/4B$. The quadrature weights, w_j, are derived (with a proof) in [5]. Equation (6) can be efficiently computed using an FFT, followed by the discrete Legendre Transform in $O(n(\log n)^2)$[5].

3.2 Rotation Theorem

We describe the rotation in the object domain, and the equivalent rotation of the magnitude navigator data, by the Euler angles α, β, and γ using the matrix representation:

$$M = R_z(\alpha)R_y(\beta)R_z(\gamma) , \qquad (7)$$

where R_y and R_z denote rotations about the y and z axis respectively. Note this is a nonstandard definition of the Euler angles, but it simplifies the estimation problem, as we describe below. Let $g(\alpha, \beta, \gamma) \in SO(3)$ be an element of the rotation group in 3D space. The rotation theorem of spherical harmonics [8] states that a rotation $g(\alpha, \beta, \gamma)$ of $f(\theta, \phi)$ induces a linear transformation of $f(l, m)$ according to:

$$\hat{f}^g(l, m) = \sum_{|p| \leq l} U_l^{pm}(g) \hat{f}(l, p) , \qquad (8)$$

where $\hat{f}^g(l, m)$ indicates the discrete spherical harmonic transform after the rotation. The weighting $U_l^{pm}(g)$ is given by:

$$U_l^{pm}(g(\alpha, \beta, \gamma)) = \exp^{-\imath p \alpha} P_l^{pm}(\cos \beta) \exp^{-\imath m \gamma} ,$$

where P_l^{pm} is the extended Jacobi Polynomial (sometimes called the generalized associated Legendre polynomial). Consider two sets of magnitude spherical navigator data with a rotation, $g(\alpha, \beta, \gamma)$ of object space in between them, f_S and f_T. We can compute the discrete spherical harmonic transform for both to obtain $\hat{f}_S(l, m)$ and $\hat{f}_T(l, m)$. Equation (8) can be used to define an over-constrained system of nonlinear equations in α, β, and γ. The solution to this system of equations is the estimated Euler angles. The rotation matrix resulting from the motion estimate can be computed from Eqn. (7).

3.3 Objective Function Optimization

Evaluation of Eqn. (8) is complicated by the $P_l^{pm}(\cos \beta)$ term in $U_l^{pm}(g)$ because the extended Jacobi polynomial can be unstable for large orders, l, or for angles, β, approaching $\frac{\pi}{2}$ [14]. An elegant simplification first used in quantum mechanics [6], and later in computer vision [13], is to rewrite the rotation, g, as a composition of two rotations, removing the dependence on $cos(\beta)$. The rotation $g(\alpha, \beta, \gamma)$ can be written as the composition of two rotations, $g_1 \circ g_2$, using the definition in Eqn. (7) above, where $g_1 = g(\beta + \pi, \frac{\pi}{2}, 0)$ and $g_2 = g(\alpha + \frac{\pi}{2}, \frac{\pi}{2}, \gamma + \frac{\pi}{2})$. Since Eqn. (8) is linear in $U_l^{pm}(g)$, the terms of $U_l^{pm}(g_1 \circ g_2)$ can be collected as follows:

$$U_l^{pm}(g_1 \circ g_2) = \sum_{|k| \leq l} U_l^{pk}(g_1) U_l^{km}(g_2) . \qquad (9)$$

Expanding the term under the sum over k gives:

$$U_l^{pk}(g_1) U_l^{km}(g_2) = \exp^{-\imath m(\gamma + \frac{\pi}{2})} P_l^{pk}(0) P_l^{km}(0) \exp^{-\imath k(\beta + \pi)} \exp^{-\imath p(\alpha + \frac{\pi}{2})} . \qquad (10)$$

Now the arguments to the extended Jacobi polynomials are zero. This allows them to be precomputed in a stable and efficient fashion using recursion [14].

Substitution of Eqn. (10) into Eqn. (8) gives the following non-linear equation in α, β, and γ:

$$\hat{f}^g(l,m) = \exp^{-\imath m(\gamma+\frac{\pi}{2})} \sum_{|p|\leq l} \exp^{-\imath p(\alpha+\frac{\pi}{2})} \hat{f}(l,p) \sum_{|k|\leq l} P_l^{pk}(0) P_l^{km}(0) \exp^{-\imath k(\beta+\pi)} \tag{11}$$

In the prospective motion correction application, we assume the previous navigator transform, $f_S(l,m)$, is available. To estimate the rotation we fix the largest order we will consider, $l_{\max}$, and compute the discrete spherical harmonic transform for the target (current) navigator, $f_T(l,m)$. We then form an objective function comparing the rotated source transform, f_S^g to the target. The estimate of the Euler angles of the rotation is then given by the following minimization problem:

$$\min_{\alpha,\beta,\gamma} \sum_{l\leq l_{\max}} \sum_{m\leq l} \overline{[f_S^g(l,m) - f_T(l,m)]}[f_S^g(l,m) - f_T(l,m)] , \tag{12}$$

where the overbar indicates conjugation.

The 3D minimization problem in Eqn. (12) can be separated into a 2D and 1D problem by observing that when $m = 0$, there is no dependence in Eqn. (11) on γ [13]. Thus we first minimize

$$\sum_{l\leq l_{\max}} \overline{[f_S^g(l,0) - f_T(l,0)]}[f_S^g(l,0) - f_T(l,0)] , \tag{13}$$

with respect to α and β. We then fix α and β and minimize

$$\sum_{l\leq l_{\max}} \sum_{m\leq l} \overline{[f_S^g(l,m) - f_T(l,m)]}[f_S^g(l,m) - f_T(l,m)] , \tag{14}$$

with respect to γ.

The computational complexity of evaluating the objective function depends on the choice of $l_{\max}$, assuming the discrete spherical harmonic transforms have been applied.

3.4 Numerical Implementation

Our implementation of the rotation motion recovery, which we call the SPHARM algorithm, is written in Matlab, with external calls to libraries written in C/C++. The discrete spherical harmonic transform is computed using the *SpharmonicKit* C library[1], which implements an algorithm based on an FFT and Fast Legendre Transform [10].

Several optimization methods are suitable for solving the non-linear minimization problems in Eqn. (13) and Eqn. (14). We have used the Nelder-Mead algorithm [17] in the results presented here. The evaluation of the objective functions are implemented as an external library written in C++ for efficiency.

---

[1] http://www.cs.dartmouth.edu/~geelong/sphere/

4 Implementation Results

4.1 A Simple Example

Figure 2 demonstrates the algorithm on a simulated object consisting of the unit cube in the object domain, rotated by an arbitrary $g(\pi/18, \pi/9, \pi/6)$. The analytic representation of the Fourier transform of the unit cube was sampled uniformly with $B = 128$ before and after the rotation was applied (Fig. 2c-d). The objective functions in Fig. 2e-f show that Eqn. (13) is more sensitive to β than α. This could lead to scaling problems in the minimization. However, the Nelder-Mead algorithm was able to reliably locate a minimum within 2 seconds (Sun-Blade-2000, 900 MHz UltraSPARC III) across a wide range of angles. Total average time to estimate the motion was 2.12 seconds, including the spherical harmonic transform for both the source and target navigator, with a variation of less than 0.25 seconds.

For comparison, we implemented a variation of the rotation motion recovery algorithm in Welch et al. [15]. The algorithm applies different trial rotations to the floating SNAV while searching for the minimum of a normalized least

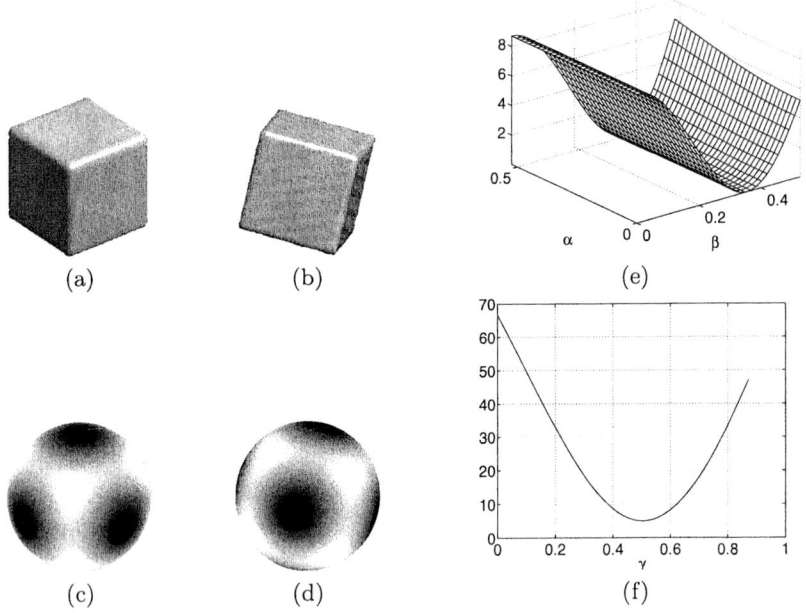

Fig. 2. Example of the unit cube. (a)-(b) cube in the object domain before and after rotation by $g(\pi/18, \pi/9, \pi/6)$. (c)-(d) SNAV before and after rotation. (e) Objective function corresponding to Eqn. (13). (f) Objective function corresponding to Eqn. (14). Note that objective function in (e) is much more sensitive to β than α. Using a cutoff of $l_{max} = 10$, the L-2 norm between the actual rotation matrix and the estimated rotation matrix was 6.1e-06

squares cost function using a multi-scale downhill simplex (ms-DHS) approach [18]. The cost function is computed by first converting 3-D Cartesian coordinates of the SNAV (x, y, z) to 2-D latitude and longitude (θ, ϕ) coordinates. Second, 2-D Delaunay triangulation is performed to generate triangular meshes of non-uniformly sampled (scattered) SNAV coordinates in the (θ, ϕ) coordinate system. Third, these triangular meshes are used for scatter data interpolation through nearest triangle search to determine the magnitude values of the new trial SNAV elements after a trial rotation is applied during the search for the best rotation angle. Finally, the cost function is computed between the reference SNAV and the trial SNAV. The algorithm was written entirely in Matlab.

For the example in Fig. 2, the ms-DHS algorithm took 22 seconds to find a minimum, approximately ten times longer than the SPHARM algorithm. Such a wall-clock comparison alone is unfair because of different optimizations possible. Examining the code profile however indicates that the majority of the time spent in the ms-DHS simplex algorithm is in the interpolation, which must be conducted at each iteration. In contrast, the most time consuming portion of the SPHARM algorithm is the evaluation of the objective function, which does not require interpolation. In addition, the choice of l_{max} restricts the terms in Eqn. (13) and Eqn. (14) required, further reducing the computation time.

The unit cube example was also used to characterize the SPHARM algorithm with respect to noise level, angular dependency, sampling rate, and execution speed. It was found the execution speed is independent of the rotation angle to be recovered. Accuracy of the rotation recovery was measured using the L-2 norm of the difference between the estimated rotation matrix and the known (applied) rotation matrix. Cutoff values of l_{max} above 10 does not appreciable increase the accuracy, but does increase the computation time. The algorithm can recover arbitrary rotations up to 45 degrees in any Euler angle or combination. The algorithm with no noise works with a sampling rate, B, as low as 16. Increasing the noise requires an increase in the sampling rate. At a sampling rate of $B = 128$, the algorithm can recover rotations with an accuracy less than 0.05 with noise levels as high as 20 percent (defined as the percent noise as a fraction of the maximum signal). The l_{max} cutoff had no appreciable effect on noise immunity.

4.2 Simulated Navigators

To evaluate the behavior of the algorithm in a more realistic k-space, an SNAV simulator was written using the T1 digital brain phantom from the McConnell Brain Imaging Centre at McGill University [19]. The magnitude of the Fourier transform of the T1 volume (1x1x1 mm voxel size) was sampled using a uniform grid ($B = 128$). Zero mean, independent, identically distributed Gaussian noise was added to the simulated navigators with different variances. To simulate rotations, the data was rotated in image space by a rigid transformation, using sinc interpolation, prior to acquiring the simulated SNAV. The error between the recovered and applied rotation is computed using the L-2 norm of the matrix difference between them.

Figure 3 shows the effect of the SNAV radius (no noise was added), which determines the signal amplitude, using a Monte Carlo simulation of Euler rota-

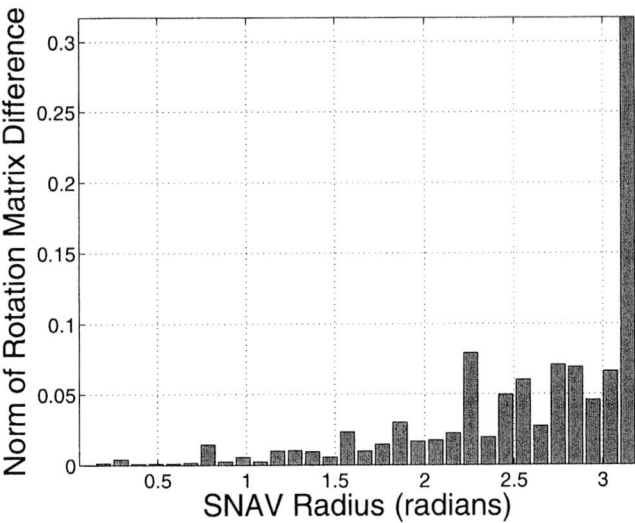

Fig. 3. SNAV brain simulation experiment. Average rotation error versus SNAV radius in digital frequency. Signal strength decreases as the radius increases leading to increased error. There were 10 repetitions of the simulations for each radius with Euler angles uniformly distributed in [0, 10] degrees

tion angles uniformly distributed between zero and ten degrees. The L-2 norm of the matrix difference between the simulated and recovered rotation matrix increased appreciably at an SNAV radius of 0.8 radians (in digital frequency), indicating the effect of decreased signal strength.

Figure 4 shows the effect of SNR on the rotation recovery, again using a Monte Carlo simulation of rotations (angles uniformly drawn from [0, 10] degrees). Similar to the unit cube example, the algorithm performs well below SNR ratios of 20 percent.

4.3   In-Vivo Experiments

A *in-vivo* study was conducted to demonstrate the rotation motion recovery using the SPHARM algorithm. We acquired SNAVs from a human volunteer after obtaining informed consent using a 1.5 T GE TwinSpeed MR Scanner (General Electric Healthcare, Milwaukee WI). The scanner is equipped with high performance gradients supporting a 40 mT/m magnitude and a 150 T/m/s slew rate. A head coil with a maximum 125 kHz sampling rate was used for both RF transmission and signal reception. The SNAVs were acquired using a constant velocity trajectory with coordinates given by:

$$k_x[n] = R\cos\left(\frac{2\pi Tn}{N}\right)\sin\left(\frac{\pi n}{N}\right)$$
$$k_y[n] = R\sin\left(\frac{2\pi Tn}{N}\right)\sin\left(\frac{\pi n}{N}\right)$$

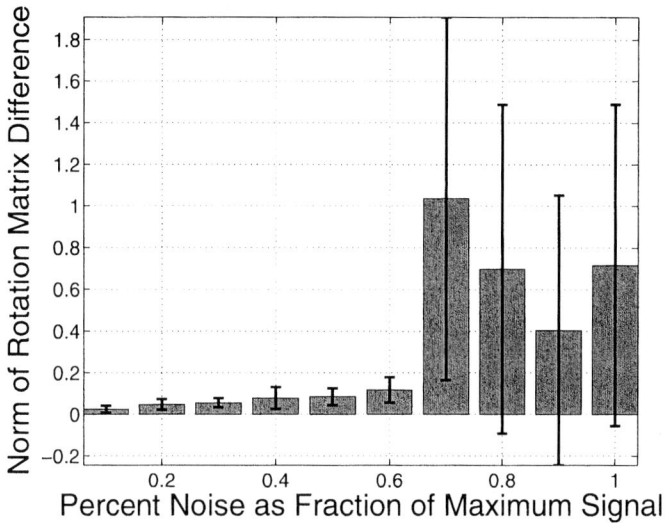

Fig. 4. SNAV brain simulation experiment. Average and standard deviation of the rotation error versus noise percent of the maximum signal strength. There were 10 repetitions of the simulations for each noise level with Euler angles uniformly distributed in [0, 10] degrees

$$k_z[n] = R \cos\left(\frac{\pi n}{N}\right),$$

where n is the sample index, $N = 5120$ points, and $T = 36$ threads. A 62.5 kHz receiver bandwidth was used, with an SNAV radius of 0.345 cm^{-1}. A total of 16 repeated SNAV signals were acquired to evaluate the effect of averaging and signal SNR. At the end of each acquisition, the subject was asked to rotate their head a small arbitrary increment. Another SNAV was acquired at this new position. This process was repeated 8 times, while the subject's head was at a different position for each trial. We treated the 7 sequential pairs of navigators ((trial-1,trial-2) (trial-2,trial-3) etc.) as the source and target respectively. The SNAV data was converted to a uniform sampling of the sphere, required by the fast spherical harmonic transform, using a Delaunay triangulation. This process took approximately 2 seconds and would add to the total rotation recovery computation time in the prospective application.

There is no gold standard for comparison or error estimation for the in-vivo experiments. However, the rotations recovered were reasonable given the instructions to the volunteer to move in small increments. Manual inspection of the objective functions was also used to verify the optimization procedure was successful. Figure 5 shows the rotations recovered for the 7 cases when the signal averages was varied between no averaging, 8 averages, and 16 averages. Trials 2, 3, and 7 with no averaging had norms beyond those expected, given the small head movements. Thus averaging is recommended to give sufficient SNR to support rotational motion recovery using the SPHARM algorithm.

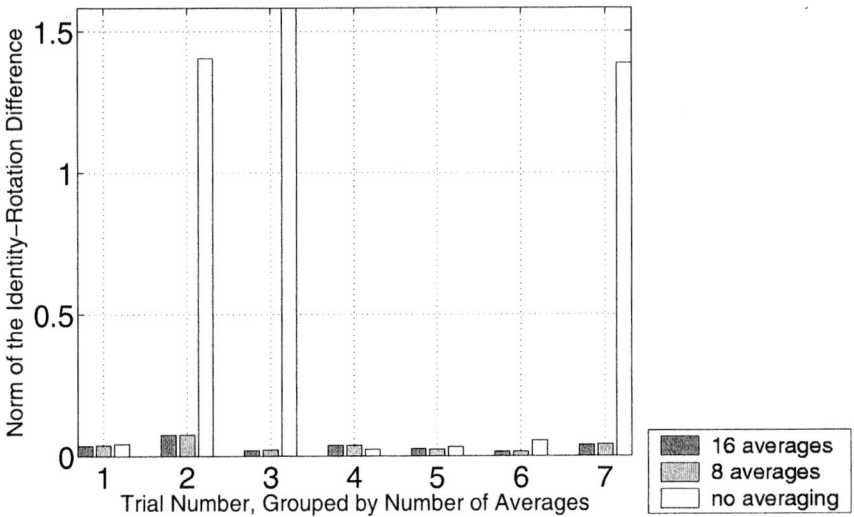

Fig. 5. In-vivo experiment, L-2 norm of identity minus rotation matrix versus the trial number, grouped by the number of signal averages. The failures in trials 2, 3, and 7 with no averaging is likely due to insufficient SNR

5 Conclusions

In this paper, we have proposed and demonstrated an approach to registration of spherical navigators that is significantly more efficient than previous methods. In this new approach, we treat the spherical navigator as a function defined on a sphere and use the harmonic transform of this function to recover rotational motion. Our simulated and preliminary *in-vivo* results indicate the algorithm is appropriate for use in prospective motion correction. Future work will focus on integrating the implementation into the navigator sequence and reducing the number of signal averages required.

The proposed approach to spherical navigator registration has applications in motion compensation and automated slice prescription for repeated small field of view acquisitions (e.g spectroscopy) within a single subject.

References

1. N. Ari: Prospective motion correction with chemically selective spherical navigator echoes for functional magnetic resonance imaging. Dissertation, Wake Forest University, 2004.
2. B.B. Biswal, J.S. Hyde: Contour-based registration technique to differentiate between task-activated and head motion-induced signal variations in fMRI. Magnetic Resonance in Medicine 38 (3): 470-476 1997.
3. G.S. Chirikjian, A.B. Kyatkin: Engineering Applications of NonCommunative Harmonic Analysis. CRC Press, 2001.

4. M.S. Cohen, R.M. Weisskoff: Ultra-fast imaging. Magnetic Resonance Imaging 9 (1): 1-37 1991.
5. J.R. Driscoll, D.M. Healy: Computing Fourier-transforms and convolutions on the 2-sphere. Advances in Applied Mathematics 15 (2): 202-250 1994.
6. A.R. Edmonds: Angular Momentum in Quantum Mechanics. Princeton University Press. 1960.
7. Z.W. Fu,Y. Wang, R.C. Grimm, P.J. Rossman, J.P. Felmlee, S.J. Riederer, R.L. Ehman: Orbital navigator echoes for motion measurements in magnetic-resonance-imaging. Magnetic Resonance in Medicine 34 (5): 746-753 1995.
8. J.D. Goldstein. The effect of coordinate system rotations on spherical harmonic expansions - a numerical-method. Journal of Geophysical Research 89 (B6): 4413-4418 1984.
9. M.W. Grouch, D.A. Turner, W. D. Erwin: Respiratory gating in magnetic-resonance-imaging - improved image quality over nongated images for equal scan time. Clinical Imaging 15 (3): 196-201 1991.
10. D.M. Healy, P.J. Kostelec, D. Rockmore: Towards safe and effective high-order Legendre transforms with applications to FFTs for the 2-sphere. Advances in Computational Mathematics 21 (1-2): 59-105 2004.
11. X.P. Hu, S. G. Kim: Reduction of signal fluctuation in functional MRI using navigator echoes. Magnetic Resonance in Medicine 31 (5): 495-503 1994.
12. C.C Lee, C.R. Jack, R.C. Grimm, P.J. Rossman, J.P. Felmlee, R.L. Ehman, S.J. Riederer: Real-time adaptive motion correction in functional MRI. Magnetic Resonance in Medicine 36 (3): 436-444 1996.
13. A. Makadia, K. Daniilidis: Direct 3D rotation estimation from spherical images via a generalized shift theorem. In Proceedings. 2003 IEEE Computer Society Conference Computer Vision and Pattern Recognition, Volume: 2, 18-20 June 2003 Pages:II - 217-24 vol.2.
14. G. Masters, K. Richards-Dinger: On the efficient calculation of ordinary and generalized spherical harmonics. Geophys. J. Int. 135: 307-309 1998.
15. E.B. Welch, A. Manduca, R.C. Grimm, H.A. Ward, C.R. Jack: Spherical navigator echoes for full 3D rigid body motion measurement in MRI. Magnetic Resonance in Medicine 47 (1): 32-41 2002.
16. B. Zitova, J. Flusser: Image registration methods: a survey. Image and Vision Computing 21 (11): 977-1000 2003.
17. J.A. Nelder and R. Mead: A simplex method for function minimization. Comput. J. 7: 308-313 1965.
18. J. Nocedal and S. J. Wright: Numerical Optimization. Springer-Verlag, Rensselaer, NY, 1999.
19. D.L. Collins and A.P. Zijdenbos and V. Kollokian and J.G. Sled and N.J. Kabani and C.J. Holmes and A.C. Evans: Design and construction of a realistic digital brain phantom. IEEE Trans. on Medical Imaging 17(3): 463-468 1998.

Tunneling Descent Level Set Segmentation of Ultrasound Images

Zhong Tao[1] and Hemant D. Tagare[1,2]

[1] Dept. of Electrical Engineering, Yale University,
New Haven CT 06520
[2] Dept. of Diagnostic Radiology,
Yale University, New Haven CT 06520

Abstract. The presence of speckle in ultrasound images causes many spurious local minima in the energy function of active contours. These minima trap the segmentation prematurely under gradient descent and cause the algorithm to fail. This paper presents a substantially new reformulation of Tunneling Descent, which is a <u>deterministic</u> technique to escape from unwanted local minima. In the new formulation, the evolving curve is represented by level sets, and the evolution strategy is obtained as a sequence of constrained minimizations.

The algorithm is used to segment the endocardium in 115 short axis cardiac ultrasound images. All segmentations are achieved without tweaking the energy function or numerical parameters. Experimental evaluation of the results shows that the algorithm overcomes multiple local minima to give segmentations that are considerably more accurate than conventional techniques.

1 Introduction

Classical active contours evolving under gradient descent are poor at the task of segmenting ultrasound images. The problem is the presence of *speckle* in the images. Speckle is a spatial random process and it introduces spurious local minima in the active contour energy function. Evolving under gradient descent, active contours get trapped in the spurious minima, which are often far from the true solution.

Clearly, what is needed is an evolution strategy that avoids getting trapped in spurious local minima. In this paper, we present such a strategy in the framework of a level set algorithm. We call the evolution strategy *tunneling descent*, since it "tunnels out" of spurious minima and keeps the energy minimization going.

The algorithm has two nice properties:

1. It is <u>deterministic</u> and is faster than stochastic techniques for escaping from local minima.
2. It segments ultrasound images <u>without</u> any parameter tweaking. We have successfully segmented 115 images with literally the same algorithm.

Tunneling descent has been completely reformulated in this paper (an older version was reported in [4]). The old algorithm was a heuristic extension of Bayesian sequential decision theory. The new algorithm is reformulated as a deterministic sequential constrained optimization problem. This change is not only conceptual, but has also led to a significantly different mathematical formulation. For example, the constraints of equations (8), (9),and (10) are completely new. Considerable effort was involved in getting the constraints just right so that the resulting optimization problem would have a simple structure. The constraints now allow the use of convex programming as a numerical technique. This is a well known numerically stable optimization problem, and the current algorithm benefits from it.

All of the 115 segmentations are of the blood-tissue boundary of the left ventricle. We loosely refer to this boundary as the *endocardium*. The statistics of speckle in tissue and blood are considerably different and it is this difference that enables us to find the boundary. We pose endocardium segmentation as an estimation problem in a maximum-a-posterior (m.a.p.) framework.

2 Background, Literature Review, and Notation

2.1 The Ultrasound Signal and Segmentation

An ultrasound image records the backscatter from a propagating acoustic wave. Random scatterers in the medium give rise to *speckle* in the ultrasound signal, which is manifest as a spatial random process in the image. There are a wide range of theoretical results for the first-order statistics of ultrasound images, e.g. [1, 2]. Empirical models for ultrasound distributions have been proposed, e.g. [3]. They are sufficient for the task of segmentation, and we use them here.

The results of empirical modelling of cardiac short axis ultrasound images [3] can be summarized as follows:

1. As an approximation, the first order gray levels in blood and tissue in short-axis cardiac images can be modelled by Gamma distributions:

$$p_0(I \mid \alpha_0, \beta_0) = \frac{I^{\alpha_0 - 1}}{\Gamma(\alpha_0)\beta_0^{\alpha_0}} e^{\frac{-I}{\beta_0}}, \quad \text{(blood)} \tag{1}$$

and

$$p_1(I \mid \alpha_1, \beta_1) = \frac{I^{\alpha_1 - 1}}{\Gamma(\alpha_1)\beta_1^{\alpha_1}} e^{\frac{-I}{\beta_1}}, \quad \text{(tissue)}. \tag{2}$$

Here, I is the gray level in blood or tissue, α_0, α_1 are the shape parameters of the Gamma distributions for blood and tissue, and β_0, β_1 are the scale parameters of the Gamma distributions for the blood and tissue.

The Gamma distribution is only a convenient model. Other distributions can also be used, as long as they are scalable and can model the overall shape of the histograms in real images. The main point of this paper, which is tunneling descent with level sets, is independent of the choice of the distribution.

2. Further, the shape parameters α_0, α_1 can be fixed [3]. The values of β_0 and β_1 vary from image to image, but their ratio has a well defined mean and variance. A simple model is to assume that the log prior of β_0, β_1 is

$$\log p_\beta(\beta_0, \beta_1) \propto \frac{-1}{2\sigma_\beta^2}(\log \frac{\beta_1}{\beta_0} - \mu_\beta)^2 \tag{3}$$

where we have dropped all terms that are independent of β_0, β_1.

The values of $\alpha_0, \alpha_1, \mu_\beta, \sigma_\beta$ used in our experiments are given in Section 7.

The literature on ultrasound segmentation is vast, and due to lack of space, we only review a small representative set. Since speckle makes ultrasound segmentation difficult, a number of researchers have developed speckle suppression techniques, e.g. order statistical filters [6], and adaptive filters [7]. Classical computer-vision approaches, such as multiresolution texture analysis [8] and edge and line detectors [9] have also been proposed for ultrasound segmentation. Multi-frame spatio-temporal approaches to ultrasound segmentation are reported in [12].

As mentioned before, active contour models perform poorly with ultrasound images. Many attempts have been made to improve their performance, e.g. Active Shape Models [10, 11].

Some words about notation. We will take the domain of the image to be a square in the plane. The interior of the square is Π. We only consider simple closed curves in Π. If C is any such curve, then Ω_C refers to the "inside" region of the curve. This is the union of the set of points of C and the interior region of C. The complement of Ω_C in Π is denoted $\widetilde{\Omega_C}$. We use this notation consistently, so that curves $D, E, F, \cdots$ have inside regions $\Omega_D, \Omega_E, \Omega_F, \cdots$ etc.

3 M.A.P. Active Contours

As in equations (1-2), assume that $p_0(I \mid \alpha_0, \beta_0)$ and $p_1(I \mid \alpha_1, \beta_1)$ are models of the first-order distributions of gray levels inside and outside the true boundary, and that the parameters α_0, α_1 are known but β_0, β_1 are unknown. Then, $L(C, \beta_0, \beta_1)$, which is the posterior log-likelihood that curve C is the boundary and β_0, β_1 are the parameters of the data, can be easily shown to be:

$$L(C, \beta_0, \beta_1) = -\int_{\Omega_C} \log \frac{p_1(I \mid \alpha_1, \beta_1)}{p_0(I \mid \alpha_0, \beta_0)} dA - \lambda \oint_C ds + \log p_\beta(\beta_0, \beta_1), \tag{4}$$

where $\lambda > 0$, and the second and third terms are priors on C and β_1, β_2. The values of C, β_0, β_1 that maximize the posterior log-likelihood are the *m.a.p. estimates* of the boundary and the distribution parameters.

In the active contour framework, it is common to define the *energy function* by $E(C, \beta_0, \beta_1) = -L(C, \beta_0, \beta_1)$ and speak of minimizing the energy function instead of maximizing the log-likelihood.

In the level set method, the curve $C \subset \Pi$ is represented by the zero level set of a Lipschitz function $\phi : \Pi \to \mathbf{R}$, which is negative in Ω_C, zero in C and positive in $\widetilde{\Omega_C}$.

Since the level set function ϕ defines the curve C, the energy function can be expressed in terms of ϕ using the Heaviside function H, and the one-dimensional Dirac function δ_0, defined as:

$$H(z) = \begin{cases} 1 \text{ if } z \geq 0, \\ 0 \text{ if } z < 0, \end{cases} \qquad \delta_0(z) = \tfrac{d}{dz} H(z). \tag{5}$$

Then, the energy is given by :

$$E(\phi, \beta_0, \beta_1)$$
$$= \int_\Pi (1 - H(\phi)) \log \frac{p_1(I \mid \alpha_1, \beta_1)}{p_0(I \mid \alpha_0, \beta_0)} dA + \lambda \int_\Pi \delta_0(\phi) |\nabla \phi| dA - \log p_\beta(\beta_0, \beta_1) \tag{6}$$

The usual strategy for minimizing energy is gradient descent, which is given by

$$\frac{\partial \phi}{\partial t} = -\rho \nabla_\phi E(\phi, \beta_0, \beta_1) = \rho [\log \frac{p_1(I \mid \alpha_1, \beta_1)}{p_0(I \mid \alpha_0, \beta_0)} + \lambda div(\frac{\nabla \phi}{|\nabla \phi|})] \delta_0(\phi),$$
$$\frac{\partial (\beta_0, \beta_1)}{\partial t} = -\rho \nabla_{(\beta_0, \beta_1)} E(\phi, \beta_0, \beta_1), \tag{7}$$

where, ρ is the step size, ∇_ϕ is the grdient with respect to ϕ, and $\nabla_{(\beta_0, \beta_1)}$ is the gradient with respect to (β_0, β_1). The evolving ϕ becomes stationary at a local minimum of the energy. The zero level set of ϕ is taken to be the evolving contour and its stationary location as the final segmentation.

When used with real life ultrasound images, the evolving contour under gradient descent almost always stops prematurely away from the boundary. Some examples are shown in Fig. 1. In each figure, the smaller circle is the initialization and the larger curve is the final segmentation. The segmentations are very inaccurate and clearly demonstrate the problem with gradient descent.

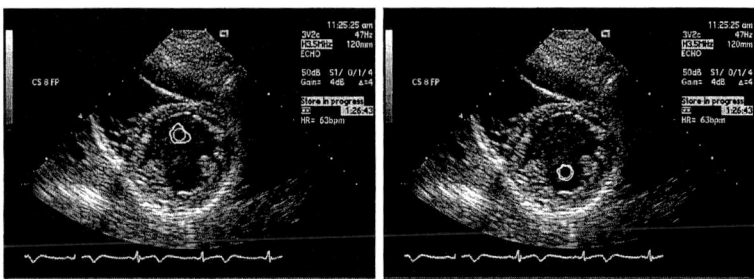

Fig. 1. The contour is trapped in spurious local minima

4 Escaping from Local Minima

We now make a key observation: *When the active contour is initialized in blood it is almost always trapped in a local minimum within the blood.*

To escape from this minima, we need an evolution strategy that monotonically grows the contour so that it evolves out of the minima towards the boundary. Actually, what is needed is a strategy that does the following:

- The contour starts from its initialization and grows monotonically.
- Among many possible ways of growing monotonically, whenever the growth is consistent with decreasing the energy, the contour chooses the direction with maximum decrease.
- At a local minimum, where all changes increase the energy, *the contour continues to grow*. It grows in the direction that gives the *least increase* in the energy, until the contour escapes from the local minimum and resumes lowering its energy again.

Thus the contour grows, alternately decreasing or increasing its energy. The lowest energy curve obtained from the *entire evolution* is the best estimate of the boundary. We call this evolution strategy *tunneling descent*. A mathematical formulation of the strategy is given below in section 5. The key idea is to *replace gradient descent by a sequence of constrained minimizations that monotonically grow the curve.*

There is one subtle point that arises in this evolution. A continuous growth of the contour will evolve it out of all local minima – spurious as well as the correct one. A *stopping rule* is necessary to stop the evolution once it has grown past the real boundary. A stopping rule is given below as well.

There is a superficial resemblance of tunneling descent to "balloons," which is the strategy of growing an active contour by adding a constant outwards expanding force to it. One major difference between the two strategies is that adding a fixed outwards expanding force alters the effective energy function of a balloon. If the change is substantial, the balloon may penetrate inside the tissue boundary before becoming stationary. On the other hand, tunneling descent *always minimizes the original energy function*. Further, a balloon requires the user to estimate the correct amount of the expanding force. The correct force is often image dependent and considerable "tweaking" is required to get it right. On the other hand, tunneling requires no tweaking.

5 Tunneling Descent

To convert the idea of the previous section into an algorithm we need to define clearly what it means for one curve to be monotonically larger than another nearby curve. We use the following notion: A curve D is monotonically larger than curve C, if (1) no part of D is inside C, i.e. $\Omega_C \subset \Omega_D$, (2) the area of D is greater than the area of C, (3) D is close to C (Fig. 2). Suppose ϕ and ψ are

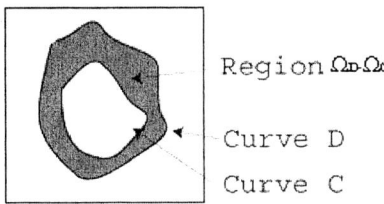

Fig. 2. Curve D is monotonically larger from curve C

the level set functions of C and D, then the constraints written in terms of the level set functions are respectively :

$$\psi(x,y) \leq \phi(x,y), \ \forall (x,y) \in \Pi \tag{8}$$

$$\int_\Pi (1 - H(\psi))dxdy \geq \int_\Pi (1 - H(\phi - \Delta_1))dA, \ \Delta_1 > 0, \tag{9}$$

$$\int_\Pi (\psi - \phi)^2 dxdy \leq \Delta_2, \ \Delta_2 > 0,, \tag{10}$$

The constraint (8) implies that D lies outside C (i.e. $\Omega_C \subset \Omega_D$). The constraint (9) says that the area of Ω_D is greater than the area of Ω_C, and constraint (10) prevents D having long finger-like extensions (especially when ϕ and ψ are distance functions). In our algorithm C and D are close to each other, and we replace constraint (9) by its linearized version

$$\int_\Pi \delta_0(\phi - \Delta_1)[\psi - (\phi - \Delta_1)]dA \leq 0. \tag{11}$$

For any level set function ϕ, let $M(\phi)$ be the set of all level set functions ψ that satisfy the above constraints. Using $M(\phi)$, we can precisely formulate tunneling descent. Assume for the time being that β_0 and β_1 are fixed, so that the energy function $E(\phi, \beta_0, \beta_1)$ is only a function of ϕ. Tunnelling descent begins with an initial level set function ϕ_0 and creates from it a sequence of functions $\phi_1, \phi_2, \ldots, \phi_n, \ldots$ by the following minimization:

$$\phi_n = \arg \min_{\phi \in M(\phi_{n-1})} E(\phi, \beta_0, \beta_1). \tag{12}$$

That is, ϕ_n minimizes the energy function amongst all possible $\phi \in M(\phi_{n-1})$. Hence, whenever it is possible to decrease the energy, tunneling descent will do so. Further, if the energy can only be increased, then tunneling descent will find the level set function that gives the least increase. This is exactly the strategy we want.

The energy sequence produced by tunneling descent $E(\phi_0), E(\phi_1), \cdots, E(\phi_n)$ will have subsequences where the energy is decreasing and subsequences where the energy is increasing. Define

$$\omega_n = \phi_k, \ \text{where}, \ k = \arg \min_{i=1,\cdots,n} E(\phi_i). \tag{13}$$

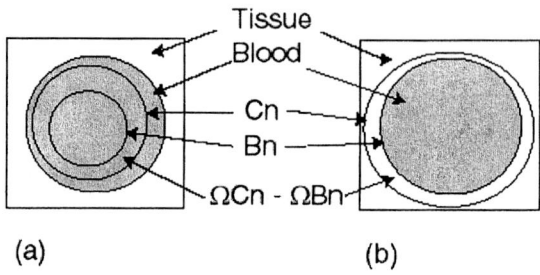

Fig. 3. Illustration of the Stopping Rule

That is, ω_n is the level set function with the least energy amongst ϕ's till the nth iteration. Hence, the zero level set of ω_n is the best estimate of the boundary at the nth iteration. For future reference, note that since the zero level set curves of $\phi_0, \cdots, \phi_n$ are monotonically getting larger, the zero level set of $\omega_n (= \phi_k)$ is always inside that of ϕ_n.

5.1 The Stopping Rule

As mentioned before, a stopping rule is necessary to terminate the evolution generated by tunneling descent. Recall that the stopping rule should terminate the sequence when the zero level set of ϕ_n has passed the real boundary and penetrated into tissue.

Let C_n denote the zero level set of ϕ_n and B_n be the zero level set of ω_n. To create the stopping rule, consider two cases: First, C_n is in blood (Fig. 3a). Then the current best estimate of the boundary B_n (which is inside C_n) is also in blood, i.e. the region $\Omega_{C_n} - \Omega_{B_n}$ is all blood. Second, C_n is outside the boundary (Fig. 3b). Here B_n is likely to be at or close to the boundary since the real boundary is close to the minimum of the energy. Thus, $\Omega_{C_n} - \Omega_{B_n}$ is mostly tissue. Therefore, we can construct a stopping rule by testing whether the gray levels in $\Omega_{C_n} - \Omega_{B_n}$ are from tissue or blood.

The likelihood ratio test for this is

$$\int_{\Omega_{C_n} - \Omega_{B_n}} \log \frac{p_1(I(x,y) \mid \alpha_1, \beta_1)}{p_0(I(x,y) \mid \alpha_0, \beta_0)} dA > T,$$

for some positive threshold $T > 0$.. This can be written in terms of the level set functions as

$$\int_\Pi (1 - H(\phi_n)) H(\psi) \log \frac{p_1(I(x,y) \mid \alpha_1, \beta_1)}{p_0(I(x,y) \mid \alpha_0, \beta_0)} dA > T, \qquad (14)$$

If the test is successful at n, then the region between C_n and B_n contains tissue, so the sequence is terminated and B_n is declared to be the boundary. Else the sequence continues to $n + 1$ and the test is applied again.

To sum up, tunneling descent works as follows:

1. Initialize a level set function ϕ with its zero level set, C_0, in the blood region. Set $n = 0$.
2. Set $n = n+1$. Generate ϕ_n using equation (12).
3. Find ω_n according to equation (13), and apply the stopping rule of equation (14). If the rule passes, terminate with ω_n with its zero level set B_n as the boundary. Else go to 2.

5.2 Simultaneous Parameter Estimation

So far we assumed that the parameters β_0, β_1 were known. We now remove that assumption, so that the energy function $E(\phi, \beta_0, \beta_1)$ is a function of ϕ and the parameters. Tunneling descent with parameter estimates is just ordinary tunneling descent with parameters estimated simultaneously in the minimization.

Tunneling descent is initialized with $\phi_0, \beta_{0,0}, \beta_{1,0}$ and it generates the sequence $\{\phi_n, \beta_{0,n}, \beta_{1,n}\}$ for $n \geq 1$ by

$$\phi_n = \arg\min_{\phi \in M(\phi_{n-1})} E(\phi, \beta_{0,n-1}, \beta_{1,n-1})$$

$$\{\beta_{0,n}, \beta_{1,n}\} = \arg\min_{\beta_0, \beta_1} E(\phi_n, \beta_0, \beta_1). \qquad (15)$$

As before, let ϕ_k be the smallest energy level set function in $\phi_0, \cdots, \phi_n$ and set $\omega_n = \phi_k$ and $(\beta_{0,n}^{min}, \beta_{1,n}^{min}) = (\beta_{0,k}, \beta_{0,k})$. We take these to be the best estimates of the boundary and the parameters till the nth iteration.

Finally, the stopping rule of equation (14) becomes

$$\int_\Pi (1 - H(\phi_n))H(\omega_n) \log \frac{p_1(I(x,y) \mid \alpha_1, \beta_{1,n}^{min})}{p_0(I(x,y) \mid \alpha_0, \beta_{0,n}^{min})} dA > T. \qquad (16)$$

5.3 Shrinking Tunneling Descent

As formulated so far, tunneling descent monotonically grows the initialized curve to find the boundary. However, there are no obstructions to creating an algorithm that monotonically shrinks the contour instead. The contour is now initialized outside the desired boundary (i.e. in tissue) and shrinks.

Two modifications are required for shrinking tunneling descent: First, a increasing level set function sequence has to be generated, and this is done by requiring that $M(\phi)$ be the set of functions ψ that satisfy:

$$\psi(x,y) \geq \phi(x,y), \ \forall (x,y) \in \Pi$$

$$\int_\Pi \delta_0(\phi + \Delta_1)[\psi - (\phi + \Delta_1)] dx dy \geq 0, \ \Delta_1 > 0,$$

$$\int_\Pi (\psi - \phi)^2 dx dy \leq \Delta_2, \ \Delta_2 > 0,,$$

Second, the stopping rule has to be modified to test whether the gray levels in $\Omega_{B_n} - \Omega_{C_n}$ come from the blood distribution:

$$\int H(\phi_n)(1 - H(\omega_n)) \log \frac{p_0(I(x,y) \mid \alpha_0, \beta_{0,n}^{\min})}{p_1(I(x,y) \mid \alpha_1, \beta_{1,n}^{\min})} dA > T. \tag{17}$$

6 Numerical Technique

The three constraints (equation(8),(11),(10)) can be easily analyzed to show that $M(\phi_n)$ is convex set for all n. Thus the minimization in equation (12) is a constrained optimization problem over a convex set. We use the gradient projection method [13] for the numerical minimization. The gradient projection step itself is done by using the classic Dykstra's Algorithm [14]. The details of the constrained minimization can be found in [17]. Following [15], the Heaviside function in equation (5) is approximated by the arc-tan function.

7 Experiments

We extensively tested tunneling descent on 115 clinical short-axis cardiac images with satisfactory results. The images were acquired from different subjects with an Acuson Sequoia $C256$ imaging system. The initial zero level set is in the blood pool and propagated outwards by tunneling descent in 37 images. In the remaining 78 images, the initial zero level set is within myocardial tissue and propagated inwards by shrinking tunneling descent.

The numerical values of all constants used in the experiment are given in Table 1. The constants α_0, α_1 are the shape parameters of the Gamma distributions of the gray levels in the blood pool and tissue. The constants μ_β and σ_β are used in the prior for β's. The constant λ occurs in equation (6). The constant Δ_1 and Δ_2 are described in equations (11) and (10), and T is the threshold in the stopping rule (equation (16)). All the outward propagating contours had the same constants, as did all the inward propagating contours. These constants are empirically set by running the algorithms on a small number of training images (different from the 115 images for test), and the algorithm is robust with respect to these parameters. The more detailed study of the effect of changing T is reported in [16].

Table 1. Values of constants used in experiments

	α_0	α_1	μ_β	σ_β	λ	Δ_1	Δ_2	T
Tun. Desc.	3.2	7.8	2.35	1.18	0.5	0.1	50	150
Shrink. Tun. Desc.	3.2	7.8	2.35	1.18	0.5	1	200	200

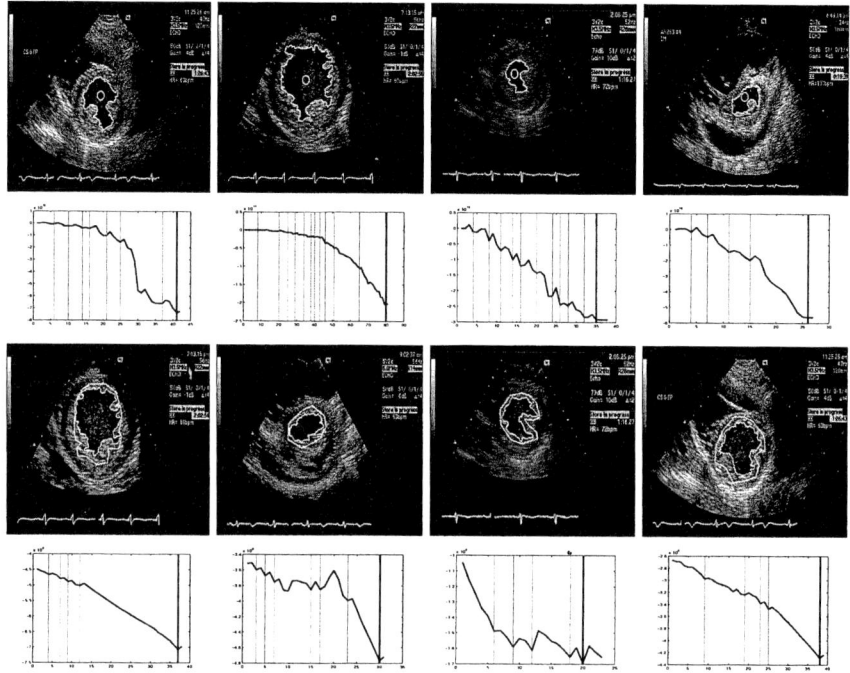

Fig. 4. Segmentation by Tunneling Descent and Shrinking Tunneling Descent

7.1 Segmentation Results

Tunneling descent segmented all 115 images successfully. We wish to emphasize *no parameter tweaking* was involved in any segmentation. Quite literally, the same algorithm worked on all images.

The first row of Fig. 4 shows four examples of the zero level set initialized in blood. In each figure of the first row, the initialization is the round shaped contour, and the final contour found by tunneling descent. Figures in the second row plot the energy $E(\phi_n, \beta_{0,n}, \beta_{1,n})$ as a function of n for the descent. The local minima in the energy function are indicated by vertical lines. Similarly, the third and the forth row of Fig. 4 show the segmentations by shrinking tunneling descent and the corresponding energy functions, where the contours are initialized in myocardial tissue. These figures shows that tunneling descent escaped through multiple local minima to find the endocardium. Gradient descent would have been trapped in any one of these.

For each of the 115 segmentations, the number of local minima that were overcome to find the endocardium were recorded. The average number of local minima overcome per image for tunneling descent was 6.5 with a standard deviation of 4.6. The average number of local minima overcome per image for shrinking tunneling descent was 2.5 with a standard deviation of 2.1. This shows clearly the need for an algorithm to escape from local minima.

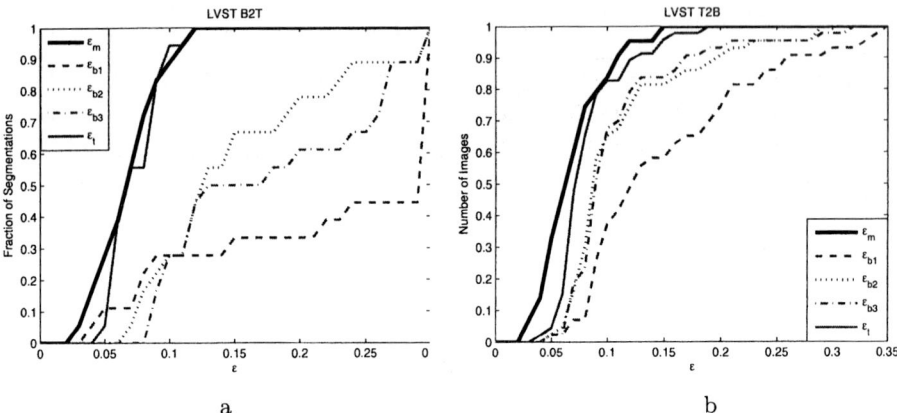

Fig. 5. Cumulative Error Comparison of Different Segmentation Methods

7.2 Validation

We further compared 19 tunneling descent results and 46 shrinking tunneling descent results with 2 sets of manual segmentations.

Given two curves C_1, C_2, we measured the extent of non overlap of the curves as 1 minus the ratio of the overlap area of the two curves to the average area of the two curves:

$$\epsilon = 1 - \frac{Area(\Omega_{C_1} \cap \Omega_{C_2})}{(Area(\Omega_{C_1}) + Area(\Omega_{C_2}))/2}$$

In any given image, we measured ϵ_m, the difference between the manual segmentations, and ϵ_t the mean of the ϵ's between the boundary found by tunneling descent and the two manual segmentations.

Since tunneling descent is superficially similar to "balloons" we also implemented a standard gradient descent active contour with a balloon force. Because the proper balloon force is usually unknown, we used three different values. For each balloon, we measured the mean difference between the balloon and the manual segmentations and these (for the three balloon forces) are denoted $\epsilon_{b1}, \epsilon_{b2}, \epsilon_{b3}$.

Fig. 5 shows the *cumulative distribution* of ϵ, i.e. for each value on the x-axis the plot gives the corresponding fraction of segmentations for which the measured ϵ was less than this value. In the figures, the thick solid lines are for ϵ_m, and the thin solid lines for ϵ_t and the other lines, dashed or dotted, for $\epsilon_{b1}, \epsilon_{b2}$ and ϵ_{b3}. Fig. 5-a shows the case of blood initialization. Tunneling descent is substantially more accurate than balloons, and its performance is close to manual segmentations. Fig. 5-b shows the comparison of tissue initialization. Although balloon performs better than before, tunneling descent still significantly outperforms balloon.

8 Conclusion

We reformulated tunneling descent and proposed a level set algorithm for it. The algorithm overcomes spurious local minima and reliably finds the endocardium in ultrasound images without tweaking.

Acknowledgments

This research was supported by the grant R01-LM06911 from the N.L.M.

References

1. R. F. Wagner, S. W. Smith, J. M. Sandrick, H. Lopez, "Statistics of speckle in ultrasound B-scans", *I.E.E.E. Trans. Son. Ultra.*, Vol. 30, pp. 156-163, Jan. 1983.
2. P. M. Shankar, "A general statistical model for ultrasonic scattering from tissues", *IEEE Trans. Ultrasonic, Ferro., Freq. Contr.*, Vol. 47, No. 3, pp. 727-736, May 2000.
3. Z. Tao, J. Beaty, C. C. Jaffe, H. D. Tagare, "Gray level models for segmentating myocardium and blood in cardiac ultrasound images". *Proceedings ISBI2002.*
4. Z. Tao, C. C. Jaffe, H. D. Tagare, "Tunneling Descent: A new algorithm for active aontour segmentation of ultrasound images", *Proceedings, IPMI 2003.*
5. C. B. Butkhardt, "Speckle in ultrasound B-mode scans", *I.E.E.E. Trans. Son. Ultra.*, Vol. SU-25, pp. 1-6, Jan. 1978.
6. M. Belohlacek and J. F. Greenleaf, "Detection of cardiac boundaries in echocardiographic images using a customized order statistics filter," Ultrasonic Imaging, 19, No. 2, pp. 127-137, April 1997.
7. J.C. Bamber and C. Daft, "Adaptive filtering for reduction of speckle in ultrasonic pulse-echo images," *Ultrasonics*, pp. 41-44, Jan. 1986.
8. R. Muzzolini, Y. Yang and R. Pierson, "Multiresolution texture segmentation with application to diagnostic ultrasound images," *IEEE Trans. Med. Img.* Vol. 12, No. 1, March 1993.
9. N. Czerwinski, D. L. Jones and W. D. O'Brien Jr., "Line and boundary detection in speckle images-Application to medical ultrasound," *IEEE Trans. Med. Img.*, pp. 126 -136, Vol.8, No. 2, Feb. 1999.
10. A. D. Parker, A. Hill, C. J. Taylor, T. F. Cootes, X. Y. Jin, D. G. Gibson, "Application of point distribution models to the automated analysis of echocardiograms," *Computers in Cardiology, 1994*, pp. 25-28, Sept. 1994.
11. A. Hill, C. J. Taylor, "Model-based image interpretation using genetic algorithms," *Image and Vision Computing*, Vol. 10, No. 5, June 1992.
12. M. Mulet-Parada, J. A. Noble, "Intensity-invariant 2D+T acoustic boundary detection", *Proceedings, Workshop on Biomedical Image Analysis 1998*, June 1998.
13. Dimitri P. Bertsekas "Nonlinear Programming", Athena Scientific, 1996.
14. Chris Perkins, "A convergence analysis of Dykstra's algorithm for phlyhedral sets", SIAM. J. Numer. Anal., Vol. 40, No.2, 2002, pp. 792-804.
15. T. Chan, L. A. Vese, "Active contours without edges", IEEE Trans. Image Processing, Vol. 10, No. 2, Febuary 2001.
16. Z. Tao, H. D. Tagare, "Stopping rules for active contour segmentation of ultrasound images", Proceedings, SPIE Medical Imaging 2005.
17. Z. Tao, H. D. Tagare, "Tunneling descent for M.A.P. active contour segmentation", Technical Report No. 05.01, 2005.

Multi-object Segmentation Using Shape Particles

Marleen de Bruijne and Mads Nielsen

IT University of Copenhagen, Denmark
marleen@itu.dk

Abstract. Deformable template models, in which a shape model and its corresponding appearance model are deformed to optimally fit an object in the image, have proven successful in many medical image segmentation tasks. In some applications, the number of objects in an image is not known a priori. In that case not only the most clearly visible object must be extracted, but the full collection of objects present in the image.

We propose a stochastic optimization algorithm that optimizes a distribution of shape particles so that the overall distribution explains as much of the image as possible. Possible spatial interrelationships between objects are modelled and used to steer the evolution of the particle set by generating new shape hypotheses that are consistent with the shapes currently observed.

The method is evaluated on rib segmentation in chest X-rays.

1 Introduction

Statistical shape models are widely applied in image segmentation [1, 2, 3], and are powerful tools especially in the case of missing or locally ambiguous boundary evidence. Most approaches perform a local optimization after the shape model has been initialized on the average position in the image. Alternatively, the best result of a set of local optimizations with different initializations can be selected. In the case of multiple objects, one would typically construct a combined model of all objects and optimize all shapes simultaneously in the image.

In some cases, modelling all objects jointly is not desirable. There may be not enough training data available to construct a sufficiently flexible and accurate model, rotation or scaling of one object with respect to another may introduce unwanted non-linearities in the model, and optimization in a high dimensional space is computationally more expensive. Moreover, if the number of objects present in the image is unknown it is impossible to define corresponding points in all images.

This paper presents a solution to the problem of segmenting an unknown number of (similar) objects. The segmentation is represented by a distribution of shape 'particles' that evolves under the influence of image terms and interaction between neighboring shapes. The particle cloud evolution is similar to Monte Carlo methods known as 'Condensation', 'particle filtering', or 'factored sampling', which have been applied to object localization and tracking [4, 5, 6]. However, the definition of the image term is different in this case in which multiple objects are modelled with the same particle distribution.

In a previous paper, we proposed the use of particle filtering to optimize shape-classification templates on a probability map obtained from pixel classification. Shape particles are weighted by their likelihood and the particle distribution is evolved using weighted resampling and a small amount of random perturbation in each iteration. In this way, particles representing unlikely shapes vanish while successful particles multiply. The initial sparse sampling evolves into a δ-peak at the maximum likelihood solution [7].

In the current paper we seek to optimize not just one object, but the entire shape distribution. The segmentation is represented as the maximum likelihood (soft) classification of the distribution of shape particles. The weights of the particles are adjusted so that the classification obtained from the shape set approximates the observed pixel classification as best as possible. The shape set thus evolves into the maximum likelihood shape collection.

Spatial consistency of the total segmentation can be enforced by neighbor interactions between particles. In the particle diffusion step each particle is allowed to produce hypotheses for neighboring shapes on basis of its own shape and position and a learned conditional shape model. This is especially useful in regular shape patterns such as the spine or the rib cage. If one vertebra or rib is found in the image, there is a high probability that a second vertebra or rib is present with approximately the same shape but a few centimeters higher or lower.

We applied this method to segmenting the ribs in the lung fields in chest radiographs. Rib segmentations are used for instance as a frame of reference for localizing abnormalities such as lung nodules, and to eliminate false positives in abnormality detection that frequently occur at crossings of posterior and anterior parts of the ribs. Classical approaches which fit geometrical models to edges in the image may miss some ribs and detect other ribs twice [8]. Loog [9] combined gray value features and contextual features in an iterative classification scheme, thus learning an implicit model of local rib structure. Although this produced significantly smoother and more accurate results than pixel classification based on intensity features alone, in some cases ribs were completely missed or the clavicles mistaken for ribs. The fact that consecutive ribs often have similar shapes and are regularly spaced calls for a global shape model describing the relations between different ribs, but construction and optimization of a global shape model is problematic since the number of ribs visible in the lung fields can vary. Ramachandran et al [10] showed that a pre classification of training images by the number of visible spaces between the ribs significantly improves the success of active shape model (ASM) segmentation.

In this work we do not model the full rib cage, but instead model separate ribs and fit those to the image in a consistent pattern using a model of spatial interrelationships between neighboring rib shapes. Neighbor relations between successive ribs in the same lung field as well as between the ribs at the same height in the opposite lung field are modelled.

Section 2 explains the main ideas behind the estimation of a maximum likelihood shape collection whereas Section 3 explains further how these ideas can be brought into practice. Section 4 gives more details on all ingredients required for multiple object segmentation and the algorithm proposed. Specific choices for rib segmentation and experiments on chest X-rays are described in Section 5. Sections 7 and 8 provide a discussion and conclusions.

2 Image Explanation as Maximum Likelihood

The standard approaches of fitting a shape model to an image can be written in Bayesian formulation as
$$p(S|I) \propto p(I|S)p(S)$$
where the shape S is searched for in the image I either as maximum a posteriori (MAP) estimate maximizing $p(S|I)$ or as maximum likelihood estimate (ML) maximizing $p(I|S)$. In both cases the maximum likelihood term may be evaluated as an object fit assuming an appropriate spatially independent noise model, maximizing
$$\log p(I|S) \propto \int_{\Omega(S)} U(I(x), S(x,\theta))dx \tag{1}$$
where x are the image coordinates, θ contains the shape model parameters to be optimized, U is the local log-likelihood function, and $\Omega(S)$ is the spatial domain of $S(\cdot,\theta)$. In the following we will generalize this to a collection of shapes.

Let $\mathcal{S}$ denote a collection of N shape instances:
$$\mathcal{S} = \{S_1, S_2, \ldots, S_N\}$$
Now one straightforward generalization of the likelihood term (Eq. 1) is the sum of the individual terms:
$$\sum_i \int_{\Omega(S_i)} U(I(x), S_i(x,\theta))dx$$
However, this sum of model fits of individual shapes is not the same as the likelihood of the collection of shapes. Optimization of θ with respect to this sum would result in all shapes fitting to the one object with the strongest image evidence. This is due to a simplification made in single-shape modelling that the integration area is only over the shape model. For a proper ML-estimation, all data must be modelled, and the integration domain is the full image domain. The collection likelihood then reads:
$$\log p(I|\mathcal{S}) \propto \int_{\Omega(\mathcal{S})} U(I(x), \mathcal{S}(x,\theta))dx$$
Hence, in every position in the image, it is necessary to take all (overlapping) shapes into account.

3 Computational Approach

Let us assume, that the data $I(x)$ takes values in a discrete set $C = \{c_1, c_2, \ldots, c_K\}$ where c_i can be integer pixel values or, as in the example below, pixel classes. Let us now for simplicity assume that in a given pixel, the pixel class due to the individual shapes is given deterministically and independent of the other shapes in the collection, so that

$$p(c_j|\mathcal{S}) = \sum_i p(c_j|S_i)p(S_i) = \sum_i \delta(c(S_i(x)), c_j)p(S_i) \qquad (2)$$

In the simple case where all the overlapping shapes are equally probable, this is simply the fraction of overlapping shapes that vote for the class c_i.

Let us now represent the shape collection $\mathcal{S}$ by a weighted set of shape instances S_i with shape parameters θ_i. The weights α_i denote the relative probability of these shape instances. In order to estimate the maximum likelihood shape collection, we must simultaneously optimize over $S_i = S(\theta_i)$ and α_i.

This optimization can be achieved by particle filtering iterating over

$$\begin{aligned} \alpha &= \arg\max_\alpha\ p(I|\theta, \alpha) \\ \theta &= \text{sampling}\ p(S|\mathcal{S}) \end{aligned} \qquad (3)$$

The first equation may be solved for analytically or obtained by stochastic optimization. If an infinite number of particles $S(\theta_i)$ were available, $\mathcal{S}(\theta, \alpha)$ is the maximum likelihood shape collection after this first optimization. To make the optimization efficient, we start out with a sparse sampling in $p(S)$ and condense this distribution around likely shape collections by the sampling step in Eq. 3. This sampling may be realized by first sampling in $p(S_i) = \alpha_i$ and then in $p(S|S_i)$. The distribution $p(S|S_i)$ represents the belief in S being a true shape in the image when the shape S_i has been observed in the collection.

If the variance of $p(S|S_i)$ decreases to zero in successive iterations the choice of distribution does not influence the point of convergence, as long as $p(S_1|S_2) = p(S_2|S_1)$ and the distribution can explore the full solution. The algorithm is guaranteed to converge to the maximum likelihood solution for a collection of shapes. The proof is analogous to the proof for the individual shape fitting by particle filtering [7].

However, the rate of convergence can be improved by choosing $p(S|S_i)$ so as to explore the solution space most effectively. Here, knowledge of spatial relationships between different objects can be exploited by letting a selected particle S_i produce a plausible hypothesis for a neighboring shape. $p(S|S_i)$ could then be a mixture of densities describing both the uncertainty in the observation S_i and the conditional densities $p(Sn|S_i)$ of all possible neighbors Sn given the observation S_i.

If the variance in $p(S|S_i)$ does not vanish during iteration, the distribution converges to the maximum likelihood shape collection convolved with $p(S|S_i)$.

4 Implementation

This section describes in more detail all ingredients needed to perform multi-object shape model segmentation, viz. a shape model, an image appearance model, possible neighbor relations, and an optimization algorithm.

4.1 Shape Model

To constrain the shape of possible solutions, any kind of shape model from which samples can be drawn can be inserted here. We will use the popular linear point distribution models (PDM) as proposed by Cootes and Taylor [1] to model the object shape variations observed in a training set.

Shapes are defined by the coordinates of a set of landmark points which correspond between different shape instances. A principal component analysis on a collection of aligned example shapes yields the so-called modes of shape variation which describe a joint displacement of all landmarks. Each shape can then be approximated by a linear combination of the mean shape and these modes of variation. Usually only a small number of modes is needed to capture most of the variation in the training set.

4.2 Neighbor Interaction

As was described in Section 3, the interaction between neighboring shapes can be introduced in the step of perturbation of the degenerate particle set after resampling. This requires $P(S_1|S_2)$, the probability distribution of the expected neighbor of a given shape. In the case where both shapes are modelled with a linear PDM, this is given by the Gaussian conditional density

$$P(S_1|S_2) = \mathcal{N}(\mu, K)$$

with

$$\mu = \Sigma_{12}\Sigma_{22}^{-1}S_2$$
$$K = \Sigma_{11} - \Sigma_{12}\Sigma_{22}^{-1}\Sigma_{21}$$

and Σ_{ij} are obtained from the covariance matrix of the combined model

$$\Sigma = \begin{bmatrix} \Sigma_{11} & \Sigma_{12} \\ \Sigma_{21} & \Sigma_{22} \end{bmatrix}$$

as

$$\Sigma_{ij} = \frac{1}{n-1}\sum_{n}(S_{in} - \bar{S}_i)(S_{jn} - \bar{S}_j)^T.$$

Alternatively, one could leave out the interaction between particles (i.e. perturbed particles are always similar to the particle that produced them) to obtain a segmentation of an unknown number of objects with unknown spatial interrelations.

Both approaches are tested on the rib data.

4.3 Image Observation Model

In the following, we will use class probability density measurements rather than discrete classes as the image observations as given in Equation 2. The class probability is obtained using a pixel classifier trained to distinguish between foreground and background pixels on the basis of local image descriptors. We have used a k-NN classifier and the outputs of a set of Gaussian derivative filters at multiple scales as image features.

Class probabilities in a pixel x are then defined by

$$P(\omega|x) = \frac{k_\omega}{k},$$

where k_ω among the k nearest neighbors of x belong to class ω.

We still assume that the pixel class due to the individual shapes is given deterministically, that is, each shape S_i is associated with a fixed class template $T_i(x, \omega)$ that defines to which class each pixel belongs. Typically, there will be two classes, one object and one background class. The aim is thus to produce a shape distribution, expressed as a weighted set of shape particles, of which the maximum likelihood classification $M(x, \omega)$ is as similar as possible to the observed (soft) classification of the image $C(x, \omega)$.

4.4 Algorithm

The algorithm for the desired optimization over θ and α looks as follows:

- Sample N shape particles S_i randomly from the prior distribution $p(S)$
- Repeat:
  1. Compute weight α_i for each particle ($\sum_i \alpha_i = 1$):

     Initialize:

     Particles S_i receive a weight α_i according to their overlap with the observed classification C, normalized for size. If several particles vote for the same class in the same pixel, they share the weight between them:

     $$\alpha_i = \frac{1}{\sum_{x,\omega} T_i(x,\omega)} \sum_{x,\omega} \frac{C(x,\omega) \times T_i(x,\omega)}{H(x,\omega)}$$

     $$H(x,\omega) = \sum_s \frac{T_i(x,\omega)}{\sum_{x,\omega} T_i(x,\omega)}$$

     Optimize α_i:

     In random permutation over particles S_i, with decreasing step size $d\alpha$:
     (a) select particle S_i
     (b) increase α_i by $d\alpha$, decrease $\alpha_{\neg i}$ so that $\sum_s \alpha_i = 1$

(c) $M(x,\omega,\alpha) = \frac{\sum_s \alpha_i T_i(x,\omega)}{\sum_{s,\omega} \alpha_i T_i(x,\omega)}$

(d) $f = \sum_{x,\omega} M(x,\omega,\alpha) \times C(x,\omega)$

(e) if f increased accept new α

2. Produce a new particle set through weighted sampling with replacement according to α_i
3. Perturb the particles from the new sample set by sampling from $p(S|S_i)$

5 Rib Segmentation Using Shape Particle Filtering

A set of leave-one-out experiments was performed on 30 standard digitized posterior-anterior chest radiographs of size 256 × 256, taken from the publicly available JSRT (Japanese Society of Radiological Technology) database [11]. This section describes the specific choices made for rib segmentation.

5.1 Shape Models

The proposed algorithm can simultaneously detect and segment an unknown number of similar objects. This could include several different types of objects as well.

For the rib application we have constructed two shape models, one for the left ribs and one for the right ribs. The size and shape of a rib in an X-ray image is strongly correlated with the position in the image. We therefore do not perform a full Procrustes alignment as would usually be preferred in shape model based segmentation. Instead, we translate each image such that the top of the lung fields (minimal y coordinate) and the horizontal center (median x-coordinate) coincide. Since the task of lung field segmentation is much less cumbersome than rib segmentation [8], we will assume that these coordinates are (approximately) known in a new image.

The lung fields and the part of the ribs that is visible in the lung fields have been manually delineated in all images. Ribs are subsequently described by landmarks equidistantly interpolated between the four corner points where a rib intersects the lung field. Ribs that have fewer than 4 corner points are not taken into account in model construction, but they can still be segmented as a variation in position of the ribs is automatically included in the model.

The spatial relations that are modelled are the first neighbor relationships between consecutive ribs in the same lung field and between the ribs that are at the same height in the both lung fields. Thus, in the particle perturbation step, a rib shape from the shape collection can either produce a perturbed version of itself or of its upper, lower, or left/right neighbor.

A linear PDM of the two shapes concatenated in one shape vector is constructed as described in Section 4. The models for a single rib, the combined models and an example of a conditional model as used in neighbor interaction are shown in Figure 1.

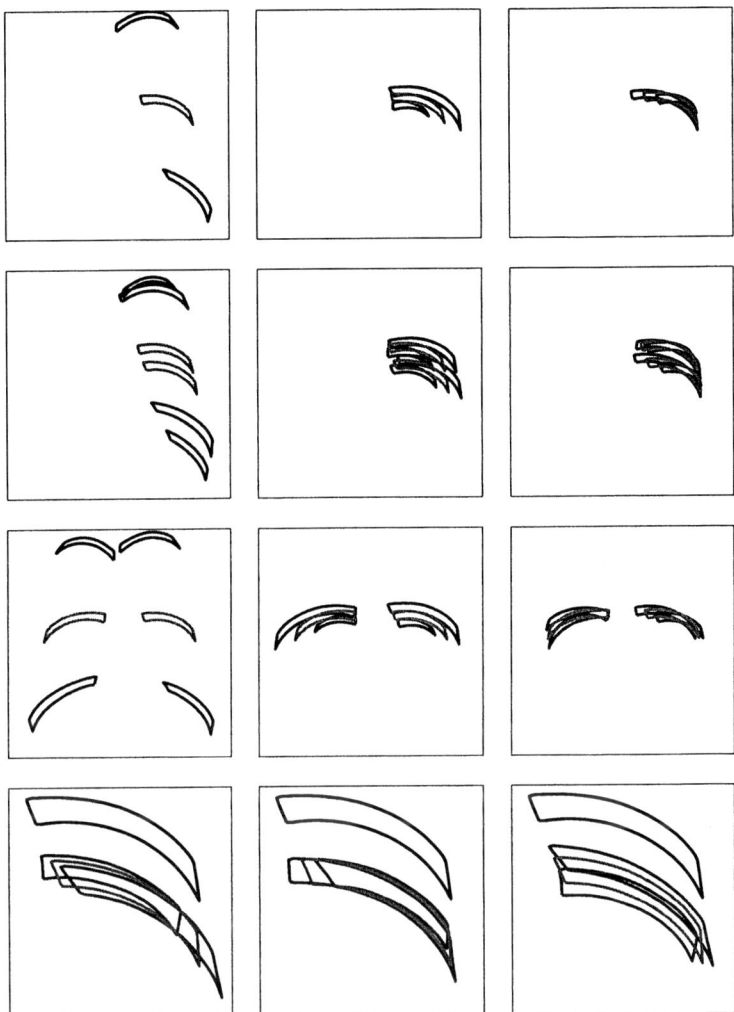

Fig. 1. Examples of the shape-and-pose models constructed for rib segmentation. From left to right, the first three modes of shape variation are visualized with the mean shape in black and the mean shape ± 2 standard deviations in gray, except for row 4 which shows the mean shape ± 4 standard deviations. From top to bottom: 1. Right rib model 2. Right successive ribs model 3. Opposite ribs model 4. Model of the lower rib conditioned on the mean shape of the upper rib. The axes of the plots correspond to the true image size for rows 1–3; row 4 is a close-up

5.2 Settings

We use a set of Gaussian derivative filters at multiple scales as image features and a k-NN classifier for probability estimation. Features include the original image and the derivatives up to the third order computed at a scale of 1, 2, and 4 pixels, resulting in a 21 dimensional feature space. The set of samples is normalized to unit variance for each feature, and k-NN classification is performed with an approximate k-NN classifier [12] with k=25. These settings were selected because they previously yielded good results on lung field classification [7] and have not been adjusted for rib classification.

Class templates as defined for each shape have two classes; inside the rib and outside the rib but within the lung fields. The template is defined by the interior of a rib shape plus a border of 5 background pixels (approximately half the thickness of a rib), so that most of the ribs can be described without overlapping the rib class of one shape template with the background class of another shape's template.

In the experiments presented here, the algorithm was run for 10 iterations without checking for convergence. The number of particles used for filtering is 1000, starting with 500 left ribs and 500 right ribs. The noise added in the particle perturbation step is of standard deviation $\sigma_d = 0.05\,\sigma$, with σ the standard deviation of the prior shape models. The prior for producing itself or one of its three first neighbors is chosen as uniform; each case occurs with a probability of 0.25.

6 Results

An example of segmentations obtained, with and without neighbor interactions, is given in Figure 2. Overall, segmentations using shape set filtering are spatially more consistent than the original pixel classification which includes spurious pix-

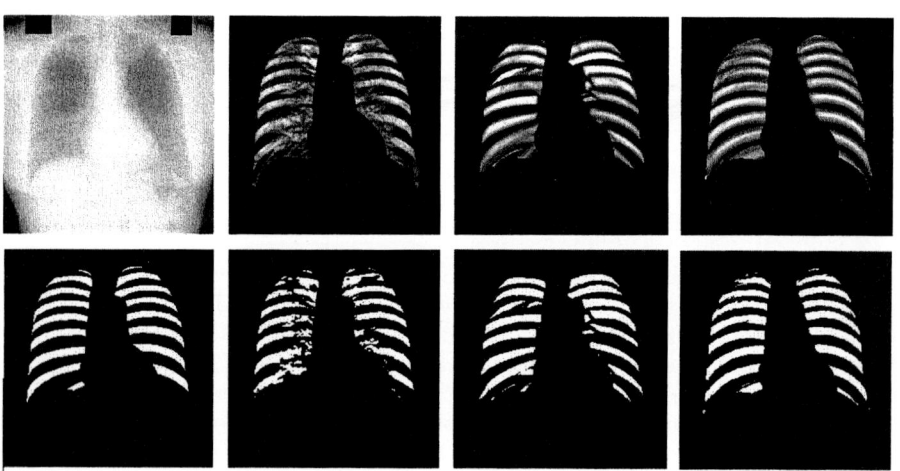

Fig. 2. Examples of segmentations obtained. The top row shows the original X-rays and the different soft classifications; the bottom row shows the hard classifications obtained by thresholding the soft classification at 0.5. From left to right: Ground truth, original pixel classification, shape set filtering without neighbor interaction; shape set filtering with neighbor interaction

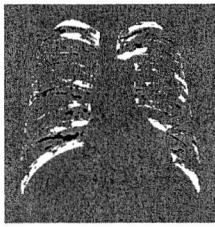 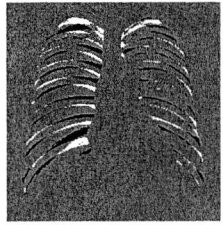

Fig. 3. Typical segmentation errors by pixel classification (left) and shape set filtering with user interaction (right). False positives are in black, false negatives in white, correct classification in gray

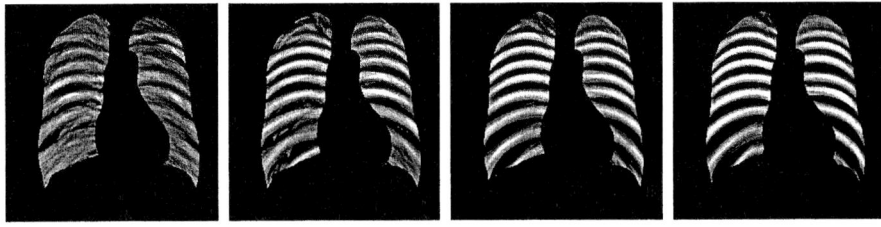

Fig. 4. Evolution of the shape set classification. From left to right: First, third, fifth, and tenth iteration

els and shows holes in the ribs. Without neighbor interaction, shape filtering may overlap crossing rib shapes to reconstruct the holes in the original classification. Shape set filtering with neighbor interaction finds the correct consistent rib pattern in most cases.

The error rate of shape set filtering with neighbor interaction is 18.7%, which is not significantly different from the error for the original pixel classification (19.1%, $p = 0.6$). Shape collection filtering without neighbor interaction performs worse (21.7%, $p < 0.0001$).

Figure 3 shows an example of the type of misclassifications by standard pixel classification compared to the proposed method. In general, shape filtering makes fewer gross errors like missing a rib completely or classifying the clavicles as ribs. There are, however, more errors near the rib boundaries which indicates that incorrect shapes have been forced on the segmentation. This may be either caused by an incorrect shape model or by a too strong neighbor interaction. Furthermore, the ribs in the lung tops — which is a problematic area for pixel classification — are difficult to segment also with our method.

The process of evolving the particle set is illustrated in Figure 4.

7 Discussion

In the current paper we have optimized a collection of shapes on the output of a pixel classifier based on local image descriptors. Such an approach was shown to be successful for single-object segmentation in several medical imaging applications [7]. The incorporation of shape constraints improves the spatial coherence of the pixel classification. However, as the shapes try to adhere to the pixel classification, the results will not be correct if the initial pixel classification results are far from the correct solution. An iterative method in which the method presented here, optimizing a shape collection to match the classification, is alternated with a pixel classification step in which the current shape collection is used as a prior, would likely improve the results.

Further improvements can be expected if more advanced shape models are used. Currently, a large variation in rib shape and position is modelled with a simple linear model, without optimizing point correspondences. This frequently results in 'illegal' shapes being produced. Although this problem is less severe in the case of a large set of shapes, it may result in blurred and less consistent classification, especially in the less regular top and bottom parts of the lungs.

In addition, in this work the variance in the particle perturbation step was kept constant during iteration. This means that in each iteration new hypotheses of neighboring particles are introduced in the shape collection. If the observed shape did not have a neighbor in that location or the neighbor has a different shape, the weight for these particles will be small, but this still results in a smearing out of the end result and occasionally in an extra rib being detected at the top and the bottom of the lung fields. This could be remedied by adjusting the interaction prior to reflect the fact that ribs in the lung tops are less likely to have an upper neighbor than those in the bottom of the lung fields, or by decreasing the variance of the perturbation density $p(S|S_i)$ over time.

Interaction between neighbors is currently realized by sampling in $p(S|S_i)$ after a new sample set of particles has been selected by sampling proportionally to the image likelihood weights α_i. Thus, the weight of a particle is determined by image forces and interaction between particles is achieved only by successful particles producing hypotheses for their neighbors. A stronger constraint of spatial consistency can be enforced by accepting a particle in the next iteration with a probability proportionally to its consistency with the rest of the current shape collection. We are currently investigating the advantages of various schemes.

Although we have for simplicity assumed that the position of the lung fields in the image is known approximately, in a previous paper we successfully applied shape particle filtering to segmentation of the lung fields [7]. Rather than first segmenting the lungs and subsequently finding ribs *near* the lungs the two tasks could be elegantly combined by filtering ribs and lungs simultaneously where the rib model is conditioned on the lung shapes. This would yield a more constrained shape-and-pose model for the ribs and may lead to better segmentations.

8 Conclusions

We propose a stochastic optimization algorithm which is capable of segmenting an unknown number of similar objects in an image. This method finds spatially more consistent segmentations than pixel classification without shape constraints. Interaction between neighboring shapes enforces consistency in regular patterns of similar shapes and improves upon the results without interaction in segmenting the ribs in chest radiographs.

Acknowledgments

The authors would like to thank B. van Ginneken and M. Loog of the Image Sciences Institute, Utrecht, The Netherlands, for providing the data sets and manual segmentations used in this study.

References

1. T. Cootes, C. Taylor, D. Cooper, and J. Graham, "Active shape models – their training and application," *Computer Vision and Image Understanding* **61**(1), pp. 38–59, 1995.
2. T. Cootes, G. Edwards, and C. Taylor, "Active appearance models," *IEEE Transactions on Pattern Analysis and Machine Intelligence* **23**(6), pp. 681–684, 2001.
3. A. Jain, Y. Zhong, and M. Dubuisson-Jolly, "Deformable template models: A review," *Signal Processing* **71**(2), pp. 109–129, 1998.
4. M. Isard and A. Blake, "Visual tracking by stochastic propagation of conditional density," in *ECCV, LNCS* **1064**, pp. 343–356, Springer, 1996.
5. A. Doucet, N. de Freitas, and N. Gordon, eds., *Sequential Monte Carlo methods in practice*, Springer-Verlag, New York, 2001.
6. J. Sullivan, A. Blake, M. Isard, and J. MacCormick, "Object localization by Bayesian correlation," in *ICCV*, pp. 1068–1075, IEEE Computer Society Press, 1999.
7. M. de Bruijne and M. Nielsen, "Shape particle filtering for image segmentation," in *MICCAI, LNCS* **3216**, pp. I:186–175, Springer, 2004.
8. B. van Ginneken, B. ter Haar Romeny, , and M. Viergever, "Computer aided diagnosis in chest radiography: A survey," *IEEE Transactions on Medical Imaging* **20**(12), pp. 1228–1241, 2001.
9. M. Loog, *Supervised Dimensionality Reduction and Contextual Pattern Recognition in Medical Image Processing.* PhD thesis, Utrecht University, 2004.
10. J. Ramachandran, M. Pattichis, and P. Soliz, "Pre-classification of chest radiographs for improved active shape model segmentation of ribs," in *Southwest Symposium on Image Analysis and Interpretation*, IEEE Computer Society Press, 2003.
11. J. Shiraishi, S. Katsuragawa, J. Ikezoe, T. Matsumoto, T. Kobayashi, K. Komatsu, M. Matsui, H. Fujita, Y. Kodera, , and K. Doi, "Development of a digital image database for chest radiographs with and without a lung nodule: Receiver operating character- istic analysis of radiologists' detection of pulmonary nodules," *American Journal of Roentgenology* **174**, pp. 71–74, 2000.
12. S. Arya, D. Mount, N. Netanyahu, R. Silverman, and A. Wu, "An optimal algorithm for approximate nearest neighbor searching," *Journal of the ACM* (45), pp. 891–923, 1998.

Author Index

Abd-Elmoniem, Khaled Z.   639
Agnus, Vincent   443
Alexander, Daniel C.   76
Amini, Amir A.   431
Ari, Narter   738
Arsigny, Vincent   27
August, Jonas   713
Awate, Suyash P.   677
Ayache, Nicholas   27

Barillot, Christian   333
Bazin, Pierre-Louis   234
Becher, Harald MD   222
Becker, James   493
Behar, Kevin L.   369
Beichel, Reinhard   114
Bischof, Horst   114
Brady, Michael   126
Bresson, Xavier   311

Çetin, Müjdat   553
Chan, Raymond   553
Chandar, Venkat   553
Chapman, Brian E.   603
Charnoz, Arnaud   443
Chen, Danny Z.   406
Chen, Yunmei   246
Cheng, Lishui   418
Chen, Xiaohua   126
Christensen, Gary E.   468
Chung, Albert C.S.   210
Chung, Moo K.   627
Ciofolo, Cybèle   333
Cointepas, Yann   52
Constantinesco, Andre   52
Cootes, Tim   1
Cosman, Eric R.   39
Cuzol, Anne   456

D'Agostino, Emiliano   689
Davatzikos, Christos   101
Davis, Simon   493
de Bruijne, Marleen   762
Deriche, Rachid   591

Ehlgen, Alexander MD   222
Evans, Alan C.   627

Fan, Xian   418
Farag, Aly A.   529
Faugeras, Olivier   591
Fessler, Jeffrey A.   174
Fillard, Pierre   27
Fischl, Bruce   393
Frangi, Alejandro F.   321

Gan, Rui   210
Gee, James C.   162
Geng, Alex   493
Geng, Xiujuan   468
Gerig, Guido   15
Glaunès, Joan   381
Golestani, Narly   52
Golland, Polina   88
Grimson, Eric   393
Guo, Weihong   246

Hagmann, Patric   311
Hammers, Alexander   689
Han, Qiong   701
Hassouna, M. Sabry   529
Hege, Hans-Christian   578
Heimann, Tobias   566
Hellier, Pierre   456
Hoffman, Eric A.   664
Holmvang, Godtfred   553
Huang, Sung-Cheng   493

Insana, Michael F.   516

Jain, Vidit   615
Jeong, Ja-Yeon   701
Jian, Bing   504
Jonasson, Lisa   311
Joshi, Anand A.   186
Joshi, Sarang C.   15, 701
Joshi, Shantanu H.   541

Kanade, Takeo   713
Kang, Ning   64
Karl, William C.   345

Karssemeijer, Nico 258
Kholmovski, Eugene G. 603
Kraft, Robert A. 738
Kumar, Dinesh 468
Kybic, Jan 299

Lamb, Hildo J. 321
Lamecker, Hans 578
Le Bihan, Denis 52
Leahy, Richard M. 186
Learned-Miller, Erik G. 615
Leberl, Franz 114
Lee, Kyoung Mu 357
Lee, Sang Uk 357
Lehericy, Stéphane 591
Lelieveldt, Boudewijn P.F. 321
Lenglet, Christophe 591
Leow, Alex 493
Li, Kang 406
Litvin, Andrew 345
Liu, Huafeng 197
Liu, Yijun 246
Lo, Jonathan Lok-Chuen 126

Maes, Frederik 689
Mai, Van 270
Malandain, Grégoire 443
Mangin, Jean-Francois 52
Manniesing, Rashindra 138
Marroquin, José L. 504
Marsland, Stephen 1
Maurer, Calvin R. 150
McLennan, Geoffrey 664
Meinzer, Hans-Peter 566
Mémin, Etienne 456
Merck, Derek 701
Meyer, Charles R. 174
Meyer, François G. 652
Millington, Steven 406
Mio, Washington 541
Moore, Niall 126

Narayanan, Ramkrishnan 174
Nicolau, Stéphane 443
Nielsen, Mads 762
Niessen, Wiro 138
Noble, J. Alison 222

Osman, Nael F. 639
Ou, Wanmei 88

Pallier, Christophe 52
Papademetris, Xenophon 369
Park, Hyunjin 174
Parker, Dennis L. 603
Pennec, Xavier 27
Perrin, Muriel 52
Petrovic, Vladimir 1
Pfefferbaum, Adolf 150
Pham, Dzung L. 234
Pizer, Stephen M. 701
Poupon, Cyril 52
Prince, Jerry L. 480, 639

Rangarajan, Anand 725
Rao, Murali 246
Reddy, Vivek 553
Reiber, Johan H.C. 321
Rieul, Bernard 52
Rivière, Denis 52
Robbins, Steve 627
Rohlfing, Torsten 150
Rohr, Karl 286
Rose, Stephen E. 64
Rousson, Mikaël 591
Rudrapatna, Mamatha 270

Schestowitz, Roy 1
Seghers, Dieter 689
Ségonne, Florent 393
Shattuck, David W. 186
Shen, Dinggang 101
Shen, Xilin 652
Shi, Pengcheng 197
Shim, Hackjoon 357
Shkarin, Pavel 369
Smutek, Daniel 299
Snoeren, Peter R. 258
Soler, Luc 443
Sonka, Milan 114, 406, 664
Sowmya, Arcot 270
Sridhar, Mallika 516
Srivastava, Anuj 541
Staib, Lawrence H. 369
Stuber, Matthias 639
Suetens, Paul 689
Suinesiaputra, Avan 321
Sullivan, Edith V. 150
Sun, Walter 553

Author Index

Tagare, Hemant D.   750
Tajine, Mohamed   443
Tao, Zhong   750
Taylor, Chris J.   1
Terriberry, Timothy B.   15
Thiran, Jean-Philippe   311
Thompson, Paul M.   27, 186, 493
Tian, Yi   197
Toga, Arthur   493
Tosun, Duygu   480
Twining, Carole J.   1

Ugurbil, Kamil   591

Vaillant, Marc   381
Vandermeulen, Dirk   689
Vemuri, Baba C.   504
Vemuri, Prashanthi   603

Wang, Qian   689
Wang, Yuehuan   431
Wedeen, Van J.   311
Wells III, William M.   39
Wenckebach, Thomas H.   578

Whitaker, Ross T.   677
Williams, Quentin   222
Williams, Tomos   566
Willsky, Alan   553
Wilson, Peter   270
Wolf, Ivo   566
Wu, Xiaodong   406
Wyatt, Christopher L.   738

Xue, Zhong   101

Yan, Xiaolu   246
Yang, Jie   418
Yun, Il Dong   357
Yushkevich, Paul A.   162

Zeng, Qingguo   246
Zhang, Hui   162
Zhang, Jie   725
Zhang, Jun   64
Zhang, Wei   258
Zhang, Xiangwei   664
Zhu, Yuemin   418

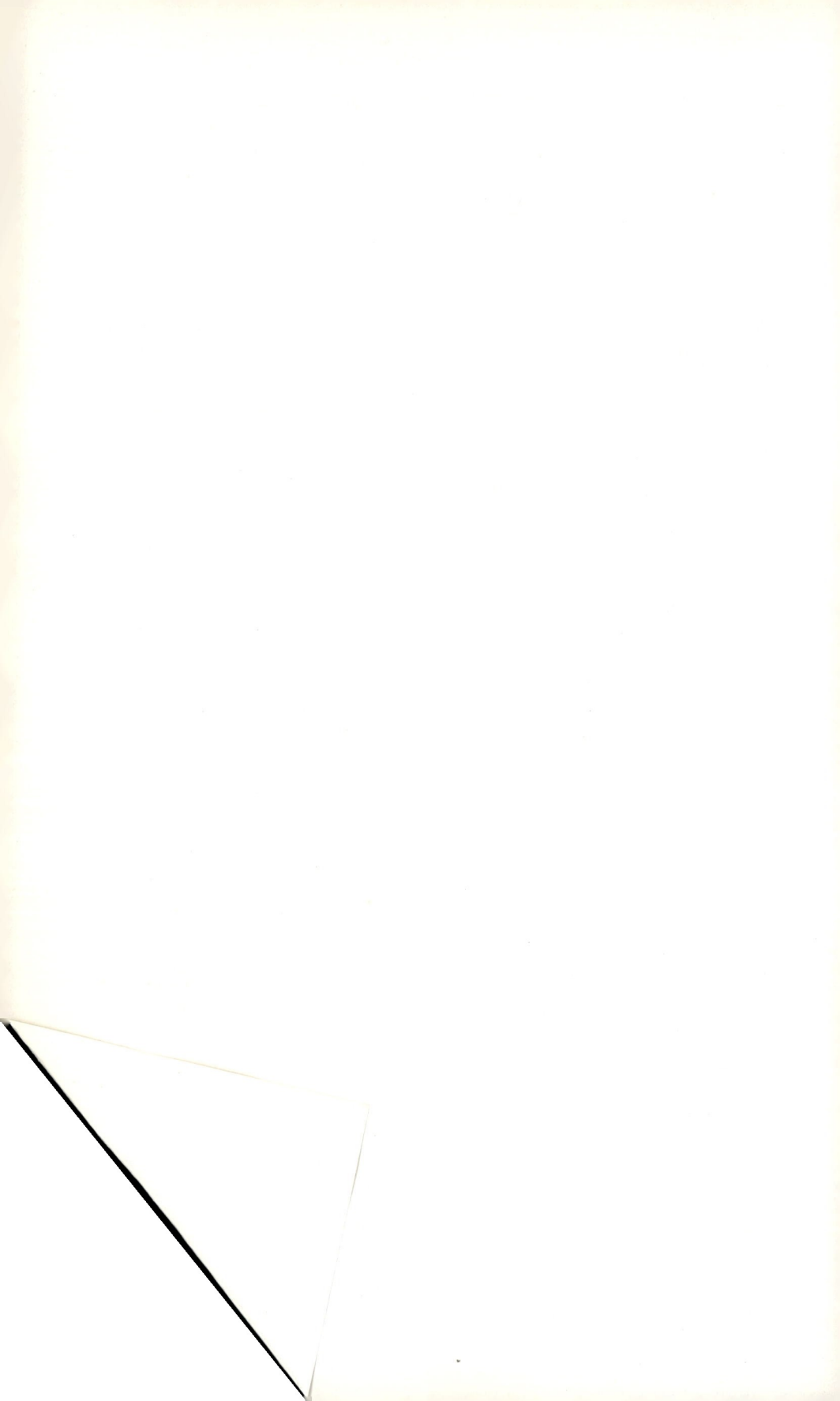

Lecture Notes in Computer Science

For information about Vols. 1–3470

please contact your bookseller or Springer

Vol. 3573: S. Etalle (Ed.), Logic Based Program Synthesis and Transformation. VIII, 279 pages. 2005.

Vol. 3572: C. De Felice, A. Restivo (Eds.), Developments in Language Theory. XI, 409 pages. 2005.

Vol. 3570: A. S. Patrick, M. Yung (Eds.), Financial Cryptography and Data Security. XII, 376 pages. 2005.

Vol. 3569: F. Bacchus, T. Walsh (Eds.), Theory and Applications of Satisfiability Testing. XII, 492 pages. 2005.

Vol. 3567: M. Jackson, D. Nelson, S. Stirk (Eds.), Database: Enterprise, Skills and Innovation. XII, 185 pages. 2005.

Vol. 3565: G.E. Christensen, M. Sonka (Eds.), Information Processing in Medical Imaging. XXI, 777 pages. 2005.

Vol. 3562: J. Mira, J.R. Álvarez (Eds.), Artificial Intelligence and Knowledge Engineering Applications: A Bioinspired Approach, Part II. XXIV, 636 pages. 2005.

Vol. 3561: J. Mira, J.R. Álvarez (Eds.), Mechanisms, Symbols, and Models Underlying Cognition, Part I. XXIV, 532 pages. 2005.

Vol. 3560: V.K. Prasanna, S. Iyengar, P.G. Spirakis, M. Welsh (Eds.), Distributed Computing in Sensor Systems. XV, 423 pages. 2005.

Vol. 3559: P. Auer, R. Meir (Eds.), Learning Theory. XI, 692 pages. 2005. (Subseries LNAI).

Vol. 3557: H. Gilbert, H. Handschuh (Eds.), Fast Software Encryption. XI, 443 pages. 2005.

Vol. 3556: H. Baumeister, M. Marchesi, M. Holcombe (Eds.), Extreme Programming and Agile Processes in Software Engineering. XIV, 332 pages. 2005.

Vol. 3555: T. Vardanega, A. Wellings (Eds.), Reliable Software Technology – Ada-Europe 2005. XV, 273 pages. 2005.

Vol. 3553: T.D. Hämäläinen, A.D. Pimentel, J. Takala, S. Vassiliadis (Eds.), Embedded Computer Systems: Architectures, Modeling, and Simulation. XV, 476 pages. 2005.

Vol. 3552: H. de Meer, N. Bhatti (Eds.), Quality of Service – IWQoS 2005. XV, 400 pages. 2005.

Vol. 3551: T. Härder, W. Lehner (Eds.), Data Management in a Connected World. XIX, 371 pages. 2005.

Vol. 3548: K. Julisch, C. Kruegel (Eds.), Intrusion and Malware Detection and Vulnerability Assessment. X, 241 pages. 2005.

Vol. 3547: F. Bomarius, S. Komi-Sirviö (Eds.), Product Focused Software Process Improvement. XIII, 588 pages. 2005.

Vol. 3543: L. Kutvonen, N. Alonistioti (Eds.), Distributed Applications and Interoperable Systems. XI, 235 pages. 2005.

Vol. 3541: N.C. Oza, R. Polikar, J. Kittler, F. Roli (Eds.), Multiple Classifier Systems. XII, 430 pages. 2005.

Vol. 3540: H. Kalviainen, J. Parkkinen, A. Kaarna (Eds.), Image Analysis. XXII, 1270 pages. 2005.

Vol. 3537: A. Apostolico, M. Crochemore, K. Park (Eds.), Combinatorial Pattern Matching. XI, 444 pages. 2005.

Vol. 3536: G. Ciardo, P. Darondeau (Eds.), Applications and Theory of Petri Nets 2005. XI, 470 pages. 2005.

Vol. 3535: M. Steffen, G. Zavattaro (Eds.), Formal Methods for Open Object-Based Distributed Systems. X, 323 pages. 2005.

Vol. 3533: M. Ali, F. Esposito (Eds.), Innovations in Applied Artificial Intelligence. XX, 858 pages. 2005. (Subseries LNAI).

Vol. 3532: A. Gómez-Pérez, J. Euzenat (Eds.), The Semantic Web: Research and Applications. XV, 728 pages. 2005.

Vol. 3531: J. Ioannidis, A. Keromytis, M. Yung (Eds.), Applied Cryptography and Network Security. XI, 530 pages. 2005.

Vol. 3530: A. Prinz, R. Reed, J. Reed (Eds.), SDL 2005: Model Driven. XI, 361 pages. 2005.

Vol. 3528: P.S. Szczepaniak, J. Kacprzyk, A. Niewiadomski (Eds.), Advances in Web Intelligence. XVII, 513 pages. 2005. (Subseries LNAI).

Vol. 3527: R. Morrison, F. Oquendo (Eds.), Software Architecture. XII, 263 pages. 2005.

Vol. 3526: S.B. Cooper, B. Löwe, L. Torenvliet (Eds.), New Computational Paradigms. XVII, 574 pages. 2005.

Vol. 3525: A.E. Abdallah, C.B. Jones, J.W. Sanders (Eds.), Communicating Sequential Processes. XIV, 321 pages. 2005.

Vol. 3524: R. Barták, M. Milano (Eds.), Integration of AI and OR Techniques in Constraint Programming for Combinatorial Optimization Problems. XI, 320 pages. 2005.

Vol. 3523: J.S. Marques, N. Pérez de la Blanca, P. Pina (Eds.), Pattern Recognition and Image Analysis, Part II. XXVI, 733 pages. 2005.

Vol. 3522: J.S. Marques, N. Pérez de la Blanca, P. Pina (Eds.), Pattern Recognition and Image Analysis, Part I. XXVI, 703 pages. 2005.

Vol. 3521: N. Megiddo, Y. Xu, B. Zhu (Eds.), Algorithmic Applications in Management. XIII, 484 pages. 2005.

Vol. 3520: O. Pastor, J. Falcão e Cunha (Eds.), Advanced Information Systems Engineering. XVI, 584 pages. 2005.

Vol. 3519: H. Li, P. J. Olver, G. Sommer (Eds.), Computer Algebra and Geometric Algebra with Applications. IX, 449 pages. 2005.

Vol. 3518: T.B. Ho, D. Cheung, H. Liu (Eds.), Advances in Knowledge Discovery and Data Mining. XXI, 864 pages. 2005. (Subseries LNAI).

Vol. 3517: H.S. Baird, D.P. Lopresti (Eds.), Human Interactive Proofs. IX, 143 pages. 2005.

Vol. 3516: V.S. Sunderam, G.D.v. Albada, P.M.A. Sloot, J.J. Dongarra (Eds.), Computational Science – ICCS 2005, Part III. LXIII, 1143 pages. 2005.

Vol. 3515: V.S. Sunderam, G.D.v. Albada, P.M.A. Sloot, J.J. Dongarra (Eds.), Computational Science – ICCS 2005, Part II. LXIII, 1101 pages. 2005.

Vol. 3514: V.S. Sunderam, G.D.v. Albada, P.M.A. Sloot, J.J. Dongarra (Eds.), Computational Science – ICCS 2005, Part I. LXIII, 1089 pages. 2005.

Vol. 3513: A. Montoyo, R. Muñoz, E. Métais (Eds.), Natural Language Processing and Information Systems. XII, 408 pages. 2005.

Vol. 3512: J. Cabestany, A. Prieto, F. Sandoval (Eds.), Computational Intelligence and Bioinspired Systems. XXV, 1260 pages. 2005.

Vol. 3510: T. Braun, G. Carle, Y. Koucheryavy, V. Tsaoussidis (Eds.), Wired/Wireless Internet Communications. XIV, 366 pages. 2005.

Vol. 3509: M. Jünger, V. Kaibel (Eds.), Integer Programming and Combinatorial Optimization. XI, 484 pages. 2005.

Vol. 3508: P. Bresciani, P. Giorgini, B. Henderson-Sellers, G. Low, M. Winikoff (Eds.), Agent-Oriented Information Systems II. X, 227 pages. 2005. (Subseries LNAI).

Vol. 3507: F. Crestani, I. Ruthven (Eds.), Information Context: Nature, Impact, and Role. XIII, 253 pages. 2005.

Vol. 3506: C. Park, S. Chee (Eds.), Information Security and Cryptology – ICISC 2004. XIV, 490 pages. 2005.

Vol. 3505: V. Gorodetsky, J. Liu, V.A. Skormin (Eds.), Autonomous Intelligent Systems: Agents and Data Mining. XIII, 303 pages. 2005. (Subseries LNAI).

Vol. 3504: A.F. Frangi, P.I. Radeva, A. Santos, M. Hernandez (Eds.), Functional Imaging and Modeling of the Heart. XV, 489 pages. 2005.

Vol. 3503: S.E. Nikoletseas (Ed.), Experimental and Efficient Algorithms. XV, 624 pages. 2005.

Vol. 3502: F. Khendek, R. Dssouli (Eds.), Testing of Communicating Systems. X, 381 pages. 2005.

Vol. 3501: B. Kégl, G. Lapalme (Eds.), Advances in Artificial Intelligence. XV, 458 pages. 2005. (Subseries LNAI).

Vol. 3500: S. Miyano, J. Mesirov, S. Kasif, S. Istrail, P. Pevzner, M. Waterman (Eds.), Research in Computational Molecular Biology. XVII, 632 pages. 2005. (Subseries LNBI).

Vol. 3499: A. Pelc, M. Raynal (Eds.), Structural Information and Communication Complexity. X, 323 pages. 2005.

Vol. 3498: J. Wang, X. Liao, Z. Yi (Eds.), Advances in Neural Networks – ISNN 2005, Part III. XLIX, 1077 pages. 2005.

Vol. 3497: J. Wang, X. Liao, Z. Yi (Eds.), Advances in Neural Networks – ISNN 2005, Part II. XLIX, 947 pages. 2005.

Vol. 3496: J. Wang, X. Liao, Z. Yi (Eds.), Advances in Neural Networks – ISNN 2005, Part II. L, 1055 pages. 2005.

Vol. 3495: P. Kantor, G. Muresan, F. Roberts, D.D. Zeng, F.-Y. Wang, H. Chen, R.C. Merkle (Eds.), Intelligence and Security Informatics. XVIII, 674 pages. 2005.

Vol. 3494: R. Cramer (Ed.), Advances in Cryptology – EUROCRYPT 2005. XIV, 576 pages. 2005.

Vol. 3493: N. Fuhr, M. Lalmas, S. Malik, Z. Szlávik (Eds.), Advances in XML Information Retrieval. XI, 438 pages. 2005.

Vol. 3492: P. Blache, E. Stabler, J. Busquets, R. Moot (Eds.), Logical Aspects of Computational Linguistics. X, 363 pages. 2005. (Subseries LNAI).

Vol. 3489: G.T. Heineman, I. Crnkovic, H.W. Schmidt, J.A. Stafford, C. Szyperski, K. Wallnau (Eds.), Component-Based Software Engineering. XI, 358 pages. 2005.

Vol. 3488: M.-S. Hacid, N.V. Murray, Z.W. Raś, S. Tsumoto (Eds.), Foundations of Intelligent Systems. XIII, 700 pages. 2005. (Subseries LNAI).

Vol. 3486: T. Helleseth, D. Sarwate, H.-Y. Song, K. Yang (Eds.), Sequences and Their Applications - SETA 2004. XII, 451 pages. 2005.

Vol. 3483: O. Gervasi, M.L. Gavrilova, V. Kumar, A. Laganà, H.P. Lee, Y. Mun, D. Taniar, C.J.K. Tan (Eds.), Computational Science and Its Applications – ICCSA 2005, Part IV. LXV, 1362 pages. 2005.

Vol. 3482: O. Gervasi, M.L. Gavrilova, V. Kumar, A. Laganà, H.P. Lee, Y. Mun, D. Taniar, C.J.K. Tan (Eds.), Computational Science and Its Applications – ICCSA 2005, Part III. LXV, 1340 pages. 2005.

Vol. 3481: O. Gervasi, M.L. Gavrilova, V. Kumar, A. Laganà, H.P. Lee, Y. Mun, D. Taniar, C.J.K. Tan (Eds.), Computational Science and Its Applications – ICCSA 2005, Part II. LXV, 1316 pages. 2005.

Vol. 3480: O. Gervasi, M.L. Gavrilova, V. Kumar, A. Laganà, H.P. Lee, Y. Mun, D. Taniar, C.J.K. Tan (Eds.), Computational Science and Its Applications – ICCSA 2005, Part I. LXV, 1234 pages. 2005.

Vol. 3479: T. Strang, C. Linnhoff-Popien (Eds.), Location- and Context-Awareness. XII, 378 pages. 2005.

Vol. 3478: C. Jermann, A. Neumaier, D. Sam (Eds.), Global Optimization and Constraint Satisfaction. XIII, 193 pages. 2005.

Vol. 3477: P. Herrmann, V. Issarny, S. Shiu (Eds.), Trust Management. XII, 426 pages. 2005.

Vol. 3476: J. Leite, A. Omicini, P. Torroni, P. Yolum (Eds.), Declarative Agent Languages and Technologies II. XII, 289 pages. 2005. (Subseries LNAI).

Vol. 3475: N. Guelfi (Ed.), Rapid Integration of Software Engineering Techniques. X, 145 pages. 2005.

Vol. 3474: C. Grelck, F. Huch, G.J. Michaelson, P. Trinder (Eds.), Implementation and Application of Functional Languages. X, 227 pages. 2005.

Vol. 3472: M. Broy, B. Jonsson, J.-P. Katoen, M. Leucker, A. Pretschner (Eds.), Model-Based Testing of Reactive Systems. VIII, 659 pages. 2005.